Gr
Ba al
En y

Edited by

David G

Mount Zion
Endocrino
Chief, Divisi
Department
University of

Dolores Shoback, MD

Professor of Medicine
Department of Medicine
University of California, San Francisco
Staff Physician, Endocrine-Metabolism Section,
Department of Medicine
San Francisco Veterans Affairs Medical Center

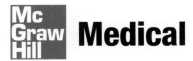

Medical

New York   Chicago   San Francisco   Lisbon   London   Madrid   Mexico City
Milan   New Delhi   San Juan   Seoul   Singapore   Sydney   Toronto

Greenspan's Basic & Clinical Endocrinology, Ninth Edition

1 2 3 4 5 6 7 8 9 0   CTP/CTP   15 14 13 12 11

ISBN 978-0-07-162243-1
MHID 0-07-162243-8
ISSN 0891-2068

Notice

This book was set in Garamond by Glyph International.
The editors were James F. Shanahan and Peter J. Boyle.
The production supervisor was Catherine H. Saggese.
Project management was provided by Rajni Pisharody, Glyph International.
The designer was Elise Lansdon.
The illustration manager was Armen Ovsepyan.
China Translation & Printing Services, Ltd., was printer and binder.

International Edition ISBN 978-0-07-176743-9; MHID 0-07-176743-6. Copyright © 2011. Exclusive rights by The McGraw-Hill Companies, Inc., for manufacture and export. This book cannot be re-exported from the country to which it is consigned by McGraw-Hill. The International Edition is not available in North America.

Contents

5. The Posterior Pituitary (Neurohypophysis)   115

Alan G. Robinson, MD

6. Growth   129

Dennis Styne, MD

7. The Thyroid Gland   163

David S. Cooper, MD & Paul W. Ladenson, MA (Oxon.), MD

8. Metabolic Bone Disease   227

Dolores Shoback, MD, Deborah Sellmeyer, MD, & Daniel D. Bikle, MD, PhD

Authors

Mark Anderson, MD, PhD
Associate Professor, Robert B. Friend and Michelle M. Friend Endowed Chair in Diabetes Research, Diabetes Center and Department of Medicine, University of California, San Francisco
manderson@diabetes.ucsf.edu
Hormones & Hormone Action

David C. Aron, MD, MS
Professor, Department of Medicine and Department of Epidemiology and Biostatistics, Division of Clinical and Molecular Endocrinology, School of Medicine, Case Western Reserve University; Associate Chief of Staff/ Education, Louis Stokes Cleveland Department of Veterans Affairs Medical Center, Cleveland, Ohio
david.aron@med.va.gov
Evidence-Based Endocrinology & Clinical Epidemiology; Hypothalamus & Pituitary Gland; Glucocorticoids & Adrenal Androgens

Martina L. Badell, MD
Department of Gynecology and Obstetrics, Emory University, Atlanta, Georgia
mbadell@emory.edu
The Endocrinology of Pregnancy

Daniel D. Bikle, MD, PhD
Professor of Medicine and Dermatology, Veterans Affairs Medical Center and University of California, San Francisco
daniel.bikle@ucsf.edu
Metabolic Bone Disease

Glenn D. Braunstein, MD
Chairman, Department of Medicine, Cedars-Sinai Medical Center; The James R. Klinenberg, MD, Chair in Medicine, Professor of Medicine, David Geffen School of Medicine at University of California, Los Angeles
glenn.braunstein@cshs.org
Testes

Ty B. Carroll, MD
Assistant Professor, Endocrinology Center, Department of Medicine, Medical College of Wisconsin, Milwaukee
tcarroll@mcw.edu
Glucocorticoids & Adrenal Androgens

Marcelle I. Cedars, MD
Professor and Director, Division of Reproductive Endocrinology, Department of Obstetrics, Gynecology and Reproductive Sciences, University of California, San Francisco
marcelle.cedars@ucsfmedctr.org
Female Reproductive Endocrinology & Infertility

Orlo H. Clark, MD
Professor of Surgery, Department of Surgery, University of California, San Francisco
clarko@surgery.ucsf.edu
Endocrine Surgery

Felix A. Conte, MD
Professor of Pediatrics Emeritus, University of California, San Francisco
felixconte@yahoo.com
Disorders of Sex Determination & Differentiation

David S. Cooper, MD
Professor of Medicine, Division of Endocrinology and Metabolism, Johns Hopkins University School of Medicine; Baltimore, Maryland
dscooper@jhmi.edu
The Thyroid Gland

James W. Findling, MD
Professor of Medicine, Director of Community Endocrine Services, Medical College of Wisconsin, Milwaukee
jfindling@mcw.edu
Hypothalamus & Pituitary Gland; Glucocorticoids & Adrenal Androgens

Paul A. Fitzgerald, MD
Clinical Professor of Medicine, Division of Endocrinology, Department of Medicine, University of California, San Francisco
paul.fitzgerald@ucsf.edu
Adrenal Medulla & Paraganglia

Janet L. Funk, MD
Associate Professor of Medicine, Division of Endocrinology, Department of Medicine, University of Arizona, Tucson
jfunk@u.arizona.edu
Humoral Manifestations of Malignancy

David G. Gardner, MD, MS
Mount Zion Health Fund Distinguished Professor of Endocrinology and Medicine; Chief, Division of Endocrinology and Metabolism, Department of Medicine; and Diabetes Center, University of California, San Francisco
dgardner@diabetes.ucsf.edu
Hormones & Hormone Action; Multiple Endocrine Neoplasia; Endocrine Emergencies

Michael S. German, MD
Professor and Justine K. Schreyer Endowed Chair in Diabetes
    Research, Department of Medicine, Division of
    Endocrinology and Diabetes Center, University of
    California, San Francisco
mgerman@biochem.ucsf.edu
Pancreatic Hormones & Diabetes Mellitus

Stephen E. Gitelman, MD
Professor of Clinical Pediatrics, Division of Pediatric
    Endocrinology, Department of Pediatrics, University of
    California, San Francisco
sgitelma@peds.ucsf.edu
Hypoglycemic Disorders

Susan L. Greenspan, MD
Professor of Medicine and Director, Osteoporosis Prevention
    and Treatment Center, University of Pittsburgh Medical
    Center; Director, Bone Health Program, Magee Women's
    Hospital; Director, Clinical and Translational Research
    Center, UPMC Braddock, Pittsburgh, Pennsylvania
greenspans@dom.pitt.edu
Geriatric Endocrinology

Melvin M. Grumbach, MD, DM Hon causa (Geneva), D Hon causa
    (Rene Descartes, Paris), D Hon causa (Athens)
Edward B. Shaw Professor of Pediatrics and Chairman
    Emeritus, Department of Pediatrics, University of
    California, San Francisco
grumbach@peds.ucsf.edu
Disorders of Sex Determination & Differentiation

Carl Grunfeld, MD, PhD
Professor of Medicine, University of California, San Francisco;
    Chief, Metabolism and Endocrine Sections, Veterans Affairs
    Medical Center, San Francisco
carl.grunfeld@ucsf.edu
AIDS Endocrinopathies

Juan Carlos Jaume, MD
Assistant Professor, Division of Endocrinology, Diabetes and
    Metabolism, Department of Medicine, University of
    Wisconsin-Madison; Chief, Endocrinology, Diabetes, and
    Metabolism Section, Veterans Affairs Medical Center,
    Madison, Wisconsin
jcj@medicine.wisc.edu
Endocrine Autoimmunity

Bradley R. Javorsky, MD
Assistant Professor of Medicine, Endocrinology Center,
    Medical College of Wisconsin, Menomonee Falls
bjavorsky@mcw.edu
Hypothalamus and Pituitary Gland

Alka M. Kanaya, MD
Associate Professor of Medicine, Epidemiology & Biostatistics,
    University of California, San Francisco
alka.kanaya@ucsf.edu
Obesity

John P. Kane, MD, PhD
Professor of Medicine, Biochemistry, and Biophysics, and
    Associate Director, Cardiovascular Research Institute,
    University of California, San Francisco
john.kane@ucsf.edu
Disorders of Lipoprotein Metabolism

Mary Korytkowski, MD
Professor of Medicine, University of Pittsburgh School of
    Medicine, Pittsburgh, Pennsylvania
mtk7@pitt.edu
Geriatric Endocrinology

Paul W. Ladenson, MA (Oxon), MD
John Eager Howard Professor of Endocrinology and
    Metabolism; Professor of Medicine, Pathology, Oncology,
    Radiology and Radiological Sciences, and International
    Health; Distinguished Service Professor; and Director,
    Division of Endocrinology and Metabolism, Johns Hopkins
    University School of Medicine, Baltimore, Maryland
ladenson@jhmi.edu
The Thyroid Gland

Geeta Lal, MD, MSc, FRCS(C), FACS
Assistant Professor of Surgery, Division of Surgical Oncology
    and Endocrine Surgery, Department of Surgery, University
    of Iowa Hospitals and Clinics, Iowa City
geeta-lal@uiowa.edu
Endocrine Surgery

Grace Lee, MD
Assistant Professor of Medicine, Department of Medicine,
    University of California, San Francisco
grace.lee.2@ucsf.edu
AIDS Endocrinopathies

Mary J. Malloy, MD
Professor (Emeritus), Department of Pediatrics and Medicine,
    Director, Pediatric Lipid Clinic and Co-Director, Adult
    Lipid Clinic, University of California, San Francisco
mary.malloy@ucsf.edu
Disorders of Lipoprotein Metabolism

Umesh Masharani, MB, BS, MRCP(UK)
Professor of Clinical Medicine, Division of Endocrinology and
    Metabolism, University of California, San Francisco
umesh.masharani@ucsf.edu
*Pancreatic Hormones & Diabetes Mellitus; Hypoglycemic
    Disorders*

Robert A. Nissenson, PhD

Senior Research Career Scientist, Endocrine Research Unit, Veterans' Affairs Medical Center, San Francisco, Professor, Department of Medicine and Physiology, University of California, San Francisco

robert.nissenson@ucsf.edu

Hormones & Hormone Action

Neil M. Resnick, MD

Thomas Detre Professor of Medicine, Chief, Division of Geriatric Medicine, and Director, University of Pittsburgh Institute on Aging, University of Pittsburgh School of Medicine, Pittsburgh, Pennsylvania

kimee@dom.pitt.edu

Geriatric Endocrinology

Alan G. Robinson, MD

Professor of Medicine, Associate Vice Chancellor, Medical Sciences and Executive Associate Dean, David Geffen School of Medicine at UCLA, University of California, Los Angeles

robinson@ucla.edu

The Posterior Pituitary (Neurohypophysis)

Mitchell P. Rosen, MD

Assistant Professor, Department of Obstetrics and Gynecology, Division of Reproductive Endocrinology, University of California, San Francisco

rosenm@obgyn.ucsf.edu

Female Reproductive Endocrinology & Infertility

Deborah Sellmeyer, MD

Associate Professor, Division of Endocrinology and Metabolism, Department of Medicine, Johns Hopkins University School of Medicine, Baltimore, Maryland

bone@jhmi.edu

Metabolic Bone Disease

Dolores Shoback, MD

Professor of Medicine, Department of Medicine, University of California, San Francisco; Staff Physician, Endocrine-Metabolism Section, Department of Medicine, San Francisco Veterans Affairs Medical Center, San Francisco, California

dolores.shoback@ucsf.edu

Metabolic Bone Disease; Humoral Manifestations of Malignancy

Dennis Styne, MD

Professor and Rumsey Chair, Department of Pediatrics, Section of Endocrinology, University of California, Davis, Sacramento

dmstyne@ucdavis.edu

Growth; Puberty

Robert N. Taylor, MD, PhD

Leach-Hendee Professor and Vice-Chairman for Research, Department of Gynecology and Obstetrics, Emory University, Atlanta, Georgia

robert.n.taylor@emory.edu

The Endocrinology of Pregnancy

J. Blake Tyrrell, MD

Clinical Professor of Medicine; Chief, Endocrine Clinic, Division of Endocrinology and Metabolism, University of California, San Francisco

blaket@medicine.ucsf.edu

Hypothalamus & Pituitary Gland; Glucocorticoids & Adrenal Androgens

Christian Vaisse, MD PhD

Associate Professor of Medicine, Department of Medicine, Diabetes Center, University of California, San Francisco

vaisse@medicine.ucsf.edu

Obesity

William F. Young, Jr, MD, MSc

Professor of Medicine, Mayo Clinic College of Medicine, Mayo Clinic, Rochester, Minnesota

young.william@mayo.edu

Endocrine Hypertension

Preface

This represents the ninth edition of *Greenspan's Basic & Clinical Endocrinology*—the first in an all-color format, which we hope will add to the value of the text for our readers. Each of the individual chapters has been revised and updated to contain the most current information in the field. We have introduced two entirely new chapters on Endocrine Hypertension (Chapter 10) and Obesity (Chapter 20) and added five new authors to our existing chapters.

Once again, we hope that you will find this text useful in dealing with the expanding world of basic and clinical endocrinology, and we trust that you will find it a valuable tool for education of trainees and the treatment of endocrine patients.

David G. Gardner, MD, MS
Dolores Shoback, MD
San Francisco, CA

Hormones and Hormone Action

David G. Gardner, MD, Mark Anderson, MD, PhD, and
Robert A. Nissenson, PhD

ACTH	Adrenocorticotropin	**GR**	Glucocorticoid receptor
AD1	Activation domain 1	**GRB2**	Growth factor receptor–bound protein-2
AD2	Activation domain 2	**GRE**	Glucocorticoid response element
AF-1	Activator function-1	**GRIP**	Glucocorticoid receptor–interacting protein
AF-2	Activator function-2	**GSK3**	Glycogen synthase kinase-3
Akt	Protein kinase B	**GTF**	General transcription factor
AMH	Anti-müllerian hormone	**GTP**	Guanosine triphosphate
ANP	Atrial natriuretic peptide	**HRE**	Hormone response element
AP-1	Activator protein-1	**HSP**	Heat shock protein
β-ARK	β-Adrenergic receptor kinase	**ID**	Receptor–repressor interaction domain
BNP	B-type natriuretic peptide	**IGF**	Insulin-like growth factor
cAMP	Cyclic adenosine-3′,5′-monophosphate	**I-κB**	Inhibitor of nuclear factor kappa B
CARM	Coactivator-associated arginine methyltransferase	**IKK**	Inhibitor of nuclear factor kappa B kinase
		IP$_3$	Inositol 1,4,5-trisphosphate
CBP	CREB-binding protein	**IP$_4$**	Inositol 1,3,4,5-tetrakis-phosphate
cGMP	Cyclic guanosine-3′,5′-monophosphate	**ISRE**	Interferon-stimulated response element
CNP	C-type natriuretic peptide	**JAK**	Janus kinase
CREB	cAMP response element-binding protein	**KHD**	Kinase homology domain
DAG	Diacylglycerol	**LBD**	Ligand-binding domain
DBD	DNA-binding domain	**LH**	Luteinizing hormone
DRIP	Vitamin D receptor–interacting protein	**MAPK**	Mitogen-activated protein kinase
EGF	Epidermal growth factor	**MEK**	MAPK kinase
ER	Estrogen receptor	**MR**	Mineralocorticoid receptor
ERK	Extracellular signal–regulated kinase	**MSH**	Melanocyte-stimulating hormone
FAD	Flavin adenine dinucleotide	**N-Cor**	Nuclear receptor corepressor
FGF	Fibroblast growth factor	**NF-κB**	Nuclear factor kappa B
FMN	Flavin mononucleotide	**NO**	Nitric oxide
FOX A1	Forkhead transcription factor A1	**NOS**	Nitric oxide synthase
GAP	GTPase-activating protein	**NPR**	Natriuretic peptide receptor
GAS	Interferon gamma activated sequences	**NR**	Nuclear receptor
GDP	Guanosine diphosphate	**NRPTK**	Nonreceptor protein tyrosine kinase
GH	Growth hormone	**PAK**	p21-activated kinase
GHR	Growth hormone receptor	**P/CAF**	p300/CBP-associated factor
GLUT 4	Glucose transporter type 4	**P/CIP**	p300/CBP cointegrator-associated protein

PDE	Phosphodiesterase
PDGF	Platelet-derived growth factor
PDK	Phosphatidylinositol-3,4,5-triphosphate-dependent kinase
PHP-1a	Pseudohypoparathyroidism type 1a
PI-3K	Phosphoinositide-3-OH kinase
PIP$_2$	Phosphatidylinositol-4,5-bisphosphate
PIP$_3$	Phosphatidylinositol-3,4,5-trisphosphate
PI(3,4)P2	Phosphatidylinositol-3,4,5-bisphosphate
PKA	Protein kinase A
PKB	Protein kinase B
PKC	Protein kinase C
PKG	cGMP-dependent protein kinase
PLCβ	Phospholipase C beta
PLCγ	Phospholipase C gamma
PLC$_{PC}$	Phosphatidylcholine-selective phospholipase
POL II	RNA polymerase II
PPARγ	Peroxisome proliferator–activated receptor
PR	Progesterone receptor
PTH	Parathyroid hormone
RANK	Receptor activator of nuclear factor kappa B
RAR	Retinoic acid receptor
RE	Response element
RGS	Regulators of G protein signaling

RSK	Ribosomal S6 kinase
RXR	Retinoid X receptor
SH2	src homology domain type 2
SIE	Sis-inducible element
SMRT	Silencing mediator for RXR and TR
SOCS	Suppressor of cytokine signaling
SOS	Son-of-sevenless
SR	Steroid receptor
SRC	Steroid receptor coactivator
SRE	Serum response element
SRF	Serum response factor
STAT	Signal transducer and activator of transcription
SWI/SNF	ATP-dependent chromatin remodeling complex
TBP	TATA-binding protein
TGF-β	Transforming growth factor beta
TPA	12-O-tetradecanoyl-phorbol 13-acetate
TR	Thyroid hormone receptor
TRAF	Tumor necrosis factor receptor–associated factor
TRAP	Thyroid hormone receptor–associated protein
TRE	TPA response element
TSH	Thyroid-stimulating hormone
VDR	Vitamin D receptor

Hormones are signaling molecules that traffic information from one cell to another, typically through a soluble medium like the extracellular fluid. Hormones fall into one of a number of different hormonal classes (eg, steroids, monoamines, peptides, proteins, eicosanoids) and signal through a variety of general (eg, nuclear vs cell surface) and specific (eg, tyrosine kinase vs phosphoinositide turnover) mechanisms in target cells.

Hormones produced in one tissue may promote activity in a target tissue at some distance from the point of secretion. In this case the hormone travels through the bloodstream, often bound to a plasma protein, to access the target tissue. In addition, hormones may act locally following secretion; either on a neighboring cell (paracrine effect), on the secretory cell itself (autocrine effect), or without actually being released from the secretory cell (intracrine effect) (Figure 1–1).

Identification of a tissue as a target for a particular hormone requires the presence of receptors for the hormone in cells of the target tissue. These receptors, in turn, are linked to effector mechanisms that lead to the physiological effects associated with the hormone.

RELATIONSHIP TO THE NERVOUS SYSTEM

Many features of the endocrine system, for example, the use of ligands and receptors to establish communication between cells, are shared by the nervous system. In fact, from a functional standpoint, the two systems are probably related from an evolutionary standpoint. However, there are some important differences between the two systems. While the nervous system uses a highly compartmentalized, closed system of cables to connect cells at some distance from one another, the endocrine system relies on circulating plasma to carry newly released hormone to its targets in the periphery. As a result, the time constants for signal delivery are quite different between the two—virtually instantaneous for the nervous system but delayed, by virtue of circulation times, for the endocrine system. Thus, while neural responses are typically measured in seconds, endocrine responses are measured in minutes to hours—thereby accommodating different needs in the organism. A second difference relates to the nature of the ligand–receptor interaction. In the nervous system, the affinity of receptor for ligand is relatively low. This allows for rapid dissociation of ligand from receptor and, if that ligand is degraded locally, a rapid cessation of biological effect. Despite this rapid dissociation, the secretory neuron is able to maintain receptor occupancy by keeping concentrations of the ligand high around the target neuron. It does this through pulsatile release of secretory granules into an incredibly small volume (ie, that determined by the volume in the synaptic cleft). The endocrine system, on the other hand, has a very large volume of distribution for many of its ligands (eg, circulating blood

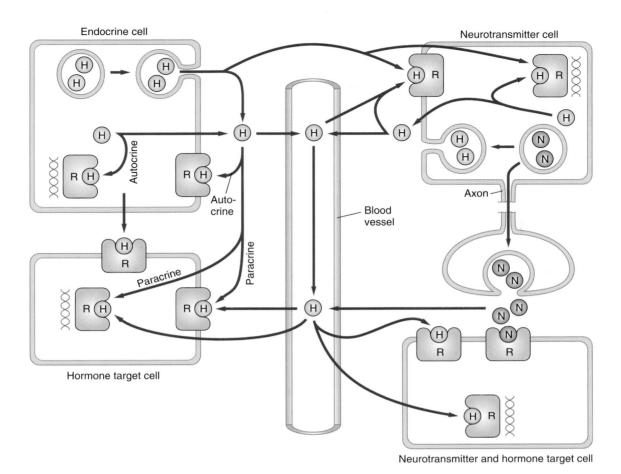

FIGURE 1–1 Actions of hormones and neurotransmitters. Endocrine and neurotransmitter cells synthesize hormones and release them by specialized secretory pathways or by diffusion. Hormones can act at the site of production either following release (autocrine) or without release (intracrine) from the producer cell. They can also act on neighboring target cells, including neurotransmitter-producing cells, without entering the circulation (paracrine). Finally, they can access target cells through the circulation (hormonal). Neurotransmitters that access the extracellular compartment, including circulating plasma, can act as paracrine or hormonal regulators of target cell activity (H, hormone; N, neurotransmitter; R, receptor).

volume). Maintaining ligand concentrations analogous to those present in the synaptic cleft would require prodigious secretory capacity. The endocrine system circumvents this problem by selecting ligand–receptor interactions of much higher affinity (100-10,000 fold higher binding affinity) than those used in the nervous system. In effect, the nervous system is structured to deliver high ligand concentrations to relatively low-affinity receptors, allowing it to activate and inactivate biological effects quickly and in a relatively well-defined topography. Its effects are short lived. The endocrine system, on the other hand, uses high-affinity receptors to extract and retain ligand from a relatively "dilute" pool in circulating plasma. Its biological effects are longlasting. It has sacrificed the rapid response to accommodate a wider area of signal distribution and prolongation of the biological effect. Thus, the systems are not only related but complementary in the respective roles that they play in contributing to normal physiological function.

CHEMICAL NATURE OF HORMONES

Hormones vary widely in terms of their chemical composition. Specific examples include proteins (eg, adrenocorticotrophin), peptides (eg, vasopressin), monoamines (eg, norepinephrine), amino acid derivatives (eg, triiodothyronine), steroids (eg, cortisol), and lipids (eg, prostaglandins). Proteins can be glycosylated (eg, thyroid-stimulating hormone) and/or dimerized (eg, follicle-stimulating hormone) to generate full biological activity. In general, protein, peptide, monoamine, and lipophilic hormones tend to exert their effects primarily through protein receptors at the cell membrane, while thyroid hormone and steroids tend to operate in the cell nucleus. However, there are increasing numbers of exceptions to these rules (eg, triiodothyronine activates classic thyroid hormone receptors in the nuclear compartment, and the trace amine receptor [TAR1]) on the cell surface and estradiol appears to activate both nuclear and plasma membrane receptors). It is likely that the biological "effect" of a given hormone reflects a composite of receptor activity located in several different cellular compartments.

ENDOCRINE GLANDS AND TARGET ORGANS

Endocrine glands are traditionally defined as the ductless glandular structures that release their hormonal secretions into the extracellular space where they eventually access circulating plasma. Classic endocrine glands include organs like the pituitary gland, thyroid gland, parathyroid glands, pancreatic islets, adrenal glands, ovaries, and testes. It is now clear that hormones can be secreted from nontraditional endocrine organs and play critical roles in the regulation of physiological homeostasis. Examples of the latter include the heart (natriuretic peptides), kidney (erythropoietin and renin), adipose tissue (leptin and adiponectin), and gut (cholecystokinin and incretins). Once in the circulation, hormones bind to receptors on target tissues to elicit their biological effects. Target tissues for some hormones (eg, glucocorticoids) are numerous reflecting the ubiquitous distribution of glucocorticoid receptors, while those for other tissues have a more limited distribution (eg, androgens).

REGULATION OF HORMONE LEVELS IN PLASMA

Hormone levels in plasma determine the effective ligand concentration at the level of the hormone receptors in peripheral target cells. Thus, regulation of hormone levels plays an important role in the control of the biological effects that the hormone exerts.

Hormone Biosynthesis

New hormone synthesis is one of the principal mechanisms used to raise hormone levels in circulating plasma. In the case of protein or peptide hormones this usually reflects increased expression of the gene encoding the hormone (ie, increased production of the mRNA encoding the hormone) with subsequent increase in hormone synthesis. In the case of steroid or thyroid hormones it reflects increased sequestration of precursors for hormone synthesis (eg, cholesterol for steroid hormones or iodide for thyroid hormone) as well as increased activity of those enzymatic proteins responsible for executing the individual catalytic events required for hormone production—typically the latter may involve a rate-limiting step in the synthetic cascade (eg, 1-alpha hydroxylase activity in the synthesis of 1,25-dihydroxyvitamin D).

Precursor Processing

Processing of hormone precursors participates to varying degrees in controlling circulating hormone levels. Most peptide and protein hormones require some degree of processing to generate the mature hormonal product (eg, conversion of proinsulin to insulin) and impairment in the processing activity can alter the ratio of precursor to product in plasma. In other cases, a critical processing event is part of the secretory process itself (eg, cleavage of thyroxine from thyroglobulin) and impaired processing can result in a dramatic reduction in immunoreactivity as well as bioactivity of the mature hormone. In addition, protein hormones may require posttranslational modification (eg, glycosylation) or assembly (eg, heterodimerization) prior to secretion in order to optimize biological activity.

Hormone Release

Many hormones (eg, peptides, proteins, and monoamines) are stored in secretory granules in endocrine cells. Release of these granules is promoted by signaling events triggered by exogenous regulators termed secretagogues. This often requires activation of a second messenger system (see discussion under "Receptors") like cyclic AMP generation or intracellular calcium mobilization in the endocrine cell. Steroid hormones, on the other hand, are not stored to a significant degree in the hormone-producing cells. In this case synthesis rather than hormone release appears to play the dominant role in controlling hormone levels in circulating plasma.

Hormone Binding in Plasma

Hormones in plasma can circulate either in a free form, uncomplexed with other molecules, or bound to other molecules like plasma proteins. It is the uncomplexed or free form of the hormone that represents the biologically active fraction of hormone in the plasma compartment, and it is this fraction which homeostatic regulatory mechanisms work to preserve. However, binding of hormone to plasma proteins does play an important role in endocrine physiology. First, it provides a reservoir of hormone that exchanges with the free hormone fraction according to the laws of mass action (see under "Receptors"). This makes plasma hormone concentrations less dependent on hormone synthesis and release, effectively stabilizing those concentrations over extended periods of time. This also serves to guarantee a uniform distribution of hormone concentration in capillary beds perfusing target tissues (Figure 1–2). Second, it slows the metabolism or turnover of the hormone by sequestering it away from degradative enzymes or filtration by the kidney.

Hormone Metabolism

Metabolism of hormones also plays an important role in regulating hormone concentrations. In some cases metabolism is responsible for converting precursors with less hormonal activity to products with greater activity (eg, conversion of 25-hydroxyvitamin D to 1,25-dihydroxyvitamin D and conversion of androstenedione to testosterone). In other cases, metabolism leads to degradation and inactivation of the hormone with a cessation of hormone activity. This type of degradation is often specific to the hormonal class under examination. Steroids, for example, are catalytically converted to inactive metabolites and/or sulfated to promote excretion. Thyroid hormones are subjected

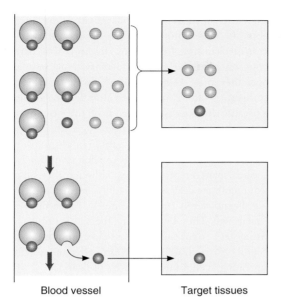

Blood vessel   Target tissues

FIGURE 1–2 Role of plasma binding in delivery of hormones to peripheral tissues. Example shows a hormone that is bound (small red circles) to a plasma protein (large circles) and a hormone that is not protein bound (small orange circles). With the bound hormone, only the free fraction is available for tissue uptake. As the free fraction is depleted, additional hormone dissociates from the plasma-binding protein, making hormone available to more distal portions of the tissue. In contrast, all hormones that are not protein bound are quickly extracted in the proximal part of the tissue.

to deiodination which strips them of their biological activity. Protein and peptide hormones are internalized by target, as well as nontarget, cells and degraded in intracellular lysosomes. In general, the more avid the degradative mechanisms, the shorter the plasma half-life of the hormone.

Regulation of Hormone Levels

Hormone levels can be modulated through regulatory factors affecting any of the steps listed earlier; however, the bulk of the acute "fine-tuning" of hormone levels occurs at the level of hormone secretion and synthesis. Many, if not most, hormone levels are controlled either directly or indirectly by the biological activity that they serve to control. For example, parathyroid hormone (PTH) secretion which responds to low extracellular calcium levels, mobilizes calcium out of bone which, in turn, signals back to the parathyroid gland to turn off PTH secretion. This negative feedback inhibition is a hallmark of endocrine regulation. The end product or negative regulator can either be an inorganic ion or metabolite (eg, calcium for PTH) or a hormonal product in the endocrine cascade (eg, thyroid hormone for TSH). Not all feedback is negative in nature and positive feedback loops (eg, mid-cycle estradiol-induced luteinizing hormone secretion) also play important roles in governing physiological homeostasis.

HORMONE ACTION

Hormones produce their biologic effects through interaction with high-affinity receptors that are, in turn, linked to one or more effector systems within the cell. These effectors involve many different components of the cell's metabolic machinery, ranging from ion transport at the cell surface to stimulation of the nuclear transcriptional apparatus. Steroids and thyroid hormones exert their effects in the cell nucleus, although regulatory activity in the extranuclear compartment has also been documented. Peptide hormones and neurotransmitters, on the other hand, trigger a plethora of signaling activity in the cytoplasmic and membrane compartments while at the same time exerting parallel effects on the transcriptional apparatus. The discussion that follows will focus on the primary signaling systems employed by selected hormonal agonists and attempt to identify examples where aberrant signaling results in human disease.

RECEPTORS

The biologic activity of individual hormones is dependent on their interactions with specific high-affinity receptors on the surfaces or in the cytoplasm or nuclei of target cells. The receptors, in turn, are linked to signaling effector systems responsible for generating the observed biologic response. Receptors, therefore, convey not only specificity of the response (ie, cells lacking receptors lack responsiveness to the hormone) but also the means for activating the effector mechanism. In general, receptors for the peptide hormones and neurotransmitters are aligned on the cell surface and those for the steroid hormones, thyroid hormone, and vitamin D are found in the cytoplasmic or nuclear compartments.

Interactions between the hormone ligand and its receptor are governed by the laws of mass action:

$$[H]+[R] \underset{k_{-1}}{\overset{k_{+1}}{\rightleftharpoons}} [HR]$$

where $[H]$ is the hormone concentration, $[R]$ is the receptor concentration, $[HR]$ is the concentration of the hormone–receptor complex, and k_{+1} and k_{-1} are the rate constants for $[HR]$ formation and dissociation, respectively. Thus, at equilibrium,

$$K_{+1}[H][R] = k_{-1}[HR]$$

or

$$\frac{[H][R]}{HR} = \frac{k_{-1}}{k_{+1}} = K_D$$

where K_D is the equilibrium dissociation constant that defines the affinity of the hormone–receptor interaction (ie, lower the dissociation constant, higher the affinity). Assuming that total receptor concentration $R_0 = [HR] + [R]$, this equation can be rearranged to give

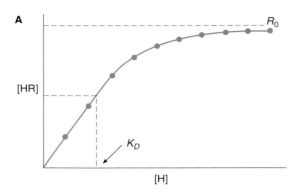

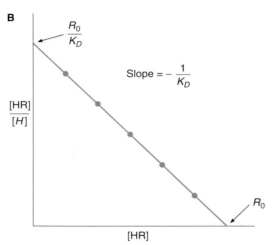

FIGURE 1–3 Ligand saturation **(A)** and Scatchard analysis **(B)** of a hypothetical hormone receptor interaction. K_D represents the dissociation constant; R_0 the total receptor concentration; [HR] and [H] the bound and free ligand, respectively. Note in **A** that the K_D is the concentration [H] at which half of available receptors are occupied.

$$\frac{[\text{HR}]}{[\text{H}]} = -\left(\frac{[\text{HR}]}{K_D}\right) + \frac{R_0}{K_D}$$

This is the Scatchard equation and states that when bound over free ligand (ie, [HR]/[H]) is plotted against bound ligand (ie, [HR]), the slope of the line is defined by $1/K_D$, the y-intercept by R_0/K_D, and the x-intercept by R_0 (Figure 1–3). When [HR] = $R_0/2$, [H] = K_D; therefore, the K_D is also the concentration of hormone [H] at which one-half of the available receptors are occupied. Thus, knowledge of bound and free ligand concentrations, which can be determined experimentally, provides information regarding the affinity of the receptor for its ligand and the total concentration of receptor in the preparation.

Agents that bind to receptors with high affinity are classified as either agonists or antagonists based on the functional outcome of this receptor–ligand interaction. Agonists are ligands that trigger the effector mechanisms and produce biologic effects. Antagonists bind to the receptor but do not activate the effector mechanisms. Because they occupy receptor and block association with the

agonist, they antagonize the functional activity of the latter. Partial agonists bind to the receptor but possess limited ability to activate the effector mechanisms. In different circumstances, partial agonists demonstrate variable biologic activity. For example, when used alone, they may display weak activating activity, whereas their use together with a full agonist may lead to inhibition of function because the latter is displaced from the receptor molecule by a ligand with lower intrinsic activity.

In some systems, receptors are available in a surplus, which is severalfold higher than that required to elicit a maximal biologic response. Such spare receptor systems, although they superficially appear redundant, are designed to rectify a mismatch between low circulating ligand levels and a relatively low-affinity ligand–receptor interaction. Thus, by increasing the number of available receptors, the system is guaranteed a sufficient number of liganded receptor units to activate downstream effector systems fully, despite operating at subsaturating levels of ligand.

NEUROTRANSMITTER AND PEPTIDE HORMONE RECEPTORS

As mentioned above, neurotransmitter and peptide hormones interact predominantly with receptors expressed on the plasma membrane at the cell surface. The K_D of a neurotransmitter for its receptor is typically higher than that of a hormone for its receptor, reflecting a higher k_{off} rate constant (see earlier). Neurotransmitter receptor occupancy is driven by the extraordinarily high concentrations of ligand that can be achieved in the synaptic cleft, and occupancy of the hormone receptor is driven by its high affinity for ligand. The high k_{off} of the neurotransmitter–receptor interaction guarantees that the effect is rapid in onset but of short duration, whereas the lower k_{off} of the hormone–receptor interaction guarantees that the effect is slow in onset but difficult to extinguish, kinetics that are more appropriate for the hormonal functions of these ligands.

The neurotransmitter and peptide receptors can be divided into several major groups (Table 1–1 and Figure 1–4). The first includes the so-called serpentine or "seven-transmembrane-domain" receptors. These receptors each contain an amino terminal extracellular domain followed by seven hydrophobic amino acid segments, each of which is believed to span the membrane bilayer (Figure 1–4). The seventh of these, in turn, is followed by a hydrophilic carboxyl terminal domain that resides within the cytoplasmic compartment. As a group, they share a dependence on the G protein transducers (see discussed later) to execute many of their biologic effects. A second group includes the single-transmembrane-domain receptors that harbor intrinsic tyrosine kinase activity. This includes the insulin, insulin-like growth factor (IGF), and epidermal growth factor (EGF) receptors. A third group, which is functionally similar to the second group, is characterized by a large, extracellular binding domain followed by a single membrane-spanning segment and a cytoplasmic tail. These receptors do not possess intrinsic tyrosine kinase activity but appear to function through interaction with soluble transducer molecules which do possess such activity. Prolactin and growth

TABLE 1–1   Major subdivisions (with examples) of the neurotransmitter-peptide hormone receptor families.[a]

Seven-Transmembrane Domain
β-Adrenergic
PTH
LH
TSH
GRH
TRH
ACTH
MSH
Glucagon
Dopamine
α₂-Adrenergic (–)
Somatostatin (–)

Single-Transmembrane Domain
Growth factor receptors
   Insulin
   IGF
   EGF
   PDGF
Cytokine receptors
   Growth hormone
   Prolactin
   Erythropoietin
   CSF
Guanylyl cyclase-linked receptors
   Natriuretic peptides

[a]Receptors have been subdivided based on shared structural and functional similarities. Minus (–) sign denotes a negative effect on cyclase activity.

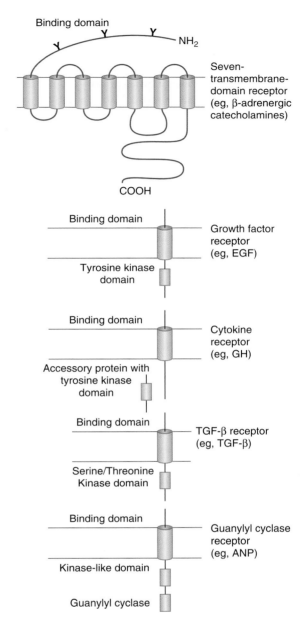

FIGURE 1–4 Structural schematics of different classes of membrane-associated hormone receptors. Representative ligands are presented in parentheses (ANP, atrial natriuretic peptide; EGF, epidermal growth factor; GH, growth hormone; TGF-β, transforming growth factor beta).

hormone are included in this group. Another group are the transforming growth factor beta (TGF-β) family members which signal through serine/threonine kinase domains in their cytoplasmic tails. A fifth group, which includes the natriuretic peptide receptors, operates through activation of a particulate guanylyl cyclase and synthesis of cGMP. The cyclase is covalently attached at the carboxyl terminal portion of the ligand-binding domain and thus represents an intrinsic part of the receptor molecule.

G PROTEIN–COUPLED RECEPTORS

G protein–coupled receptors constitute a large superfamily of molecules capable of responding to ligands of remarkable structural diversity—ranging from photons to large polypeptide hormones. These receptors share overall structural features, most notably seven membrane-spanning regions connected by intracellular and extracellular loops (see Figure 1–4). The receptors are oriented such that the amino terminal domain is extracellular, whereas the carboxyl terminal tail is cytoplasmic. The membrane-spanning segments interact with one another, forming an irregular cylindrical bundle around a central cavity within the molecule. G protein–coupled receptors can assume at least two conformations with differing orientations of the membrane-spanning segments relative to one another. One orientation is favored in the absence of an agonist ligand, and in this orientation the receptor does not activate a G protein (inactive conformation). The second

orientation is stabilized by the binding of an appropriate agonist ligand, and in this conformation the receptor activates a cognate G protein (active conformation). All G protein–coupled receptors are thought to undergo a similar conformational switch on agonist binding, producing a structural change in the cytoplasmic domain that promotes G protein activation. Some small agonists, such as catecholamines, are able to enter the cavity formed by the transmembrane segments, thereby directly stabilizing the active receptor conformation. Other agonists, such as large polypeptide hormones, bind primarily to the extracellular domain of their G protein–coupled receptors. This indirectly results in movement of the transmembrane region of the receptor and stabilization of the active receptor conformation.

Until recently, it was thought that G protein–coupled receptors function exclusively as monomers. Many G protein–coupled receptors are now known to dimerize either with themselves (homodimerization) or with other G protein–coupled receptors (heterodimerization). In some cases, dimerization is important for efficient receptor biosynthesis and membrane localization. In other cases, dimerization is important for optimal ligand affinity, specificity, or receptor signaling.

Heritable mutations in a variety of G protein–coupled receptors are known to be associated with disease. Loss-of-function phenotypes result from mutations that eliminate one or both receptor alleles, or that result in the synthesis of signaling-defective receptors. Gain-of-function phenotypes generally result from point mutations that produce constitutively active receptors (ie, stably assume the active receptor conformation even in the absence of an agonist ligand). Examples of such G protein–coupled receptor disorders relevant to endocrinology are described below and discussed in greater detail elsewhere in this book.

G PROTEIN TRANSDUCERS

G protein–coupled receptors initiate intracellular signaling by activating one (or in some cases multiple) G proteins. G proteins are a family of heterotrimeric proteins that regulate the activity of effector molecules (eg, enzymes, ion channels) (Table 1–2), resulting ultimately in biological responses. The identity of a G protein is defined by the nature of its α subunit, which is largely responsible for effector activation. The major G proteins involved in hormone action (and their actions on effectors) are G_s (stimulation of adenylyl cyclase), G_i (inhibition of adenylyl cyclase; regulation of calcium and potassium channels), and $G_{q/11}$ (stimulation of phospholipase C [PLC] β). The β and γ subunits of G proteins are tightly associated with one another and function as a dimer. In some cases, the $\beta\gamma$ subunit dimer also regulates effector function.

G proteins are noncovalently tethered to the plasma membrane and are thus proximate to their cognate receptors and to their effector targets. The basis for specificity in receptor–G protein interactions has not been fully defined. It is likely that specific structural determinants presented by the cytoplasmic loops of the G protein–coupled receptor determine the identity of the G proteins that are activated. It is the nature of the α subunit of the G protein that is critical for receptor recognition. There are about a dozen different G protein α subunits and hundreds of distinct G protein–coupled receptors. Thus, it is clear that a particular G protein is activated by a large number of different receptors. For example, G_s is activated by receptors for ligands as diverse as β-adrenergic catecholamines and large polypeptide hormones such as luteinizing hormone (LH). LH is thereby able to stimulate adenylyl cyclase and raise intracellular levels of

TABLE 1–2 G protein subunits selectively interact with specific receptor and effector mechanisms.

G Protein Subunit	Associated Receptors	Effector
α_s	β-Adrenergic TSH Glucagon	Adenylyl cyclase Ca^{2+} channels K^+ channels
α_i	α_2-Adrenergic Muscarinic (type II)	Adenylyl cyclase Ca^{2+} channels K^+ channels
α_q	α_1-Adrenergic	PLCβ
β/α		Adenylyl cyclase (+ or –) PLC Supports βARK-mediated receptor phosphorylation and desensitization

cAMP in cells that express LH receptors (eg, Leydig cells of the testis).

Figure 1–5 is a schematic representation of the molecular events associated with activation of G proteins by G protein–coupled receptors. In the basal, inactive state, the G protein is an intact heterotrimer with guanosine diphosphate (GDP) bound to the α subunit. Agonist binding to a G protein–coupled receptor promotes the physical interaction between the receptor and its cognate G protein. This produces a conformational change in the G protein, resulting in the dissociation of GDP.

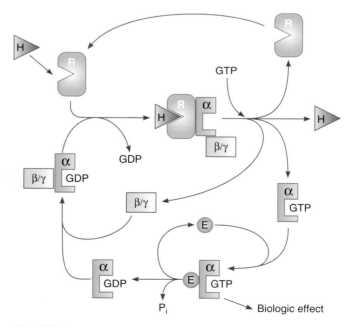

FIGURE 1–5 G protein–mediated signal transduction. α and β/γ subunits of a representative G protein are depicted (see text for details) (E, effector; H, hormonal ligand; R, hormone receptor).

This in turn allows the binding of GTP (which is present at a much higher concentration in cells than is GDP) to the α subunit. Dissociation of the GTP-bound α subunit from the βγ dimer then occurs, allowing these subunits to activate their effector targets. Dissociation of the hormone–receptor complex also occurs. The duration of activation is determined by the intrinsic GTPase activity of the G protein α subunit. Hydrolysis of GTP to GDP terminates the activity and promotes reassociation of the αβγ trimer, returning the system to the basal state. The GTPase activity of G protein α subunits can be increased by the action of proteins termed "regulators of G protein signaling" (RGS proteins).

EFFECTORS

Numerous effectors have been linked to the G protein–coupled receptors. A number of these are presented in Table 1–2. A great many other G proteins—not dealt with here—are coupled to physical or biochemical stimuli but have very limited involvement

in hormone action. As discussed, adenylyl cyclase, perhaps the best-studied of the group, is activated by G_s (Figure 1–6). This activation results in a transient increase in intracellular cAMP levels. The cAMP binds to the inhibitory regulatory subunit of inactive protein kinase A (PKA) and promotes its dissociation from the complex, thereby permitting enhanced activity of the catalytic subunit. The latter phosphorylates a variety of cellular substrates, among them the hepatic phosphorylase kinase that initiates the enzymatic cascade which results in enhanced glycogenolysis. It also phosphorylates and activates the cAMP response element–binding protein (CREB), which mediates many of the known transcriptional responses to cAMP (and to some extent calcium) in the nuclear compartment. Other transcription factors are also known to be phosphorylated by PKA.

PLC beta (PLCβ) is a second effector system that has been studied extensively. The enzyme is activated through G_q-mediated transduction of signals generated by a wide array of hormone–receptor complexes, including those for angiotensin II, α-adrenergic agonists, and endothelin. Activation of the enzyme leads to

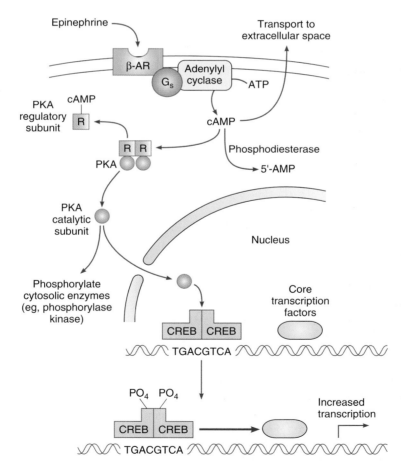

FIGURE 1–6 β-Adrenergic receptor signaling in the cytoplasmic and nuclear compartments. The cAMP response element–binding protein (CREB) is depicted bound to a consensus CRE in the basal state. Phosphorylation of this protein leads to activation of the juxtaposed core transcriptional machinery.

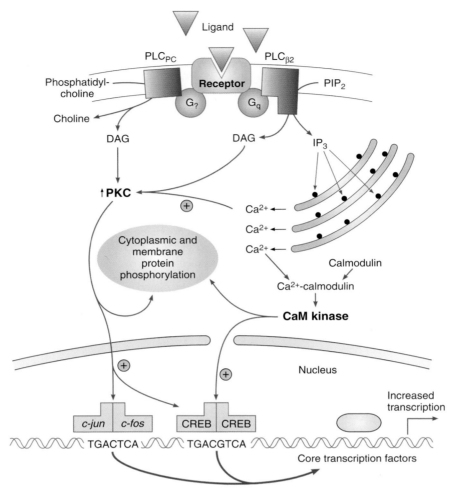

FIGURE 1–7 PLCβ-coupled receptor signaling in the cytoplasmic and nuclear compartments (DAG, diacylglycerol; PC, phosphatidylcholine; PKC, protein kinase C; PLC, phospholipase).

cleavage of phosphoinositol 4,5-bisphosphate in the plasma membrane to generate inositol 1,4,5-trisphosphate (IP_3) and diacylglycerol (DAG) (Figure 1–7). The former interacts with a specific receptor present on the endoplasmic reticulum membrane to promote release of Ca^{2+} into the cytoplasmic compartment. The increased calcium, in turn, may activate protein kinases, promote secretion, or foster contractile activity. Depletion of intracellular calcium pools by IP_3 results in enhanced uptake of calcium across the plasma membrane (perhaps through generation of IP_4 [1,3,4,5-tetrakisphosphate]), thereby activating a second, albeit indirect, signaling mechanism that serves to increase intracellular calcium levels even further. DAG functions as an activator of several protein kinase C (PKC) isoforms within cells. Several different isoforms of PKC (eg, α, β, γ) exist in a given cell type. A number of these are calcium dependent, a property which, given the IP_3 activity mentioned above, provides the opportunity for a synergistic interaction of the two signaling pathways driven by PLCβ activity. However, not all PKC activity derives from the breakdown of PIP_2 substrate. Metabolism of phosphatidylcholine by PLC_{PC} (phosphatidyl choline-selective phospholipase) leads to the generation of phosphocholine and DAG. This latter pathway is believed to be responsible for the more protracted elevations in PKC activity seen following exposure to agonist.

Other phospholipases may also be important in hormone-dependent signaling. Phospholipase D employs phosphatidylcholine as a substrate to generate choline and phosphatidic acid. The latter may serve as a precursor for subsequent DAG formation. As with PLC_{PC} above, no IP_3 is generated as a consequence of this reaction. Phospholipase A_2 triggers release of arachidonic acid, a precursor of prostaglandins, leukotrienes, endoperoxides, and thromboxanes, all signaling molecules in their own right. The relative contribution of these other phospholipases to hormone-mediated signal transduction and the role of the specific lipid breakdown products (eg, phosphocholine, phosphatidic acid) in conveying regulatory information remains an area of active research.

Activation of effectors by G protein–coupled receptors is subject to regulatory mechanisms that prevent overstimulation of cells by an agonist ligand. At the level of the receptor, two regulatory events are known to occur. One is desensitization, wherein initial

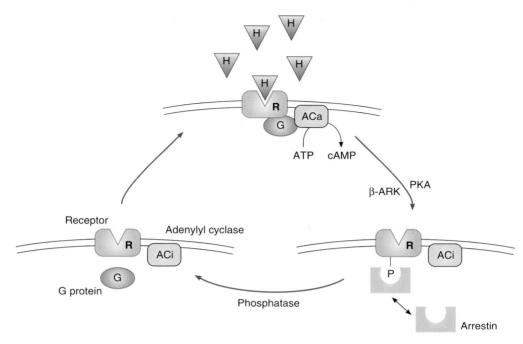

FIGURE 1–8 Kinase-dependent desensitization of the ligand–receptor complex. Schema shown is that for the β-adrenergic receptor, but similar systems probably exist for other types of G protein–linked receptors (ACa, active adenylyl cyclase; ACi, inactive adenylyl cyclase; β-ARK, β-adrenergic receptor kinase; PKA, protein kinase A).

stimulation of a receptor by its agonists leads to a loss of the ability of the receptor to subsequently elicit G protein activation. This is shown schematically in Figure 1–8 for the β-adrenergic receptor. A similar regulatory mechanism exists for many G protein–coupled receptors. Agonist binding to the receptor produces G protein activation and results also in activation of a kinase (termed G protein–coupled receptor kinase, GRK) that phosphorylates the cytoplasmic domain of the receptor. By virtue of this phosphorylation, the receptor acquires high affinity for a member of the arrestin family of proteins. The name "arrestin" derives from the observation that the receptor is no longer capable of interacting with a G protein when arrestin is bound. Thus, the phosphorylated receptor becomes uncoupled from its G protein, preventing signaling to the effector. The receptor remains inactive until a phosphatase acts to restore the receptor to its unphosphorylated state.

Many G protein–coupled receptors are also susceptible to agonist-induced downregulation, resulting in a reduced level of cell surface receptors following exposure of cells to an agonist. This can result from agonist-induced internalization of receptors, followed by trafficking of receptors to lysosomes where degradation occurs. In addition, chronic exposure of cells to an agonist may result in signaling events that suppress the biosynthesis of new receptors, thereby lowering steady-state receptor levels. Together, these regulatory events ensure that the cell is protected from excessive stimulation in the presence of sustained high levels of an agonist.

Recently, it has become clear that these events that serve to dampen G protein signaling can also have important positive roles in promoting cell signaling. For example, arrestin association with G protein–coupled receptors can produce activation of specific pathways such as the MAP kinase pathway, and this occurs independently of G protein signaling. In addition, internalized G protein–coupled receptors can in some cases retain the ability to signal, and the effects may differ from those produced when activation occurs at the plasma membrane.

DISORDERS OF G PROTEINS AND G PROTEIN–COUPLED RECEPTORS

Two bacterial toxins are capable of covalently modifying specific G protein α subunits, thereby altering their functional activity. Cholera toxin is a protein that binds to receptors present on all cells, resulting in the internalization of the enzymatic subunit of the toxin. The toxin enzyme is an ADP-ribosyl transferase that transfers ADPribose from NAD to an acceptor site (Arg[201]) on the α subunit of G_s. This covalent modification greatly inhibits the GTPase activity of α_s, enhancing the activation of adenylyl cyclase by extending the duration of the active GTP-bound form of the G protein. Even in the absence of an active G protein–coupled receptor, GDP dissociates (albeit very slowly) from the G protein. Thus, cholera toxin will eventually activate adenylyl cyclase activity even without agonist binding to a G protein–coupled receptor. The result is a large and sustained activation of adenylyl cyclase. When this occurs in intestinal epithelial cells, the massive increase in cAMP results in the increased water and salt secretion characteristic of cholera.

Pertussis toxin is also an ADP-ribosyl transferase. However, in this case, the substrates are α subunits of different G proteins, most notably G_i and G_o. The ADPribose moiety is transferred to a cysteine residue near the carboxyl terminus of the α subunit, a region required for interaction with activated G protein–coupled receptors. Once ADP-ribosylated by pertussis toxin, these G proteins are no longer able to interact with activated receptors and are thus stuck in an inactive (GDP-bound) conformation. Inhibition of receptor-mediated activation of G_i and G_o accounts for many of the clinical manifestations of pertussis infection.

Genetic mutations in G protein α subunits are seen in a number of human diseases. Acquired activating mutations in $α_s$ can produce a variety of phenotypes depending on the site of expression of the mutant protein. In McCune-Albright syndrome, the mutation occurs in a subset of neural crest cells during embryogenesis. All of the descendants of these cells, including certain osteoblasts, melanocytes, and ovarian or testicular cells, express the mutant protein. The result is a form of genetic mosaicism in which the consequence of unregulated production of cAMP in particular tissues is evident (ie, the progressive bone disorder polyostotic fibrous dysplasia, the abnormal skin pigmentation referred to as café au lait spots, gonadotropin-independent precocious puberty). In cells where cAMP is linked to cell proliferation (eg, thyrotropes, somatotropes), a subset of patients with benign tumors has been shown to have acquired activating mutations in $α_s$. Activating mutations in one of the G_i proteins that is coupled to cell proliferation, $α_{i2}$, have been reported in a subset of adrenal and ovarian tumors.

Loss-of-function mutations in $α_s$ are associated with the hereditary disorder pseudohypoparathyroidism type 1 (PHP-1a). This disorder, first described by Fuller Albright, is the first documented example of a human disease attributable to target cell resistance to a hormone. Affected patients display biochemical features of hypoparathyroidism (eg, hypocalcemia, hyperphosphatemia) but have markedly increased circulating levels of parathyroid hormone (PTH) and display target cell resistance to PTH. Many hormone receptors couple to adenylyl cyclase via G_s, yet patients with PHP-1a generally display only subtle defects in responsiveness to other hormones (eg, TSH, LH). The explanation for this lies in the fascinating genetics of this disorder. In brief, affected patients have one normal and one mutated $α_s$ allele. The mutated allele fails to produce an active form of the protein. Tissues in these patients are expected to express about 50% of the normal level of $α_s$, a level sufficient to support signaling to adenylyl cyclase. However, in certain tissues, the $α_s$ gene is subject to genetic imprinting such that the paternal allele is expressed poorly or not at all. In individuals harboring inactivating mutations, if the paternal allele has the mutation, all cells express about 50% of the normal level of $α_s$ (derived from the normal maternal allele). However, if the maternal allele has the mutation, then the cells in which paternal imprinting occurs express low levels or no $α_s$. One of the major sites of this paternal imprinting is in the proximal renal tubule, an important target tissue for the physiologic actions of PTH. This accounts for the clinical resistance to PTH seen in PHP-1a and accounts also for the fact that only a subset of patients with haploinsufficiency of

$α_s$ are resistant to PTH. Interestingly, essentially all patients with haploinsufficiency of $α_s$ display Albright hereditary osteodystrophy, a developmental disorder with phenotypic manifestations affecting a variety of tissues. This indicates that even a partial loss of adenylyl cyclase signaling is incompatible with normal development.

Mutations in the genes encoding G protein–coupled receptors are being increasingly recognized as important in the pathogenesis of endocrine disorders. Loss-of-function mutations generally need to be homozygous (or compound heterozygous) in order to result in a significant disease phenotype. This is probably due to the fact that most cells have a complement of receptors which exceeds what is needed for maximal cellular response (spare receptors). Thus, a 50% reduction in the amount of a cell surface receptor may have little influence on the ability of a target cell to respond. However, in some situations, haploinsufficiency of a G protein–coupled receptor can produce a clinical phenotype. For instance, heterozygous loss-of-function mutations in the G protein–coupled calcium-sensing receptor results in the autosomal dominant disorder familial hypocalciuric hypercalcemia due to mild dysregulation of PTH secretion and renal calcium handling. Homozygous loss-of-function of the calcium-sensing receptor results in severe neonatal hyperparathyroidism due to the loss of the ability of plasma calcium to suppress PTH secretion and promote renal calcium clearance. Syndromes of hormone resistance have also been reported in patients lacking expression of functional G protein–coupled receptors for vasopressin, ACTH, and TSH. Loss of functional expression of the PTH receptor results in Blomstrand chondrodysplasia, a disorder that is lethal due to the inability of PTH-related protein (a PTH receptor agonist) to promote normal cartilage development.

Mutations that render G protein–coupled receptors constitutively active (in the absence of an agonist ligand) are seen in a number of endocrine disorders. Generally speaking, such mutations produce a disease phenotype resembling that seen with excessive levels of the corresponding hormone agonist. Thus, activating mutations in the TSH receptor produce neonatal thyrotoxicosis, and activating mutations in the LH receptor result in pseudoprecocious puberty or testotoxicosis. Activating mutations in the PTH receptor result in Jansen type metaphyseal chondrodysplasia; a disorder characterized by hypercalcemia and increased bone resorption (mimicking the effects of excess PTH on bone) and delayed cartilage differentiation (mimicking the effects of excess PTH-related protein on cartilage). A theoretical approach to treating disorders resulting from constitutively active G protein–coupled receptors would be administration of "inverse agonists," agents that stabilize receptors in their inactive conformation. Although inverse agonists have been identified for a number of G protein–coupled receptors, they have yet to be successfully employed as therapeutics. Molecular analysis of G protein–coupled receptors has revealed that point mutations, in addition to producing constitutive activity, can alter the specificity of ligand binding or the ability of the receptor to become desensitized. It is almost certain that such mutations will be found to provide the basis for some perhaps more subtle endocrinopathies.

GROWTH FACTOR RECEPTORS

The growth factor receptors differ from those described earlier both structurally and functionally. Unlike the G protein–associated receptors, these proteins span the membrane only once and acquire their signaling ability, at least in part, through activation of tyrosine kinase activity, which is intrinsic to the individual receptor molecules. The insulin and IGF receptors fall within this group as do those for the autocrine or paracrine regulators platelet-derived growth factor (PDGF), fibroblast growth factor (FGF), and EGF. Signaling is initiated by the association of ligand (eg, insulin) with the receptor's extracellular domain (Figure 1–9) and

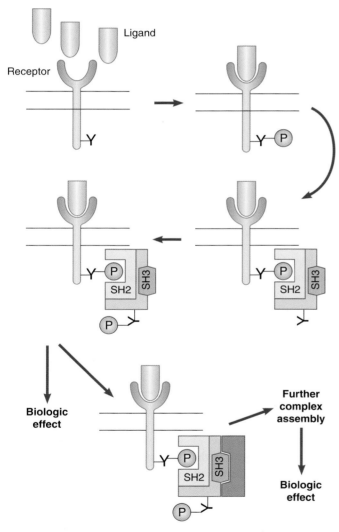

FIGURE 1–9 Signaling by tyrosine kinase–containing growth factor receptor. Receptors depicted here as monomers for simplicity; typically dimerization of receptors follows association with ligand. Autophosphorylation of one or more critically positioned tyrosine residues in the receptor leads to association with accessory proteins or effectors through SH2 domains present on the latter. In some cases, an SH3 domain present on the same protein leads to recruitment of yet other proteins leading to further complex assembly.

subsequent receptor dimerization. This results in phosphorylation of tyrosines both on the receptor itself as well as on nonreceptor substrates. It is assumed that phosphorylation of these substrates results in a cascade of activation events, similar to those described for the G protein–coupled systems, which contribute to perturbations in intracellular pathways. The autophosphorylation of the receptor molecules themselves has been studied extensively and provided some intriguing insights into the mechanisms that underlie signal transduction by this group of proteins.

Tyrosine phosphorylation takes place at specific locations in the receptor molecule. Once phosphorylated, these sites associate, in highly specific fashion, with a variety of accessory proteins that possess independent signaling capability. These include PLCγ, phosphoinositol (PI) 3′ kinase, GTPase-activating protein (GAP), growth factor receptor–bound protein-2 (GRB2), and the Src family nonreceptor tyrosine kinases. These interactions are fostered by the presence of highly conserved type 2 *src* homology (based on sequence homology to the *src* proto-oncogene) domains (SH2) in each of the accessory molecules. Each individual SH2 domain displays specificity for the contextual amino acids surrounding the phosphotyrosine residues in the receptor molecule. In the PDGF receptor, for example, the SH2 domain of PLCγ associates selectively with Tyr^{977} and Tyr^{989}, whereas that of PI 3′ kinase associates with Tyr^{708} and Tyr^{719}. Thus, diversity of response is controlled by contextual sequences around individual phosphotyrosine residues that determine the types of accessory proteins brought into the signaling complex. These protein–protein interactions may provide a means of directly activating the signaling molecule in question, perhaps through a change in steric conformation. Alternatively, they may facilitate the sequestration of these accessory proteins in or near the plasma membrane compartment, in close proximity to key substrates (eg, membrane lipids in the case of PLCγ) or other important regulatory proteins.

Some of these associations trigger immediate signaling events, but others (eg, GRB2) may act largely to provide the scaffolding needed to construct a more complex signaling apparatus (Figure 1–10). In the case of GRB2, another accessory protein (son-of-sevenless; SOS) associates with the receptor–GRB2 complex through a type 3 *src* homology (SH3) domain present in the latter. This domain recognizes a sequence of proline-rich amino acids present in the SOS protein. SOS, in turn, facilitates assembly of the Ras–Raf complex, which permits activation of downstream effectors such as mitogen-activated protein kinase (MAPK) kinase (MEK). This latter kinase, which possesses both serine-threonine and tyrosine kinase activity, activates the p42 and p44 MAPKs (also called extracellular signal–regulated kinases; ERKs). ERK acts on a variety of substrates within the cell, including the RSK kinases, which, in turn, phosphorylate the ribosomal S_6 protein and thereby stimulates protein synthesis. These phosphorylation reactions (and their amplification in those instances where the MAPK substrate is a kinase itself) often lead to protean changes in the phenotype of the target cells.

The liganded growth factor receptors, including the insulin receptor, may also signal through the phosphoinositide 3-OH kinase (PI-3K). SH2 domains of the p85 regulatory subunit of PI-3K associate with the growth factor receptor through specific

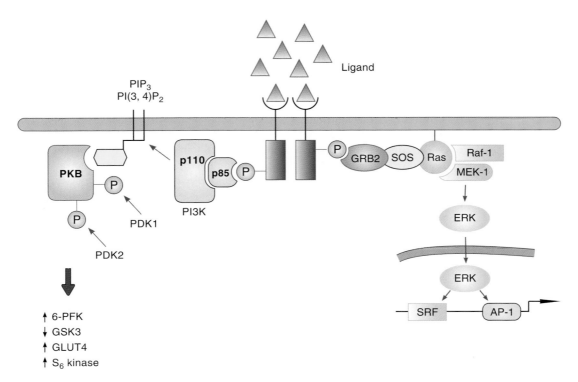

FIGURE 1–10 Growth factor–dependent pathway. Assembly of the components involved in the Ras/Raf/MEK/MAPK and PI-3K/PKB–signaling mechanisms.

phosphotyrosine residues (Tyr^{740} and Tyr^{751} in the PDGF receptor) in a manner similar to that described above for GRB2 (see Figure 1–10). This leads to activation of the p110 catalytic subunit of PI-3K and increased production of phosphatidylinositol-3,4,5-trisphosphate (PIP_3) and phosphatidylinositol-3,4-bisphosphate ($PI[3,4]P_2$). These latter molecules sequester protein kinase B (also known as Akt) at the cell membrane through association with the plekstrin homology domains in the amino terminal of the kinase molecule. This in turn leads to phosphorylation of PKB at two separate sites (Thr^{308} in the active kinase domain and Ser^{473} in the carboxyl terminal tail) by PIP_3-dependent kinases (PDK1 and PDK2). These phosphorylations result in activation of PKB. In the case of insulin-sensitive target cells, downstream targets of activated PKB (eg, following insulin stimulation) include 6-phosphofructo-2-kinase (increased activity), glycogen synthase kinase-3 (GSK3) (decreased activity), the insulin-responsive glucose transporter GLUT 4 (translocation and increased activity), and p70 S6 kinase (increased activity). This leads to increased glycolysis, increased glycogen synthesis, increased glucose transport, and increased protein synthesis, respectively. There is also a growing body of evidence suggesting that PKB may protect cells from programmed cell death through phosphorylation of key proteins in the apoptotic pathway.

It has been reported that G protein–coupled receptors may also activate the Raf-MEK-ERK cascade, although in this case the signal traffics through a nonreceptor protein tyrosine kinase (NRPTK such as Src and Fyn) rather than the traditional growth factor receptor–linked tyrosine kinases. The details of the mechanism are incompletely understood, but it appears to require the participation of β-arrestin (discussed earlier) as an adaptor molecule linking the G protein receptor to the NRPTK. Interestingly, this implies that β-arrestin, which terminates coupling between the receptor and G protein, actually promotes coupling between the desensitized receptor and downstream effectors traditionally associated with growth factor–dependent activation.

CYTOKINE RECEPTORS

These include the receptors for a variety of cytokines, erythropoietin, colony-stimulating factor, GH, and prolactin. These cell membrane receptors have a single internal hydrophobic stretch of amino acids, suggesting that they span the membrane but once (see Figure 1–4). They can be composed of monomers or heterodimers of different molecules.

Growth Hormone and Prolactin Receptors

Receptors for GH and prolactin are prototypical cytokine receptors (Figure 1–11). Interestingly, alternative splicing of the GH receptor gene primary transcript results in a foreshortened "receptor" that lacks the membrane anchor and carboxyl terminal domain of the protein. This "receptor" is secreted and serves to bind GH in the extracellular space (eg, circulating plasma). Unlike the growth factor receptors described above, GH receptors lack a

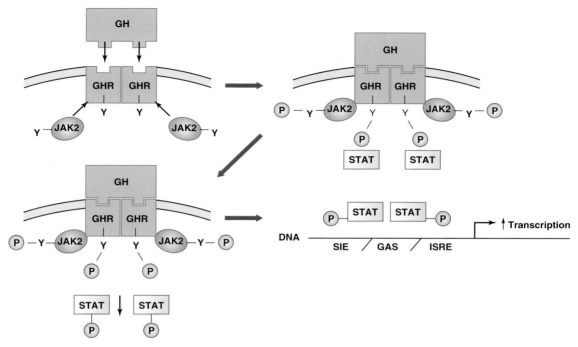

FIGURE 1–11 Signaling by the growth hormone receptor (GHR). Different portions of a single growth hormone molecule associate with homologous regions of two independent GHR molecules. This is believed to lead to the recruitment of Janus kinase 2 (JAK2), which phosphorylates the GHR, providing a docking site for STAT. The latter is phosphorylated, dissociates from the liganded receptor complex, and migrates to the nucleus, where it associates with binding elements of target genes and regulates transcription.

tyrosine kinase domain. Different domains of a single GH molecule associate with homologous regions of two independent GH receptors, promoting dimerization of the receptors and subsequent association with and activation of Janus kinase (JAK) 2. JAK2 undergoes autophosphorylation and concurrently tyrosine phosphorylates the GH receptors. The latter provide a docking site for the signal transducer and activator of transcription (STAT) factors; STAT 5a and 5b appear to be particularly relevant to GH and prolactin action. The STATs are phosphorylated, dissociate from the GH receptor, migrate to the nucleus, and bind to specific STAT-binding DNA regulatory elements (SIE/ISRE/GAS) responsible for transcriptional control of GH target genes such as IGF-1. There are a number of different STAT family members, and there is specificity of certain cytokine receptors for certain STAT family members. This helps direct the specificity of signaling by each type of receptor. STAT signaling is also regulated by a family of inhibitors referred to as suppressor of cytokine signaling (SOCS) proteins. SOCS proteins bind to JAK and STAT proteins and target them for degradation. SOCS proteins are induced after cytokine/hormone binding and help to autoregulate signaling in this pathway.

TGF-β Receptors

These receptors bind a variety of ligands that include the cytokine transforming growth factor beta (TGF-β) and the hormones inhibin, activin, and anti-müllerian hormone (AMH). The ligands for these receptors are typically homo- or heterodimers of subunits that have a highly conserved, cysteine-dependent structure. TGF-β family receptors bind to ligands through a heterodimeric receptor consisting of two transmembrane subunits known as type I and type II receptors (Figure 1–12). There are a number of different type I and type II receptor subunits in this family and type I/type II pairs can form between several different family members. Both type I and type II receptors have an intracellular serine/threonine kinase domain. The type II receptor is constitutively phosphorylated and active, while the type I receptor is not. The ligands in this family initially bind the type II receptor. The type I receptor is recruited to the complex where the type II receptor kinase phosphorylates and activates the type I receptor, which then further propagates the signal. Downstream in the signaling pathway are a group of phosphorylation targets called the Smad proteins. These proteins, upon phosphorylation, can migrate to the nucleus to activate and/or repress transcription of target genes.

TNF-Receptors

The tumor necrosis factor (TNF) family of receptors is a large group of cytokine receptors that bind to both soluble and cell-membrane-associated ligands. One important member of this family is the receptor activator of nuclear factor kappa B (RANK) which plays a critical function in the regulation of bone physiology (see Chapter 8). These receptors consist of a trimeric complex of three single transmembrane receptors that bind to ligand. The cytoplasmic tail of many TNF-receptors

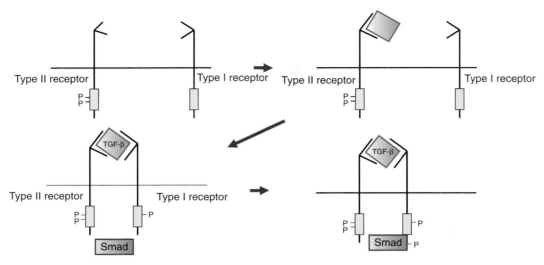

FIGURE 1–12 Signaling by the TGF-β receptors. TGF-β ligand first docks with the type II receptor which has an intracellular serine/threonine kinase domain that is constitutively active. After ligand binding, the type I receptor is then recruited to the complex and the type II receptor can phosphorylate the intracellular serine/threonine kinase domain of the type I receptor. This then propagates the signal downstream leading to the phosphorylation and activation of Smad proteins which can migrate to the nucleus and activate or repress gene transcription.

(including RANK) interacts with a family of adapter molecules called TNF receptor–associated factors (TRAFs) that further activate a number of downstream pathways, the most of important of which is the activation of nuclear factor kappa B (NF-κB) (Figure 1–13). Activation of NF-κB is a central event in many if not all inflammatory responses and leads to the induction of many molecules including those involved in apoptotic, cytokine, and chemokine pathways. TNF-receptor signaling leads to the activation of NF-κB through phosphorylation of the heterotrimeric I-κB kinase (IKK) complex, which then phosphorylates the inhibitor of NF-κB (I-κB). I-κB complexes with NF-κB in the cytosol and keeps it inactive; however, when I-κB is phosphorylated it dissociates from the complex and undergoes degradation through the ubiquitin-dependent proteasome pathway. NF-κB then translocates to the nucleus where it regulates gene transcription.

GUANYLYL CYCLASE–LINKED RECEPTORS

Activation of guanylyl cyclase–dependent signaling cascades can occur through two independent mechanisms. The first involves activation of the soluble guanylyl cyclase, a heme-containing enzyme that is activated by the gas nitric oxide (NO) generated in the same or neighboring cells. NO is produced by the enzyme nitric oxide synthase. NO synthase exists as three different isozymes in selected body tissues. Constitutive forms of NO synthase (NOS) are produced in endothelial (NOS-3) and neuronal (NOS-1) cells. The endothelial enzyme possesses binding sites for FAD and FMN as well as calcium and appears to require calcium for optimal activity. Agents such as bradykinin and acetylcholine, which interact with receptors on the surface of endothelial cells

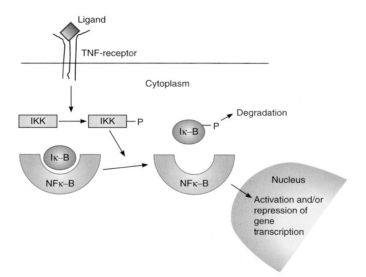

FIGURE 1–13 TNF receptor signaling. TNF binds to a trimolecular cell surface receptor which transmits a downstream signal that leads to the phosphorylation and activation of the I-κB kinase (IKK). IKK phosphorylates the inhibitor of NF-κB (I-κB) which is then tagged for degradation through a ubiquitin-dependent proteosomal pathway. This allows NF-κB to migrate to the nucleus where it can carry out activation or repression of gene transcription.

and increase intracellular calcium levels, trigger an increase in constitutive NO synthase activity with consequent generation of NO and activation of soluble guanylyl cyclase activity in neighboring vascular smooth muscle cells (Figure 1–14). Thus, in this instance, the cGMP-dependent vasodilatory activity of acetylcholine requires sequential waves of signaling activity in two different cell types to realize the ultimate physiologic effect.

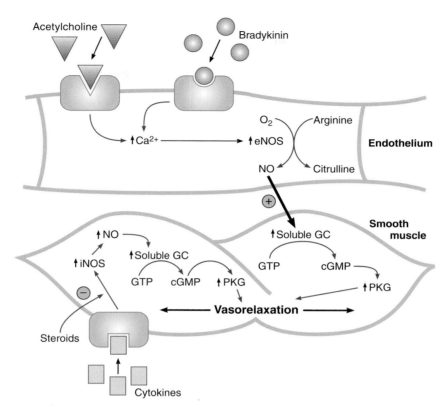

FIGURE 1–14 Signaling through the endothelial (e) and inducible (i) nitric oxide synthases (NOS) in the vascular wall. Activation of eNOS in the endothelial cell or iNOS in the vascular smooth muscle cell leads to an increase in NO and stimulation of soluble guanylyl cyclase (GC) activity. Subsequent elevations in cGMP activate cGMP-dependent protein kinase (PKG) and promote vasorelaxation.

The inducible (i) form of NO synthase (NOS-2) is found predominantly in inflammatory cells of the immune system, although it has also been reported to be present in smooth muscle cells of the vascular wall. Unlike the endothelial form of NO synthase, expression of iNO synthase is low in the basal state. Treatment of cells with a variety of cytokines triggers an increase in new iNO synthase synthesis (hence, the inducible component of iNO synthase activity), probably through activation of specific *cis* elements in the iNO synthase promoter. Thus, hormones, cytokines, or growth factors with the capacity for induction of iNO synthase activity may direct at least a portion of their signaling activity through a cGMP-dependent pathway.

A third mechanism for increasing cGMP levels within target cells involves the activation of particulate guanylyl cyclases (Figure 1–15). From an endocrine standpoint, this involves predominantly the natriuretic peptide receptors (NPR). NPR-A is a single-transmembrane-domain receptor (about 130 kDa) with a large extracellular domain that provides ligand recognition and binding. This is followed by a hydrophobic transmembrane domain and a large intracellular domain that harbors the signaling function. The amino terminal portion of this intracellular region contains an ATP-binding kinase homology domain (KHD) that is involved in regulating cyclase activity, whereas the carboxyl terminal domain contains the catalytic core of the particulate guanylyl cyclase. It is believed that association of ligand with the extracellular domain leads to a conformational change in the receptor that arrests the tonic inhibitory control of the kinase-like domain and permits activation of guanylyl cyclase activity. Recent studies suggest that the small GTPase Rac can directly activate the catalytic domain through its effector kinase PAK (p21-activated kinase). NPR-B, the product of a separate gene, has a similar topology and a relatively high level of sequence homology to the NPR-A gene product; however, while NPR-A responds predominantly to the cardiac atrial natriuretic peptide (ANP) and brain natriuretic peptide (BNP), NPR-B is activated by the C-type NP (CNP), a peptide found in the central nervous system, endothelium, and reproductive tissues but not in the heart. Thus, segregated expression of the ligand and its cognate receptor convey a high level of response specificity to these two systems despite the fact that they share a common final effector mechanism. Noteworthy, both NPR-A and NPR-B require a high degree of phosphorylation in the kinase homology domain to retain sensitivity to agonist. Dephosphorylation, perhaps through agonist-triggered exposure of the phosphoserine residues to regulatory phosphatase activity in the target cell, results in receptor desensitization. In humans, homozygous mutation of the *NPR-B* genes results in acromesomelic dysplasia, Maroteaux type (AMDM), a rare form of autosomal recessive, short-limbed dwarfism.

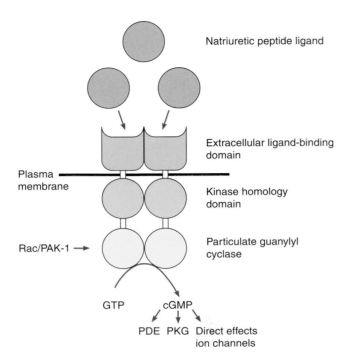

FIGURE 1–15. Signaling by particulate guanylyl cyclase. Ligand (ANP or BNP for the type A natriuretic peptide receptor or CNP for the type B receptor) associates with the extracellular domain of the receptor. This effects a change in the receptor that reduces affinity for ligand and alters conformation of the kinase homology domain (KHD) which, in turn, reverses tonic inhibition of particulate guanylyl cyclase activity at the carboxy terminal portion of the receptor. Rac and PAK-1 are thought to activate the receptor through a more direct interaction with the guanylyl cyclase domain. Increased cyclase activity increases cellular cGMP levels which increase protein kinase G (PKG) activity through a mechanism similar to that described for cAMP (see Figure 1–6), regulates phosphodiesterase (PDE) activity, and alters the ion transport properties of the target cell.

NUCLEAR ACTION OF PEPTIDE HORMONES

Although the initial targets of peptide hormone receptor signaling appear to be confined to the cytoplasm, it is clear that these receptors can also have profound effects on nuclear transcriptional activity. They accomplish this through the same mechanisms they use to regulate enzymatic activity in the cytoplasmic compartment (eg, through activation of kinases and phosphatases). In this case, however, the ultimate targets are transcription factors that govern the expression of target genes. Examples include hormonal activation of c-Jun and c-Fos nuclear transcription factors that make up the heterodimeric AP-1 complex. This complex has been shown to alter the expression of a wide variety of eukaryotic genes through association with a specific recognition element, termed the phorbol ester (TPA) response element (TRE), present within the DNA sequence of their respective promoters. Other growth factor receptors that use the MAPK-dependent signaling mechanism appear to target the serum response factor (SRF) and its

associated ternary complex proteins. Posttranslational modification of these transcription factors is believed to amplify the signal that traffics from this complex, when associated with the cognate serum response element (SRE), to the core transcriptional apparatus. The cAMP-dependent activation of protein kinase A results in the phosphorylation of a nuclear protein CREB (cAMP response element–binding protein) at Ser[119], an event that results in enhanced transcriptional activity of closely positioned promoters. The latter requires the participation of an intermediate CREB-binding protein (CBP). CBP is a coactivator molecule that functionally tethers CREB to proteins of the core transcriptional machinery. Interestingly, CBP may also play a similar role in nuclear receptor (NR) signaling (see "Nuclear Receptors"). GH is known to induce the phosphorylation of an 84-kDa and a 97-kDa protein in target cells. These proteins have been shown to associate with the sis-inducible element (SIE) in the *c-fos* promoter and to play a role in signaling cytokine activity that traffics through this element. It remains to be demonstrated that these proteins play a similar functional role in mediating GH-dependent effects. Several recent studies have provided evidence suggesting that a number of peptide hormones and growth factors may bind to high-affinity receptors in the cell nucleus. The role these receptors play—if any—in contributing to the signaling profile of these peptides remains undefined.

NUCLEAR RECEPTORS

The NRs, which include those for the glucocorticoids, mineralocorticoids, androgens, progesterone, estrogens, thyroid hormone, and vitamin D, differ from the receptors of the surface membrane described above in that they are soluble receptors with a proclivity for using transcriptional regulation as a means of promoting their biologic effects. Thus, although some receptors are compartmentalized in the cytoplasm (eg, glucocorticoid receptor), whereas others are confined to the nucleus (eg, thyroid hormone receptor), they all operate within the nuclear chromatin to initiate the signaling cascade. These receptors can be grouped into two major subtypes based on shared structural and functional properties. The first, the steroid receptor family, includes the prototypical glucocorticoid receptor (GR) and the receptors for mineralocorticoids (MR), androgens (AR), and progesterone (PR). The second, the thyroid receptor family, includes the thyroid hormone receptor (TR) and the receptors for estrogen (ER), retinoic acid (RAR and RXR), and vitamin D (VDR) as well as the peroxisome proliferator–activated receptor (PPAR). There are also so-called orphan receptors that bear structural homology to members of the extended NR family. For most of these, the "ligand" is unknown, and their functional roles in the regulation of gene expression have yet to be determined. In total, there are 48 nuclear receptors and orphan receptors in humans.

STEROID RECEPTOR FAMILY

Steroid receptors (ie, GR, MR, AR, and PR), under basal conditions, exist as cytoplasmic, multimeric complexes that include the heat shock proteins (HSP) 90, 70, and 56. ER, although

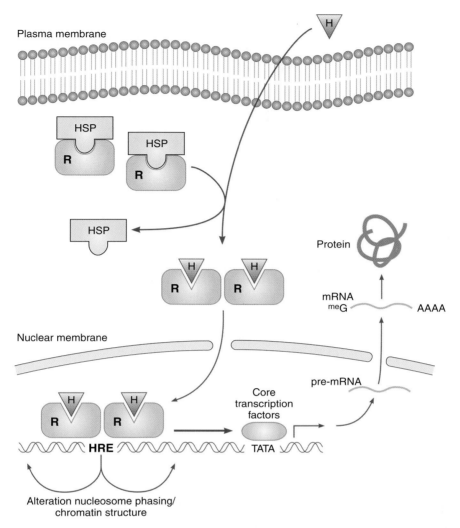

FIGURE 1–16 Signaling through the steroid receptor complex. Similar mechanisms are employed by members of the *TR* gene family, though most of the latter are concentrated in the nuclear compartment and are not associated with the heat shock protein complex (HSP) prior to binding ligand (^{me}G, methyl guanosine).

demonstrating similar association with HSP, is largely confined to the nuclear compartment. Association of the steroid ligand with the receptor results in dissociation of the HSP. This in turn exposes a nuclear translocation signal previously buried in the receptor structure and initiates transport of the receptor to the nucleus, where it associates with the hormone response element (Figure 1–16).

Each of the family members has been cloned and sequenced, and crystallographic structures have been obtained for many of them. Consequently, we know a great deal about their structure and function (Figure 1–17). Each has an extended amino terminal domain of varying length and limited sequence homology to other family members. In at least some receptors, this region, which has been termed AF-1, is believed to participate in the transactivation function through which the individual receptors promote increased gene transcription. Significant variability in the length of the amino terminal regions of the different receptors suggests potential differences in their respective mechanisms for transcriptional

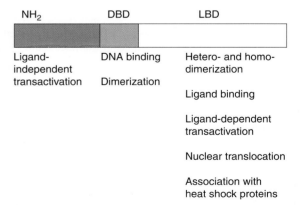

FIGURE 1–17 Structural schematic of a representative steroid receptor molecule. Separate designations are given to the amino terminal (NH$_2$), DNA-binding (DBD), and ligand-binding (LBD) domains. Functional activity associated with each of these individual domains, as determined by mutagenesis studies, is indicated below each individual domain.

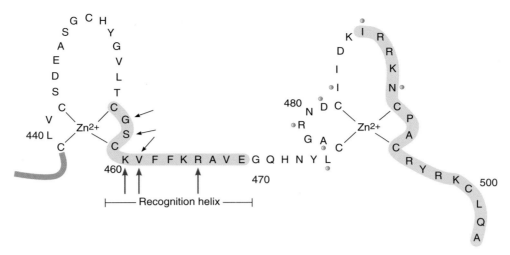

FIGURE 1–18 Schema of the two zinc fingers, together with coordinated zinc ion, which make up the DNA-binding domain of the gluco-corticoid receptor (amino acids are numbered relative to the full-length receptor). Shaded regions denote two alpha helical structures which are oriented perpendicularly to one another in the receptor molecule. The first of these, the recognition helix, makes contact with bases in the major groove of the DNA. Red arrows identify amino acids which contact specific bases in the glucocorticoid response element (GRE). Black arrows identify amino acids that confer specificity for the GRE; selective substitutions at these positions can shift receptor specificity to other response elements. Dots identify amino acids making specific contacts with the phosphate backbone of DNA. (Modified from Luisi BF et al. Reprinted, with permission, from *Nature*. 1991;352:498. Copyright 1991 by Macmillan Magazines Ltd.)

regulation. The amino terminal is followed by a basic region that has a high degree of sequence homology in both the steroid and thyroid receptor gene families. This basic region encodes two zinc finger motifs (Figure 1–18) that have been shown to establish contacts in the major groove of the cognate DNA recognition element (see the discussion later). Based on crystallographic data collected for the DNA-binding region of the GR, we know that the amino acid sequence lying between the first and second fingers (ie, recognition helix) is responsible for establishing specific contacts with the DNA. The second finger provides the stabilizing contacts that increase the affinity of the receptor for DNA. The DNA-binding region also harbors amino acid residues that contribute to the dimerization of monomers contiguously arrayed on the DNA recognition element. Following the basic region is the carboxyl terminal domain of the protein. This domain is responsible for binding of the relevant ligand, receptor dimerization or heterodimerization, and association with the heat shock proteins. It also contributes to the ligand-dependent transactivation function (incorporated in a subdomain termed AF-2) that drives transcriptional activity. Interestingly, in selected cases, nonligands have been shown to be capable of activating steroid receptors. Dopamine activates the progesterone receptor and increases PR-dependent transcriptional activity, probably through a phosphorylation event, which elicits a conformational change similar to that produced by the association of the receptor with progesterone.

The DNA-binding regions of these receptors contact DNA through a canonical HRE, which is described in Table 1–3. Interestingly, each receptor in the individual subfamily binds to the same recognition element with high affinity. Thus, specificity

TABLE 1–3   DNA recognition elements for major classes of nuclear hormone receptors.[a]

Element	Recognition Sequence	Receptor
HRE	AGAACANNNTGTTCT	Glucocorticoid Mineralocorticoid Progesterone Androgen
ERE	AGGTCANNNTGACCT	Estrogen
TRE	AGGTCA(N)$_n$AGGTCA	Vitamin D Thyroid hormone Retinoic acids PPAR ligands

[a]Elements represent consensus sequences selected to emphasize the modular nature of the half-sites and their capacity for palindrome generation. Sequences read in the 5′ to 3′ direction. N denotes a spacer nucleoside (either A, G, C, or T). Half-sites are identified by the overlying arrows. The TRE is arrayed as a direct repeat but may also exist as a palindrome or an inverted palindrome. A variable number of spacer nucleotides are positioned between the two direct repeats, depending on the type of hormone receptor. Three, four, and five nucleosides (ie, n = 3, 4, or 5) are preferred for binding of the VDR, TR, or RAR, respectively.

of hormone action must be established either by contextual DNA sequence lying outside the recognition element or by other, nonreceptor DNA-protein interactions positioned in close proximity to the element. Interestingly, the GR, as well as some other NRs (eg, ER), are capable of binding to DNA sequence lacking the classic HRE. Originally described in the mouse proliferin gene promoter, these composite elements associate with heterologous complexes containing GR, as well as with components of the AP-1 transcription factor complex (ie, c-Jun and c-Fos). They display unique regulatory activity at the level of contiguously positioned promoters. One such composite element, for example, directs very specific transcriptional effects depending on whether the GR or the MR is included in the complex.

Several steroids, particularly the glucocorticoids and estrogens, have been reported to have independent effects on the stability of target gene transcripts. At this point, it is unclear what role the hormone receptors play in this process and whether transcript stabilization is tied mechanistically to the enhancement of transcriptional activity.

THYROID RECEPTOR FAMILY

Included in this group are the TR, RAR, RXR, ER, PPAR, and VDR. They share a high degree of homology to the proto-oncogene c-*erb*A and high affinity for a common DNA recognition site (Table 1–3). With the exception of the ER, they do not associate with the HSPs, and they are constitutively bound to chromatin in the cell nucleus. Specificity of binding for each of the individual receptors is, once again, probably conferred by a contextual sequence surrounding this element, the orientation of the elements (eg, direct repeats or inverted repeats or palindromes), the polarity (ie, 5′ in contrast to 3′ position on two successive repeats), and the number and nature of the spacing nucleotides separating the repeats.

The ER binds to its RE as a homodimer, whereas the VDR, RAR, RXR, and TR prefer binding as heterodimers. The nature of the heterodimeric partners has provided some intriguing insights into the biology of these receptors. The most prevalent TR-associated partners appear to be the retinoid X receptors. These latter receptors, which as homodimers form high-affinity associations with 9-*cis*-retinoic acid, also form heterodimeric complexes in the unliganded state with VDR and RAR. In the individual cases in which it has been examined, heterodimerization with RXR amplifies both the DNA binding and the functional activity of these other receptors. Thus, the ability to form such heterodimeric complexes may add significantly to the flexibility and potency of these hormone receptor systems in regulating gene expression. Interestingly, the positioning (5′ vs 3′) of the participant proteins on the RE is important in determining the functional outcome of the association. In most of those situations linked to transcriptional activation, RXR seems to prefer the upstream (5′) position in the dimeric complex. Thus, diversity of response is engendered by the selection of recognition elements (eg, monomeric vs dimeric vs oligomeric sites) and by the choice and positioning of the dimeric partner (eg, homodimer vs heterodimer) where applicable.

The crystallographic structures of the ligand-binding domains (LBDs) of several members of the TR family have been described. These include the dimeric unliganded RXRα, monomeric liganded RARγ, monomeric liganded TRα, dimeric agonist (ie, estradiol)—and antagonist (ie, raloxifene)—liganded ERα, liganded VDR, and liganded PPARγ. A composite LBD displays

a common folding pattern with 12 alpha helices (numbered by convention H1-H12) and a conserved beta turn. Some variability exists in that there is no H2 in RARγ and a short H2′ helix is present in PPARγ, but the overall structural configuration is preserved. The dimeric interface is formed through interaction of amino acids located in helices 7 to 10, with the strongest influence exerted by H10. These interactions appear to be important for both homodimeric as well as heterodimeric interactions. Binding of ligand has been shown to occur through what has been termed a "mousetrap" mechanism. In the unliganded state, H12, which contains the carboxyl terminal activation domain AF-2, is displaced away from the ligand-binding pocket (Figure 1–19). Association of agonist ligand (eg, estradiol in the case of the ER) with the hydrophobic core of the receptor leads to a repositioning of H12 over the ligand-binding cavity, where it stabilizes receptor–ligand interactions and closes the "mousetrap." Binding of an antagonist ligand such as raloxifene, which because of its structure engenders steric hindrance in the ligand-binding pocket, prevents closure of H12 into the normal agonist position. Instead, H12 folds into an alternative location between H4 and H3, a conformation that suppresses the activation function of the receptor (discussed later). Crystal structure of a full-length nuclear receptor pair (in this case PPAR gamma and RXR alpha) shows that the PPAR gamma protein dominates its heterodimeric partner, dictating the overall structure of the complex.

The mechanistic underpinnings of transcriptional regulation by the NRs have been partially elucidated (Figure 1–20). In the unliganded state, the receptor dimers are associated with a macromolecular complex containing the repressor proteins N-CoR or SMRT, a transcriptional corepressor Sin3, and a histone deacetylase RPD3. N-CoR and SMRT each use two independent receptor interaction domains (IDs) to associate with the NRs (one repressor; two receptors). Each ID contains an amino acid sequence (L/IXXI/VI, where I = isoleucine, L = leucine, V = valine, X = any amino acid), which interacts with helices 4, 5, and 6 of the NR LBD. Histone acetylation is typically associated with activation of gene transcription (presumably reflecting decompaction of chromatin surrounding the transcriptional unit), so the presence of histone deacetylase activity in the complex is thought to promote a transcriptionally quiescent state. Addition of ligand leads to a change in receptor conformation that no longer favors interaction with the corepressor (a shift in position of helix 12 in the LBD prevents corepressor interaction and promotes coactivator assembly into the complex) and promotes both ATP-dependent chromatin remodeling and assembly of an activator complex containing p160 coactivator proteins (eg, SRC-1, GRIP-1, or P/CIP) and, secondarily, the CREB-binding protein (CBP) and the histone acetylase P/CAF. The net accrual of histone acetylase activity (CBP and P/CIP as well as P/CAF possess acetylase activity) leads to acetylation of chromatin proteins (eg, histones) as well as components of the core transcriptional machinery, resulting in chromatin decompaction and a net increase in transcriptional activity. Interaction of the NRs with the coactivators in this complex takes place through LXXLL motifs (where L = leucine and X = any amino acid) present in the coactivator proteins. Each coactivator

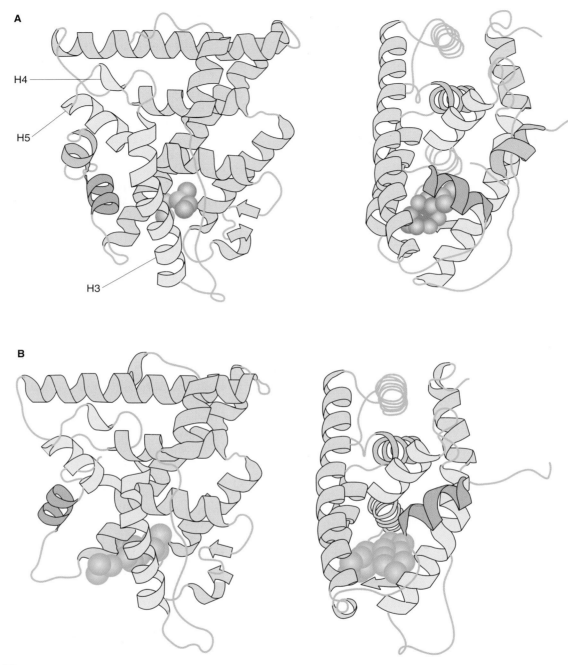

FIGURE 1–19 Three-dimensional structures for the agonist- and antagonist-occupied ERα LBD. **(A)** Orthogonal views of the agonist diethylstilbestrol-ERα LBD-NR Box II peptide complex. Coactivator peptide and LBD are presented as ribbon diagrams. Peptide is colored medium orange, helix (H) 12 (ERα residues 538-546) is colored dark orange. Helices 3, 4, and 5 are colored light pink. Diethylstilbestrol is depicted in red in a space-filling format. **(B)** Orthogonal views of the antagonist 4-hydroxytamoxifen-ERα LBD complex. Color scheme is the same as in panel A. 4-Hydroxytamoxifen is shown in green in a space-filling format. Note that NR Box II is absent in this structure. **(C)** Schematic representation of the mechanism underlying agonist-dependent activation of nuclear hormone receptor. In the presence of agonist, helix 12 (the terminal helix in the LBD) folds across the ligand-binding pocket, stabilizing ligand–receptor interaction and promoting a conformation conducive for coactivator association. In the presence of antagonist, steric hindrance precludes folding of helix 12 across the ligand-binding pocket. Instead, it positions itself in the region typically occupied by the coactivator, thereby blocking the activation function of the receptor. (Reprinted, with permission, from Shiau AK, Barstad D, Loria PM, et al. The structural basis of estrogen receptor/coactivator recognition and the antagonism of this interaction by tamoxifen. *Cell*. 1998;95:927. Copyright 1998 by Cell Press.)

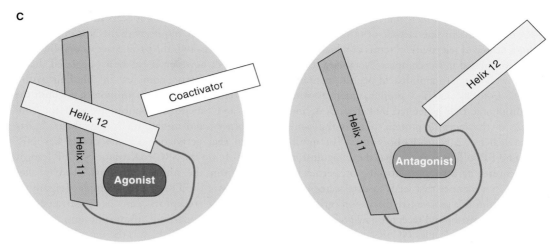

FIGURE 1–19 (*Continued*)

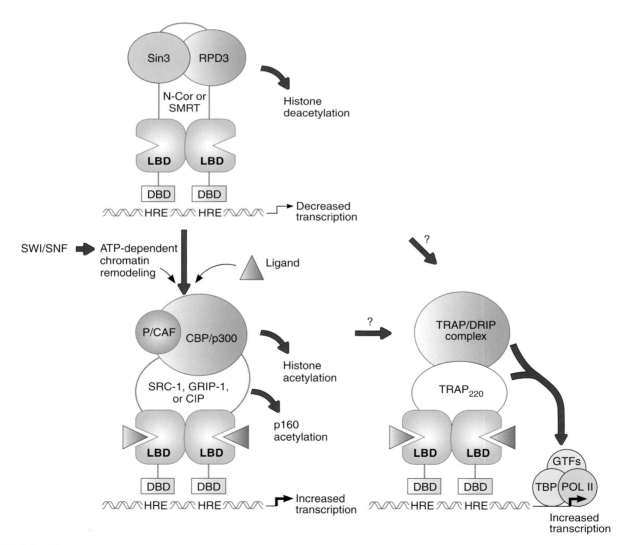

FIGURE 1–20 Interaction of corepressor (top) versus coactivator (bottom) molecules with the ligand-binding domain of a representative nuclear receptor (See text for details.). The temporal order of p160 versus DRIP/TRAP–binding remains undetermined.

may have several of these motifs, which preferentially associate with different NRs, other transcription factors, or other coactivators. This allows for a degree of selectivity in terms of which regulatory proteins are incorporated in the complex. Notably, a recent structural analysis showed that a 13-amino-acid peptide, containing an LXXLL motif from the GRIP-1 protein, interacts with TRβ through a hydrophobic cleft generated by helices 3, 4, and 12 (including AF-2) in the receptor protein. This is the same cleft that is occupied by helix 12, which harbors an LXXLL motif, in the raloxifene-bound ERα. This suggests that the antagonist in the latter instance acquires its activation-blocking properties by repositioning helix 12 in a manner that leads to displacement of the coactivator protein from this groove (see discussion earlier). It also appears that the antagonist-bound receptor may preferentially associate with the corepressor molecules NCoR and SMRT. SRC also interacts with the AF-1 domain, suggesting a potential mechanism for maximizing synergistic activity between AF-1 and AF-2 domains in the receptors. The importance of SRC1 in thyroid hormone action is underscored by the finding that SRC1 knockout mice display significant thyroid hormone resistance in peripheral tissues.

CBP is thought to function as a pivotal component of the NR regulatory complex. While the p160 class of coactivators interact directly with the NRs (primary coactivator), CBP associates primarily with the p160 coactivators, thereby establishing an indirect link to the receptors (secondary coactivator). CBP also has the ability to establish weaker, primary associations with the receptor proteins. As noted above, CBP functions as a central integrator of transcriptional regulatory signals from multiple pathways, including the cAMP-dependent activation of the transcription factor CREB. Recent evidence suggests that an additional level of regulatory control may be involved in selectively amplifying NR-dependent transcriptional activity. An enzyme called coactivator-associated arginine methyltransferase 1 (CARM1) associates with CBP and methylates the protein. This results in a reduction in CREB-dependent gene activation and, secondarily, an increase in NR-dependent gene transcription. This switching mechanism effectively refocuses the transcriptional machinery on expression of NR-dependent gene expression. CARM1 also interacts with all three members of the SRC family. It binds to the AD2 domain at the carboxy terminus of the p160 coactivators (by contrast, CBP associates with the AD1 domain located in the midregion of the molecule). CARM1 in this context promotes methylation of the p160 coactivator and dissociation of the CARM1-SRC complex from NR-associated DNA, effectively clearing the promoter of the transcriptional regulatory complex.

More recently, another family of coactivator complexes has been identified as playing an important role in NR signaling. The human TR-associated protein (TRAP) and vitamin D receptor–interacting protein (DRIP) complexes are the best characterized to date. These complexes, which contain in the neighborhood of 25 individual proteins, are thought to serve as a functional bridge between the liganded NR bound to DNA and the general transcription factors (GTFs) (eg, TBP, TFIIB, RNA polymerase II, and TAFs) involved in formation of the preinitiation complex, a function previously assigned to the Mediator complex in yeast.

The TRAP220 subunit appears to establish the relevant contacts, through LXXLL motifs, with the NRs in promoting this assembly. Their role vis-à-vis the p160 coactivators alluded to earlier remains undefined; however, it has been suggested that they succeed the p160 coactivator complex in binding with liganded NRs positioned on target gene promoters, establish the requisite structural and functional connections with the core transcriptional machinery, and initiate mRNA synthesis. It has also been suggested that acetylation of one of the key NR-binding motifs (LXXLL) on the SRC coactivator by CBP leads to dissociation of SRC from the nuclear receptors, thereby allowing access for assembly of the TRAP/DRIP complex (Figure 1–20).

Nuclear receptors can be posttranslationally modified through acetylation, ubiquitination, and phosphorylation. Phosphorylation, which is the most extensively studied of these modifications, can affect virtually all nuclear receptors. Phosphorylation by kinases associated with the general transcriptional machinery (eg, cyclin-dependent kinase 7) or major intracellular signaling pathways (eg, Akt) may serve to recruit coactivators into the complex, thereby facilitating transcriptional regulation. Coactivator molecules or other factors recruited into the multisubunit transcription complexes may possess kinase, ubiquitin ligase, ATPase, methyltransferase, or acetylase activity which can target either nuclear receptors or other coregulators. Thus, in addition to their ability to provide the scaffolding for transcription complex assembly, they also possess the enzymatic capacity to fine tune the transcriptional activity of the complex. In addition to their effects on transcription, coactivators have been suggested to be involved in transcript elongation, RNA splicing, and mRNA transport.

Recent studies have shown that a significant portion of ER DNA-binding sites in MCF7 lines (breast cancer cell line) are topographically linked to, or in some cases directly overlap with, those for the forkhead box transcription factor A1 (FOX A1). FOX A1 has been referred to as a pioneer factor that aids in positioning ER (or AR) at specific sites on DNA. FOX A1 is recruited to specific epigenetic markers in chromatin; in the case of MCF7 cells this is a lysine 4 methylation on histone 3. This, in turn, directs ER binding to nearby regions on the DNA. Similar findings have been reported with the AR, albeit with different epigenetic chromatin markers.

Although the glucocorticoid receptor is encoded by a single gene, TR is encoded by two genes (α and β). TR α1 and TR β1 appear to be the dominant forms of TR in the body. Although considerable overlap exists in their tissue distribution, TR α1 is enriched in skeletal muscle, brown fat, and the central nervous system, and TR β1 is found in the liver, kidney, and central nervous system. They are believed to signal most of the developmental and thermogenic effects of thyroid hormone in the whole animal. TR β2, a splice variant of the TR β gene, is found in the rodent pituitary gland, where it may subserve a specific regulatory function (eg, control of TSH secretion). TR α2, an alternatively spliced product of the TR α gene, lacks the hormone-binding domain at the carboxyl terminal of the molecule and thus is not a true thyroid hormone receptor. Under certain experimental conditions, TR α2 can block the activity of other members of the TR family, but its physiologic role, if one exists, remains undefined.

Similar heterogeneity exists in the retinoid receptor family. There are three isoforms for both the RXR and RAR. Collectively, these receptors are thought to play an important role in morphogenesis, but the function of the individual isoforms remains only partially understood. There are two ER isoforms. ERα appears to signal the bulk of traditional estrogenic activity. ERβ is found in a variety of different tissues and possesses antiproliferative activity that may serve to dampen the effects of liganded ER.

NONGENOMIC EFFECTS OF THE STEROID HORMONES

Although steroids exert most of their biologic activity through direct genomic effects, there are several lines of evidence suggesting that this does not provide a complete picture of steroid hormone action. There are several examples that, for kinetic or experimental reasons, do not fit the classic paradigm associated with a transcriptional regulatory mechanism. Included within this group are the rapid suppression of ACTH secretion following steroid administration, the modulation of oocyte maturation and neuronal excitability by progesterone, the stimulation of endothelial nitric oxide synthase (through interaction of ERα with the p85 subunit of PI-3K) by estrogen, the inhibition of type II deiodinase and stimulation of mitochondrial oxygen consumption by thyroid hormone, and regulation of calcium channel function by $1,25\text{-}(OH)_2$ vitamin D. Recent studies have demonstrated the presence of conventional estrogen receptors on the plasma membrane of target cells. The relationship of these receptors to their nuclear counterparts and their role in signaling estrogen-dependent activity (genomic vs nongenomic) is being actively investigated. The PR displays a novel ability to interact with the SH3 domains of the Src family tyrosine kinases, thereby accessing the Ras/Raf/MEK-1/ERK signaling pathway (discussed earlier). Although we still do not completely understand the mechanisms underlying these nongenomic effects, their potential importance in mediating steroid or thyroid hormone action may, in selected instances, approach that of their more conventional genomic counterparts.

Neurosteroids represent another class of nontraditional hormonal agonists with unique biologic activity. Some of these are native steroids (eg, progesterone), whereas others are conjugated derivatives or metabolites of the native steroids (eg, dihydroprogesterone). These agonists have been identified in the central nervous system and in some instances shown to have potent biologic activity. It is believed that they operate through interaction with the receptor for γ-aminobutyric acid, a molecule that increases neuronal membrane conductance to chloride ion. This has the net effect of hyperpolarizing the cellular membrane and suppressing neuronal excitability. Interactions that promote receptor activity would be predicted to produce sedative-hypnotic effects in the whole animal, whereas inhibitory interactions would be expected to lead to a state of central nervous system excitation.

STEROID AND THYROID HORMONE RECEPTOR RESISTANCE SYNDROMES

Heritable defects in these receptors have been linked to the pathophysiology of a number of hormone-resistance syndromes. These syndromes are characterized by a clinical phenotype suggesting hormone deficiency, by elevated levels of the circulating hormone ligand, and increased (or inappropriately detectable) levels of the relevant trophic regulatory hormone (eg, ACTH, TSH, FSH, or LH). Point mutations in the zinc fingers of the DNA-binding domain as well the ligand-binding domain of the vitamin D receptor lead to a form of vitamin D–dependent rickets (type II) characterized by typical rachitic bone lesions, secondary hyperparathyroidism, and alopecia. It is inherited as an autosomal recessive disorder. Molecular defects scattered along the full length of the androgen receptor, although concentrated in the ligand-binding domain, have been linked to syndromes characterized by varying degrees of androgen resistance ranging from infertility to the full-blown testicular feminization syndrome. Clinical severity, in this case, is thought to be related to the severity of the functional impairment that the mutation imposes on the receptor. Because the androgen receptor is located on the X chromosome, these disorders are inherited in an X-linked fashion. Defects in the glucocorticoid receptor are less common, perhaps reflecting the life-threatening nature of derangements in this system. However, mutations have been identified that impact negatively on receptor function. Clinical presentations in these cases have been dominated by signs and symptoms referable to glucocorticoid deficiency (eg, fatigue, asthenia) and adrenal androgen (eg, hirsutism and sexual precocity) and mineralocorticoid (low renin hypertension) overproduction. This presumably results from defective steroid-mediated suppression of ACTH secretion and adrenal hyperplasia as the former rises in a futile attempt to restore glucocorticoid activity at the periphery. Resistance to thyroid hormone has been linked to a large number of mutations scattered along the full length of the β form of the receptor, although, once again, there is a concentration of mutations in the ligand-binding domain, particularly along the rim of the coactivator-binding pocket. No mutations in the α form of the receptor have been linked to a hormone-resistant phenotype. The clinical presentation of thyroid hormone resistance extends from the more typical mild attention-deficit syndromes to full-blown hypothyroidism with impaired growth. Different target tissues harboring the mutant receptors display variable sensitivity to thyroid hormone, with some tissues (eg, pituitary) displaying profound resistance and others (eg, heart) responding in a fashion suggesting hyperstimulation with thyroid hormone (ie, thyrotoxicosis). The latter effects (eg, tachycardia) may reflect the predominance of the normal α isoform, as opposed to defective β TR isoform, in the target tissue (eg, heart). These syndromes are rather unique in that they are inherited as autosomal dominant disorders, presumably reflecting the ability of the mutated receptors to interfere with receptors produced from the normal allele, either by binding to the RE with higher affinity than the wild-type receptors and precluding access of the latter to target genes or by forming inactive heterodimers with the wild-type receptor proteins. A number of patients with thyroid hormone resistance have been described that lack mutations in the TR. In two cases, the defect has been assigned to defects in the transport and intracellular metabolism of thyroid hormone. Defects in the ER are rare, perhaps reflecting the critical role estrogens play in regulating lipoprotein metabolism. However, one male patient who harbors a mutation within the ligand-binding domain of the ER has been described. His clinical presentation was characterized by infertility as well as osteopenia, suggesting important roles for estrogens in the maintenance of spermatogenesis as well as bone growth even in male subjects. A novel mutation in the PPARγ receptor leads to a phenotype that clearly resembles that of patients with the metabolic syndrome (ie, severe insulin resistance, diabetes mellitus, and hypertension). A syndrome of mineralocorticoid resistance, or pseudohypoaldosteronism, has been described in a number of independent kindreds. Pseudohypoaldosteronism type I is characterized by neonatal renal salt wasting, dehydration, hypotension, hyperkalemia, and hyperchloremic metabolic acidosis despite the presence of elevated aldosterone levels. Heterozygous mutations in the MR are responsible for a milder form of the disease which is inherited in an autosomal dominant pattern with abnormalities largely confined to the kidney. A more severe form of the disease with generalized systemic involvement is inherited in an autosomal recessive pattern and appears to be due to loss-of-function mutations in genes encoding subunits of the amiloride-sensitive epithelial sodium channel. Of equivalent interest is the recent identification of an activating mineralocorticoid receptor mutation (Ser_{810}-to-Leu_{810}). This mutation results in severe early-onset hypertension that is markedly exacerbated by pregnancy. The mutation leads to constitutive activation of the MR and alters the specificity of ligand binding such that traditional MR antagonists, like progesterone, function as partial agonists. This latter property presumably accounts for the dramatic increase in blood pressure during pregnancy.

REFERENCES

Hormones and Hormone Action

Funder JW. Receptors, hummingbirds and refrigerators. *News Physiol Sci.* 1987;2:231.

G Protein Receptors

Barki-Harrington L, Rockman HA. β-Arrestins: multifunctional cellular mediators. *Physiology.* 2008;23:17. [PMID: 18268361]

Lania AG, Mantovani G, Spada A. Mechanisms of disease: mutations of G proteins and G-protein-coupled receptors in endocrine diseases. *Nat Clin Pract Endocrinol Metab.* 2006;2:681. [PMID: 17143315]

Métayé T, Gibelin H, Perdrisot R, Kraimps JL. Pathophysiological roles of G-protein-coupled receptor kinases. *Cell Signal.* 2005;17:917. [PMID: 15894165]

Schöneberg T, Schulz A, Biebermann H, Hermsdorf T, Rompler H, Sangkuhl K. Mutant G-protein-coupled receptors as a cause of human diseases. *Pharmacol Ther.* 2004;104:173. [PMID: 1556674]

Weinstein LS, Chen M, Xie T, Liu J. Genetic diseases associated with heterotrimeric G proteins. *Trends Pharmacol Sci.* 2006;27:260. [PMID: 16600389]

G Protein Effectors

Cazzolli R, Shemon AN, Fang MQ, Hughes WE. Phospholipid signaling through phospholipase D and phosphatidic acid. *IUBMB Life.* 2006;58:457. [PMID: 16916782]

Kiselyov K, Shin DM, Muallem S. Signaling specificity in GPCR-dependent Ca^{2+} signaling. *Cell Signal.* 2003;15:243. [PMID: 12531423]

Luttrell LM. Transmembrane signaling by G protein-coupled receptors. *Methods Mol Biol.* 2006;332:3. [PMID: 16878684]

Werry TD, Sexton PM, Christopoulos A. "Ins and outs" of seven-transmembrane receptor signaling to ERK. *Trend Endocrinol Metab.* 2005;16:26. [PMID: 15620546]

Woehler A, Ponimaskin EG. G protein-mediated signaling: same receptor, multiple effectors. *Curr Mol Pharmacol.* 2009;2:237. [PMID: 20021461]

Tyrosine Kinase–Coupled and Cytokine Receptors

Belfiore A, Frasca F, Pandini G, Sciacca L, Vigneri R. Insulin receptor isoforms and insulin receptor/insulin-like growth factor receptor hybrids in physiology and disease. *Endocr Rev.* 2009;30:586. [PMID: 19752219]

Hupfeld CJ, Olefsky JM. Regulation of receptor tyrosine kinase signaling by GRKs and beta-arrestins. *Annu Rev Physiol.* 2007;69:561. [PMID: 17002595]

Kikani CK, Dong LQ, Liu F. "New"-clear functions of PDK1: beyond a master kinase in the cytosol? *J Cell Biochem.* 2005;96:1157. [PMID: 16187290]

LeRoith D, Yakar S. Mechanisms of disease: metabolic effects of growth hormone and insulin-like growth factor 1. *Nat Clin Pract Endocrinol Metab.* 2007;3:302. [PMID: 17315038]

Leung K-C. Regulation of cytokine receptor signaling by nuclear hormone receptors: a new paradigm for receptor interaction. *DNA Cell Biol.* 2004;23:463. [PMID: 15307949]

Guanylyl Cyclase-Linked Receptors

Dudzinski DM, Igarashi J, Greif D, Michel T. The regulation and pharmacology of endothelial nitric oxide synthases. *Annu Rev Pharmacol Toxicol.* 2006;46:235. [PMID: 16402905]

Garbers DL, Chrisman TD, Wiegn P, et al. Membrane guanylyl cyclase receptors: an update. *Trends Endo Metab.* 2006;17:251. [PMID: 16815030]

Gardner DG, Chen S, Glenn DJ, Grigsby CL. Molecular biology of the natriuretic peptide system: implications for physiology and hypertension. *Hypertension.* 2007;49:419. [PMID: 17283251]

Kuhn M. Function and dysfunction of mammalian membrane guanylyl cyclase receptors: lessons from genetic mouse models and implications for human disease. *Handb Exp Pharmacol.* 2009;191:47. [PMID: 19089325]

Nuclear Receptors

Chrousos GP, Kino T. Glucocorticoid signaling in the cell. Expanding clinical implications to complex human behavioral and somatic disorders. *Ann NY Acad Sci.* 2009;1179:153. [PMID: 19906238]

Cornell W, Nam K. Steroid hormone binding receptors: application of homology modeling, induced fit docking, and molecular dynamics to study structure-function relationships. *Curr Top Med Chem.* 2009;9:844. [PMID: 19754398]

Ito M, Roeder RG. The TRAP/SMCC/mediator complex and thyroid hormone receptor function. *Trends Endocrinol Metab.* 2001;12:127. [PMID: 11306338]

Knouff C, Auwerx J. Peroxisome proliferators-activated receptor-gamma calls for activation in moderation: lessons from genetics and pharmacology. *Endocr Rev.* 2004;25:899. [PMID: 15583022]

Lonard DM, O'Malley B. Nuclear receptor coregulators: judges, juries, and executioners of cell regulation. *Mol Cell.* 2007;27:691. [PMID: 17803935]

O'Malley B. The year in basic science: nuclear receptors and coregulators. *Mol Endo.* 2008;22:2751. [PMID: 18845672]

Ordonez-Moran P, Munoz A. Nuclear receptors: genomic and non-genomic effects converge. *Cell Cycle.* 2009;8:1675. [PMID: 19448403]

Rochel N, Moras D. Ligand binding domain of vitamin D receptors. *Curr Top Med Chem.* 2006;6:1229. [PMID: 16848737]

Yang J, Young MJ. The mineralocorticoid receptor and its coregulators. *J Mol Endocrinol.* 2009;43:53. [PMID 19617444]

Endocrine Autoimmunity

2

Juan Carlos Jaume, MD

AADC	Aromatic L-amino acid decarboxylase	**IPEX**	Immunodeficiency, polyendocrinopathy, and enteropathy, x-linked
ACA	Antibodies recognizing the adrenal cortex	**LFA**	Lymphocyte function-associated antigen
ADCC	Antibody-dependent cell-mediated cytoxicity	**MHC**	Major histocompatibility complex
AICD	Activation-induced cell death	**NALP1**	NACHT leucine-rich-repeat protein 1
AIRE	Autoimmune regulator gene	**NALP5**	NACHT leucine-rich-repeat protein 5
APECED	Autoimmune polyendocrinopathy-candidiasis-ectodermal dystrophy	**NK**	Natural killer (cells)
APS	Autommune polyglandular syndrome	**NOD**	Nonobese diabetic (mice)
BB	Bio breeding	**SCA**	Steroid-producing cell antibodies
BCR	B-cell receptor	**SCID**	Spontaneous combined immunodeficiency
cAMP	Cyclic adenosine monophosphate	**TAP**	Transporter associated with antigen processing
CaSR	Calcium-sensing receptor	**TBI**	Thyrotropin-binding inhibition
CD	Cluster of differentiation	**TCR**	T-cell receptor
CTLA	Cytotoxic T lymphocyte antigen	**TD**	Thymus-dependent
DPT	Diabetes Prevention Trial	**Tg**	Thyroglobulin
FOXP3	Forkhead box P3	**TI**	Thymus-independent
GABA	Gamma-aminobutyric acid	**TNF**	Tumor necrosis factor
GAD	Glutamic acid decarboxylase	**TPO**	Thyroperoxidase
HLA	Human leukocyte antigen	**TSH**	Thyroid-stimulating hormone
IA-2	Islet cell antigen-2 (tyrosine phosphatase)	**TSH-R**	Thyrotropin receptor
IFN	Interferon	**TSI**	Thyroid-stimulating immunoglobulin
IL	Interleukin	**VNTR**	Variable number of tandem repeats

Epidemiologic analysis of a large population reported that about 1 of 30 (3.2%) people in the United States (more than 8.5 million individuals) are currently affected by autoimmune diseases. Graves disease, type 1 diabetes, pernicious anemia, rheumatoid arthritis, Hashimoto thyroiditis, and vitiligo are the most prevalent such conditions, accounting for 93% of affected individuals. A more global approach at calculating prevalence led to a corrected estimate between 7.6% and 9.4% of the world's population as affected by autoimmune diseases (2.5 in 30 people worldwide).

These autoimmune diseases have traditionally been looked upon as forming a spectrum. At one end are found organ-specific diseases with organ-specific targets. Hashimoto thyroiditis is an example in which a specific lesion affects the thyroid (lymphocytic infiltration, destruction of follicular cells) and autoantibodies are produced with absolute specificity for thyroid proteins. At the other end of the spectrum are the systemic autoimmune diseases, broadly belonging to the class of rheumatologic disorders. Systemic lupus erythematosus is an example of a disease characterized by widespread pathologic changes and a collection of autoantibodies to DNA and other nuclear constituents of all cells. Many organ-specific autoimmune diseases are autoimmune endocrinopathies. Furthermore, most endocrine glands are subject to autoimmune attack including the adrenals (autoimmune Addison disease), gonads (autoimmune oophoritis), pancreas (type 1 diabetes), pituitary (autoimmune hypophysitis), and thyroid (autoimmune thyroid disease) (Table 2–1).

TABLE 2–1 Some autoimmune endocrinopathies, antigens, and autoantibodies.

Disease	Gland	Autoantigen	Autoantibody
Autoimmune (lymphocytic) hypophysitis Granulomatous hypophysitis	Pituitary	Pituitary cytosolic protein	Antipituitary
Graves disease	Thyroid	TSH-R, TPO	TSI, TBII, anti-TPO
Hashimoto thyroiditis	Thyroid	TPO, Tg	Anti-TPO, anti-Tg
Autoimmune (idiopathic) hypoparathyroidism	Parathyroid	CaSR, NALP5	Antiparathyroid
Type 1 diabetes mellitus	Pancreas (β cells)	GAD65, IA-2, insulin	Anti-GAD, anti-IA-2 (ICA), antiinsulin
Type B insulin resistance with acanthosis nigricans (rare)	Adipocytes, muscle cells	Insulin receptor	Insulin receptor blocking
Autoimmune Addison disease (autoimmune adrenal failure)	Adrenal	21-Hydroxylase 17α-Hydroxylase P450scc	Anti-21-hydroxylase (ACA) Anti-17α-hydroxylase and anti-P450scc (SCA)
Autoimmune oophoritis (premature ovarian failure)	Ovaries	Not yet identified unequivocally, 17α-hydroxylase P450scc	Also SCA in association with adrenal insufficiency
Autoimmune orchitis Male infertility (some forms)	Testes	Sperm	Antisperm

By far the most common autoimmune endocrine diseases are those involving the thyroid and type 1 diabetes. When the target is the thyroid gland and the clinical manifestation is hypothyroidism (Hashimoto thyroiditis), the prevalence is about 1%. When the manifestation is hyperthyroidism (Graves disease), the prevalence is about 0.4%. Both thyroid autoimmune disorders affect women preferentially. When the targets of the autoimmune response are the β cells of the pancreas, the clinical presentation is type 1 diabetes. The prevalence of type 1 diabetes is close to that of Graves disease (0.2%-0.5%); however, it has no gender predilection.

Basic immunologic concepts as they apply to clinical autoimmune endocrine diseases as sole entities and as polyglandular failure syndromes are reviewed in this chapter.

BASIC IMMUNE COMPONENTS AND MECHANISMS

The immune system is constantly confronted with a variety of molecules and recognizes them as either self or foreign. The adaptive immune system has evolved to recognize virtually any foreign molecule, either in existence or yet to come. The repertoire of immune recognition molecules randomly formed by gene rearrangements is not limited by the genetic information encoded in the genome (Figure 2–1). As a result, an enormously wide array of immune recognition molecules is acquired by the human immune system. By way of illustration, the theoretical diversity of T-cell receptors (T-cell recognition molecules) by random rearrangements reaches 10^{15}. This mechanism of rearrangement also applies

to B-cell recognition molecules (ie, immunoglobulins). The random mechanism of gene rearrangement, however, produces immune recognition molecules that react with self components. Potentially dangerous immune cells carrying self-reactive recognition molecules are eliminated (negatively selected) during development of T lymphocytes in the thymus and of B lymphocytes in the bone marrow. It appears that only immune cells which react with foreign antigen strongly and with self antigen very weakly are positively selected and comprise the peripheral immune cell repertoire. This selection mechanism of immune cells is termed "central tolerance." Self-reactive immune cells that skip central tolerance and reach the periphery are managed by other control mechanisms against autoimmunity and are either eliminated, rendered unresponsive, or suppressed ("peripheral tolerance"). Failures in these mechanisms of immunologic regulation, as proposed by Mackay and Burnet in 1964, are central features of the concept of autoimmunity.

IMMUNE RECOGNITION AND RESPONSE

T and B lymphocytes are the fundamental and predominant immune cells. T lymphocyte precursors (pre-T cells) originate in the bone marrow and migrate to the thymus, where they undergo maturation and differentiation. At early stages, they express several T-cell surface molecules but still have genomic (not rearranged) configuration of their T-cell receptors (TCRs). These pre-T cells, destined to become T cells with TCR α/β chains (T α/β cells), pass through a critical phase during which self-reactive T cells are deleted by negative selection (see T-Cell Tolerance, later in this chapter). Few pre-T cells will express other types of chains on their

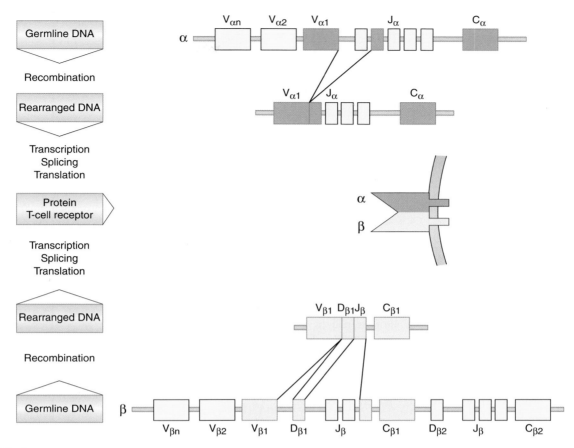

FIGURE 2–1 Rearrangement of the T-cell receptor (TCR) α and β genes to form a functionally diverse receptor. During T-cell development, the TCR α and β gene segments rearrange by somatic recombination so that one of the V_α segments pairs with a single J_α segment, and a V_β segment pairs with a single D_β and J_β segment. The C (constant) segments are brought together with the rearranged segments by transcription and splicing to generate the functional mRNA that will be translated into the α and β protein chains that compose the TCR.

TCR (T γ/δ cells). T α/β cells differentiate into either mature CD4 or CD8 cells. These now mature lymphocytes migrate to T-cell areas of peripheral lymphoid organs and exert their function as helper (T_H) or cytotoxic (T_C) cells when activated.

B lymphocytes mature and differentiate in the bone marrow and then migrate to the B-cell areas of lymphoid organs. Influenced by factors derived from T_H cells previously activated by professional antigen-presenting cells (APCs) such as macrophages, some B cells differentiate to become immunoglobulin M (IgM)-producing cells (plasma cells). Most of the other activated B cells that do not differentiate into plasma cells revert to the resting state to become memory B cells. When memory B cells are further activated, two events occur: isotype switching (immunoglobulin class switching) and hypermutation of the immunoglobulin-variable region to further increase diversity and specificity (affinity maturation).

Activation of B cells requires recognition of the antigen as a whole, while T cells require recognition of antigenic peptides bound to major histocompatibility complex (MHC) molecules on the surfaces of professional APCs. Therefore, T-cell recognition is said to be MHC restricted.

The human MHC (human leukocyte antigen; HLA) consists of a linked set of genes encoding major glycoproteins involved in antigen presentation (Figure 2–2). The complex locates to the short arm of chromosome 6 and divides into three separate regions: class I, class II, and class III genes. The class I "classic" region encodes HLA-A, HLA-B, and HLA-C loci; the nonclassic or class I-related region encodes HLA-E, HLA-F, and HLA-G loci and other immunity-related genes such as CD1. The class II region (HLA-D) encodes HLA-DP, HLA-DQ, and HLA-DR loci and other genes related to antigen processing, transport, and presentation, such as, transporter associated with antigen processing (TAP). The class III region encodes genes for tumor necrosis factors α and β (TNF-α and TNF-β); complement factors C2, C4, and B; and the steroidogenic enzyme 21-hydroxylase. MHC class I (classic) molecules are found on all somatic cells, whereas MHC class I nonclassic antigens are expressed only on some (eg, HLA-F on fetal liver, HLA-G on placental tissues). CD1 molecules are expressed on Langerhans cells, dendritic cells, macrophages, and B cells (all professional APCs). MHC class II molecules are exclusively expressed on these professional APCs. However, virtually all cells except mature erythrocytes can express MHC class II

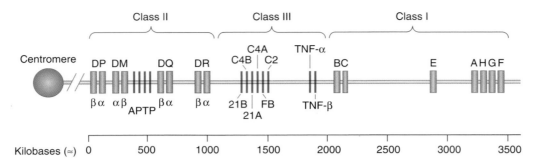

FIGURE 2–2 Gene organization of the human major histocompatibility complex or human leukocyte antigen (HLA) complex. Regions encoding the three classes of MHC proteins are on top. APTP denotes a cluster of genes within the class II region, encoding genes related to antigen processing, transport, and presentation. Class III region encodes genes unrelated to class I or class II not involved in antigen presentation (TNF-α and -β, complement factors C2, C4, B, and 21-hydroxylase and others).

molecules under particular conditions (eg, stimulation with interferon-γ [IFN-γ]). As a general rule, MHC class I molecules present peptides derived from endogenous antigens that have access to cytosolic cell compartments (eg, virus) to CD8 T_C cells. On the other hand, MHC class II molecules present peptides derived from antigens internalized by endocytosis into vesicular compartments (eg, bacteria) to CD4 T_H cells. MHC class II molecules also bind peptides derived from many membrane-bound self antigens.

APCs process and present antigen in order to activate T cells utilizing MHC-peptide presentation (Figure 2–3). T cells require at least two signals to become activated. The interaction of a TCR expressed on antigen-specific T cells and the antigenic peptide–MHC complex expressed on APCs provides the first signal. The second signal is delivered primarily by the interaction between costimulatory molecules CD80 (B7.1) and CD86 (B7.2) on APCs and CD28 on T cells. These two signals induce proliferation of T cells, production of interleukin-2 (IL-2), and expression of the antiapoptotic protein Bcl-xL. T_H cells and T_C cells are effector cells that require both signals in order to become activated. However, T_C cells also need the "help" provided by T_H cells. Until recently, it was thought that T_H and T_C cells needed to interact with the same APC simultaneously and that cytokines (such as IL-2) produced by the T_H cell would then act on the T_C cell to facilitate its response. New studies suggest that the interaction between another costimulatory molecule, CD40 ligand (CD154), present on T cells, and CD40, present on APCs, may provide an alternative explanation. It appears that T_H cells–recognizing antigenic peptides presented by APCs deliver a signal through the CD154–CD40 complex that "licenses" APCs to directly stimulate T_C cells (Figure 2–4). Thus, there is no need for simultaneous interactions of T_H and T_C cells while encountering the APC. CD154–CD40 interaction also enhances expression of CD80 and CD86 as well as secretion of cytokines (IL-1, -6, -8, -10, and -12 and TNF-α).

Yet another molecule on T cells, the CD28 homolog cytotoxic T lymphocyte antigen 4 (CTLA-4 or CD152), functions to suppress T-cell responses (see Figure 2–3). CD152 is expressed at low

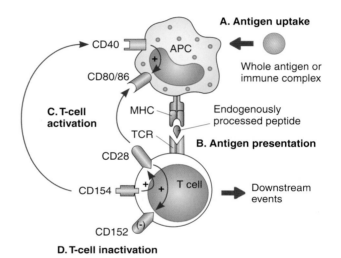

FIGURE 2–3 Antigen recognition by T cells. From top to bottom: **A. Antigen uptake:** Incorporation of antigen (via phagocytosis, pinocytosis, or FcR-mediated endocytosis of immune complex). **B. Antigen presentation:** APCs deliver an antigen-specific signal through the MHC-peptide–TCR interaction on T cells (MHC I coupled to CD8 interacts with T_C cells, MHC II coupled to CD4 interacts with T_H cells). **C. T-cell activation:** The required second signal is provided via CD80/86 (B7.1; B7.2)–CD28 that induces the expression of CD154 (CD40 L) first and CD152 (CTLA-4) later on. Binding of CD154 on T cells with CD40 on APCs enhances expression of CD80/86. The APC–CD80/86 increased expression and consequent binding of CD28 on T cells perpetuates the activation and proliferation of these effector cells (downstream events). **D. T-cell inactivation:** CD152 (expressed 48-72 hours after T-cell activation) will preferentially bind to CD80/86 on APCs because of its higher affinity, displacing CD28 and in turn suppressing T-cell activity.

to undetectable levels on resting T cells. It is upregulated by the ligation of CD28 on T cells with CD80/86 on APCs, or by IL-2. CD152 and CD28 on T cells share the same counterreceptors, namely, CD80/86 on APCs. However, CD152 has a 20-fold higher affinity than CD28 for their ligands.

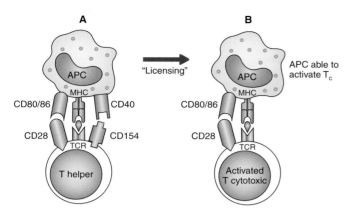

FIGURE 2–4 Licensed APCs directly activate T_C cells. According to the traditional model, T_H cells and T_C cells recognize antigen on the same APC. The APC-activated T_H cell produces IL-2, which contributes to the activation of T_C cells while in simultaneous interaction with the same APC. According to the proposed new model **(A)**, APCs are licensed to activate T_C cells by T_H or other stimuli (lipopolysaccharides, IFN-γ, viruses). APCs first interact with T_H cells. The association of CD154 (CD40 L) on the T_H cell and CD40 on the APC allows (or licenses) the latter to activate T_C cells directly **(B)**. Thus, once licensed, APCs are capable of activating cytotoxic T cells without the need of simultaneous interaction with T_H cells.

The integration of all these interactions may be as follows (see Figure 2–3): After processing antigen, APCs deliver an antigen-specific first signal through the MHC-peptide–TCR interaction on T cells. A second signal is provided by a costimulatory interaction of the CD80/86–CD28 complex that induces the expression of CD154 first and then CD152. Binding of CD154 on T_H cells with CD40 on APCs enhances expression of CD80/86 and licenses APCs for direct activation of T_C cells. Other inflammatory cytokines as well as lipopolysaccharides and viruses may do the same. The increased expression of APC–CD80/86 and consequent binding of CD28 on T cells then perpetuates the activation and proliferation of these effector cells. However, the expression of CD152 48 to 72 hours after T-cell activation leads to the preferential binding of this molecule to CD80/86 on APCs because of its higher affinity for CD80/86. This may displace CD28 from CD80/86 and, in turn, suppress T-cell activity. This sequence of complex events is probably simplistic relative to what nature has to offer. A new B7 family of receptors has been reported: some with positive costimulatory capacity, many with a role in downregulating immune responses, yet others with dual functions. For some of these pathways such as B7H3/H4 (expressed in APCs with unknown counterreceptor on T cells), very little is known, but even for those pathways that have been extensively studied, such as the CD80/86:CD28/CTLA-4 (mentioned above); B7h:ICOS (inducible costimulator) and PD-L1/PD-L2:PD1, new insights are still being generated. The intricacies of controlling T-cell activation are enhanced by the complexity of the costimulatory pathways, such that there are multiple possible receptor–ligand interactions.

Activation and differentiation of B cells often require two signals also. Naive B cells are triggered by antigen but may also require accessory signals that come from activated T_H cells. Some antigens can directly activate naive B cells without the need for T_H cells (eg, lipopolysaccharides from gram-negative bacteria or polymeric protein structures). The former type of B-cell activation (MHC class II-restricted T cell help) is called thymus-dependent (TD). The latter type is called thymus-independent (TI). T_H cells also control isotype switching and initiate somatic hypermutation of antibody variable-region genes (see Tolerance, later). Interaction between CD154 on T_H cells and CD40 on B cells and the cytokines produced by T_H cells are essential for isotype switching and formation of germinal centers in peripheral lymphoid organs. The immunoglobulin isotype switching is critical for the generation of functional diversity of a humoral immune response. Somatic hypermutation (point mutations of the variable-region genes of immunoglobulins during the course of an immune response) is necessary for the affinity maturation of antibodies.

Overall, the immune response is a combination of effector mechanisms that function to eliminate pathogenic organisms. These effector mechanisms include, as **innate immunity**, phagocytosis (by macrophages, neutrophils, monocytes, and dendritic cells) and cytotoxicity (by natural killer [NK] cells); and as **adaptive immunity**, antibody-dependent complement-mediated cytotoxicity, antibody-dependent cell-mediated cytotoxicity (ADCC), cytotoxicity by T γ/δ cells that recognize heat shock proteins on target cells, and cytotoxicity by CD8 or CD4 T_C cells. CD8 and CD4 T_C cells are activated by the described recognition of specific antigenic peptides bound to class I (for CD8), class II (for CD4) MHC molecules on the APCs and classically by IL-2 from nearby activated CD4 T_H cells. These cells kill the target by either secreting cytotoxins (perforin, granzyme) or by inducing apoptosis through the Fas–FasL (Fas ligand) interaction (killer cells carrying FasL molecules activate programmed cell death in target cells expressing Fas molecules). FasL or CD95L is a type II transmembrane protein that belongs to the TNF family. The binding of FasL with its receptor induces apoptosis. FasL–Fas receptor interactions play an important role in the regulation of the immune system.

The specificity of the immune response is crucial if self-reactivity is to be avoided. In order to ensure that lymphocyte responses and the downstream effector mechanisms they control are directed exclusively against foreign antigens and not against "self" components, a number of safety-check barriers must be negotiated before autoreactive lymphocytes can differentiate and proliferate.

TOLERANCE

T-Cell Tolerance

T cells developing in the thymus (pre-T cells) are destined to become T α/β cells through rearrangement of the TCR β gene initially, followed by the TCR α gene (Figure 2–5). If unproductive rearrangements of TCR genes occur (nonfunctional TCR α or β proteins), apoptosis of these pre-T cells follows (Figure 2–5A).

A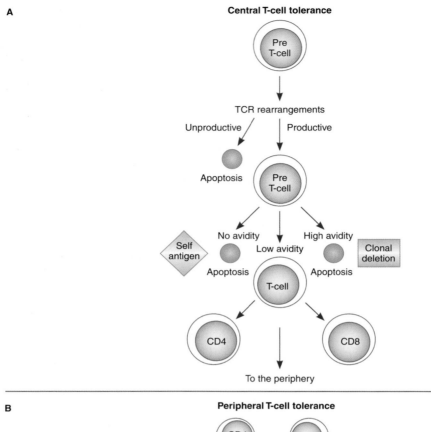

B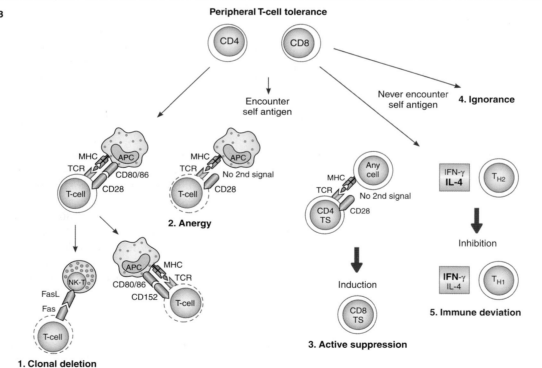

FIGURE 2–5   **A. Central T-cell tolerance:** Mechanisms of central tolerance (at the thymus level) are depicted. From top to bottom, pre-T cells first rearrange their TCR. Unproductive (nonfunctional) rearrangements lead to apoptosis, while productive ones engage pre-T cells in self-antigen recognition. Clonal deletion indicates elimination of cells based on their high or no avidity for self antigen (apoptosis). Surviving low-avidity cells reach the periphery as mature CD4 and CD8 cells. **B. Peripheral T-cell tolerance:** May be accomplished through any of the five depicted mechanisms. **1. Clonal deletion:** After encountering self antigen in the context of self-MHC molecules and simultaneous delivery of a second signal (CD80/86–CD28) by APCs (top left), autoreactive T cells become activated. These activated T cells express Fas molecules on their

If functional rearrangements of TCR α and β proteins occur, cells express TCR α/β dimer and CD3 molecules at low levels on the cell surface. TCR-rearranged cells proliferate 100-fold. Positive and negative selection occurs based on the ability of the rearranged TCR α/β to recognize antigenic peptides in association with self-MHC molecules on thymic epithelial and dendritic cells. Negative selection (clonal deletion) appears to take place in the thymus medulla, where pre-T cells–bearing TCRs specific for self peptides bound to self-MHC molecules are deleted. At least 97% of developing T cells undergo apoptosis within the thymus (central tolerance). Positively selected pre-T cells increase expression of TCR α/β, express either CD4 or CD8, and become mature T cells. These mature T cells exit the thymus and go to the periphery. CD4 T cells are activated in the periphery in an MHC class II-restricted fashion, while CD8 T cells are activated in an MHC class I-restricted fashion.

A differential avidity model in which the fate of T cells is determined by the intrinsic affinity of TCRs for their ligands has been advanced to explain the paradox between positive and negative selection. According to this model, T cells with high avidity for MHC-self peptide complexes would be eliminated (negative selection), whereas T cells with low avidity to MHC-self peptide complexes would be positively selected. If the avidity is close to zero, T cells would not be selected (for lack of effective signal to survive). The biochemical factor or factors that signal survival (low avidity of TCR binding) versus apoptosis (triggered by high avidity interactions) have yet to be found.

Costimulatory interactions between CD28 and CD80/86 and between CD154, CD40, and adhesion molecules, such as lymphocyte function-associated antigen-1 (LFA-1), are also involved in preferential deletion of self-reactive T cells in the medullary region of the thymus. It is known that negative selection is not 100% effective and that some potentially autoreactive T cells do escape to the periphery. Not all self peptides would be presented to pre-T cells during their development in the thymus. Self peptides derived from secluded proteins (ie, intracytoplasmic enzymes) only timely expressed after rigid regulatory control (ie, puberty) in endocrine glands are believed to be a likely source. Therefore, the peripheral immune system must maintain tolerance through complementary control mechanisms.

"Peripheral tolerance" (Figure 2–5B) may be maintained by the induction of unresponsiveness to self antigen (anergy) or by the induction of regulatory T cells (T regs), such as suppressor T cells (active suppression). Peripheral clonal deletion (apoptosis) of

autoreactive T cells that have escaped from the thymus may play an important role in limiting rapidly expanding responses, but there are many examples where autoreactive T cells persist. Some autoreactive T cells may never encounter the self antigen because it may be sequestered from the immune system (ignorance). Lastly, immune deviation, whereby noninflammatory T$_{H2}$ responses suppress an autoreactive inflammatory T$_{H1}$ response, inducing peripheral tolerance, deserves further discussion. T$_{H1}$ cells, which regulate cell-mediated responses, secrete IFN-γ and small amounts of IL-4. In contrast, T$_{H2}$ cells, which provide help for antibody production, secrete abundant IL-4 and little IFN-γ. A prevailing concept in human autoimmunity is that T$_{H1}$ responses are believed to dominate. It has been shown in animal models that induction of T$_{H2}$ responses ameliorates T$_{H1}$ responses. Hence, unbalanced T$_{H1}$ immune deviation may lead to a breakage of peripheral tolerance. However, evidence to the contrary exists in some endocrinopathies. (See autoimmune response in the section on Autoimmune Aspects of Thyroid Disease, later in the chapter.)

Clonal deletion and anergy occur through apoptosis at the site of activation or after passage through the liver. High antigen dose and chronic stimulation induce peripheral elimination of both CD4 and CD8 T cells. Activated T cells express Fas molecules on their surfaces but are resistant to FasL-mediated apoptosis because of the simultaneous expression of Bcl-xL (apoptosis-resistance molecules), induced by CD28 ligation during activation (see Immune Recognition and Response, earlier in the chapter). Several days after activation, when Bcl-xL has declined, CD4 cells become susceptible to Fas-mediated apoptosis (activation-induced cell death; AICD). A similar mechanism via p75 tumor necrosis factor (TNF) receptor has been shown for CD8 cells. Therefore, autoreactive T cells might be deleted by apoptosis induced by chronic stimulation with self antigens, present abundantly in the periphery. However, autoreactive T cells specific for very rare self antigens may be difficult to eliminate.

Anergy also results from the lack of a second costimulatory signal. When nonhematopoietic cells stimulated by IFN-γ present antigen in an MHC class II-restricted fashion (as thyrocytes do in AITD), autoreactive T cells may be rendered unresponsive because of the absence of a CD28–CD80/86-mediated signal (nonhematopoietic cells do not express CD80/86 as professional APCs do). However, even if the two signals are provided, anergy may result from the lack of T$_H$ cell-originated cytokines (IL-2, -4, -7, etc). It has also been shown that in vivo T-cell anergy may be

surface but are resistant to Fas ligand (FasL)-mediated apoptosis because of the simultaneous expression of Bcl-xL (not shown) induced by CD28 ligation during activation. Several days after activation, when Bcl-xL presence has declined, CD4 cells become susceptible to FasL-mediated apoptosis. Natural killer cells (NK-T) may then accomplish the task of eliminating these autoreactive T cells. **2. Anergy:** Anergy may be induced via CD80/86–CD152 interaction 48 to 72 hours following activation or may result from the lack of a second costimulatory signal from APCs presenting self antigen (nonprofessional APCs). **3. Active suppression:** Active suppression is thought to occur when nonhematopoietic cells (stimulated by IFN-γ) present antigen in an MHC class II–restricted fashion to CD4 T-suppressor cells (T$_S$, also known as CD4 + CD25 + FOXP3 + regulatory T cells, T regs). Before becoming unresponsive, these cells may induce specific CD8 T$_S$ cells. In turn, these CD8 T$_S$ cells may suppress antigen-specific autoreactive T cells. **4. Ignorance (top right):** Some autoreactive T cells may never encounter self antigen because it may be sequestered from the immune system. Although they may persist in the circulation, they never become activated. **5. Immune deviation:** Under specific circumstances, noninflammatory T$_{H2}$ responses could suppress inflammatory (autoreactive) T$_{H1}$ responses (see text).

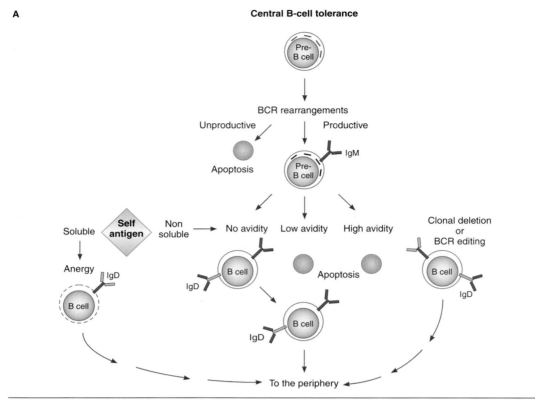

A   **Central B-cell tolerance**

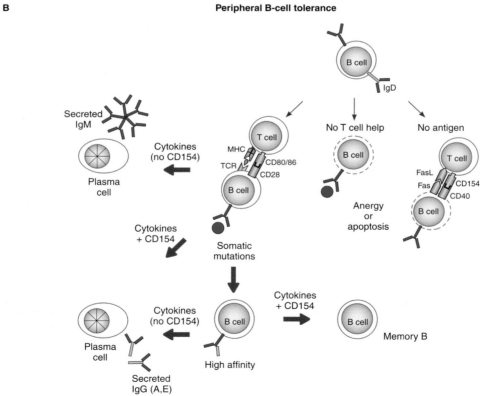

B   **Peripheral B-cell tolerance**

FIGURE 2-6 A. Central B-cell tolerance: As T cells do in the thymus, B-cells rearrange their B-cell receptor (BCR) in the bone marrow. Unproductive rearrangements drive pre-B cells to apoptosis. Functional rearrangements allow expansion and expression of IgM. Next, similar to T-cell clonal deletion, immature B cells that strongly bind self antigens in the bone marrow are eliminated by apoptosis. Some autoreactive immature B cells, instead of becoming apoptotic, however, resume rearrangements of their L-chain genes, attempting to reassemble new allelic

induced by CD80/86–CD152 interaction (see also Immune Recognition and Response, discussed earlier).

T-cell **active suppression** is considered to be a major regulatory mechanism of peripheral tolerance; however, its mode of action is still under study. As mentioned above, nonhematopoietic cells stimulated by IFN-γ present antigen in an MHC class II-restricted fashion to T cells and render them anergic. These nonhematopoietic cells (nonprofessional APCs) may also present to CD4 T-suppressor cells (T_S, also known as CD4 + CD25 + FOXP3 + regulatory T cells, T regs). Before becoming unresponsive, these cells may induce specific CD8 T suppressor (T_S) cells. In turn, these CD8 T_S cells may regulate (via T-cell-suppressor factors or cytotoxicity) autoreactive T cells (see also Figure 2–5B).

B-Cell Tolerance

Instead of the thymus, the bone marrow provides the setting for central B-cell tolerance. Pre-B cells rearrange their B-cell receptor (BCR or membrane-bound immunoglobulin) early in development. The immunoglobulin heavy (H) chain genes rearrange first, followed by light (L) chain gene rearrangement. Unproductive rearrangements and pairings leading to formation of nonfunctional immunoglobulin drive pre-B cells to apoptosis (Figure 2–6A). Functional rearrangements (functional BCRs) allow immature B-cell expansion and expression of IgM and CD21 (a marker of functionality). Only one-third of the precursor cells reach this stage. The random rearrangement of the V, D, and J segments of immunoglobulin genes during this period inevitably generates self-recognizing immunoglobulins. Negative selection of autoreactive B cells occurs at the immature B cell stage on the basis of the avidity of the BCR for self antigens. Similar to the T-cell clonal deletion, immature B cells that strongly bind antigens in the bone marrow are eliminated by apoptosis. Some autoreactive immature B cells, instead of undergoing apoptosis, resume rearrangements of their L-chain genes in an attempt to reassemble new κ or λ genes. This procedure, called **BCR editing**, permanently inactivates the autoreactive immunoglobulin genes. Soluble antigens, presumably because they generate weaker signals through the BCR of immature B cells, do not cause apoptosis but render cells unresponsive to stimuli (anergy). These anergic B cells migrate to the periphery, where they express IgD. They may be activated under special circumstances, making anergy less than sufficient as a mechanism of enforcing tolerance. Only immature B cells in the bone marrow with no avidity for antigens (membrane-bound or soluble)

become mature B cells with the capacity to express both IgM and IgD. As with T cells, 97% of developing B cells undergo apoptosis within the bone marrow. Also, and as with T cells, **central clonal deletion, anergy,** and **BCR editing** eliminates autoreactive B cells, recognizing bone marrow-derived self antigens.

Peripheral B-cell tolerance (Figure 2–6B) is also crucial for protection against autoimmunity. It appears that in the absence of antigen, mature B cells are actively eliminated in the periphery by activated T cells via Fas–FasL and CD40–CD154 interactions. In the presence of specific antigen but without T-cell help, antigen recognition by BCRs induces apoptosis or anergy of mature B cells. If antigen and specific T-cell help are provided—that is, if antigen bound to the BCR is internalized, processed, and presented in an MHC class II-restricted fashion to a previously activated T_H cell specific for the same antigen—two events occur. One, the B cell becomes an IgM-secreting plasma cell, and—in the presence of the appropriate cytokines and after expression of CD40 (for T_H cell CD154 interaction)—class switching occurs. Two, further somatic hypermutation of the immunoglobulin variable region genes of such mature B cells, which changes affinity of BCRs for antigens, also occurs in germinal centers (see also Immune Recognition and Response, discussed earlier). Mutants with low-affinity receptors undergo apoptosis, while enhanced-affinity BCRs are positively selected. In the presence of CD40 ligation of CD154, antigen-stimulated B cells become memory B cells (see Figure 2–6B).

The ability of mature B cells to capture very low quantities of antigen via high-affinity BCRs allows them to amplify their antigen-presenting capacity to more than 1000 times that of other professional APCs. This particular property may become critical in the development of chronic organ-specific autoimmune diseases in which the source of antigen is limited. Thus, autoreactive B cells that happen to escape the control mechanisms described could amplify and perpetuate autoimmune responses in patients with failing endocrine organs when tissue destruction has left only minute amounts of residual antigen.

AUTOIMMUNITY IS MULTIFACTORIAL

Although the breakage of self-tolerance seems to be a central pathogenic step in the development of autoimmune diseases, autoimmunity is a multifactorial event. Specifically, defects in apoptosis-related molecules (Fas–FasL) of thymic dendritic cells

κ or λ genes (BCR editing). Soluble self antigens presumably generate weaker signals through the BCR of immature B cells; they do not cause apoptosis but make cells unresponsive to stimuli (anergy). These anergic B cells migrate to the periphery, expressing IgD, and may be activated under special circumstances. Only immature B cells with no avidity for antigens become mature B cells, expressing both IgM and IgD. These are the predominant cells that make it to the periphery. **B. Peripheral B-cell tolerance:** In the "absence" of antigen (top right), mature B cells are actively eliminated by activated T cells via Fas–FasL and CD40–CD154 interactions. In the "presence" of specific self antigen but "without T-cell help," antigen recognition by BCRs induces apoptosis or anergy on mature B cells. If self antigen and specific autoreactive T-cell help are provided, two events develop (center): (1) The B cell becomes an IgM-secreting plasma cell (top left), and, in the presence of the appropriate cytokines after expression of CD40 (for T_H cell CD154 interaction), class switching occurs (bottom left). (2) Further somatic hypermutation of the Ig-variable region genes, which changes affinity of BCRs, occurs. Mutants with low-affinity receptors undergo apoptosis, while improved-affinity BCRs are positively selected. In the presence of CD40 ligation of CD154, antigen-stimulated B cells become memory B cells. These two events are the same as in foreign antigen recognition.

have been shown to impair central clonal deletion. Also, in the periphery, similar defects (Fas–FasL, CD152) on T cell-APC molecules may prevent apoptosis of autoreactive T cells. However, it is difficult to consider these general defects as causative of organ-specific disorders. Furthermore, clonal ignorance of T cells cannot be maintained if antigens sequestered from the immune system are released in blood or if cryptic epitopes of antigens that have never been recognized by the immune system are presented to T cells for recognition (after tissue destruction, for example). Defects of active suppression (T regs dysfunction, CTLA-4 downregulation), immune deviation (T_{H1}/T_{H2} imbalance), and defects in B-cell tolerance may all be involved in the pathogenesis of autoimmune diseases. How and why loss of immune self-tolerance occurs is not completely understood. Both genetic and environmental factors appear to be necessary.

GENETIC FACTORS IN AUTOIMMUNITY

Epidemiologic studies demonstrate that susceptibility to most autoimmune diseases has a significant genetic component. In type 1 diabetes, for example, there is a clear association between race and susceptibility to disease—the incidence is approximately 40 times higher in Finland than in Japan. Family studies also demonstrate a strong underlying genetic component. The lifetime risk of developing type 1 diabetes in the United States general population is 0.4%, whereas in relatives of diabetics the risk is substantially higher (4% for parents, 5%-7% for siblings, 20% for HLA-identical siblings, 25%-40% for monozygotic twins).

The inheritance pattern of autoimmune disorders is complex. These disorders are polygenic, arising from several independently segregating genes. The most consistent genetic marker for autoimmune diseases to date is the MHC genotype. Considering again genetic susceptibility to type 1 diabetes, up to 95% of Caucasians developing diabetes express the HLA alleles DR3 or DR4— compared to about 40% of normal individuals. Individuals heterozygous for both DR3 and DR4 have the highest risk. It has been shown that the DQ rather than DR genotype is a more specific marker of susceptibility and that the association of both markers is due to the fact that they are products of closely linked genes. But what is more important than the fact that HLA genes are linked to diabetes is that HLA haplotypes are no longer simply undefined genetic markers. It has been shown that the polymorphisms of the DQ molecules are critical for high-affinity recognition of autoantigens (eg, islet cell antigens) by TCRs. HLA-DQ structure analysis suggests that the lack of aspartic acid at position 57 (Asp^{57}) on the DQ β chain allows the autoantigen (processed peptide) to fit better in the antigen-binding groove formed by this molecule. To the contrary, the presence of Asp^{57} allows the formation of a salt bridge with a conserved arginine at position 76 on the DQ α chain, preventing the accommodation of the immunogenic peptide recognized by the TCR. Several autoimmune diseases have been linked to HLA-DQβ1 genes, including type 1 diabetes, celiac disease, bullous pemphigoid, autoimmune hepatitis, and premature ovarian failure, and the structure of the DQβ1 molecule may be the reason for the increased susceptibility. Other

candidate genes associated with autoimmune endocrinopathies are discussed further under the single and polyglandular syndromes.

ENVIRONMENTAL FACTORS IN AUTOIMMUNITY

Environmental factors also play a critical role in the pathogenesis of autoimmune disease. The strongest evidence for this statement comes from studies of monozygotic twins, which show that concordance rates for autoimmune disorders are imperfect (never 100%). As mentioned above, in type 1 diabetes, identical twins show less than 50% concordance.

The environmental factors thought to have greatest influence on disease development include infectious agents, diet, and toxins. In type 1 diabetes, viruses have been strong suspects. Up to 20% of children prenatally infected with rubella develop type 1 diabetes. Children with congenital rubella also have an increased incidence of other autoimmune disorders, including thyroiditis and dysgammaglobulinemia. The mechanisms by which these pathogens may induce autoimmune responses include molecular mimicry and direct tissue injury. The hypothesis of molecular mimicry suggests that immune responses directed at infectious agents can cross-react with self antigens, causing tissue or organ destruction. Support for this concept is found in well-known clinical syndromes such as rheumatic fever (immune responses directed against streptococcal M protein seem to cross-react with cardiac myosin, inducing clinical myocarditis). In autoimmune diabetes, the best-studied example of molecular mimicry is the B4 coxsackievirus protein P2-C. Coxsackie B4 virus has also been epidemiologically implicated in the development of type 1 diabetes. There is a striking amino acid sequence similarity between P2-C viral protein and the enzyme glutamic acid decarboxylase (GAD), found in pancreatic β cells (see Autoimmune Aspects of Type 1 Diabetes, discussed later).

The importance of diet in the development of autoimmune diseases remains controversial. An association between early exposure to cow's milk proteins and the risk of type 1 diabetes has been observed in several epidemiologic studies. For example, one study demonstrated that primary immunity to insulin is induced in infancy by oral exposure to cow's milk insulin, but the relevance of this observation is still unknown. On the other hand, selected antigens (from bovine serum albumin to porcine insulin) have been administered orally to mice with a broad spectrum of autoimmune disorders, including nonobese diabetic (NOD) mice, with favorable outcomes. Those data in mice were so compelling that oral tolerance trials in humans have been conducted or are ongoing. Unfortunately, the results of already completed trials in other autoimmune diseases have been disappointing. Three large, randomized, controlled trials designed to delay or prevent type 1 diabetes—the two Diabetes Prevention Trial (DPT-1 and 2) and the European Diabetes Nicotinamide Intervention Trial—have failed to demonstrate a treatment effect. Thus, it should not be concluded that it is impossible to delay or prevent type 1 diabetes; rather, it may require testing of more potent interventions or combinations of therapies, guided by better understanding of the immunopathogenesis of the disease, to demonstrate attenuation or amelioration of the destructive immune process leading to type 1 diabetes.

SINGLE-GLAND AUTOIMMUNE SYNDROMES

Organ-specific autoimmune endocrine disorders may present as single entities or may cluster in polyglandular syndromes. Most endocrine glands are susceptible to autoimmune attack. Some are affected more frequently than others (see Table 2–1).

AUTOIMMUNE ASPECTS OF THYROID DISEASE

Autoimmune thyroid disease can present in a polarized fashion with Graves disease (thyroid hyperfunction) at one end and Hashimoto thyroiditis (thyroid failure) at the other. This functional subdivision is clinically useful. However, both diseases have a common autoimmune origin.

Genes and Environment

Major susceptibility genes in autoimmune thyroid disease have yet to be identified. Although certain HLA alleles (mainly HLA-DR3 and DQA1*0501) have been shown to be present more frequently in Graves disease than in the general population, this association has frequently been challenged. In fact, no consistent association has been found between Graves disease and any known HLA polymorphism. Furthermore, the risk of developing Graves disease in HLA-identical siblings (7%) is not significantly different from that in control populations. HLA-DR5, -DR3, -DQw7 in Caucasian, HLA-DRw53 in Japanese, and HLA-DR9 in Chinese patients were found to be associated with Hashimoto thyroiditis. However, genetic linkage between Hashimoto thyroiditis and a specific HLA locus has not been demonstrated consistently. Overall, the HLA loci are likely to provide less than 5% of the genetic contribution to autoimmune thyroid disease, confirming the relative importance of non-HLA-related genes in susceptibility. For example, it has been shown that the inheritance pattern of autoantibodies to thyroperoxidase (TPO) is genetically transmitted. Other candidates are currently under study. However, autoimmune thyroid disease linkage to CTLA-4, HLA, IgH chain, TCR, thyroglobulin (Tg), TPO, and thyrotropin receptor (TSH-R) genes has been excluded. Recently, using positional genetics of a candidate gene, Graves disease susceptibility was mapped to a noncoding 6.13 kb 3′ region of CTLA-4, the common allelic variation of which was correlated with lower messenger RNA levels of the soluble alternatively spliced form of CTLA-4 (sCTLA-4). sCTLA-4 is known to be present in human serum. It can bind CD80/86 molecules on APCs and inhibit T-cell proliferation in vitro. The reduction in the level of sCTLA-4 could potentially lead to reduced blocking of CD80/86, causing increased activation through CD28 of autoreactive T cells.

An important environmental factor influencing the natural history of autoimmune thyroid disease is that of iodine intake (dietary, or present in drugs such as amiodarone or in x-ray contrast media). There is considerable evidence that iodine adversely affects both thyroid function and antibody production in those with occult or overt autoimmune thyroid disease.

Autoimmune Response

In Graves disease, thyrocytes are the differentiated carriers of TSH-Rs and the target cells of autoantibodies and probably the autoimmune response. The development of autoantibodies that functionally stimulate the TSH-R mimicking the action of TSH was the first example of antibody-mediated activities of a hormone receptor in humans. Autoantibodies that may stimulate the calcium-sensing receptor (CaSR) (another G-protein–coupled receptor) and signal the inhibition of PTH production have been described in autoimmune hypoparathyroidism. Similarly, stimulating antibodies that bind to the adrenocorticotropin (ACTH) receptor may be involved in the pathogenesis of primary pigmented nodular adrenocortical disease (also referred to as nodular adrenal dysplasia).

In Graves disease, antibodies to the TSH-R present with different types of activity. Thyroid-stimulating immunoglobulins (TSIs), the cause of the hyperthyroidism, are detected by a bioassay that measures cAMP production in a cell line that expresses TSH-Rs. TSH-R autoantibodies (stimulating, blocking, or neutral) can be identified by their ability to prevent TSH binding to the TSH-R (TSH-binding inhibition immunoglobulins, TBII). No direct immunoassay for the measurement of TSH-R autoantibodies is available yet, and its development may be difficult because TSH-R autoantibodies are present at very low concentrations in patients with the disease.

A particular feature of Graves disease is its early clinical presentation. Unlike other autoimmune endocrinopathies (type 1 diabetes, Hashimoto thyroiditis, autoimmune Addison disease), in which much of the target organ has to be destroyed before the disease is manifested, Graves hyperthyroidism often presents with an enlarged and active gland. Minimal lymphocytic infiltration is present when hyperthyroidism (due to the presence of TSH-R-stimulating antibodies) develops. This unique feature may ultimately allow early immune intervention in preference to current ablative therapeutic options.

Another peculiar feature of Graves disease is the helper T-cell response observed in this disease. The activation of antibody-producing B cells by T_H lymphocytes in Graves disease is well recognized. At present, a prevailing concept of human autoimmunity suggests that as in acute allograft rejection, "deviation" toward a T_{H1} response dominates its pathogenesis. Counterdeviation toward T_{H2} is thought to be a consequence of tolerance induction and has been postulated as a potential therapeutic approach. Graves disease seems to challenge that concept. Analysis of TSH-R-specific T-cell clones from patients with Graves disease has provided direct evidence for polarization of T_H responses; however, instead of T_{H1} deviation, T_{H0} and T_{H2} responses have been observed. As mentioned before, T_{H1} cells, which regulate cell-mediated responses, secrete mainly IFN-γ and small amounts of IL-4. In contrast, T_{H2} cells that regulate antibody production (such as TSH-R autoantibodies in Graves disease) preferentially produce IL-4 and little IFN-γ. T cells expressing both IL-4 and IFN-γ are known as T_{H0} cells. These experimental results suggest that in Graves disease T_{H0} to T_{H2} cell responses appear to be dominant. Hence, in human autoimmunity, Graves disease appears to be an exception to the usual T_H cell pattern.

In Hashimoto thyroiditis, the hallmark of the humoral immune response is the presence of autoantibodies to TPO. Although the effector mechanism for TPO (or thyroglobulin [Tg]) autoantibodies is still controversial, under special circumstances (at least in vitro) the autoantibodies are themselves cytotoxic agents or activators of cytotoxic T lymphocytes. Furthermore, in secondary T-cell responses, antibodies may play a critical role in antigen processing or presentation to T cells. In short, macrophages internalize (and subsequently process) antigen by phagocytosis and antigen-antibody complex uptake via Fc receptors. B cells have membrane-bound antibodies (B-cell receptors; BCRs) which provide a much more powerful system for antigen capture. Indeed, recombinant TPO-specific membrane-bound autoantibody captures antigen and allows presentation efficiently. Antibody binding also modulates antigen processing of immune complexes, enhancing or suppressing the presentation of different T-cell peptides. Hence, APCs (internalizing immune complexes through Fc receptors) and B cells (capturing antigen through BCRs) can influence the secondary T-cell response that perpetuates autoimmune disease. The potential role of autoantibodies in modulating presentation of T-cell determinants in thyroid (and diabetes) autoimmunity is being explored.

Animal Models of Autoimmune Thyroid Disease

The classic immunologic approach to development of an animal model of an autoimmune disease is to immunize the animal with soluble antigen in adjuvant. For autoimmune thyroid disease, the induction of thyroiditis in rabbits using human Tg was one of the earliest attempts to do this—by Rose and coworkers in 1956. In subsequent studies, mice immunized with human or murine Tg developed experimental autoimmune thyroiditis. Immunization with TPO (human or porcine) induces thyroid autoantibodies and, as in the case of Tg, causes thyroiditis to develop in particular MHC strains of mice. However, unlike spontaneous thyroiditis in chickens, none of the immunized mouse models of thyroiditis develop hypothyroidism.

In 1996, Shimojo and coworkers developed a mouse model that clearly mimics some of the major features of Graves disease. This was achieved by the ingenious approach of immunizing mice with fibroblasts stably transfected with the cDNA for the human TSH-R and syngeneic MHC class II (Figure 2–7). Most of the animals had moderately high TBII activity in their sera, and about 25% were clearly thyrotoxic, with elevated T_4 and T_3 values, detectable TSI activity, and thyroid hypertrophy. For the first time, therefore, an animal model was established in which a significant number of affected subjects have the immunologic and

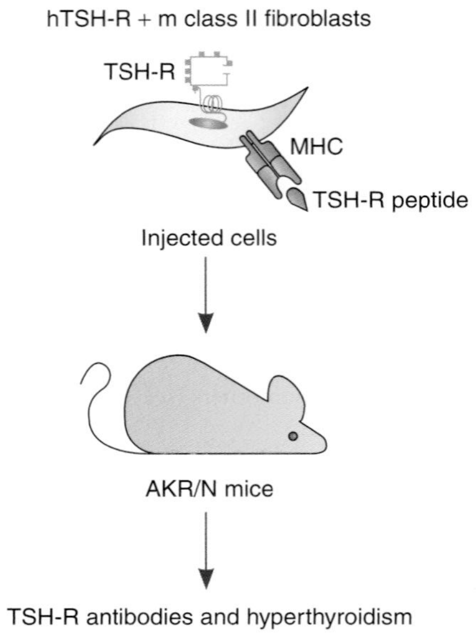

FIGURE 2–7   Animal model for Graves disease. This first animal model of Graves-like disease was achieved by injecting AKR/N mice with syngeneic (MHC-identical) fibroblasts dually transfected with mouse MHC class II (H2-k) and human TSH-R cDNA. About 25% of the animals developed endocrinologic (hyperthyroidism) and immunologic (TSI, TBII) features of Graves disease.

endocrinologic features of Graves hyperthyroidism. More recently, other models have become available. The general rule for induction of an antibody response to the TSH-R in the form of TSI and consequent Graves disease appears to be the need to express the antigen in a native form in an MHC class II carrying cell. Thus, TSH-R-transfected B cells (M12 cell line), TSH-R-adenovirus-infected dendritic cells, and even naked TSH-R DNA or TSH-R adenovirus parenterally delivered and probably captured and expressed by MHC class II expressing cells, have been used to induce TSI and Graves-like disease. However, the focal thyroiditis that accompanies human Graves, as well as the extrathyroidal manifestations that define the disease, have never been reliably reproduced in any of these models. Nevertheless, these models open up new ways of investigating the pathogenesis of Graves disease.

AUTOIMMUNE ASPECTS OF TYPE 1 DIABETES

Most type 1 diabetes results from autoimmune destruction of pancreatic β cells in a process that can span several years. This results in glucose intolerance and clinical disease when the majority of β cells have been destroyed. The destruction is marked by circulating antibodies to pancreatic β cells and by massive infiltration of mononuclear lymphocytes into the islets of Langerhans while pancreatic β cells remain. The lymphocytes disappear when the β cells are gone. Although insulin is available for replacement therapy, type 1 diabetes remains a chronic disorder of major socioeconomic impact, especially because it mainly afflicts the young. Elucidation of the molecular mechanisms underlying this destruction—and the development of methods to prevent autoimmunity—may ultimately lead to effective treatment. Such developments, however, require animal models of type 1 diabetes that closely resemble the disease in humans.

Genes and Environment

The susceptibility to develop type 1 diabetes is associated with certain alleles of the MHC class II locus that have been statistically linked to a variety of autoimmune disorders. The most recent analyses indicate that in Caucasians, HLA-DR3, DQ2 (DQB1*0201) and HLA-DR4 (DRB1*0401), DQ8 (DQB1*0302) haplotypes are most strongly associated with type 1 diabetes. In Asian populations, DRB1*0405 is the major susceptibility haplotype. In contrast, the DR2, DQ6 (DQB1*0602) haplotype is negatively associated with type 1 diabetes. More importantly, susceptibility requires both HLA-DQ β chain alleles to be negative for aspartic acid at position 57 (Asp^{57}) in the amino acid sequence. Studies of different populations have shown a linear relationship between the incidence of type 1 diabetes and the estimated frequency of homozygous absence of Asp^{57}.

Non-HLA candidate genes consistently associated with type 1 diabetes include the "variable number of tandem repeats" (VNTR) polymorphisms in the insulin gene and the CTLA-4 gene (CD152). The VNTR polymorphisms are located adjacent to defined regulatory sequences that influence insulin gene expression. Of immunologic importance, CTLA-4 gene (see Immune Recognition and Response, discussed earlier) is the other non-HLA candidate gene consistently found to be associated with type 1 diabetes.

Although environmental factors definitely play a role in the development of type 1 diabetes (eg, Coxsackie B4 virus, mumps virus, rubella virus, Kilham rat virus in the bio breeding [BB]-rat; or cow's milk formula exposure), more studies are needed to establish a definite etiologic link.

Autoimmune Response

The autoantibodies associated with β cell destruction can be present up to several years before the clinical onset of disease and are thus excellent markers of disease risk. Furthermore, they have served as important tools to identify human pancreatic β cell autoantigens. In 1990, Baekkeskov and coworkers identified a 64-kDa islet cell protein as the smaller isoform of the enzyme that synthesizes γ-aminobutyrate (GABA): glutamic acid decarboxylase (GAD65). This autoantigen was shown to be recognized by 70% to 80% of prediabetic and newly diagnosed type 1 diabetic patients' sera. A second component of the 64-kDa antigen was shown to be a putative tyrosine phosphatase, termed IA-2. IA-2 is recognized by 60% to 70% of prediabetic and newly diagnosed type 1 diabetic patients. Together, GAD65 and IA-2 autoantibodies detect over 90% of individuals who develop type 1 diabetes and can be used to detect individuals at risk several years before the clinical onset of disease.

Although autoantibody responses to GAD65 are not easily detected, there is strong evidence to suggest that GAD65 is an important T-cell autoantigen in the NOD mouse. Thus, GAD65 is the earliest known target of the autoimmune T-cell response in the NOD mouse. Administration of the protein in a tolerogenic form prevents disease in NOD mice. In contrast, induction of tolerance to other potential autoantigens in this model (such as carboxypeptidase H and hsp60) does not prevent disease. The NOD mouse does not develop autoimmunity to the IA-2 molecule and thus distinguishes itself from the human disease with regard to this target antigen (see Models, discussed later).

Insulin is a third well-characterized autoantigen in type 1 diabetes. Insulin autoantibodies can be detected in about 50% of newly diagnosed children with type 1 diabetes. Insulin-specific T-cell clones can transfer disease in the NOD mouse. Furthermore, administration of whole insulin, insulin B chain, or an insulin peptide epitope in a tolerogenic form can protect against disease in NOD mice. Because animals receiving insulin or insulin B chain continue to have intra-islet insulitis—in contrast to young NOD mice treated with GAD65 in a tolerogenic way—it has been suggested that insulin reactivity is more distal in disease progression. Additional but less well-characterized proteins have been implicated as targets of autoantibodies in type 1 diabetes in humans.

Autoantibodies, although they are good markers of disease, do not seem to be directly involved in destruction of pancreatic β cells. Adoptive transfer of diabetes to NOD mice with spontaneous, combined immunodeficiency (NOD-SCID) lacking B cells, can be mediated by T cells alone. However, because β-cell-deficient NOD mice do not develop disease, it is possible that B lymphocytes function as important APCs in the islet to perpetuate an ongoing autoimmune response and thus are essential for presentation of rare antigens such as GAD65 and IA-2. (See also autoimmune response in the section on Autoimmune Aspects of Thyroid Disease, discussed earlier.)

An important question is whether GAD65, IA-2, and insulin are major target antigens of T-cell mediated β-cell destruction that results in type 1 diabetes in humans. Proliferative and cytotoxic T-cell responses to GAD65 are detected in the peripheral blood of newly diagnosed type 1 diabetes patients, but their pathogenicity has not been addressed. Induction of neonatal tolerance to GAD65 specifically prevents diabetes in the NOD mouse model. The role of IA-2 in destructive autoimmunity to the pancreatic β cell in humans is suggested by the high predictive value of IA-2 antibodies for clinical onset of diabetes.

Both GAD65 and IA-2 are neuroendocrine proteins, which are expressed at significant levels in the brain and β cell. Stiff-man syndrome—a very rare neurologic disorder in humans with a high coincidence of diabetes—is characterized by a strong autoantibody response to GAD65, the titer of which is several orders of magnitude higher than in diabetes. It has been suggested that impairment of GABA-secreting neurons in stiff-man syndrome is mediated by GAD65 autoantibodies, whereas development of type 1 diabetes is associated with a cellular immune response to GAD65. The low incidence of stiff-man syndrome compared with type 1 diabetes (only one in 10^4 type 1 diabetic patients develops stiff-man syndrome, whereas 40% of stiff-man syndrome patients develop type 1 diabetes) probably reflects in part the protection of GABAergic neurons by the blood–brain barrier and the absence of MHC class II antigen expression in normal neurons. The cellular localization of IA-2 expression in brain is not known, and there are no known disorders of the central nervous system that involve autoimmunity to IA-2.

In the NOD mouse, the destruction of pancreatic β cells requires both the CD4 T-helper (T_H) cells and CD8 cytotoxic (T_C) cells. Whereas T_H cells seem to be required for the development of an autoimmune response to the islets and generation of intrainsulitis, T_C cells are probably the effector cells of β-cell destruction. Furthermore, there is evidence that in the CD4 lineage, the T_{H1} subset is important for development of disease in the NOD mouse. T_{H1} cells are induced by IL-12 and are biased toward secreting IFN-γ and IL-2. In contrast, there is evidence that the T_{H2} cytokine IL-4 exerts a dominant-negative effect on diabetes progression in the NOD mouse. In humans, low autoantibody titers associated with type 1 diabetes and high titers associated with a protective haplotype (DR2) suggest that a strong T_{H2} response can be inhibitory for β-cell destruction. A role for T_{H1} cells in human disease is also suggested by results of cytokine profiles of peripheral human NK cells in identical twins which are discordant for the development of diabetes. This is different from the observed T_H responses in Graves disease (see Autoimmune Aspects of Thyroid Disease, discussed earlier).

Recently, it has been suggested that it is not the presence of autoantibodies to GAD65 but the absence of the corresponding anti-idiotypic antibodies that defines type 1 diabetes. Anti-idiotypic antibodies bind to the idiotype (binding region) of other antibodies. Investigators found that while diabetes patients are positive for GAD65 antibodies because they lack certain anti-idiotypic antibodies, healthy individuals are negative for GAD65 antibodies because of the very presence of anti-idiotypic antibodies directed against GAD65 antibodies in their serum.

Animal Models of Autoimmune Diabetes Mellitus

The nonobese diabetic (NOD) mouse has been invaluable for studies of molecular mechanisms of autoimmunity directed toward the pancreatic β cells and the development of diabetes. It has several features, however, which distinguish it from the human disease. The incidence of diabetes is two to three times higher in female than in male NODs, whereas in humans there is a slight preponderance of type 1 diabetes in males. Furthermore, while the induction of organ-specific autoimmunity and inflammation in humans may be caused by human pathogens or toxins, autoimmunity seems to be the default mechanism in the NOD mouse. Thus, mice in clean, pathogen-free environments have a high incidence of disease, whereas a variety of regimens that stimulate the immune system of the mouse, such as viral infection or injection of complete Freund adjuvant, prevent disease. To date, more than 125 treatments for successful prevention or delay of diabetes in the NOD mouse have been identified, but none have been identified for humans.

The bio breeding (BB) rat develops spontaneous T-cell-mediated diabetes. The BB-rat disease is significantly different from the human disease in that it is accompanied by autoantibodies to lymphocytes and a severe lymphocytopenia, which is essential for development of β-cell autoimmunity and diabetes in this model.

In an attempt to develop better models of diabetes, "humanized" transgenic mice that express diabetes-prone **human MHC class II** molecules were developed. Since these animals did not develop spontaneous diabetes, they were backcrossed into the NOD background. However, backcrossing to NOD once again prevented the development of diabetes. Other animal models of type 1 diabetes, some of them *carrying* **human MHC class II** diabetes-susceptibility genes, were developed by expression of ectopic molecules in the islets using the rat insulin promoter (RIP). In some of these models, diabetes needed to be induced by immunization with, for example, insulin peptides or lymphocytic choriomeningitis virus. However, none of these models fully reflect the human disease in that the immune attack was initiated against target human β-cell autoantigen(s) in an MHC class II–restricted fashion, without the need for *aberrant protein(s)* (foreign to the pancreatic β-cell) expression.

Although some of the models of type 1 diabetes described have been very useful for studies of basic immunologic mechanisms associated with pancreatic β-cell autoimmunity, other models of type 1 diabetes closer to what occurs in humans are needed if immunoprevention and immunomodulatory techniques are to be tested. At a minimum, human susceptibility genes and human target antigens need to coexist in an animal model to mimic human autoimmune responses.

AUTOIMMUNE ASPECTS OF OTHER ENDOCRINOPATHIES

Autoimmune Adrenal Failure

Autoimmune Addison disease seldom develops as a single-gland syndrome. In about 50% of cases, the disease is associated with other gland and organ failure. Anderson and coworkers described the existence of adrenal-specific autoantibodies for the first time in 1963. Using immunofluorescence techniques on sections of human, bovine, or monkey adrenals, antibodies specifically recognizing the adrenal cortex (ACA) were described. Steroid-producing cell autoantibodies (SCA) reactive with cells of the adrenals, gonads, and placenta were described by Anderson and coworkers in 1968. SCAs are detected predominantly in ACA-positive patients with Addison disease who have premature ovarian failure in the context of autoimmune polyglandular syndrome type I (APS-I; see Autoimmune Polyglandular Syndromes, discussed later).

Steroid 21-hydroxylase has been identified as a major adrenal autoantigen in ACA-positive patients with Addison disease. Using a sensitive assay based on the immune precipitation of radiolabeled recombinant 21-hydroxylase, workers in one study reported positive testing in sera from 72% of patients with isolated Addison

TABLE 2–2 Adrenal autoantibodies in different syndromes.

Autoantibodies	Addison Disease(%)	APS-I[a] (%)	APS-II[b] (%)	ACA(+)[c] (%)
21-Hydroxylase	72	92	100	80
17α-Hydroxylase	5	55	33	20
P450scc	9	45	36	20

[a]APS-I: Autoimmune polyglandular syndrome type I: Autoimmune polyendocrinopathy, candidiasis, and ectodermal dystrophy.

[b]APS-II: Autoimmune polyglandular syndrome type II: Adrenal insufficiency, thyroid disease, and diabetes mellitus.

[c]ACA(+): Adrenal cortex antibody-positive without clinically overt Addison disease.

disease, 92% of patients with APS-I, 100% of patients with APS-II, and 80% of patients who were positive for ACA by immunofluorescence but did not have clinically overt Addison disease (apparently healthy blood donors showed 2.5% positivity) (Table 2–2). Another study measured ACA in 808 children with organ-specific autoimmune diseases without adrenal insufficiency. ACAs were detectable in 14. Ten of these ACA-positive children (also positive for 21-hydroxylase antibodies) and 12 ACA-negative children were prospectively followed with adrenocortical function testing and antibodies. Overt Addison disease developed in 9 (90%) ACA/21-hydroxylase antibody-positive children within 3 to 121 months, and the one remaining child had subclinical hypoadrenalism throughout an extra 24-month observation period. The progression to adrenal failure was not related to ACA titer, sex, baseline adrenal function (subclinical insufficiency vs. normal function), type of associated autoimmune disease, or HLA status. Although ACA 21-hydroxylase antibodies appear to be highly predictive in children, in adults the cumulative risk of developing Addison disease in patients with other organ-specific autoimmune diseases and positive ACA 21-hydroxylase antibodies is about 32%. Steroid 17α-hydroxylase is another adrenal autoantigen. 17α-Hydroxylase antibodies were found in 5% of patients with isolated Addison disease, 55% of patients with APS-I, 33% of patients with APS-II, and 20% of sera from patients who were positive for ACA but did not have clinically overt Addison disease (see Table 2–2). Antibodies against another adrenal autoantigen, cytochrome P450 side-chain cleavage enzyme (P450scc), were found to be present in 9% of patients with isolated Addison disease, 45% of patients with APS-I, 36% of patients with APS-II, and 20% of sera from patients who were positive for ACA but did not have clinically overt Addison disease (see Table 2–2). The prevalence of P450scc antibodies in these groups of patients was always lower than that of 21-hydroxylase antibodies but similar to that of 17α-hydroxylase antibodies. Furthermore, almost all sera that were positive for 17α-hydroxylase or P450scc antibodies were also positive for 21-hydroxylase antibodies. In addition, a comparison of SCAs measured by immunofluorescence with 17α-hydroxylase and P450scc antibody measurements suggested that 17α-hydroxylase and P450scc are the major components of the SCA antigen just as 21-hydroxylase is the major component of ACA antigen.

Overall, immune responses in autoimmune adrenal disease may involve other antigens, but reactivity to the three described, particularly 21-hydroxylase, appears to predominate. Although inhibition of enzymatic activity by these antibodies has been shown in vitro, no clear relationship to the pathogenesis of the clinical syndrome has yet been established.

Autoimmune Oophoritis and Orchitis

An autoimmune origin for premature ovarian failure with concomitant Addison disease or oophoritis can be based on the following human and animal data: (1) the presence of autoantibodies to SCA in most cases, (2) the characterization of shared autoantigens between the adrenals and the ovaries (ie, 17α-hydroxylase and P450scc), (3) the histologic features of the ovaries (lymphocyte and plasma cell infiltrate involving steroid-producing cells), and (4) animal models of the syndrome. There is some evidence of autoimmunity in idiopathic premature ovarian failure not associated with Addison disease (cellular immune abnormalities, presence of various ovarian antibodies in some patients, and associations with type 1 diabetes and myasthenia gravis); however, the absence of histologic confirmation makes the autoimmune pathogenesis less credible.

Less is known about the autoimmune pathogenesis of human orchitis. Animal models, however, have shown that infectious or traumatic injury to the testes can induce autoimmune responses in this immune-privileged tissue (defined as sites where antigens are not presented to the host immune system; see Tolerance, discussed earlier).

Autoimmune Hypophysitis

Autoimmune hypophysitis (also called lymphocytic hypophysitis) should be considered in the differential diagnosis of pituitary abnormalities in women (8:1 female:male ratio) during the latter half of pregnancy and in the first 6 months postpartum, as well as in patients with coexisting autoimmune disorders, for example, thyroiditis, adrenalitis, autoimmune hypoparathyroidism, or atrophic gastritis. More than 380 cases have been described since the original report in 1962. Antipituitary antibodies have been detected in a minority of patients. Owing to the lack of markers for the disease, the diagnosis can only be confirmed with histologic examination. Nevertheless, because of the usually transient endocrine and compressive features of this condition, conservative management based on clinical suspicion may prevent the consequences of unnecessary pituitary surgery. Granulomatous hypophysitis—another form of autoimmune hypophysitis—appears to have a similar autoimmune pathogenesis but more commonly affects postmenopausal women and men. The presence of regulatory T cells in this form of hypophysitis, however, makes the autoimmune pathogenesis less clear.

Autoimmune Hypoparathyroidism

Autoimmune hypoparathyroidism, also called idiopathic hypoparathyroidism, is one of the major components of APS type I (APS-I;

see next section). It also presents as a sporadic disease, sometimes associated with Hashimoto thyroiditis in women. The fact that autoimmune hypoparathyroidism presents in association with other autoimmune diseases and also the presence of autoantibodies reactive with parathyroid tissue in many affected patients suggests an autoimmune pathogenesis. Parathyroid autoantibodies have been reported to show a complement-dependent cytotoxic effect on cultured bovine parathyroid cells. At least one major parathyroid autoantigen has been identified as the CaSR. The CaSR is of great importance in the regulation of parathyroid hormone secretion and renal tubular calcium reabsorption. This receptor is a member of the 7-membrane-spanning domain G protein–coupled receptor family. It is also expressed in thyroid C cells, the pituitary, the hypothalamus, and in other regions of the brain. The relationship of the autoimmune response directed against the receptor to the pathogenesis of the disease is not clear. However, antibody-mediated stimulation of the CaSR with consequent inhibition of PTH synthesis and secretion has been suggested. The prevalence of the CaSR antibodies in clinically diagnosed idiopathic hypoparathyroidism was found to be 56% in one study. Measurement of these antibodies may have value in predicting the development of autoimmune hypoparathyroidism in patients with autoimmune endocrinopathies who are at risk. Furthermore, hypercalcemia in a patient with multiple autoimmune disorders, responsive to glucocorticoids, has been recently described as secondary to the presence of a blocking IgG4 autoantibody directed against the CaSR and apparently capable of blocking the inhibitory actions of the ligand calcium (see also Chapter 8).

AUTOIMMUNE POLYGLANDULAR SYNDROMES

Associations of multiple autoimmune endocrine disorders have been classified in different syndromes. APS type I and type II (APS-I and -II) can be clearly separated clinically (Table 2–3). Some authors have attempted to subdivide APS-II (ie, APS-II and -III) on the basis of the association of some autoimmune disorders but not others. Little information is gained, however, by making this subdivision in terms of understanding pathogenesis or prevention of future endocrine failure in patients or their relatives. Other autoimmune associations, not always described in syndromes, are also classically recognized. Vitiligo, for example, seems to accompany multiple autoimmune endocrinopathies. There is now convincing evidence of linkage between *NALP1* (*NACHT leucine-rich-repeat protein 1*), a gene involved in immune regulation, and the presence of vitiligo associated with at least one endocrine autoimmune disease including but not limited to type 1 diabetes, Addison disease, and thyroiditis.

AUTOIMMUNE POLYGLANDULAR SYNDROME I (APS-I)

APS-I is an autosomal recessive disorder with 25% incidence among siblings of affected individuals. Also known as APECED, or autoimmune polyendocrinopathy-candidiasis-ectodermal

dystrophy, APS-I is characterized by the triad of chronic mucocutaneous candidiasis, autoimmune hypoparathyroidism, and adrenal insufficiency (only two are required in the index case for the diagnosis, and only one in the siblings). Chronic mucocutaneous candidiasis (involving oral mucosa and nails or, less frequently, the esophagus) is usually first manifested as the initial problem early in life. In most individuals, the development of autoimmune hypoparathyroidism, a major clinical phenotype, usually follows. Specifically for hypoparathyroidism, the presence of antibodies to *NALP5* (*NACHT leucine-rich-repeat protein 5*), a gene highly expressed in parathyroid and ovary, have been recently described. In one study these antibodies were detected in 49% of patients with known APS-I and hypothyroidism (see also Chapter 8). Addison disease is another component of the triad that can manifest prior to, concomitantly with, or following hypoparathyroidism. Lifelong surveillance is important since decades may elapse between the development of one feature of the disorder and the onset of another. There is no female preponderance in this syndrome, and it is not HLA-associated. APS-I may occur sporadically or in families. The genetic locus responsible for the disease has been mapped to the long arm of chromosome 21 (21q22.3). The haplotype analysis of this region in different populations has shown that APS-I is linked to different mutations in a gene identified as the autoimmune regulator *(AIRE)*. AIRE encodes a putative nuclear protein with transcription factor motifs (including two zinc finger motifs). It is expressed in different tissues but particularly in the thymus. The mechanism by which mutations of this putative transcription factor lead to the diverse manifestations of APS-I is still unknown. In mice, however, the absence of the analogous protein "aire" influences ectopic expression of peripheral tissue antigens in thymic medullary epithelial cells (MECs), resulting in the development of an autoimmune disorder similar to APS-I and establishing aire/AIRE as an important factor in the induction of central tolerance. Other immune response-related genes as well as environmental factors probably play a role in development of the syndrome. Several studies of large cohorts of patients from different ethnic backgrounds have reported the appearance of chronic candidiasis at different sites in all patients. Hypoparathyroidism and Addison disease present with similar high frequency (see Table 2–3). The occurrence of the diagnostic triad reportedly presents in 57% of patients. Female hypogonadism, presenting as total or partial failure of pubertal development or as premature ovarian failure in adults, has been reported in up to 60% of patients. Male hypogonadism is less frequent (14%). Type 1 diabetes is not as frequent as in APS-II, but if present, usually develops early (under 21 years of age). Autoimmune hypothyroidism (atrophic thyroiditis) is also less frequent than in APS-II; however, thyroid autoantibodies may be present in many euthyroid patients. Other manifestations are described in Table 2–3. Acute autoimmune hepatitis is reportedly less common than chronic hepatitis, which appears to be present in most individuals. Autoantibodies to aromatic L-amino acid decarboxylase (AADC) are associated with chronic active autoimmune hepatitis and vitiligo, which are found in APS-I. These antibodies, if present, can be helpful in making the

TABLE 2–3 Comparison of the different components of autoimmune polyglandular syndromes.

Characteristics	Type I	Type II
Inheritance	Autosomal recessive	Polygenic
Genetic association or linkage	Linked to AIRE	Some HLA association
Gender	Equal distribution	Female preponderance
Age at onset	Infancy	Age 20-40
Endocrine disorders		
Addison disease	60%-72%	70%
Hypoparathyroidism	Common (79%-96%)	Rare (late onset)
Autoimmune thyroid disease	Less frequent (about 5%)	More frequent (about 70%)
Type 1 diabetes	14% (lifetime)	>50%
Primary hypogonadism	60% female, 14% male	About 5%
Hypophysitis	Not reported	Reported
Dermatologic		
Chronic mucocutaneous candidiasis	Often at onset (about 100%)	Not reported
Alopecia	Common (about 29%)	Reported
Vitiligo	About 13%	About 5%
Dermatitis herpetiformis	Not reported	Reported
Gastrointestinal		
Celiac disease	None (only steatorrhea)	Present in 2%-3%
Autoimmune hepatitis	About 12%	Not reported
Hematologic		
Pernicious anemia	About 13%	As common as in APS-I
Pure red cell hypoplasia	Reported	Not reported
Idiopathic thrombocytopenic purpura	Not reported	Reported
Ectodermal		
Enamel hypoplasia	All reported	Not reported
Nail dystrophy		
Tympanic membrane calcification		
Neurologic		
Myasthenia gravis	None reported	All reported
Stiff-man syndrome		
Parkinson disease		
Other		
Asplenism	Reported	Not reported
Keratopathy	Reported	Not reported
Progressive myopathy	Reported	Not reported
IgA deficiency	Not reported	Reported
Serositis	Not reported	Reported
Idiopathic heart block	Not reported	Reported
Goodpasture syndrome	Not reported	Reported

diagnosis. Autoantibodies against tryptophan hydroxylase have been associated with gastrointestinal dysfunction in APS-I. Autoantibodies to the H^+-K^+-ATPase and to intrinsic factor are associated with pernicious anemia, and autoantibodies to tyrosinase are associated with vitiligo. Other autoantibodies associated with the single gland disorders that make up this polyglandular syndrome have been discussed above.

AUTOIMMUNE POLYGLANDULAR SYNDROME II (APS-II)

APS-II is the most common of the polyglandular failure syndromes. It affects women in a 3:1 ratio to men. APS-II is diagnosed when at least two of the following are present: adrenal insufficiency, autoimmune thyroid disease (thyroiditis with hypothyroidism or

Graves disease with hyperthyroidism), and type 1 diabetes. Historically, Schmidt (1926) first described the association of Addison disease and thyroiditis. Carpenter and coworkers in 1964 included type 1 diabetes in the syndrome. Other components of APS-II include the following (see Table 2–3): primary hypogonadism, myasthenia gravis, celiac disease, pernicious anemia, alopecia, vitiligo, and serositis. The most frequent association appears to be with type 1 diabetes (over 50%) and autoimmune thyroid disease (70% in some series). Adrenal insufficiency may be concurrent, may be delayed in onset for up to two decades, or may never manifest. Some diabetic patients (2%-3%) develop celiac disease. Gluten-free diet is usually effective. If the celiac disease is untreated, hypocalcemia (not due to hypoparathyroidism), osteopenia, and occasionally gastrointestinal lymphoma may occur.

Although this syndrome and its components aggregate in families, there is no identifiable pattern of inheritance. Susceptibility is probably determined by multiple gene loci (HLA being the strongest) that interact with environmental factors. Many of the disorders of APS-II are associated (some genetically linked) with the HLA haplotype identified in single organ disorders. HLA-A1, -B8, -DR3 and -DR4, DQA1*0501, and DQB1*0201 have all been described as associated with APS-II.

MANAGEMENT OF AUTOIMMUNE POLYGLANDULAR SYNDROMES

Hormonal replacement therapy remains the only form of treatment of the APS. The clinical management of these disorders mandates early diagnosis of associated components. Since the age at onset of associated disorders is clinically unpredictable, long-term follow-up is needed. Endocrine disorders are treated as they develop and are diagnosed. Hormonal treatments for the specific gland failures are described elsewhere in this book. However, specific combinations of endocrine organ failure require specific management. For example, thyroxine replacement can precipitate life-threatening adrenal failure in a patient with untreated Addison disease. Furthermore, hypoglycemia or decreasing insulin requirements in a patient with type 1 diabetes may be the earliest symptom/sign of adrenal insufficiency. Hypocalcemia, seen in APS-II, is more commonly due to celiac disease than hypoparathyroidism. Treatment of mucocutaneous candidiasis with ketoconazole in patients with APS-I may induce adrenal insufficiency in a failing gland (ketoconazole is a global P450 cytochrome inhibitor). These antifungal drugs may also elevate liver enzymes, making the diagnosis of autoimmune hepatitis—requiring treatment with immunosuppressants—more difficult in these patients.

Screening of affected individuals as well as their relatives is the only way of preventing morbidity and mortality. Annual measurement of TSH is recommended as cost-effective in first-degree relatives of patients with type 1 diabetes. Autoantibody measurements may help in the preclinical assessment of several disorders. Complete blood counts, electrolytes, calcium and phosphorus levels, thyroid and liver function tests, blood smears (including RBC indices), and vitamin B_{12}/plasma methylmalonic acid measurements are all recommended in the follow-up of APS-I. For APS-II patients with type 1 diabetes, thyroid disease and celiac disease coexist with sufficient frequency to justify not only TSH measurement but also screening for endomysial antibodies containing transglutaminase antibodies, which are prevalent in celiac disease.

IMMUNODEFICIENCY, POLYENDOCRINOPATHY, AND ENTEROPATHY, X-LINKED SYNDROME

Another autoimmune polyglandular failure syndrome, immunodeficiency, polyendocrinopathy, and enteropathy, x-linked (IPEX) syndrome, is characterized by development of overwhelming systemic autoimmunity in the first year of life resulting in the observed triad of watery diarrhea, eczematous dermatitis, and endocrinopathy seen most commonly as type 1 diabetes mellitus. Most children have other autoimmune phenomena including Coombs positive anemia, autoimmune thrombocytopenia, autoimmune neutropenia, and tubular nephropathy. The majority of affected males die within the first year of life of either metabolic derangements or sepsis; a few survive into the second or third decade.

Diagnosis is based on clinical findings. FOXP3 is the only gene currently known to be associated with IPEX syndrome. Approximately 50% of males with IPEX syndrome have mutations identified in FOXP3. Genetic testing is clinically available. FOXP3 is expressed primarily in lymphoid tissues (thymus, spleen, and lymph nodes), particularly in CD4+ CD25+ regulatory T lymphocytes. In mice, it is required for the development and suppressive function of this important regulatory T-cell population. In humans, it is not expressed at baseline in CD4+ CD25- or CD8+ T cells but is expressed upon T-cell activation. The FOXP3 protein is absent (due to nonsense, frameshift, or splicing mutations) in individuals with severe, early-onset IPEX syndrome. Some individuals with FOXP3 point mutations express a protein that appears to have decreased function, thereby leading to a milder form of the disease. Peripheral blood mononuclear cells from individuals with IPEX syndrome show an excess production of the Th2 cytokines IL-4, IL-5, IL-10, and IL-13 and decreased production of the Th1 cytokine IFN-γ.

Treatment options include: immunosuppressive agents (eg, cyclosporin A, tacrolimus) alone or in combination with steroids; sirolimus (rapamycin) for persons in whom tacrolimus therapy is toxic or ineffective; granulocyte colony-stimulating factor (G-CSF, filgrastim) for autoimmune neutropenia; nutritional support; and standard treatment of diabetes mellitus and autoimmune thyroid disease. If performed early, bone marrow transplantation (BMT) using nonmyeloablative conditioning regimens can resolve clinical symptoms. If the family-specific mutation is known, FOXP3 sequence analysis in at-risk males can be undertaken immediately after birth to permit early diagnosis and BMT before significant organ damage occurs; otherwise, monitoring at-risk males for symptoms is needed to enable early diagnosis and treatment.

IPEX syndrome is inherited in an x-linked manner. The risk to siblings of the proband depends on the carrier status of the mother. If the mother of the proband is a carrier, the chance of transmitting the disease-causing mutation in each pregnancy is 50%. Males who inherit the mutation will be affected; females who inherit the mutation are carriers and will not be affected. Affected males pass the disease-causing mutation to all of their daughters and none of their sons. Prenatal testing for pregnancies at risk is possible for families in which the disease-causing mutation has been identified.

POEMS SYNDROME (OSTEOSCLEROTIC MYELOMA)

The POEMS (polyneuropathy, organomegaly, endocrinopathy, M spike, skin abnormalities) syndrome, which is frequently seen as a concomitant of Castelman disease (giant cell lymph node hyperplasia), includes a variety of endocrinopathies of the adrenal, thyroid, pituitary, gonads, parathyroids, and pancreas.

The POEMS syndrome displays a number of endocrinopathies in the setting of lymphoproliferative disorders and presumed B-cell dysfunction. Aside from one report in which 2 of 11 patients with monoclonal gammopathy and some form of autoimmunity had POEMS, the endocrinological manifestations of POEMS are not yet established as autoimmune in origin. When associated with Castleman, Kaposi-associated herpes virus (HHV8) may be implicated in the pathogenesis of the lymphoproliferation and the gammopathy.

Two-thirds of patients with POEMS reportedly had at least one endocrine abnormality at presentation. During the course of disease, endocrine abnormalities developed in another 10% of patients with POEMS. Hypogonadism seems to be the most common endocrine abnormality. Elevated levels of follicle-stimulating hormone (FSH) in the absence of primary hypogonadism have been reported. One-third of patients reportedly have erectile dysfunction with low serum testosterone levels. Fourteen percent of patients have hypothyroidism requiring therapy. An additional 12% had mild increases in TSH levels but normal thyroxine levels in one series. Sixteen percent of patients with POEMS have abnormalities of the adrenal-pituitary axis at presentation; with 5% of patients developing adrenal insufficiency later in the course of their disease. Three percent of patients have diabetes mellitus. Serum levels of parathyroid hormone were increased in three of four patients in whom it was measured in one series of 99 POEMS patients. Finally and although still hypothetical for POEMS, autoantibody-mediated mechanisms of disease (Graves disease) have been described in patients with other gammopathies.

REFERENCES

Cooper GS, Bynum ML, Somers EC. Recent insights in the epidemiology of autoimmune diseases: improved prevalence estimates and understanding of clustering of diseases. *J Autoimmun.* 2009 Oct 8;33:197-207. [Epub ahead of print] [PMID: 19819109].

Elagin RB, Balijepalli S, Diacovo MJ, Baekkeskov S, Jaume JC. Homing of GAD65 specific autoimmunity and development of insulitis requires expression of both DQ8 and human GAD65 in transgenic mice. *J Autoimmun.* 2009;33:50. [PMID: 19289270].

Janeway CA, Jr, Travers P, Walport M, Shlomchik MJ, eds. *Immunobiology: The Immune System in Health and Disease.* 6th ed. New York: Garland Science; 2005.

Jaume JC, Parry SL, Madec AM, Sonderstrup G, Baekkeskov S. Suppressive effect of glutamic acid decarboxylase 65-specific autoimmune B lymphocytes on processing of T cell determinants located within the antibody epitope. *J Immunol.* 2002;169:665. [PMID: 12097368].

Khoury S, Sayegh M. The roles of the new negative T cell costimulatory pathways in regulating autoimmunity. *Immunity.* 2004;20:529. [PMID: 15142522].

Lanzavecchia A. Immunology. Licence to kill. *Nature.* 1998;393:413. [PMID: 9623994].

McLachlan SM, Nagayama Y, Rapoport B. Insight into Graves hyperthyroidism from animal models. *Endocr Rev.* 2005;26:800. [PMID: 15827111].

Mirocha S, Elagin RB, Salamat S, Jaume JC. T regulatory cells distinguish two types of primary hypophysitis. *Clin Exp Immunol.* 2009;155:403. [PMID: 19077086].

Roitt IM, Delves PJ. *Roitt's Essential Immunology.* 10th ed. Oxford: Blackwell Science; 2001.

Skyler JS, Krischer JP, Wolfsdorf J, et al. Effects of oral insulin in relatives of patients with type 1 diabetes: The Diabetes Prevention Trial—Type 1. *Diab Care.* 2005;28:1068. [PMID: 15855569].

Evidence-Based Endocrinology and Clinical Epidemiology

David C. Aron, MD, MS

ARR	Absolute risk reduction	**PiD**	Positivity in disease
CI	Confidence interval	**QALY**	Quality-adjusted life year
CV	Coefficient of variation	**RCT**	Randomized controlled trial
EBM	Evidence-based medicine	**ROC**	Receiver-operating characteristic
ER	Event rate	**RRR**	Relative risk reduction
NiH	Negativity in health	**USPSTF**	U.S. Preventive Services Task Force
NNT	Number needed to treat		

The individual practitioner faces a multiplicity of potential diagnoses, limitations in diagnostic capacity, subclinical disease identified by tests rather than by clinical manifestations, and rapid changes in scientific knowledge. The paradigm of clinical decision-making based on the assumption that all that is needed to guide clinical practice is personal experience (however unsystematic), understanding of pathophysiology, and thorough training plus common sense is insufficient to address these challenges. Moreover, the integration of relevant research findings into clinical practice has been haphazard; the lag time between development of scientific knowledge and introduction into practice can be many years, and there is marked variation in practice. A systematic approach based on principles of clinical epidemiology can help address some of these issues. This quantitative approach has formed the primary, albeit not the only, basis of the evidence-based medicine movement. This movement posits that understanding certain rules of evidence is necessary to interpret the literature correctly and that physicians who practice based on the above understanding will provide superior care. This chapter will summarize some of the principles of clinical epidemiology and evidence-based endocrinology and some of their limitations.

CLINICAL EPIDEMIOLOGY

Clinical epidemiology consists of the application of epidemiologic principles and methods to problems encountered in clinical medicine. Clinical epidemiology emphasizes a quantitative approach and is therefore concerned with counts of clinical events. Its applications are paramount (1) in diagnostic testing and how the results modify the probability of a particular disorder being present and (2) in treatment decisions in which the potential benefits and harms must be addressed. The techniques of clinical epidemiology have become increasingly important as practitioners confront the complexity of contemporary medical practice.

DIAGNOSTIC TESTING: TEST CHARACTERISTICS

The appropriate choice and interpretation of diagnostic tests, whether biochemical assays, radiologic procedures, or clinical findings, have always been essential to the clinical practice of endocrinology. These tests, when introduced in the medical literature, are accompanied by varying degrees of validation. The clinician's assessment of the utility of tests, now even more important with the emphasis on cost-effectiveness, can be improved by knowledge of test EBM principles. We review some of these concepts as they apply to diagnosis and management of endocrine disorders, including the topics of test characteristics such as sensitivity and specificity, receiver-operating characteristic (ROC) curves, likelihood ratios, predictive values, and diagnostic accuracy.

The evaluation of endocrine function begins with a clinical question. The more vague the question, the more difficult it is to obtain a clear answer. Part of this step involves a clinical judgment about the likelihood of the disease prior to obtaining a test and its results. This pretest probability is combined with the performance characteristics of the test and its use (sensitivity and specificity, ROC curves, likelihood ratios, predictive values, and diagnostic accuracy) in order for proper interpretation. Variation is inherent in biological systems. Therefore, diagnostic tests must take into account not only variability of the tests themselves and how they are performed but also variability in the populations in whom the tests were developed, both with the disease and without the disease. Key aspects in the analysis of a test include reproducibility (precision) and accuracy. **Reproducibility** describes how close the test comes to producing the same results every time and depends on such factors as intraobserver and interobserver variability (as in the assessment of a physical finding or x-ray) and, in the case of biochemical tests, characteristics such as intra-assay and interassay coefficients of variation (CVs). Although studies utilizing radioimmunoassays and other assays routinely report intra-assay and interassay CVs, few papers publish multiple results performed on the same patient (intraindividual variation). There have also been relatively few studies on the reliability of measurements (ie, the degree of intraindividual variation). One study found that the minimum number of replicate measurements necessary to achieve satisfactory reliability of the mean of basal levels was 3 for plasma cortisol and 18 for salivary cortisol. Responses to dynamic tests required fewer replicates to achieve the same reliability (one to two samples).

Reproducibility depends on the conditions under which the test is performed. Clinicians must be aware of the distinction between efficacy and effectiveness when translating published results into practice. As applied to diagnostic testing, efficacy refers to the degree to which the test has been shown scientifically to accomplish the desired outcome. In contrast, effectiveness refers to the degree to which the test achieves this outcome in actual clinical practice. Most large studies have been performed in research venues and thus are efficacy studies, whereas the effectiveness of most tests in practice has not been extensively evaluated. In comparing one's own results with a published report or laboratory normal range, it is important to take into account those conditions (eg, test performed in a hospital vs a physician's office).

Accuracy describes how close the test comes to producing results that are a true measure of the phenomenon of interest; systematic bias of a highly reproducible test may produce the same incorrect result every time. Like reproducibility, accuracy depends on the conditions under which the test is performed; accuracy in the clinical practice setting may differ from that in the experimental setting where many extraneous influences are controlled.

When interpreting a test, the result is usually compared to a normal range. Frequently, the normal range is developed by using a reference population assumed (or preferably shown) to be disease free. For example, when designing a test to be used in the diagnosis of Cushing syndrome, the reference group should be made up of individuals who have clinical features suggestive of Cushing syndrome but who in fact do not have the disorder. However, reference groups may be made up of individuals who are readily accessible and not more appropriate comparisons. It is also important to note that in establishing a normal range based on a Gaussian or normal distribution, encompassing the mean ± two standard deviations, 5% of disease-free individuals have a result outside the limits of normal. (It is important to note that the definition of normal based on a Gaussian distribution of values is only one of a number of definitions of normal. Some others include the one most representative or most common in a class, the one most suited to survival, and the one that carries no penalty [ie, no risk].) Figure 3–1 illustrates a normal range and a range in a population with disease. A result outside normal limits is not equivalent to disease. Moreover, values within the normal range do not necessarily exclude disease. Values in the population of individuals with disease are determined separately, and the overlap with the normal range is assessed.

Sensitivity and Specificity

Ideally, a diagnostic test has no overlap between the results of individuals with the disease and those without the disease. The reality, however, is different. Test characteristics that describe this overlap are sensitivity and specificity, and they are typically illustrated in a 2 × 2 table. As shown in Figure 3–2, sensitivity and specificity are collectively known as **operating characteristics**. Sensitivity refers to the ability to identify correctly individuals with a disease. The sensitivity of a sign or symptom (or diagnostic test) is the proportion of patients with disease who has a positive test result, sign, or symptom. In contrast, specificity refers to the ability to identify correctly individuals without a disease. The specificity of a test is the proportion of healthy patients who have a negative test result or who lack that sign or symptom.

Thus, the **sensitivity** of a test equals the number of individuals with disease who have a positive test (true positive [TP] divided by the number of individuals with disease (true positives plus false negatives [FN]), whereas **specificity** equals the number of individuals without the disease who have a negative test (true negatives) divided by the number of individuals without disease (true negatives plus false positives [FP]). Sensitivity is sometimes termed **PiD** or positivity in disease, and specificity is sometimes termed **NiH** or negativity in health. In theory, sensitivity and specificity are characteristics of the test itself and not of the patients on whom the test is applied. However, this may not be correct in practice. The sensitivity of a test may be affected by the stage or severity of the disease. The specificity of a test may depend on the characteristics of the reference population. The nature of the groups used to establish the cut-points that differentiate normal from abnormal must be appropriate and should be specified in any report of a diagnostic test. The value chosen for a cutoff point

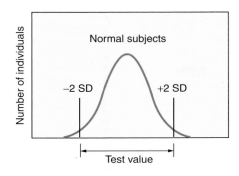

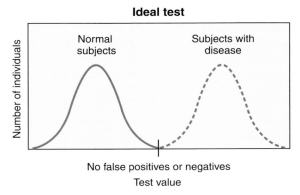

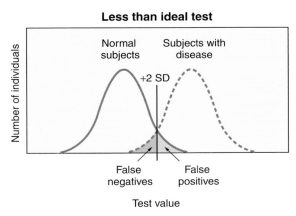

FIGURE 3-1 Defining a normal range and diagnostic testing. The top panel shows the Gaussian (normal) distribution of test values in a population of individuals. The middle panel illustrates two such curves that describe the findings in an ideal test. In this case, there is no overlap in the results between normal subjects and subjects with disease (ie, there are no false-positive results and no false-negative results). The bottom panel illustrates the results for a less-than-ideal test. Normal subjects with test values above the given threshold have abnormal results (ie, false-positive results), whereas some subjects with disease have test values below that threshold (ie, normal or false-negative results).

also affects the sensitivity and specificity. To assist the clinician in assessing a report on a diagnostic test, a series of questions has been proposed (Table 3–1).

The overnight dexamethasone suppression test is commonly used as a screening test in the diagnosis of Cushing syndrome, and its use illustrates some of the issues in diagnostic testing. As shown in Figure 3–3, combining the results of a number of studies indicates a sensitivity of 98.1% and specificity of 98.9%. However, the individual studies varied, with sensitivities ranging from 83% to 100% and specificities from 77% to 100%. Moreover, the studies used different cortisol assays, doses of dexamethasone, and criteria for a positive test. Caution must be exercised in drawing conclusions from the combining of such data. In order to apply the sensitivity and specificity of a test derived from one study sample to a different population, the test cannot deviate from methods used (eg, dose of dexamethasone, type of cortisol assay, timing of dexamethasone administration, and cortisol assay) when the optimal cutoff was determined, and the sample studied must be similar to the new population to be tested. To meet this latter prerequisite, the sample studied must account for variability of diseased individuals. This requires that subjects with disease be defined using the best available gold standard (independent of the test in question) and include a broad enough cross-section of those with disease (eg, mild versus severe disease, different etiologies of disease, as well as age, sex, and race) to establish a reliable range of measurements. The characteristics of the reference sample of subjects without the disease are equally important. Although the 1-mg overnight dexamethasone suppression test is still believed to have excellent, albeit less than 100% sensitivity, it has serious problems with specificity, and false-positive results have been described with a variety of drugs as well as medical, surgical, and psychiatric conditions.

One additional method of reporting the performance of a test is diagnostic accuracy. This can also be derived from the 2 × 2 table. Diagnostic accuracy is defined as the ability of a test to identify correctly those with the disease and those without the disease:

$$\text{Diagnostic accuracy} \frac{(TP+TN)}{(TP+TN+FP+FN)}$$

From Crapo composite data on the 1-mg overnight dexamethasone suppression test, the diagnostic accuracy is calculated as 98.7%. In addition to the characteristics of the study subjects, the number of subjects included in the sample is also critical to assess the accuracy of the test. Each operating characteristic determined in a study should be accompanied by a **confidence interval (CI)**—a range of values calculated from sample size and standard error which expresses a degree of confidence (usually 90%, 95%, or 99%) that the unknown true sensitivity or specificity lies in that interval. CIs are a measure of the precision of an estimate. The range of a CI depends on two factors: (1) the number of observations; and (2) the spread in the data (commonly measured as a standard deviation). The fewer the number of observations, the larger the range of the CI, and the greater the standard deviation of the data, the larger the range of the CI.

In addition to the limitations on the operating characteristics based on the samples from which the data are derived, sensitivity and specificity are not independent of each other. They vary with the cutoff level chosen to represent positive and negative test results. In general, as sensitivity increases, specificity decreases and

		Disease	
		+ Present	− Present
Test result	+	a True positive (TP)	b False positive (FP)
	−	c False negative (FN)	d True negative (TN)

Sensitivity = a/(a + c) = TP/(TP + FN)

Specificity = d/(b + d) = TN/(TN + FP)

Positive predictive value = a/(a + b) = (TP/TP + FP)

Negative predictive value = d/(c + d) = TN/(TN + FN)

Diagnostic accuracy = (a + d)/(a + b + c + d) = (TP+ TN)/(TP + FP + TN + FN)

Pretest (prior) probability = (a + c)/(a + b + c + d) = (TP + FN)/(TP + FP + TN + FN)

Likelihood ratio for a positive test result (LR+):

    = [a/(a + c)]/[b/b(b + d)] = TP rate/FP rate = [TP/(TP + FN)/(FP/TN + FP)] =

    = sensitivity/(1 − specificity)

Likelihood ratio for a negative test result (LR−):

    = [c/(a + c)]/[d/(b + d)] = FN rate/TN rate = [FN/(TP + FN)]/[TN + FP)] =

    = (1 − sensitivity)/specificity

FIGURE 3-2 This 2 × 2 table graphically depicts how tests can be performed in individuals with and without a disease.

as specificity increases, sensitivity decreases. This phenomenon is depicted graphically in an ROC curve.

Receiver-Operating Characteristic Curves

An ROC curve graphically illustrates the trade-off between the false-negative and false-positive rates for different cutoff points of a diagnostic test. In an ROC curve, the true-positive rate (sensitivity) is plotted on the vertical axis and the false-positive rate (1–specificity) is plotted on the horizontal axis for different cutoff

TABLE 3-1   Guide for evaluating studies of test performance.

Question #1	Is the study population described well enough?
Question #2	Does the spectrum of illness in the study population differ from that of my patients (eg, spectrum bias)?
Question #3	Was a positive result on the index test a criterion for referral to have the gold standard test?
Question #4	Was there blinding of those who interpreted the index test and those who interpreted the gold standard test (eg, test review bias)?
Question #5	Was the gold standard test an adequate measure of the true state of the patient?

Reprinted with permission from Jaeschke R, Guyatt G, Sackett DL. Users' guide to the medical literature. III. How to use an article about a diagnostic test. A. Are the results of the study valid? *JAMA.* 1994;271:389-391; and Jaeschke R, Guyatt G, Sackett DL. Users' guide to the medical literature. III. How to use an article about a diagnostic test. B. What are the results and will they help me in caring for my patients? *JAMA.* 1994:271:703.

points for the test. The dotted diagonal line in Figure 3–4 corresponds to a test that is positive or negative just by chance (ie, the true-positive rate equals the false-positive rate). Such a test provides no useful information. Ideally, a test would provide results that could be plotted on one point in the top left corner—100% true-positive rate and 100% true-negative rate. The closer an ROC curve is to the upper left-hand corner of the graph, the more accurate it is, because the true-positive rate is 1 and the false-positive rate is 0. As the criterion for a positive test becomes more stringent, the point on the curve corresponding to sensitivity and specificity (point A) moves down and to the left (lower sensitivity, higher specificity); if less evidence is required for a positive test, the point on the curve corresponding to sensitivity and specificity (point B) moves up and to the right (higher sensitivity, lower specificity). Analysis of the area between the actual results and the straight line indicates how good the test is. The greater the area under the curve, the better the test.

Depending on the purpose of the test, the curves may be used to decide an optimal cutoff level for a single test. For example, with a screening test, high sensitivity is typically desired, and the trade-off is lower specificity. The cutoff point may also be chosen depending on health costs (morbidity and mortality associated with an error in diagnosis), financial costs, or need for maximal information (the operating position giving the greatest increase in posttest probability).

ROC curves may also be used to compare two or more tests by comparing the areas under the curves, which represent the inherent accuracy of each test. An example of the comparison of the performance of different tests for the diagnosis of pheochromocytoma is given in Figure 3–5. It is important to remember, however,

		Cushing syndrome	
		Present	Absent
1-mg overnight dexamethasone suppression	No suppression	151	5
	Suppression	3	461

Sensitivity = 151/(151 + 3) = 98.1%

Specificity = 461/(5 + 461) = 98.9%

A

		Cushing syndrome	
		Present	Absent
1-mg overnight dexamethasone suppression	No suppression	151	101
	Suppression	3	858

Specificity = 858/(101 + 858) = 89.5%

B

		Cushing syndrome	
		Present	Absent
1-mg overnight dexamethasone suppression	No suppression	151	96
	Suppression	3	397

Specificity = 397/(96 + 397) = 80.5%

C

FIGURE 3–3 Diagnosis of Cushing syndrome with the 1-mg overnight dexamethasone suppression test: test characteristics with normal controls (**Panel A**); all controls (**Panel B**); and "obese" and "other" controls (**Panel C**). These data show how the specificity of the test is affected by the types of control subjects. (Reproduced with permission from Crapo L. Cushing's syndrome: a review of diagnostic tests. *Metabolism.* 1979;28:955.)

that ROC curves are only as good as the operating characteristics from which they are generated.

Finally, determining cost-effective diagnostic strategies requires careful evaluation not only of a test in isolation, but also in the context of the other information available and the likelihood of disease. This is the essence of Bayesian models of decision-making. In this model, the physician updates his or her belief in a hypothesis with each new item of information, with different weights given to the new information depending on its operating characteristics. Consideration must be given to the question of the value added by a test or procedure. This can be assessed with ROC curves and statistical models.

Predictive Values, Likelihood Ratios, and Diagnostic Accuracy

Sensitivity and specificity are important test characteristics, yet the clinician wants to know how to interpret a test result. Predictive values help in this regard. As shown in Figure 3–6, the **positive predictive value** is the proportion of patients with a positive test who actually have the disease. Similarly, the **negative predictive value** is the proportion of those with a negative test who do not have the disease. Because each of these values are calculated using results from both individuals with and without the disease in question, the prevalence of the disease has a great impact on the values. For any given sensitivity and specificity, the lower the prevalence of disease (or the lower the pretest probability), the more false-positive results there are (Figure 3–6).

The **likelihood ratio**, which is derived from sensitivity and specificity, is an expression of the odds that a sign, symptom, or test result is expected in a patient with a given disease as opposed to one without the disease. Two forms of the likelihood ratio exist, the likelihood ratio for a positive finding and the likelihood ratio for a negative finding. Calculations are shown in Figure 3–2. Likelihood ratios offer some advantages over sensitivity and specificity. They are the most useful in calculating posttest probabilities given prevalence (a probability) and likelihood ratios. A convenient nomogram for this has been published (Figure 3–7).

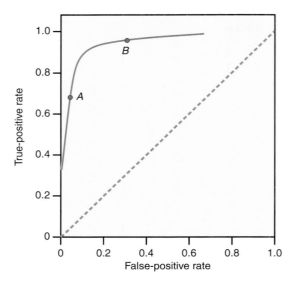

FIGURE 3–4 Receiver-operating characteristic (ROC) curve. In an ROC curve, the true-positive rate (sensitivity) is plotted on the vertical axis, and the false-positive rate (1 – specificity) is plotted on the horizontal axis for different cutoff points for the test. The dotted diagonal line corresponds to a test that is positive or negative just by chance (ie, the true-positive rate equals the false-positive rate). The closer an ROC curve is to the upper left-hand corner of the graph, the more accurate it is, because the true-positive rate is 1 and the false-positive rate is 0. As the criterion for a positive test becomes more stringent, the point on the curve corresponding to sensitivity and specificity (**point A**) moves down and to the left (lower sensitivity, higher specificity); if less evidence is required for a positive test, the point on the curve corresponding to sensitivity and specificity (**point B**) moves up and to the right (higher sensitivity, lower specificity). Analysis of the area between the actual results and the straight line indicates how good the test is. The greater the area under the curve, the better the test.

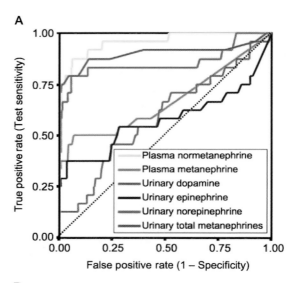

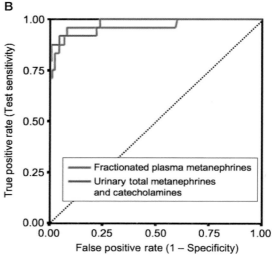

FIGURE 3–5 Receiver-operating characteristic (ROC) curves for diagnostic tests for pheochromocytoma. Receiver-operating characteristic (ROC) curve. In an ROC curve, the true-positive rate (sensitivity) is plotted on the vertical axis, and the false-positive rate (1 - specificity) is plotted on the horizontal axis for different cutoff points for the test. A diagonal line drawn for the points where true positive rate = false positive rate corresponds to a test that is positive or negative just by chance. The closer an ROC curve is to the upper left-hand corner of the graph, the more accurate it is, because the true-positive rate is 1 and the false positive rate is 0. As the criterion for a positive test becomes more stringent, the point on the curve corresponding to sensitivity and specificity moves down and to the left (lower sensitivity, higher specificity); if less evidence is required for a positive test, the point on the curve corresponding to sensitivity and specificity moves up and to the right (higher sensitivity, lower specificity). Analysis of the area between the actual results and the line representing chance alone indicates how good the test is. The greater the area under the curve, the better the test. The area under the curve from plasma-free metanephrines exceeds that of other tests indicating that it is more accurate overall.

AN APPROACH TO DIAGNOSIS IN PRACTICE

In approaching a case, the clinician makes a series of inferences about the nature of a patient's condition and proceeds toward a working diagnosis along with some alternatives—generation of a differential diagnosis. Although one could create a listing of all possible causes of the patient's complaint (ie, a possibilistic differential diagnosis), experienced clinicians generate a differential diagnosis that is a combination of probabilistic (ie, considering first those disorders that are more likely), prognostic (ie, considering first those disorders that are more serious if missed), and pragmatic (ie, considering first those disorders that are most responsive to treatment). The clinician then refines the diagnostic hypotheses, sometimes using clues from the history and physical examination and often with the use of laboratory or radiologic tests. In so doing, the clinician tries to reduce the inherent uncertainty so that the most appropriate course of treatment can be prescribed.

Disease prevalence or pretest probability	0.1%	1%	10%	50%	90%
Positive predictive value	0.89%	8.33%	50.0%	90.0%	98.78%
Negative predictive value	99.99%	99.89%	98.78%	90%	50.0%

FIGURE 3-6 Positive and negative predictive values as a function of disease prevalence, assuming test sensitivity and specificity of 90% for each.

The first step in this process is to understand the concept of probability. A probability is an expression of likelihood and thus represents an opinion of the relative frequency with which an event is likely to occur. In the case of diagnosis, probability is a numerical expression of the clinician's uncertainty about a diagnosis; expressing a clinical opinion in subjective terms such as *likely* and *possible* is fraught with imprecision and misunderstanding. Certainty that a disease is present is assigned a probability of one, certainty that a disease is not present is assigned a probability of zero, and a clinician's opinion of the disease being present or absent usually falls somewhere in between. Of course, probabilities are derived from different data sources that vary in their reliability and application to a given patient, such as the clinician's experience (remembered cases), research studies, and population-based epidemiologic studies. Therefore, some degree of uncertainty is inherent in a given probability, and the confidence with which one can rely on a given probability depends to a large extent on the data underlying it.

The diagnostic approach to minimizing uncertainty requires four steps. First, the clinician starts with an estimate of probability based on initial clinical impressions. This starting point is dubbed the *pretest* or a priori probability and is a number between zero and one that expresses the likelihood of disease. For example, a clinician who sees a large population of patients with diabetes mellitus may think that a 55-year-old patient with polyuria, polydipsia, weight loss, and fatigue has a probability of 0.70 of having diabetes mellitus (ie, if there were 100 such individuals, 70 would have diabetes).

Second, the clinician determines the threshold probability for treatment. The treatment threshold probability is defined as the probability of disease at which one is indifferent between giving treatment and withholding treatment. Establishing a treatment threshold probability takes into account the costs (not just in the monetary sense) and benefits of treating or not treating. Because probability is predicated on the lack of certainty about the presence or absence of disease, it is inevitable that some patients who are not diseased receive treatment and others who are diseased do not receive treatment. Third, if the pretest probability is greater than the threshold probability, the clinician chooses to treat; if it is less than the threshold probability, the clinician opts not to treat. If the clinician is not comfortable enough about the presence or absence of disease, he or she may choose to order further tests with the objective of getting closer to certainty. The fourth step involves taking information gained from the test and using it to update the pretest probability. The updated, or *posttest*, probability can also serve as a new *pretest* probability for the next step in hypothesis testing (Figure 3-8).

Treatment threshold probability depends on the effectiveness of treatment, including its adverse effects. In general, treatment threshold probability is generally low when treatment has a high benefit for diseased patients and/or a low risk of harm for nondiseased patients. Likewise, the treatment threshold probability is generally high when there is a high risk to nondiseased patients and/or a low benefit to diseased patients. For example, an endocrinologist evaluating an incidentally found pituitary microadenoma would need to be as certain as possible that the patient suffered from hormone hypersecretion before recommending surgical resection because of the high risk of harm to nondiseased patients relative to the benefit to diseased patients. The same principles apply to diagnostic testing. There is a test-threshold defined as the probability of disease at which one is indifferent between performing a test and not performing a test. Depending on the circumstances, one would treat without performing the test or not perform the test and ignore the issue entirely.

Tests can be combined in the hope that diagnostic accuracy is enhanced. Two tests can be performed in parallel (simultaneously) or in series (sequentially). When two tests are performed in parallel, a positive result in either test establishes the diagnosis; when

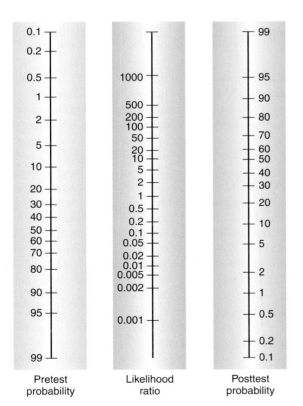

FIGURE 3-7 Nomogram for likelihood ratios. (Adapted from Fagan TJ. Letter: nomogram for Bayes theorem. *N Engl J Med.* 1975;293;257. Reprinted, with permission, of *The New England Journal of Medicine.* Copyright 1975, Massachusetts Medical Society.)

Positive test result

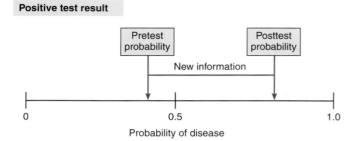

Negative test result

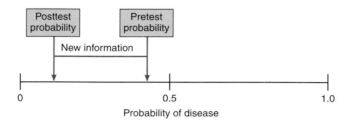

Determining to treat or not to treat based on probability

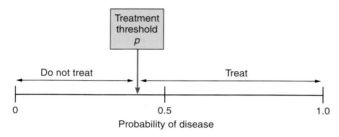

FIGURE 3–8 Adjusting probabilities with new information and treatment thresholds. The top panel shows a pretest probability of disease of approximately 0.4. With the new information provided by a test, the probability rose to approximately 0.7. The middle panel shows the same pretest probability, but a negative test result reduced the probability of disease to approximately 0.15. The treatment threshold probability is the probability above which one would treat. The actual threshold value depends on the morbidity and mortality of disease and the adverse effects (morbidity and mortality) of treatment.

two tests are performed in series, positive results in both tests are required to make the diagnosis. Thus, parallel testing increases sensitivity at the cost of specificity, whereas series testing increases specificity at the cost of sensitivity. For this approach to be better than one test alone, the second test has to provide information not provided by the first test. A common practice is to repeat the same test. This approach may be quite logical when the disorder is intermittently active (eg, intermittent Cushing syndrome) or when there is concern about the way the first test was performed. When tests are performed in series, the first test is usually the one with the higher sensitivity so that as many patients with the

disease are discovered. False-positive results are then identified by a second test with higher specificity. Another approach to sequential testing uses as the first test the one with highest specificity so that fewer patients without the disease go on to further testing. This approach makes sense when the second test is associated with more morbidity. Adjusting cut-points for the first test can make it 100% specific (at the cost of some sensitivity). This approach has been used frequently in tests related to Cushing syndrome. One caveat applies to the method of choosing the cutoff point. In addition to considering whether the patients without the disease are an appropriate control group, attention should be paid to sample size. Caution must be exercised when applying test characteristics derived from small samples.

CLINICAL EPIDEMIOLOGIC PRINCIPLES APPLIED TO TREATMENT DECISIONS

Critical to decision-making is the appropriate interpretation of the results of clinical trials and the impact of treatments on clinical events. The use of a 2 × 2 table can facilitate this process (Figure 3–9).

The **event rate (ER)** is the rate of occurrence of the outcome of interest. The **relative risk reduction (RRR)** is the proportional reduction in rates of bad outcomes between experimental and control participants in a trial, and it can be calculated as:

$$\text{RRR} \quad \frac{1 - \text{Relative risk of experimental treatment}}{\text{Relative risk of control treatment}}$$

RRR is usually reported accompanied by a 95% CI. **Absolute risk reduction (ARR)** is the absolute arithmetic difference in rates of poor outcomes between experimental and control participants in a trial and is usually accompanied by a 95% CI. Another way to think about this is to ask how many patients would have to be treated in order to prevent one negative outcome or achieve one additional favorable outcome. This is termed **number needed to treat (NNT)**, and it is calculated as 1/ARR and accompanied by a 95% CI. An example is provided (see Figure 3–9) from the results of a clinical trial. In the United Kingdom Prospective Diabetes Study (UKPDS-38), hypertensive patients with type 2 diabetes were randomized to tight versus less tight blood pressure control. The patients with tight blood pressure control had fewer diabetes-related complications and fewer deaths due to diabetes compared to the patients with less tight blood pressure control. Over a period of 8 years of treatment, 15.9% of patients in the less tight control group had died of diabetes complications compared with 10.9% in the tight control group.

To apply these statistics in clinical decision-making to patients, it is necessary to calculate ARR, RRR, and NNT. The RRR of 32% indicates that approximately one-third of the expected deaths were prevented by tight control of blood pressure. However, although the RRR may be similar across different risk groups, the ARRs are not. ARRs become smaller when event rates are low, whereas RRR remains constant. Thus, RRR can be misleading.

		Outcome	
		Negative outcome	Positive outcome
Treatment group	Experimental	a	b
	Control	c	d

Relative risks

RRa—risk rate of the negative outcome occurring in the experimental group = a/(a + b)

RRb—risk rate of the negative outcome occurring in the control group = c/(c + d)

RR—the relative risk of the negative outcome occurring in experimental treatment compared tc control treatment = RRa/RRb = {a/(a + b)}/{c/(c + d)}

Relative risk reduction (RRR) = (1 − RR) X 100%

Absolute risk reduction (ARR) = RRb − RRa

Number needed to treat (NNT) = 1/ARR

EXAMPLE:

Figure 2 X 2 Table for UKPDS Trial of Tight Control of Blood Pressure in Patients with Diabetes

		Outcome—Deaths from diabetes	
		Negative outcome —Death	Positive outcome —Alive
Treatment group	Experimental (n = 758)	82	676
	Control (n = 390)	62	328

RRa—10.8%

RRb—15.9%

RR—0.68

RRR—32%

ARR—5.1%

NNT—20

FIGURE 3–9 A 2 × 2 table for treatment groups and outcomes.

The lower the ER in the control group, the larger the difference between RRR and ARR. In other words, the benefits of treatment as reflected in ARR are usually greater in patients at higher risk of negative outcomes than in patients at lower risk of negative outcomes.

The RRR fails to discriminate absolute treatment effects that are clinically significant from those that are trivial. The NNT is 20, so that one would need to treat 20 patients for 8 years with tight blood pressure control to prevent one death from diabetes. NNT can be readily used to compare different treatments. In this case, RRR was 32% and ARR was 5.1%. If a different treatment with the same RRR of 32% has an ARR of 0.51%, the NNT would be 196, indicating that a much greater effort would be needed to achieve one additional favorable outcome. This might or might not be worth the effort, depending on a variety of factors. One method by which treatment thresholds can be determined is with the method of decision analysis.

DECISION ANALYSIS

Decision analysis is a mathematical tool designed to facilitate complex clinical decisions in which many variables must be considered simultaneously. This analytical procedure selects among available diagnostic or therapeutic options based on the probability and predetermined value (utility) of all possible outcomes of those options. Decision analysis provides a systematic framework for organizing all data relevant to the decision so that relevant uncertainties are less likely to be overlooked. Performing a decision analysis requires clear definition of the relationship between possible courses of action and their associated outcomes and assignment of numerical values to various courses of action. In so doing, decision analysis simplifies comparisons among different strategies.

There is substantial variation in duration and severity of disease between individuals. Choosing a treatment option in the setting of unpredictable effects is a difficult problem, and expected value decision-making is a useful tool. When individual outcomes are uncertain, expected value is the result that is expected *on average*. In preparing to perform a decision analysis, one first must define the problem with a clear statement of the strategies to be examined. Two or more strategies may be included. Clinical decisions have effects over different time frames. An important step in defining a decision problem is to decide the time horizon for outcomes to be evaluated. For example, if strategies for diabetes treatment are to be compared, a period of weeks to months may be appropriate for evaluating the risk of hypoglycemic episode. However, this relatively short time horizon would not be appropriate when the study outcome is diabetic retinopathy, where a time horizon of years would be a better choice. After choosing the problem and a single time horizon, carrying out a formal analysis typically involves six general steps:

1. Construction of a decision tree that maps out all the possibilities
2. Determination and assignment of probabilities
3. Assignment of utilities to each potential outcome
4. Determination of the expected utility
5. Choosing the course of action with the highest expected utility
6. Evaluation of the sensitivity of the chosen course of action to changes in probabilities and utilities

In a decision tree, the term decision alternative refers to one of the potential strategies to be analyzed (Figure 3–10). Each alternative should be listed. Figure 3–11 shows a sample decision tree that outlines strategies of medical versus surgical treatment for disease. The decision itself is represented by a box called a decision node. All of the possible outcomes for each decision alternative are listed. An event that has outcomes under the control of chance is denoted by a chance node. The symbol for a chance node is a circle. The series of events leading to the clinical outcomes is represented by a series of chance nodes and decision nodes. The decision tree is usually written from left to right, with the initial decision node on the far left and the final outcomes on the far right. A final outcome is represented by a terminal node. There may be any number of outcomes at a chance node. The listed outcomes should include all possible outcomes, and they must not overlap. In addition to this assumption of mutual exclusivity, structuring a tree in this fashion assumes that the probability of occurrence of one event does not influence the probability of occurrence of another event(s). The decision tree structure should be as similar as possible for all strategies, because differences may lead to a structural bias in the analysis.

The decision tree described above is relatively simple, and this approach cannot readily represent complex, dynamic clinical situations with recurring events. More elaborate models, such as Markov models, can be used to represent the passage through multiple health states. Patients may transition from one health state to another with some probability within a specified time period or model cycle. Like each terminal node in a static decision tree, each health state in the Markov model is associated with a specific clinical measure, utility, or cost. A key assumption of the Markov model is that the future is determined only by the individual's present health state; events prior to that health state or how long it took to arrive there do not affect the individual's future, a simplifying assumption that may not hold true for some health problems.

One strength of the decision analysis process is that it may be used for a variety of outcome measures. The outcome measure of interest determines the information needed for analysis. For example, one may use clinical measures such as survival following total thyroidectomy for differentiated thyroid cancer, preservation of vision after laser photocoagulation, or meeting a target level for glycosylated hemoglobin. Economic measures provide measures of

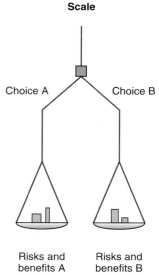
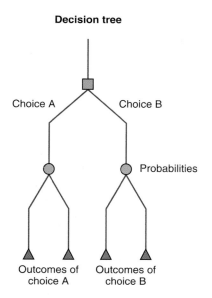

FIGURE 3–10 Balancing outcomes and a decision tree.

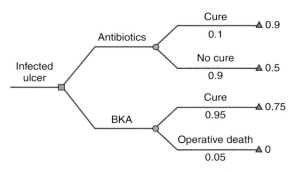

FIGURE 3–11 A decision tree with probabilities and utilities. This sample decision tree outlines strategies of medical versus surgical treatment—below-knee amputation (BKA) for a particular disease. The decision node (open square) represents the decision itself. All of the possible outcomes for each decision alternative are listed emanating from an open circle or chance node. The events are governed by chance. The series of events leading to the clinical outcomes is represented by a series of chance nodes and decision nodes. Terminal nodes (triangles) denote the outcomes. Probabilities and utilities are listed. For example, if one chooses antibiotics, there is a 10% chance of cure, whereas if one chooses surgery, there is a 95% chance of cure. However, although surgery has a higher cure rate, one is left with an amputation. Having a BKA has lower utility (eg, 0.75) compared with antibiotic treatment (eg, 0.9). The predicted outcome is $(0.1 \times 0.9) + (0.9 \times 0.5)$ or 0.54 for antibiotics vs $(0.95 \times 0.74) + (0.05 \times 0)$ or 0.71 for surgery. This indicates that on the *average*, surgery is a better choice.

cost and resource use. When cost measures are included, it is important to consider whose perspective is represented; analyses may reflect the viewpoint of society as a whole, payers, or patients.

A detailed analysis of costs may be used for cost-effectiveness analysis or cost–utility analysis. Utility measures reflect outcome preferences. For an individual, utilities represent quality of life preferences. They are quantitative values used to summarize multiple dimensions, which may be conflicting. For example, decision-makers frequently must choose among strategies that have differing effects on length of life and quality of life and involving trade-offs between the two. Utilities are traditionally scored on a scale from 0 to 1. The ideal situation, often perfect health, is scored as a 1. The worst situation, death, is scored as a 0, and this assumes that there are no utilities worse than death. Intermediate states are assigned values between 0 and 1. For example, living with diabetes mellitus may receive a score of 0.80—less than perfect, but preferable to death. Among the assumptions underlying this approach are: stability of estimates of utilities, that is, the estimates obtained prior to experiencing an event will not change after the event has been experienced; and the it-does-not-matter-how-you-get-there assumption (ie, death or other outcomes have the same utility regardless of the route a patient takes in getting there).

There are different ways to obtain utility values for different health states. One relatively simple method is the visual analog scale, in which a subject is asked to rate a given health state on a scale from 0 to 100. There also are more specific ways of determining utility. The standard gamble approach was developed by von

Neumann and Morgenstern as a method for assessing utility. One advantage of this method is that it incorporates the participant's attitudes about risk taking, because the process involves consideration of a hypothetical gamble. For example, consider a 74-year-old diabetic man with known coronary artery disease and a chronically infected lower extremity ulcer. His physicians suggest a below-the-knee amputation (BKA), but they also discuss the option of a course of antibiotics instead of surgery. Assume that antibiotics have a 10% cure rate and that an amputation has a 95% cure rate. To assess utility from the patient's perspective, it is necessary to list all of the possible outcomes; rank the outcome states in the order of preference; assign a utility of 1 to the most preferred outcome and 0 to the least preferred outcome; and formulate situations where a patient is indifferent about choosing between a gamble (between outcomes of known utility) and a sure thing (involving an outcome with unknown utility). This is how the utility of each intermediate outcome is determined. For example, suppose the patient decides that a cure with antibiotics is an appealing outcome. This outcome is compared to those with known utilities—perfect health and death. When asked to choose between a cure with antibiotics and a gamble in which he has a 90% chance of achieving perfect health and a 10% chance of dying, he is unable to choose (indifferent). Thus, the utility for the outcome of cure with antibiotics is 0.9. However, a surgical cure with an amputation is a less appealing scenario. The utility for an amputation is only 0.75. By a similar process, the utility of a failure of antibiotics necessitating an amputation is 0.5. The utility scores can then be incorporated into a decision tree (see Figure 3–11). The expected utility for each decision alternative may be obtained by adding each (utility × probability) value. The utility for each outcome is on the right. The probabilities are below the outcome branches. The utility for antibiotic treatment = $(0.1 \times 0.9) + (0.9 \times 0.5) = 0.54$, whereas the utility for BKA = $(0.95 \times 0.75) + (0.05 \times 0) = 0.71$. In terms of the patient's quality of life, the expected value of amputation is greater than the expected value of antibiotic treatment. Different utilities for these health states would alter the analyses.

The time trade-off method is another way of determining utility. The utility may be described as a number between 0 and 1. For example, a subject may consider 10 years with pain from diabetic neuropathy equivalent to 5 years in perfect health. The utility of diabetic neuropathy would be 0.5. Alternatively, the utility may be expressed in quality-adjusted life years (QALYs). To determine the number of QALYs associated with an outcome, the time horizon for the outcome state is specified. Often, this is a patient's life expectancy in a particular outcome state. The number of years in full health that the subject sees as equivalent to the specified time with that outcome is the corresponding number of QALYs.

Determine the Probability of Each Chance Event

Once the decision tree structure is formed, the probability of each chance event may be determined. In general, this is best performed by taking a systematic review of published, peer-reviewed literature. However, this approach assumes that probabilities derived from a period in the past accurately reflect the probabilities in the future. Moreover, it assumes that the probabilities derived from other settings apply to the one in question. However, all these probabilities must reflect actual practice. For example, if decision analysis is being used to determine the best strategy for specific individual patients, the probabilities must be those of the site when the care is to be delivered. At times, not all of the information needed for the decision tree is available. This frequently occurs during analysis of a relatively new practice. If possible, primary data may be collected or secondary data may be analyzed. Expert opinion may be used in the absence of relevant data. At a given chance node, the sum of probabilities equals one.

Deciding on a Strategy: Averaging Out and Folding Back the Tree

The goal of decision analysis is to identify the strategy that leads to the most favorable expected outcome. To calculate the expected outcome, one starts at the outcome measures (typically the far right). Each group of branches, which start at a single chance node, is reduced to a single numerical value by multiplying each outcome measure by the probability associated with that outcome and adding all of the values. This is the process of folding back the decision tree. This process is repeated until there is a single numerical value for each strategy at the initial decision node. At this point, the expected outcome for each strategy has been calculated. The strategy with the more favorable outcome is the preferred strategy.

Discounting Future Events

A greater value is placed on current events than future events. It is better to pay $100 in 10 years rather than pay $100 now. Similarly, if one is to have a disease, it is preferable to have a disease in the future than to have it today. The value of a future event then depends on how far in the future it occurs. Discounting refers to calculating the present value of an outcome that occurs in the future. The discount rate is the annual rate at which costs are discounted, which is usually the rate of interest that money would bring if it were invested.

Sensitivity Analysis

Sensitivity analysis is an important part of the decision analysis process that tests the stability or robustness of a conclusion over a range of structural assumptions, value judgments, and estimates of probability. The initial analysis, or base case analysis, uses the best estimates for each part of the model. In sensitivity analysis, a plausible range of values is determined for each portion of the model. Variables that have the most influence on the model are determined. Different time horizons or perspectives may be considered. The objective is to see whether conclusions change when possibilities within a reasonable range are included.

Cost-Effectiveness Analysis Using Decision Analysis

Cost-effectiveness analysis is the use of decision analysis to compare strategies in terms of their cost per unit of output. Output is an outcome such as years of life, utility, or cases of disease prevented.

Cost-effectiveness ratios are interpreted by comparing them to ratios for other strategies. An incremental cost-effectiveness ratio indicates how much additional money needs to be spent for a better, but more expensive strategy to generate one additional unit of outcome.

Of practical importance, there usually is a limit to the amount of money a policy-maker is willing to spend to gain one QALY; this is termed the willingness-to-pay threshold. Cost–utility analysis is a specific type of cost-effectiveness analysis that uses QALYs (or other measures of utility) as the effectiveness end-point. By convention, cost–utility analyses are often called cost-effectiveness analyses. However, not all cost-effectiveness studies use the cost–utility methodology. Because they use QALYs as an end-point, cost–utility analyses generate information that may be compared across disease states. It is important to note that although they are useful in providing a common metric among outcomes, a number of stringent assumptions must be made to compare cost-effectiveness analyses. Principles for assessing decision analysis have been developed by the evidence-based medicine (EBM) group and are shown in Table 3–2. Representative decision analyses related to endocrine disorders are shown in Table 3–3.

OTHER ASPECTS OF CLINICAL EPIDEMIOLOGY

The methods of clinical epidemiology have been applied to risk, prognosis, the assessment of studies of different designs, and many other issues in clinical medicine. Readers are referred to standard texts.

EVIDENCE-BASED ENDOCRINOLOGY

The definition of evidence-based medicine (EBM) has evolved over time. A 2005 definition states that EBM requires the integration

TABLE 3–2 Users' guide to decision analyses.

I. Are the results of the study valid?
    Were all important strategies and outcomes included?
    Was an explicit and sensible process used to identify, select, and combine the evidence into probabilities?
    Were the utilities obtained in an explicit and sensible way from credible sources?
    Was the potential impact of any uncertainty in the evidence determined?

II. What are the results?
    In the baseline analysis, does one strategy result in a clinically important gain for patients? If not, is the result a "toss-up"?
    How strong is the evidence used in the analysis?
    Could the uncertainty in the evidence change the result?

III. Will the results help me in caring for my patients?
    Do the probability estimates fit my patients' clinical features?
    Do the utilities reflect how my patients would value the outcomes of the decision?

Richardson WS, Detsky AS for the Evidence-Based Medicine Working Group; based on the *Users' Guides to Evidence-Based Medicine* and reproduced with permission from *JAMA.* 1995 Apr 26;273:1292-1295 and 1995 May 24;273:1610-1613. Copyright 1995, American Medical Association.

TABLE 3–3 Representative decision analyses in endocrinology.

Study	Clinical Problem and Strategies	Time Horizon	Outcome Measures	Results
Diabetes				
DCCT	Conventional vs intensive insulin therapy in approximately 120,000 persons with IDDM in the United States who meet DCCT inclusion criteria	Lifetime	Years free from diabetic complica-tions Cost per life-year	Intensive insulin therapy results in a gain of 920,000 y of sight, 691,000 y free from ESRD, 678,000 y free from lower extremity amputation, and 611,000 y of life at a cost of $4 billion. Cost per life-year gained is $28,661.
CDC	Screening for type 2 DM with routine medical contact at age 25 vs age 45	Lifetime	Cost per life-year Cost per QALY	IC-ER for early screening was $236,449 per life-year gained and $56,649 per QALY gained. Early screening is more cost-effective in younger persons and African Americans.
Vijan	Prevention of blindness and ESRD in patients with type 2 DM with lowering hemoglobin A1c by 2 % points to a lower limit of 7	Lifetime	Risk of developing blindness and ESRD	Patients with early onset of type 2 diabetes benefit from near-normal glycemic control. Moderate control prevents most of the studied complications in patients with later onset of disease
Hoerger	Screening for type 2 DM in all people vs only screening those with hypertension	Lifetime	Cost per QALY	Screening in people with hypertension is more cost-effective. Targeted screening for people age 55-75 is most cost-effective.
Gillies	Different strategies for screening and prevention of type 2 DM in adults	Lifetime	Cost per QALY	Screening for type 2 DM and impaired glucose tolerance, with appropriate intervention for those with impaired glucose tolerance, in an above average risk population aged 45 seems to be cost-effective.
Golan	To preserve kidney function in patients with DM type 2, strategies of treating all patients with ACE inhibitors vs screening for microalbuminuria vs screening for gross proteinuria	Lifetime	Cost per QALY	Screening for gross proteinuria has the highest cost and lowest benefit. Compared with microalbuminuria, treating all patients with an ACE-inhibitor was beneficial with an IC-ER of $7500 per QALY gained.
Gaede	Intensified vs conventional multifactorial intervention in type 2 DM	Lifetime	Cost per QALY	From a health-care perspective in Denmark, intensive therapy was more cost-effective than conventional treatment. Assuming that persons in both arms were treated in a primary care setting, intensive therapy was both cost- and life-saving.
Thyroid				
Danese	In asymptomatic adults, screening for mild thyroid failure every 5 y starting at age 35 vs no screening	Lifetime	Cost per QALY	Screening was cost-effective with a cost per QALY gained of $9223 for women and $22,595 for men.
Vidal-Trécan	Four strategies to treat solitary toxic thyroid adenoma in a 40-y-old woman: (A) Primary radioactive iodine (B) Primary surgery after euthyroidism achieved by ATDs (C) ATDs followed by surgery or (D) ATDs followed by radioactive iodine. C and D were used if severe reaction to ATDs occurred	Lifetime	Cost per QALY	Surgery was the most effective and least costly strategy. Primary radioactive iodine was more effective if surgical mortality exceeded 0.6%.
Nasuti	Evaluation of FNA by a cytopathologist with on-site processing vs standard processing at the University of Pennsylvania Medical Center	Short term	Cost	By avoiding nondiagnostic specimens, an estimated cost savings of $404,525 per year may be achieved with on-site FNA review.
McCartney	Analysis of different thyroid nodule biopsy guideline criteria	Short term	Utility (expected value)	As a general approach to 10-14 mm thyroid nodules, routine FNA appears to be the least desirable compared with observation alone or FNA of nodules with ultrasonographic risk factors.
Cheung	Calcitonin measurement in the evaluation of thyroid nodules in the United States	Lifetime	Cost per life years saved	Routine serum calcitonin screening in patients undergoing evaluation for thyroid nodules appears to be comparable in cost-effectiveness to other screening procedures, eg, mammography, colonoscopy, TSH.

(Continued)

TABLE 3–3 Representative decision analyses in endocrinology. (*Continued*)

Study	Clinical Problem and Strategies	Time Horizon	Outcome Measures	Results
Other				
King	Four strategies to manage incidental pituitary microadenoma in an asymptomatic patient: (1) Expectant management (2) PRL screening (3) Screening for PRL, insulin-like growth factor I, and (4) MRI follow-up	Lifetime	Cost per QALY	PRL test may be the most cost-effective strategy. Compared to expectant management, the IC-ER for PRL was $1428. The IC-ER for the extended screening panel was $69,495. MRI follow-up was less effective and more expensive.
Sawka	Three strategies to evaluate pheochromocytoma in patients with refractory hypertension, suspicious symptoms, adrenal mass, or history of pheochromocytoma: (A) Fractionated plasma metanephrines with imaging if abnormal (B) 24-h urinary metanephrines or catecholamines with imaging if abnormal (C) Plasma metanephrines if modestly elevated, urine studies to decide on imaging	Short term	Cost per pheochromocytoma detected	Strategy C is least costly and has reasonable sensitivity in patients with moderate pretest probability for pheochromocytoma.
Col	For menopausal symptom relief in healthy, white, 50-y-old women with intact uteri, use of hormone therapy vs no hormone therapy	2 y	Survival QALE	Hormone therapy is associated with lower survival but gains in QALE. Benefits depend on severity of menopausal symptoms and CVD risk.
Smith	For 60-y-old men with erectile dysfunction, sildenafil vs no drug therapy	Lifetime	Cost per QALY gained	From the societal perspective, cost per QALY gained with sildenafil is less than $50,000 if treatment-related morbidity is less than 0.55% per year, treatment success rate is greater than 40.2%, or cost of sildenafil is less than $244 per month.

DCCT, Diabetes Control and Complications Trial; IDDM, insulin-dependent diabetes mellitus; ESRD, end-stage renal disease; DM, diabetes mellitus; QALY, quality-adjusted life year; IC-ER, incremental cost-effectiveness ratio; ACE, angiotensin-converting enzyme; CVD, cardiovascular disease; ATDs, antithyroid drugs; FNA, fine-needle aspiration; PRL, prolactin; MRI, magnetic resonance imaging; QALE, quality-adjusted life expectancy.

- DCCT. Lifetime benefits and costs of intensive therapy as practiced in the diabetes control and complications trial The Diabetes Control and Complications Trial Research Group. *JAMA*. 1996;276(17):1409-1415.
- The CDC Diabetes Cost-Effectiveness Study Group. The cost-effectiveness of screening for type 2 diabetes. *JAMA*. 1998;280(20):1757-1763.
- Vijan S, Hofer TP, Hayward RA. Estimated benefits of glycemic control in microvascular complications in type 2 diabetes. *Ann Intern Med*. 1997;127(9):788-795.
- Hoerger TJ, Harris R, Hicks KA, Donahue K, Sorensen S, Engelgau M. Screening for type 2 diabetes mellitus: a cost-effectiveness analysis. *Ann Intern Med*. 2004;140(9):689-699.
- Gillies CL, Lambert PC, Abrams KR, et al. Different strategies for screening and prevention of type 2 diabetes in adults: cost effectiveness analysis. *BMJ*. 2008;336:1180-1185.
- Golan L, Birkmeyer JD, Welch HG. The cost-effectiveness of treating all patients with type 2 diabetes with angiotensin-converting enzyme inhibitors. *Ann Intern Med*. 1999;131(9):660-667.
- Gaede P, Valentine WJ, Palmer AJ, et al. Cost-effectiveness of intensified versus conventional multifactorial intervention in type 2 diabetes. *Diabetes Care*. 2008;31(8):1510-1515.
- Danese MD, Powe NR, Sawin CT, Ladenson PW. Screening for mild thyroid failure at the periodic health examination: a decision and cost-effectiveness analysis. *JAMA*. 1996;276(4):285-292.
- Vidal-Trecan GM, Stahl JE, Durand-Zaleski I. Managing toxic thyroid adenoma: a cost-effectiveness analysis. *Eur J Endocrinol*. 2002;146(3):283-294.
- Nasuti JF, Gupta PK, Baloch ZW. Diagnostic value and cost-effectiveness of on-site evaluation of fine-needle aspiration specimens: review of 5,688 cases. *Diagn Cytopathol*. 2002;27(1):1-4.
- McCartney CR, Stukenborg GJ. Decision analysis of discordant thyroid nodule biopsy guideline criteria. *J Clin Endocrinol Metab*. 2008;93(8):3037-3044.
- Cheung K, Roman SA, Wang TS, Walker HD, Sosa JA. Calcitonin measurement in the evaluation of thyroid nodules in the United States: a cost-effectiveness and decision analysis. *J Clin Endocrinol Metab*. 2008;93(6):2173-2180.
- King JT, Jr, Justice AC, Aron DC. Management of incidental pituitary microadenomas: a cost-effectiveness analysis. *J Clin Endocrinol Metab*. 1997;82(11):3625-3632.
- Sawka AM, Gafni A, Thabane L, Young WF, Jr. The economic implications of three biochemical screening algorithms for pheochromocytoma. *J Clin Endocrinol Metab*. 2004;89(6):2859-2866.
- Col NF, Weber G, Stiggelbout A, Chuo J, D'Agostino R, Corso P. Short-term menopausal hormone therapy for symptom relief: an updated decision model. *Arch Intern Med*. 2004;164(15):1634-1640.
- Smith KJ, Roberts MS. The cost-effectiveness of sildenafil. *Ann Intern Med*. 2000;132(12):933-937.

of the best research evidence with clinical expertise and patient's unique values and circumstances. The best research evidence refers to valid and clinically relevant research, often from the basic sciences of medicine, but especially from patient-centered clinical research. Clinical expertise refers to the ability to use physicians' clinical skills and past experience to rapidly identify each patient's unique health state and diagnosis, their individual risks and benefits of potential interventions, and their personal circumstances and expectations. Patient values consist of the unique preferences, concerns, and expectations each patient brings to a clinical encounter that must be integrated into clinical decisions if they are to serve the patient. Patient circumstances refer to the patient's individual clinical state and the clinical setting.

The five steps of EBM as defined in 1997 are discussed below. Entire textbooks are devoted to the principles of EBM. In this chapter, we will briefly review these five steps and focus on how EBM views evidence and review some of the limitations.

Step One: Translation of the Clinical Problem into Answerable Questions

One of the fundamental skills required for practicing EBM is the asking of well-built clinical questions. To benefit patients and clinicians, such questions need to be both directly relevant to patients' problems and phrased in ways that direct a literature search to relevant and precise answers. In practice, well-built clinical questions usually contain four elements: patient, intervention, comparison, and outcome. The patient refers to the individual to whom the evidence will be applied (eg, a hypertensive patient with diabetes). (The evidence-based approach can also be applied to a group to inform policy.) The intervention is the diagnostic test or therapy being considered for application to the particular patient (or group) (eg, tight control of blood pressure). The comparison is that intervention to which a new intervention being considered is to be compared (eg, less tight control of blood pressure). The outcome is the end point of interest to the physician or patient (eg, stroke, myocardial infarction, or death from diabetes). Background questions relate to general information or basic facts about a disease, and this information can usually be found in reliable textbooks, whether published in book form or on-line. However, more involved clinical questions, especially those that require the most up-to-date information about diagnosis, prognosis, or treatment, have been termed foreground questions and require a different approach.

Step Two: Finding the Best Evidence

The finding of best research evidence from the medical literature is a critical feature of the EBM approach and is an iterative process that involves medical informatics. Given the enormous breadth and depth of the medical literature, with more than two million articles published each year in about 20,000 biomedical journals (with more being established each year), efficient strategies must be used to take advantage of the best original journal articles, reviews and synopses of primary studies, and practice guidelines, along with textbooks, both traditional and innovative. Among the useful sources of information are PubMed, which allows sophisticated search strategies of the MEDLINE database. A variety of tools have been developed to facilitate this process. However, these are beyond the scope of this chapter, and readers are referred to references on the subject. Certain journals are specifically devoted to critically appraised articles (eg, ACP Journal Club, BMJ Evidence-Based Medicine). It is important to remember, however, that the presence of the label *evidence based* does not ensure that the information meets the highest standards. Systematic reviews are another useful source for evidence. In addition to the professional journals, such reviews are available from both governmental agencies (eg, Agency for Healthcare Research and Quality) and nongovernmental agencies (eg, the Cochrane Collaboration). Standards have been developed for reporting systematic reviews: preferred reporting items for systematic reviews and meta-analyses (PRISMA). Among the issues addressed specifically is that of publication bias and its potential effects on the results. Publication bias reflects, among other things, the tendency to not publish studies with negative findings.

Step Three: Appraising the Evidence for its Validity and Usefulness

Critical appraisal is the process of systematically examining research evidence to assess its validity, results, and relevance before using it to inform a decision. There are three basic questions to be addressed in evaluating any kind of research: (1) Is it valid? (2) Is it important? and (3) Is it applicable to my patient? This involves assessment of the study's methods in order to assess the internal validity of the conclusions. Once criteria for internal validity are satisfied, then the importance of the finding can be assessed. It is critical that statistical significance not be equated with clinical significance. Assuming the finding is important, it is necessary to consider the study's relevance to the patient (ie, the external validity of the study). A series of guides has been developed to help the clinician to critically appraise different types of studies. An example is shown in Table 3–4. Underlying this appraisal process is the EBM model of the hierarchy of evidence.

TABLE 3–4   Users' guides for an article about therapy.

I. Are the results of the study valid?
Primary Guides
Was the assignment of patients to treatments randomized?
Were all patients who entered the trial properly accounted for and attributed at its conclusion?
Was follow-up complete?
Were patients analyzed in the groups to which they were randomized?
Secondary Guides
Were patients, health workers, and study personnel "blind" to treatment?
Were the groups similar at the start of the trial?
Aside from the experimental intervention, were the groups treated equally?
II. What were the results?
How large was the treatment effect?
How precise was the estimate of the treatment effect?
III. Will the results help me in caring for my patients?
Can the results be applied to my patient care?
Were all clinically important outcomes considered?
Are the likely treatment benefits worth the potential harms and costs?

Guyatt GH, Sackett D, Cook DJ, for the Evidence Based Medicine Working Group. Based on the *Users' Guides to Evidence-Based Medicine* and reproduced with permission from *JAMA.* 1993;270:2598-2601 and 1994;271:59-63. Copyright 1995, American Medical Association.

A. Hierarchies of evidence Any empirical observation about the apparent relation between events constitutes evidence. This includes the thoughtful observations of an experienced clinician, the observations derived from physiologic experiments, and the results of large, randomized clinical trials. Methodological safeguards to protect against systematic error (bias) are inherent in experimental design. In this way, experiments differ from clinical observations. Different study designs lend themselves to different safeguards, and these safeguards vary in their efficacy both in theory and in practice.

The EBM approach uses a hierarchy of study designs based on their inherent safeguards. A hierarchy is shown in Table 3–5. In this hierarchy, randomized controlled trials (RCTs) are given the highest weight, followed by quasi-experimental studies (ie, no-RCTs), followed by other study designs, and finally opinions of authorities and unsystematic clinical observations. Evidence from the top of the hierarchy should have greater impact in clinical decision-making than observations from the lower levels. There is disagreement about what the hierarchy should be. Some have an N of 1 randomized trial (the equivalent of an RCT with one subject) at the top of the hierarchy, whereas others place meta-analyses of randomized trials at the top. However, the term *evidence* is not synonymous with evidence from RCTs (or whatever study design occupies at the preferred level of the hierarchy). Rather, it is preferred to use that sort of evidence when it is available. Evidence from other sources is still evidence and may be more than sufficient. For example, the introduction of thyroid replacement therapy for hypothyroidism or insulin therapy for type 1 diabetes has never been subjected to RCTs.

While recognizing the central role of evaluating the quality of the evidence in decision-making, the U.S. Preventive Services Task Force (USPSTF) has developed a different approach to address some of the shortcomings of the EBM approach. The USPSTF adopted three major changes to the process. First, a rating of internal validity was added to the study criterion for judging individual studies. A well-designed cohort or case-control study could be more compelling than an inadequately powered or poorly conducted RCT. Second, evidence was explicitly assessed at three different levels—the level of the individual study, both in terms of internal and external validity; the body of evidence supporting a given linkage in the analytic framework; and, because of the focus of the USPSTF, the level of evidence for the entire

preventive service. Third, the magnitude of effect was separated from the assessment of quality. Both benefit and harm are considered in assessing the magnitude of the effect(s). Overall, the USPSTF grades the quality of the overall evidence for a service on a three-point scale (good, fair, poor) and grades its recommendations according to one of five classifications (A, B, C, D, I) reflecting the strength of evidence and magnitude of net benefit (benefits minus harms) (Table 3–6). This approach of assessing both the quality of evidence and strength of recommendations has been expanded to include practice guidelines: grading of recommendations, assessment, development, and evaluation (GRADE) system. Although a discussion of practice guidelines is beyond the scope of this chapter, it is important to recognize that they vary widely in quality, strength of evidence, and bias. Before a practitioner bases a decision on a practice guideline, the basis of that guideline must be clear.

B. Other evidence-related issues Notwithstanding these improvements, there are three other major issues concerning the evidence. First, it is important to recognize that all of this evidence is essentially quantitative in nature. Thus, the EBM definition of evidence is relatively narrow and excludes information important to clinicians; many qualitative factors are involved in clinical decision-making concerning individual patients. Second, there are problems in the evidence in terms of the quality and scope of the data (eg, the soft data that clinicians usually use); the scope of the topics (average patients, gray zones of practice, lack of RCTs); sources of authority, which however explicit, require judgment; and potential abuses (eg, key findings could be ignored). Third, there is the issue of applying results in populations (ie, average results) to individuals.

Steps Four and Five: Applying the Results in Practice and Evaluating Performance

Knowledge of the best available evidence of treatment is not enough to recommend a particular course of action. Underlying this issue is heterogeneity of treatment effects. **Treatment effect heterogeneity** is the term given to the phenomenon in which the same treatment produces different results in different patients. For the average effect observed in a clinical trial to occur with certainty in one patient, all patients in the trial must have had that average response. Yet average response may also reflect a large response in some and small or no response or even harm in others. Part of clinical decision-making involves addressing this phenomenon to individualize therapy in the most effective way. To do so, four major factors about the patient must be taken into account: (1) baseline probability of incurring a disease-related adverse event (risk without treatment or susceptibility/prognosis), (2) responsiveness to the treatment, (3) vulnerability to the adverse side-effects of the treatment, and (4) utilities for different outcomes. When lacking good data on a patient's individual level of risk, responsiveness, and vulnerability, the average treatment effect as reported in good clinical trials provides the most reasonable guide for decision-making. However, it is important that physicians evaluate the results in their own patients so that the course can be modified when necessary.

TABLE 3–5   A hierarchy of evidence.

1. Evidence obtained from at least one properly designed randomized controlled trial.
2a. Evidence obtained from well-designed controlled trials without randomization.
2b. Evidence obtained from well-designed cohort or case-control analytical studies, preferably from more than one center or research group.
2c. Evidence from comparisons between times or places with or without the intervention. Dramatic results in uncontrolled experiments could be included in this section.
3. Opinions of respected authorities, based on clinical experience, descriptive studies, or reports on expert committees.

TABLE 3–6 The USPSTF grading system for recommendations reflecting the strength of evidence and magnitude of net benefit (benefits minus harms).

Grade	Definition	Suggestions for Practice
A	The USPSTF recommends the service. There is high certainty that the net benefit is substantial.	Offer or provide this service.
B	The USPSTF recommends the service. There is high certainty that the net benefit is moderate or there is moderate certainty that the net benefit is moderate to substantial.	Offer or provide this service.
C	The USPSTF recommends against routinely providing the service. There may be considerations that support providing the service in an individual patient. There is at least moderate certainty that the net benefit is small.	Offer or provide this service only if other considerations support the offering or providing the service in an individual patient.
D	The USPSTF recommends against the service. There is moderate or high certainty that the service has no net benefit or that the harms outweigh the benefits.	Discourage the use of this service.
I Statement	The USPSTF concludes that the current evidence is insufficient to assess the balance of benefits and harms of the service. Evidence is lacking, of poor quality, or conflicting, and the balance of benefits and harms cannot be determined.	Read the clinical considerations section of USPSTF Recommendation Statement. If the service is offered, patients should understand the uncertainty about the balance of benefits and harms.

Levels of Certainty Regarding Net Benefit

Level of Certainty*	Description
High	The available evidence usually includes consistent results from well-designed, well-conducted studies in representative primary care populations. These studies assess the effects of the preventive service on health outcomes. This conclusion is therefore unlikely to be strongly affected by the results of future studies.
Moderate	The available evidence is sufficient to determine the effects of the preventive service on health outcomes, but confidence in the estimate is constrained by such factors as: • The number, size, or quality of individual studies. • Inconsistency of findings across individual studies. • Limited generalizability of findings to routine primary care practice. • Lack of coherence in the chain of evidence. As more information becomes available, the magnitude or direction of the observed effect could change, and this change may be large enough to alter the conclusion.
Low	The available evidence is insufficient to assess effects on health outcomes. Evidence is insufficient because of: • The limited number or size of studies. • Important flaws in study design or methods. • Inconsistency of findings across individual studies. • Gaps in the chain of evidence. • Findings not generalizable to routine primary care practice. • Lack of information on important health outcomes. More information may allow estimation of effects on health outcomes.

*The USPSTF defines certainty as "likelihood that the USPSTF assessment of the net benefit of a preventive service is correct." The net benefit is defined as benefit minus harm of the preventive service as implemented in a general, primary care population. The USPSTF assigns a certainty level based on the nature of the overall evidence available to assess the net benefit of a preventive service.

U.S. Preventive Services Task Force Ratings. Strength of recommendations and quality of evidence. *Guide to Clinical Preventive Services.* 3rd ed. Periodic Updates, 2000–2003. Rockville, MD: Agency for Healthcare Research and Quality; http://www.uspreventiveservicestaskforce.org/uspstf/grades.htm

Practicing and perfecting the art of medicine demands recognition that uncertainty permeates all clinical decisions. How clinicians make decisions, whether diagnostic or therapeutic, by combining the art and the science is a complicated matter replete with unknowns. There is a variety of modes of clinical problem-solving ranging from automatic decisions in which a clinician makes a decision without consciously considering alternatives or even specific features of the problem to rational decision-making using simplified strategies to take into account probabilities and values of outcomes to formal decision analysis. The potential deficiencies of automatic decisions (nondecisions one might say) are obvious. Formal decision analyses, even if accepted as gold standards (which they are not), are beyond practical use for the vast majority of clinicians, so that we are left with simplified processes to combine likelihoods and values. However, even in striving to reduce uncertainty and coming up with the best course of action for the patient, it is critical to recognize that uncertainty will always be with us. In using a quantitative approach, we can only become more certain about the probability of the outcome. We cannot guarantee the desired outcome.

REFERENCES

General

Greenberg RS, Daniels SR, Flanders WD, et al. *Medical Epidemiology*. New York, NY: McGraw-Hill Medical; 2005.

Grobbee DE, Hoes AW. *Clinical Epidemiology: Principles, Methods, and Applications for Clinical Research*. London: Jones & Bartlett Publishing; 2009.

Guyatt G, Rennie D, Meade M, Cook D. *Users' Guides to the Medical Literature: Essentials of Evidence-Based Clinical Practice*. 2nd ed (*JAMA* & Archives Journals). New York, NY: McGraw-Hill; 2008.

Janicek M. *The Foundations of Evidence-Based Medicine*. New York, NY: Parthenon Publishing Group; 2003.

Jenicek M, Hitchcock DL. *Evidence-Based Practice: Logic and Critical Thinking in Medicine*. Chicago, IL: AMA Press; 2005.

Mayer D. *Essential Evidence-Based Medicine*. New York, NY: Cambridge Medicine; 2009.

Muennig P. *Cost-Effectiveness in Health: A Practical Approach*. New York, NY: John Wiley and Sons; 2009.

Montori VM, ed. *Evidence-Based Endocrinology*. Tolowa: Humana Press Inco; 2006.

Strauss SE, Richardson WS, Glasziou P, Haynes, RB. *Evidence-Based Medicine*. 3rd ed. Churchill Livingstone; 2005.

Diagnostic Testing and Treatment Decisions (Clinical Decision Making and Decision Analysis)

Hunink M, Glasziou P. *Decision Making in Health and Medicine: Integrating Evidence and Values*. New York, NY: Cambridge University Press; 2001.

Montori VM, Wyer P, Newman TB, et al. Evidence-Based Medicine Teaching Tips Working Group: Tips for learners of evidence-based medicine. 5. The effect of spectrum of disease on the performance of diagnostic tests. *CMAJ*. 2005;173:385. [PMID: 16103513]

Schwartz A, Bergus G. *Medical Decision Making: A Physician's Guide*. New York, NY: Cambridge University Press; 2008.

Evidence-Based Medicine: General

Berwick D. Broadening the view of evidence-based medicine. *Qual Saf Health Care*. 2005;14:315. [PMID: 16195561]

Daly J. *Evidence-Based Medicine and the Search for a Science of Clinical Care*. California: University of California Press/Milbank Memorial Fund; 2005.

Greenhalgh T. Integrating qualitative research into evidence based practice. *Endocrinol Metab Clin North Am*. 2002;31:583. [PMID: 12227121]

Translation of the Clinical Problem into Answerable Questions

Bergus GR, Randall CS, Sinift SD. Does the structure of clinical questions affect the outcome of curbside consultations with specialty colleagues? *Arch Fam Med*. 2000;9:541. [PMID: 10862217]

Villanueva EV, Burrows EA, Fennessy PA, Rajendran M, Anderson JN. Improving question formulation for use in evidence appraisal in a tertiary care setting: a randomised controlled trial. *BMC Med Inf Decis Making*. 2001;I:4. [PMID: 11716797]

Finding the Best Evidence

Haynes RB, Walker-Dilks CJ. Evidence-based endocrinology: finding the current best research evidence for practice in endocrinology. *Endocrinol Metab Clin North Am*. 2002;31:527. [PMID: 12227117]

Richter B, Clar C. Systematic reviews in endocrinology: the Cochrane Metabolism and Endocrine Disorders Review Group. *Endocrinol Metab Clin North Am*. 2002;31:613. [PMID: 12227123]

Critical Appraisal and Applying the Results

Glasziou P, Vandenbroucke J, Chalmers I. Assessing the quality of research. *BMJ*. 2004;328:39. [PMID: 14703546]

Haynes RB, Devereaux PJ, Guyatt GH. Clinical expertise in the era of evidence-based medicine and patient choice. *ACP J Club*. 2002;136:[a11]. [PMID: 11874303]

Helfand M, Morton SC, Guallar E, Mulrow C. A guide to this supplement. Challenges of summarizing better information for better health: the evidence-based practice center experience. *Ann Intern Med*. 2005;142(suppl):1033.

Ioannidis JP, Haidich AB, Pappa M, et al. Comparison of evidence of treatment effects in randomized and nonrandomized studies. *JAMA*. 2001;286:821. [PMID: 11497536]

Liberati A, Altman DG, Tetzlaff J, et al. The PRISMA statement for reporting systematic reviews and meta-analyses of studies that evaluate health care interventions: explanation and elaboration. *Ann Intern Med*. 2009;151:W-65. www.annals.org. [PMID: 1000100]

Montori VM, Jaeschke R, Schünemann HJ, et al. Users' guide to detecting misleading claims in clinical research reports. *BMJ*. 2004;329:1093. [PMID: 15528623]

U.S. Preventive Services Task Force Ratings. Strength of Recommendations and Quality of Evidence. *Guide to Clinical Preventive Services*. 3rd ed. Periodic Updates, 2000-2003. Rockville, MD: Agency for Healthcare Research and Quality. http://www.ahrq.gov/clinic/3rduspstf/ratings.htm.

van Dam HA, van der Horst F, van den Borne B, et al. Provider–patient interaction in diabetes care: effects on patient self-care and outcomes. A systematic review. *Patient Educ Couns*. 2003;51:17. [PMID: 12915276]

Whitney SN, McGuire AL, McCullough LB. A typology of shared decision making, informed consent, and simple consent. *Ann Intern Med*. 2003;140:54. [PMID: 14706973]

Practice Guidelines

Aron D, Pogach L. Transparency standards for diabetes performance measures. *JAMA*. 2009;301:210. [PMID: 19141769]

Boyd CM, Darer J, Boult C, et al. Clinical practice guidelines and quality of care for older patients with multiple comorbid diseases: implications of pay for performance. *JAMA*. 2005;294:716-724. [PMID: 16091574]

Brozek JL, Akl EA, Jaeschke R, et al. Grading quality of evidence and strength of recommendations in clinical practice guidelines. Part 1 of 3. An overview of the GRADE approach and grading quality of evidence about interventions. *Allergy*. 2009;64:669. [PMID: 19210357]

Guyatt GH, Oxman AD, Vist G, et al. Rating quality of evidence and strength of recommendations GRADE: an emerging consensus on rating quality of evidence and strength of recommendations. *BMJ*. 2008;336:924. [PMID: 18436948]

Guyatt GH, Oxman AD, Kunz R, et al. Rating quality of evidence and strength of recommendations: what is "quality of evidence" and why is it important to clinicians? *BMJ*. 2008;336:995. [PMID: 18456631]

Guyatt GH, Oxman AD, Kunz R, et al. Rating quality of evidence and strength of recommendations: incorporating considerations of resources use into grading recommendations. *BMJ*. 2008;336:1170. [PMID: 18497416]

Guyatt GH, Henry D, Hill S, et al. Rating quality of evidence and strength of recommendations: going from evidence to recommendations. *BMJ*. 2008;336:1049. [PMID: 18467413]

Jaeschke R, Guyatt GH, Dellinger P, et al. Use of GRADE grid to reach decisions on clinical practice guidelines when consensus is elusive. *BMJ*. 2008;337:a744. [PMID: 18669566]

McGoey L. Sequestered evidence and the distortion of clinical practice guidelines. *Persp Biol Med*. 2009;52:203. [PMID: 19395820]

Qaseem A, Vijan S, Snow V, Cross JT, Weiss KB, Owens DK. Clinical Efficacy Assessment Subcommittee of the American College of Physicians. Glycemic control and type 2 diabetes mellitus: the optimal hemoglobin A1c targets: a guidance statement from the American College of Physicians. *Ann Intern Med*. 2007;147:417. [PMID: 17876024]

Schünemann HJ, Oxman AD, Brozek J. Grading quality of evidence and strength of recommendations for diagnostic tests and strategies. *BMJ*. 2008;336:1106. [PMID: 18483053]

Shaneyfelt TM, Centor RM. Reassessment of clinical practice guidelines: go gently into that good night. *JAMA*. 2009;301:868. [PMID: 19244197]

Internet Sites Related to Evidence-Based Medicine

Center for Health Evidence. http://www.cebm.net/

Center for Evidence Based Medicine. http://www.ahrq.gov/clinic/epc/

Evidence-Based Medicine Web Resources. University of Washington Health Sciences Library. http://healthlinks.washington.edu/howto/ebmtable.html

Health Information Resource Unit, McMaster University. http://hiru.mcmaster.ca/

Hypothalamus and Pituitary Gland

Bradley R. Javorsky, MD, David C. Aron, MD, MS, James W. Findling, MD, and J. Blake Tyrrell, MD

ACTH	Adrenocorticotropic hormone		**IRMA**	Immunoradiometric assay
ADH	Antidiuretic hormone (vasopressin)		**KAL1**	Kallmann syndrome 1
CLIP	Corticotropin-like intermediate lobe peptide		**LH**	Luteinizing hormone
CRH	Corticotropin-releasing hormone		**β-LPH**	β-Lipotropin
CRHBP	Corticotropin-releasing hormone-binding protein		**Met-Enk**	Methionine-enkephalin
FGF8	Fibroblast growth factor 8		**MEN**	Multiple endocrine neoplasia
FGFR1	Fibroblast growth factor receptor 1		**MSH**	Melanocyte-stimulating hormone
FSH	Follicle-stimulating hormone		**Pit-1**	Pituitary-specific positive transcription factor 1
GABA	Gamma-aminobutyric acid		**POMC**	Pro-opiomelanocortin
GH	Growth hormone (somatotropin)		**PROK2**	Prokineticin 2
GHBP	Growth hormone–binding protein		**PROKR2**	Prokineticin receptor 2
GHRH	Growth hormone–releasing hormone		**Prop-1**	Prophet of Pit-1
GHS-R	Growth hormone secretagogue receptor		**PRL**	Prolactin
GnRH	Gonadotropin-releasing hormone		**PTTG**	Pituitary tumor transforming gene
hCG	Human chorionic gonadotropin		**SHBG**	Sex hormone–binding globulin
hMG	Human menopausal gonadotropin		**SIADH**	Syndrome of inappropriate secretion of antidiuretic hormone
hPL	Human placental lactogen		**TRH**	Thyrotropin-releasing hormone
ICMA	Immunochemiluminescent assay		**TSH**	Thyroid-stimulating hormone (thyrotropin)
IGF	Insulin-like growth factor		**VIP**	Vasoactive intestinal peptide

The hypothalamus and pituitary gland form a unit that exerts control over the function of several endocrine glands—thyroid, adrenals, and gonads—as well as a wide range of physiologic activities. This unit is highly conserved across vertebrate species and constitutes a paradigm of neuroendocrinology—brain–endocrine interactions. The actions and interactions of the endocrine and nervous systems, whereby the nervous system regulates the endocrine system and endocrine activity modulates the activity of the central nervous system, constitute the major regulatory mechanisms for virtually all physiologic activities. These neuroendocrine interactions are also important in pathogenesis. This chapter will review the normal functions of the pituitary gland, the neuroendocrine control mechanisms of the hypothalamus, and the disorders of those mechanisms.

Nerve cells and endocrine cells, which are both involved in cell-to-cell communication, share certain characteristic features—secretion of chemical messengers (neurotransmitters or hormones) and electrical activity. A single chemical messenger—peptide or amine—can be secreted by neurons as a neurotransmitter or neural hormone and by endocrine cells as a classic hormone. Examples of such multifunctional chemical messengers are shown in Table 4–1. The cell-to-cell communication may occur by four

TABLE 4–1 Neuroendocrine messengers: substances that function as neurotransmitters, neural hormones, and classic hormones.

	Neurotransmitter (Present in Nerve Endings)	Hormone Secreted by Neurons	Hormone Secreted by Endocrine Cells
Dopamine	+	+	+
Norepinephrine	+	+	+
Epinephrine	+		+
Somatostatin	+	+	+
Gonadotropin-releasing hormone (GnRH)	+	+	+
Thyrotropin-releasing hormone (TRH)	+	+	
Oxytocin	+	+	+
Vasopressin	+	+	+
Vasoactive intestinal peptide	+	+	
Cholecystokinin (CCK)	+		+
Glucagon	+		+
Enkephalins	+		+
Pro-opiomelanocortin derivatives	+		+
Other anterior pituitary hormones	+		+

mechanisms: (1) autocrine communication via messengers that diffuse in the interstitial fluid and act on the cells that secreted them, (2) neural communication via synaptic junctions, (3) paracrine communication via messengers that diffuse in the interstitial fluid to adjacent target cells (without entering the bloodstream), and (4) endocrine communication via circulating hormones (Figure 4–1). The two major mechanisms of neural regulation of endocrine function are direct innervation and neurosecretion (neural secretion of hormones). The adrenal medulla, kidney, parathyroid gland, and pancreatic islets are endocrine tissues that receive direct autonomic innervation (see Chapters 9, 10, 11). An example of neurosecretory regulation is the hormonal secretion of certain hypothalamic nuclei into the portal hypophysial vessels, which

regulate the hormone-secreting cells of the anterior lobe of the pituitary. Another example of neurosecretory regulation is the posterior lobe of the pituitary gland, which is made up of the endings of neurons whose cell bodies reside in hypothalamic nuclei. These neurons secrete vasopressin and oxytocin into the general circulation.

Anatomy and Embryology

The anatomic relationships between the pituitary and the main nuclei of the hypothalamus are shown in Figure 4–2. The posterior lobe of the pituitary (neurohypophysis) is of neural origin, arising embryologically as an evagination of the ventral hypothalamus and the third ventricle. The neurohypophysis consists of the axons and

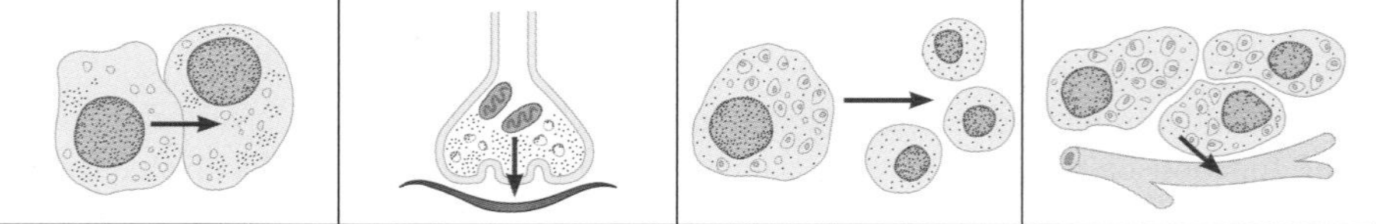

	Gap junctions	Synaptic	Paracrine	Endocrine
Message transmission	Directly from cell to cell	Across synaptic cleft	By diffusion in interstitial fluid	By circulating body fluids
Local or general	Local	Local	Locally diffuse	General
Specificity depends on	Anatomic location	Anatomic location and receptors	Receptors	Receptors

FIGURE 4–1 Intercellular communication by chemical mediators.

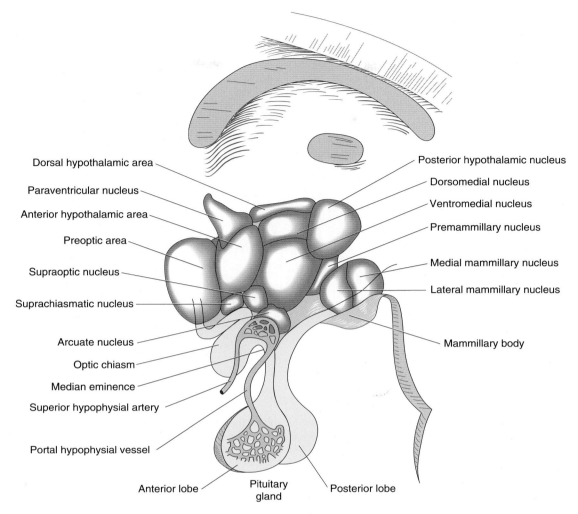

Dorsal hypothalamic area

Paraventricular nucleus

Anterior hypothalamic area

Preoptic area

Supraoptic nucleus

Suprachiasmatic nucleus

Arcuate nucleus

Optic chiasm

Median eminence

Superior hypophysial artery

Portal hypophysial vessel

Anterior lobe

Pituitary gland

Posterior lobe

Posterior hypothalamic nucleus

Dorsomedial nucleus

Ventromedial nucleus

Premammillary nucleus

Medial mammillary nucleus

Lateral mammillary nucleus

Mammillary body

FIGURE 4–2 The human hypothalamus, with a superimposed diagrammatic representation of the portal hypophysial vessels. (Reproduced, with permission, from Ganong WF. *Review of Medical Physiology*. 15th ed. McGraw-Hill; 1993).

nerve endings of neurons whose cell bodies reside in the supraoptic and paraventricular nuclei of the hypothalamus and supporting tissues. This hypothalamic-neurohypophysial nerve tract contains approximately 100,000 nerve fibers. Repeated swellings along the nerve fibers ranging in thickness from 1 to 50 μm constitute the nerve terminals.

The human fetal anterior pituitary anlage is initially recognizable at 4 to 5 weeks of gestation, and rapid cytologic differentiation leads to a mature hypothalamic-pituitary unit at 20 weeks. The anterior pituitary (adenohypophysis) originates from Rathke pouch, an ectodermal evagination of the oropharynx, and migrates to join the neurohypophysis. The portion of Rathke pouch in contact with the neurohypophysis develops less extensively and forms the intermediate lobe. This lobe remains intact in some species, but in humans its cells become interspersed with those of the anterior lobe and develop the capacity to synthesize and secrete pro-opiomelanocortin (POMC) and adrenocorticotropic hormone (ACTH). Remnants of Rathke pouch may persist at the boundary of the neurohypophysis, resulting in small colloid cysts.

In addition, cells may persist in the lower portion of Rathke pouch beneath the sphenoid bone, the pharyngeal pituitary. These cells have the potential to secrete hormones and have been reported to undergo adenomatous change.

The pituitary gland itself lies at the base of the skull in a portion of the sphenoid bone called the sella turcica (Turkish saddle). The anterior portion, the tuberculum sellae, is flanked by posterior projections of the sphenoid wings, the anterior clinoid processes. The dorsum sellae forms the posterior wall, and its upper corners project into the posterior clinoid processes. The gland is surrounded by dura, and the roof is formed by a reflection of the dura attached to the clinoid processes, the diaphragma sellae. The arachnoid membrane and, therefore, cerebrospinal fluid are prevented from entering the sella turcica by the diaphragma sellae. The pituitary stalk and its blood vessels pass through an opening in this diaphragm. The lateral walls of the gland are in direct apposition to the cavernous sinuses and separated from them by dural membranes. The optic chiasm lies 5 to 10 mm above the diaphragma sellae and anterior to the stalk (Figure 4–3).

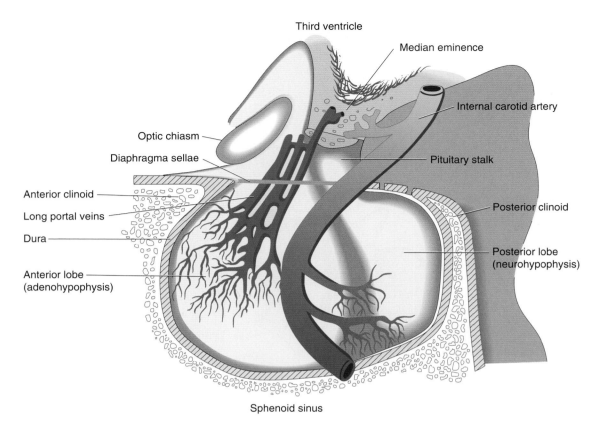

FIGURE 4–3 Anatomic relationships and blood supply of the pituitary gland. (Reproduced, with permission, from Frohman LA. Diseases of the anterior pituitary. In: Felig P, Baxter JD, Frohman LA, eds. *Endocrinology and Metabolism*. 3rd ed. McGraw-Hill; 1995).

The size of the pituitary gland, of which the anterior lobe constitutes two-thirds, varies considerably. It measures approximately $15 \times 10 \times 6$ mm and weighs 500 to 900 mg; it may double in size during pregnancy. The sella turcica tends to conform to the shape and size of the gland, and for that reason there is considerable variability in its contour.

Blood Supply

The anterior pituitary is the most richly vascularized of all mammalian tissues, receiving 0.8 mL/g/min from a portal circulation connecting the median eminence of the hypothalamus and the anterior pituitary. Arterial blood is supplied from the internal carotid arteries via the superior, middle, and inferior hypophysial arteries. The superior hypophysial arteries form a capillary network in the median eminence of the hypothalamus that recombines in long portal veins draining down the pituitary stalk to the anterior lobe, where they break up into another capillary network and re-form into venous channels. The pituitary stalk and the posterior pituitary are supplied directly from branches of the middle and inferior hypophysial arteries (see Figures 4–2 and 4–3).

Venous drainage of the pituitary, the route through which anterior pituitary hormones reach the systemic circulation, is variable, but venous channels eventually drain via the cavernous sinus posteriorly into the superior and inferior petrosal sinuses to the jugular bulb and vein (Figure 4–4). The axons of the neurohypophysis

terminate on capillaries that drain via the posterior lobe veins and the cavernous sinuses to the general circulation. The hypophysial portal system of capillaries allows control of anterior pituitary function by the hypothalamic hypophysiotropic hormones secreted into the portal hypophysial vessels. This provides a short, direct connection to the anterior pituitary from the ventral hypothalamus and the median eminence (Figure 4–5). There may also be retrograde blood flow between the pituitary and hypothalamus, providing a possible means of direct feedback between pituitary hormones and their neuroendocrine control centers.

Pituitary Development and Histology

Anterior pituitary cells were originally classified as acidophils, basophils, and chromophobe cells based on staining with hematoxylin and eosin. Immunocytochemical and electron microscopic techniques now permit classification of cells by their specific secretory products: somatotrophs (growth hormone [GH]-secreting cells), lactotrophs (prolactin [PRL]-secreting cells), thyrotrophs (cells secreting thyroid-stimulating hormone [thyrotropin; TSH]), corticotrophs (cells-secreting ACTH [corticotropin] and related peptides), and gonadotrophs (luteinizing hormone [LH]– and follicle-stimulating hormone [FSH]–secreting cells). The development of the pituitary gland and the emergence of the distinct cell types from common primordial cells are controlled by a limited set of transcription factors, most notably Prop1 and Pit1

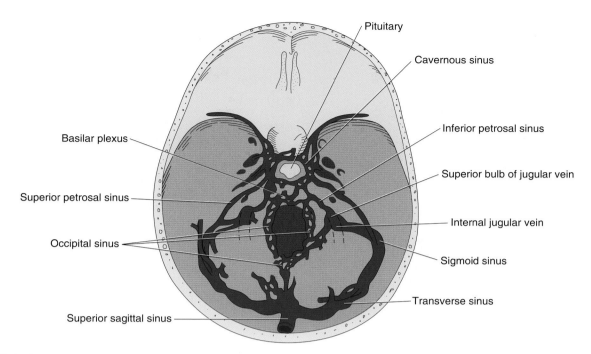

FIGURE 4–4 Venous drainage of the pituitary gland—the route by which adenohypophysial hormones reach the systemic circulation. (Reproduced, with permission, from Findling JW, et al. Selective venous sampling for ACTH in Cushing's syndrome: differentiation between Cushing's disease and the ectopic ACTH syndrome. *Ann Intern Med*. 1981;94:647).

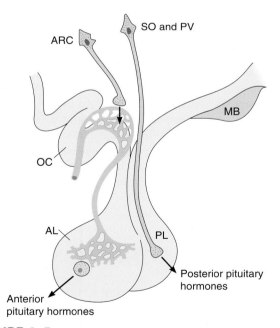

FIGURE 4–5 Secretion of hypothalamic hormones. The hormones of the posterior lobe (PL) are released into the general circulation from the endings of supraoptic and paraventricular neurons, whereas hypophysiotropic hormones are secreted into the portal hypophysial circulation from the endings of arcuate and other hypothalamic neurons (AL, anterior lobe; ARC, arcuate and other nuclei; MB, mamillary bodies; OC, optic chiasm; PV, paraventricular nucleus; SO, supraoptic nucleus).

(Figure 4–6). The individual hormone-secreting cells emerge in a specific order and from distinct lineages. Abnormalities of pituitary and lineage–specific transcription factors have been associated with the development of hypopituitarism. Although traditionally the pituitary has been conceptualized as a gland with distinct and highly specialized cells that respond to specific hypothalamic and peripheral hormones, it has become clear that local (ie, paracrine) factors also play a role in normal pituitary physiology.

A. Somatotrophs The GH-secreting cells are acidophilic and usually located in the lateral portions of the anterior lobe. Granule size by electron microscopy is 150 to 600 nm in diameter. These cells account for about 50% of the adenohypophysial cells.

B. Lactotrophs The PRL-secreting cell is a second but distinct acidophil-staining cell randomly distributed in the anterior pituitary. These cells account for 10% to 25% of anterior pituitary cells. Granule size averages approximately 550 nm on electron microscopy. There are two types of lactotrophs: sparsely granulated and densely granulated. These cells proliferate during pregnancy as a result of elevated estrogen levels and account for the twofold increase in gland size.

C. Thyrotrophs These TSH-secreting cells, because of their glycoprotein product, are basophilic and also show a positive reaction with periodic acid-Schiff stain. Thyrotrophs are the least common pituitary cell type, making up less than 10% of adenohypophysial cells. The thyrotroph granules are small (50-100 nm), and these cells

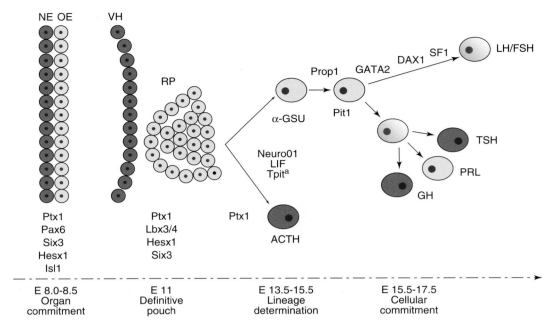

FIGURE 4–6 Transcription factors involved in the early development of mouse pituitary, including Tpit.
Tpit is expressed on embryonic day E 11.5, followed by expression of POMC-producing cells by E 12.5 (DAX1, dosage sensitive sex-reversal-adrenal hypoplasia congenital critical region on the X chromosome 1; GATA2, GATA-binding protein 2, zinc-finger transcription factor; α-GSU, alpha subunit of pituitary glycoprotein hormones; Hesx1, homeobox gene expressed in embryonic stem cells 1; Isl1, islet 1 transcription factor; LH/FSH, luteinizing hormone/follicle-stimulating hormone; Lhx3/4, LIM-domain transcription factor 3/4; LIF, leukemia inhibiting factor; NE, neural epithelium; Neuro01, neurogenic basic helix-loop-helix transcription factor 01; OE, oral ectoderm; Pax6, paired box containing transcription factor 6; Pit1, pituitary transcription factor 1; PRL, prolactin; Prop1, prophet of Pit1; Ptx1, pituitary homeobox 1; RP, Rathke pouch; SF1, steroidogenic factor 1; Six3, sine oculis-like homeobox transcription factor 3; Tpit, T-box pituitary transcription factor; VH, ventral hypothalamus). (From Asteria C. T-Box and isolated ACTH deficiency. *Eur J Endocrinol.* 2002;146:463).

are usually located in the anteromedial and anterolateral portions of the gland. During states of primary thyroid failure, the cells demonstrate marked hypertrophy, increasing overall gland size.

D. Corticotrophs   ACTH and its related peptides (see below) are secreted by basophilic cells that are embryologically of intermediate lobe origin and usually located in the anteromedial portion of the gland. Corticotrophs represent 15% to 20% of adenohypophysial cells. Electron microscopy shows that these secretory granules are about 360 nm in diameter. In states of glucocorticoid excess, corticotrophs undergo degranulation and a microtubular hyalinization known as Crooke hyaline degeneration.

E. Gonadotrophs   LH and FSH originate from basophil-staining cells, whose secretory granules are about 200 nm in diameter. These cells constitute 10% to 15% of anterior pituitary cells, and they are located throughout the entire anterior lobe. They become hypertrophied and cause the gland to enlarge during states of primary gonadal failure such as menopause, Klinefelter syndrome, and Turner syndrome.

F. Other cell types   Some cells, usually chromophobes, contain secretory granules but do not exhibit immunocytochemical staining for the major known anterior pituitary hormones. These cells have been called null cells; they may give rise to (apparently) nonfunctioning adenomas. Some may represent undifferentiated primitive secretory cells, and others (eg, glia-like or folliculostellate cells) may produce one or more of the many paracrine factors that have been described in the pituitary. Mammosomatotrophs contain both GH and PRL; these bihormonal cells are most often seen in pituitary tumors. Human chorionic gonadotropin is also secreted by the anterior pituitary gland, but its cell of origin and physiologic significance are uncertain. The six known major anterior pituitary hormones are listed in Table 4–2.

HYPOTHALAMIC HORMONES

The hypothalamic hormones can be divided into those secreted into hypophysial portal blood vessels and those secreted by the neurohypophysis directly into the general circulation. The hypothalamic nuclei, their neurohormones, and their main functions are shown in Table 4–3. The structures of the eight major hypothalamic hormones are shown in Table 4–4.

Hypophysiotropic Hormones

The hypophysiotropic hormones that regulate the secretion of anterior pituitary hormones include growth hormone–releasing

TABLE 4–2 Major adenohypophysial hormones and their cellular sources.

Cellular Source and Histologic Staining	Main Hormone Products	Structure of Hormone	Main Functions
Somatotroph (acidophil)	GH; also known as STH or somatotropin	191 amino acids, 22-kDa protein, mainly nonglycosylated	Stimulates the production of IGF-1 (the mediator of the indirect actions of GH); also exerts direct actions on growth and metabolism.
Lactotroph or mammotroph (acidophil)	PRL	198 amino acids, 23-kDa protein, mainly nonglycosylated (Note: most of the decidually produced PRL is glycosylated)	Stimulation of milk production (protein and lactose synthesis, water excretion, and sodium retention); inhibits gonadotropin; immunomodulator
Corticotroph (small cells with basophil granules with strong PAS positivity, indicating the presence of glycoproteins)	Derivatives of POMC, mainly ACTH and β-LPH	POMC: glycosylated polypeptide of 134 amino acid residues ACTH: simple peptide of 39 amino acid residues, 4.5 kDa β-LPH: simple peptide of 91 amino acid residues, 11.2 kDa	ACTH: stimulation of glucocorticoids and sex steroids in the zona fasciculata and zona reticularis of the adrenal cortex, inducing hyperplasia and hypertrophy of the adrenal cortex β-LPH: weak lipolytic and opioid actions
Thyrotroph (large cells with basophil granules with PAS positivity)	TSH	Glycoprotein hormone consisting of a shared α (89 amino acid) and a TSH-specific β (112 amino acid) subunit Total size: 28 kDa	Stimulation of all aspects of thyroid gland function: hormone synthesis, secretion, hyperplasia, hypertrophy, and vascularization
Gonadotroph (small cells with basophil granules with periodic acid-Schiff positivity)	LH: named after its effect in females; is identical to the ICSH (interstitial cell stimulating hormone) originally described in males	Glycoprotein hormone consisting of a shared α and an LH-specific β (115 amino acid) subunit Total size: 29 kDa	Females: stimulates steroid hormone synthesis in theca interna cells, lutein cells, and hilar cells; promotes luteinization and maintains corpus luteum Males: stimulates steroid hormone production in Leydig cells
	FSH	Glycoprotein hormone consisting of a shared α and an FSH-specific β (115 amino acid) subunit. Total size: 29 kDa	Females: targets the granulosa cells to promote follicular development; stimulates aromatase expression and inhibin secretion Males: targets the Sertoli cells to promote spermatogenesis and to stimulate inhibin secretion

Modified from Kacsoh B. *Endocrine Physiology*. McGraw-Hill; 2000.

hormone (GHRH), somatostatin, dopamine, thyrotropin-releasing hormone (TRH), corticotropin-releasing hormone (CRH), and gonadotropin-releasing hormone (GnRH). The location of the cell bodies of the hypophysiotropic hormone–secreting neurons is depicted in Figure 4–7. Most of the anterior pituitary hormones are controlled by stimulatory hormones, but GH and especially PRL are also regulated by inhibitory hormones. Some hypophysiotropic hormones are multifunctional. The hormones of the hypothalamus are secreted episodically and not continuously, and in some cases there is an underlying circadian rhythm.

A. GHRH GHRH stimulates GH secretion by, and is trophic for, somatotrophs. GHRH-secreting neurons are located in the arcuate nuclei (see Figure 4–2), and axons terminate in the external layer of the median eminence. The major isoform of GHRH is 44 amino acids in length. It was isolated from a pancreatic tumor in a patient with clinical manifestations of GH excess (acromegaly) associated with somatotroph hyperplasia (see discussion later in the chapter). GHRH is synthesized from a larger precursor of 108 amino acids. Other secretory products derived from this precursor have also been found. Full biologic activity of these releasing factors appears to reside in the 1 to 29 amino acid sequence of the amino terminal portion of the molecule. Human GHRH is a member of a homologous family of peptides that includes secretin, glucagon, vasoactive intestinal peptide (VIP), and others. The half-life of GHRH is approximately 3 to 7 minutes.

B. Somatostatin Somatostatin inhibits the secretion of GH and TSH. Somatostatin-secreting cells are located in the periventricular region immediately above the optic chiasm (see Figure 4–2) with nerve endings found diffusely in the external layer of the median eminence.

Somatostatin, a tetradecapeptide, has been found not only in the hypothalamus but also in the D cells of the pancreatic islets, the gastrointestinal mucosa, and the C cells (parafollicular cells) of the thyroid. The somatostatin precursor has 116 amino acids.

TABLE 4–3 The hypothalamic nuclei and their main functions.

Nucleus	Location	Major Neurohormones or Function
Supraoptic	Anterolateral, above the optic tract	ADH: osmoregulation, regulation of ECF volume Oxytocin: regulation of uterine contractions and milk ejection
Paraventricular	Dorsal anterior periventricular	Magnocellular paraventricular nucleus (PVN): ADH, oxytocin: same functions as above Parvocellular PVN TRH: regulation of thyroid function CRH: regulation of adrenocortical function, regulation of the sympathetic nervous system and adrenal medulla, regulation of appetite ADH: coexpressed with CRH, regulation of adrenocortical function VIP: prolactin-releasing factor (?)
Suprachiasmatic	Above the optic chiasm, anteroventral periventricular zone	Regulator of circadian rhythms and pineal function (zeitgeber [pacemaker]): VIP, ADH neurons project mainly to the PVN
Arcuate	Medial basal hypothalamus close to the third ventricle	GHRH: stimulation of growth hormone GnRH: regulation of pituitary gonadotropins (FSH and LH) Dopamine: functions as PIH Somatostatin: inhibition of GHRH release Regulation of appetite (neuropeptide Y, agouti-related transcript, α-MSH, cocaine- and amphetamine-related transcript)
Periventricular	Anteroventral	Somatostatin: inhibition of growth hormone secretion by direct pituitary action: most abundant SRIF location
Ventromedial	Ventromedial	GHRH (as above) Somatostatin: inhibition of GHRH release Functions as a satiety center
Dorsomedial	Dorsomedial	Focal point of information processing: receives input from ventromedial nucleus (VMN) and lateral hypothalamus and projects to the PVN
Lateral hypothalamus	Lateral hypothalamus	Functions as a hunger center (melanin-concentrating hormone, anorexins)
Preoptic area	Preoptic area	Main regulator of ovulation in rodents; only a few GnRH neurons in primates
Anterior hypothalamus	Anterior hypothalamus	Thermoregulation: cooling center Anteroventral third ventricular region: regulation of thirst
Posterior hypothalamus	Posterior hypothalamus	Thermoregulation: heating center

Modified from Kacsoh B. *Endocrine Physiology.* McGraw-Hill; 2000.

Processing of the carboxyl terminal region of preprosomatostatin results in the generation of the tetradecapeptide somatostatin 14 and an amino terminal extended form containing 28 amino acid residues (somatostatin 28). Somatostatin 14 is the major species in the hypothalamus, whereas somatostatin 28 is found in the gut. In addition to its profound inhibitory effect on GH secretion, somatostatin also has important inhibitory influences on many other hormones, including insulin, glucagon, gastrin, secretin, and VIP. This inhibitory hypothalamic peptide plays a role in the physiologic secretion of TSH by augmenting the direct inhibitory effect of thyroid hormone on the thyrotrophs; administration of anti-somatostatin antibodies results in a rise in circulating TSH level. Somatostatin has a half-life of 2 to 3 minutes.

C. Dopamine   Dopamine, the primary PRL-inhibitory hormone, is found in the portal circulation and binds to dopamine receptors on lactotrophs. It has a short half-life, on the order of 1 to 2 minutes. The hypothalamic control of PRL secretion, unlike that of the other pituitary hormones, is predominantly inhibitory.

Thus, disruption of the hypothalamic-pituitary connection by stalk section, hypothalamic lesions, or pituitary autotransplantation increases PRL secretion. Dopamine-secreting neurons (tuberoinfundibular dopaminergic system) are located in the arcuate nuclei, and their axons terminate in the external layer of the median eminence, primarily in the same area as the GnRH endings (laterally) and to a lesser extent medially (see Figure 4–2). The neurotransmitter gamma-aminobutyric acid (GABA) and cholinergic pathways also appear to inhibit PRL release.

D. Prolactin-releasing factors   The best-studied factor with PRL-releasing activity is TRH (see discussion later), but there is little evidence for a physiologic role. PRL increase associated with sleep, during stress, and after nipple stimulation or suckling is not accompanied by an increase in TRH or TSH. Another hypothalamic peptide, VIP, stimulates PRL release in humans. Serotonergic pathways may also stimulate PRL secretion, as demonstrated by the increased PRL secretion after the administration of serotonin precursors and by the reduction of secretion following treatment with serotonin antagonists.

TABLE 4–4 Hypothalamic hormones.

Hormone	Structure
Posterior pituitary hormones	
Arginine vasopressin	⌐—S————S—⌐ Cys-Tyr-Phe-Gln-Asn-Cys-Pro-Arg-Gly-NH$_2$
Oxytocin	⌐—S————S—⌐ Cys-Tyr-Ile-Gln-Asn-Cys-Pro-Leu-Gly-NH$_2$
Hypophysiotropic hormones	
Thyrotropin-releasing hormone (TRH)	(pyro)Glu-His-Pro-NH$_2$
Gonadotropin-releasing hormone (GnRH)	(pyro)Glu-His-Trp-Ser-Tyr-Gly-Leu-Arg-Pro-Gly-NH$_2$
Somatostatin[a]	⌐—S—————————S—⌐ Ala-Gly-Cys-Lys-Asn-Phe-Phe-Trp-Lys-Thr-Phe-Thr-Ser-Cys
Growth hormone–releasing hormone (GHRH)	Tyr-Ala-Asp-Ala-Ile-Phe-Thr-Asn-Ser-Tyr-Arg-Lys-Val-Leu-Gly-Gln-Leu-Ser- Ala-Arg-Lys-Leu-Leu-Gln-Asp-Ile-Met-Ser-Arg-Gln-Gln-Gly-Glu-Ser-Asn-Gln- Glu-Arg-Gly-Ala-Arg-Ala-Arg-Leu-NH$_2$
Prolactin-inhibiting hormone (PIH, dopamine)	HO, HO— benzene ring —CH$_2$CH$_2$NH$_2$
Corticotropin-releasing hormone (CRH)	Ser-Gln-Glu-Pro-Pro-Ile-Ser-Leu-Asp-Leu-Thr-Phe-His-Leu-Leu-Arg-Glu-Val- Leu-Glu-Met-Thr-Lys-Ala-Asp-Gln-Leu-Ala-Gln-Gln-Ala-His-Ser-Asn-Arg-Lys- Leu-Leu-Asp-Ile-Ala-NH$_2$

[a]In addition to the tetradecapeptide shown here (somatostatin 14), an amino terminal–extended molecule (somatostatin 28), and a 12-amino-acid form (somatostatin 28 [1-12]) are found in most tissues.

E. Thyrotropin-releasing hormone TRH, a tripeptide, is the major hypothalamic factor regulating TSH secretion. Human TRH is synthesized from a large precursor of 242 amino acids that contains six copies of TRH. TRH-secreting neurons are located in the medial portions of the paraventricular nuclei (see Figure 4–2), and their axons terminate in the medial portion of the external layer of the median eminence. The half-life of TRH is approximately 6 minutes.

F. Corticotropin-releasing hormone CRH, a 41-amino-acid peptide, stimulates the secretion of ACTH and other products of its precursor molecule, POMC. CRH is synthesized from a precursor of 196 amino acids. The half-life of CRH follows a biphasic pattern in plasma lasting approximately 6 to 10 minutes and 40 to 50 minutes. Both antidiuretic hormone (ADH) and angiotensin II potentiate CRH-mediated secretion of ACTH. In contrast, oxytocin inhibits CRH-mediated ACTH secretion. CRH-secreting neurons are found in the anterior portion of the paraventricular nuclei just lateral to the TRH-secreting neurons; their nerve endings are found in all parts of the external layer of the median eminence. CRH is also secreted from human placenta. The level of this hormone increases significantly during late pregnancy and delivery. In addition, a specific CRH-binding protein (CRHBP) has been described in both serum and in intracellular locations within a variety of cells. It is likely that CRHBPs modulate the actions and plasma half-life of CRH. Since the 1990s, three proteins homologous to CRH, termed urocortins, and two different receptors, have been identified. In addition to the role of CRH in the physiologic response to stress, this family of peptides appears to play a significant role in energy balance.

G. Gonadotropin-releasing hormone The secretion of LH and FSH is controlled by a single stimulatory hypothalamic hormone, GnRH. This is achieved through differences in the size and frequency of GnRH release as well as feedback from estrogens and androgens; low-frequency pulses favor FSH release while high-frequency pulses result in LH release. GnRH is a linear decapeptide that stimulates only LH and FSH; it has no effect on other pituitary hormones except in some patients with acromegaly and Cushing disease (see discussion later). The precursor of GnRH—proGnRH—contains 92 amino acids. ProGnRH also contains the sequence of a 56-amino-acid polypeptide called GnRH-associated peptide. This secretory product exhibits PRL-inhibiting activity, but its physiologic role is unknown. GnRH-secreting neurons are located primarily in the preoptic area of the anterior hypothalamus, and their nerve terminals are found in the lateral portions of the external layer of the median eminence adjacent to the pituitary stalk (see Figure 4–2). GnRH has a half-life of 2 to 4 minutes.

Neuroendocrinology: The Hypothalamus as Part of a Larger System

The hypothalamus is involved in many nonendocrine functions such as regulation of body temperature, thirst, and food intake

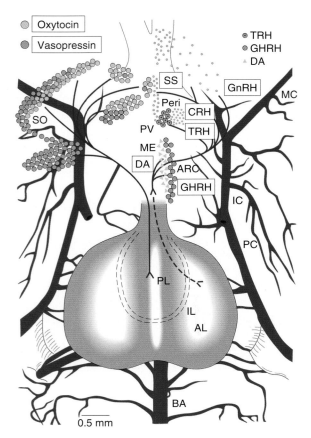

FIGURE 4–7 Location of cell bodies of hypophysiotropic hormone-secreting neurons projected on a ventral view of the hypothalamus and pituitary of the rat. (AL, anterior lobe; ARC, arcuate nucleus; BA, basilar artery; IC, internal carotid; IL, intermediate lobe; MC, middle cerebral; ME, median eminence; PC, posterior cerebral; Peri, periventricular nucleus; PL, posterior lobe; PVL and PVM, lateral and medial portions of the paraventricular nucleus; SO, supraoptic nucleus.) The names of the hormones are enclosed in the boxes (SS, somatostatin; DA, dopamine). (Courtesy of LW Swanson and ET Cunningham Jr.)

and is connected with many other parts of the nervous system. The brain itself is influenced by both direct and indirect hormonal effects. Steroid and thyroid hormones cross the blood–brain barrier and produce specific receptor-mediated actions (see Chapters 1, 7, and 9). Peptides in the general circulation, which do not cross the blood–brain barrier, elicit their effects indirectly (eg, insulin-mediated changes in blood–glucose concentration). In addition, communication between the general circulation and the brain may take place via the circumventricular organs, which are located outside the blood–brain barrier (see later). Moreover, hypothalamic hormones in extrahypothalamic brain function as neurotransmitters or neurohormones. They are also found in other tissues where they function as hormones (endocrine, paracrine, or autocrine). For example, somatostatin-containing neurons are widely distributed in the nervous system. They are also found in the pancreatic islets (D cells), the gastrointestinal

mucosa, and the C cells of the thyroid gland (parafollicular cells). Somatostatin is not only secreted into the general circulation as well as locally—it is also secreted into the lumen of the gut, where it may affect gut secretion. A hormone with this activity has been called a **lumone**. Hormones common to the brain, pituitary, and gastrointestinal tract include not only TRH and somatostatin but also VIP and peptides derived from POMC.

Hypothalamic function is regulated both by hormone-mediated signals (eg, negative feedback) and by neural inputs from a wide variety of sources. These nerve signals are mediated by neurotransmitters including acetylcholine, dopamine, norepinephrine, epinephrine, serotonin, GABA, and opioids. The hypothalamus can be considered a final common pathway by which signals from multiple systems reach the anterior pituitary. For example, cytokines that play a role in the response to infection, such as the interleukins, are also involved in regulation of the hypothalamic-pituitary-adrenal axis. This system of immunoneuroendocrine interactions is important in the organism's response to a variety of stresses.

The hypothalamus also sends signals to other parts of the nervous system. For example, while the major nerve tracts of the magnocellular neurons containing vasopressin and oxytocin terminate in the posterior pituitary, nerve fibers from the paraventricular and supraoptic nuclei project toward many other parts of the nervous system. In the brain stem, vasopressinergic neurons are involved in the autonomic regulation of blood pressure. Similar neurons project to the gray matter and are implicated in higher cortical functions. Fibers terminating in the median eminence permit release of ADH into the hypophysial-portal system; delivery of ADH in high concentrations to the anterior pituitary may facilitate its involvement in the regulation of ACTH secretion. Magnocellular neurons also project to the choroid plexus, where they may release ADH into the cerebrospinal fluid. In addition to magnocellular neurons, the paraventricular nuclei contain cells with smaller cell bodies—**parvicellular neurons**. Such neurons are also found in other regions of the nervous system and may contain other peptides such as CRH and TRH.

The Hypothalamus and the Control of Appetite

With the growing appreciation of adipose tissue as an endocrine organ, as well as the increasing problem of obesity and its associated health risks, understanding how energy balance and appetite are regulated has become a major topic of study. In 1901, Frohlich observed that some tumors affecting the pituitary and hypothalamus were associated with excess subcutaneous fat and hypogonadism. Subsequent lesioning experiments by Hetherington and Ranson in the 1940s established the hypothalamus as a fundamental site in the regulation of appetite. These experiments introduced the classic *dual center* model of food intake where the ventromedial hypothalamic nucleus functions as a *satiety center* and the lateral hypothalamic area serves as a *feeding center*. Subsequent studies have led to refinements of this model.

Growing evidence points to the pivotal role of the arcuate nucleus in the integration of feeding signals and energy reserves. It has special access to circulating hormones via the underlying median eminence, an area rich with fenestrated capillaries, that is, it is not protected by the blood–brain barrier (see Figure 4–2). Two populations of neurons involved in the regulation of feeding are located within the arcuate nucleus: one that inhibits food intake via the expression of neuropeptides POMC and cocaine- and amphetamine-regulated transcript, and one that stimulates food intake via expression of neuropeptide Y and agouti-related peptide. The arcuate nucleus projects to second-order neuronal populations including the paraventricular nucleus, dorsomedial nucleus, ventromedial nucleus, and lateral hypothalamic area, which then activate downstream pathways controlling appetite and energy expenditure.

Circulating markers of adiposity (leptin, adiponectin, insulin), and hormones from the gastrointestinal tract (ghrelin, peptide YY, glucagon-like peptide 1, cholecystokinin, oxyntomodulin, pancreatic polypeptide) converge on the hypothalamus and brain stem to signal adequacy of short- and long-term energy stores. Alterations in the levels or tissue sensitivity of these hormones may underlie disorders of weight regulation such as obesity, and could prove useful as therapeutic targets (see also Chapter 20).

The Pineal Gland and the Circumventricular Organs

The circumventricular organs are secretory midline brain structures that arise from the ependymal cell lining of the ventricular system (Figure 4–8). These organs are located adjacent to the third ventricle—subfornical organ, subcommissural organ, organum vasculosum of the lamina terminalis, pineal, and part of the median eminence—and at the roof of the fourth ventricle—area postrema (see Figure 4–8). The tissues of these organs have relatively large interstitial spaces and have fenestrated capillaries which, being highly permeable, permit diffusion of large molecules from the general circulation; elsewhere in the brain tight capillary endothelial junctions prevent such diffusion—the blood–brain barrier. For example, angiotensin II (see Chapter 10) is involved in the regulation of water intake, blood pressure, and secretion of vasopressin. In addition to its peripheral effects, circulating angiotensin II acts on the subfornical organ resulting in an increase in water intake.

The pineal gland, considered by the 17th century French philosopher René Descartes to be the seat of the soul, is located at the roof of the posterior portion of the third ventricle. The pineal gland in humans and other mammals has no direct neural connections with the brain except for sympathetic innervation via the superior cervical ganglion. The pineal gland secretes melatonin, an indole synthesized from serotonin by 5-methoxylation and *N*-acetylation (Figure 4–9). The pineal releases melatonin into the general circulation and into the cerebrospinal fluid. Melatonin secretion is regulated by the sympathetic nervous system and is increased in response to hypoglycemia and darkness. The pineal also contains other bioactive peptides and amines including TRH,

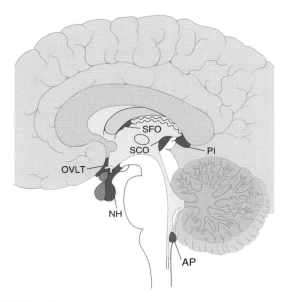

FIGURE 4–8 Circumventricular organs. The neurohypophysis (NH) and adjacent median eminence, the organum vasculosum of the lamina terminalis (OVLT), the subfornical organ (SFO), and the area postrema (AP) are shown projected on a sagittal section of the human brain. The pineal (PI) and the subcommissural organ (SCO) are also shown but probably do not function as circumventricular organs. (Reproduced, with permission, from Ganong WF. *Review of Medical Physiology*. 15th ed. McGraw-Hill; 1993).

somatostatin, GnRH, and norepinephrine. The physiologic roles of the pineal remain to be elucidated, but they appear to involve regulation of gonadal function and development and chronobiologic rhythms.

The pineal gland may be the site of origin of pineal cell tumors (pinealomas) or germ cell tumors (germinomas). Neurologic signs and symptoms are the predominant clinical manifestations; examples include increased intracranial pressure, visual abnormalities, ataxia, and Parinaud syndrome—upward gaze palsy, absent pupillary light reflex, paralysis of convergence, and wide-based gait. Endocrine manifestations result primarily from deficiency of hypothalamic hormones (diabetes insipidus, hypopituitarism, or disorders of gonadal development). Treatment involves surgical removal or decompression, radiation therapy, and hormone replacement (discussed later).

ANTERIOR PITUITARY HORMONES

The six major anterior pituitary hormones—ACTH, GH, PRL, TSH, LH, and FSH—may be classified into three groups: ACTH-related peptides (ACTH itself, lipotropin [LPH], melanocyte-stimulating hormone [MSH], and endorphins); the somatomammotropin proteins (GH and PRL); and the glycoproteins (LH, FSH, and TSH). The chemical features of these hormones are set forth in Table 4–2.

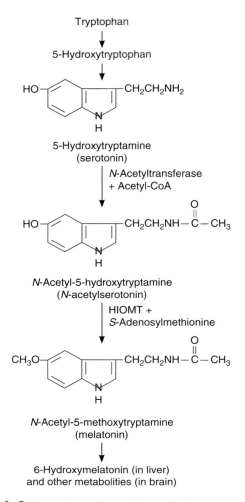

Tryptophan

5-Hydroxytryptophan

5-Hydroxytryptamine
(serotonin)

N-Acetyltransferase
+ Acetyl-CoA

N-Acetyl-5-hydroxytryptamine
(N-acetylserotonin)

HIOMT +
S-Adenosylmethionine

N-Acetyl-5-methoxytryptamine
(melatonin)

6-Hydroxymelatonin (in liver)
and other metabolites (in brain)

FIGURE 4–9 Formation and metabolism of melatonin
(HIOMT, hydroxyindole-O-methyltransferase.) (Reproduced, with
permission, from Ganong WF. *Review of Medical Physiology*. 15th ed.
McGraw-Hill; 1993).

ADRENOCORTICOTROPIC HORMONE AND RELATED PEPTIDES

Biosynthesis

ACTH is a 39-amino-acid peptide hormone (MW 4500) processed from a large precursor molecule, POMC (MW 28,500). Within the corticotroph, a single mRNA directs the synthesis and processing of POMC into smaller, biologically active fragments (Figure 4–10), which include β-LPH, α-MSH, β-MSH, β-endorphin, and the amino terminal fragment of POMC. Most of these peptides are glycosylated, which accounts for differences in the reporting of molecular weights. These carbohydrate moieties are responsible for the basophilic staining of corticotrophs.

Two of these fragments are contained within the structure of ACTH: α-MSH is identical to ACTH 1 to 13, and corticotropin-like intermediate lobe peptide (CLIP) represents ACTH 18 to 39 (see Figure 4–10). Although these fragments are found in species with developed intermediate lobes (eg, the rat), they are not secreted as separate hormones in humans. β-LPH, a fragment with 91 amino acids (1-91), is secreted by the corticotroph in equimolar quantities with ACTH. Within the β-LPH molecule exists the amino acid sequence for β-MSH (41-58), γ-LPH (1-58), and β-endorphin (61-91).

Function

ACTH stimulates the secretion of glucocorticoids, mineralocorticoids, and androgens—all steroids from the adrenal cortex (see Chapters 9 and 10). The amino terminal end (residues 1-18) is responsible for this biologic activity. ACTH binds to receptors on the adrenal cortex and induces steroidogenesis through a cAMP-dependent mechanism.

The hyperpigmentation observed in states of ACTH hypersecretion (eg, Addison disease, Nelson syndrome) appears to be primarily due to ACTH binding to the MSH receptor, because

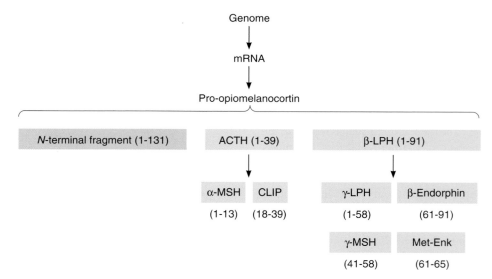

FIGURE 4–10 The processing of pro-opiomelanocortin (MW 28,500) into its biologically active peptide hormones. Abbreviations are expanded in the text.

α-MSH and β-MSH do not exist as separate hormones in humans.

The physiologic function of β-LPH and its family of peptide hormones, including β-endorphin, is not completely understood. However, both β-LPH and β-endorphin have the same secretory dynamics as ACTH.

Measurement

The development of immunoradiometric and immunochemiluminescent assays (IRMAs and ICMAs, respectively) has provided a sensitive and practical clinical ACTH assay for the evaluation of pituitary-adrenal disorders. The basal morning concentration ranges from 9 to 52 pg/mL (2-11 pmol/L). Its short plasma half-life (7-12 minutes) and episodic secretion cause wide and rapid fluctuations both in its plasma concentration and in that of cortisol.

Although β-LPH has a longer half-life than ACTH and is more stable in plasma, its measurement has not been extensively utilized. Current data suggest that the normal concentration of β-LPH is 10 to 40 pg/mL (1-4 pmol/L).

Secretion

The physiologic secretion of ACTH is mediated through neural influences by means of a complex of hormones, the most important of which is CRH (Figure 4–11).

CRH stimulates ACTH in a pulsatile manner: diurnal rhythmicity causes a peak before awakening and a decline as the day progresses. The diurnal rhythm is a reflection of neural control and provokes concordant diurnal secretion of cortisol from the adrenal cortex (Figure 4–12). This episodic release of ACTH is

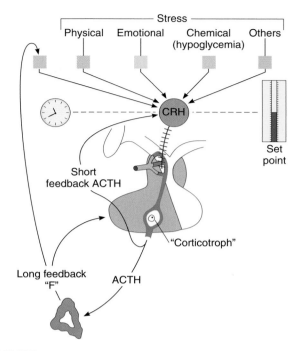

FIGURE 4–11 The hypothalamic-pituitary-adrenal axis, illustrating negative feedback by cortisol (F) at the hypothalamic and pituitary levels. A short negative feedback loop of ACTH on the secretion of corticotropin-releasing hormone (CRH) also exists. (Reproduced, with permission, from Gwinup G, Johnson B. Clinical testing of the hypothalamic-pituitary-adrenocortical system in states of hypo- and hypercortisolism. *Metabolism.* 1975;24:777).

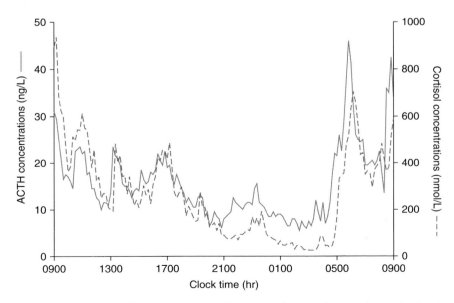

FIGURE 4–12 The episodic, pulsatile pattern of ACTH secretion and its concordance with cortisol secretion in a healthy human subject during a 24-hour period. (Previously unpublished, used with permission, from Johannes D. Veldhuis, MD.)

independent of circulating cortisol levels (ie, the magnitude of an ACTH impulse is not related to preceding plasma cortisol levels). An example is the persistence of diurnal rhythm in patients with primary adrenal failure (Addison disease). ACTH secretion also increases in response to feeding in both humans and animals.

Many stresses stimulate ACTH, often superseding the normal diurnal rhythmicity. Physical, emotional, and chemical stresses such as pain, trauma, hypoxia, acute hypoglycemia, cold exposure, surgery, depression, and interleukin-1 and vasopressin administration have all been shown to stimulate ACTH and cortisol secretion. The increase in ACTH levels during stress is mediated by vasopressin as well as CRH. Although physiologic cortisol levels do not blunt the ACTH response to stress, exogenous corticosteroids in high doses suppress it.

Negative feedback of cortisol and synthetic glucocorticoids on ACTH secretion occurs at both the hypothalamic and pituitary levels via two mechanisms: fast feedback is sensitive to the rate of change in cortisol levels, whereas slow feedback is sensitive to the absolute cortisol level. The first mechanism is probably nonnuclear; that is, this phenomenon occurs too rapidly to be explained by the influence of corticosteroids on nuclear transcription of the specific mRNA responsible for ACTH. Recent studies suggest fast feedback is mediated by a novel membrane-associated glucocorticoid receptor that stimulates a rapid synthesis and retrograde release of endocannabinoids, thereby suppressing synaptic excitation. Slow feedback, occurring later, may be explained by a nuclear-mediated mechanism and a subsequent decrease in synthesis of ACTH. This latter form of negative feedback is the type probed by the clinical dexamethasone suppression test. In addition to the negative feedback of corticoids, ACTH also inhibits its own secretion (short-loop feedback).

GROWTH HORMONE

Biosynthesis

GH or somatotropin is a 191-amino-acid polypeptide hormone (MW 21,500) synthesized and secreted by the somatotrophs of the anterior pituitary. Its larger precursor peptide, pre-GH (MW 28,000), is also secreted but has no physiologic significance.

Function

The primary function of GH is promotion of linear growth. Its basic metabolic effects serve to achieve this result, but most of the growth-promoting effects are mediated by insulin-like growth factor 1 (IGF-I; previously known as somatomedin C). The metabolic and biologic effects of GH and IGF-I are shown in Tables 4–5 and 4–6 (see also Chapter 6).

GH, via IGF-I, increases protein synthesis by enhancing amino acid uptake and directly accelerating the transcription and translation of mRNA. In addition, GH tends to decrease protein catabolism by mobilizing fat as a more efficient fuel source: it directly causes the release of fatty acids from adipose tissue and enhances their conversion to acetyl-CoA, from which energy is derived. This protein-sparing effect is an important mechanism by which GH promotes growth and development.

TABLE 4–5 Metabolic effects of GH and IGF-1 In vivo.

Function, Parameter Group	Function, Parameter Subgroup	GH	IGF-1
Carbohydrate metabolism	Glucose uptake in extrahepatic tissues	Decrease[a]	Increase
	Hepatic glucose output	Increase	Decrease
	Hepatic glycogen stores	Increase (jointly with glucocorticoids and insulin)	
	Plasma glucose	Increase	Decrease
	Insulin sensitivity	Decrease	Increase
Lipid metabolism	Lipolysis in adipocytes, plasma-free fatty acid levels	Increase	Decrease
	Plasma ketone bodies	Increase	Decrease
Protein metabolism (muscle, connective tissue)	Amino acid uptake	Increase (?)	Increase
	Protein synthesis	Increase (?)	Increase
	Nitrogen excretion	Decrease (?)	Decrease

[a]In GH-deficient patients, administration of GH results in a short-lived insulin-like action. During this time, glucose uptake by peripheral (extrahepatic) tissues increases.

Modified from Kacsoh B. *Endocrine Physiology*. McGraw-Hill; 2000.

GH also affects carbohydrate metabolism. In excess, it decreases carbohydrate utilization and impairs glucose uptake into cells. This GH-induced insulin resistance appears to be due to a postreceptor impairment in insulin action. These events result in glucose intolerance and secondary hyperinsulinism.

Measurement

GH has a plasma half-life of 10 to 20 minutes. The healthy adult secretes approximately 400 μg/d (18.6 nmol/d); in contrast, young adolescents secrete about 700 μg/d (32.5 nmol/d). The early morning GH concentration in fasting unstressed adults is less than 2 ng/mL (90 pmol/L). There are no significant sex differences.

About half of circulating GH is bound to specific GH-binding proteins (GHBPs) that function to reduce oscillations in GH levels (due to its pulsatile secretion) and prolong plasma GH half-life. GHBPs include a high-affinity GHBP (corresponding to the extracellular portion of the GH receptor formed through proteolytic cleavage) and a low-affinity species. Measurement of serum concentrations of the high-affinity GHBP provides an index of GH receptor concentrations. For example, individuals with Laron dwarfism, a form of GH insensitivity characterized by mutations in the GH receptor, usually have abnormally low levels of GHBP.

TABLE 4–6 Main biologic effect of the GH-IGF-1 axis.

Target, Source	Parameter	Effect
Blood and plasma (liver, bone, and bone marrow actions)	IGF-1, acid-labile subunit	Increased by GH only
	IGF-binding protein-3	Increased by both GH and IGF-1
	Alkaline phosphatase (bone specific)	Increase (mainly IGF-1)
	Fibrinogen	Increase
	Hemoglobin, hematocrit	Increase (mainly IGF-1 action on bone marrow)
Cartilage, bone	Length (before epiphysial closure), width (periosteal and perichondrial growth)	Stimulation (mainly IGF-1)
Visceral organs (liver, spleen, thymus, thyroid), tongue and heart	Growth	Stimulation, organomegaly (both GH and IGF-1)
Renal 25-hydroxyvitamin D 1α-hydroxylase activity	Plasma calcitriol	Increase (mainly GH), promotes positive calcium balance
Kidney	GFR	Increase (IGF-1)
Skin	Hair growth	Stimulation (IGF-1?)
	Sweat glands	Hyperplasia, hypertrophy, hyperfunction (GH?)
	Dermis	Thickening (both GH and IGF-1)

Modified from Kacsoh B. *Endocrine Physiology*. McGraw-Hill; 2000.

Concentrations of IGF-I are determined by radioreceptor assays or radioimmunoassays. Determining the levels of these mediators of GH action may result in more accurate assessment of the biologic activity of GH (see Chapter 6).

Secretion

The secretion of GH is predominantly mediated by two hypothalamic hormones: GHRH and somatostatin (GH-inhibiting hormone), both of which contribute to the episodic pattern of GH secretion. These hypothalamic influences are tightly regulated by an integrated system of neural, metabolic, and hormonal factors. Table 4–7 summarizes the many factors that affect GH secretion in physiologic, pharmacologic, and pathologic states.

A. Growth hormone–releasing hormone GHRH binds to specific receptors, stimulating cAMP production by somatotrophs and stimulating both GH synthesis and secretion. The effects of GHRH are partially blocked by somatostatin. The administration of GHRH to normal humans leads to rapid release of GH (within minutes); levels peak at 30 minutes and are sustained for 60 to 120 minutes.

Other peptide hormones such as ADH, ACTH, and α-MSH may act as GH-releasing factors when present in pharmacologic amounts. Even TSH and GnRH often cause GH secretion in patients with acromegaly; however, it is not certain whether any of these effects are mediated by the hypothalamus or represent direct effects on the somatotroph. Regulation of GHRH is primarily under neural control (see discussion later), but there is also short-loop negative feedback by GHRH itself.

B. Somatostatin Somatostatin, a tetradecapeptide, is a potent inhibitor of GH secretion. It decreases cAMP production in GH-secreting cells and inhibits both basal and stimulated GH secretion. Somatostatin secretion is increased by elevated levels of GH and IGF-I. Long-acting analogs of somatostatin have been used therapeutically in the management of GH excess and in conditions such as pancreatic and carcinoid tumors that cause diarrhea.

C. Growth hormone secretagogues Non-GHRH secretagogues act to release GH, not through the GHRH receptor, but through a separate receptor, the growth hormone secretagogue receptor (GHS-R). A number of synthetic secretagogues, both peptides and nonpeptides, have been described. **Ghrelin**, a circulating peptide made by endocrine cells in the stomach, was identified in 1999 as the endogenous ligand for GHS-R. Its location in the stomach suggests a new mechanism for regulation of GH secretion.

D. Neural control The neural control of basal GH secretion results in irregular and intermittent release associated with sleep and varying with age. Peak levels occur 1 to 4 hours after the onset of sleep (during stages 3 and 4) (Figure 4–13). These nocturnal sleep bursts, which account for nearly 70% of daily GH secretion, are greater in children and tend to decrease with age. Glucose infusion does not suppress this episodic release. Emotional, physical, and chemical stress, including surgery, trauma, exercise, electroshock therapy, and pyrogen administration, provoke GH release. In addition, impairment of secretion leading to growth failure has been well documented in children with severe emotional deprivation (see Chapter 6).

E. Metabolic control The metabolic factors affecting GH secretion include all fuel substrates: carbohydrate, protein, and fat. Glucose administration, orally or intravenously, lowers GH in

TABLE 4–7 Factors affecting GH secretion.

Increase	Decrease[a]
Physiologic	
Sleep	Postprandial hyperglycemia
Exercise	Elevated free fatty acids
Stress (physical or psychologic)	
Postprandial	
Hyperaminoacidemia	
Hypoglycemia (relative)	
Pharmacologic	
Hypoglycemia	Hormones
Absolute: insulin or 2-deoxyglucose	Somatostatin
Relative: postglucagon	Growth hormone
Hormones	Progesterone
GHRH	Glucocorticoids
Ghrelin	Neurotransmitters, etc
Peptide (ACTH, α-MSH, vasopressin)	Alpha-adrenergic
Estrogen	antagonists
Neurotransmitters, etc	(phentolamine)
Alpha-adrenergic agonists	Beta-adrenergic agonists
(clonidine)	(isoproterenol)
Beta-adrenergic antagonists	Serotonin agonists
(propranolol)	(methysergide)
Serotonin precursors	Dopamine antagonists
Dopamine agonists (levodopa,	(phenothiazines)
apomorphine, bromocriptine)	
GABA agonists (muscimol)	
Potassium infusion	
Pyrogens (pseudomonas	
endotoxin)	
Pathologic	
Protein depletion and starvation	Obesity
Anorexia nervosa	Acromegaly; dopamine
Ectopic production of GHRH	agonists
Chronic renal failure	Hypothyroidism
Acromegaly	Hyperthyroidism
TRH	
GnRH	

[a]Suppressive effects of some factors can be demonstrated only in the presence of a stimulus.

Modified and reproduced, with permission, from Frohman LA. Diseases of the anterior pituitary. In: *Endocrinology and Metabolism.* Felig P, et al, ed. McGraw-Hill, 1981.

healthy subjects and provides a simple physiologic maneuver useful in the diagnosis of acromegaly (see discussed below). In contrast, hypoglycemia stimulates GH release. This effect depends on intracellular glycopenia, because the administration of 2-deoxyglucose (a glucose analog that causes intracellular glucose deficiency) also increases GH. This response to hypoglycemia depends on both the rate of change in blood glucose and the absolute level attained.

A protein meal or intravenous infusion of amino acids (eg, arginine) causes GH release. Paradoxically, states of protein-calorie malnutrition also increase GH, possibly as a result of decreased IGF-I production and lack of inhibitory feedback.

Fatty acids suppress GH responses to certain stimuli, including arginine and hypoglycemia. Fasting stimulates GH secretion, possibly as a means of mobilizing fat as an energy source and preventing protein loss.

F. Effects of other hormones Responses to stimuli are blunted in states of cortisol excess and during hypo- and hyperthyroidism. Estrogen enhances GH secretion in response to stimulation.

G. Effects of neuropharmacologic agents Many neurotransmitters and neuropharmacologic agents affect GH secretion. Biogenic amine agonists and antagonists act at the hypothalamic level and alter GHRH or somatostatin release. Dopaminergic, alpha-adrenergic, and serotonergic agents all stimulate GH release.

Dopamine agonists such as levodopa, apomorphine, and bromocriptine increase GH secretion, whereas dopaminergic antagonists such as phenothiazines inhibit GH. The effect of levodopa, a precursor of both norepinephrine and dopamine, may be mediated by its conversion to norepinephrine, because its effect is blocked by the alpha-adrenergic antagonist phentolamine. Moreover, phentolamine suppresses GH release in response to other stimuli such as hypoglycemia, exercise, and arginine, emphasizing the importance of alpha-adrenergic mechanisms in modulating GH secretion.

Beta-adrenergic agonists inhibit GH, and beta-adrenergic antagonists such as propranolol enhance secretion in response to provocative stimuli.

PROLACTIN

Biosynthesis

PRL is a 198-amino-acid polypeptide hormone (MW 22,000) synthesized and secreted from the lactotrophs of the anterior pituitary. Despite evolution from an ancestral hormone common to GH and human placental lactogen (hPL), PRL shares only 16% of its residues with the former and 13% with hPL. A precursor molecule (MW 40,000-50,000) is also secreted and may constitute 8% to 20% of the PRL plasma immunoreactivity in healthy persons and in patients with PRL-secreting pituitary tumors. PRL and GH are structurally related to members of the cytokine-hematopoietin family that include erythropoietin, granulocyte-macrophage colony stimulating factor (GM-CSF), and interleukins IL-2 to IL-7.

Function

PRL stimulates lactation in the postpartum period (see Chapter 16). During pregnancy, PRL secretion increases and, in concert with many other hormones (estrogen, progesterone, hPL, insulin, and cortisol), promotes additional breast development in preparation for milk production. Despite its importance during pregnancy, PRL has not been demonstrated to play a role in the development of normal breast tissue in humans. During pregnancy, estrogen enhances breast development but blunts the effect of PRL on lactation; the decrease in both estrogen and progesterone after parturition allows initiation of lactation. Accordingly, galactorrhea may accompany the discontinuance of oral contraceptives or

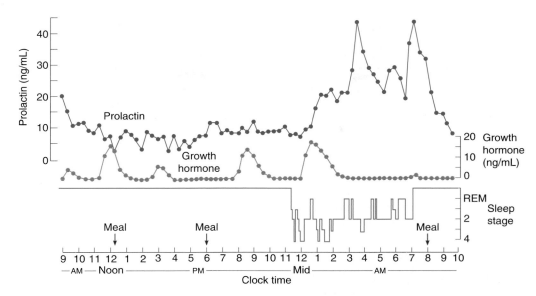

FIGURE 4–13 Sleep-associated changes in prolactin (PRL) and growth hormone (GH) secretion in humans. Peak levels of GH occur during sleep stages 3 or 4; the increase in PRL is observed 1 to 2 hours after sleep begins and is not associated with a specific sleep phase. (Reproduced, with permission, from Sassin JF, et al. Human prolactin: 24-hour pattern with increased release during sleep. *Science.* 1972;177:1205).

estrogen therapy. Although basal PRL secretion falls in the postpartum period, lactation is maintained by persistent breast suckling.

PRL levels are very high in the fetus and in newborn infants, declining during the first few months of life.

Although PRL does not appear to play a physiologic role in the regulation of gonadal function, hyperprolactinemia in humans leads to hypogonadism. In women, initially there is a shortening of the luteal phase; subsequently, anovulation, oligomenorrhea or amenorrhea, and infertility occur. In men, PRL excess leads to decreased testosterone synthesis and decreased spermatogenesis, which clinically present as decreased libido, impotence, and infertility. The exact mechanisms of PRL inhibition of gonadal function are unclear, but the principal one appears to be alteration of hypothalamic-pituitary control of gonadotropin secretion. Basal LH and FSH levels are usually normal; however, their pulsatile secretion is decreased and the midcycle LH surge is suppressed in women. Gonadotropin reserve, as assessed by administration of exogenous GnRH, is usually normal. PRL also has a role in immunomodulation; extrapituitary synthesis of PRL occurs in T lymphocytes (among other sites), and PRL receptors are present on T and B lymphocytes and macrophages. PRL modulates and stimulates both immune cell proliferation and survival.

Measurement

The PRL secretory rate is approximately 400 μg/d (18.6 nmol/d). The hormone is cleared by the liver (75%) and the kidney (25%), and its half-time of disappearance from plasma is about 25 to 50 minutes.

Basal levels of PRL in adults vary considerably, with a mean of 13 ng/mL (0.6 nmol/L) in women and 5 ng/mL (0.23 nmol/L) in

men. The upper range of normal in most laboratories is 15 to 20 ng/mL (0.7-0.9 nmol/L).

PRL is measured using a highly specific immunoradiometric assay. However, when PRL levels are extremely high, which can occur with some PRL-secreting tumors, this assay may be susceptible to the "hook effect." PRL levels are erroneously reported as normal or modestly elevated due to saturation of available assay antibodies. Appropriate sample dilutions (ie, 1:100) will avoid this artifact.

In some patients a form of PRL with molecular mass greater than 150 kDa predominates. This is termed macroprolactinemia and consists of aggregates of monomeric PRL as well as PRL-immunoglobulin G complexes. These complexes may have reduced biological activity and can be measured using polyethylene glycol precipitation of serum samples.

Secretion

The hypothalamic control of PRL secretion is predominantly inhibitory, and dopamine is the most important inhibitory factor. The physiologic, pathologic, and pharmacologic factors influencing PRL secretion are listed in Table 4–8.

A. Prolactin-releasing factors TRH is a potent PRL-releasing factor that evokes release of PRL at a threshold dose similar to that which stimulates release of TSH. An exaggerated response of both TSH and PRL to TRH is observed in primary hypothyroidism, and their responses are blunted in hyperthyroidism. In addition, PRL secretion is also stimulated by VIP and serotonergic pathways.

B. Episodic and sleep-related secretion PRL secretion is episodic. An increase is observed 60 to 90 minutes after sleep

TABLE 4–8   Factors affecting prolactin secretion.

Increase	Decrease
Physiologic	
Pregnancy	
Nursing	
Nipple stimulation	
Exercise	
Stress (hypoglycemia)	
Sleep	
Seizures	
Neonatal	
Pharmacologic	
TRH	Dopamine agonists
Estrogen	(levodopa, apomorphine,
Vasoactive intestinal peptide	bromocriptine,
Dopamine antagonists	pergolide)
(phenothiazines, haloperidol,	GABA
risperidone, metoclopramide,	
reserpine, methyldopa, amoxapine,	
opioids)	
Monoamine oxidase inhibitors	
Cimetidine (intravenous)	
Verapamil	
Licorice	
Pathologic	Pseudohypoparathyroidism
Pituitary tumors	Pituitary destruction or
Hypothalamic/pituitary stalk lesions	removal
Neuraxis irradiation	Lymphocytic hypophysitis
Chest wall lesions	
Spinal cord lesions	
Hypothyroidism	
Chronic renal failure	
Severe liver disease	

begins but—in contrast to GH—is not associated with a specific sleep phase. Peak levels are usually attained between 4 and 7 AM (see Figure 4–13). This sleep-associated augmentation of PRL release is not part of a circadian rhythm, like that of ACTH; it is related strictly to the sleeping period regardless of when it occurs during the day.

C. Other stimuli   Stresses, including surgery, exercise, hypoglycemia, and acute myocardial infarction, cause significant elevation of PRL levels. Nipple stimulation in nonpregnant women also increases PRL. This neurogenic reflex may also occur from chest wall injury such as mechanical trauma, burns, surgery, and herpes zoster of thoracic dermatomes. This reflex discharge of PRL is abolished by denervation of the nipple or by spinal cord or brain stem lesions.

D. Effects of other hormones   Many hormones influence PRL release. Estrogens augment basal and stimulated PRL secretion after 2 to 3 days of use (an effect that is of special clinical importance in patients with PRL-secreting pituitary adenomas); glucocorticoids tend to suppress TRH-induced PRL secretion; and thyroid hormone administration may blunt the PRL response to TRH.

E. Effects of pharmacologic agents (Table 4–8)   Many pharmacologic agents alter PRL secretion. Dopamine agonists (eg, bromocriptine) decrease secretion, forming the basis for their use in states of PRL excess. Dopamine antagonists (eg, receptor blockers such as phenothiazines and metoclopramide) and dopamine depletors (eg, reserpine) augment PRL release. Serotonin agonists enhance PRL secretion; serotonin receptor blockers suppress PRL release associated with stress and with nursing.

THYROTROPIN

Biosynthesis

TSH is a glycoprotein (MW 28,000) composed of two noncovalently linked alpha and beta subunits. The structure of the alpha subunit of TSH is identical to that of the other glycoprotein molecules—FSH, LH, and human chorionic gonadotropin (hCG)—but the beta subunits differ in these glycoproteins and is responsible for their biologic and immunologic specificity. The peptides of these subunits appear to be synthesized separately and united before the carbohydrate groups are attached. The intact molecule is then secreted, as are small amounts of nonlinked subunits.

Function

The beta subunit of TSH attaches to high-affinity receptors in the thyroid, stimulating iodide uptake, hormonogenesis, and release of T_4 and T_3. This occurs through activation of adenylyl cyclase and the generation of cAMP. TSH secretion also causes an increase in gland size and vascularity by promoting mRNA and protein synthesis. (For a more detailed description, see Chapter 7.)

Measurement

TSH circulates unbound in the blood with a half-life of 35 to 50 minutes. With ultrasensitive IRMAs for measuring TSH concentration, the normal range is usually 0.5 to 4.7 µU/mL (0.5-4.7 mU/L). These new assays are helpful in the diagnosis of primary hypothyroidism and hyperthyroidism; however, TSH levels alone cannot be used to evaluate pituitary or hypothalamic hypothyroidism.

The alpha subunit can be detected in about 80% of normals, with a range of 0.5 to 2 ng/mL. Plasma alpha subunit levels increase after administration of TRH in normal subjects, and basal levels are elevated in primary hypothyroidism, primary hypogonadism, and in patients with TSH-secreting, gonadotropin-secreting, or pure alpha subunit-secreting pituitary adenomas.

Secretion

The secretion of TSH is controlled by both stimulatory (TRH) and inhibitory (somatostatin) influences from the hypothalamus and in addition is modulated by the feedback inhibition of thyroid hormone on the hypothalamic-pituitary axis.

A. TRH   The response of TSH to TRH is modulated by the circulating concentration of thyroid hormones. Small changes in serum levels (even within the physiologic range) cause substantial

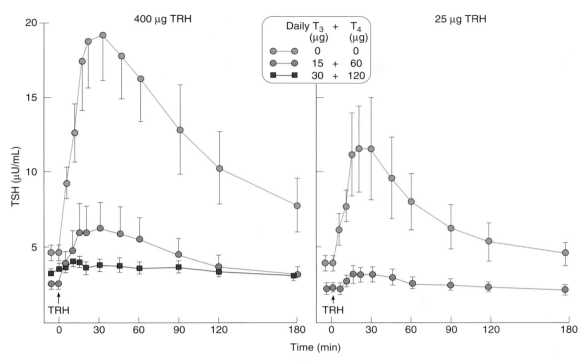

FIGURE 4–14 Administration of small doses of T_3 (15 µg) and T_4 (60 µg) to healthy subjects inhibits the TSH response to two doses (400 µg, left; 25 µg, right) of TRH (protirelin). (Reproduced, with permission, from Snyder PJ, Utiger RD. Inhibition of thyrotropin-releasing hormone by small quantities of thyroid hormones. *J Clin Invest.* 1972;51:2077).

alterations in the TSH response to TRH. As shown in Figure 4–14, the administration of T_3 (15 µg) and T_4 (60 µg) to healthy persons for 3 to 4 weeks suppresses the TSH response to TRH despite only small increases in circulating T_3 and T_4 levels. Thus, the secretion of TSH is inversely proportional to the concentration of thyroid hormone.

The set point (the level at which TSH secretion is maintained) is determined by TRH. Deviations from this set point result in appropriate changes in TSH release. Administration of TRH increases TSH within 2 minutes, and this response is blocked by previous T_3 administration; however, larger doses of TRH may overcome this blockade—suggesting that both T_3 and TRH act at the pituitary level to influence TSH secretion. In addition, T_3 and T_4 inhibit mRNA for TRH synthesis in the hypothalamus, indicating that a negative feedback mechanism operates at this level also.

B. Somatostatin This inhibitory hypothalamic peptide augments the direct inhibitory effect of thyroid hormone on the thyrotrophs. Infusion of somatostatin blunts the early morning TSH surge and suppresses high levels of TSH in primary hypothyroidism. Octreotide acetate, a somatostatin analog, has been used successfully to inhibit TSH secretion in patients with TSH-secreting pituitary tumors.

C. Neural control In addition to these hypothalamic influences on TSH secretion, neurally mediated factors may be important. Dopamine physiologically inhibits TSH secretion.

Intravenous dopamine administration decreases TSH in both healthy and hypothyroid subjects as well as blunts the TSH response to TRH. Thus, as expected, dopaminergic agonists such as bromocriptine inhibit TSH secretion and dopaminergic antagonists such as metoclopramide increase TSH secretion in euthyroid subjects.

D. Effects of cortisol and estrogens Glucocorticoid excess has been shown to impair the sensitivity of the pituitary to TRH and may lower serum TSH to undetectable levels. However, estrogens increase the sensitivity of the thyrotroph to TRH; women have a greater TSH response to TRH than men do, and pretreatment of men with estradiol increases their TRH-induced TSH response. (See also Chapter 7.)

GONADOTROPINS: LUTEINIZING HORMONE AND FOLLICLE-STIMULATING HORMONE

Biosynthesis

LH and FSH are glycoprotein gonadotropins composed of alpha and beta subunits and secreted by the same cell. The specific beta subunit confers on these hormones their unique biologic activity, as it does with TSH and hCG. The biologic activity of hCG, a placental glycoprotein, closely resembles that of LH. Human menopausal gonadotropin (hMG, menotropins)—an altered mixture of pituitary gonadotropins recovered from the urine of postmenopausal women—is a preparation with FSH-like activity. Menotropins and hCG are used clinically for induction of spermatogenesis or ovulation (see Chapters 12 and 13).

Function

LH and FSH bind to receptors in the ovary and testis and regulate gonadal function by promoting sex steroid production and gametogenesis.

In men, LH stimulates testosterone production from the interstitial cells of the testes (Leydig cells). Maturation of spermatozoa, however, requires both LH and FSH. FSH stimulates testicular growth and enhances the production of an androgen-binding protein by the Sertoli cells, which are a component of the testicular tubule necessary for sustaining the maturing sperm cell. This androgen-binding protein promotes high local concentrations of testosterone within the testis, an essential factor in the development of normal spermatogenesis (see Chapter 12).

In women, LH stimulates estrogen and progesterone production from the ovary. A surge of LH in the midmenstrual cycle is responsible for ovulation, and continued LH secretion subsequently stimulates the corpus luteum to produce progesterone by enhancing the conversion of cholesterol to pregnenolone. Development of the ovarian follicle is largely under FSH control, and the secretion of estrogen from this follicle is dependent on both FSH and LH.

Measurement

The normal levels of LH and FSH vary with the age of the subject (see Appendix). They are low before puberty and elevated in postmenopausal women. A nocturnal rise of LH in boys and the cyclic secretion of FSH and LH in girls usually herald the onset of puberty before clinical signs are apparent. In women, LH and FSH vary during the menstrual cycle; during the initial phase of the cycle (follicular), LH steadily increases, with a midcycle surge that initiates ovulation. FSH, on the other hand, initially rises and then decreases during the later follicular phase until the midcycle surge, which is concordant with LH. Both LH and FSH levels fall steadily after ovulation (see Chapter 13).

LH and FSH levels in men are similar to those in women during the follicular phase. The alpha subunit, shared by all the pituitary glycoprotein hormones, can also be measured (see TSH) and will rise following GnRH administration.

Secretion

The secretion of LH and FSH is controlled by GnRH, which maintains basal gonadotropin secretion, generates the phasic release of gonadotropins for ovulation, and determines the onset of puberty. As noted above, the size and frequency of GnRH pulses determine the ratio of gonadotropin secretion: low-frequency pulses favor FSH release while high-frequency pulses result in LH release. Many other factors are involved in regulation of this axis. For example, activins and follistatins are paracrine

factors that exert opposing effects on gonadotrophs. Leptin, a hormone made in adipocytes in proportion to fat stores, is involved in regulation of this axis and may help to explain the suppression of gonadotropin secretion that accompanies caloric restriction.

A. Episodic secretion   In both males and females, secretion of LH and FSH is episodic, with secretory bursts that occur each hour and are mediated by a concordant episodic release of GnRH. The amplitude of these secretory surges is greater in patients with primary hypogonadism. The pulsatile nature of GnRH release is critical for sustaining gonadotropin secretion. A continuous, prolonged infusion of GnRH in women evokes an initial increase in LH and FSH followed by prolonged suppression of gonadotropin secretion. This phenomenon may be explained by downregulation of GnRH receptors on the pituitary gonadotrophs. Consequently, long-acting synthetic analogs of GnRH may be used clinically to suppress LH and FSH secretion in conditions such as precocious puberty.

B. Positive feedback   Circulating sex steroids affect GnRH secretion and thus LH and FSH secretion by both positive and negative (inhibitory) feedback mechanisms. During the menstrual cycle, estrogens provide a positive influence on GnRH effects on LH and FSH secretion, and the rise in estrogen during the follicular phase is the stimulus for the LH and FSH ovulatory surge. This phenomenon suggests that the secretion of estrogen is to some extent influenced by an intrinsic ovarian cycle. Progesterone amplifies the duration of the LH and FSH surge and augments the effect of estrogen. After this midcycle surge, the developed egg leaves the ovary. Ovulation occurs approximately 10 to 12 hours after the LH peak and 24 to 36 hours after the estradiol peak. The remaining follicular cells in the ovary are converted, under the influence of LH, to a progesterone-secreting structure, the corpus luteum. After about 12 days, the corpus luteum involutes, resulting in decreased estrogen and progesterone levels and then uterine bleeding (see Chapter 13).

C. Negative feedback   Negative feedback effects of sex steroids on gonadotropin secretion also occur. In women, primary gonadal failure or menopause results in elevations of LH and FSH, which can be suppressed with long-term, high-dose estrogen therapy. However, a shorter duration of low-dose estrogen may enhance the LH response to GnRH. In men, primary gonadal failure with low circulating testosterone levels is also associated with elevated gonadotropins. However, testosterone is not the sole inhibitor of gonadotropin secretion in men, since selective destruction of the tubules (eg, by cyclophosphamide therapy) results in azoospermia and elevation of only FSH.

Inhibin, a polypeptide (MW 32,000) secreted by the Sertoli cells of the seminiferous tubules, is the major factor that inhibits FSH secretion by negative feedback. Inhibin consists of separate alpha and beta subunits connected by a disulfide bridge. Androgens stimulate inhibin production; this peptide may help to locally regulate spermatogenesis (see Chapter 12).

ENDOCRINOLOGIC EVALUATION OF THE HYPOTHALAMIC-PITUITARY AXIS

The precise assessment of the hypothalamic-pituitary axis has been made possible by radioimmunoassays of the major anterior pituitary hormones and their specific target gland hormones. In addition, provocative testing using synthetic or purified hormones (eg, ACTH, ovine CRH, glucagon, insulin) can be used to assess hypothalamic-pituitary reserve and excess.

This section describes the principles involved in testing each pituitary hormone as well as special situations (eg, drugs, obesity) that may interfere with pituitary function or pituitary testing. Specific protocols for performing and interpreting diagnostic procedures are outlined at the end of this section and in Table 4–9. The clinical manifestations of either hypo- or hypersecretion of anterior pituitary hormones are discussed in subsequent sections.

EVALUATION OF ADRENOCORTICOTROPIC HORMONE

ACTH deficiency leads to secondary adrenocortical insufficiency, characterized by decreased secretion of cortisol and the adrenal androgens; aldosterone secretion, controlled primarily by the renin-angiotensin axis, is usually maintained. In contrast, excessive ACTH secretion leads to adrenal hyperfunction (Cushing syndrome, discussed in a later section of this chapter and in Chapter 9).

Plasma ACTH Levels

Basal ACTH measurements are usually unreliable indicators of pituitary function, because its short plasma half-life and episodic secretion result in wide fluctuations in plasma levels (see Figure 4–12). Therefore, the interpretation of plasma ACTH levels requires the simultaneous assessment of cortisol secretion by the adrenal cortex. These measurements are of greatest utility in differentiating primary and secondary adrenocortical insufficiency and in establishing the etiology of Cushing syndrome (see the later section on Cushing disease and also Chapter 9).

Evaluation of ACTH Deficiency

In evaluating ACTH deficiency, measurement of basal cortisol levels is also generally unreliable. Because plasma cortisol levels are usually low in the late afternoon and evening, reflecting the normal diurnal rhythm, samples drawn at these times are of virtually no value for this diagnosis. Plasma cortisol levels are usually highest in the early morning; however, there is considerable overlap between adrenal insufficiency and normal subjects. A plasma cortisol level less than 5 µg/dL (138 nmol/L) at 8 AM strongly suggests the diagnosis—and the lower the level, the more likely the diagnosis. Conversely, a plasma cortisol greater than 20 µg/dL (552 nmol/L) virtually excludes the diagnosis. Similarly, salivary cortisol levels less than 1.8 ng/mL (5 nmol/L) at 8 AM strongly suggest adrenal insufficiency, while levels in excess of 5.8 ng/mL (16 nmol/L) greatly reduce the probability of the diagnosis.

Consequently, the diagnosis of ACTH hyposecretion (secondary adrenal insufficiency) must be established by provocative testing of the reserve capacity of the hypothalamic-pituitary axis.

Adrenal Stimulation

Because adrenal atrophy develops as a consequence of prolonged ACTH deficiency, the initial and most convenient approach to evaluation of the hypothalamic-pituitary-adrenal axis is assessment of the plasma cortisol response to synthetic ACTH (cosyntropin). In normal individuals, injection of cosyntropin (250 µg) causes a rapid increase (within 30 minutes) of cortisol to at least 18 to 20 µg/dL (496-552 nmol/L), and this response usually correlates with the cortisol response to insulin-induced hypoglycemia. A subnormal cortisol response to ACTH confirms adrenocortical insufficiency. However, a normal response does not directly evaluate the ability of the hypothalamic-pituitary axis to respond to stress (see Chapter 9). Thus, patients withdrawn from long-term glucocorticoid therapy may have an adequate increase in cortisol following exogenous ACTH that precedes complete recovery of the hypothalamic-pituitary-adrenal axis. Therefore, such patients should receive glucocorticoids during periods of stress for at least 1 year after steroids are discontinued, unless the hypothalamic-pituitary axis is shown to be responsive to stress as described below.

The more physiologic dose administered in the 1 µg ACTH test is designed to improve its sensitivity in detection of secondary adrenal insufficiency. The cortisol response to 1 µg of synthetic ACTH correlates better with the cortisol response to insulin-induced hypoglycemia in patients with complete chronic secondary adrenal insufficiency. However, the results in partial secondary adrenal insufficiency are less reliable and technical difficulties make the test impractical for routine use. Thus, the standard 250 µg ACTH test remains the procedure of choice (see discussion later and Chapter 9).

Pituitary Stimulation

Direct evaluation of pituitary ACTH reserve can be performed by means of insulin-induced hypoglycemia, metyrapone administration, or CRH stimulation. These studies are unnecessary if the cortisol response to rapid ACTH stimulation is subnormal.

A. Insulin-induced hypoglycemia The stimulus of neuroglycopenia associated with hypoglycemia (blood glucose <40 mg/dL) evokes a stress-mediated activation of the hypothalamic-pituitary-adrenal axis. Subjects should experience adrenergic symptoms (diaphoresis, tachycardia, weakness, headache) associated with the fall in blood sugar. In normal persons, plasma cortisol increases to more than 18 to 20 µg/dL (496-552 nmol/L), indicating normal ACTH reserve. Although plasma ACTH also rises, its determination has not proved to be as useful, because pulsatile secretion requires frequent sampling, and the normal response is not well standardized. Although insulin-induced hypoglycemia most reliably predicts ACTH secretory capacity in times of stress, it is rarely performed at present, because the procedure

TABLE 4–9 Endocrine tests of hypothalamic-pituitary function.

	Method	Sample Collection	Possible Side Effects; Contraindications	Interpretation
Rapid ACTH stimulation test (cosyntropin test)	Administer synthetic ACTH (1-24) (cosyntropin), 250 μg intravenously or intramuscularly. The test may be performed at any time of the day or night and does not require fasting. The low-dose test is performed in the same manner except that 1 μg of synthetic ACTH (1-24) is administered.	Obtain samples for plasma cortisol at 0 and 30 min or at 0 and 60 min.	Rare allergic reactions have been reported.	A normal response is a peak plasma cortisol level >18-20 μg/dL (496-552 nmol/L).
Insulin hypoglycemia test	Give nothing by mouth after midnight. Start an intravenous infusion with normal saline solution. Regular insulin is given intravenously in a dose sufficient to cause adequate hypoglycemia (blood glucose <40 mg/dL). The dose is 0.1-0.15 unit/kg (healthy subjects); 0.2-0.3 unit/kg (obese subjects or those with Cushing syndrome or acromegaly); 0.05 unit/kg (patients with suspected hypopituitarism).	Collect blood for glucose determinations every 15 min during the study. Samples of GH and cortisol are obtained at 0, 30, 45, 60, 75, and 90 min.	A physician must be in attendance. Symptomatic hypoglycemia (diaphoresis, headache, tachycardia, weakness) is necessary for adequate stimulation and occurs 20-35 min after insulin is administered in most patients. If severe central nervous system signs or symptoms occur, intravenous glucose (25-50 mL of 50% glucose) should be given immediately; otherwise, the test can be terminated with a meal or with oral glucose. This test is contraindicated in the elderly or in patients with cardiovascular or cerebrovascular disease and seizure disorders.	Symptomatic hypoglycemia and a fall in blood glucose to <40 mg/dL (2.2 mmol/L) will increase GH to a maximal level >5 ng/mL; some investigators regard an increment of 6 ng/mL (280 pmol/L) as normal. Plasma cortisol should increase to a peak level of at least 18-20 μg/dL (496-552 nmol/L).
Metyrapone test	Metyrapone is given orally between 11 and 12 PM with a snack to minimize gastrointestinal discomfort. The dose is 30 mg/kg.	Blood for plasma 11-deoxycortisol and cortisol determinations is obtained at 8 AM the morning after metyrapone is given.	Gastrointestinal upset may occur. Adrenal insufficiency may occur. Metyrapone should not be used in sick patients or those in whom primary adrenal insufficiency is suspected.	Serum 11-deoxycortisol should increase to >7 μg/dL (0.19 μmol/L). Cortisol should be <10 μg/dL (0.28 μmol/L) in order to ensure adequate inhibition of 11β-hydroxylation.
GHRH-arginine infusion test	The patient should be fasting after midnight. Give GHRH, 1 μg/kg intravenously over 1 min followed by arginine hydrochloride, 0.5 g/kg intravenously, up to a maximum of 30 g over 30 min.	Blood for plasma GH determinations is collected at 0, 30, 60, 90, and 120 min.	Mild flushing, a metallic taste, or nausea and vomiting may occur. This test is contraindicated in patients with severe liver disease, renal disease, or acidosis.	The lower limit of normal for the peak GH response is 6 ng/mL (280 pmol/L) although most normals reach levels of >10-15 ng/mL (460-700 pmol/L).
Glucagon stimulation test	The patient should be fasting after midnight. Give glucagon 1 mg intramuscularly.	Blood for plasma GH and capillary blood glucose at 0, 30, 60, 90, 120, 150, and 180 min.	Nausea and late hypoglycemia. This test is contraindicated in malnourished patients or patients who have not eaten for >48 h.	GH rises to >3 μg/L in normal individuals. Glucose usually rises to peak around 90 min, then gradually declines.
Glucose growth hormone suppression test	The patient should be fasting after midnight; give glucose, 75-100 g orally.	GH and glucose should be determined at 0, 30, and 60 min after glucose administration.	Patients may complain of nausea after the large glucose load.	GH levels are suppressed to <2 ng/mL (90 pmol/L) in healthy subjects. Failure of adequate suppression or a paradoxic rise may be seen in acromegaly, starvation, protein-calorie malnutrition, and anorexia nervosa.
TRH test	Fasting is not required, but since nausea may occur, it is preferred. Give protirelin, 500 μg intravenously over 15-30 s. The patient should be kept supine, since slight hypertension or hypotension may occur. Protirelin is supplied in vials of 500 μg, although 400 μg will evoke normal responses.	Blood for determination of plasma TSH and PRL is obtained at 0, 30, and 60 min. An abbreviated test utilizes samples taken at 0 and 30 min only. A maximum TSH response takes 45 min or less.	No serious complications have been reported. Most patients complain of a sensation of urinary urgency and a metallic taste in the mouth; other symptoms include flushing, palpitations, and nausea. These symptoms occur within 1-2 min of the injection and last 5 min at most.	Normal TSH response: ≥ 6 μU/mL (≥6 mU/L) in women and men aged <49 ≥ 2 μU/mL(≥ 2 mU/L) in men aged 40-79 Normal PRL response varies with gender and age.

(Continued)

TABLE 4–9 Endocrine tests of hypothalamic-pituitary function. (*Continued*)

	Method	Sample Collection	Possible Side Effects; Contraindications	Interpretation
GnRH test	The patient should be at rest but need not be fasting. Give GnRH (gonadorelin), 100 µg intravenously, over 15 s.	Blood samples for LH and FSH determinations are taken at 0, 30, and 60 min. Since the FSH response is somewhat delayed, a 90-min specimen may be necessary.	Side effects are rare, and no contraindications have been reported.	This response is dependent on sex and the time of the menstrual cycle. Table 4–9 illustrates the mean maximal change in LH and FSH after GnRH administration. An increase of LH of 1.3-2.6 µg/L (12-23 IU/L) is considered to be normal; FSH usually responds more slowly and less markedly. FSH may not increase even in healthy subjects.
Clomiphene test	Clomiphene is administered orally. For women, give 100 mg daily for 5 d (beginning on day 5 of the cycle if the patient is menstruating); for men, give 100 mg daily for 7-10 d.	Blood for LH and FSH determinations is drawn before and after clomiphene is given.	This drug may stimulate ovulation, and women should be advised accordingly.	In women, LH and FSH levels peak on the fifth day to a level above the normal range. After the fifth day, LH and FSH levels decline. In men, LH should double after 1 wk; FSH will also increase, but to a lesser extent.
CRH test	CRH (1 µg/kg) is given intravenously as a bolus injection.	Blood samples for ACTH and cortisol are taken at 0, 15, 30, and 60 min.	Flushing often occurs. Transient tachycardia and hypotension have also been reported.	The ACTH response is dependent on the assay utilized and occurs 15 min after CRH is administered. The peak cortisol response occurs at 30-60 min and is usually >10 µg/dL (276 nmol/L).
Low-dose dexamethasone suppression test	Dexamethasone (1 mg) is given between 11 PM and midnight.	Blood samples for cortisol and dexamethasone are taken at 8 AM the next morning.	Side effects are rare. Compliance is sometimes an issue. Some medications and patient variability can affect dexamethasone metabolism.	Cortisol should suppress to <1.8 µg/dL in normal individuals. This cutoff has a high sensitivity, but specificity is compromised.

requires a physician's presence and is contraindicated in elderly patients, patients with cerebrovascular or cardiovascular disease, and those with seizure disorders. It should be used with caution in patients in whom diminished adrenal reserve is suspected, because severe hypoglycemia may occur; in these patients, the test should always be preceded by the ACTH adrenal stimulation test.

B. Metyrapone stimulation   Metyrapone administration is an alternative method for assessing ACTH secretory reserve. Metyrapone inhibits P450c11 (11β-hydroxylase), the enzyme that catalyzes the final step in cortisol biosynthesis (see Chapter 9). The inhibition of cortisol secretion interrupts negative feedback on the hypothalamic-pituitary axis, resulting in a compensatory increase in ACTH. The increase in ACTH secretion stimulates increased steroid biosynthesis proximal to P450c11, and the increase can be detected as an increase in the precursor steroid (11-deoxycortisol) in plasma. The overnight test is pre-

ferred because of its simplicity; it is performed by administering 30 mg/kg of metyrapone orally at midnight. Plasma 11-deoxycortisol is determined the following morning and rises to more than 7 µg/dL (0.2 nmol/L) in healthy individuals. Again the test should be used cautiously in patients with suspected adrenal insufficiency and should be preceded by a rapid ACTH stimulation test (see discussion earlier). The traditional 3-day metyrapone test should not be used at present because of the risk of precipitating adrenal insufficiency. The overnight metyrapone test is most useful in patients with partial secondary adrenal insufficiency in whom the rapid ACTH stimulation test is normal or borderline. It has been shown to correlate well with the response to insulin-induced hypoglycemia. Metyrapone may be obtained directly from the Novartis Pharmaceutical Corporation, East Hanover, New Jersey.

C. CRH stimulation   Ovine CRH administered intravenously is used to assess ACTH secretory dynamics. In healthy subjects,

CRH (1 μg/kg) provokes a peak ACTH response within 15 minutes and a peak cortisol response within 30 to 60 minutes. This dose may be associated with mild flushing, occasional shortness of breath, tachycardia, and hypotension. Patients with primary adrenal insufficiency have elevated basal ACTH levels and exaggerated ACTH responses to CRH. Secondary adrenal insufficiency results in an absent ACTH response to CRH in patients with pituitary corticotroph destruction; however, in patients with hypothalamic dysfunction, there is a prolonged and augmented ACTH response to CRH with a delayed peak. Because of overlap between the responses of normal individuals and those with partial secondary adrenal insufficiency, the CRH test is less useful than the procedures described above.

ACTH Hypersecretion

ACTH hypersecretion is manifested by adrenocortical hyperfunction (Cushing syndrome). The diagnosis and differential diagnosis of ACTH hypersecretion and hypercortisolism are outlined in a later section on Cushing disease and also in Chapter 9. The low-dose dexamethasone suppression test is used to establish the presence of hypercortisolism regardless of its cause. Dexamethasone 1 mg is taken orally between 11 PM and midnight. The following morning at 8 AM, a blood sample is obtained for cortisol (and dexamethasone level if available or cortisol does not suppress). Cortisol values less than 1.8 μg/dL are normal. Sensitivity using this cutoff is good though specificity is compromised. Patient compliance, individual differences in dexamethasone metabolism, drugs that affect metabolism of dexamethasone, and medical conditions that alter cortisol secretion (acute illness, anxiety, depression, alcoholism) may influence the accuracy of this test.

EVALUATION OF GROWTH HORMONE

The evaluation of GH secretory reserve is important in the assessment of children with short stature and in adults with suspected hypopituitarism. Provocative tests are necessary because basal levels of GH are usually low and, therefore, do not distinguish between normal and GH-deficient patients. Special attention must be given to the methodology and the laboratory standards of GH measurement. Newer IRMAs give results that are 30% to 50% lower than older radioimmunoassays.

Insulin-Induced Hypoglycemia

The most reliable stimulus of GH secretion is insulin-induced hypoglycemia. In normal individuals, GH levels increase to more than 5 ng/mL after adequate hypoglycemia is achieved. Because 10% of normal individuals fail to respond to hypoglycemia, other stimulatory tests may be necessary.

GHRH-Arginine Test

Both forms of human GHRH (GHRH-40 and GHRH-44) have been used to evaluate GH secretory capacity. A dose of GHRH (1 μg/kg) combined with a 30-minute infusion of arginine

(0.5 g/kg to a maximum of 20 g) promptly stimulates GH; the mean peak is 10 to 15 ng/mL (460-700 pmol/L) at 30 to 60 minutes in healthy subjects. The results are comparable to those achieved with insulin-induced hypoglycemia. Unfortunately, GHRH is no longer available in the United States.

Glucagon Stimulation Test

Glucagon can also be used to evaluate GH secretory capacity. A dose of glucagon (1 mg) is given intramuscularly and GH levels are measured every 30 minutes for 3 to 4 hours. In adults with GH deficiency, peak GH levels fail to rise above 3 ng/mL.

Tests with Levodopa, Arginine, and Other Stimuli

Stimulation testing with levodopa, arginine infusion alone, or propranolol, is less reliable in the diagnosis of GH deficiency.

GH Hypersecretion

The evaluation of GH hypersecretion is discussed in the section on acromegaly and is most conveniently assessed by GH suppression testing with oral glucose and measurement of IGF-I levels.

EVALUATION OF PROLACTIN

PRL secretion by the pituitary is the most resistant to local damage, and decreased PRL secretory reserve indicates severe intrinsic pituitary disease.

PRL hypersecretion is a common endocrine problem. Macroprolactinemia can be assessed using polyethylene glycol precipitation of serum samples. Additional evaluation of hyperprolactinemia is discussed in the section on prolactinomas.

EVALUATION OF THYROID-STIMULATING HORMONE

Basal Measurements

The laboratory evaluation of TSH secretory reserve begins with an assessment of target gland secretion; thyroid function tests (free thyroxine [FT_4]) should be obtained. Normal thyroid function studies in a clinically euthyroid patient indicate adequate TSH secretion, and no further studies are warranted. Laboratory evidence of hypothyroidism requires measurement of a TSH level. With primary thyroid gland failure, the TSH level is elevated; low or normal TSH in the presence of hypothyroidism suggests hypothalamic-pituitary dysfunction (see Chapter 7).

TRH Test

Because accurate methods for determining TSH and FT_4 readily establish the diagnosis of hypothyroidism in virtually all patients, the TRH test is rarely indicated today (TRH is also not currently commercially available).

EVALUATION OF LH AND FSH

Testosterone and Estrogen Levels

The evaluation of gonadotropin function also requires assessment of target gland secretory function, and measurement of gonadal steroids (testosterone in men, estradiol in women) is useful in the diagnosis of hypogonadism. In women, the presence of regular menstrual cycles is strong evidence that the hypothalamic-pituitary-gonadal axis is intact. Estradiol levels rarely fall below 50 pg/mL (180 pmol/L), even during the early follicular phase. A level of less than 30 pg/mL (110 pmol/L) in the presence of oligomenorrhea or amenorrhea is indicative of gonadal failure. In men, serum testosterone (normal range, 300-1000 ng/dL; 10-35 nmol/L) is a sensitive index of gonadal function (see Chapters 12 and 13).

LH and FSH Levels

In the presence of gonadal insufficiency, high LH and FSH levels are a sign of primary gonadal failure; low or normal LH and FSH suggest hypothalamic-pituitary dysfunction (hypogonadotropic hypogonadism).

GnRH Test

LH and FSH secretory reserves may be assessed with the use of synthetic GnRH (gonadorelin). Administration of GnRH causes a prompt increase in plasma LH and a lesser and slower increase in FSH. However, in most patients, the GnRH test provides no more useful information than is obtained by measurement of basal gonadotropin and gonadal steroid levels. Thus, this test is uncommonly performed.

PROBLEMS IN EVALUATION OF THE HYPOTHALAMIC-PITUITARY AXIS

This section briefly outlines some of the disorders and conditions that may cause confusion and lead to misinterpretation of pituitary function tests. The effects of drugs are described in the next section.

Obesity

GH dynamics are impaired in many severely obese patients; all provocative stimuli, including insulin-induced hypoglycemia, arginine, levodopa, and glucagon plus propranolol, often fail to provoke GH secretion. The GH response to GHRH is also impaired in obesity and improves with weight loss. Obesity is also a common cause of hypogonadotropic hypogonadism in adult men.

Diabetes Mellitus

Although glucose normally suppresses GH secretion, most individuals with type 1 diabetes have normal or elevated GH levels that often do not rise further in response to hypoglycemia or arginine. Levodopa increases GH in some diabetic patients, and even a dopamine infusion (which produces no GH change in nondiabetic subjects, because it does not cross the blood–brain barrier), stimulates GH in diabetic patients. Despite the increased GH secretion in patients with inadequately controlled diabetes, the GH response to GHRH in insulin-dependent diabetic patients is similar to that of nondiabetic subjects. IGF-I levels are low in insulin-deficient diabetes despite the elevated GH levels.

Uremia

Basal levels of GH, PRL, LH, FSH, TSH, and free cortisol tend to be elevated, for the most part owing to prolongation of their plasma half-life. GH may paradoxically increase following glucose administration and is often hyperresponsive to a hypoglycemic stimulus. Although the administration of TRH (protirelin) has no effect on GH secretion in healthy subjects, the drug may increase GH in patients with chronic renal failure. The response of PRL to TRH is blunted and prolonged. Gonadotropin response to synthetic GnRH usually remains intact. Dexamethasone suppression of cortisol may be impaired.

Starvation and Anorexia Nervosa

GH secretion increases with fasting and malnutrition, and such conditions may cause a paradoxical increase in GH following glucose administration. Severe starvation, such as occurs in patients with anorexia nervosa, may result in low levels of gonadal steroids. LH and FSH responses to GnRH may be intact despite a state of functional hypogonadotropic hypogonadism. Cortisol levels may be increased and fail to suppress adequately with dexamethasone. PRL and TSH dynamics are usually normal despite a marked decrease in circulating total thyroid hormones (see Chapter 7).

Depression

Depression may alter the ability of dexamethasone to suppress plasma cortisol and may elevate cortisol secretion; the response to insulin-induced hypoglycemia usually remains intact. In addition, late-evening salivary cortisol levels usually remain normal and are not elevated as seen in patients with Cushing syndrome. The ACTH response to CRH is blunted in endogenous depression. Some depressed patients also have abnormal GH dynamics: TRH may increase GH, and hypoglycemia or levodopa may fail to increase GH. These patients may also show blunted TSH responses to TRH.

EFFECTS OF PHARMACOLOGIC AGENTS ON HYPOTHALAMIC-PITUITARY FUNCTION

Glucocorticoid excess impairs the GH response to hypoglycemia, the TSH response to TRH, and the LH response to GnRH. Estrogens tend to augment GH dynamics as well as the PRL and TSH response to TRH. Estrogens increase plasma cortisol secondary to a rise in corticosteroid-binding globulin and may result in inadequate suppression with dexamethasone.

Phenytoin enhances the metabolism of dexamethasone, making clinical testing in patients of this agent difficult to interpret. Phenothiazines may blunt the GH response to hypoglycemia and levodopa and frequently cause hyperprolactinemia. The many other pharmacologic agents that increase PRL secretion are listed in Table 4–8.

Narcotics, including heroin, morphine, and methadone, may all raise PRL levels and suppress GH and cortisol response to hypoglycemia.

In chronic alcoholics, alcohol excess or withdrawal may increase cortisol levels and cause inadequate dexamethasone suppression and an impaired cortisol increase after hypoglycemia.

ENDOCRINE TESTS OF HYPOTHALAMIC-PITUITARY FUNCTION

Methods for performing endocrine tests and their normal responses are summarized in Table 4–9. The indications for and the clinical utility of these procedures are described in the preceding section and will be mentioned again in the section on pituitary and hypothalamic disorders.

NEURORADIOLOGIC EVALUATION

Symptoms of pituitary hormone excess or deficiency, headache, or visual disturbance lead the clinician to consider a hypothalamic-pituitary disorder. In this setting, accurate neuroradiologic assessment of the hypothalamus and pituitary is essential in confirming the existence and defining the extent of hypothalamic-pituitary lesions. However, the diagnosis of such lesions should be based on both endocrine and radiologic criteria, because variability of pituitary anatomy in the normal population may lead to false-positive interpretations. Furthermore, patients with pituitary microadenomas may have normal neuroradiologic studies. Imaging studies must be interpreted in light of the fact that 10% to 20% of the general population harbor nonfunctional and asymptomatic pituitary microadenomas.

Magnetic Resonance Imaging

MRI is the current procedure of choice for imaging the hypothalamus and pituitary. It has superseded the use of computed tomography (CT) because it allows better definition of normal structures and has better resolution in defining tumors. Arteriography is rarely utilized at present except in patients with intrasellar or parasellar aneurysms.

Imaging is performed in sagittal and coronal planes at 1.5 to 2 mm intervals. This allows clear definition of hypothalamic and pituitary anatomy and can accurately visualize lesions as small as 3 to 5 mm. The use of the heavy-metal contrast agent gadolinium allows even more precise differentiation of small pituitary adenomas from normal anterior pituitary tissue and other adjacent structures as shown in Figure 4–15.

A. Normal anatomy   The normal anterior pituitary is 5 to 7 mm in height and approximately 10 mm in its lateral dimensions. The superior margin is flat or concave but may be upwardly convex with a height of 10 to 12 mm in healthy menstruating young women. The floor of the sella turcica is formed by the bony roof of the sphenoid sinus, and its lateral margins are formed by the dural membranes of the cavernous sinuses, which contain the carotid arteries and the third, fourth, and sixth cranial nerves. The posterior pituitary appears on MRI as a high-signal-intensity structure, the "posterior pituitary bright spot," which is absent in patients with diabetes insipidus. The pituitary stalk, which is normally in the midline, is 2 to 3 mm in diameter and 5 to 7 mm in length. The pituitary stalk joins the inferior hypothalamus below the third ventricle and posterior to the optic chiasm. All of these normal structures are readily visualized with MRI; the normal pituitary and the pituitary stalk show increased signal intensity with gadolinium.

B. Microadenomas   These lesions, which range from 2 to 10 mm in diameter, appear as low-signal-intensity lesions on MRI and do not usually enhance with gadolinium. Adenomas less than 5 mm in diameter may not be visualized and do not usually alter the normal pituitary contour. Lesions greater than 5 mm in diameter create a unilateral convex superior gland margin and usually cause deviation of the pituitary stalk toward the side opposite the adenoma.

MRI scans must be interpreted with caution, because minor abnormalities occur in 10% of patients who have had incidental high-resolution scans but no clinical pituitary disease. These abnormalities may represent the clinically insignificant pituitary abnormalities that occur in 10% to 20% of the general population, and they may also be due to small intrapituitary cysts, which usually occur in the pars intermedia. Artifacts within the sella turcica associated with the bones of the skull base may also result in misinterpretation of imaging studies. Finally, many patients with pituitary microadenomas have normal high-resolution MRI scans. Therefore, despite increased accuracy of neuroradiologic diagnosis, the presence or absence of a small pituitary tumor and the decision concerning its treatment must be based on the entire clinical picture.

C. Macroadenomas   Pituitary adenomas greater than 10 mm in diameter are readily visualized with MRI scans, and the scan also defines the adjacent structures and degree of extension of the lesion. Thus, larger tumors show compression of the normal pituitary and distortion of the pituitary stalk. Adenomas larger than 1.5 cm frequently have suprasellar extension, and MRI scans show compression and upward displacement of the optic chiasm. Less commonly, there is lateral extension and invasion of the cavernous sinus.

D. Other uses   High-resolution MRI scanning is also a valuable tool in the diagnosis of empty sella syndrome, hypothalamic tumors, and other parasellar lesions.

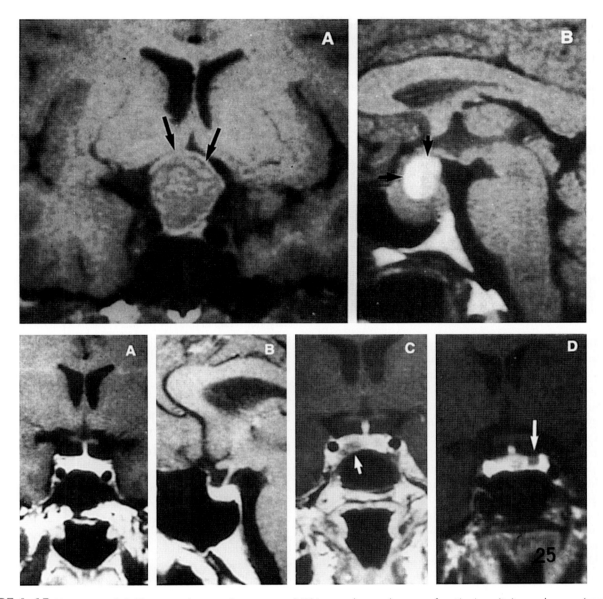

FIGURE 4–15 **Upper panel: A:** The coronal magnetic resonance (MR) image shows a large nonfunctioning pituitary adenoma (arrows) with pronounced suprasellar extension and chiasmal compression. **B:** A sagittal MR image of another large pituitary adenoma shows spontaneous hemorrhage within the suprasellar portion of the adenoma (arrows). (Photographs courtesy of David Norman, MD. Reproduced, with permission, from *West J Med.* 1995;162:342, 350.)

Lower panel: Gadolinium-enhanced MR images are shown of the pituitary gland. **A and B:** Coronal and sagittal images show the normal, uniformly enhancing pituitary stalk and pituitary gland. **C:** A pituitary microadenoma appears as a low-intensity lesion in the inferior aspect of the right lobe of the gland (arrow). **D:** The pituitary microadenoma appears as a low-intensity lesion between the left lobe of the pituitary and the left cavernous sinus (arrow). (Photographs courtesy of David Norman, MD.)

PITUITARY AND HYPOTHALAMIC DISORDERS

Hypothalamic-pituitary lesions present with a variety of manifestations, including pituitary hormone hypersecretion and hyposecretion, sellar enlargement, and visual loss. The approach to evaluation should be designed to ensure early diagnosis at a stage when the lesions are amenable to therapy.

Etiology and Early Manifestations

In adults, the most common cause of hypothalamic-pituitary dysfunction is a pituitary adenoma, of which the great majority are hypersecreting. Thus, the earliest symptoms of such tumors are due to endocrinologic abnormalities—hypogonadism is the most frequent manifestation—and these precede sellar enlargement and local manifestations such as headache and visual loss, which are late manifestations seen only in patients with larger tumors or suprasellar extension.

In children, pituitary adenomas are uncommon; the most frequent structural lesions causing hypothalamic-pituitary dysfunction are craniopharyngiomas and other hypothalamic tumors. These also usually manifest as endocrine disturbances (low GH levels, delayed puberty, diabetes insipidus) prior to the development of headache, visual loss, or other central nervous system symptoms.

Common and Later Manifestations

A. Pituitary hypersecretion   PRL is the hormone most commonly secreted in excess amounts by pituitary adenomas, and it is usually elevated in patients with hypothalamic disorders and pituitary stalk compression as well. Thus, PRL measurement is essential in evaluating patients with suspected pituitary disorders and should be performed in patients presenting with galactorrhea, gonadal dysfunction, secondary gonadotropin deficiency, or enlargement of the sella turcica. Hypersecretion of GH or ACTH leads to the more characteristic syndromes of acromegaly and Cushing disease (see discussion later).

B. Pituitary insufficiency   Although panhypopituitarism is a classic manifestation of pituitary adenomas, it is present in less than 20% of patients in current large series because of earlier diagnosis of these lesions.

The earliest clinical manifestation of a pituitary adenoma in adults is hypogonadism secondary to elevated levels of PRL, GH, or ACTH and cortisol. The hypogonadism in these patients is due to interference with the secretion of GnRH rather than to destruction of anterior pituitary tissue. Thus, patients with hypogonadism should first be screened with FSH and LH measurements to exclude primary gonadal failure (elevated FSH or LH) and those with hypogonadotropic hypogonadism should have serum PRL levels measured and be examined for clinical evidence of GH or ACTH and cortisol excess.

In children, short stature is the most frequent clinical presentation of hypothalamic-pituitary dysfunction; in these patients, GH deficiency should be considered (see Chapter 6).

TSH or ACTH deficiency is relatively unusual and, if present, usually indicates panhypopituitarism. Thus, patients with secondary hypothyroidism or hypoadrenalism should undergo a complete assessment of pituitary function and neuroradiologic studies, because panhypopituitarism and large pituitary tumors are common in this setting. PRL measurement is again essential, because prolactinomas are the most frequent pituitary tumors in adults.

C. Enlarged sella turcica   Patients may present with enlargement of the sella turcica, which may be noted on radiographs performed for head trauma or on sinus series. These patients usually have either a pituitary adenoma or empty sella syndrome. Other less common causes include craniopharyngioma, lymphocytic hypophysitis, and carotid artery aneurysm. Evaluation should include clinical assessment of pituitary dysfunction and measurements of PRL and thyroid and adrenal function. Pituitary function is usually normal in the empty sella syndrome; this diagnosis can be confirmed by MRI. Patients with clinical or laboratory evidence of pituitary dysfunction usually have a pituitary adenoma.

D. Visual field defects   Patients presenting with bitemporal hemianopsia or unexplained visual field defects or visual loss should be considered to have a pituitary or hypothalamic disorder until proven otherwise. The initial steps in diagnosis should be neuro-ophthalmologic evaluation and neuroradiologic studies with MRI, which will reveal the tumor if one is present. These patients should also have PRL measurements and be assessed for anterior pituitary insufficiency, which is especially common with large pituitary adenomas.

In addition to causing visual field defects, large pituitary lesions may extend laterally into the cavernous sinus, compromising the function of the third, fourth, or sixth cranial nerve, leading to diplopia.

E. Diabetes insipidus   Diabetes insipidus is a common manifestation of hypothalamic lesions and metastases to the pituitary, but is rare in primary pituitary lesions. Diagnostic evaluation is described in Chapter 5. In addition, all patients should undergo radiologic evaluation and assessment of anterior pituitary function.

EMPTY SELLA SYNDROME

Etiology and Incidence

Empty sella syndrome occurs when the subarachnoid space extends into the sella turcica, partially filling it with cerebrospinal fluid. This process causes remodeling and enlargement of the sella turcica and flattening of the pituitary gland.

Primary empty sella syndrome resulting from congenital incompetence of the diaphragma sellae (Figure 4–16) is common, with an incidence in autopsy series ranging from 5% to 23%. It is the most frequent cause of enlarged sella turcica. An empty sella is also commonly seen after pituitary surgery or radiation therapy and may also occur following postpartum pituitary infarction (Sheehan syndrome). In addition, both PRL-secreting and GH-secreting pituitary adenomas may undergo subclinical hemorrhagic infarction and cause contraction of the overlying suprasellar cistern downward into the sella. Therefore, the presence of an empty sella does not exclude the possibility of a coexisting pituitary tumor.

Clinical Features

A. Symptoms and signs   Most patients are middle-aged obese women. Many have systemic hypertension; benign intracranial hypertension may also occur. Although 48% of patients complain of headache, this feature may have only initiated the evaluation (ie, skull x-rays), and its relationship to the empty sella is probably coincidental. Serious clinical manifestations are uncommon. Spontaneous cerebrospinal fluid rhinorrhea and visual field impairment may occur rarely.

Normal

Empty sella

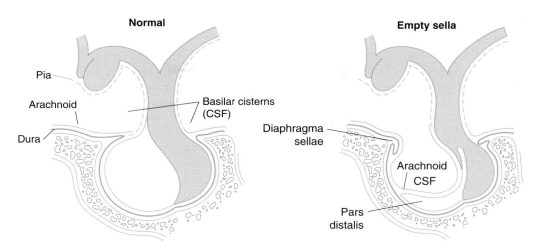

FIGURE 4–16 Representation of the normal relationship of the meninges to the pituitary gland **(left)** and the findings in the empty sella **(right)** as the arachnoid membrane herniates through the incompetent diaphragma sellae. (Reproduced, with permission, from Jordan RM, Kendall JW, Kerber CW. The primary empty sella syndrome: analysis of the clinical characteristics, radiographic features, pituitary function, and cerebrospinal fluid adenohypophysial hormone concentrations. *Am J Med*. 1977;62:569).

B. Laboratory findings   Tests of anterior pituitary function are almost always normal, although some patients have hyperprolactinemia. Endocrine function studies should be performed to exclude pituitary hormone insufficiency or a hypersecretory pituitary microadenoma.

Diagnosis

The diagnosis of empty sella syndrome can be readily confirmed by MRI, which demonstrates the herniation of the diaphragma sellae and the presence of cerebrospinal fluid in the sella turcica.

HYPOTHALAMIC DYSFUNCTION

Hypothalamic dysfunction is most often caused by tumors, of which craniopharyngioma is the most common in children, adolescents, and young adults. In older adults, primary central nervous system tumors and those arising from hypothalamic (epidermoid and dermoid tumors) and pineal structures (pinealomas) are more common. Other causes of hypothalamic-pituitary dysfunction are discussed below in the section on hypopituitarism.

Clinical Features

A. Craniopharyngioma   Craniopharyngiomas are thought to originate from metaplasia of remnant epithelial cell rests in Rathke pouch and the craniopharyngeal duct during development. The differential diagnosis includes Rathke cleft cysts and arachnoid cysts. Rathke cleft cysts are a common incidental finding within the pituitary, but may present with symptoms similar to craniopharyngiomas. Although Rathke cleft cysts and craniopharyngiomas are both thought to arise from Rathke pouch during development, craniopharyngiomas tend to be more aggressive and are more likely to recur after resection.

The initial symptoms of craniopharyngioma in children and adolescents are predominantly endocrinologic; however, these manifestations are frequently unrecognized, and at diagnosis more than 80% of patients have hypothalamic-pituitary endocrine deficiencies. These endocrine abnormalities may precede presenting symptoms by months or years; GH deficiency is most common, with about 50% of patients having growth retardation and approximately 70% decreased GH responses to stimulation at diagnosis. Gonadotropin deficiency leading to absent or arrested puberty is usual in older children and adolescents; TSH and ACTH deficiencies are less common, and diabetes insipidus is present in about 15%.

Symptoms leading to the diagnosis are frequently neurologic and due to the mass effect of the expanding tumor. Symptoms of increased intracranial pressure such as headache and vomiting are present in about 40% of patients; decreased visual acuity or visual field defects are the presenting symptoms in another 35%. MRI confirms the tumor in virtually all patients; in 95%, the tumor is suprasellar.

In adults, craniopharyngiomas have similar presentations; that is, the diagnosis is usually reached as a result of investigation of complaints of headache or visual loss. However, endocrine manifestations—especially hypogonadism, diabetes insipidus, or other deficiencies of anterior pituitary hormones—usually precede these late manifestations. MRI readily demonstrates the tumors, which in adults are almost always both intrasellar and suprasellar. The appearance is typically of a heterogeneous, cystic mass that enhances with contrast. Calcifications may also be present.

B. Other tumors   Other hypothalamic or pineal tumors and primary central nervous system tumors involving the hypothalamus have variable presentations in both children and adults. Thus, presentation is with headache, visual loss, symptoms of increased intracranial pressure, growth failure, various degrees of hypopituitarism, or diabetes insipidus. Endocrine deficiencies usually precede neurologic manifestations. Hypothalamic tumors in childhood may present with precocious puberty.

C. Other manifestations of hypothalamic dysfunction

Lesions in the hypothalamus can cause many other abnormalities, including disorders of consciousness, behavior, thirst, appetite, and temperature regulation. These abnormalities are usually accompanied by hypopituitarism and diabetes insipidus.

Somnolence can occur with hypothalamic lesions, as can a variety of changes in emotional behavior. Decreased or absent thirst may occur and predispose these patients to dehydration. When diminished thirst accompanies diabetes insipidus, fluid balance is difficult to control. Hypothalamic dysfunction may also cause increased thirst, leading to polydipsia and polyuria that may mimic diabetes insipidus. Obesity is common in patients with hypothalamic tumors because of hyperphagia, decreased satiety, and decreased activity. Frohlich syndrome, or adiposogenital dystrophy, is characterized by obesity, growth retardation, and delayed development of sexual organs. Anorexia and weight loss are unusual manifestations of these tumors.

Temperature regulation can also be disordered in these patients. Sustained or, less commonly, paroxysmal hyperthermia can occur following acute injury due to trauma, hemorrhage, or craniotomy. This problem usually lasts less than 2 weeks. Poikilothermia, the inability to adjust to changes in ambient temperature, can occur in patients with bilateral hypothalamic lesions. These patients most frequently exhibit hypothermia but can also develop hyperthermia during hot weather. A few patients manifest sustained hypothermia due to anterior hypothalamic lesions.

Diagnosis

Patients with suspected hypothalamic tumors should undergo MRI to determine the extent and nature of the tumor. Complete assessment of anterior pituitary function is necessary in these patients, because deficiencies are present in the great majority (see section on Hypopituitarism below), and the evaluation will establish the requirements for replacement therapy. PRL levels should also be determined, because most hypothalamic lesions cause hyperprolactinemia either by hypothalamic injury or by damage to the pituitary stalk.

Treatment

Treatment depends on the type of tumor. Because complete resection of craniopharyngioma is usually not feasible, this tumor is best managed by limited neurosurgical removal of accessible tumor and decompression of cysts, followed by radiotherapy. Patients treated by this method have a recurrence rate of approximately 20%; with surgery alone, the recurrence rate approximates 80%.

Other hypothalamic tumors are usually not completely resectable; however, biopsy is indicated to arrive at a histologic diagnosis.

HYPOPITUITARISM

Hypopituitarism is manifested by diminished or absent secretion of one or more pituitary hormones. The development of signs and symptoms is often slow and insidious, depending on the rate of onset and the magnitude of hypothalamic-pituitary damage—factors that are influenced by the underlying pathogenesis. Hypopituitarism is either a primary event caused by destruction of the anterior pituitary gland or a secondary phenomenon resulting from deficiency of hypothalamic stimulatory factors normally acting on the pituitary. In general, acquired loss of anterior pituitary function follows the sequence of GH, LH/FSH, TSH, ACTH, and PRL. Treatment and prognosis depend on the extent of hypofunction, the underlying cause, and the location of the lesion in the hypothalamic-pituitary axis.

Etiology

The etiologic considerations in hypopituitarism are diverse. As shown below, a helpful mnemonic device is the phrase "nine Is": invasive, infarction, infiltrative, injury, immunologic, iatrogenic, infectious, idiopathic, and isolated. Most of these lesions may cause pituitary or hypothalamic failure (or both). Establishing the precise cause of hypopituitarism is helpful in determining treatment and prognosis.

A. Invasive

Space-occupying lesions cause hypopituitarism by destroying the pituitary gland or hypothalamic nuclei or by disrupting the hypothalamic-hypophysial portal venous system. Large pituitary adenomas cause hypopituitarism by these mechanisms, and pituitary function may improve after their removal. Small pituitary tumors—microadenomas (<10 mm in diameter)—characteristically seen in the hypersecretory states (excess PRL, GH, ACTH) do not directly cause pituitary insufficiency. Craniopharyngioma, the most common tumor of the hypothalamic-pituitary region in children, frequently impairs pituitary function by its compressive effects. Primary central nervous system tumors, including meningioma, chordoma, optic glioma, epidermoid tumors, and dermoid tumors, may decrease hypothalamic-pituitary secretion by their mass effects. Metastatic lesions to this area are common (especially breast carcinoma) but rarely result in clinically obvious hypopituitarism. Anatomic malformations such as basal encephalocele and parasellar aneurysms cause hypothalamic-pituitary dysfunction and may enlarge the sella turcica and mimic pituitary tumors.

B. Infarction

Ischemic damage to the pituitary has long been recognized as a cause of hypopituitarism. In 1914, Simmonds reported pituitary necrosis in a woman with severe puerperal sepsis and in 1937 Sheehan published his classic description of its occurrence following postpartum hemorrhage and vascular collapse. The mechanism for the ischemia in such cases is not certain. Hypotension along with vasospasm of the hypophysial arteries is currently believed to compromise arterial perfusion of the anterior pituitary. During pregnancy, the pituitary gland may be more sensitive to hypoxemia because of its increased metabolic needs or more susceptible to the prothrombotic effects of the hyperestrogenic state. Some investigators have noted that the hypopituitarism does not always correlate with the degree of hemorrhage but that there is good correlation between the pituitary lesion and severe disturbances of the clotting mechanism (as in patients with placenta previa). Ischemic pituitary necrosis has also been reported to occur with greater frequency in patients with diabetes mellitus.

The extent of pituitary damage determines the rapidity of onset as well as the magnitude of pituitary hypofunction. The gland has a great secretory reserve, and more than 75% must be destroyed before clinical manifestations are evident. The initial clinical feature in postpartum necrosis may be failure to lactate after parturition; failure to resume normal menstrual periods is another clue to the diagnosis. However, the clinical features of hypopituitarism are often subtle, and years may pass before pituitary insufficiency is recognized following an ischemic insult.

Spontaneous hemorrhagic infarction of a pituitary tumor (pituitary apoplexy) frequently results in partial or total pituitary insufficiency. Pituitary apoplexy is often a fulminant clinical syndrome manifested by severe headache, visual impairment, ophthalmoplegias, meningismus, and an altered level of consciousness. Pituitary apoplexy is usually associated with a pituitary tumor; it may also be related to diabetes mellitus, radiotherapy, or open heart surgery. Acute pituitary failure with hypotension may result, and rapid mental deterioration, coma, and death may ensue. Emergency treatment with corticosteroids (see Chapter 24) and transsphenoidal decompression of the intrasellar contents may be lifesaving and may prevent permanent visual loss. Most patients who have survived pituitary apoplexy have developed multiple adenohypophysial deficits, but infarction of the tumor in some patients may cure the hypersecretory pituitary adenoma and its accompanying endocrinopathy. Pituitary infarction may also be a subclinical event (silent pituitary apoplexy), resulting in improvement of pituitary hormone hypersecretion without impairing the secretion of other anterior pituitary hormones.

C. Infiltrative Hypopituitarism may be the initial clinical manifestation of infiltrative disease processes such as sarcoidosis, hemochromatosis, and Langerhan histiocytosis.

1. **Sarcoidosis**—The most common intracranial sites of involvement of sarcoidosis are the hypothalamus and pituitary gland. At one time, the most common endocrine abnormality in patients with sarcoidosis was thought to be diabetes insipidus; however, many of these patients actually have centrally mediated disordered control of thirst that results in polydipsia and polyuria, which in some cases explains the abnormal water metabolism. Deficiencies of multiple anterior pituitary hormones have been well documented in sarcoidosis and are usually secondary to hypothalamic insufficiency. Granulomatous involvement of the hypothalamic-pituitary unit is occasionally extensive, resulting in visual impairment, and therefore, may simulate the clinical presentation of a pituitary or hypothalamic tumor.

2. **Hemochromatosis**— Hypopituitarism, particularly hypogonadotropic hypogonadism, is a prominent manifestation of iron storage disease—either primary (hereditary) hemochromatosis or transfusional iron overload. Hypogonadism occurs in most such cases and is often the initial clinical feature of iron excess; complete iron studies should be considered in any patient presenting with unexplained hypogonadotropic hypogonadism. If the diagnosis is established early, hypogonadism in hemochromatosis may be reversible with iron depletion. Pituitary deficiencies of TSH, GH, and ACTH may occur later in the course of the disease and are not reversible by iron chelation therapy.

3. **Langerhan histiocytosis**— In this disorder, the infiltration of multiple organs by well-differentiated histiocytes, is often heralded by the onset of diabetes insipidus and anterior pituitary hormone deficiencies. Most histologic and biochemical studies have indicated that this infiltrative process involves chiefly the hypothalamus, and hypopituitarism occurs only as a result of hypothalamic damage.

D. Injury Severe head trauma may cause anterior pituitary insufficiency and diabetes insipidus. Posttraumatic anterior hypopituitarism may be due to injury to the anterior pituitary, the pituitary stalk, or the hypothalamus. Pituitary insufficiency with growth retardation has been described in battered children who suffer closed head trauma with subdural hematoma.

E. Immunologic Lymphocytic hypophysitis resulting in anterior hypopituitarism is a distinct entity, occurring most often in women during pregnancy or in the postpartum period. It may present as a mass lesion of the sella turcica with visual field disturbances simulating pituitary adenoma. An autoimmune process with extensive infiltration of the gland by lymphocytes and plasma cells destroys the anterior pituitary cells. These morphologic features are similar to those of other autoimmune endocrinopathies (eg, thyroiditis, adrenalitis, and oophoritis). About 50% of patients with lymphocytic hypophysitis have other endocrine autoimmune disease, and circulating pituitary autoantibodies have been found in several cases. It is presently uncertain how this disorder should be diagnosed and treated. It must be considered in the differential diagnosis of women with pituitary gland enlargement and hypopituitarism during pregnancy or the postpartum period.

Lymphocytic hypophysitis may result in isolated hormone deficiencies (especially ACTH or prolactin). Consequently, women with this type of hypopituitarism may continue to menstruate while suffering from secondary hypothyroidism or hypoadrenalism.

F. Iatrogenic Both surgical and radiation therapy to the pituitary gland may compromise its function. The anterior pituitary is quite resilient during transsphenoidal microsurgery, and despite extensive manipulation during the search for microadenomas, anterior pituitary function is usually preserved. The dose of conventional radiation therapy presently employed to treat pituitary tumors is 4500 to 5000 cGy and results in a 50% to 60% incidence of hypothalamic and pituitary insufficiency. Such patients most frequently have modest hyperprolactinemia (PRL 30-100 ng/mL [1.3-4.5 nmol/L]) with GH and gonadotropin failure; TSH and ACTH deficiencies are less common. Heavy particle (proton beam) irradiation and gamma knife radiosurgery for pituitary tumors results in a 15% to 55% incidence of hypopituitarism. Irradiation of tumors of the head and neck (nasopharyngeal cancer, brain tumors) and prophylactic cranial irradiation in leukemia may also cause hypopituitarism. The clinical onset of pituitary failure in such patients is usually insidious and results from both pituitary and hypothalamic injury.

G. Infectious Although many infectious diseases, including tuberculosis, syphilis, and mycotic infections, have been implicated as causative agents in pituitary hypofunction, antimicrobial drugs have now made them rare causes of hypopituitarism.

H. Idiopathic In some patients with hypopituitarism, no underlying cause is found. These may be isolated (see discussion later) or multiple deficiencies. Familial forms of hypopituitarism characterized by a small, normal, or enlarged sella turcica have been described. Both autosomal recessive and X-linked recessive inheritance patterns have been reported. A variety of complex congenital disorders may include deficiency of one or more pituitary hormones (eg, Prader-Willi syndrome, septo-optic dysplasia). Although progress has been made into understanding the genetic basis for some of these disorders, the pathogenesis remains uncertain.

I. Isolated Isolated (monotropic) deficiencies of the anterior pituitary hormones have been described. Some of these have been associated with mutations in the genes coding for the specific hormones. Others, particularly GH deficiency, have been associated with mutations in genes necessary for normal pituitary development as noted.

1. **GH deficiency**—In children, congenital monotropic GH deficiency may be sporadic or familial. These children, who may experience fasting hypoglycemia, have a gradual deceleration in growth velocity after 6 to 12 months of age. Diagnosis must be based on failure of GH responsiveness to provocative stimuli and the demonstration of normal responsiveness of other anterior pituitary hormones. Monotropic GH deficiency and growth retardation have also been observed in children suffering severe emotional deprivation. This disorder is reversed by placing the child in a supportive psychosocial milieu. A more detailed description of GH deficiency and growth failure is provided in Chapter 6.

2. **ACTH deficiency**—Monotropic ACTH deficiency is rare and is manifested by the signs and symptoms of adrenocortical insufficiency. LPH deficiency has also been noted in such patients. The defect in these patients may be due to primary failure of the corticotrophs to release ACTH and its related peptide hormones or may be secondary to impaired secretion of CRH by the hypothalamus. Most acquired cases of monotropic ACTH deficiency are presumed to be due to lymphocytic hypophysitis.

3. **Gonadotropin deficiency**—Isolated deficiency of gonadotropins is not uncommon. Kallmann syndrome initially described in the 1940s, is characterized by an isolated defect in GnRH secretion associated with maldevelopment of the olfactory center with hyposmia or anosmia; X-linked recessive, autosomal dominant, and autosomal recessive patterns of inheritance are seen. Sporadic cases occur, and other neurologic defects such as color blindness and nerve deafness have been reported. At least five Kallmann syndrome genes have been identified: KAL1, FGFR1, FGF8, PROKR2, and PROK2. KAL1 mutations are responsible for the X-linked form of the disease and result in decreased expression of the extracellular glycoprotein anosmin-1. This in turn interferes with the normal embryonic development and migration of GnRH-secreting neurons. Because anterior pituitary function is otherwise intact, young men with isolated hypogonadotropic hypogonadism develop a eunuchoid appearance, since testosterone deficiency results in failure of epiphysial closure (see Chapter 12). In women, a state of hypogonadotropic hypogonadism manifested by oligomenorrhea or amenorrhea often accompanies weight loss, emotional or physical stress, and athletic training. Anorexia nervosa and marked obesity both result in hypothalamic dysfunction and impaired gonadotropin secretion. Hypothalamic hypogonadism has also been observed in overtrained male athletes. Sickle cell anemia also causes hypogonadotropic hypogonadism due to hypothalamic dysfunction and results in delayed puberty. Clomiphene treatment has been effective in some cases. Isolated gonadotropin deficiency may also be seen in the polyglandular autoimmune syndrome; this deficiency is related to selective pituitary gonadotrope failure from autoimmune hypophysitis. Other chronic illnesses (eg, poorly controlled diabetes, malnutrition) may result in gonadotropin deficiency. Isolated deficiencies of both LH and FSH without an obvious cause such as those described have been reported but are rare. In addition, acquired partial gonadotropin deficiency may occur in middle-aged men. The cause and exact frequency of this disorder are unknown.

4. **TSH deficiency**—Monotropic TSH deficiency is rare and can be caused by a reduction in either hypothalamic TRH secretion (tertiary hypothyroidism) or pituitary TSH secretion (secondary hypothyroidism). These defects have reported in association with gene mutations, empty sella, lymphocytic hypophysitis, and pituitary tumors. Some patients with chronic renal failure also appear to have impaired TSH secretion.

5. **Prolactin deficiency**—PRL deficiency almost always indicates severe intrinsic pituitary damage, and panhypopituitarism is usually present. However, isolated PRL deficiency has been reported after lymphocytic hypophysitis. Deficiencies of TSH and PRL have been noted in patients with pseudohypoparathyroidism.

6. **Multiple hormone deficiencies isolated from other pituitary damage**—Multiple hormone deficiencies result from abnormal pituitary development related to abnormalities of the genes encoding the transcription factors, PIT-1 (TSH, GH, and PRL) and PROP-1 (TSH, GH, PRL, LH, FSH, and ACTH).

Clinical Features

The onset of pituitary insufficiency is usually gradual, and the classic course of progressive hypopituitarism is an initial loss of GH and gonadotropin secretion followed by deficiencies of TSH, then ACTH, and finally PRL.

A. Symptoms Impairment of GH secretion causes decreased growth in children but may be clinically occult in adult patients. GH deficiency is associated with a decreased sense of well-being and a lower health-related quality of life. Decreased muscle mass and increased fat mass can also be seen, although this may be difficult to discern in any given individual.

Hypogonadism, manifested by amenorrhea in women and decreased libido or erectile dysfunction in men, may antedate the clinical appearance of a hypothalamic-pituitary lesion. The only symptom of PRL deficiency is failure of postpartum lactation.

Hypothyroidism caused by TSH deficiency generally simulates the clinical changes observed in primary thyroid failure; however, it is usually less severe, and goiter is absent. Cold intolerance, dry skin, mental dullness, bradycardia, constipation, hoarseness, and anemia have all been observed; gross myxedematous changes are uncommon.

ACTH deficiency causes adrenocortical insufficiency, and its clinical features resemble those of primary adrenal failure. Weakness, nausea, vomiting, anorexia, weight loss, fever, and hypotension may occur. The zona glomerulosa and the renin-angiotensin system are usually intact; therefore, the dehydration and sodium depletion seen in Addison disease are uncommon. However, these patients are susceptible to hypotension, shock, and cardiovascular collapse, because glucocorticoids are necessary to maintain vascular reactivity, especially during stress. In addition, because of their gradual onset, the symptoms of secondary adrenal insufficiency may go undetected for prolonged periods, becoming manifest only during periods of stress. Hypoglycemia aggravated by GH deficiency may occur with fasting and has been the initial presenting feature of some patients with isolated ACTH deficiency. In contrast to the hyperpigmentation that occurs during states of ACTH excess (Addison disease, Nelson syndrome), depigmentation and diminished tanning have been described as a result of ACTH insufficiency. In addition, lack of ACTH-stimulated adrenal androgen secretion will cause a decrease in body hair if gonadotropin deficiency is also present.

B. Signs Abnormal findings on physical examination may be subtle and require careful observation. Patients with hypopituitarism are not cachectic. A photograph of a cachectic patient with "Simmonds syndrome" that appeared in some older textbooks of endocrinology caused confusion. That particular patient probably suffered from anorexia nervosa and was found to have a normal pituitary gland at postmortem examination.

Patients with pituitary failure are usually slightly overweight. The skin is fine, pale, and smooth, with fine wrinkling of the face. Body and pubic hair may be deficient or absent, and atrophy of the genitalia may occur. Postural hypotension, bradycardia, decreased muscle strength, and delayed deep tendon reflexes occur in more severe cases. Neuro-ophthalmologic abnormalities depend on the presence of a large intrasellar or parasellar lesion.

C. Laboratory and other findings These may include anemia (related to thyroid and androgen deficiency and chronic disease), hypoglycemia, hyponatremia (related to hypothyroidism and hypoadrenalism, which cause inappropriate water retention, not sodium loss), and low-voltage bradycardia on electrocardiographic testing. Hyperkalemia, which is common in primary

adrenal failure, is not present. Adult GH deficiency is associated with decreased red blood cell mass, increased LDL cholesterol, and decreased bone mass.

Diagnosis

A. Assessment of target gland function (Figure 4–17) If endocrine hypofunction is suspected, pituitary hormone deficiencies must be distinguished from primary failure of the thyroid, adrenals, or gonads. Basal determinations of each anterior pituitary hormone are useful only if compared to target gland secretion. Baseline laboratory studies should include thyroid function tests (free T_4) and determination of serum testosterone levels. Testosterone is a sensitive indicator of hypopituitarism in women as well as in men. In women, a substantial decrease in testosterone is commonly observed in pituitary failure related to hypofunction of the two endocrine glands responsible for its production—the ovary and the adrenal. Adrenocortical reserve should initially be evaluated by a rapid ACTH stimulation test.

B. Evaluation of prolactin Because hyperprolactinemia (discussed later), regardless of its cause, leads to gonadal dysfunction, serum PRL should be measured early in the evaluation of hypogonadism.

C. Differentiation of primary and secondary hypofunction Subnormal thyroid function as shown by appropriate tests, a low serum testosterone level, or an impaired cortisol response to the rapid ACTH stimulation test requires measurement of basal levels of specific pituitary hormones. In primary target gland hypofunction, such as autoimmune polyglandular syndromes types 1 and 2 (APS 1 and 2), TSH, LH, FSH, or ACTH will be elevated. Low or normal values for these pituitary hormones suggest hypothalamic-pituitary dysfunction.

D. Stimulation tests Provocative endocrine testing may then be employed to confirm the diagnosis and to assess the extent of hypofunction. At present, these tests are not required in most patients.

Treatment

A. ACTH Treatment of secondary adrenal insufficiency, like that of primary adrenal failure, must include glucocorticoid support (see Chapter 9). Hydrocortisone (15-25 mg/d orally) or prednisone (5-7.5 mg/d orally) in two or three divided doses provides adequate glucocorticoid replacement for most patients. The minimum effective dosage should be given in order to avoid iatrogenic hypercortisolism. Increased dosage is required during periods of stress such as illness, surgery, or trauma. Patients with only partial ACTH deficiency may need steroid treatment only during stress. A two- to threefold increase in steroid dosage during the stressful situation should be recommended, followed by gradual tapering as the stress resolves. Unlike primary adrenal insufficiency, ACTH deficiency does not usually require mineralocorticoid therapy. Patients with adrenal insufficiency should wear

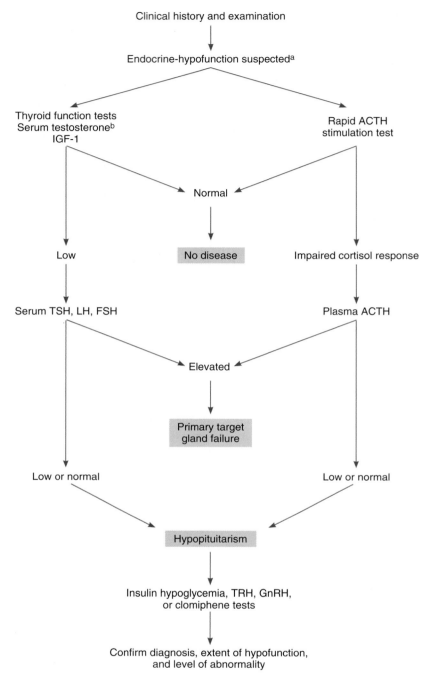

Clinical history and examination

Endocrine-hypofunction suspected[a]

Thyroid function tests
Serum testosterone[b]
IGF-1

Rapid ACTH
stimulation test

Normal

Low

No disease

Impaired cortisol response

Serum TSH, LH, FSH

Plasma ACTH

Elevated

Primary target
gland failure

Low or normal

Low or normal

Hypopituitarism

Insulin hypoglycemia, TRH, GnRH,
or clomiphene tests

Confirm diagnosis, extent of hypofunction,
and level of abnormality

[a]Evaluate GH in children (see text).
[b]Measure prolactin if hypogonadism suspected.

FIGURE 4–17 Diagnostic evaluation of hypothalamic-pituitary-target gland hypofunction.

medical alert bracelets so they may receive prompt treatment in case of emergency.

B. TSH The management of patients with secondary hypothyroidism must be based on clinical grounds and the circulating concentration of serum thyroxine (see Chapter 7). The treatment of secondary and tertiary hypothyroidism is identical to that for primary thyroid failure. Full oral replacement dose of levothyroxine sodium is 1.6 μg/kg daily (0.1-0.15 mg/d is usually adequate). Response to therapy is monitored clinically and with measurement of serum free thyroxine levels, which should be maintained in the mid to upper range of normal. Measurement of TSH levels is obviously of no value in the management of these patients.

Caution: Because thyroid hormone replacement in patients with hypopituitarism may aggravate even partial adrenal insufficiency, the adrenal hormone deficiency should be treated first.

C. Gonadotropins   The object of treatment of secondary hypogonadism is to replace sex steroids and restore fertility (see Chapters 12 and 13).

1. **Estrogens and progesterone**—In premenopausal women, estrogen replacement is essential. Adequate estrogen treatment maintains secondary sex characteristics (eg, vulvar and vaginal lubrication), prevents osteoporosis, and abolishes vasomotor symptoms, with an improvement in sense of well-being. Many estrogen preparations are available (eg, oral estradiol, 1-2 mg daily; conjugated estrogens, 0.3-1.25 mg orally daily; or transdermal estradiol, 0.05-0.1 mg daily). Estrogens should be cycled with a progestin compound (eg, medroxyprogesterone, 5-10 mg orally daily during the last 10 days of estrogen therapy each month) to induce withdrawal bleeding and prevent endometrial hyperplasia. Many oral contraceptive pill combinations are also clinically available.

2. **Ovulation induction**—Ovulation can often be restored in women with hypothalamic-pituitary dysfunction (see Chapter 13). In patients with gonadal failure of hypothalamic origin, clomiphene citrate may cause a surge of gonadotropin secretion resulting in ovulation. Pulsatile subcutaneous injections of GnRH with an infusion pump can also be used to induce ovulation and fertility in women with hypothalamic dysfunction. Combined treatment with FSH (human menopausal gonadotropins; menotropins) and LH (chorionic gonadotropin) can be utilized to provoke ovulation in women with intrinsic pituitary failure. This form of therapy is expensive, and multiple births are a risk (see Chapter 13).

3. **Androgens in women**—Because of a deficiency of both ovarian and adrenal androgens, some women with hypopituitarism have diminished libido despite adequate estrogen therapy. Although experience is limited, small doses of long-acting androgens (testosterone enanthate, 25-50 mg intramuscularly every 4-8 weeks) may be helpful in restoring sexual activity without causing hirsutism. In addition, some reports have suggested that oral dehydroepiandrosterone (DHEA) in doses of 25 to 50 mg/d may restore plasma testosterone levels to normal. A transdermal delivery system is being evaluated for use in women, but efficacy appears to be modest and the long-term safety is unknown.

4. **Androgens in men**—The treatment of male hypogonadism is discussed in Chapter 12. Testosterone gels (available in packets in doses of 2.5, 5, or 10 g, or from a metered-dose pump in 1.25 g increments) and testosterone patches (in doses of 2.5 or 5 mg) are applied daily. A transbuccal formulation is administered at a dose of 30 mg twice daily. Other therapeutic preparations include intramuscular testosterone enanthate or cypionate in doses of 100 mg every week or 200 mg every 2 weeks. Testosterone undecanoate is an intramuscular preparation available in several countries that can be given every 3 months. Oral testosterone preparations available in the United States are rarely used out of concern for hepatic side effects.

5. **Spermatogenesis**—Spermatogenesis can be achieved in many patients with the combined use of hCG and recombinant FSH. If pituitary insufficiency is of recent onset, therapy with hCG alone may restore both fertility and adequate gonadal steroid production. Pulsatile GnRH infusion pumps have also been used to restore fertility in male patients with secondary hypogonadism.

D. Growth hormone (also see chapter 6)   Human GH (hGH) produced by recombinant DNA technology is available for use in children with hypopituitarism and for adults with GH deficiency and known pituitary disease. Some studies indicate improvement in body composition, bone density, psychologic well-being, and functional status with GH therapy. However, the long-term benefits and risks remain to be established. In adults, GH is usually administered subcutaneously, once per day in a dosage of 2 to 5 μg/kg. Monitoring of effectiveness is accomplished by measurement of IGF-I, and the dosage of GH is adjusted accordingly (up to about 10 μg/kg/d). Side effects (eg, edema, paresthesias, arrhythmias, glucose intolerance, diabetes) should be assessed. Contraindications to GH therapy include the presence of diabetic retinopathy, active malignancy, intracranial hypertension, or airway obstruction in individuals with Prader-Willi syndrome.

PITUITARY ADENOMAS

Advances in endocrinologic and neuroradiologic research in recent years have allowed earlier recognition and more successful therapy of pituitary adenomas. Prolactinomas are the most common type, accounting for about 60% of primary pituitary tumors; GH hypersecretion occurs in approximately 20%; and ACTH excess in 10%. Hypersecretion of TSH, the gonadotropins, or alpha subunits is unusual. Nonfunctional tumors currently represent only 10% of all pituitary adenomas, and some of these may in fact be gonadotropin-secreting or alpha subunit-secreting adenomas. The differential diagnosis of nonpituitary sellar and parasellar masses is listed in Table 4–10.

Early clinical recognition of the endocrine effects of excessive pituitary secretion, especially the observation that PRL excess causes secondary hypogonadism, has led to early diagnosis of pituitary tumors before the appearance of late manifestations such as sellar enlargement, panhypopituitarism, and suprasellar extension with visual impairment.

Pituitary **microadenomas** are defined as intrasellar adenomas less than 1 cm in diameter that present with manifestations of hormonal excess without sellar enlargement or extrasellar extension. Panhypopituitarism does not occur, and such tumors can usually be treated successfully.

Pituitary **macroadenomas** are those larger than 1 cm in diameter and cause generalized sellar enlargement. Tumors 1 to 2 cm in diameter confined to the sella turcica can usually be successfully treated; however, larger tumors—especially those with suprasellar, sphenoid sinus, or lateral extensions—are much more difficult to manage. Panhypopituitarism and visual loss increase in frequency with tumor size and suprasellar extension.

Insights into the pathogenesis and biologic behavior of pituitary tumors have been gained from studies of pituitary tumor

TABLE 4-10 Differential diagnosis of sellar and parasellar masses (excluding pituitary adenomas).

Benign tumors
Craniopharyngioma
Rathke cleft cyst
Meningioma
Enchondroma
Arachnoid cyst
Dermoid cyst

Empty sella

Nonadenomatous pituitary hyperplasia
Lactotroph hyperplasia during pregnancy
Somatotroph hyperplasia from ectopic GHRH-secreting tumor
Thyrotroph, gonadotroph hyperplasia

Malignant tumors
Sarcoma
Chordoma
Germ cell tumor (ectopic pinealoma)

Metastatic lesions (breast, lung)

Gliomas
Optic glioma
Astrocytoma
Oligodendroglioma
Ependymoma

Vascular lesions

Granulomatous, inflammatory, infectious
Lymphocytic hypophysitis
Sarcoidosis
Histiocytosis X
Tuberculosis
Pituitary abscess

clonality and somatic mutations. Analyses of allelic X inactivation of specific genes has shown that most pituitary adenomas are monoclonal, a finding most consistent with a somatic mutation model of tumorigenesis; polyclonality of tumors would be expected if tonic stimulation by hypothalamic-releasing factors were the mechanism underlying neoplastic transformation. In fact, transgenic animals expressing GHRH have exhibited pituitary hyperplasia but not pituitary adenomas. One somatic mutation has been found in 30% to 40% of GH-secreting tumors (but not in leukocytes from the same patients). Point mutations in the alpha subunit of the GTP-binding protein responsible for activation of adenylyl cyclase result in constitutive stimulation of pituitary cell growth and function. In studies of anterior pituitary cell ontogeny, PIT-1 has been identified as a transcription factor important in pituitary differentiation. The restriction of its expression to somatotrophs, lactotrophs, and thyrotrophs may account for the plurihormonal expression seen in some tumors. A host of other candidate genes have been described, including the pituitary tumor transforming gene (PTTG). Overexpression of this gene has been found in all pituitary tumor types and may promote tumorigenesis through cell cycle disruption, stimulation of fibroblast growth factor secretion, and abnormal chromatid separation. Several genetic syndromes are associated with pituitary tumors including multiple endocrine neoplasia type 1, McCune-Albright syndrome, Carney syndrome, and familial acromegaly.

Treatment

Pituitary adenomas are treated with surgery, irradiation, or drugs to suppress hypersecretion by the adenoma or its growth. The aims of therapy are to correct hypersecretion of anterior pituitary hormones, to preserve normal secretion of other anterior pituitary hormones, and to remove or suppress the adenoma itself. These objectives are currently achievable in most patients with pituitary microadenomas; however, in the case of larger tumors, multiple therapies are frequently required and may be less successful.

A. Surgical treatment The transsphenoidal microsurgical approach to the sella turcica, now done endoscopically in most centers, is the procedure of choice; transfrontal craniotomy is required only in the rare patient with massive suprasellar extension of the adenoma. In the transsphenoidal procedure, the surgeon approaches the pituitary from the nasal cavity through the sphenoid sinus, removes the anterior-inferior sellar floor, and incises the dura. The adenoma is selectively removed; normal pituitary tissue is identified and preserved. Success rates approach 90% in patients with microadenomas. Major complications, including postoperative hemorrhage, cerebrospinal fluid leak, meningitis, and visual impairment, occur in less than 5% of patients and are most frequent in patients with large or massive tumors. Transient diabetes insipidus lasting a few days to 1 to 2 weeks occurs in approximately 15%; permanent diabetes insipidus is rare. A transient form of the syndrome of inappropriate secretion of antidiuretic hormone (SIADH) with symptomatic hyponatremia occurs in 10% of patients within 5 to 14 days of transsphenoidal pituitary microsurgery. These abnormalities of water balance can occur within days of each other making medical management difficult. A *triphasic response* of diabetes insipidus, SIADH, and diabetes insipidus is occasionally encountered and thought to be due to early hypothalamic dysfunction, followed by release of ADH from the degenerating pituitary, and then depletion of ADH stores. Surgical hypopituitarism is rare in patients with microadenomas but approaches 5% to 10% in patients with larger tumors. The perioperative management of such patients should include glucocorticoid administration in stress doses (see Chapter 9) and postoperative assessment of daily weight, fluid balance, and electrolyte status to look for evidence of diabetes insipidus. Mild diabetes insipidus is managed by giving fluids orally; in more severe cases—urine output greater than 5 to 6 L/24 h—ADH therapy in the form of desmopressin, or DDAVP, can be administered intranasally, orally, subcutaneously, or parenterally (see Chapter 5). SIADH is managed by fluid restriction; however, in more severe cases, hypertonic saline may be required. ADH receptor antagonists (tolvaptan is given orally and conivaptan is administered intravenously) are also now available for use in some patients (see section on SIADH).

B. Radiotherapy Pituitary irradiation should be reserved for patients who have had incomplete resection of larger pituitary adenomas and whose tumors are not amenable to, or have failed, medical therapy.

1. **Conventional irradiation**—Conventional irradiation using high-energy sources, in total doses of 4000 to 5000 cGy given in daily doses of 180 to 200 cGy, is most commonly employed. The response to radiation therapy is slow, and 5 to 10 years may be required to achieve the full effect (see section on Acromegaly). Treatment is ultimately successful in about 80% of patients with acromegaly but in only about 55% to 60% of patients with Cushing disease. The response rate in prolactinomas is not precisely known, but tumor progression is prevented in most patients. Morbidity during radiotherapy is minimal, although some patients experience malaise and nausea, and serous otitis media may occur. Hypopituitarism is common, and the incidence increases with time following radiotherapy—about 50% to 60% at 5 to 10 years. Rare late complications include damage to the optic nerves and chiasm, seizures, and radionecrosis of brain tissue. Recent studies from the United Kingdom have shown that conventional radiotherapy is a major risk factor for excess mortality in acromegaly.

2. **Gamma knife radiosurgery**—This form of radiotherapy utilizes stereotactic CT-guided cobalt-60 gamma radiation to deliver high radiation doses to a narrowly focused area. Remission rates have been reported in the range of 43% to 78%. An adequate distance of the pituitary tumor from the optic chiasm is needed to prevent radiation-induced damage. Repeat treatments put patients at higher risk of new visual or third, fourth, or sixth cranial nerve deficits.

3. **Proton stereotactic radiotherapy**—Experience with this modality is limited. In one study, 52% of patients with Cushing disease had clinical remission. A similar rate of new pituitary hormone deficiencies was seen, although no visual complications or brain injury was reported.

C. Medical treatment Medical management of pituitary adenomas became feasible with the availability of bromocriptine, a dopamine agonist that suppresses both PRL and tumor growth in patients with prolactinomas. Somatostatin analogs are useful in the therapy of acromegaly and some TSH-secreting adenomas. Specifics of the use of these and other medications are discussed later.

Posttreatment Follow-Up

Patients undergoing transsphenoidal microsurgery should be reevaluated 4 to 8 weeks postoperatively to document that complete removal of the adenoma and correction of endocrine hypersecretion has been achieved. Prolactinomas are assessed by basal PRL measurements, GH-secreting tumors by glucose suppression testing and IGF-I levels, and ACTH-secreting adenomas by measurement of urine-free cortisol and the response to low-dose dexamethasone suppression (see later). Other anterior pituitary hormones—TSH, ACTH, and LH/FSH—should also be assessed as described earlier in the section on endocrine evaluation. In patients with successful responses, yearly evaluation should be performed to watch for late recurrence; late hypopituitarism does not occur after microsurgery. MRI is not necessary in patients with normal postoperative pituitary function but should be utilized in patients with persistent or recurrent disease.

TABLE 4–11 Indications for prolactin measurement.

Galactorrhea
Enlarged sella turcica
Suspected pituitary tumor
Hypogonadotropic hypogonadism
Unexplained amenorrhea
Unexplained male hypogonadism or infertility

Follow-up of patients treated by pituitary irradiation is also essential, because the response to therapy may be delayed and the incidence of hypopituitarism increases with time. Yearly endocrinologic assessment of both the hypersecreted hormone and the other pituitary hormones is recommended.

1. PROLACTINOMAS

PRL hypersecretion is the most common endocrine abnormality due to hypothalamic-pituitary disorders, and PRL is the hormone most commonly secreted in excess by pituitary adenomas.

The understanding is that PRL hypersecretion causes not only galactorrhea but also gonadal dysfunction, and the use of PRL measurements in screening such patients has permitted recognition of these PRL-secreting tumors before the development of sellar enlargement, hypopituitarism, or visual impairment. Thus, plasma PRL should be measured in patients with galactorrhea, suspected hypothalamic-pituitary dysfunction, or sellar enlargement and in those with unexplained gonadal dysfunction, including amenorrhea, infertility, decreased libido, or impotence (Table 4–11).

Pathology

PRL-secreting pituitary adenomas arise most commonly from the lateral wings of the anterior pituitary, but with progression they fill the sella turcica and compress the normal anterior and posterior lobes. Tumor size varies greatly from microadenomas to large invasive tumors with extrasellar extension. Most patients have microadenomas (ie, tumors <1 cm in diameter at diagnosis).

Prolactinomas usually appear chromophobic on routine histologic study, reflecting the inadequacy of the techniques used. The cells are small and uniform, with round or oval nuclei and scanty cytoplasm, and secretory granules are usually not visible with routine stains. The stroma contains a diffuse capillary network.

Electron microscopic examination shows that prolactinoma cells characteristically contain secretory granules that usually range from 100 to 500 nm in diameter and are spherical. Larger granules (400-500 nm), which are irregular or crescent-shaped, are less commonly seen. The cells show evidence of secretory activity, with a large Golgi area, nucleolar enlargement, and a prominent endoplasmic reticulum. Immunocytochemical studies of these tumors have confirmed that the secretory granules indeed contain PRL.

Clinical Features

The clinical manifestations of PRL excess are the same regardless of the cause (see later). The classic features are galactorrhea and amenorrhea in women and decreased libido or impotence in men. Although the sex distribution of prolactinomas is approximately equal, microadenomas are much more common in women, presumably because of earlier recognition of the endocrine consequences of PRL excess.

A. Galactorrhea   Galactorrhea occurs in the majority of women with prolactinomas and is much less common in men. It is usually not spontaneous, or may be present only transiently or intermittently. The absence of galactorrhea despite markedly elevated PRL levels is probably due to concomitant deficiency of the gonadal hormones required to initiate lactation (see Chapter 16).

B. Gonadal dysfunction

1. **In women**—Amenorrhea, oligomenorrhea with anovulation, or infertility is present in approximately 90% of women with prolactinomas. These menstrual disorders usually present concurrently with galactorrhea if it is present but may either precede or follow it. The amenorrhea is usually secondary and may follow pregnancy or oral contraceptive use. Primary amenorrhea occurs in the minority of patients who have onset of hyperprolactinemia during adolescence. The necessity of measuring PRL in patients with unexplained primary or secondary amenorrhea is emphasized by several studies showing that hyperprolactinemia occurs in as many as 20% of patients with neither galactorrhea nor other manifestations of pituitary dysfunction. A number of these patients have been shown to have prolactinomas.

Gonadal dysfunction in these women is due to interference with the hypothalamic-pituitary-gonadal axis by the hyperprolactinemia and except in patients with large or invasive adenomas is not due to destruction of the gonadotropin-secreting cells. This has been documented by the return of menstrual function following reduction of PRL levels to normal by drug treatment or surgical removal of the tumor. Although basal gonadotropin levels are frequently within the normal range despite reduction of sex steroid levels in hyperprolactinemic patients, PRL inhibits both the normal pulsatile secretion of LH and FSH and the midcycle LH surge, resulting in anovulation. The positive feedback effect of estrogen on gonadotropin secretion is also inhibited; in fact, patients with hyperprolactinemia are usually estrogen deficient.

Estrogen deficiency in women with prolactinomas may be accompanied by decreased vaginal lubrication, other symptoms of estrogen deficiency, and low bone mass as assessed by bone densitometry. Other symptoms may include weight gain, fluid retention, and irritability. Hirsutism may also occur, accompanied by elevated plasma levels of dehydroepiandrosterone (DHEA) sulfate. Patients with hyperprolactinemia may also suffer from anxiety and depression. In small clinical trials, treatment with dopamine agonists has been shown to improve psychologic well-being in such patients.

2. **In men**—In men, PRL excess may also occasionally cause galactorrhea; however, the usual manifestations are those of hypogonadism. The initial symptom is decreased libido, which may be dismissed by both the patient and physician as due to psychosocial factors; thus, the recognition of prolactinomas in men is frequently delayed, and marked hyperprolactinemia (PRL >200 ng/mL [9.1 nmol/L]) and sellar enlargement are usual. Unfortunately, prolactinomas in men are often not diagnosed until late manifestations such as headache, visual impairment, or hypopituitarism appear; virtually all such patients have a history of sexual or gonadal dysfunction. Serum testosterone levels are low, and in the presence of normal or subnormal gonadotropin levels, PRL excess should be suspected as should other causes of hypothalamic-pituitary-gonadal dysfunction (see section on Hypopituitarism). Impotence also occurs in hyperprolactinemic males. Its cause is unclear, because testosterone replacement may not reverse it if hyperprolactinemia is not corrected. Male infertility accompanied by reduction in sperm count is a less common initial complaint.

C. Tumor progression   In general, the growth of prolactinomas is slow; several studies have shown that most microadenomas do not change significantly in size, and macroadenomas tend to grow very slowly.

Differential Diagnosis

The many conditions associated with hyperprolactinemia are listed in Table 4–8. Pregnancy, hypothalamic-pituitary disorders, primary hypothyroidism, and drug ingestion are the most common causes.

Hypothalamic lesions frequently cause PRL hypersecretion by decreasing the secretion of dopamine that tonically inhibits PRL release; the lesions may be accompanied by panhypopituitarism. Similarly, traumatic or surgical section of the pituitary stalk leads to hyperprolactinemia and hypopituitarism. Nonfunctional pituitary macroadenomas frequently cause mild hyperprolactinemia by compression of the pituitary stalk or hypothalamus.

Pregnancy leads to a physiologic increase in PRL secretion; the levels increase as pregnancy continues and may reach 200 ng/mL (9.1 nmol/L) during the third trimester. Following delivery, basal PRL levels gradually fall to normal over several weeks but increase in response to breast feeding. Hyperprolactinemia persisting for 6 to 12 months or longer following delivery is an indication for evaluation. PRL levels are also high in normal neonates.

Several systemic disorders lead to hyperprolactinemia. Primary hypothyroidism is a common cause, and measurement of thyroid function, and especially TSH, should be part of the evaluation. In primary hypothyroidism, there is hyperplasia of both thyrotrophs and lactotrophs, presumably due to TRH hypersecretion. This may result in significant pituitary gland enlargement, which may be mistaken for a PRL-secreting pituitary tumor. The PRL response to TRH is usually exaggerated in these patients. PRL may also be increased in liver disease, particularly in patients with severe cirrhosis, and in patients with chronic renal failure.

PRL excess and galactorrhea may also be caused by breast disease, nipple stimulation, disease or injury to the chest wall, and spinal cord lesions. These disorders increase PRL secretion by stimulation of afferent neural pathways. Artifactual elevations in PRL levels may be observed in the presence of anti-PRL antibodies or of macroprolactinemia. In the latter, a high-molecular-weight complex of PRL molecules maintains immunologic activity, but minimal or no bioactivity. Macroprolactinemia can be assessed with polyethylene glycol precipitation of serum samples.

The most common cause of hyperprolactinemia is drug ingestion, and a careful history of drug intake must be obtained. Elevated PRL levels, galactorrhea, and amenorrhea may occur following estrogen therapy or oral contraceptive use, but their persistence should suggest prolactinoma. Many other drugs also cause increased PRL secretion and elevated plasma levels (see Table 4–8). PRL levels are usually less than 200 ng/mL (9 nmol/L), and the evaluation should focus on discontinuation of the drug or medication and reevaluation of the patient after several weeks. In patients in whom drug withdrawal is not feasible, neuroradiologic studies, if normal, usually exclude prolactinoma.

Diagnosis

A. General evaluation The evaluation of patients with galactorrhea or unexplained gonadal dysfunction with normal or low plasma gonadotropin levels should first include a history regarding menstrual status, pregnancy, fertility, sexual function, and symptoms of hypothyroidism or hypopituitarism. Current or previous use of medication, drugs, or estrogen therapy should be documented. Basal PRL levels, gonadotropins, thyroid function tests, and TSH levels should be established, as well as serum testosterone in men. Liver and kidney function should be assessed. A pregnancy test should be performed in women with amenorrhea.

Patients with galactorrhea but normal menses may not have hyperprolactinemia and usually do not have prolactinomas. If the PRL level is normal, they may be reassured and followed with sequential PRL measurements. Those with elevated levels require further evaluation as described later.

B. Specific diagnosis When other causes of hyperprolactinemia have been excluded, the most likely cause of persistent hyperprolactinemia is a prolactinoma, especially if there is associated hypogonadism. Because currently available suppression and stimulation tests do not distinguish PRL-secreting tumors from other causes of hyperprolactinemia, the diagnosis must be established by the assessment of both basal PRL levels and neuroradiologic studies. Patients with large tumors and marked hyperprolactinemia usually present little difficulty. With very rare exceptions, basal PRL levels greater than 200 to 300 ng/mL (9.1-13.7 nmol/L) are virtually diagnostic of prolactinoma. In addition, because there is a general correlation between the PRL elevation and the size of the pituitary adenoma, these patients usually have sellar enlargement and obvious macroadenomas. Similarly, if the basal PRL level is between 100 and 200 ng/mL (4.5 and 9.1 nmol/L), the cause is usually prolactinoma. These patients may have either micro- or macroadenomas; however, with basal levels of PRL greater than 100 ng/mL (4.5 nmol/L), the PRL-secreting tumor is usually radiologically evident, and again the diagnosis is generally straightforward. Patients with mild to moderate hyperprolactinemia (20-100 ng/mL [0.9-4.5 nmol/L]) present the greatest difficulty in diagnosis, because both PRL-secreting microadenomas and the many other conditions causing hyperprolactinemia (see Table 4–8) cause PRL hypersecretion of this degree. In such patients, MRI frequently demonstrates a definite pituitary microadenoma. Scans showing only minor or equivocal abnormalities should be

interpreted with caution, because of the high incidence of false-positive scans in the normal population (see Neuroradiologic Evaluation, above). Because the diagnosis cannot be either established or excluded in patients with normal or equivocal neuroradiologic studies, they require further evaluation or serial assessment (see later). Dilutions of prolactin samples can be performed in patients with modest prolactin elevation or macroadenomas to rule out interference from the high-dose *hook effect*; large quantities of antigen can impair antigen-antibody binding, resulting in erroneously low prolactin measurements in some immunoassays.

Treatment

Satisfactory control of PRL hypersecretion, cessation of galactorrhea, and return of normal gonadal function can be achieved in most patients with PRL-secreting microadenomas. In patients with hyperprolactinemia, ovulation should not be induced without careful assessment of pituitary anatomy, because pregnancy may cause further expansion of these tumors as discussed later.

Although most microadenomas do not progress, treatment of these patients is recommended to restore normal estrogen levels and fertility and to prevent early osteoporosis secondary to persistent hypogonadism. In addition, medical or surgical therapy is more successful in these patients than in those with larger tumors. All patients with PRL-secreting macroadenomas should be treated, because of the risks of further tumor expansion, hypopituitarism, and visual impairment. Patients with persistent hyperprolactinemia and hypogonadism and normal neuroradiologic studies—that is, those in whom prolactinoma cannot be definitely established— may be managed by observation if hypogonadism is of short duration. However, in patients whose hypogonadism has persisted for more than 6 to 12 months, dopamine agonists should be used to suppress PRL secretion and restore normal gonadal function. In women with macroprolactinomas, replacement estrogen therapy should be initiated only after PRL hypersecretion has been controlled by dopamine agonist therapy since estrogen stimulates lactotroph hyperplasia and may increase tumor size. In this regard, periodic measurement of serum PRL should be performed in women with microadenomas on estrogen therapy who are not also receiving dopamine agonist therapy.

A. Dopamine agonists Bromocriptine became available in the United States more than 30 years ago and was the first effective medical therapy for pituitary adenomas; however, cabergoline is more potent, much longer acting, and better tolerated. Cabergoline has, therefore, become the dopamine agonist of choice in the therapy of prolactinomas.

1. **Bromocriptine**—Bromocriptine stimulates dopamine receptors and has effects at both the hypothalamic and pituitary levels. It is effective therapy for a PRL-secreting pituitary adenoma and directly inhibits PRL secretion by the tumor. Doses of 2.5 to 5 mg daily are often effective. However, at present, cabergoline is the therapy of choice

2. **Cabergoline**—Cabergoline, a newer nonergot dopamine agonist, is administered once or twice a week and has a better side-effect profile than bromocriptine. It is as effective as

bromocriptine in reducing macroadenoma size and is more effective in reducing PRL levels. It has been used successfully in most patients previously intolerant or resistant to bromocriptine. Cabergoline should be started at a dosage of 0.25 mg twice per week and increased if necessary to 0.5 mg twice per week. Although several recent studies have demonstrated associations between cabergoline and cardiac valve disease in patients treated for Parkinson disease, clinically relevant valve disease in patients treated for prolactinoma appears to be rare, likely because doses used to manage symptoms of Parkinsonism are often 20 to 30 times higher and administered daily rather than twice weekly. The risk also appears to be related to the affinity of different dopamine agonists for valvular serotonin (5-HT2B) receptors. Until larger, prospective safety studies are available, some authorities recommend echocardiographic evaluation in patients who are expected to need long-term treatment, especially at high doses.

a. **Microadenomas**—Cabergoline is successful in about 90% of patients, and very few are intolerant or resistant. Correction of hyperprolactinemia allows recovery of normal gonadal function; ovulation and fertility are restored, so that mechanical contraception should be advised if pregnancy is not desired. Bromocriptine induces ovulation in most female patients who wish to become pregnant. In these patients with microadenomas, the risk of major expansion of adenoma during the pregnancy is less than 2%; however, both the patient and the physician must be aware of this potential complication. Current data do not indicate an increased risk of multiple pregnancy, abortion, or fetal malformations in pregnancies occurring in women taking dopamine agonists; however, patients should be instructed to discontinue these drugs at the first missed menstrual period and obtain a pregnancy test. Although no late toxicity has yet been reported other than the side effects noted above, questions about possible long-term risk are currently unanswered. Maternal hyperprolactinemia should not be harmful to the developing fetus; prolactin increases normally during pregnancy and does not appear to cross the placenta.

b. **Macroadenomas**—Dopamine agonists are effective in controlling hyperprolactinemia in patients with PRL-secreting macroadenomas even when basal PRL levels are markedly elevated. Dopamine agonists may be used either as initial therapy or to control residual hyperprolactinemia in patients unsuccessfully treated with surgery or radiotherapy. Dopamine agonists should not be used to induce ovulation and pregnancy in women with untreated macroadenomas, because the risk of tumor expansion and visual deficits in the later part of pregnancy is approximately 15% to 25%. These patients should first have tumor volume decreased with medical therapy or be treated with surgery prior to induction of ovulation.

Dopamine agonists normalize PRL secretion in about 60% to 70% of patients with macroadenomas and also reduce tumor size in about the same percentage of patients. Reduction of tumor size may occur within days to weeks following institution of therapy. The drugs have been used to restore vision in patients with major suprasellar extension and chiasmal compression.

c. **Long-Term Remission**—Current studies suggest that 30% to 40% of patients with micro- and macroadenomas will remain in long-term remission after withdrawal of cabergoline therapy of 2 to 3 years duration provided that they have normalization of PRL levels and tumor shrinkage. Larger macroadenomas (>2.0 cm) are likely to recur, and long-term dopamine agonist therapy should be continued in these patients.

B. Surgical treatment   Transsphenoidal microsurgery is the surgical procedure of choice in patients with prolactinomas.

1. **Microadenomas**—In patients with microadenomas, remission, as measured by restitution of normal PRL levels, normal menses, and cessation of galactorrhea, is achieved in 85% to 90% of cases. Success is most likely in patients with basal PRL levels under 200 ng/mL (9.1 nmol/L) and duration of amenorrhea of less than 5 years. In these patients, the incidence of surgical complications is less than 2%, and hypopituitarism is a rare complication. Thus, in this group of patients with PRL-secreting microadenomas, PRL hypersecretion can be corrected, gonadal function restored, and secretion of TSH and ACTH preserved. Recurrence rates vary considerably in reported series. In our experience, approximately 85% of patients have had long-term remissions, and 15% have had recurrent hyperprolactinemia.

2. **Macroadenomas**—Transsphenoidal microsurgery is considerably less successful in restoring normal PRL secretion in patients with macroadenomas; many clinicians would treat these patients with dopamine agonists alone. The surgical outcome is directly related to tumor size and the basal PRL level. Thus, in patients with tumors 1 to 2 cm in diameter without extrasellar extension and with basal PRL levels less than 200 ng/mL (9.1 nmol/L), transsphenoidal surgery is successful in about 80% of cases. In patients with higher basal PRL levels and larger or invasive tumors, the success rate—defined as complete tumor resection and restoration of normal basal PRL secretion—is 25% to 50%. Although progressive visual loss or pituitary apoplexy is a clear indication for surgery, the great majority of these patients should be treated with dopamine agonists.

C. Radiotherapy   Conventional radiation therapy is reserved for patients with PRL-secreting macroadenomas who have persistent hyperprolactinemia and who have not responded to attempts to control their pituitary adenomas with surgery or dopamine agonists. In this group of patients, radiotherapy with 4000 to 5000 cGy prevents further tumor expansion, although PRL levels usually do not fall into the normal range. Impairment of anterior pituitary function occurs in approximately 50% to 60% of patients. Experience with gamma knife radiosurgery in prolactinomas is limited and rates of remission and reduction in tumor volume have been reported with varying degrees of success.

Selection of Therapy for Prolactinomas

The selection of therapy for prolactinomas depends on the wishes of the patient, the patient's plans for pregnancy and tolerance of medical therapy, and the availability of a skilled neurosurgeon.

A. Microadenomas   All patients should be treated to prevent the occasional tumor progression, loss of bone mass, and the other effects of prolonged hypogonadism. Medical therapy with cabergoline effectively restores normal gonadal function and fertility, and pregnancy carries only a small risk of tumor expansion. Those patients who respond should be treated for 2 to 3 years, and then the drug should be withdrawn to determine if long-term remission will occur. Patients who have recurrence of hyperprolactinemia after cabergoline withdrawal may resume the drug or choose to have surgical excision. Transsphenoidal adenectomy, either initially or after a trial of dopamine agonist therapy, carries little risk when performed by an experienced neurosurgeon and offers a high probability of long-term remission.

B. Macroadenomas Primary surgical therapy in these patients usually does not result in long-term remission, so medical therapy is the primary therapy of choice, particularly when the patient's PRL levels are greater than 200 ng/mL (9.1 nmol/L) and the tumor is larger than 2 cm. Although transsphenoidal microsurgery rapidly decreases tumor size and decompresses the pituitary stalk, the optic chiasm, and the cavernous sinuses, there is usually residual tumor and hyperprolactinemia. Thus, these patients require additional therapy with dopamine agonists. Although tumor growth and PRL secretion can be controlled by medical therapy in most patients, therapeutic failure can result from drug intolerance, poor compliance, or resistance. Radiation therapy is reserved for postsurgical patients with residual adenomas who are not controlled with dopamine agonists.

2. ACROMEGALY AND GIGANTISM

GH-secreting pituitary adenomas are second in frequency to prolactinomas and cause the classic clinical syndromes of acromegaly and gigantism.

The characteristic clinical manifestations are the consequence of chronic GH hypersecretion, which in turn leads to excessive generation of IGF-I, the mediator of most of the effects of GH (see Chapter 6). Although overgrowth of bone is the classic feature, GH excess causes a generalized systemic disorder with deleterious effects and an increased mortality rate, although deaths are rarely due to the space-occupying or destructive effects of pituitary adenoma per se.

Acromegaly and gigantism are virtually always secondary to a pituitary adenoma. Ectopic GHRH secretion has been identified as another cause of GH hypersecretion and acromegaly in a few patients with carcinoid or islet cell tumors. Reports of intrapituitary GHRH-secreting gangliocytomas in direct contiguity with GH-secreting somatotroph adenomas and a report of a GHRH-secreting hypothalamic hamartoma in a patient with acromegaly provide a link between ectopic and eutopic GHRH production. Ectopic secretion of GH per se is very rare but has been documented in a few lung tumors.

In adults, GH excess leads to acromegaly, the syndrome characterized by local overgrowth of bone, particularly of the skull and mandible. Linear growth does not occur, because of prior fusion of the epiphyses of long bones. In childhood and adolescence, the onset of chronic GH excess leads to gigantism. Most of these patients have associated hypogonadism, which delays epiphysial closure and the combination of IGF-I excess and hypogonadism leads to a striking acceleration of linear growth. Most patients with gigantism also have features of acromegaly if GH hypersecretion persists through adolescence and into adulthood.

Pathology

Pituitary adenomas causing acromegaly are usually more than 1 cm in diameter when the diagnosis is established. These tumors arise from the lateral wings of the anterior pituitary; less than 10% are diagnosed as microadenomas.

GH-secreting adenomas are of two histologic types: densely and sparsely granulated. However, there appears to be no difference in the degree of GH secretion or clinical manifestations in these patients. About 15% of GH-secreting tumors also contain lactotrophs, and these tumors thus hypersecrete both GH and PRL.

Etiology and Pathogenesis

In most cases, excessive pituitary GH secretion is a primary pituitary disorder. A somatic mutation in the G_s protein leading to excessive cAMP production has been identified in 40% of GH-secreting adenomas. Pituitary adenomas are present in virtually all patients and are usually greater than 1 cm in diameter; hyperplasia alone is rare, and nonadenomatous anterior pituitary tissue does not exhibit somatotroph hyperplasia when examined histologically. In addition, there is a return of normal GH levels and dynamic control of GH secretion following selective removal of the pituitary adenoma.

Pathophysiology

In acromegaly, GH secretion is increased and its dynamic control is abnormal. Secretion remains episodic; however, the number, duration, and amplitude of secretory episodes are increased, and they occur randomly throughout the 24-hour period. The characteristic nocturnal surge is absent, and there are abnormal responses to suppression and stimulation. Thus, glucose suppressibility is lost (see Diagnosis, later), and GH stimulation by hypoglycemia is usually absent. TRH and GnRH may cause GH release, whereas these substances do not normally stimulate GH secretion. Dopamine and dopamine agonists such as bromocriptine and apomorphine, which normally stimulate GH secretion, paradoxically cause GH suppression in about 70% to 80% of patients with acromegaly.

Most of the deleterious effects of chronic GH hypersecretion are caused by its stimulation of excessive amounts of IGF-I (see Chapter 6), and plasma levels of this protein are increased in acromegaly. The growth-promoting effects of IGF-I (DNA, RNA, and protein synthesis) lead to the characteristic proliferation of bone, cartilage, and soft tissues and increase in size of other organs to produce the classic clinical manifestations of acromegaly. The insulin resistance and carbohydrate intolerance seen in acromegaly appear to be direct effects of GH and not due to IGF-I excess.

Clinical Features

The sex incidence of acromegaly is approximately equal; the mean age at diagnosis is approximately 40 years; and the duration of symptoms is usually 5 to 10 years before the diagnosis is established.

Acromegaly is a chronic disabling and disfiguring disorder with increased late morbidity and mortality if untreated. Although spontaneous remissions have been described, the course is slowly progressive in the great majority of cases.

A. Symptoms and signs Early manifestations (Table 4–12) include soft tissue proliferation, with enlargement of the hands and feet and coarsening of the facial features. This is usually accompanied by increased sweating, heat intolerance, oiliness of the skin, fatigue, and weight gain.

At diagnosis, most patients have classic manifestations, and acral and soft tissue changes are always present. Bone and cartilage changes affect chiefly the face and skull. These changes include thickening of the calvarium; increased size of the frontal sinuses, which leads to prominence of the supraorbital ridges; enlargement of the nose; and downward and forward growth of the mandible, which leads to prognathism and widely spaced teeth. Soft tissue

growth also contributes to the facial appearance, with coarsening of the features and facial and infraorbital puffiness. The hands and feet are predominantly affected by soft tissue growth; they are large, thickened, and bulky, with blunt, spade-like fingers (Figure 4–18) and toes. A bulky, sweaty handshake frequently suggests the diagnosis, and there are increases in ring, glove, and shoe sizes. There is generalized thickening of the skin, with increased oiliness and sweating. Acne, sebaceous cysts, and fibromata mollusca (skin tags and papillomas) are common, as is acanthosis nigricans of the axillae and neck and hypertrichosis in women.

These bony and soft tissue changes are accompanied by systemic manifestations, which include hyperhidrosis, heat intolerance, lethargy, fatigue, and increased sleep requirement. Sleep apnea, both obstructive and central, is very common in patients with acromegaly. This has particular importance for the anesthesiologist who must take special precautions to protect the airway during surgery. Moderate weight gain usually occurs. Paresthesias, usually due to carpal tunnel compression, occur in 70%; sensorimotor neuropathies occur uncommonly. Bone and cartilage overgrowth leads to arthralgias and in longstanding cases to degenerative arthritis of the spine, hips, and knees. Photophobia of unknown cause occurs in about half of cases and is most troublesome in bright sunlight and during night driving.

GH excess leads to generalized visceromegaly, clinically evident as thyromegaly and enlargement of the salivary glands. Enlargement of other organs is usually not clinically detectable.

Hypertension occurs in about 25% of patients and cardiomegaly in about 15%. Cardiac enlargement may be secondary to hypertension, atherosclerotic disease, or, rarely, to acromegalic cardiomyopathy. Renal calculi occur in 11% secondary to the hypercalciuria induced by GH excess.

Other endocrine and metabolic abnormalities are common and may be due either to GH excess or to mechanical effects of the pituitary adenoma. Glucose intolerance and hyperinsulinism occur in 50% and 70% of patients, respectively, owing to GH-induced insulin resistance. Overt clinical diabetes occurs in a minority, and diabetic ketoacidosis is rare. Hypogonadism occurs in 60% of female and 46% of male patients and is of multifactorial origin; tumor growth and compression may impair pituitary gonadotropin secretion, and associated hyperprolactinemia (see later) or the PRL-like effect of excessive GH secretion may impair gonadotropin and gonadal function. In men, low total plasma testosterone levels may be due to GH suppression of sex hormone–binding globulin (SHBG) levels; in these cases, plasma-free testosterone levels may be normal, with normal gonadal function. With earlier diagnosis, hypothyroidism and hypoadrenalism due to destruction of the normal anterior pituitary are unusual and are present in only 13% and 4% of patients, respectively. Galactorrhea occurs in about 15% and is usually caused by hyperprolactinemia from a pituitary adenoma with a mixed cell population of somatotrophs and lactotrophs. Gynecomastia of unknown cause occurs in about 10% of men. Although acromegaly may be a component of multiple endocrine neoplasia (MEN) type 1 syndrome, it is distinctly unusual, and concomitant parathyroid hyperfunction or pancreatic islet cell tumors are rare.

TABLE 4–12 Clinical manifestations of acromegaly in 100 patients.

Manifestations of GH excess	
Acral enlargement	100[a]
Soft tissue overgrowth	100
Hyperhidrosis	88
Lethargy or fatigue	87
Weight gain	73
Paresthesias	70
Joint pain	69
Photophobia	46
Papillomas	45
Hypertrichosis	33
Goiter	32
Acanthosis nigricans	29
Hypertension	24
Cardiomegaly	16
Renal calculi	11
Disturbance of other endocrine functions	
Hyperinsulinemia	70
Glucose intolerance	50
Irregular or absent menses	60
Decreased libido or impotence	46
Hypothyroidism	13
Galactorrhea	13
Gynecomastia	8
Hypoadrenalism	4
Local manifestations	
Enlarged sella	90
Headache	65
Visual deficit	20

[a]Percentage of patients in whom these features were present.

Adapted from Tyrrell JB, Wilson CB. Pituitary syndromes. In: Friesen SR, ed. *Surgical Endocrinology: Clinical Syndromes.* Lippincott; 1978.

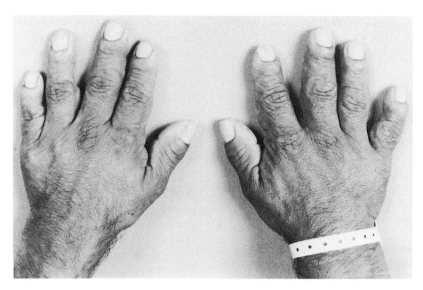

FIGURE 4-18 Markedly increased soft tissue bulk and blunt fingers in a middle-aged man with acromegaly.

When GH hypersecretion is present for many years, late complications occur, including progressive cosmetic deformity and disabling degenerative arthritis. In addition, the mortality rate is increased; after age 45, the death rate in acromegaly from cardiovascular and cerebrovascular atherosclerosis, respiratory diseases, and colon cancer is two to four times that of the normal population. Death rates tend to be higher in patients with hypertension, cardiovascular disease, or clinical diabetes mellitus.

Space-occupying manifestations of the pituitary adenoma are also common in acromegaly (eg, 65% of patients have headache). Although visual impairment was usually present in older series, it now occurs in only 15% to 20%, because most patients are now diagnosed because of the manifestations of GH excess.

B. Laboratory findings In addition to elevations in IGF-I and GH, postprandial plasma glucose may be elevated, and serum insulin is increased in 70% of cases. Elevated serum phosphate (due to increased renal tubular resorption) and hypercalciuria appear to be due to direct effects of GH or IGF-I.

C. Imaging studies Plain films (Figure 4–19) show sellar enlargement in 90% of cases. Thickening of the calvarium, enlargement of the frontal and maxillary sinuses, and enlargement of the jaw can also be seen. Radiographs of the hand show increased soft tissue bulk, "arrowhead" tufting of the distal phalanges, increased width of intra-articular cartilages, and cystic changes of the carpal bones. Radiographs of the feet show similar changes,

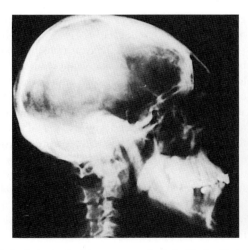
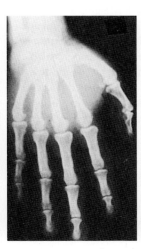
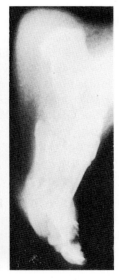

FIGURE 4-19 Radiologic signs in acromegaly. **Left:** Skull with enlarged sella turcica and frontal sinuses, thickening of the calvarium, and enlargement of the mandible. **Center:** Hand with enlarged sesamoid bone and increased soft tissue shadows. **Right:** Thickened heel pad. (Reproduced, with permission, from Levin SR. Manifestations and treatment of acromegaly. *Calif Med.* 1972;116:57).

and there is increased thickness of the heel pad (normal, <22 mm).

Diagnosis

Acromegaly is usually clinically obvious and can be readily confirmed by assessment of GH secretion; basal fasting GH levels (normal, 1-5 ng/mL [46-232 pmol/L]) are greater than 10 ng/mL (465 pmol/L) in more than 90% of patients and range from 5 ng/mL (232 pmol/L) to greater than 500 ng/mL (23,000 pmol/L), with a mean of approximately 50 ng/mL (2300 pmol/L). However, single measurements are not entirely reliable, because GH secretion is episodic in acromegaly and because other conditions may increase GH secretion (see discussed later).

A. Glucose suppression   Suppression with oral glucose is the simplest and most specific dynamic test for acromegaly. In healthy subjects, oral administration of 100 g of glucose causes a reduction of the GH level to less than 1 ng/mL (47 pmol/L) at 60 minutes. In acromegaly, GH levels may decrease, increase, or show no change; however, they do not decrease to less than 1 ng/mL (47 pmol/L), and this lack of response establishes the diagnosis.

Supersensitive GH assays have been developed and are becoming commercially available. With these assays, normal individuals may suppress GH levels to less than 0.1 ng/mL. Thus, the criteria expressed above may need to be adjusted in the near future.

B. IGF-I measurement   Measurement of IGF-I (see Chapter 6) is a useful means of establishing the diagnosis of GH hypersecretion. IGF-I results must be interpreted according to age- and sex-adjusted normative data. IGF-I levels directly reflect GH activity. IGF-I has a long half-life, so that IGF-I levels fluctuate much less than GH levels. IGF-I levels are elevated in virtually all patients with acromegaly (normal ranges vary widely in different laboratories, and some commercial assays are not reliable).

C. Tumor localization   Radiographic localization of the pituitary adenoma causing acromegaly is usually straightforward (see Neuroradiologic Evaluation, above). In virtually all patients, tumor location and size can be shown by MRI; 90% have tumors greater than 1 cm in diameter that are readily visualized. In the rare patient with normal neuroradiologic studies, an extrapituitary ectopic source of GH or GHRH should be considered. If scans suggest diffuse pituitary enlargement or hyperplasia, ectopic GHRH should also be suspected.

Differential Diagnosis

A. Other causes of GH or IGF-I hypersecretion   The presence of clinical features of GH excess, elevated GH and IGF-I secretion, and abnormal GH dynamics, together with the demonstration of a pituitary tumor by neuroradiologic studies, are diagnostic of acromegaly. However, other conditions associated with GH hypersecretion must be considered in the differential diagnosis. These include anxiety, exercise, acute illness, chronic renal failure, cirrhosis, starvation, protein-calorie malnutrition, anorexia nervosa, and type I (insulin-dependent) diabetes mellitus. Estrogen therapy may increase GH responsiveness to various stimuli. These conditions may be associated with abnormal GH suppressibility by glucose and by abnormal GH responsiveness to TRH; however, patients with these conditions do not have clinical manifestations of GH excess and are thus readily differentiated from patients with acromegaly. In addition, the conditions listed above do not lead to elevation of IGF-I concentrations. Use of testosterone or the contraceptive depot medroxyprogesterone acetate has been associated with modest elevations in IGF-I.

B. Ectopic GH or GHRH secretion   These rare patients with acromegaly due to ectopic secretion of GH or GHRH have typical clinical manifestations of acromegaly. This may occur in lung carcinoma, carcinoid tumors, and pancreatic islet cell tumors. These syndromes should be suspected in patients with a known extrapituitary tumor who have GH excess or in those with clinical and biochemical features of acromegaly who have radiologic procedures that show normal pituitary glands or that suggest diffuse pituitary enlargement or hyperplasia.

Treatment

All patients with acromegaly should undergo therapy to halt progression of the disorder and to prevent late complications and excess mortality. The objectives of therapy are removal or destruction of the pituitary tumor, reversal of GH hypersecretion, and maintenance of normal anterior and posterior pituitary function. These objectives are currently attainable in most patients, especially those with smaller tumors and only moderate GH hypersecretion. In patients with large tumors who have marked GH hypersecretion, several therapies are usually required to achieve normal GH secretion.

The criteria for an adequate response to therapy continue to evolve. Recent reports described increased late mortality in patients with GH levels by radioimmunoassay greater than 2.5 ng/mL (116 pmol/L) after therapy. Therefore, current guidelines for remission are a fasting GH of 1 ng/mL (47 pmol/L) or less and a glucose-suppressed GH of 1 ng/mL (47 pmol/L) or less accompanied by a normal level of IGF-I.

The initial therapy of choice is transsphenoidal microsurgery because of its high success rate, rapid reduction of GH levels, the low incidence of postoperative hypopituitarism, and the low surgical morbidity rate. Patients with persisting GH hypersecretion after surgery should currently be treated medically with somatostatin analogs, dopamine agonists, or a GH receptor antagonist. Radiation therapy should be reserved for those patients with inadequate responses to surgery and medical therapy.

A. Surgical treatment   Transsphenoidal selective adenoma removal is the procedure of choice; craniotomy is necessary in the rare patient in whom major suprasellar extension precludes the transsphenoidal approach. Successful reduction of GH levels is achieved in approximately 60% to 80% of patients. In those with small or moderate-sized tumors (<2 cm), success is achieved in more than 80%, whereas in those with larger tumors and basal

GH levels greater than 50 ng/mL (2325 pmol/L)—and particularly in those with major extrasellar extension of the adenoma—successful responses occur in only 30% to 60%. Recurrence rates in those with a successful initial response are low (about 5% of patients at our institution). Surgical complications (discussed earlier) occur in less than 2%.

B. Medical treatment   Octreotide acetate, a somatostatin analog, was the first effective medical therapy for patients with acromegaly. However, the drug required high doses (100-500 μg) given subcutaneously three times daily. Its use in acromegaly has been superseded by sustained-release somatostatin analogs with activities lasting up to 1 month. Preparations include octreotide LAR and lanreotide acetate given by injection every 4 weeks. Octreotide LAR normalizes GH and IGF-I levels in 75% of patients when used at doses of 20 to 40 mg/mo; however, tumor reduction occurs in a much smaller percentage. These long-acting agents have become the therapy of choice for patients with residual GH hypersecretion following surgery. Side effects of this class of agents consist mainly of gastrointestinal symptoms and the development of gallstones. Impaired glucose tolerance has been reported in some studies. The dopamine agonist cabergoline normalizes IGF-I levels in about 30% of acromegalic patients when used at doses of 1 to 2 mg/wk. However, it has not been commonly used as sole therapy. When cabergoline is added to somatostatin analog therapy, the number of patients with normalization of GH and IGF-I levels is increased.

Pegvisomant, the latest medical therapy for acromegaly, is a GH receptor antagonist. In doses of 10 to 20 mg/d given by subcutaneous injection, it reduces IGF-I levels to normal in more than 90% of patients. Although there are concerns regarding the continued excess GH secretion and possible tumor progression, serious problems have not arisen to date. Pegvisomant is effective, but its use is limited by cost and the need for daily injection. Therefore, it is currently used mainly in those patients who have failed therapy with surgery and somatostatin analogs.

C. Radiotherapy   Conventional supervoltage irradiation in doses of 4500 to 5000 cGy, although ultimately successful in 60% to 80% of patients, should not be used, because GH levels may not return to normal until 10 to 15 years after therapy. In one series, GH levels were under 10 ng/mL (460 pmol/L) in only 38% of patients at 2 years posttreatment; however, at 5 and 10 years, 73% and 81% had achieved such levels. The incidence of hypopituitarism is appreciable, and in this series hypothyroidism occurred in 19%, hypoadrenalism in 38%, and hypogonadism in approximately 50% to 60% of patients as a consequence of radiotherapy. Gamma knife radiosurgery has also been used for tumors confined to the sella. Current series, although limited, suggest remission rates of about 50% to 70% at 2 years following therapy.

Response to Treatment

In patients with successful reduction in GH hypersecretion, there is cessation of bone overgrowth. In addition, these patients experience considerable clinical improvement, including reduction in soft tissue bulk of the extremities, decreased facial puffiness, increased energy, and cessation of hyperhidrosis, heat intolerance, and oily skin. Bony changes typically do not regress. Headache, carpal tunnel syndrome, arthralgias, sleep apnea, and photophobia are also reversible with successful therapy. Glucose intolerance and hyperinsulinemia as well as hypercalciuria are also reversed in most cases.

Recent studies have also shown that the excess mortality associated with acromegaly can be reversed if GH levels are normalized.

Posttreatment Follow-Up

Posttreatment assessment includes evaluation of GH secretion, anterior pituitary function, and tumor size. Patients undergoing surgery should be seen 4 to 8 weeks after the operation for assessment of GH secretion and pituitary function. Those with persistent GH hypersecretion (>1 ng/dL [47 pmol/L]) should receive further therapy with somatostatin analogs. Patients with postoperative GH levels under 1 ng/mL (47 pmol/L) should have follow-up GH and IGF-I determinations at 6-month intervals for 2 years and yearly thereafter to rule out recurrences. Recurrent elevations in IGF-I should prompt a repeat MRI of the sella. Late hypopituitarism after surgery alone does not occur. GH replacement therapy in patients with history of acromegaly and hypopituitarism is controversial and further studies are needed.

3. ACTH-SECRETING PITUITARY ADENOMAS: CUSHING DISEASE

In 1932, Harvey Cushing documented the presence of small basophilic pituitary adenomas in six of eight patients with clinical features of adrenocortical hyperfunction. Years later, ACTH hypersecretion was identified from such tumors and found to be the cause of bilateral adrenal hyperplasia. Pituitary ACTH hypersecretion (Cushing disease) is now recognized as the most common cause of spontaneous hypercortisolism (Cushing syndrome) and must be distinguished from the other forms of adrenocorticosteroid excess—ectopic ACTH syndrome and adrenal tumors (see Chapter 9).

Pathology

ACTH-secreting pituitary tumors exist in virtually all patients with Cushing disease. These tumors are usually benign microadenomas under 10 mm in diameter; 50% are 5 mm or less in diameter, and microadenomas as small as 1 mm have been described. These tumors in Cushing disease are either basophilic or chromophobe adenomas and may be found anywhere within the anterior pituitary. Rarely, ACTH-secreting tumors are large, with invasive tendencies, and malignant tumors have rarely been reported.

Histologically, the tumors are composed of compact sheets of uniform, well-granulated cells (granule size, 200-700 nm by electron microscopy) with a sinusoidal arrangement and a high content of ACTH and its related peptides (β-LPH, β-endorphin). A zone of perinuclear hyalinization (Crooke changes) is frequently observed as a result of exposure of the corticotroph cells to prolonged hypercortisolism. A specific ultrastructural finding in these adenomas is the deposition of bundles of perinuclear microfilaments that encircle the nucleus; these are the ultrastructural equivalent of Crooke hyaline changes seen on light microscopy. In contrast to the adenoma's cells, ACTH content in the portion of the anterior pituitary not involved with the tumor is decreased.

Diffuse hyperplasia of anterior pituitary corticotrophs or adenomatous hyperplasia, presumed to result from hypersecretion of CRH, occurs rarely.

The adrenal glands in Cushing disease are enlarged, weighing 12 to 24 g (normal, 8-10 g). Microscopic examination shows a thickened cortex due to hyperplasia of both the zona reticularis and zona fasciculata; the zona glomerulosa is normal. In some cases, ACTH-secreting pituitary adenomas cause bilateral nodular hyperplasia; the adrenals show diffuse bilateral cortical hyperplasia and the presence of one or more nodules that vary from microscopic to several centimeters in diameter, with multiple small nodules being the most common.

Pathogenesis

The weight of current evidence is that Cushing disease is a primary pituitary disorder and that hypothalamic abnormalities are secondary to hypercortisolism. The endocrine abnormalities in Cushing disease are as follows: (1) hypersecretion of ACTH, with bilateral adrenocortical hyperplasia and hypercortisolism; (2) absent circadian periodicity of ACTH and cortisol secretion; (3) absent responsiveness of ACTH and cortisol to stress (hypoglycemia or surgery); (4) abnormal negative feedback of ACTH secretion by glucocorticoids; and (5) subnormal responsiveness of GH, TSH, and gonadotropins to stimulation.

Evidence that Cushing disease is a primary pituitary disorder is based on the high frequency of pituitary adenomas, the response to their removal, and the interpretation of hypothalamic abnormalities as being secondary to hypercortisolism. In addition, molecular studies have found that nearly all corticotroph adenomas are monoclonal. These findings suggest that ACTH hypersecretion arises from a spontaneously developing pituitary adenoma and that the resulting hypercortisolism suppresses the normal hypothalamic-pituitary axis and CRH release, thereby abolishing the hypothalamic regulation of circadian variability and stress responsiveness.

Analysis of the response to therapy by pituitary microsurgery sheds some light on the pathogenesis of Cushing disease. Selective removal of pituitary microadenomas by transsphenoidal microsurgery corrects ACTH hypersecretion and hypercortisolism in most patients. After selective removal of the pituitary adenoma, the following return to normal: the circadian rhythmicity of ACTH and cortisol, the responsiveness of the hypothalamic-pituitary axis to hypoglycemic stress, and the dexamethasone suppressibility of cortisol secretion.

Clinical Features

Cushing disease presents with the signs and symptoms of hypercortisolism and adrenal androgen excess (see Chapter 9). The onset of these features is usually insidious, developing over months or years. Obesity (with predominantly central fat distribution), hypertension, glucose intolerance, and gonadal dysfunction (amenorrhea or impotence) are common features. Other common manifestations include moon (rounded) facies, plethora, osteopenia, proximal muscle weakness, easy bruisability, psychologic disturbances, violaceous striae, hirsutism, acne, poor wound healing, and superficial fungal infections. Unlike patients with the classic form of ectopic ACTH syndrome, patients with Cushing disease rarely have hypokalemia, weight loss, anemia, or hyperpigmentation. Virilization, observed occasionally in patients with adrenal carcinoma, is unusual in Cushing disease. Clinical symptoms related to the ACTH-secreting primary tumor itself, such as headache or visual impairment, are rare because of the small size of these adenomas.

The usual age range is 20 to 40 years, but Cushing disease has been reported in infants and in patients over 70. There is a female:male ratio of approximately 8:1. In contrast, the ectopic ACTH syndrome occurs more commonly in men (male:female ratio of 3:1).

Diagnosis

The initial step in the diagnosis of an ACTH-secreting pituitary adenoma is the documentation of endogenous hypercortisolism, which is confirmed by increased urine-free cortisol secretion, abnormal cortisol suppressibility to low-dose dexamethasone, and/or abnormal late night salivary cortisol measurement. The differentiation of an ACTH-secreting pituitary tumor from other causes of hypercortisolism must be based on biochemical studies, including the measurement of basal plasma ACTH levels and central venous sampling, to detect a central to peripheral gradient of ACTH levels (see Chapter 9). The diagnosis and differential diagnosis of Cushing syndrome are presented in Chapter 9.

Treatment

Transsphenoidal microsurgery is the procedure of choice in Cushing disease. A variety of other therapies—operative, radiologic, pharmacologic—are discussed below.

A. Surgical treatment   Selective transsphenoidal resection of ACTH-secreting pituitary adenomas is the initial treatment of choice. At operation, meticulous exploration of the intrasellar contents by an experienced neurosurgeon is required. The tumor, which is usually found within the anterior lobe tissue, is selectively removed, and normal gland is left intact.

In about 85% of patients with microadenomas, selective microsurgery is successful in correcting hypercortisolism. Surgical damage to anterior pituitary function is rare, but most patients develop transient secondary adrenocortical insufficiency requiring postoperative glucocorticoid support until the hypothalamic-pituitary-adrenal axis recovers, usually in 2 to 18 months. The role of total hypophysectomy is currently unclear, however; hemihypophysectomy based on central venous sampling lateralization is successful in only about 50% to 70% of patients.

By contrast, transsphenoidal surgery is successful in only 25% of the 10% to 15% of patients with Cushing disease with pituitary macroadenomas or in those with extrasellar extension of tumor.

Transient diabetes insipidus occurs in about 10% of patients, but other surgical complications (eg, hemorrhage, cerebrospinal fluid rhinorrhea, infection, visual impairment, permanent diabetes insipidus) are rare. Hypopituitarism occurs only in patients who undergo total hypophysectomy.

Before the introduction of pituitary microsurgery, bilateral total adrenalectomy was the preferred treatment of Cushing disease and may still be employed in patients in whom other therapies are unsuccessful. Total adrenalectomy, which can now be performed laparoscopically, corrects hypercortisolism but produces permanent hypoadrenalism, requiring lifelong glucocorticoid and mineralocorticoid therapy. The ACTH-secreting pituitary adenoma persists and may progress, causing hyperpigmentation and invasive complications (Nelson syndrome; see below). Persistent hypercortisolism may occasionally follow total adrenalectomy as ACTH hypersecretion stimulates adrenal remnants or congenital rests.

B. Radiotherapy Conventional radiotherapy of the pituitary is of benefit in patients who have persistent or recurrent disease following pituitary microsurgery. In these patients, reported remission rates are 55% to 70% at 1 to 3 years after radiotherapy.

Gamma knife radiosurgery achieves remission rates of 65% to 75%. However, as noted above, both forms of radiotherapy cause late loss of pituitary function in more than 50% of patients and visual deficits can occur with damage to the optic chiasm or cranial nerves.

C. Medical treatment Drugs that inhibit adrenal cortisol secretion are useful in Cushing disease, often as adjunctive therapy (see Chapter 9). No drug currently available successfully suppresses pituitary ACTH secretion.

Ketoconazole, an imidazole derivative, has been found to inhibit adrenal steroid biosynthesis. It inhibits the cytochrome P450 enzymes P450scc and P450c11. In daily doses of 600 to 1200 mg, ketoconazole has been effective in the management of Cushing syndrome. Hepatotoxicity is common, however, but may be transient. **Metyrapone**, which inhibits P450c11, and **aminoglutethimide**, which inhibits P450scc, have also been utilized to reduce cortisol hypersecretion. Metyrapone is only available directly through the manufacturer and aminoglutethimide is no longer manufactured in the United States.

The use of these drugs is accompanied by increased ACTH levels that may overcome the enzyme inhibition. In addition, they cause gastrointestinal side effects that may limit their effectiveness. More effective control of hypercortisolism with fewer side effects is obtained by combined use of these agents. Adequate data are not available on the long-term use of these drugs as the sole treatment of Cushing disease. Thus, ketoconazole and aminoglutethimide ordinarily are used while awaiting a response to therapy or in the preparation of patients for surgery.

The adrenolytic drug **mitotane** results in adrenal atrophy predominantly of the zonae fasciculata and reticularis. Remission of hypercortisolism is achieved in approximately 80% of patients with Cushing disease, but most relapse after therapy is discontinued. Mitotane therapy is limited by the delayed response, which may take weeks or months, and by the frequent side effects, including severe nausea, vomiting, diarrhea, somnolence, and skin rash.

The anesthesia induction agent **etomidate** inhibits P450c11. It must be given intravenously and is generally reserved for life-threatening cases of hypercortisolism resistant to conventional therapy or when oral medications are contraindicated.

Pharmacologic inhibition of ACTH secretion in Cushing disease has also been attempted with cyproheptadine, bromocriptine, and cabergoline. However, few patients have had successful responses, and the use of these agents is not recommended.

4. NELSON SYNDROME

The clinical appearance of an ACTH-secreting pituitary adenoma following bilateral adrenalectomy as initial therapy for Cushing disease was first described by Nelson and coworkers in 1958. However, with the evolution of pituitary microsurgery as the initial therapy for Cushing disease, the Nelson syndrome is now a rare occurrence.

Pathogenesis

It now seems likely that Nelson syndrome represents the clinical progression of a preexisting adenoma after the restraint of hypercortisolism on ACTH secretion and tumor growth is removed. Thus, following adrenalectomy, the suppressive effect of cortisol is no longer present, ACTH secretion increases, and the pituitary adenoma may progress.

Incidence

Prior to the development of transsphenoidal surgery, when bilateral adrenalectomy was the initial therapy for Cushing disease, the incidence of Nelson syndrome ranged from 10% to 78% depending on what criteria were used for diagnosis (see Chapter 9). In one series, approximately 30% of patients adrenalectomized for Cushing disease developed classic Nelson syndrome with progressive hyperpigmentation and an obvious ACTH-secreting tumor; another 50% developed evidence of a microadenoma without marked progression; and about 20% never developed a progressive tumor. The reasons for these differences in clinical behavior are uncertain. Prophylactic pituitary radiotherapy is controversial. At present, when adrenalectomy is utilized only in those patients who fail pituitary microsurgery, the incidence of Nelson syndrome is less than 10%. Nevertheless, continued examination, including plasma ACTH levels and MRI, is required following bilateral adrenalectomy in patients with Cushing disease.

Clinical Features

The pituitary tumors in patients with classic Nelson syndrome can be among the most aggressive and rapidly growing of all pituitary tumors. These patients present with hyperpigmentation and with manifestations of an expanding intrasellar mass lesion. Visual field defects, headache, cavernous sinus invasion with extraocular muscle palsies, and even malignant changes with local or distant metastases may occur. Pituitary apoplexy may also complicate the course of these tumors.

Diagnosis

Plasma ACTH levels are markedly elevated, usually over 1000 pg/mL (222 pmol/L) and often as high as 10,000 pg/mL (2220 pmol/L). MRI defines the extent of the tumor.

Treatment

Pituitary surgery by the transsphenoidal approach is the initial mode of treatment. Complete resection is usually not possible, because of the large size of these tumors. Conventional radiotherapy or gamma knife radiosurgery is employed postoperatively in patients with residual tumor or extrasellar extension.

5. THYROTROPIN-SECRETING PITUITARY ADENOMAS

TSH-secreting pituitary adenomas are rare tumors manifested as hyperthyroidism with goiter in the presence of elevated TSH. Patients with TSH-secreting tumors are often resistant to routine ablative thyroid therapy, requiring large, often multiple doses of ^{131}I and several operations for control of thyrotoxicosis. Histologically, the tumors are chromophobe adenomas. They are often very large and cause visual impairment, which alerts the physician to a pituitary abnormality. Patients with these tumors do not have extrathyroidal systemic manifestations of Graves disease such as ophthalmopathy or dermopathy.

The diagnosis is based on findings of hyperthyroidism (elevated T_4 or T_3) with elevated serum TSH and alpha subunit, and neuroradiologic studies consistent with pituitary tumor. The differential diagnosis includes those patients with primary hypothyroidism (thyroid failure) that develops major hyperplasia of pituitary thyrotrophs and lactotrophs with sellar enlargement and occasional suprasellar extension. These patients can be identified by symptoms of hypothyroidism and low thyroid hormone levels. Thyroid hormone resistance may be more difficult to exclude as T_4 and T_3 levels can also be elevated. These patients, however, tend to be clinically euthyroid or hypothyroid, have a family history of thyroid hormone resistance, and generally do not present with sellar masses. Alpha subunit levels in these patients are usually not elevated.

Treatment should be directed initially at the adenoma via the transsphenoidal microsurgical approach. However, additional therapy is usually required because of the large size of these adenomas.

Somatostatin analogs normalize TSH and T_4 levels in more than 70% of these patients when given in doses similar to those used for the treatment of acromegaly (see discussion earlier). Shrinkage of the tumor has been observed in about 40% of patients.

If tumor growth and TSH hypersecretion cannot be controlled by surgery and somatostatin analogs, the next step is pituitary irradiation. In addition, such patients may also require ablative therapy of the thyroid with either ^{131}I or surgery to control their thyrotoxicosis.

6. GONADOTROPIN-SECRETING PITUITARY ADENOMAS

Although many pituitary adenomas synthesize gonadotropins (especially FSH) and their subunits, only a minority of these patients have elevated serum levels of FSH or LH. The majority of these tumors produce FSH and the alpha subunit, but tumors secreting both FSH and LH and a tumor secreting only LH have been described.

Gonadotropin-secreting pituitary adenomas are usually large chromophobe adenomas presenting with visual impairment. Most patients have hypogonadism and many have panhypopituitarism. Hormonal evaluation reveals elevated FSH in some patients accompanied by normal LH values. Basal levels of the alpha subunit may also be elevated. The presence of elevation of both FSH and LH should suggest primary hypogonadism. TRH stimulation leads to an increase in FSH secretion in 33% and an increase in LH-β in 66% of patients.

Therapy for gonadotropin-secreting adenomas has been directed at surgical removal. Because of their large size, adequate control of the tumor is difficult to achieve, and radiotherapy is usually required.

7. ALPHA SUBUNIT-SECRETING PITUITARY ADENOMAS

Excessive quantities of the alpha subunit of the glycoprotein pituitary hormones have been observed in association with the hypersecretion of many anterior pituitary hormones (TSH, GH, PRL, LH, FSH). However, pure alpha subunit hypersecretion has been identified in several patients with large invasive chromophobe adenomas and partial panhypopituitarism. Thus, the determination of the alpha subunit may be a useful marker in patients with presumed "nonfunctioning" pituitary adenomas.

8. NONFUNCTIONAL PITUITARY ADENOMAS

"Nonfunctional" chromophobe adenomas once represented approximately 80% of all primary pituitary tumors; however, with clinical application of radioimmunoassay of anterior pituitary hormones, these tumors currently account for only about 10% of all pituitary adenomas. Thus, the great majority of these chromophobe adenomas have now been documented to be PRL-secreting; a smaller number secrete TSH or the gonadotropins.

Nonfunctional tumors are usually large when the diagnosis is established; headache and visual field defects are the usual presenting symptoms. However, endocrine manifestations are usually present for months to years before the diagnosis is made, with gonadotropin deficiency being the most common initial symptom.

Hypothyroidism and hypoadrenalism are also common, but the symptoms are subtle and may be missed.

Evaluation should include MRI and visual field testing; endocrine studies should include assessment of pituitary hormones and end-organ function to determine whether the adenoma is hypersecreting or whether hormonal replacement is needed.

Because these tumors are generally large, both surgery and radiation therapy are usually required to prevent tumor progression or recurrence. In the absence of an endocrine index of tumor hypersecretion such as PRL excess, serial scans at yearly intervals are required to assess the response to therapy and to detect possible recurrence.

9. PITUITARY CARCINOMA

Pituitary carcinomas are extremely rare with fewer than 200 cases reported and defined by the distant metastases of a pituitary tumor. Most present as hormone-producing invasive macroadenomas with symptoms of mass effect. ACTH- and PRL-secreting tumors are most common. Metastases may present many years after diagnosis of the primary pituitary tumor. Survival rates are low and treatment may include additional surgery, radiotherapy, or chemotherapy.

REFERENCES

Neuroendocrinology

Anderson JR, Antoun N, Burnet N, et al. Neurology of the pituitary gland. *J Neurol Neurosurg Psychiat.* 1999;66:703. [PMID: 10329742]

Ben-Jonathan N, Hnasko R. Dopamine as a prolactin (PRL) inhibitor. *Endocr Rev.* 2001;22:724. [PMID: 11739329]

Burgess R, Lunyak V, Rosenfeld MG. Signaling and transcriptional control of pituitary development. *Curr Opin Gene Develop.* 2002;12:534. [PMID: 12200158]

Burrows HL, Douglas KR, Seasholtz AF, Camper SA. Genealogy of the anterior pituitary gland: tracing a family tree. *Trends Endocrinol Metab.* 1999;10:343. [PMID: 10511693]

Coppari R, Ramadori G, Elmquist JK. The role of transcriptional regulators in central control of appetite and body weight. *Nat Clin Pract Endocrinol Metab.* 2009;5:160. [PMID: 19229236]

Davies T, Marians R, Latif R. The TSH receptor reveals itself. *J Clin Invest.* 2002;110:209. [PMID: 12122107]

Elmquist JK. Hypothalamic pathways underlying the endocrine, autonomic, and behavioral effects of leptin. *Int J Obes Relat Metab Disord.* 2001;25:S78. [PMID: 11840221]

Fauquier T, Lacampagne A, Travo P, Bauer K, Mollard P. Hidden face of the anterior pituitary. *Trends Endocrinol Metab.* 2002;13:304. [PMID: 12163233]

Le Roith D, Bondy C, Yakar S, Liu JL, Butler A. The somatomedin hypothesis. *Endocr Rev.* 2001;22:53. [PMID: 11159816]

Moller M, Baeres FM. The anatomy and innervation of the mammalian pineal gland. *Cell Tissue Res.* 2002;309:139. [PMID: 12111544]

Muccioli G, Tschop M, Papotti M, Deghenghi R, Heiman M, Ghigo E. Neuroendocrine and peripheral activities of ghrelin: implications in metabolism and obesity. *Eur J Pharmacol.* 2002;440:235. [PMID: 12007539]

Richard D, Lin Q, Timofeeva E. The corticotropin-releasing factor family of peptides and CRF receptors: their roles in the regulation of energy balance. *Eur J Pharmacol.* 2002;12:189. [PMID: 12007535]

Sheng HZ, Westphal H. Early steps in pituitary organogenesis. *Trends Genet.* 1999;15:236. [PMID: 10354584]

Tasker JG. Rapid glucocorticoid actions in the hypothalamus as a mechanism of homeostatic integration. *Obesity.* 2006;14:259S. [PMID: 17021378]

van Vliet-Ostaptchouk JV, Hofker MH, Van Der Schouw YT. Genetic variation in the hypothalamic pathways and its role on obesity. *Obes Rev.* 2009;10:593. [PMID: 19712437]

Zigman JM, Elmquist JK. Minireview: from anorexia to obesity—the yin and yang of body weight control. *Endocrinology.* 2003;144:3749. [PMID: 12933644]

Pituitary Function Testing and Neuroradiology

Biller BM, Samuels MH, Zagar A, et al. Sensitivity and specificity of six tests for the diagnosis of adult GH deficiency. *J Clin Endocrinol Metab.* 2002;87:2067. [PMID: 11994342]

Gasco V, Corneli G, Rovere S, et al. Diagnosis of adult GH deficiency. *Pituitary.* 2008;11:121. [PMID: 18404387]

Kazlauskaite R, Evans AT, Villabona CV, et al. Corticotropin tests for hypothalamic-pituitary-adrenal insufficiency: a metaanalysis. *J Clin Endocrinol Metab.* 2008;93:4245. [PMID: 18697868]

Patronas N, Bulakbasi N, Stratakis CA, et al. Spoiled gradient recalled acquisition in the steady state technique is superior to conventional postcontrast spin echo technique for magnetic resonance imaging detection of adrenocorticotropin-secreting pituitary tumors. *J Clin Endocrinol Metab.* 2003;88:1565. [PMID: 12679440]

Raff H. Utility of salivary cortisol measurements in Cushing's syndrome and adrenal insufficiency. *J Clin Endocrinol Metab.* 2009;94:3647. [PMID: 19602555]

Smith TP, Kavanagh L, Healy ML, McKenna TJ. Technology insight: measuring prolactin in clinical samples. *Nat Clin Pract Endocrinol Metab.* 2007;3:279. [PMID: 17315036]

Pituitary Adenomas: General

Al-Brahim NY, Asa SL. My approach to pathology of the pituitary gland. *J Clin Pathol.* 2006;59:1245. [PMID: 17142570]

Asa SL, Ezzat S. The pathogenesis of pituitary tumors. *Annu Rev Pathol.* 2009;4:97. [PMID: 19400692]

Brada M, Jankowska P. Radiotherapy for pituitary adenomas. *Endocrinol Metab Clin N Am.* 2008;37:263. [PMID: 18226740]

Dekkers OM, Pereira AM, Romijn JA. Treatment and follow-up of clinically nonfunctioning pituitary macroadenomas. *J Clin Endocrinol Metab.* 2008;93:3717. [PMID: 18682516]

Elston MS, McDonald KL, Clifton-Bligh RJ, Robinson BG. Familial pituitary tumor syndromes. *Nat Rev Endocrinol.* 2009;5:453. [PMID: 19564887]

Ezzat S, Asa SL, Couldwell WT, et al. The prevalence of pituitary adenomas: a systematic review. *Cancer.* 2004;101:613. [PMID: 15274075]

Jagannathan J, Kanter AS, Sheehan JP, Jane JA Jr, Laws ER Jr. Benign brain tumors: sellar/parasellar tumors. *Neurol Clin.* 2007;25:1231. [PMID 17964033]

Komninos J, Vlassopoulou V, Protopapa D, et al. Tumors metastatic to the pituitary gland: case report and literature review. *J Clin Endocrinol Metab.* 2004;89:574. [PMID: 14764764]

Krikorian A, Aron D. Evaluation and management of pituitary incidentalomas—revisiting an acquaintance. *Nat Clin Pract Endocrinol Metab.* 2006;2:138. [PMID 16932273]

Lopes MB, Scheithauer BW, Schiff D. Pituitary carcinoma: diagnosis and treatment. *Endocrine.* 2005;28:115. [PMID: 16311418]

Vance ML. Pituitary adenoma: a clinician's perspective. *Endocr Pract.* 2008;14:757. [PMID: 18996799]

ACTH: Cushing Disease

Assié G, Bahurel H, Bertherat J, et al. The Nelson's syndrome... revisited. *Pituitary.* 2004;7:209. [PMID: 16132203]

Findling JW, Raff H. Cushing's syndrome: important issues in diagnosis and management. *J Clin Endocrinol Metab.* 2006;91:3746. [PMID: 16868050]

Jehle S, Walsh JE, Freda PU, Post KD. Selective use of bilateral inferior petrosal sinus sampling in patients with adrenocorticotropin-dependent Cushing's syndrome prior to transsphenoidal surgery. *J Clin Endocrinol Metab.* 2008;93:4624. [PMID: 18796519]

Nieman LK, Biller BM, Findling JW, et al. The diagnosis of Cushing's syndrome: an Endocrine Society Clinical Practice Guideline. *J Clin Endocrinol Metab.* 2008;93:1526. [PMID:18334580]

Sonino N, Boscaro M. Medical therapy for Cushing's disease. *Endocrinol Metab Clin North Am.* 1999;28:211. [PMID: 10207692]

Vance ML. Cushing's disease: radiation therapy. *Pituitary.* 2009;12:11. [PMID: 18437577]

Growth Hormone: Acromegaly

Freda PU, Post KD, Powell JS, Wardlaw SL. Evaluations of disease status with sensitive measures of growth hormone secretion in 60 postoperative patients with acromegaly. *J Clin Endocrinol Metab.* 1998;83:3808. [PMID: 9814451]

Melmed S. Acromegaly pathogenesis and treatment. *J Clin Invest.* 2009;119:3189. [PMID: 19884662]

PRL: Prolactinoma

Gibney J, Smith TP, McKenna TJ. Clinical relevance of macroprolactin. *Clin Endocrinol (Oxf).* 2005;62:633. [PMID: 15943822]

Molitch ME. Medication-induced hyperprolactinemia. *Mayo Clin Proc.* 2005;80:1050. [PMID: 16092584]

Schade R, Andersohn F, Suissa S, Haverkamp W, Garbe E. Dopamine agonists and the risk of cardiac-valve regurgitation. *N Engl J Med.* 2007;356:29. [PMID: 17202453]

Schlechte JA. Long-term management of prolactinomas. *J Clin Endocrinol Metab.* 2007;92:2861. [PMID: 17682084]

Vilar L, Freitas MC, Naves LA, et al. Diagnosis and management of hyperprolactinemia: results of a Brazilian multicenter study with 1234 patients. *J Endocrinol Invest.* 2008;31:436. [PMID: 18560262]

Gonadotropins (LH/FSH): Gonadotropin-Secreting Pituitary Tumors

Shomali ME, Katznelson L. Medical therapy for gonadotroph and thyrotroph tumors. *Endocrinol Metab Clin North Am.* 1999;28:223. [PMID: 10207693]

Snyder PJ. Extensive personal experience: gonadotroph adenomas. *J Clin Endocrinol Metab.* 1995;80:1059. [PMID: 7714066]

TSH-Secreting Pituitary Tumors

Brucker-Davis F, Oldfield EH, Skarulis MC, Doppman JL, Weintraub BD. Thyrotropin-secreting pituitary tumors: diagnostic criteria, thyroid hormone sensitivity, and treatment outcome in 25 patients followed at the National Institutes of Health. *J Clin Endocrinol Metab.* 1999;84:476. [PMID: 10022404]

Laws ER, Vance ML, Jane JA, Jr. TSH adenomas. *Pituitary.* 2006;9:313. [PMID: 17080266]

Shomali ME, Katznelson L. Medical therapy for gonadotroph and thyrotroph tumors. *Endocrinol Metab Clin North Am.* 1999;28:223. [PMID: 10207693]

Hypopituitarism and Other Hypothalamic-Pituitary Disorders

Bihan H, Christozova V, Dumas JL, et al. Sarcoidosis: clinical, hormonal, and magnetic resonance imaging (MRI) manifestations of hypothalamic-pituitary disease in 9 patients and review of the literature. *Medicine.* 2007;86:259. [PMID: 17873755]

Carpinteri R, Patelli I, Casanueva FF, Giustina A. Pituitary tumours: inflammatory and granulomatous expansive lesions of the pituitary. *Best Pract Res Clin Endocrinol Metab.* 2009;23:639. [PMID19945028]

Cohen LE, Radovick S, Wondisford FE. Transcription factors and hypopituitarism. *Trends Endocrinol Metab.* 1999;10:326. [PMID: 10481164]

Hardelin JP, Dode C. The complex genetics of Kallmann syndrome: KAL1, FGFR1, FGF8, PROKR2, PROK2, et al. *Sex Dev.* 2008;2:181. [PMID: 18987492]

Molitch ME, Gillam MP. Lymphocytic hypophysitis. *Horm Res.* 2007;68:145. [PMID: 18174733]

Schneider HJ, Kreitschmann-Andermahr I, Ghigo E, Stalla GK, Agha A. Hypopituitarism. *Lancet.* 2007;369:1461. [PMID: 17467517]

Schneider HJ, Kreitschmann-Andermahr I, Ghigo E, Stalla GK, Agha A. Hypothalamopituitary dysfunction following traumatic brain injury and aneurysmal subarachnoid hemorrhage: a systematic review. *JAMA.* 2007;298:1429. [PMID: 17895459]

Vance ML, Mauras N. Growth hormone therapy in adults and children. *N Engl J Med.* 1999;341:1206. [PMID: 10519899]

5

The Posterior Pituitary (Neurohypophysis)

Alan G. Robinson, MD

ACTH	Adrenocorticotropic hormone	**PAVP**	Plasma vasopressin concentration
ADH	Antidiuretic hormone	**pOsm**	Plasma osmolality
AIDS	Acquired immunodeficiency syndrome	**SIADH**	Syndrome of inappropriate antidiuretic hormone secretion
AVP	Arginine vasopressin	**V$_{1-3}$**	Vasopressin receptor, types 1-3
CSW	Cerebral salt wasting		
DDAVP	Desamino, D-8 arginine vasopressin		

PHYSIOLOGY OF HORMONE FUNCTION

Vasopressin is the water-retaining hormone in all mammals and along with thirst is the primary regulator of osmolality. Pressure and volume are primarily regulated by changes in sodium balance mediated via renin, angiotensin, and aldosterone. The relative importance of vasopressin in regulation of osmolality versus regulation of pressure is reflected in the sensitivity to changes in osmolality versus changes in pressure/volume. Figure 5–1 illustrates the exquisite sensitivity of the osmostat to as little as a 1% change in osmolality. The regulation of vasopressin secretion by baroreceptors, however, involves many concurrent and synergistic sympathetic inputs, and decrease in volume or pressure of 10% to 15% is necessary before there is a measurable increase in plasma vasopressin.

The exquisite sensitivity in the relation of plasma osmolality to urine osmolality and urine volume is illustrated in Figure 5–2. While the normal range of plasma osmolality encompasses a range of approximately 10 mOsm/L, for any individual, the set-point is much more narrow. Small changes in osmolality produce a corresponding and linear change in plasma vasopressin. As illustrated in Figure 5–2, the normal range of plasma osmolality and plasma vasopressin produces a corresponding linear increase in urine osmolality from maximally dilute to maximally concentrated. This entire range from maximally dilute urine to maximally concentrated urine is accomplished by a narrow range of plasma vasopressin (from approximately 1 to 5 pg/mL). In unusual circumstances, plasma osmolality can rise higher than the normal range, and there

is a corresponding increase in plasma vasopressin, but urine osmolality plateaus at the concentration of the renal inner medulla. When urine in the collecting duct is iso-osmotic with the urine in the inner medulla, maximum urine concentration is achieved. While the relation of plasma osmolality, plasma vasopressin, and urine osmolality are linear, the relation of these to urine volume is not linear. Rather, there is a logarithmic relationship between urine volume and urine osmolality. The total urine volume required to excrete a fixed quantity of urine osmolytes changes relatively little until plasma vasopressin and urine concentration are nearly absent, then urine volume increases dramatically from a few liters per day to 18 to 20 L/d.

In the kidney, fluid is conserved by reabsorption of sodium and fluid in the distal and the proximal tubules and then reabsorption of water in the collecting duct. The counter-current multiplier system in the loop of Henle generates a high osmolality in the renal medulla. Vasopressin acts on principal cells in the collecting duct by V$_2$ receptors that stimulate the expression of intracellular water channels, aquaporin-2. When vasopressin binds to the V$_2$ receptor, adenylate cyclase is activated to produce cyclic AMP which stimulates both the production of new aquaporin-2 protein and the transfer of existing aquaporin-2 from the cytoplasm into the cell membrane. In the cell membrane, aquaporins act as water channels in the hydrophobic lipid bilayer so that water moves down the osmotic gradient from the collecting duct into the principal cell. Aquaporins-3 and -4 are involved in moving water out of the principal cell into the medullary extracellular fluid and from there into the circulation. In response to changes in vasopressin,

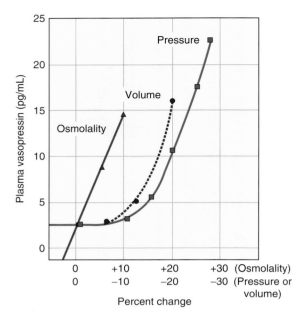

FIGURE 5–1 Vasopressin secretion in response to percentage increases in osmolality or decreases in pressure or volume. (Redrawn, with permission, from Robertson GL, Berl T. Water metabolism. In: Brenner BM, Rector FC, Jr, eds. *The Kidney*. vol. 1. 3rd ed. Philadelphia, PA: WB Saunders; 1986: 385.)

aquaporin-2 can be quickly shuttled in and out of the membrane producing rapid changes in water reabsorption and concentration of urine.

Volume/pressure regulation by vasopressin operates through V_1 receptors on blood vessels. These receptors cause contraction of smooth muscle to raise blood pressure and, secondarily reduce intravascular volume.

V_2 receptors also stimulate antihemophilic and von Willebrand factors. There is a third type receptor (V_3) on anterior pituitary cells that stimulates ACTH. These functions are not further considered in this chapter.

In most physiologic situations, changes in osmolality and volume are additive or synergistic in producing the appropriate physiologic response. For example, most cases of dehydration result in greater loss of water than solute. This produces an increase in plasma osmolality and a decrease in volume that act together to stimulate thirst and the secretion of vasopressin, which promotes retention of water. Similarly, excess ingestion of hypotonic fluid produces a decrease in plasma osmolality and an increase in plasma volume, both of which decrease plasma vasopressin and result in excretion of dilute urine. The normal regulation of osmolality is an elegant and simple system. Fluid ingested and water produced from metabolized food is in excess of true need. The retained water causes a small decrease in plasma osmolality with a small decrease in vasopressin and an excretion of the ingested fluid. If the water intake is not sufficient to supply body needs, plasma osmolality rises, producing concentrated urine to reduce fluid loss, and stimulates thirst that induces drinking to replenish body fluid.

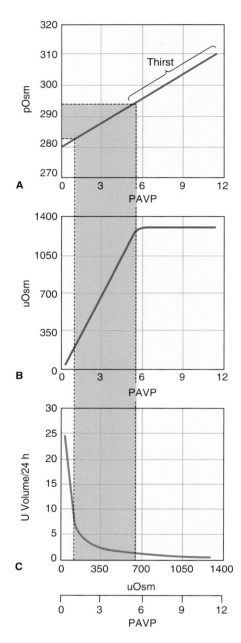

FIGURE 5–2 Normal physiologic relationship between plasma osmolality (pOsm; mOsm/kg H_2O), plasma vasopressin (PAVP; pg/mL), urine osmolality (uOsm; mOsm/kg H_2O), and urine volume (L/d). **(A)** Changes in osmolality induce linear changes in vasopressin with a normal physiologic range of osmolality producing vasopressin levels of 0.5 to 5 pg/mL. **(B)** The physiologic range of vasopressin produces linear changes in urine osmolality. At vasopressin levels above 5 to 6 pg/mL, urine osmolality is at the maximum, determined by the osmolality of the inner medulla of the kidney. **(C)** Assuming a constant osmolar load, the relationship of volume to urine osmolality is logarithmic. The urine volume to excrete a given osmolar load at the urine osmolality in **(B)** is indicated in **C**. (Calculated from formulas in Robertson GL, Shelton RL, Athar S. The osmoregulation of vasopressin. *Kidney Int*. 1976;10:25-37.) (Copyright 2003, A.G. Robinson, University of California at Los Angeles.)

Fluid and electrolyte balance is not well regulated in elderly people. By age 80, total body water declines to as low as 50% of the level in normal young adults. Older subjects may have a decrease in glomerular filtration rate, and the collecting duct is less responsive to vasopressin. Numerous studies have indicated a decreased thirst with dehydration in elderly subjects, but also a lessened ability to excrete a water load. These age-related changes in body fluid and renal function predispose elderly people to both hypernatremia and hyponatremia. Also, elderly people are more likely to have comorbid diseases which enhance their tendency to become hyponatremic or hypernatremic. It is incumbent upon the physician to pay special attention to fluid balance in older people.

ANATOMY OF HORMONE SYNTHESIS AND RELEASE

The posterior pituitary (unlike the anterior pituitary) is not a gland but only the distal axon terminals of the hypothalamic magnocellular neurons that make up the neurohypophysis. The cell bodies of these neurons are located in paired supraoptic nuclei and paired paraventricular nuclei of the hypothalamus. The paraventricular nuclei are located on each side of the third ventricle and axons from these neurons trace laterally and anteriorly to the location of the magnocellular neurons of the supraoptic nucleus just lateral to and above the optic chiasm. Axons of the supraoptic nucleus join axons of the paraventricular nucleus and course to the basal hypothalamus where they join the axons from the other side and course through the infundibular stalk to the axon terminals in the posterior pituitary.

The anatomic location of the physiologic regulators of osmotic and pressure/volume (baroreceptor) are located in vastly different sites. Osmoreceptors that control both thirst and osmotic regulation of vasopressin are located in the hypothalamus just anterior to the third ventricle, so the entire regulation of osmotic-induced changes in thirst and vasopressin secretion resides in a small and discrete area in the hypothalamus. Increases in osmolality stimulate the osmoreceptor to send a positive signal to stimulate thirst and to release vasopressin. For volume and pressure regulation, the receptors are located in the chest. There are high-pressure arterial baroreceptors in the carotid sinus and aortic arch and low-pressure volume receptors in the atria and pulmonary venous system. The pressure/volume receptor afferent signals are carried through cranial nerves 9 and 10 and synapse in the medulla before carrying their input to the magnocellular neurons. Both excitatory and inhibitory baroreceptor influences act on the magnocellular neurons, although some evidence indicates that a predominant mechanism involves the tonic inhibition of vasopressin secretion. A decrease in pressure/volume decreases the inhibition and stimulates release of vasopressin.

Vasopressin and oxytocin are nonapeptides that are synthesized in the cell bodies of the magnocellular neurons as part of a larger precursor peptide. Like other polypeptide hormones, the precursor proteins traverse the endoplasmic reticulum and the Golgi apparatus to be packaged in secretory granules. The neurosecretory granules then travel down the long axons through the stalk of the infundibulum to the posterior pituitary where the granules are stored. During transport, peptide enzymes (peptidases) cleave the prohormone into the hormone (vasopressin or oxytocin), a carrier protein (neurophysin), and (for vasopressin only) a glycopeptide. The synthesis of oxytocin and vasopressin is in separate neurons organized in clusters within the paraventricular nuclei and supraoptic nuclei. This allows stimulation of individual neurons and independent release of individual hormones. The stimulus for secretion of vasopressin or oxytocin is by neurotransmitters acting on the appropriate magnocellular cell body. An action potential propagates along the axon, causing an influx of calcium at the axon terminal and release of the hormone content of neurosecretory granules into the perivascular space.

PATHOPHYSIOLOGY

All defined pathophysiology of the posterior pituitary is related to the function of vasopressin rather than oxytocin. Both decreased function of vasopressin and increased function of vasopressin manifest as abnormalities of water balance and depend upon action of vasopressin on the V_2 receptor of the kidney rather than the V_1 vascular receptors. The clinical presentation of low vasopressin function (diabetes insipidus) or excess vasopressin function (syndrome of inappropriate secretion of antidiuretic hormone, SIADH) is determined by the physiology of thirst. In humans thirst is well regulated to turn on when needed but not well regulated to turn off when not needed. When vasopressin is decreased or absent (diabetes insipidus), there is abnormal excretion of a large volume of dilute urine. This should cause hyperosmolality and an increase in serum sodium. However, as illustrated in Figure 5–2, an elevated plasma osmolality stimulates thirst, and a patient will drink a large volume of fluid to keep their sodium in the normal range. So, the clinical presentation of decreased vasopressin is one associated with polyuria and dilute urine together with polydipsia but with a normal serum sodium. Alternatively, when vasopressin is increased, there is abnormal concentration of urine and retention of water. The volume expansion by water dilutes serum sodium. If thirst were inhibited by hypo-osmolality as efficiently as thirst is stimulated by hyperosmolality, then the decrease in osmolality would produce a profound decrease in fluid intake, and a normal serum sodium would be maintained by the natural loss of fluid with perspiration, gastrointestinal fluid loss, and the urine output necessary to excrete ingested osmoles produced by food intake. Thirst, however, is not sufficiently inhibited, and the volume expansion not only dilutes serum sodium, but induces sodium excretion to reduce extracellular volume, which worsens the hyponatremia. So, the presentation of increased vasopressin is a chemical presentation of hyponatremia. There is concurrent concentrated urine with no change in thirst, modest volume expansion, hyponatremia, and natriuresis.

The other physiologic principles which determine some of the pathophysiology of abnormal secretion of vasopressin are: osmolality is regulated by changes in water balance, and volume is regulated by changes in sodium balance. When in conflict, volume will be preserved at the expense of osmolality. Thus, as described later, if dehydration is produced by diabetes insipidus, sodium will be retained to protect volume, even if it aggravates hypernatremia. With SIADH when sodium is diluted and extracellular volume is expanded, natriuresis is initiated to decrease extracellular volume in spite of the need to retain sodium to correct the hypo-osmolality.

DEFICIENT VASOPRESSIN: DIABETES INSIPIDUS

Diabetes insipidus is literally the excretion of a large volume of urine (diabetes) that is hypotonic, dilute, and tasteless (insipid). Patients present with polyuria. Other causes of polyuria such as osmotic diuresis that occur in diabetes mellitus or intrinsic renal disease must be excluded. Frequent urination, without an increase in urine volume, suggests a urologic abnormality. Most adults will tolerate polyuria without complaint until it exceeds 3 to 4 L/d. If polyuria is shown to be dilute, the pathophysiologic mechanisms include: (1) primary ingestion of excess fluid, (2) abnormally decreased synthesis and secretion of vasopressin, (3) increased metabolism of vasopressin, and (4) decreased end-organ response to vasopressin.

A. Ingestion of excess fluid and normal urine excretion—primary polydipsia

Primary polydipsia with ingestion of large quantities of water produces modest decreases in plasma osmolality, decreased secretion of vasopressin, and excretion of profound quantities of urine. As the volume of dilute fluid delivered to the collecting duct is approximately 18 L/d, this quantity of dilute urine can be excreted on a daily basis while maintaining serum osmolality in the normal range. Virtually any pathologic process in the hypothalamus that causes diabetes insipidus may rarely cause primary stimulation of the thirst center and primary polydipsia on an organic basis. Alternatively, primary polydipsia may occur as a behavioral abnormality in psychiatric patients in whom the excess water ingestion and urination may represent delusions tied to bodily cleansing. The large volume of urine passing through the collecting duct in these patients washes urea out of the inner medulla and reduces the inner medulla osmolality. Additionally, the chronic suppression of vasopressin release and lack of action of vasopressin on the renal collecting duct decreases the synthesis of aquaporins in the collecting duct cells, adding to the inability to concentrate the urine maximally. Each of these abnormalities returns to normal in several days to weeks after fluid ingestion is decreased to normal.

Primary polyuria may be induced in a normal person if excess fluid is administered parenterally. This occasionally occurs in postoperative cases that do not involve the pituitary. In many surgical procedures, the stress of the surgery is a stimulus to release of vasopressin, and administered fluids may be retained during the procedure. Postoperatively, the stress is released, and patients have a normal diuresis of the retained fluids. If this normal excretion of fluid is matched by increased fluids administered parenterally, the patient will continue to excrete large volumes of urine. If the administered fluid is normal saline, the patients will excrete a large

volume of isotonic urine. If the volume administered is sufficiently great, the patients will be unable to dilute or concentrate their urine above or below an iso-osmotic level regardless of therapeutic agents. The large osmotic load delivered to the kidney may make the patient unresponsive even to administered desmopressin, producing an iatrogenic therapeutic dilemma.

B. Abnormal synthesis and secretion of vasopressin
It is important to remember that the complaint of polyuria is based upon the volume of the urine not the urinary concentration. Therefore, as evident from Figure 5–2, considerable loss of ability to secrete vasopressin may occur before there is much loss of ability to concentrate the urine and even greater loss may occur before there is a noticeable increase in urine volume.

1. GENETIC ABNORMALITIES OF NEUROHYPOPHYSEAL NEURONS
Familial hypothalamic diabetes insipidus.   Familial diabetes insipidus may be caused by an autosomal dominant mutation in the vasopressin gene. Usually the mutation involves DNA sequences in the neurophysin or signal peptide region of the precursor gene rather than the region encoding vasopressin itself. These mutations cause abnormal folding of the precursor protein which produces abnormal trafficking and accumulation of a mutant prohormone in the endoplasmic reticulum. This produces alterations in packaging of the prohormone into neurosecretory granules in the Golgi apparatus. By ill-defined mechanisms, this leads to cell death of the vasopressin-producing neurons. Because the pathology in these neurons develops over time, young children may have normal urine output, and diabetes insipidus is not expressed until late childhood. An autosomal dominant form of diabetes insipidus also occurs in association with diabetes mellitus, optic atrophy, and deafness (DIDMOAD), also known as Wolfram syndrome.

2. PATHOLOGIC LESIONS OF NEUROHYPOPHYSEAL NEURONS
Solid tumors and hematologic malignancies.   The most common solid tumor to produce diabetes insipidus is craniopharyngioma. Suprasellar germinoma or pinealoma, which may be associated with precocious puberty, commonly produces diabetes insipidus. Metastatic disease to the pituitary hypothalamic area, for example, from breast or lung cancer, is more likely to produce diabetes insipidus than a deficiency of anterior pituitary hormones because the metastases lodge in the portal system of the hypothalamus where the vasopressin axons from the two sides join to form the pituitary stalk. Usually, there are widespread unidentified metastatic lesions elsewhere. Lymphoma or infiltration of the hypothalamus with leukemia are rare causes of diabetes insipidus.

Trauma or surgery.   The anatomy of the neurohypophyseal system aids our understanding of this pathology. Hormone synthesis and regulation of release is high in the hypothalamus. Surgery or trauma at the level of the pituitary traumatizes only the axon terminals. Trauma of the axon terminals may disrupt the

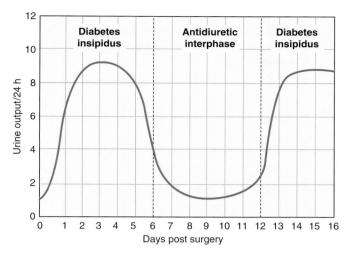

FIGURE 5–3 Illustration of the phases of urine output after section of the pituitary stalk. The *triphasic response* consists of: (1) diabetes insipidus due to axonal shock and lack of release of vasopressin; (2) an antidiuretic interphase when vasopressin leaks from the severed neurons; and (3) return of diabetes insipidus when the store of vasopressin in the posterior pituitary is depleted.

release of hormone, but usually this produces only a transient inability to secrete hormone and transient diabetes insipidus. Sectioning of the posterior pituitary stalk produces a characteristic pattern of diabetes insipidus known as the triphasic response. This is illustrated in Figure 5–3. Initial axonal shock inhibits the release of any vasopressin, and there is a period of diabetes insipidus that lasts for 5 to 10 days. Then, the severed axons in the posterior pituitary become necrotic and there is uncontrolled release of vasopressin. If excess fluid is administered during this time, the syndrome of inappropriate antidiuretic hormone is produced with hyponatremia (described later). This lasts for 5 to 10 days until all of the residual vasopressin leaks from the axon terminals when there is return of diabetes insipidus. While the classic response to stalk section is the three phases, in many clinical situations not all three phases occur. The most common occurrence after surgery in the pituitary or hypothalamus is transient diabetes insipidus that lasts a few days without subsequent sequelae. With partial damage to the pituitary stalk rather than total section, it is possible that the second phase will occur without preceding or subsequent diabetes insipidus (ie, isolated second phase). In the isolated second phase, there are sufficient normally functioning vasopressinergic neurons to avoid diabetes insipidus in the first and third phase; however, the damaged axon terminals leak vasopressin that will, when coupled with excess fluid intake, produce SIADH and hyponatremia. Characteristically, hyponatremia occurs 5 to 10 days after pituitary surgery, lasts for 5 to 10 days, and then resolves. Late occurrence of diabetes insipidus, that is, third phase without a first or second phase, is distinctly uncommon.

Patients with diabetes insipidus due to surgery or trauma may eventually recover. The level of section determines the number of magnocellular neurons that are actually killed. The higher in the stalk and the closer the section to the perikaria, the greater the number of neurons that die. Vasopressin-producing neurons whose axons terminate in the hypothalamus and serve as secretagogues for ACTH in the anterior pituitary may persist and hypertrophy after surgery or trauma. Additionally, branching of axons may develop in the hypothalamus after surgery or trauma, and these branches may generate new connections of vasopressinergic neurons to blood vessels. By these mechanisms, sufficient vasopressin function may return (usually within 1 year) to have normal fluid balance and no symptoms of diabetes insipidus.

Granulomatous disease. Langerhans cell histiocytosis is the generic term that includes severe fulminant visceral Letterer-Siwe disease, multifocal Hand-Schuller-Christian disease, and benign eosinophilic granuloma. Diabetes insipidus is part of the central nervous system involvement in these disorders and is associated with other abnormalities of the head involving the cranial bones, oral mucosa, or brain. Systemic manifestations in the lung, bone, and skin may also be present. Wegener granulomatosis and sarcoidosis may also have diabetes insipidus as a part of the central nervous system pathology.

Lymphocytic infundibulohypophysitis. It is now recognized that many cases of diabetes insipidus, that were previously termed idiopathic and for which there was no specific etiology, are probably due to lymphocytic infiltration of the neurohypophysis on an autoimmune basis. X-rays may reveal enlargement of the pituitary stalk as evidence of the lymphocytic invasion. There may be resolution of the autoimmune response with time and the stalk may return to normal size, but the diabetes insipidus is usually permanent.

Essential hypernatremia—Adipsic hypothalamic diabetes insipidus. A rare variant of diabetes insipidus involves an absent osmoreceptor function, but an intact baroreceptor function. In this form of diabetes insipidus, patients do not sense thirst and, therefore, do not drink water. This results in an elevation of serum osmolality because the osmostat does not respond to the increased osmolality by releasing vasopressin or stimulating thirst. However, vasopressin synthesis and storage are normal as demonstrated by specific tests of baroreceptor function. Characteristically, these patients do not drink water and become sufficiently dehydrated that their baroreceptors stimulate vasopressin release, they then remain in a balanced situation with an elevated serum sodium level, relatively concentrated urine, and lack of thirst.

Cerebral anoxia/brain death. Brain dead patients who are on life support often have diabetes insipidus as part of the central nervous system pathology. It is standard practice to maintain electrolyte and water balance for maximal preservation of organs for transplantation.

C. Increased metabolism of vasopressin in pregnancy to produce diabetes insipidus
During pregnancy, there is a true resetting of the osmostat at an osmolality approximately

10 mOsm/kg H_2O less than the normal pOsm–PAVP relationship. So, in Figure 5–2 (A), the pOsm–PAVP would have the same linear relationship but would be shifted downward on the graph with the increase in PAVP beginning at pOsm of 270. Both increases and decreases in plasma vasopressin occur at the lower pOsm while the uOsm and U volume response to PAVP remains the same. There is a similar change in the regulation of plasma volume. In normal pregnancy, total body water is increased by 7 to 8 L as a result of profound vasodilatation. This expanded volume is also sensed as normal with vasopressin increasing and decreasing around this new volume. Relaxin, which is produced in pregnancy, is the mediator of these effects. In pregnancy the placenta produces an enzyme, cysteine aminopeptidase, that is known as oxytocinase but similarly degrades vasopressin. Therefore, vasopressin metabolism is increased in pregnancy, markedly so from 20 to 40 weeks of gestation.

Because of the reset osmostat, a "normal" serum sodium during pregnancy may represent dehydration. There are two types of diabetes insipidus that are associated with pregnancy. In the first, the patient has a preexisting limitation of vasopressin function such as partial hypothalamic diabetes insipidus or mild nephrogenic diabetes insipidus. The ability to concentrate the urine may be limited but sufficient to maintain acceptable urine volume prepartum. During pregnancy, however, the metabolism of vasopressin is accelerated. With increased metabolism of vasopressin, these patients may then not have sufficient concentrating ability to maintain an acceptable urine volume (see vasopressin–volume relationships in Figure 5–2) and manifest diabetes insipidus that reverts to the existing asymptomatic condition when the pregnancy ends. A second form of diabetes insipidus occurs when the level of cysteine aminopeptidase is extraordinarily higher than in normal pregnancy and produces diabetes insipidus in a patient with normal pituitary and renal function. There may be other associated pathology with the latter disease such as preeclampsia, fatty liver, and coagulopathies. Diabetes insipidus in this situation also abates when the pregnancy ends and may not recur with subsequent pregnancies.

D. Decreased end organ response to vasopressin—nephrogenic diabetes insipidus

1. **Congenital nephrogenic diabetes insipidus**   There are two causes of congenital nephrogenic diabetes insipidus: (1) an X-linked recessive mutation of the V_2 receptor, which accounts for 90% of the cases; and, (2) an autosomal recessive mutation of the aquaporin-2 water channels. The X-linked disorder, of course, only occurs in males while disease due to mutations of the aquaporin-2 gene occurs in males and females. Female carriers of the X-linked V_2 receptor abnormality usually have no clinical disease nor do heterozygote carriers of the recessive aquaporin-2 mutations. Nephrogenic diabetes insipidus due to aquaporin-2 defects is produced when the child inherits a mutated gene from each parent that carries the recessive mutation.

Regardless of etiology, the presentation of nephrogenic diabetes insipidus usually occurs in the first week of life presenting with vomiting, constipation, failure to thrive, fever, and polyuria. The patients are found to be hypernatremic with low urine osmolality. When measured, vasopressin levels are elevated.

2. **Acquired nephrogenic diabetes insipidus**   The ability to produce concentrated urine depends upon hyperosmolality of the inner medulla which in turn requires normal kidney architecture with descending and ascending limbs of the loop of Henle, normal sodium transport, functional aquaporins, and intact long loop vascular structures (vasa recta) so that the hyperosmolality in the inner medulla is not washed away by normal blood flow. One form of nephrogenic diabetes insipidus is produced by renal disease that distorts the architecture of the kidney as in polycystic renal disease, infarcts, sickle cell anemia, and so forth. The polyuria associated with potassium deficiency and hypercalcemia both are associated with decreased expression of aquaporin-2. Among drugs that may produce nephrotoxicity, the most common to produce nephrogenic diabetes insipidus are lithium (commonly when used to treat bipolar disorders) and demeclocycline.

DIAGNOSTIC TESTS OF DIABETES INSIPIDUS

One can determine whether there is true polyuria by measuring the 24-hour urine output, but collecting this large volume is inconvenient. Alternatively, the patient can keep a diary, recording the time and volume of each voided urine without saving the urine for examination.

A. Dehydration test   After other causes of polyuria are eliminated, the diagnosis of diabetes insipidus is accomplished by some form of dehydration test. The dehydration test should be done in a controlled environment. The description here is for adults. Dehydration of children requires special attention and should only be done by a pediatrician. Dehydration tests should not be done in infants. The patient is weighed at the beginning of the test, and a serum sodium concentration and plasma osmolality are obtained. Nothing is allowed by mouth, and the volume and osmolality of each voided urine are recorded. The patient is weighed after each liter of urine is excreted. When two consecutive measures of urine osmolality differ by less than 10% and the patient has lost 2% of his body weight, the serum sodium concentration and plasma osmolality are again determined, and a blood sample is drawn for a determination of plasma vasopressin. The patient is then given parenterally 2 μg of desmopressin, a synthetic analogue of vasopressin described later, and urine osmolality and output are recorded for an additional 2 hours. The duration of the test varies, but in most patients a plateau in the urine osmolality will be reached by 18 hours. The test is discontinued if the patient loses 3% of the body weight. The different responses to this testing are depicted in Figure 5–4. If the patient is dehydrated and hyperosmolar and the urine is dilute when first seen, no further dehydration is necessary. Blood is drawn to measure plasma vasopressin, and the response to desmopressin is determined.

Patients with primary polydipsia are distinguished from diabetes insipidus by the concentration of the urine at a plateau which is frequently 500 to 700 mOsm/kg and by the lack of further response to administered desmopressin. Patients with

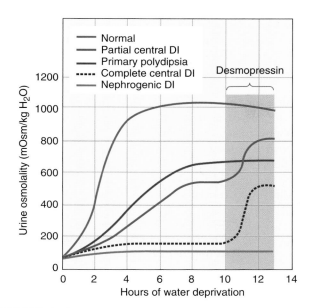

FIGURE 5–4 Urine osmolality during a dehydration test followed by administration of desmopressin to differentiate various types of diabetes insipidus and primary polydipsia as described by Miller et al. (Miller M, Dalakos T, Moses AM, Fellerman H, Streeten D. Recognition of partial defects in antidiuretic hormone secretion. *Ann Int Med.* 1970;73:721-729). See text for discussion of the differential diagnosis based on the plateau of urine osmolality with dehydration and subsequent response to administered desmopressin.

hypothalamic diabetes insipidus have undetectable or low plasma vasopressin levels at the end of dehydration, minimal concentration of the urine, and an additional increase in urine osmolality to administered desmopressin of at least 50% but often 200% to 400%. Patients with nephrogenic diabetes insipidus do not concentrate their urine similar to hypothalamic diabetes insipidus, but the levels of plasma vasopressin are high, often greater than 5 pg/mL at the end of the test. Additionally, there is no further increase in urine osmolality after the administration of desmopressin. Occasionally, patients with partial hypothalamic diabetes insipidus concentrate their urine minimally with dehydration, but their maximum urinary concentration is not achieved, and there is an additional boost with administered desmopressin. This pattern can be similar to some patients with primary polydipsia who achieve a plateau level of urine osmolality before reaching their maximum attainable urine osmolality and show a boost in urine osmolality in response to desmopressin. These patients are usually distinguished by their response to desmopressin over time. Patients with partial hypothalamic diabetes insipidus do well while those with primary polydipsia may continue to drink excessive amounts of water and develop hyponatremia.

Measurements of plasma vasopressin by clinically available assays is only of help in distinguishing nephrogenic diabetes insipidus (in which the level will be unequivocally elevated) from other causes of diabetes insipidus. Recent reports have described a radioimmunoassay of copeptin, the inactive carboxy peptide that is cleaved from the provasopressin molecule and secreted with

vasopressin and neurophysin, but the clinical usefulness has yet to be determined.

B. Imaging in diabetes insipidus Imaging of the hypothalamus is an important diagnostic tool in diabetes insipidus. The exquisite sensitivity of the kidney to vasopressin, especially with regard to urine volume, determines that even 10% of the vasopressin neurons may be sufficient to maintain homeostasis without symptoms. Because of the wide anatomic distance between the paraventricular and supraoptic nuclei, tumors that produce diabetes insipidus are either sufficiently large to destroy 90% of the vasopressin neurons or, most commonly, are located just above the diaphragma sella where the neurohypophyseal tracts of the two sides converge as they enter the pituitary stalk. Small tumors of the anterior pituitary confined to the sella are never the cause of diabetes insipidus. On T1-weighted images, the normal posterior pituitary appears as a bright spot on MRI studies. The bright spot is produced by the stored hormone in the posterior pituitary. Most normal subjects have the bright spot, although it decreases with age, and most patients with diabetes insipidus do not have a bright spot. An MRI may reveal thickening of the stalk and absence of the posterior pituitary bright spot. This is a characteristic finding of some granulomatous diseases of the neurohypophysis and of lymphocytic infundibulitis.

TREATMENT OF DIABETES INSIPIDUS

As noted above, adults with intact thirst mechanisms usually drink sufficient fluid to maintain serum sodium levels in the normal range. Babies and adults without access to fluid or patients who are unconscious may not drink and will develop severe dehydration and hypernatremia. If hypothalamic diabetes insipidus is caused by a specific disease such as a granulomatous disorder, that condition should be treated. Rarely, however, does successful treatment of the underlying disease produce remission of the diabetes insipidus.

Hypothalamic diabetes insipidus is best treated by the vasopressin analogue desmopressin (desamino, D-8 arginine vasopressin, DDAVP). In desmopressin, the amine at position 1 is removed, increasing the half-life of the compound, and at position 8, L-arginine is changed to D-arginine, markedly reducing the pressor activity. Thus, the agent is highly selective for the V_2 receptor and is nearly 2000 times more specific for antidiuresis than is the naturally occurring L-arginine vasopressin. Desmopressin is available as tablets (0.1 and 0.2 mg), a solution for nasal installation (100 µg/mL), and a parenteral solution (4 µg/mL). There is considerable individual variability in the duration of action of desmopressin, so the dosing should be adjusted for each individual. Usually, a satisfactory schedule can be achieved with 2 to 3 tablets per day or one to two intranasal doses. A parenteral preparation can be given intravenously, intramuscularly, or subcutaneously and is 5 to 20 times more potent than the intranasally administered dose. The drug is expensive, and in many patients, a smaller dose given more frequently is more cost-effective. Other agents that prolong the action of vasopressin or the release of vasopressin include chlorpropamide, carbamazepine, clofibrate, and indo-methacin, but these are not first-line therapies. Desmopressin is the only therapeutic agent recommended for treatment of diabetes insipidus in pregnancy because desmopressin is not destroyed by cysteine aminopeptidase and has minimal oxytocic activity on the uterus.

In patients with inadequate thirst, the best treatment is con-tinuous administration of desmopressin to maintain a concen-trated urine and then rigid adjustment of the amount of fluid that must be taken every 6 to 8 hours to maintain normal serum sodium.

In nephrogenic diabetes insipidus, any offending drug or elec-trolyte abnormality that might produce acquired nephrogenic diabetes insipidus should be stopped or corrected. In congenital nephrogenic diabetes insipidus, therapy is aimed at reducing urine volume through a low sodium diet and a thiazide diuretic. This causes a natriuresis which produces some contraction of the extra-cellular fluid volume, decreased glomerular filtration rate, decreased delivery of fluid to the collecting duct, and a decreased urine vol-ume. Amiloride is especially recommended in this setting because it is potassium sparing. Amiloride may also have some advantage in lithium-induced nephrogenic diabetes insipdus because amiloride decreases lithium entrance into cells in the distal tubule. Indomethacin has an antidiuretic action that especially prolongs the action of vasopressin and administered desmopressin. It also decreases urine volume in nephrogenic diabetes insipidus, but there is concern about gastrointestinal bleeding.

When diabetes insipidus occurs in patients who also have ante-rior pituitary deficiency, adequate treatment with thyroid hor-mone and hydrocortisone is essential to maintain normal renal response to desmopressin. Clinical situations such as surgical pro-cedures, treatments that require a saline diuresis, and periods when patients are not allowed fluids by mouth require careful bal-ance of antidiuretics, administered fluid, and sodium.

EXCESS VASOPRESSIN: SYNDROME OF INAPPROPRIATE ANTIDIURETIC HORMONE

Excess vasopressin becomes a clinical problem when there is con-current retention of water producing hypo-osmolality. Hypo-osmolality is common in hospitalized patients but in most cases is due to underlying illness. Statistically, hyponatremia is associated with increased morbidity and mortality because it is a measure of the severity of the underlying illness. This chapter focuses on cases in which inappropriately elevated vasopressin and water retention are the cause of the hypo-osmolality (see also Chapter 21 Humoral Manifestations of Malignancy).

The differential diagnosis of hypo-osmolality is based upon measuring the serum sodium concentration and estimating the extracellular fluid status. Sodium is the major cation of the extracellular fluid, and potassium is the major cation of the intra-cellular fluid. Water moves freely between the intracellular and extracellular fluid, so osmolality is always equivalent in both compartments. The relative balance between solute depletion and water retention, as a cause of hypo-osmolality, is complex, but in virtually all cases of clinically significant hypo-osmolality, there is some element of impaired water excretion and/or excessive water intake.

Plasma osmolality can be measured directly by freezing point depression or vapor pressure of plasma, but usually, hypo-osmolality is brought to clinical attention because of decreased concentration of sodium rather than measure of osmolality. In the extracellular fluid, the major contributions to osmolality are sodium, glucose, and blood urea nitrogen (BUN). A calculated osmolality usually correlates well with measured osmolality.

$$\text{Plasma osmolality (mOsm/kg } H_2O)$$
$$= 2 \times [Na^+] \text{ (mEq/L)} + \text{Glucose (mg/dL)}/18$$
$$+ \text{BUN (mg/dL)}/2.8$$

Occasionally, when the serum sodium concentration is mea-sured by flame photometry the measured sodium is artifactually low because flame photometry calculates the sodium in a fixed volume of plasma. If a large proportion of the plasma volume is taken up by extremely elevated levels of lipid or protein, sodium determined by flame photometry is low. Plasma osmolality deter-mined by freezing point or vapor pressure is a direct measure of particles in solution and will be normal in these situations. So the low sodium level by flame photometry is referred to as pseudohy-ponatremia. Hyperglycemia will produce hyponatremia because of the shift of water from the intracellular fluid to the extracellular fluid; however, the calculated osmolality will be normal. The serum sodium can be corrected for the glucose elevation by adding 1.6 to 2.4 mEq/L for each 100 mg/dL increase in serum glucose.

When true hypo-osmolality is found to exist, the differential diagnosis is of hyponatremia as illustrated in Table 5–1. The dis-order is divided into four major subgroups based on the extracel-lular fluid volume status and the measured urinary sodium. Extracellular fluid volume status may be determined by central venous pressure, BUN/creatinine, hematocrit, or plasma protein concentrations, but usually it is estimated by physical examination.

TABLE 5–1 Differential diagnosis of hyponatremia.

Volume	Urine Na$^+$	Diagnosis
Low (evidence of dehydration)	< 20 mEq/L	Category 1: Total body Na$^+$ depleted, normal renal response (eg, hemorrhage, GI losses)
	> 25 mEq/L	Category 2: Renal Na$^+$ loss (eg, renal disease, diuretics, CSW Addison disease)
Normal or expanded (edema may be present)	< 20 mEq/L	Category 3: Hyperaldos teronism secondary to inadequate perfusion (eg, CHF ascites, etc)
	> 40 mEq/L	Category 4: SIADH-Na$^+$ loss secondary to volume expansion

If the patient is dehydrated and the urinary sodium is low, this indicates normal physiologic response to extra renal sodium loss (with continued intake of water) such as vomiting or diarrhea. The appropriate therapy is to replace the sodium and fluid deficiency with normal saline. If the patient is dehydrated but the urinary sodium is increased, this indicates a renal loss of sodium inappropriate to the decreased volume and hyponatremia. This may be due to intrinsic renal disease, diuretic use, aldosterone deficiency (see discussion of Addison disease in Chapter 9), or cerebral salt wasting (to be discussed later). Appropriate therapy is to replace the sodium and fluid loss with normal saline but also with appropriate treatment of the underlying defect. If the extracellular fluid volume is expanded with edema or ascites and the urinary sodium is low, this indicates hyperaldosteronism, secondary to reduced or ineffective plasma volume as in cirrhosis or congestive heart failure, and the appropriate therapy is treatment of the underlying condition. Where the extracellular fluid volume appears to be normal with increased urinary sodium, this indicates the pathophysiology of inappropriate secretion of antidiuretic

hormone. Note that the urine osmolality will not be maximally dilute and that measured vasopressin will not be maximally suppressed in any of the four categories in Table 5–1. Although not appropriate to the osmolality, in the first three categories, the elevation of vasopressin is appropriate to the real or perceived decreased plasma volume. It is only in the fourth category (SIADH) that vasopressin is inappropriate both for plasma volume and osmolality. Copeptin, the inactive carboxy peptide that is cleaved from the provasopressin molecule and secreted with vasopressin and neurophysin, was mentioned earlier. Some studies have indicated that measurement of levels of this peptide might be useful in evaluating various causes of hyponatremia, but the clinical utility of such measurements is not yet established.

A. The pathophysiology of the hyponatremia in SIADH

The pathophysiology of SIADH begins with uncontrolled secretion of vasopressin. Thirst is not adequately suppressed so water intake continues. This produces volume expansion and hyponatremia in the sequence illustrated in Figure 5–5. Vasopressin

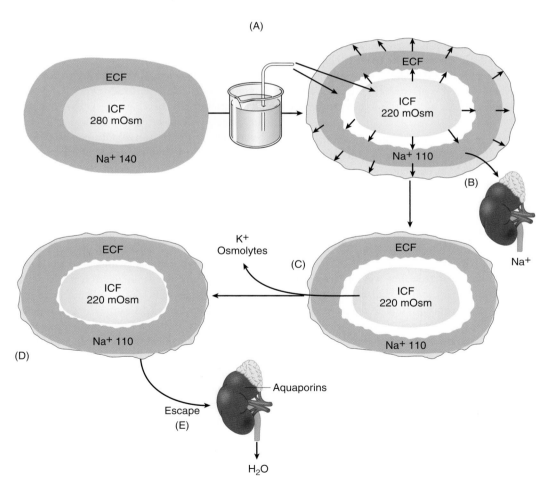

FIGURE 5–5 Illustration of the changes in intracellular fluid and extracellular fluid volumes in the pathophysiology of SIADH with the chronologic pattern of: **(A)** Expanded ECF and ICF volume with solute dilution. **(B)** Natriuresis to decrease ECF volume expansion. **(C)** Extrusion of intracellular potassium and osmolytes to decrease intracellular volume expansion. **(D)** Restoration of near normal volume in ECF and ICF. **(E)** Renal adaptation to allow excretion of more dilute urine in spite of excess vasopressin. (Copyright 2005, A.G. Robinson, University of California at Los Angeles.)

limits the excretion of water in the urine. Continued ingestion of water (part A) produces an expansion of extracellular and intracellular volume. The body attempts to bring the extracellular fluid volume back to normal by natriuresis (part B) of isotonic urine. The mechanism of natriuresis is complex and involves increased glomerular filtration, pressure natriuresis, and natriuretic factors, especially atrial natriuretic peptide and brain natriuretic peptide. This natriuresis decreases total body water and total body sodium but because it is isotonic, it contributes little to the degree of hyponatremia. Next, the body attempts to return intracellular fluid volume to normal by (part C) excreting from the intracellular fluid potassium and organic osmolytes such as glutamine, glutamate, myoinositol, aspartate, and N-acetylaspartate. In spite of the attempt to normalize extracellular and intracellular fluid, there remains a tendency for these compartments to be slightly expanded. The last adaptation (part D) is caused by this tendency for volume expansion and produces changes in the kidney to make it less responsive to the chronically inappropriate excess of vasopressin and to allow an increase in water excretion. Vasopressin retains water by increasing the number of aquaporin-2 molecules in the principal cells of the collecting duct. With chronic excess of vasopressin, the density of aquaporins in the membrane increases dramatically, producing a state of super water retention. The adaptation to chronic volume expansion is to reduce the number of aquaporins in principal cells. In this new state (part E), ingestion of sodium somewhat reexpands the extracellular fluid volume and is excreted, while ingestion of water is more easily excreted because of the renal adaptation to decrease aquaporins—therefore a new steady state.

Of the differential diagnoses of hyponatremia shown in Table 5–1, the two categories that are most difficult to differentiate are those with elevated urinary sodium concentrations. On physical examination, it may be difficult to differentiate moderately low extracellular fluid volume from normal extracellular fluid volume. In this situation, the differential diagnosis may be aided by a volume challenge of normal saline infused at a modest rate over a few hours while following urinary sodium and plasma sodium determinations. If the patient is in diagnostic category 4 (SIADH) and relatively equilibrated, the administered saline will be excreted so there will be an increase in urinary sodium and no change or a slight decrease in serum sodium concentration. If the patient is in category 2 with a renal loss of sodium, sodium from the administered saline will be retained, and the water excreted will somewhat dilute urinary sodium. This will result in a decrease in urinary sodium while the serum sodium concentration will rise. This volume challenge in difficult cases is not considered therapy, but only an assist to make the appropriate diagnosis, which will then lead to the initiation of appropriate therapy.

In diagnostic category 2 (Table 5–1), there is considerable controversy regarding the diagnosis and incidence of cerebral salt wasting (CSW). CSW is severe primary natriuresis producing volume depletion and hyponatremia. The diagnosis is only confirmed when volume depletion can be confirmed by some combination of decreased central venous pressure, decreased plasma volume, increased BUN/creatinine, or increased hematocrit and plasma protein levels. Cerebral salt wasting has been intensively studied as a cause of hyponatremia in subarachnoid hemorrhage. Natriuretic peptides are increased in subarachnoid hemorrhage, but they are also increased in well-documented SIADH. Measured plasma volume in subarachnoid hemorrhage is difficult to interpret because of the lack of sensitivity of readily available clinical measures. There may be both inappropriate secretion of vasopressin and inappropriate natriuresis in these patients with the clinical presentation depending on the relative contributions of each. It is consistent that infusion of isotonic saline does not correct the hyponatremia in SIADH but may do so with CSW. The most convincing cases of cerebral salt wasting are those that occur in hospitalized patients in whom there is a sudden unexplained increase in urine volume (not seen in SIADH) and urine sodium excretion. This has been reported in several cases of children with traumatic brain injury or brain surgery. The acute massive diuresis and natriuresis is accompanied by definitive volume contraction by the measures listed above. Most of these cases respond to replacement with normal or hypertonic saline.

B. Symptoms of hyponatremia   The symptoms of hyponatremia are largely dependent on the rapidity of the development of hyponatremia. When hyponatremia develops rapidly and is severe (serum sodium level <120 mEq/L), patients are at risk for cerebral edema with herniation of the brain stem (especially children and young women). Other complications include neurogenic pulmonary edema, seizures, coma, and respiratory arrest. Hyponatremia that develops slowly over a long period of time is surprisingly well-tolerated even at very low levels of serum sodium. Neurologic symptoms usually do not occur with sodium values above 120 mEq/L, but any degree of hyponatremia might exacerbate other comorbid conditions. Hyponatremia is usually considered chronic if hyponatremia has developed slowly and persisted for greater than 48 hours.

C. Clinical syndromes of SIADH   The clinical criteria for SIADH remain those described by Bartter and Schwartz in 1967: decreased plasma osmolality; inappropriate concentration of the urine; clinical euvolemia; increased urinary sodium excretion; and absence of other causes of euvolemic hypo-osmolality such as hypothyroidism, adrenal insufficiency, or diuretic use. The three main etiologies of SIADH are ectopic production of vasopressin by cancer (see Chapter 21), drug-induced SIADH, and lesions in the pathway of the baroreceptor system, especially central nervous system disorders and pulmonary disorders. As noted earlier, the baroreceptors consist of a diffuse system of receptors in the chest and synapses in the brain. Some of the input from them is inhibitory. Lesions which disrupt the flow of signals in the lung or in the brain may decrease this inhibitory signal and produce inappropriate secretion of vasopressin. Acquired immune deficiency syndrome (AIDS) is a recognized cause of SIADH, although dehydration, adrenal insufficiency, pneumonitis, and renal tubular toxicity associated with therapy may confound the ability to make the diagnosis of SIADH an exclusive cause of the hyponatremia. Prolonged strenuous exercise (eg, marathon running) may increase

TABLE 5–2 Major etiologies of SIADH.

Ectopic production of vasopressin by tumors
   Bronchogenic carcinoma
   Carcinoma of duodenum and pancreas
   Ureteral, prostate, bladder carcinoma
   Carcinoma of the uterus
   Thymoma
   Mesothelioma
   Lymphoma and leukemia

Drug induced
   Desmopressin and oxytocin
   Chlorpropamide
   Carbamazepine
   Clofibrate
   Ecstasy
   Selective serotonin reuptake inhibitors
   Tricyclic antidepressants
   Monoamine oxidase inhibitors
   Vinca alkaloids, cisplatin, cyclophosphamide

Disrupt neural pathways
   Pulmonary disorders: pneumonia, tuberculosis, fungal infection,
      empyema, positive pressure ventilation
   Central nervous system disorders: infection, trauma, surgery,
      hemorrhage, inflammatory diseases, degenerative diseases, porphyria

Nephrogenic SIADH
   Extremely rare mutation of the V_2 receptor producing
   chronic activation

Other etiologies
   AIDS
   Marathon running or other strenuous exercise
   Acute psychosis

secretion of vasopressin and with excessive intake of hypotonic fluid induce SIADH. A rare cause of SIADH reported in two pediatric patients is a genetic mutation of the V_2 receptor in principal cells producing unregulated activation. These patients have the manifestations of hyponatremia and SIADH but no measurable plasma vasopressin. Some elderly patients fit the criteria for SIADH without a definitive diagnosis.

Specific disorders, which have been reported to cause SIADH, are detailed in Table 5–2, but because of the diffuse regulation of the baroreceptor system and the multiple disorders that can influence vasopressin release via this system, no list should ever be considered complete.

TREATMENT OF HYPONATREMIA IN SIADH

The therapy of hyponatremia follows pari passu the symptoms of hyponatremia. When hyponatremia is known to have occurred rapidly and is severe and symptomatic, the patient should be treated quickly. When the onset is slow and the syndrome chronic, the treatment should be slow. Acute hyponatremia is arbitrarily defined as having developed over less than 48 hours. Usually, the serum sodium must be less than 120 mEq/L to produce

symptomatology. Discontinuing the administration of hypotonic fluid and the administration of hypertonic NaCl (eg, 3%), possibly with the addition of a diuretic, should be promptly considered. Often acute disorders occur in the hospital in a surgical or obstetrical setting and children and young women are at the greatest risk. For chronic hyponatremia, overly aggressive treatment may cause new and additional pathology. As shown in Figure 5–5, tissue adaptation to chronic hyponatremia results in the loss of intracellular osmolytes. In the brain these are the same osmolytes that would normally increase in neurons to protect brain volume from a sudden shift of intracellular fluid to the extracellular fluid when there is an acute increase in osmolality of the extracellular fluid. If during the treatment of hyponatremia in SIADH the extracellular fluid osmolality is rapidly increased, the brain has lost the ability to protect intracellular volume and water rapidly moves out of neurons. Brain shrinkage is thought to be the cause of a syndrome of myelinolysis which was first described in the pons—hence the term central pontine myelinolysis. The process can occur diffusely throughout the brain. The cause may be disruption of the blood–brain barrier and influx of plasma components that are toxic to the oligodendrocytes. The syndrome consists of neurologic deterioration over several days with fluctuating consciousness, convulsions, hypoventilation, and hypotension. Eventually, these patients may develop pseudobulbar palsy with difficulty in swallowing and inability to speak, even leading to quadriparesis. Recovery from this syndrome is variable, and many neurologic complications are permanent. MRI scans will demonstrate the demyelination, but usually not until 3 to 4 weeks after correction of the hyponatremia.

In chronic hyponatremia that is asymptomatic, the safest therapy is restriction of free water intake and slow correction of the hyponatremia over days. For chronic hyponatremia that has central nervous system symptoms, carefully controlled and limited increases in the osmolality should be undertaken. Coma or convulsions are obvious signs of neurologic symptoms that may be produced by hyponatremia, but nausea, vomiting, and confusion may be less specific signs of neurologic impairment. There is considerable debate in the literature about the exact rate of correction of the sodium concentration in these cases, and one should review the most up to date recommendations prior to initiating therapy. At present, general parameters of therapy are that the first 10% of increase of serum sodium might be accomplished at a rate of 0.5 to 1 mEq/L/h with a total correction not to exceed 12 mEq/L in the first 24 hours, and 18 in the first 48 hours. Active correction is stopped when the patient's symptoms are abolished, the serum sodium level is greater than 120 mEq/L, or the total magnitude of correction of 18 to 20 mEq has been achieved. Further treatment is undertaken with fluid restriction as for asymptomatic hyponatremia. While fluid intake is restricted in chronic SIADH, salt intake is not, as all of these patients have some degree of sodium loss secondary to the volume expansion and natriuresis.

The tetracycline derivative demeclocycline, known to cause nephrogenic diabetes insipidus, has been used to treat chronic SIADH. Dosages in the range of 600 to 1200 mg/d in divided doses decrease urine osmolality. Three to four days are required for the effect to reach equilibrium. Azotemia and nephrotoxicity have been reported with demeclocycline especially in patients with cirrhosis.

Any of the therapies for hyponatremia and especially fluid restriction will reduce the extracellular fluid volume and, hence, remove the volume-mediated stimulus of renal adaptation illustrated in part D of Figure 5–5 in which the kidney becomes somewhat less responsive to the excess vasopressin by reduction in the amount of aquaporin-2 water channels. When the volume stimulus is removed, there is again an increase in the density of membrane water channels, and the kidney becomes more efficient in retaining water. This accounts for the common clinical observation that fluid restriction that is initially effective may have to be increasingly severe to maintain a beneficial effect.

The most specific treatment for SIADH is to block the V_2 receptors in the kidney. There are recently approved vasopressin receptor antagonists, vaptans, that enhance renal free water excretion (aquaresis) without sodium excretion (natriuresis). Unlike the agonist desmopressin, these antagonist are nonpeptide drugs. Conivaptan is a combined V_{1A} and V_2 receptor antagonist that is available for intravenous administration to hospitalized patients. Tolvaptan is a selective V_2 receptor antagonist that can be administered orally and is approved to treat severe hyponatremia (serum Na <125 mEq/L) in patients who are symptomatic or patients who have failed to correct with fluid restriction. Clinical trials with these agents indicate they will be useful to treat hyponatremia of SIADH and of other causes. The risk of brain myelolysis caused by too rapid correction of sodium with these agents is the same as with other therapies, so the same recommendations about rates of correction of serum sodium described earlier will apply as physicians gain further experience with these agents.

SUMMARY

Table 5–3 compares and contrasts pathophysiologic entities associated with decreased vasopressin, diabetes insipidus, and excess vasopressin, SIADH.

OXYTOCIN

The anatomy and synthesis of oxytocin is similar to that described for vasopressin. While there are a number of central nervous system actions that have been attributed to oxytocin (probably acting as a neurotransmitter), the physiologic functions are limited to lactation and parturition.

A. Lactation   The hypothalamic/pituitary hormones critical to lactation are prolactin and oxytocin. Prolactin secretion from the anterior pituitary is described in Chapter 4, and its primary activity is to promote milk production. Oxytocin stimulates milk letdown associated with nursing. The milk-producing unit of the breast is the alveolar system in which clusters of milk-producing

cells are surrounded by specialized myoepithelial cells. Milk is synthesized in glandular cells of the alveoli. Oxytocin receptors are localized on glandular cells and on myoepithelial cells along the duct. Oxytocin stimulates the cells along the duct to shorten and the ducts to widen, enhancing milk flow through the ducts to the nipple. Suckling at the breast stimulates mechanoreceptors or tactile receptors that ascend through the spinal cord to the lateral cervical nucleus and eventually to the oxytocinergic magnocellular neurons in the supraoptic and paraventricular nuclei. Neurotransmitters trigger the release of oxytocin. Oxytocin is released in a pulsatile fashion producing a pumping action on the alveoli and promoting maximal emptying of milk from the alveoli. There is no evidence for a central pacemaker to regulate the secretion of oxytocin, and the mechanism of synchrony among individual oxytocinergic neurons is unknown. The importance of oxytocin in maintaining milk secretion is demonstrated in transgenic mice with a knockout of oxytocin synthesis. These animals deliver their young normally, demonstrating the redundant systems for parturition, and produce milk normally, demonstrating the role of prolactin, but are unable to release milk when the pups suckle, demonstrating the importance of oxytocin for milk letdown. The pups die of dehydration with no milk in their stomachs. Administration of oxytocin to the knockout mothers restores milk secretion, and the pups survive.

B. Parturition   Estrogen activates many events that initiate and stimulate parturition whereas progesterone inhibits these events. The uterine myometrial cells have intrinsic contraction activity and are responsive to oxytocin. During pregnancy, oxytocin is released, but oxytocinase decreases the plasma level of oxytocin, and progesterone and relaxin decrease the intrinsic contractility of the myometrium. In humans, there is a dramatic increase in uterine responsiveness to oxytocin as parturition approaches. Several hormones other than oxytocin including prostaglandins, endothelins, adrenergic agonists, corticotropin-releasing hormone, glucocorticoids, and cytokines also participate in the initiation and completion of labor. The most specific role of oxytocin may be the release of oxytocin brought about by vaginal and cervical dilatation, known as the Fergusson reflex. This may be important in stimulating uterine muscle to contract maximally and clamp down blood vessels to decrease blood loss. It is perhaps not surprising that parturition, which is so important to survival of the species, is controlled by many different pathways of cross-stimulation and feed-forward activity. The many redundant systems ensure survival of the species. Oxytocin remains the strongest stimulant to myometrial contraction, explaining its value as a therapeutic agent in inducing parturition.

C. Other actions   Other actions of oxytocin have been described in a number of species including effects on behavior of animals, effects on feeding and satiety, response to stress, stimulation of sperm transport, effects on memory, and so forth. None of these have been documented to be physiologically important in humans.

TABLE 5-3 Comparison and contrasting the pathophysiology of DI and SIADH.

Pathophysiologic	Lack of Vasopressin: Diabetes Insipidus	Excess Vasopressin: SIADH
Urine	Dilute with increased volume—polyuria	Concentrated with decreased or normal volume
Thirst	Increased and protective—polydipsia	*Not* decreased and *not* protective—normal intake
Serum sodium	Tendency to hypernatremia, but *high normal* due to polydipsia	Decreased—hyponatremia due to water retention
Initial plasma volume	Decreased by polyuria	Increased by water retention
Urine sodium	Variable	Inappropriately elevated for hyponatremia—natriuresis induced by volume expansion
Presentation	Polyuria and polydipsia	Hyponatremia (in SIADH accompanying euvolemia and natriuresis)
Differential diagnostic considerations with the presenting symptoms and laboratory data	*Excess water intake (primary polydipsia where polyuria is normal)*	*Renal Na$^+$ loss (diuretics, Addison disease, renal disease, cerebral salt wasting)* *Elevated urine Na$^+$, but plasma volume is low*
	Solute diuresis producing polyuria and polydipsia, eg, diabetes mellitus	*Volume expansion, hyper-aldosteronism (CHF, ascites, etc.), but urine Na$^+$ is low*
		ECF loss (sweating, diarrhea), but volume is decreased and urine Na$^+$ is low
Decreased or increased synthesis of vasopressin based on anatomy	Tumors with suprasellar origin or extension—infiltrative lesions of the basal hypothalamus—neurohypophyseal infundibulitis	Interruption of inhibitory input from baroreceptors in the chest or CNS
Decreased or increased synthesis based on genetics	Hereditary hypothalamic DI—autosomal recessive *AVP* gene in AVP producing neurons	Ectopic production of vasopressin by gene depression in cancer
Disruption of normal control mechanisms	Osmoreceptor system—discrete lesions in anterior hypothalamic area decrease positive signal to AVP neurons and decrease AVP	Baroreceptor system—diffuse lesions in chest, brain stem, and hypothalamus decrease negative input to AVP neurons and increase AVP
Abnormal metabolism of vasopressin	DI in pregnancy	None
Decreased or increased response of V$_2$ receptor	Nephrogenic DI—X-linked recessive mutated inactive V$_2$ receptor	Nephrogenic SIADH—mutated activated V$_2$ receptor—*rare*—unmeasurable AVP
Decreased or increased response of aquaporins	Nephrogenic DI—autosomal recessive mutated inactive aquaporin 2	None
Diagnostic laboratory tests	Elevated pOsm with low uOsm	Decreased pOsm with high uOsm (not maximally dilute)
		Urine Na$^+$ inappropriate for hyponatremia
	AVP elevated in nephrogenic DI, low in other DI	AVP elevated in SIADH but also in all differential causes of hyponatremia
	Masked by adrenal or thyroid deficiency, which inhibits free water excretion	Normal cortisol, and thyroid and no diuretic therapy; each may cause hyponatremia
Diagnostic imaging—MRI	Head, suprasellar area, tumors, infiltrates, widened stalk, absent posterior pituitary bright spot.	Chest—for any pathology, but especially for cancer; head for CNS pathology; full body for cancer
Treatment	Encourage water	Restrict water
	Diuretics cause volume contraction and reduce urine volume in nephrogenic DI	Drugs that inhibit renal action of vasopressin—demeclocycline
	Vasopressin receptor agonists—desmopressin	Vasopressin receptor antagonists—vaptans
	If hypernatramic, overaggressive treatment may rapidly decrease pOsm and produce cerebral edema	Acute onset = rapid therapy Chronic disease = slow therapy Overaggressive treatment to rapidly increase serum Na$^+$ may produce osmotic demyelination

REFERENCES

General References

Morgenthaler NG, Struck J, Jochberger S, Dunser MW. Copeptin: clinical use of a new biomarker. *Trends Endocrinol Metab.* 2008;19:43. [PMID: 18291667]

Robinson AG, Verbalis JG. The posterior pituitary gland. In: Larsen PR, Kronenberg H, Melmed S, Polonsky K, eds. *Williams Textbook of Endocrinology.* 11th ed. Philadelphia, PA: Elsevier; 2008.

Schrier RW, Cadnapaphornchai MA. Renal aquaporin water channels: from molecules to human disease. *Prog Biophys Mol Biol.* 2003;81:117. [PMID: 12565698]

Diabetes Insipidus

Bichet DG. Vasopressin receptor mutations in nephrogenic diabetes insipidus. *Semin Nephrol.* 2008;28:245. [PMID: 18519085]

Fujisawa I. Magnetic resonance imaging of the hypothalamic-neurohypophyseal system. *J Neuroendocrinol.* 2004;16:297. [PMID: 15089965]

Kalelioglu I, Kubat Uzum A, Yildirim A, Ozkan T, Gungor F, Has R. Transient gestational diabetes insipidus diagnosed in successive pregnancies: review of pathophysiology, diagnosis, treatment, and management of delivery. *Pituitary.* 2007;10:87. [PMID: 17308961]

Majzoub JA, Srivatsa A. Diabetes insipidus: clinical and basic aspects. *Pediatr Endocrinol Rev.* 2006;4:60. [PMID: 17261971]

Sands JM, Bichet DG. Nephrogenic diabetes insipidus. *Ann Intern Med.* 2006;144:186. [PMID: 16461963]

Smith D, Finucane F, Phillips J, et al. Abnormal regulation of thirst and vasopressin secretion following surgery for craniopharyngioma. *Clin Endocrinol (Oxf).* 2004;61:273. [PMID: 15272926]

Smith M. Physiologic changes during brain stem death—lessons for management of the organ donor. *J Heart Lung Transplant.* 2004;9:S217. [PMID: 15381167]

Valenti G, Procino G, Tamma G, Carmosino M, Svelto M. Minireview: aquaporin 2 trafficking. *Endocrinology.* 2005;146:5063. [PMID: 16150901]

SIADH

Bartter FC, Schwartz WB. The syndrome of inappropriate secretion of antidiuretic hormone. Am J Med 1967; 42(5):790-806. [PMID:5337379]

Ecelbarger CA, Murase T, Tian Y, Nielsen S, Knepper MA, Verbalis JG. Regulation of renal salt and water transporters during vasopressin escape. *Prog Brain Res.* 2002;139:75. [PMID: 12436927]

Feldman BJ, Rosenthal SM, Vargas, GA, et al. Nephrogenic syndrome of inappropriate antidiuresis. *N Engl J Med.* 2005;352:1884. [PMID: 15872203]

Greenberg A, Verbalis JG. Vasopressin receptor antagonists. *Kidney Int.* 2006;69:2124. [PMID: 16672911]

Hartung TK, Schofield E, Short AI, Parr MJ, Henry, JA. Hyponatraemic states following 3,4-methylenedioxymethamphetamine (MDMA, "ecstasy") ingestion. *Quart J Med.* 2002;95:431. [PMID: 12096147]

Kratz A, Siegel AJ, Verbalis JG, et al. Sodium status of collapsed marathon runners. *Arch Pathol Lab Med.* 2005;129:227. [PMID: 15679427]

Loh JA, Verbalis JG. Disorders of water and salt metabolism associated with pituitary disease. *Endocrinol Metab Clin North Am.* 2008;37:213. [PMID: 18226738]

Sterns RH, Baer J, Ebersol S, Thomas D, Lohr JW, Kamm DE. Organic osmolytes in acute hyponatremia. *Am J Physiol.* 1993;264:F833. [PMID: 8498536]

Sterns RH, Thomas DJ, Herndon RM. Brain dehydration and neurologic deterioration after rapid correction of hyponatremia. *Kidney Int.* 1989;35:69. [PMID: 2709662]

Verbalis JG, Murase T, Ecelbarger CA, Nielsen S, Knepper MA. Studies of renal aquaporin-2 expression during renal escape from vasopressin-induced antidiuresis. *Adv Exp Med Biol.* 1998;449:395. [PMID: 10026831]

Cerebral Salt Wasting

Berkenbosch JW, Lentz CW, Jimenez, DF, Tobias JD. Cerebral salt wasting syndrome following brain injury in three pediatric patients: suggestions for rapid diagnosis and therapy. *Pediatr Neurosurg.* 2002;36:75. [PMID: 11893888]

Betjes MG. Hyponatremia in acute brain disease: the cerebral salt wasting syndrome. *Eur J Intern Med.* 2002;13:9. [PMID: 11836078]

Cerda-Esteve M, Cuadrado-Godia E, Chillaron JJ, et al. Cerebral salt wasting syndrome: review. *Eur J Intern Med.* 2008;19:249. [PMID: 18471672]

Donati-Genet PC, Dubuis JM, Girardin E, Rimensberger PC. Acute symptomatic hyponatremia and cerebral salt wasting after head injury: an important clinical entity. *J Pediatr Surg.* 2001;36:1094. [PMID: 11431791]

Palmer BF. Hyponatremia in patients with central nervous system disease: SIADH versus CSW. *Trends Endocrinol Metab.* 2003;14:182. [PMID: 12714279]

Sviri GE, Feinsod M, Soustiel JF. Brain natriuretic peptide and cerebral vasospasm in subarachnoid hemorrhage. Clinical and TCD correlations. *Stroke.* 2000;31:118. [PMID: 10625725]

von Bismarck P, Ankermann T, Eggert P, Claviez A, Fritsch MJ, Krause MF.. Diagnosis and management of cerebral salt wasting (CSW) in children: the role of atrial natriuretic peptide (ANP) and brain natriuretic peptide (BNP). *Childs Nerv Syst.* 2006;22:1275. [PMID: 16607534]

Parturition

Blanks AM, Thornton S. The role of oxytocin in parturition. *Br J Obstet Gyn.* 2003;110(suppl 20):46. [PMID: 12763111]

Brown AG, Leite RS, Strauss JF, 3rd. Mechanisms underlying "functional" progesterone withdrawal at parturition. *Ann N Y Acad Sci.* 2004;1034:36. [PMID: 15731298]

Gross G, Imamura T, Muglia LJ. Gene knockout mice in the study of parturition. *J Soc Gynecol Investig.* 2000;7:88. [PMID: 10785607]

Hertelendy F, Zakar T. Prostaglandins and the myometrium and cervix. *Prostaglandins Leukot Essent Fatty Acids.* 2004;70:207. [PMID: 14683694]

Smith JG, Merrill DC. Oxytocin for induction of labor. *Clin Obstet Gynecol.* 2006;49:594. [PMID: 16885666]

Smith R. Parturition. *N Engl J Med.* 2007;356:271. [PMID: 17229954]

Young WS, 3rd, Shepard E, Amico J, et al. Deficiency in mouse oxytocin prevents milk ejection, but not fertility or parturition. *J Neuroendocrinol.* 1996;8:847. [PMID: 8933362]

Lactation

Buhimschi CS. Endocrinology of lactation. *Obstet Gynecol Clin North Am.* 2004;31:963. [PMID: 15550345]

Neville MC, Morton J, Umemura S. The transition from pregnancy to lactation. *Pediatr Clin North Am.* 2001;48:35. [PMID: 11236732]

Other Oxytocin

Marazziti D, Catena Dell'osso M. The role of oxytocin in neuropsychiatric disorders. *Curr Med Chem.* 2008;15:698. [PMID: 18336283]

Growth

Dennis Styne, MD

ACTH	Adrenocorticotropin
ALS	Acid labile subunit
cAMP	Cyclic adenosine monophosphate
CPHD	Combined pituitary hormone deficiency
EGF	Epidermal growth factor
EGF-R	Epidermal growth factor receptor
FGF	Fibroblast growth factor
FGF-R	Fibroblast growth factor receptor
GH	Growth hormone
GHBP	Growth hormone–binding protein
GHRH	Growth hormone–releasing hormone
GnRH	Gonadotropin-releasing hormone
hCG	Human chorionic gonadotropin
hCS	Human chorionic somatomammotropin
HDL	High-density lipoprotein
HESX1	Hesx1 homeodomain
hGH	Human growth hormone
IGHD	Isolated growth hormone deficiency
IGF-I	Insulin-like growth factor I
IGF-II	Insulin-like growth factor II
IGFBP	Insulin-like growth factor–binding protein

IUGR	Intrauterine growth retardation or restriction
JAK-STAT	Janus kinase-signal transducers and activators of transcription
LDL	Low-density lipoptrotein
LH	Luteinizing hormone
LS	Lower segment
MC4R	Melanocortin 4 receptor
NSD1	Nuclear receptor–binding SET domain protein 1
Pit1/POU1F1	Pituitary-specific transcription factor 1 or POU class 1 homeobox 1
PTH	Parathyroid hormone
PTPN11	Protein tyrosine phosphatase nonreceptor 11
RTA	Renal tubular acidosis
SOD	Septo-optic dysplasia
SGA	Small-for-gestational age
SHOX	Short stature homeobox
TBG	Thyroxine-binding globulin
SRIF	Somatostatin
TRH	Thyrotropin-releasing hormone
TSH	Thyrotropin
US	Upper segment

Assessment of growth in stature is an essential part of the pediatric examination. Growth is an important index of physical and mental health and of the quality of the child's psychosocial environment; chronic problems in any of these areas may be reflected in a decreased growth rate which may be a critical clue as to the onset of the condition. We shall consider influences on normal growth, the normal growth pattern, the measurement of growth, and conditions that lead to disorders of growth.

NORMAL GROWTH

INTRAUTERINE GROWTH

The growth of a fetus begins with a single fertilized cell and ends with differentiation into more than 200 cell types, length increasing by 5000-fold, surface area by 6×10^6-fold, and weight by 6×10^{12}-fold. This all to leads to an approximately 7 lb newborn. Overall, the growth of the fetus is dependent on the availability of adequate oxygen and nutrition delivered by the placenta and is orchestrated by a group of growth factors, all overseen by a basic genetic plan. Genetic factors are more important early in gestation, whereas the maternal environment attains more importance late in gestation.

The classic definition of small-for-gestational age (SGA), although somewhat arbitrary, is a birth weight 2 standard deviations below the mean or below the fifth percentile for birth weight, or birth weight below 2500 g for a term infant in the United States. The term intrauterine growth retardation or intrauterine growth restriction (IUGR) is not synonymous with SGA, because IUGR refers to decreased intrauterine growth velocity noted on ultrasound. Statistics and charts showing various percentiles of weight for gestational age are available to determine which premature infants are SGA and what weights are appropriate for gestational age. About 20% of SGA infants remain short as children and adults, in contrast to appropriate-for-gestational-age premature infants, who are smaller at birth but generally experience catch-up growth in the first 2 years. Those SGA infants who do not experience catch-up growth by 2 years of age may be candidates for growth hormone therapy. Recent studies suggest that preterm, AGA babies who show poor growth in the first 3 postnatal months follow growth patterns similar to SGA infants; thus consideration of GH therapy may be warranted as this situation receives further study.

THE PLACENTA

The placenta acting as an endocrine organ influences most aspects of fetal growth, including the supply of adequate nutrition and oxygen and regulation of hormones and growth factors. Aberrant delivery or control of any of these factors affects fetal growth; placental weight is usually directly related to birth weight.

CLASSIC HORMONES OF GROWTH AND FETAL GROWTH

The hormones that mediate postnatal growth do not necessarily play the same roles in fetal growth. Growth hormone (GH) is present in very high concentrations in the fetus, in contrast to the limited presence of GH receptors. Although this discrepancy suggests limited activity of GH in the fetus, GH does play a role in fetal growth as reflected in the average birth weight 1 standard deviation (SD) below the mean in GH-deficient infants. Infants with GH resistance due to abnormal, reduced or absent GH receptors (eg, Laron syndrome) have elevated GH and low serum insulin-like growth factor (IGF)-I levels; they also have decreased birth length and weight. Thyroid hormone deficiency does not directly affect human birth weight, but prolonged gestation can be a feature of congenital hypothyroidism, and this factor will itself increase weight. Placental lactogen exerts no effect on birth size in human beings. However, the concentration of placental-derived GH (from the *GHV* gene) is significantly decreased in the serum of a pregnant woman bearing a fetus with IUGR.

GROWTH FACTORS AND ONCOGENES IN FETAL GROWTH

Oncogenes may be responsible for neoplastic growth in postnatal life, but expression of these genes is important in the normal development of many fetal organs. Remarkably, the same oncogenes that cause postnatal neoplasia are prevented from causing tumors in the normally differentiating fetus. For example, a mutation in the *von Hippel-Lindau* gene predisposes to retinal, cerebellar, and spinal hemangioblastomas, renal cell carcinomas, and pheochromocytomas, but the normal *VHL* gene is expressed in all three germ cell layers of the embryo and in the central nervous system, kidneys, testis, and lung of the fetus, suggesting a role in normal fetal development for this gene.

INSULIN-LIKE GROWTH FACTORS, RECEPTORS, AND BINDING PROTEINS

IGF-I in the fetus is regulated by metabolic factors other than GH, in contrast to the dependence of IGF-I generation upon GH in postnatal life. One explanation is that there are fewer GH receptors in the fetus than after birth. In the human fetus, serum GH falls during later gestation owing to maturation of central nervous system's negative control, whereas serum IGF-I and IGF-binding protein (IGFBP)-3 rise during gestation, demonstrating their independence from GH stimulation.

Studies of knockout mice, which lack various growth factors or binding proteins, indicate a role for IGF-II in growth during early gestation and one for IGF-I during later gestation. Knockout of type 1 IGF receptors leads to a more profound growth failure than is found in IGF-I knockout mice alone, suggesting that factors other than IGF-I (eg, IGF-II) exert effects on fetal growth through the type 1 receptor.

Study of transgenic mice overexpressing IGFBPs supports the concepts that excess IGFBP-1 stunts fetal growth while excess IGFBP-3 leads to selective organomegaly. For example, overexpression of IGFBP-3 in mice led to organomegaly of the spleen, liver, and heart, although birth weight was not different from that of wild-type mice.

Although controversy remains over some of the data regarding IGFs and fetal growth, a summary of the complex IGF system in the fetus, based on the evidence from various species, appears to apply to the human being as follows.

1. IGFs are detectable in many fetal tissues from the first trimester onward.
2. Concentrations of IGFs in the fetal circulation increase during pregnancy, and at term the concentrations of IGF-I are directly related to birth weight.
3. In mice, disruption of the *IGF* genes leads to severe growth retardation.
4. There is a striking increase in IGFBP-1 and IGFBP-2 concentrations in amniotic fluid at the end of the first trimester.
5. The major binding proteins in the human fetus are IGFBP-1 and IGFBP-2.

6. From as early as 16 weeks, there is an inverse correlation between fetal concentrations of IGFBP-1 and birth weight.

7. In the mother, circulating concentrations of IGF-I and IGFBP-1 increase during pregnancy.

8. Maternal IGFBP-1 concentrations are elevated in severe pre-eclampsia and IUGR.

9. Fetal concentrations of IGFBP-1 are elevated in cases of IUGR, especially those associated with specific evidence of reduced uteroplacental blood flow. Production of IGFBP-1 appears to be a sensitive indicator of the short- or long-term response to reduced fetal nutrition.

INSULIN

Although insulin is a major regulatory factor for carbohydrate metabolism, many lines of evidence demonstrate that it is a growth factor as well and has importance in fetal growth. Macrosomia is a well-known effect of fetal hyperinsulinism as is found in the infant of the diabetic mother. Errors in the normal pattern of *IGF-II* gene expression from the paternal chromosome and type 2 IGF receptor (for IGF-II) from the maternally derived gene underlie the pathogenesis of Beckwith-Wiedemann syndrome. Affected infants are large and have elevated insulin concentrations. Increased weight gain in pregnant women over 40 lb leads to significantly increased risk of fetal macrosomia in gestational diabetes mellitus as well as in those with normal glucose tolerance test results.

Just as increased insulin stimulates fetal growth, syndromes of fetal insulin deficiency such as congenital diabetes mellitus, pancreatic dysgenesis, or fetal insulin resistance (eg, leprechaunism) are characterized by IUGR. Infants born to diabetic mothers with vascular disease, hypertension, and or eclampsia or preeclampsia also have IUGR and are born SGA. In that situation, it is clear that limited nutrient delivery compromises the growth of the infant.

EPIDERMAL GROWTH FACTOR

Epidermal growth factor (EGF) is involved with fetal growth, and expression varies with disordered fetal growth. Microvilli purified from the placentas of infants with IUGR have decreased or absent placental epidermal growth factor receptor (EGF-R) phosphorylation and tyrosine kinase activity. Maternal smoking decreases birth weight by an average of 200 g, with the major effect occurring late in pregnancy; the placenta responds to smoking by significant changes in its vascularity, which leads to fetal hypoxia. There are decreased numbers of EGF-Rs and a reduced affinity of these receptors for EGF in the placentas of women who are smokers. Hypertensive patients also have decreased numbers of placental EGF-Rs, which may result in IUGR.

EGF levels in amniotic fluid are normally increased near term but decreased in pregnancies complicated by IUGR—although not, conversely, increased in infants who are large for gestational age. EGF levels in the first urines to be voided by IUGR and macrosomic infants are lower than in control infants.

EGF administered to fetal monkeys results in histologic and biochemical maturation of their lungs, leading to improved air exchange and a diminished requirement for respiratory support. Surfactant apoprotein A concentration and the lecithin-sphingomyelin ratio are both significantly higher in the amniotic fluid of EGF-treated fetuses. Whereas birth weight is not affected by EGF, adrenal and gut weights, standardized for body weight, are increased significantly. Furthermore, EGF stimulates gut muscle, gut enzyme maturation, and gut size and content, improving the ability of the infant to absorb nutrients. Lastly, EGF advances the maturation of the fetal adrenal cortex, increasing the expression of 3-beta-hydroxysteroid dehydrogenase. Because EGF can be absorbed orally, this raises a question as to whether EGF could be a useful treatment for premature infants or, postnatally, for causing more rapid maturation of the neonate and improving survival in premature infants.

FIBROBLAST GROWTH FACTOR

Genetically engineered fibroblast growth factor receptor 2 (FGF-R)-deficient mice are severely growth-retarded and die before gastrulation. Aberrant FGF signaling during limb and skeletal development in the human being can lead to syndromes of dysmorphia. For example, achondroplasia is due to mutations in the transmembrane domain of the type 3 FGF-R.

GENETIC, MATERNAL, AND UTERINE FACTORS

Maternal factors, often expressed through the uterine environment, exert more influence on birth size than paternal factors. The height of the mother correlates better with fetal size than the height of the father. However, there is a genetic component to length at birth that is not sex specific. Firstborn infants are on the average 100 g heavier than subsequent infants; maternal age over 38 years leads to decreased birth weight; and male infants are heavier than female infants by an average of 150 to 200 g. Poor maternal nutrition is the most important condition leading to low birth weight and length on a worldwide basis. Chronic maternal disease and eclampsia can also lead to poor fetal growth. Maternal alcohol ingestion has severe adverse effects on fetal length and mental development and predisposes to other physical abnormalities seen in the fetal alcohol syndrome such as microcephaly, mental retardation, midfacial hypoplasia, short palpebral fissures, wide-bridged nose, long philtrum, and narrow vermilion border of the lips. Affected infants never recover from this loss of length but attain normal growth rates in the postnatal period. Abuse of other substances and chronic use of some medications (eg, phenytoin) can cause IUGR. Cigarette smoking causes not only retarded intrauterine growth but also decreased postnatal growth for as long as 5 years after parturition. Maternal infection—most commonly toxoplasmosis, rubella, cytomegalovirus infection, herpes simplex infection, and HIV infection—leads to many developmental abnormalities as well as short birth length. In multiple births, the weight of each fetus is usually less than that of the average singleton. Uterine tumors or malformations may decrease fetal growth.

CHROMOSOMAL ABNORMALITIES AND MALFORMATION SYNDROMES

Infant's with abnormal karyotypes may have malformation syndromes and may also demonstrate poor fetal or postnatal growth. In most cases, endocrine abnormalities have not been noted. For further discussion of this extensive subject, the reader is referred to other sources listed in the references at the end of this chapter.

FETAL ORIGINS OF ADULT DISEASE

The metabolic syndrome, "syndrome X," or the insulin resistance syndrome consists of (1) hypertension, (2) impaired glucose tolerance, and (3) elevated triglycerides among other features (see Chapter 17). Insulin resistance is a cardinal feature and might be the basis for most or all of these complications or may be just one feature of the syndrome, according to some. The metabolic syndrome is one of the long-lasting effects of abnormalities in fetal growth. Evidence from many international studies indicates a relationship between low birth weight or low weight at 1 year of age and chronic disease in adulthood. An opposing view is that catch-up growth, rather than low birth weight, is responsible for these defects long into the child's future.

Inanition during the last two trimesters of pregnancy, which occurred during the famine in Holland during World War II, led to an 8% to 9% decrease in birth weight; however, female infants born under these conditions later gave birth to normal-sized infants. On the other hand, in the Dutch and Leningrad famines, infants born after early gestational starvation of their mothers, but with improved maternal nutrition in late gestation were of normal size at birth. However, the female infants, born of normal size after this early gestational maternal starvation themselves gave birth to small infants (SGA of 300-500 g decrease). In other populations, women with a history of SGA tend to have SGA infants themselves, and some studies show that generations of malnutrition must be followed by generations of normal nutrition before there is correction of the birth weight of subsequent infants. The sparse environment of the fetus early in gestation in a mother with various degrees of starvation *programs* the fetal metabolism for survival of the fetus but later in life these survival techniques become maladaptive in an environment of plenty. Insulin resistance in fetal life may spare nutrients from utilization in muscle, thus leaving them available for the brain; this mechanism would serve to minimize central nervous system damage in the fetus during periods of malnutrition. The complexity of the situation is not completely understood but is the target of extensive research in vivo, in vitro, and in long-term clinical studies.

Birth weight and rate of postnatal growth (ie, catch-up growth)—not prematurity alone—are inversely related to cardiovascular mortality and the prevalence of the metabolic syndrome. It is not yet clear what the optimal nutrition is for a premature or small-for-gestational-age infant to avoid this metabolic programming.

Studies of otherwise normal but thin children, who had a history of SGA, demonstrated insulin resistance before the teenage years, supporting the concept of early metabolic programming. Present-day adults, who were born in the Netherlands during the Dutch famine who had the lowest birth weights and the lowest maternal weights (those subjects whose mothers experienced malnutrition during the last two trimesters noted above), show a degree of insulin resistance that is directly related to their degree of SGA, further documenting the relationship between fetal undernutrition and adult insulin resistance as the etiology of poor growth.

On the other hand, large infants born to mothers with diabetes mellitus often develop childhood obesity and insulin resistance even if they have a period of normal weight between 1 and 5 years of age. Remarkably, studies of the offspring of Dutch mothers exposed to famine during World War II in the first two trimesters (the time in which birth weight is least affected by maternal starvation) demonstrated a two-fold increase in the incidence of obesity at 18 years of age, compared with a 40% decrease in the incidence of obesity if the individual was exposed to famine in the last trimester (the time in which birth weight is most negatively impacted by maternal starvation).

Individuals born SGA also have variations in pubertal development and reproductive hormones. SGA girls tend to have earlier puberty, or if puberty occurs at an average age, more rapid progression of puberty or polycystic ovarian syndrome (PCOS). Adult males born SGA have increased aromatase and increased 5-alpha reductase demonstrating effects on reproduction in the male as well as the female. In sum, prenatal and early postnatal growth affects the older child and adult in many ways.

POSTNATAL GROWTH

Postnatal growth in stature follows a characteristic pattern in normal children (Figures 6–1 and 6–2). The highest overall growth rate occurs in the fetus, the highest postnatal growth rate just after birth, and a slower growth rate follows in mid-childhood (Figures 6–3 and 6–4). There are two periods characterized by brief growth spurts in childhood: the infant-childhood growth spurt between 1½ years and 3 years and the mid-childhood growth spurt between 4 and 8 years. The mid-childhood growth spurt does not occur in all children, is more frequent in boys than girls, and its presence is hereditary. After another plateau, the striking increase in stature, the pubertal growth spurt follows, causing a second peak growth velocity. The final decrease in growth rate then ensues, until the epiphyses of the long bones fuse and growth ceases.

In addition, an *adiposity rebound* of accelerating weight gain and rising body mass index (BMI) occurs in early childhood after a period of relative stability of weight gain. An early adiposity rebound is a risk factor for the development of obesity later in childhood and thereafter.

Endocrine Factors

A. Growth hormone and insulin-like growth factors   As discussed in Chapter 4, somatotropin or GH is suppressed by

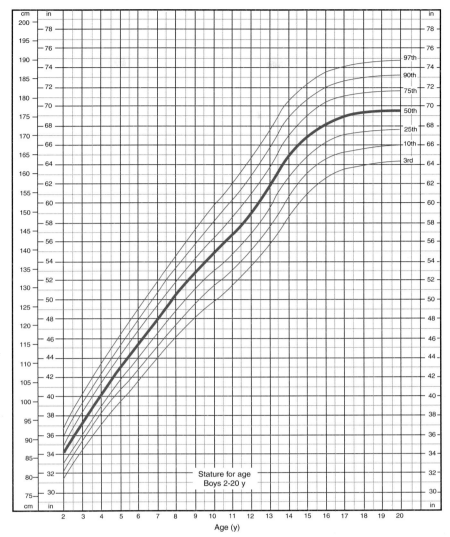

FIGURE 6-1 Growth chart for boys in most clinical situations showing the 3rd to the 97th percentiles. The lines for the 3rd and the 97th percentiles approximate those for −2.5 standard deviations and +2.5 standard deviations from the mean. (Redrawn from the original developed by the National Center for Health Statistics in collaboration with the National Center for Chronic Disease Prevention and Health Promotion. http://www.cdc.gov/growthcharts. Published May 30, 2000 [modified 11/21/00].)

hypothalamic GH release-inhibiting factor (somatostatin or SRIF) and stimulated by GH-releasing hormone (GHRH or GRF). The gene for GH is located on the long arm of chromosome 17 in a cluster of five genes: *GHN* codes for human GH (a single 191-amino-acid polypeptide chain with a molecular weight of 22 kD); *GHV* codes for a variant GH produced in the placenta; *CSH1* and *CSH2* code for prolactin; and *CSHP1* codes for a variant prolactin molecule. A 20-kD variant of pituitary GH accounts for 5% to 10% of circulating GH and is derived from the same gene, *GHN*, but results from alternative splicing. The 22-kD variant is poorly characterized but when derived from the placental gene, *GHV*, in vitro it has less diabetogenic effect but similar growth-promoting and lipolytic activity.

The effects of GH are mainly mediated by the IGFs, but GH also directly stimulates lipolysis, increased amino acid transport into tissues, and increased protein and glucose synthesis in liver. It also has direct effect on cartilage growth. GH in excess causes insulin resistance and is diabetogenic. GH is secreted in a pulsatile manner, so that serum concentrations are low much of the day, but peak during short intervals. Values are higher in the immediate neonatal period, decrease through childhood, and rise again as a result of increased pulse amplitude (but not frequency) during puberty. GH secretion falls again during aging.

GH circulates in plasma bound to a protein, the GH-binding protein (GHBP), with a sequence equivalent to that of the extracellular membrane domain of the GH receptor. The physiology of

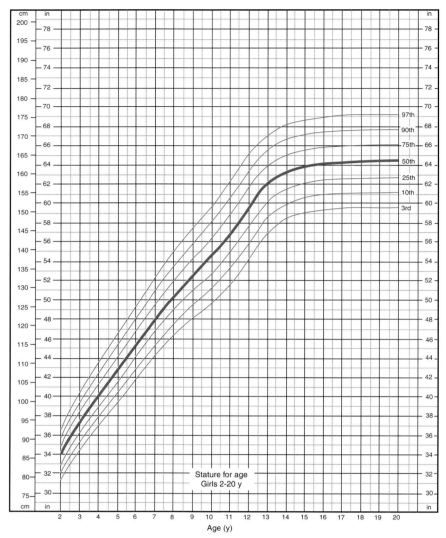

FIGURE 6–2 Growth chart for girls in most clinical situations showing the 3rd to 97th percentiles. The lines for the 3rd and the 97th percentiles approximate those for −2.5 standard deviations and +2.5 standard deviations from the mean. (Redrawn from the original developed by the National Center for Health Statistics in collaboration with the National Center for Chronic Disease Prevention and Health Promotion. http://www.cdc.gov/growthcharts. Published May 30, 2000 [modified 11/21/00].)

the GHBP appears to reflect important interrelationships between GH and GHR in terms of effects on growth. For example, obese patients have lower plasma GH concentrations but higher GHBP levels, whereas starvation raises GH concentrations and lowers GHBP levels. Patients with abnormalities of the GH receptor (eg, Laron dwarfism) also have a defect reflected in the serum GHBP concentrations; those with decreased numbers of GH receptors have decreased serum GHBP concentrations. Patients who are unable to dimerize the GH receptors to allow activation of the complex or those who have intracellular defects in the JAK-STAT system have no alteration in GHBP concentration, but are short.

GH exerts its effects on growth mainly, but not solely, through the IGFs and their binding proteins. IGF-I and IGF-II have structures similar to that of the proinsulin molecule but differ from insulin in regulation, receptors, and biologic effects. The structure of the IGFs (originally called sulfation factor and then somatomedin), the genes responsible for their production, and information about their physiology have been elucidated. Recombinant IGF is available for clinical use and some recent studies compared the effect of a GH and IGF-I combination to see if it is more beneficial than GH treatment alone. The single copy gene for prepro-IGF-I is located on the long arm of chromosome 12. Posttranslational processing produces the 70-amino acid mature form; alternative splicing mechanisms produce structural variants of the molecule. The IGF-I cell membrane receptor (the type 1 receptor) resembles the insulin receptor in its structure consisting of two alpha and two beta chains. Binding of IGF-I to type 1 receptors stimulates tyrosine kinase activity and autophosphorylation of

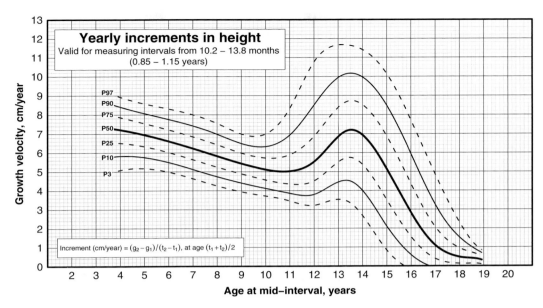

FIGURE 6–3 Incremental growth charts for boys derived from Flemish children and generally applicable to the US population. Height velocity can be compared with the percentiles labeled on each curve. Increments in height are calculated over periods of no less than 10.2 months (0.85 years) and no more than 13.8 months (1.15 years) in order to avoid the effect of seasonal variation in growth and to reduce the effect of measurement error on the estimation of yearly increment in stature. The yearly increment in stature is calculated as the difference between measurements of height $(g_2 - g_1)$ divided by the size of the interval $(t_2 - t_1)$. This formula is also shown on the charts for yearly increments in height. It is important to plot the increments at an age which corresponds to the centre of the interval, i.e. at the age $(t_1 + t_2)/2$. (Modified from Flemish Growth Charts 2004. Accessed at http://www.vub.ac.be/groeicurven/files/2-20050604-EP2-20M.pdf)

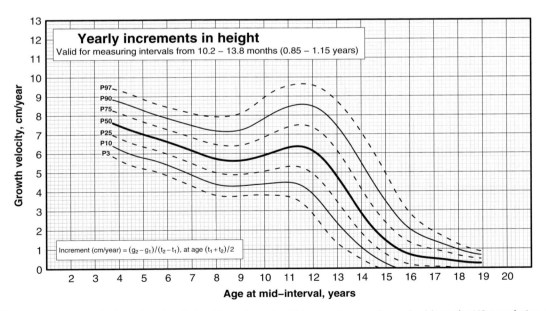

FIGURE 6–4 Incremental growth charts for girls derived from Flemish children and generally applicable to the US population. Height velocity can be compared with the percentiles labeled on each curve. Increments in height are calculated over periods of no less than 10.2 months (0.85 years) and no more than 13.8 months (1.15 years) in order to avoid the effect of seasonal variation in growth and to reduce the effect of measurement error on the estimation of yearly increment in stature. The yearly increment in stature is calculated as the difference between measurements of height $(g_2 - g_1)$ divided by the size of the interval $(t_2 - t_1)$. This formula is also shown on the charts for yearly increments in height. It is important to plot the increments at an age which corresponds to the centre of the interval, i.e. at the age $(t_1 + t_2)/2$. (Modified from Flemish Growth Charts 2004. Accessed at http://www.vub.ac.be/groeicurven/files/2-20050604-EP2-20F.pdf.)

tyrosine residues in the receptor. This leads to cell differentiation or division (or both). IGF-I receptors are downregulated by increased IGF-I concentrations, whereas decreased IGF-I concentrations increase IGF-I receptors.

IGF molecules in the circulation are mostly bound to a 6 IGFBPs. IGFBP-1 and IGFBP-3 have been most extensively studied. IGFBP-1 is a 25-kD protein and mainly inhibits IGF-I action. Serum levels of IGFBP-1 are inversely proportional to insulin levels. This protein does not appear to be regulated by GH. It is present in high concentrations in fetal serum and amniotic fluid. Newborn serum concentrations of IGFBP-1 are inversely proportional to birth weight.

IGF-I circulates bound to IGFBP-3 and an acid labile subunit (ALS) in a 150-kD complex. Abnormalities of the ALS lead to decreased growth. Serum IGFBP-3 concentrations are directly proportional to GH concentrations but also to nutritional status. In malnutrition, IGFBP-3 and IGF-I levels fall while GH rises as does IGFBP-1. IGF-I directly regulates IGFBP-3 as well. IGFBP-3 rises with advancing age through childhood, with highest values achieved during puberty; however, the pattern of change of IGF-I at puberty is different from that of IGFBP-3. The molar ratio of IGF-I to IGFBP-3 rises at puberty, suggesting that more IGF-I is free to influence growth during this period.

IGF-I is produced in most tissues and is exported to neighboring cells to act on them in a paracrine manner or on the cell of origin in an autocrine manner. Thus, serum IGF-I concentrations may not reflect the most significant actions of this growth factor. The liver is a major site of IGF-I synthesis, and much of the circulating IGF-I probably originates in the liver; serum IGF-I concentrations vary in liver disease, falling with reductions in functional hepatic mass. IGF-I is a progression factor, so that a cell which has been exposed to a competence factor such as platelet-derived growth factor (PDGF) in stage G_0 of the cell cycle and has progressed to G_1 can, with IGF-I exposure in G_1, undergo division in the S phase of the cell cycle. Aside from the stimulatory effects of IGF-I on cartilage growth, IGF-I has stimulatory effects on hematopoiesis, ovarian steroidogenesis, myoblast proliferation and differentiation, and differentiation of the lens.

IGF-I was in short supply until production by recombinant DNA technology became possible. IGF-I administration in clinical trials increased nitrogen retention and decreased blood urea nitrogen. In GH-resistant patients (Laron dwarfs), IGF-I stimulates growth in the absence of GH. IGF-I has recently been approved by the Food and Drug Administration (FDA) for use in short stature due to primary IGF-I deficiency. IGF-I may prove useful in treatment of various clinical conditions such as catabolic states, including the postoperative period and burns in addition to short stature, but experience is limited. GH is used in these situations by some authorities with some publications showing beneficial results.

IGF-II is a 67-amino acid peptide. The gene for prepro-IGF-II is located on the short arm of chromosome 11, close to the gene for preproinsulin. The type 2 IGF receptor preferentially binds IGF-II and is identical to the mannose 6-phosphate receptor, a single-chain transmembrane protein. Although most of the effects of IGF-II appear to be mediated by its interaction with the type 1 receptor, independent actions of IGF-II, via the type 2 receptor, have been described.

Plasma concentrations of the IGFs vary with age and physiologic condition. IGF-I concentrations are low at term in neonates and remain relatively low in childhood until a peak is reached during puberty, with values rising higher than at any other time in life. Serum IGF-I then decreases to adult levels, values higher than in childhood but lower than in puberty. With advancing age, serum GH and IGF-I levels decrease. IGF-I concentrations are more highly correlated in monozygotic twins than in same-sex dizygotic twins, indicating a genetic effect on regulation of IGF-I levels.

GH deficiency leads to lower serum IGF-I and IGF-II concentrations, whereas GH excess leads to elevated IGF-I but no rise in IGF-II above normal. Because serum IGF-I is lower during states of nutritional deficiency, IGF-I is not a perfect tool in the differential diagnosis of conditions of poor growth, which often include impaired nutritional state. IGF-I suppresses GH secretion by a negative feedback mechanism, so that patients who lack GH receptors (Laron dwarfs) or who are unable to produce IGF-I, have elevated GH concentrations but negligible IGF-I concentrations. Rare patients with poor growth who lack IGF-I receptors have elevated concentrations of IGF-I which exerts no biological activity.

B. Thyroid hormone   As noted above, newborns with congenital hypothyroidism are of normal length, but if untreated, they manifest exceedingly poor growth soon after birth. Infants with untreated congenital hypothyroidism suffer permanent developmental delay so early treatment is necessary. Newborn screening for congenital hypothyroidism is universal in the United States and most countries. Acquired hypothyroidism leads to a markedly decreased growth rate but no permanent intellectual defects. Bone age advancement is severely delayed in hypothyroidism, usually more so than in GH deficiency, and epiphyseal dysgenesis is seen as calcification of the epiphyses progresses. The normal decrease in the upper to lower segment ratio with age (Figure 6–5) is delayed, and therefore, the ratio is elevated, owing to poor lower limb growth in hypothyroidism.

C. Sex steroids   Gonadal sex steroids exert an important influence on the pubertal growth spurt, whereas absence of these factors is not of major importance in prepubertal growth. Gonadal and adrenal sex steroids in excess can cause a sharp increase in growth rate as well as the premature appearance and progression of secondary sexual features. If unabated, increased sex steroids mediated by estrogen will cause advancement of skeletal age, premature epiphyseal fusion, and short adult stature. The pubertal rise in gonadal steroids exerts direct and indirect effects on IGF-I production. Estradiol (secreted or aromatized from testosterone) directly stimulates the production of IGF-I from cartilage and also increases GH secretion, which stimulates IGF-I production indirectly. Both actions appear important in the pubertal growth spurt.

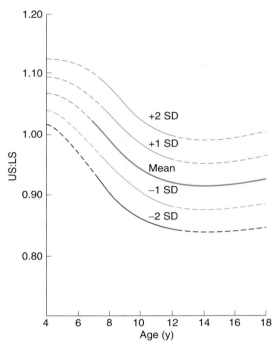

FIGURE 6–5 Normal upper:lower segment (US:LS) ratios, based on findings in 1015 white children. Values are slightly lower for black children. (Reproduced, with permission, from McKusick V. *Hereditable Disorders of Connective Tissue.* 4th ed. St. Louis: CV Mosby; 1972.)

D. Glucocorticoids Endogenous or exogenous glucocorticoids in excess quickly stop growth; this effect occurs more quickly than weight gain. The absence of glucocorticoids has little effect on growth if the individual is clinically well in other respects (eg, in the absence of hypotension or hypoglycemia).

Other Factors

A. Genetic factors Genetic factors influence adult height. There is correlation between midparental height and the child's height; appropriate methods to utilize this phenomenon and determine the target height for a child are presented in Figure 6–6. There is a change in growth. These effects are sex specific.

B. Socioeconomic factors Worldwide, the most common cause of short stature is poverty and its effects. Thus, poor nutrition, poor hygiene, and poor health influence growth both before and after birth. Parasitic infection by endemic worms is prevalent in less developed countries and severely stunts growth and depletes energy. In people of the same ethnic group and in the same geographic location, variations in stature are often attributable to socioeconomic factors. For example, Japanese individuals born and reared in North America after World War II were generally taller than Japanese-born immigrants to North America. Conversely, when factors are equal, the differences in average height between various ethnic groups are mainly genetic. The newest growth charts for children in the United States

published by the Centers for Disease Control and Prevention (CDC) in 2001 are not ethnicity specific because it is believed that the major growth differences between ethnic groups are due to socioeconomic status and nutrition rather than genetic endowments. Indeed, the World Health Organization (WHO) has developed internationally relevant growth charts for all populations.

C. Nutritional factors The influence of malnutrition accounts for much of the socioeconomic discrepancy in height noted above, but malnutrition may occur in the midst of plenty and must always be suspected in disorders of growth. Other factors may be blamed for poor growth when nutritional deficiencies are actually responsible. For example, Sherpas were thought to have short stature mainly because of genetic factors or the effects of high altitude living on the slopes of Mount Everest; however, nutritional supplementation increased stature in this group, demonstrating the effects of adequate nutrition. The developed world places a premium on appearance, and women portrayed as beautiful in the media are characteristically thin. Significant numbers of children, chiefly teenagers, voluntarily decrease their caloric intake even if they are not obese; this accounts for some cases of poor growth. Chronic disease, which hampers adequate nutrition, often leads to short stature. For example, bronchopulmonary dysplasia decreases growth to some degree because it increases metabolic demands, shifting nutrient usage away from growth; improved nutrition increases growth in these patients. Celiac disease is another common disorder that impairs growth, pubertal development, and bone acquisition.

Feeding problems in infants, resulting from inexperience of parents or poor child–parent interactions (maternal deprivation), may account for poor growth. Fad diets, such as poorly constructed vegan diets that put children at risk for vitamin B_{12} or iron deficiency, as well as major dietary manipulation, such as a severely low-fat diet, may place children at risk for deficiency of fat-soluble vitamins. Deliberate starvation of children by caregivers is an extreme form of child abuse that may be first discovered because of poor growth.

Remarkably, obesity increases IGF-I concentrations by increasing GH receptors even though GH secretion is suppressed to levels that might suggest GH deficiency. There are significant endocrine changes associated with malnutrition. Decreased GH receptors or postreceptor defects in GH action, leading to decreased production of IGF-I and decreased concentration of serum IGF-I are notable. The characteristic results of malnutrition are an elevation of serum GH and a decrease in IGF-I. IGFBP-1, a suppressor of IGF-I effects, is elevated in obesity.

D. Psychologic factors Aberrant intrafamilial dynamics, psychologic stress, or psychiatric disease can inhibit growth either by altering endocrine function or by secondary effects on nutrition (psychosocial dwarfism or maternal deprivation). It is essential to diagnose those situations that might suggest organic disease states as the management approach is very different.

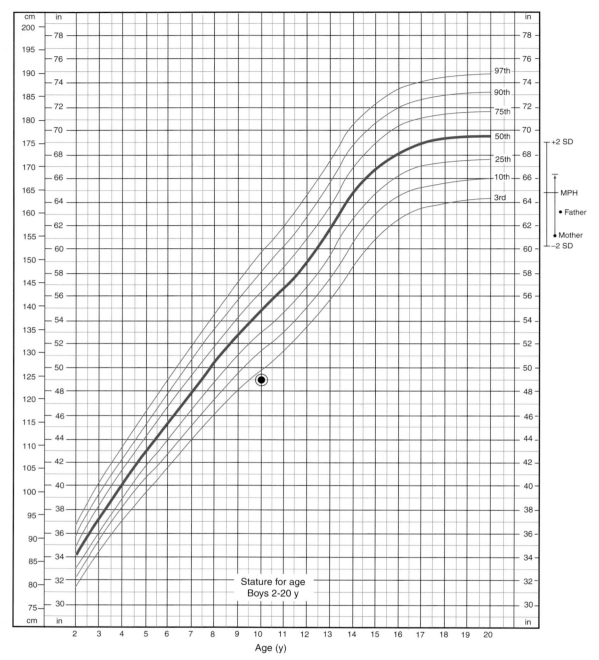

FIGURE 6–6 Determination of target height in a shorter family. This 10-year-old boy is 124 cm tall, his mother is 61 in tall (adults recall their heights in inches and feet but, if they are available, their height should be actually measured in centimeters), and the father is 63 in tall. Five inches are added to the mother's height to convert her height percentile to the equivalent percentile on a boy's chart. (If we were considering a daughter whose height is plotted on a girl's chart, the mother's height would be directly plotted and 5 in would be subtracted from the father's height to correct his height percentile to the equivalent for an adult woman.) Her corrected height and that of the father are plotted at the far right of the chart where adult heights are displayed. The midparental height is calculated by adding the father's height to the corrected mother's height, and the sum is divided by two; the result is the target height. The limits of 2 standard deviations (SDs) above and below the target height are displayed by plotting 2 SDs (~4 in above and below the target height). This process is equivalent to moving the 50th percentile for the US population to a conceptual 50th percentile for the family under consideration. It is evident that the height of the child, although below the third percentile for the United States, is within the bounds of the percentiles described by ±2 SD from the target height, and the child appears to fit within the genetic pattern of the family. The growth velocity and the degree of skeletal maturation are some of the factors necessary to evaluate this child in more detail.

E. Chronic disease Many chronic systemic diseases interfere with growth independent of poor nutrition. For example, congestive heart failure and asthma, if uncontrolled, are associated with decreased stature; in some cases, adult height is in the normal range because growth continues over a longer period of time. Children of mothers with HIV infection are often small at birth and have an increased incidence of poor postnatal growth, delayed bone age development, and reduced IGF-I concentrations. In addition, thyroid dysfunction may develop, further complicating the growth pattern. Infants born of HIV-infected mothers, who are not infected themselves, may exhibit catch-up growth.

Catch-up Growth

Correction of growth-retarding disorders may be temporarily followed by an abnormally high growth rate as the child approaches normal height for age. This catch-up growth occurs after initiation of therapy for hypothyroidism and GH deficiency, after correction of glucocorticoid excess, and after appropriate treatment of many chronic diseases such as celiac disease. Catch-up growth is usually short-lived and is followed by a more standard growth rate. Catch-up growth after small-for-gestational-age birth may not be beneficial as it is linked by some evidence to metabolic disease, particularly insulin resistance, in later life.

MEASUREMENT OF GROWTH

Accurate measurement of height is an essential part of the physical examination of children and adolescents. The onset of a chronic disease may often be determined by an inflection point in the growth chart. In other cases, a detailed growth chart indicates a normal constant growth rate in a child observed to be short for age. If careful growth records are kept, a diagnosis of constitutional delay in growth and adolescence or genetic short stature may be made in such a patient; without previous measurements, the child might be subjected to unnecessary diagnostic testing, or months of delay may occur as the child's growth is finally carefully monitored. Poor measurement technique may suggest lack of growth in a child who is growing normally, subjecting the child to unnecessary testing as well.

Height

The National Center for Health Statistics (NCHS) revised the growth charts for children in the United States in 2001 (see Figures 6–1 and 6–2). The new charts display the 3rd and 97th percentiles rather than the 5th and 95th percentiles, and SDs of height for age are also available. Charts displaying BMI by age contain data appropriate for the evaluation of obesity and underweight. All of these charts and are available online or from companies making GH or infant formulas.

But growth charts still leave 6 of 100 healthy children outside of their boundaries, with 3 of 100 below the more worrisome (to parents) *lower limits of normal*. It is both unnecessary and impractical to evaluate 3% of the population. Instead, the examining physician should determine which short children warrant further evaluation and which ones (and their parents) require only reassurance that they are healthy. When parents see that their child is below the third percentile and in a section of the chart colored differently from the *normal area*, they assume that there is a serious problem. Thus, the format of the chart can dictate parental reaction to height, because all parents want their children to be in the *normal range*. Figures 6–1 and 6–2 furnish data necessary to evaluate the height of children at various ages using percentiles or the SD method used by the WHO. SD determination is more useful in extremely short children below the second or first percentile.

Pathologic short stature is usually more than 3.5 SD below the mean, whereas the third percentile is only at 2 SD below the mean. However, a diagnosis of pathologic short stature should not be based on a single measurement. Serial measurements are required because they allow determination of growth velocity, which is a more sensitive index of the growth process than a single determination. A very tall child who develops a postnatal growth problem will not fall 3.5 SD below the mean in height for years but will fall below the mean in growth velocity soon after the onset of the disorder. As Figures 6–3 and 6–4 demonstrate, growth velocity varies at different ages, but as a rough guide, a growth rate of less than 5 cm/y between age 4 years and the onset of puberty is abnormal. In children under 4 years of age, normal growth velocity changes more strikingly with age. Healthy term newborns tend to be clustered in length measurements around 21 in (mostly owing to difficulties in obtaining accurate measurements).

In the ensuing 24 postnatal months, the healthy child's height will enter a channel on the growth chart and remain there throughout childhood. Thus, a child with constitutional delay in growth or genetic short stature, whose height is at the mean at birth and gradually falls to the 10th percentile at 1 year of age and to the 5th percentile by 2 years of age, may in fact be healthy in spite of crossing percentile lines in the journey to a growth channel at the 5th percentile. Although the growth rate may decrease during these years, it should not be less than the fifth percentile for age. A steeper decrease in growth rate may be a sign of disease. Alternatively, catch-up growth after SGA birth may not be beneficial because, as stated before, it is linked by some evidence to metabolic disease, particularly insulin resistance later in life. When a question of abnormal growth arises, previous measurements are essential. Every physician treating children should record supine length (<2 years of age) or standing height (>2 years of age) as well as weight at every office visit. As the child leaves infancy, height and growth velocity should be determined in relation to the standards for the child's age on a graphic chart with indication of the child's position (supine or standing) at measurement which is especially important at the time children switch from lying to standing. Failure to recognize a change in measurement technique as the child moves from lying to standing may falsely suggest a growth problem.

Patients who cannot be measured in the standing position (eg, because of cerebral palsy) require other approaches. The use of arm span is a possible surrogate for the measurement of height, and there are formulas available for the calculation of height based on the measurement of upper arm length, tibial length, and knee length (see below).

This discussion pre-supposes accuracy of measurements. However, it is reported that screening examinations in the real world fall short of that ideal. Forty-one percent of a presumably normal population screened at a school in England met the criteria for evaluation of abnormal growth (approximately two-thirds grew faster than the normal growth category and one-third were in the slower than normal category), leading to an unreasonable size of a referral population, all due to simple measuring error.

Relation to Midparental Height: The Target Height

There is a positive correlation between midparental height (the average of the heights of both parents) and the stature of a child. One way to use this relationship of parents' heights to the expected heights of children within a given family is to calculate target adult height range using parents' heights, correcting these heights for the sex of the child and plotting the results on the child's growth chart. There is an average 5-in difference between adult men and women in the United States. Thus, for boys, add 5 in to the mother's height, add the result to the father's height, and divide by 2. This is the target height, and it is expected that sons of these parents will reach a height within 2 SD of this target—or, for simplicity, within 4 in above or 4 in below the target height. (Two inches approximates 1 SD for adult stature.) For girls, subtract 5 in from the father's height and add the result to the mother's height and divide by 2, leading to the target height for the girl. The range for girls will also be within 4 in above and below this target. In effect, this corrects the North American growth charts for the particular family being considered. The calculated target height corresponds to the 50th percentile for the family, and the limits of the ±2 SD approximate the 5th to 95th percentile for the family. This method is useful only in the absence of disease affecting growth, and the prediction is more valid when the parents are of similar rather than of widely different heights. Figures 6–6 and 6–7 demonstrate the calculation of target height and the ranges. When there is a large discrepancy between the heights of the mother and the father, prediction of target height becomes difficult. A child may follow the growth pattern of the shorter parent more closely than the midparental height. A boy may, for example, follow the growth pattern of a short mother rather than a taller father.

A parent who spent the growing years in poverty, with chronic disease, or in an area of political unrest might have shorter adult height, due to nutritional factors or disease, that may not be passed on to the children. Of course, the height of an adopted child will have no relationship to the adoptive parents' heights. All of these factors must be determined by history.

Technique of Measurement

Length and height must be measured accurately. Hasty measurements derived from marks made on paper at an infant's foot and head while the infant is squirming on the paper on the examining table are useless. Infants must be measured on a firm horizontal surface with a permanently attached rule, a stationary plate perpendicular to the rule for the head, and a movable perpendicular plate for the feet. One person should hold the head stable while another makes sure the knees are straight and the feet are firm against the movable plate. Children over age 2 are measured standing up. Standing height is on the average 1.25 cm less than supine length, and it is essential to record the position of measurement each time during the change over from lying to standing height at 2 to 3 years of age; shifting from supine height at 2 years to standing height at 2½ years can falsely suggest an inadequate growth rate over that 6-month period.

These measurements cannot be accurately performed with the measuring rod that projects above the common weight scale; the rod is too flexible, and the scale footplate will in fact drop lower when the patient stands on it. Instead, height should be measured with the child standing back to the wall with heels at the wall, ankles together, and knees and spine straight against a vertical metal rule permanently attached to the wall or to a wide upright board. The child's head is to be horizontal with the eyes looking ahead and the chin gently elevated if necessary. Height is measured at the top of the head by a sliding perpendicular plate (or square wooden block). A Harpenden stadiometer is a mechanical measuring device capable of such accurate measurement. It is preferable to measure in the metric system, because the smaller gradations make measurements more accurate by minimizing the effect of rounding off numbers.

Growth is not constant but is characterized by short spurts and periods of slowed growth. The interval between growth measurements should be adequate to allow an accurate evaluation of growth velocity. Appropriate sampling intervals vary with age but should not be less than 3 months in childhood, with a 6-month interval being optimal.

The problem of measuring the growth rate of children with orthopedic deformities or contractures is significant, because these patients may have nutritional and/or endocrine disorders as well. The measurement of knee height, tibial length, or upper arm length correlates well with standing height ($r = 0.97$); thus, these measurements may be translated, using special linear regression equations, into total height, which is then plotted on standard growth charts. Specialized laser-calibrated devices to measure tibial length (kneeometry) are reported to be accurate for assessment of short-term growth down to weekly intervals.

In addition to height or length, other significant measurements include: (1) the frontal-occipital head circumference; (2) horizontal arm span (between the outspread middle fingertips with the patient standing against a flat backboard); and (3) the upper segment (US) to lower segment (LS) ratio. For the latter, the LS is measured from the top of the symphysis pubis vertically to the floor with the patient standing straight, and the US is determined by subtracting the LS from the standing height measurement noted above. (Normal standard US-LS ratios are shown in Figure 6–5.) These measurements become important in skeletal or reproductive disorders. Sitting height is used in some clinical studies of growth, but the sitting stadiometer is rarely available.

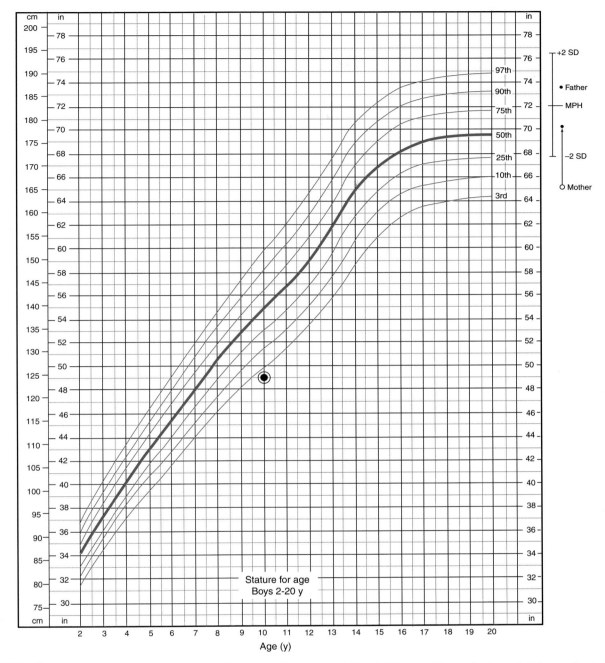

FIGURE 6–7 Determination of target height in a taller family. This 10-year-old boy is 124 cm tall just as in Figure 6–6, his mother is 65 in tall, and the father is 73.5 in tall. Five inches are added to the mother's height to convert her height percentile to the equivalent percentile on a boy's chart. (If we were considering a daughter whose height is plotted on a girl's chart, the mother's height would be directly plotted and 5 in would be subtracted from the father's height to correct his height percentile to the equivalent height percentile for an adult woman.) Her corrected height and that of the father are plotted at the far right of the chart where adult heights are displayed. The midparental height is calculated by adding the father's height to the corrected mother's height, and the sum is divided by 2; the result is the target height. The limits of 2 standard deviations (SDs) above and below the target heights are displayed by plotting 2 SDs (about 4 in. above and below the target height). This is equivalent to moving the 50th percentile for the United States population to a conceptual 50th percentile for the family under consideration. It is evident that the height of the child, which is below the third percentile for the United States, is even farther outside the bounds of the percentiles described by ±2 SD from the target height, and, thus, the child appears to fall far outside the genetic pattern of the family, and this is of clinical concern. The growth velocity and the degree of skeletal maturation are some of the other factors necessary to evaluate this analysis in more detail.

Height and Growth Rate Summary

In summary, we may consider three criteria for pathologic short stature: (1) height more than 3.5 SD below the mean for chronologic age; (2) growth rate more than 2 SD below the mean for chronologic age; and (3) height more than 2 SD below the target height when corrected for midparental height.

Weight

The measured weight should be plotted for age on standard graphs developed by the NCHS, which are available online or from various companies (http://www.cdc.gov/growthcharts/clinical_charts.htm). BMI charts displaying percentiles of BMI (weight in kilograms divided by height in meters squared) are widely available and provide an essential method to assess nutritional status.

SKELETAL (BONE) AGE

Skeletal development is a reflection of physiologic maturation. For example, menarche is better correlated with a bone age of 13 years than with a given chronologic age. However, bone age is as variable as chronologic age at the onset of puberty.

Estrogen plays the major role in advancing skeletal maturation. Patients with aromatase deficiency, who cannot convert testosterone to estradiol, and patients with estrogen receptor defects, who cannot respond to estrogen, grow taller well into their twenties without having epiphysial fusion. Bone age indicates remaining growth available to a child and can be used to predict adult height. However, bone age is not a definitive diagnostic test of any disease; it can assist in diagnosis only when considered along with other factors.

Bone age is determined by comparing the shapes and stage of fusion of epiphyses or bones on the patient's radiograph with an atlas demonstrating normal skeletal maturation for various ages. The Greulich and Pyle atlas of radiographs of the left hand and wrist is most commonly used in the United States, but other methods of skeletal age determination, such as Tanner and Whitehouse maturity scoring, are preferred in Europe. Any bone age more than 2 SD above or below the mean for chronologic age is out of the normal range. The standard deviation of bone age readings for chronological age is a full year by the mid teenage years, indicating the imprecision of prediction. Further, there appear to be ethnic differences in bone age maturation that is not reflected in the guidelines for interpretation. For newborn infants, knee and foot radiographs are compared with an appropriate bone age atlas. For late pubertal children, just before epiphyseal fusion, the knee atlas reveals whether any further growth can be expected or whether the epiphyses are fused. All the methods are imperfect, as there is great variation in bone age in relation to chronologic age even in typically developing children.

Height is predicted most often in the United States by determining bone age and height at the time the radiograph was taken and consulting the Bayley-Pinneau tables in the Greulich and Pyle skeletal atlas of the hand to determine the amount of growth left before epiphyseal fusion. Height prediction by any method becomes more accurate as the child approaches the time of epiphyseal fusion.

DISORDERS OF GROWTH

SHORT STATURE DUE TO NONENDOCRINE CAUSES

There are many causes of decreased childhood growth and short adult height (Table 6–1). The following discussion covers only the more common conditions, emphasizing those that might be included in an endocrine differential diagnosis. Shorter than average stature need not be considered a disease, because variation in stature is a normal feature of human beings, and a normal child should not be burdened with a misdiagnosis. Although the classifications described below may apply to most patients, some will still be resistant to definitive diagnosis.

1. CONSTITUTIONAL SHORT STATURE

Constitutional short stature (constitutional delay in growth and adolescence) is not a disease but rather a variation from normal for the population and is considered a slowing of the pace of development. There is usually an associated delay in pubertal development as well as a decrease in growth (see Constitutional Delay in Adolescence, Chapter 15). It is characterized by moderate short stature (usually not far below the third percentile), thin habitus, and retardation of bone age. The family history often includes similarly affected members (eg, mother with delayed menarche or father who first shaved later than peers and continued to grow past his teen years).

All other causes of decreased growth must be considered and ruled out before this diagnosis can be made with confidence. The patient may be considered physiologically (but not mentally) delayed in development. Characteristic growth patterns include normal birth length and height, with a gradual decrease in percentiles of height for age by 2 years; on the contrary, a rapid decrease in percentiles is an ominous sign of pathology. Onset of puberty is usually delayed for chronologic age but normal for skeletal age. Adult height is in the normal range but varies according to parental heights. The height is often less than the predicted height, because growth is less than expected during puberty. Aromatase inhibitors have been used in clinical studies for boys with constitutional delay in growth; they inhibit the conversion of androgens to estrogen so that bone age does not advance and growth continues longer. While this is not a treatment in general clinical use, most studies suggest that it causes no ill effects, although long-term data dealing with effects on bone mineral density as a result of the use of these agents are not available. Elevated testosterone levels and testicular enlargement result from aromatase inhibition.

TABLE 6–1 Causes of abnormalities of growth.

I. CAUSES OF SHORT STATURE

Nonendocrine Causes	Endocrine Disorders
Constitutional short stature	GH deficiency and variants
Genetic short stature	Congenital GH deficiency
Intrauterine growth retardation and SGA	Isolated GH deficiency
Syndromes of short stature	With other pituitary hormone deficiencies
Turner syndrome and its variants	With midline defects
Noonan syndrome (pseudo-Turner syndrome)	Pituitary agenesis
Laurence-Moon and Bardet-Biedl syndromes	Holoprosencephaly
	Other anomalies
Other autosomal abnormalities and dysmorphic syndromes	Acquired GH deficiency
Chronic disease	Hypothalamic-pituitary tumors
Cardiac disorders	Histiocytosis X
Left to right shunt	Central nervous system infections
Congestive heart failure	Head injuries
Pulmonary disorders	GH deficiency following cranial irradiation
Cystic fibrosis	
Asthma	Central nervous system vascular accidents
Gastrointestinal disorders	
Malabsorption	Hydrocephalus
Celiac disease	Empty sella syndrome
Disorders of swallowing	Abnormalities of GH action
Hepatic disorders	Primary IGF-1 abnormality
Hematologic disorders	Laron dwarfism
Sickle cell anemia	Pygmies
Thalassemia	IGF-1 receptor defect
Renal disorders	Psychosocial dwarfism
Renal tubular acidosis	Hypothyroidism
Chronic uremia	Glucocorticoid excess (Cushing syndrome)
Immunologic disorders	
Connective tissue disease	Endogenous
Juvenile rheumatoid arthritis	Exogenous
Chronic infection	Psuedohypoparathyroidism
Central nervous system disorders	Disorders of vitamin D metabolism
Malnutrition	
Decreased bioavailability of nutrients	Diabetes mellitus, poorly controlled
Fad diets	
Voluntary dieting	
Anorexia nervosa	
Anorexia of cancer chemotherapy	

II. CAUSES OF TALL STATURE

Nonendocrine Causes	Endocrine Disorders
Constitutional tall stature	Pituitary gigantism
Genetic tall stature	Sexual precocity
Syndromes of tall stature	Thyrotoxicosis
Cerebral gigantism	Infants of diabetic mothers
Marfan syndrome	
Homocystinuria	
Beckwith-Wiedemann syndrome	
XYY and XYYY syndromes	
Klinefelter syndrome	

2. FAMILIAL SHORT STATURE

Short stature may also occur in a familial pattern without retarded bone age or delay in puberty; this is considered **familial short stature**. Affected children are closer to the mean on the normal population growth charts after familial correction for mid-parental height by calculation of the target height (see Figures 6–6 and 6–7). Adult height depends on the mother's and father's heights. Patients with the combination of constitutional short stature and genetic short stature are quite noticeably short due to both factors, and these patients are most likely to seek evaluation. Boys are brought to consultation more often than girls. Children in these families may be born AGA but exhibit slowed growth in the first 2 postnatal years; this process is gradual in comparison to the striking changes in growth rate that are characteristic of diseases that primarily affect growth, but it may still be difficult to tell the difference without extended observation.

3. PREMATURITY AND SGA

Although the majority of SGA infants show catch-up growth, about 20% may follow a lifelong pattern of short stature. In comparison, appropriate-for-gestational-age premature infants usually catch up to the normal range of height and weight by 1 to 2 years of age. Severe premature infants with birth weights less than 800 g (that are appropriate for gestational age), however, may maintain their growth retardation at least through their third year; only follow-up studies will determine whether this group of premature infants reaches reduced adult heights. Bone age and yearly growth rate are normal in SGA patients until puberty occurs, and the patients are characteristically thin. SGA is now recognized as a risk factor for premature thelarche or early menarche, so bone age may advance more rapidly after childhood (Chapter 15).

Within this grouping are many distinctive genetic or sporadically occurring syndromes. The most common example is Russell-Silver dwarfism (OMIM #180860), characterized by small size at birth, triangular facies, and a variable degree of asymmetry of the extremities; this condition is due to epigenetic changes of DNA hypomethylation at the telomeric imprinting control region (ICR1) on chromosome 11p15, involving the *H19* and *IGF-II* genes or to maternal, uniparental disomy of chromosome 7. Intrauterine infections with *Toxoplasma gondii*, rubella virus, cytomegalovirus, herpesvirus, and HIV are noted to cause SGA. Furthermore, maternal drug usage, either illicit (eg, cocaine), legal but ill-advised (eg, alcohol during pregnancy), or legally prescribed medication (eg, phenytoin) may cause SGA. Reports of other syndromes in SGA infants can be found in sources listed in the bibliography.

Although SGA is not an endocrine cause of short stature, GH treatment is approved by the FDA and leads to increased adult height. Those SGA infants with the Δ3-isoform (genomic deletion of exon 3) of the GH receptor (GHR) are more likely catch up on GH therapy, as are girls with Turner syndrome. Remarkably, this same isoform is associated with reduced prenatal growth. The presence of this isoform does not guarantee taller adult stature even if growth velocity is greater while on GH treatment.

There are many endocrine associations with being born SGA including premature adenarche, puberty, and menarche in girls and dyslipidemia and insulin resistance in boys and girls. Girls have a predilection to develop PCOS after being SGA. GH antagonizes the action of insulin given the tendency for SGA children to have insulin resistance, there may be concerns regarding the potential additive effect. Recent studies of insulin sensitivity in SGA subjects receiving GH treatment indicate that in most cases the effects are not long lasting and do not seem to have clinical significance.

4. SYNDROMES OF SHORT STATURE

Many syndromes include short stature as a characteristic feature, and some also include SGA. Common conditions are described briefly below. Laurence-Moon, Biedl-Bardet, or Prader-Willi syndrome may combine obesity with short stature (as do the endocrine conditions, hypothyroidism, glucocorticoid excess, pseudohypoparathyroidism with Albright Hereditary Osteodystrophy (OMIM #103580), and GH deficiency). Moderately obese but otherwise normal children without these conditions tend to have slightly advanced bone age and advanced physiologic maturation with increased stature during childhood and early onset of puberty. Thus, short stature in an overweight child must be considered to have an organic cause until proven otherwise.

Turner Syndrome and Its Variants

Although classic Turner syndrome of 45,XO gonadal dysgenesis (see Chapter 14) is often correctly diagnosed, it is not always appreciated that any phenotypic female with short stature may have a variant of Turner syndrome. Thus, a karyotype determination should be performed for every short girl if no other cause for short stature is found, especially if puberty is delayed (see Chapter 15). The short stature of Turner syndrome is due to a mutation of the *short stature homeobox* (*SHOX*) gene on the short (p) arm in the pseudoautosomal region of the X chromosome (OMIM #312865). A mutation of the *SHOX* gene may also cause the Léri-Weill dyschondrosteosis form of short-limbed dwarfism (OMIM # 127300).

Noonan Syndrome (Pseudo-Turner Syndrome) (OMIM #163950)

This syndrome shares several phenotypic characteristics of Turner syndrome, including short stature, webbed neck, low posterior hairline, and facial resemblance to Turner syndrome, but the karyotype is 46,XX in the female or 46,XY in the male with Noonan syndrome, and other features clearly differentiate it from Turner syndrome. For example, in Turner syndrome, there is characteristically left-sided heart disease and in Noonan syndrome right-sided heart disease. Noonan syndrome is an autosomal dominant disorder at gene locus 12q24 (see Chapter 14). GH therapy is approved by the FDA for Noonan syndrome to increase height. About half of patients with Noonan syndrome have a mutation of the protein tyrosine phosphatase nonreceptor type 11 (PTPN11) (OMIM #176876). These children have a decreased response to GH treatment and tend to have low IGF-I and ALS with normal IGFBP-3 levels.

Prader-Willi Syndrome (OMIM #176270)

This condition is characterized by poor intrauterine movement, acromicria (small hands and feet), developmental delay, and almond-shaped eyes along with infantile hypotonia. Short stature is common but not invariable. Although hypotonia limits feeding in infancy, later insatiable hunger develops and leads to extreme obesity. Glucose intolerance and delayed puberty are characteristic. This syndrome is due to deletion of the small nuclear riboprotein polypeptide N (SNRPN) on paternal chromosome 15 (q11-13), uniparental disomy of maternal chromosome 15, or methylation of this region of chromosome 15 of paternal origin. If a mutation of the same locus is derived from the mother, Angelman syndrome results. GH therapy is approved by the FDA for Prader-Willi syndrome to improve body composition and muscle strength. There is the possibility of fatal complications of GH given in the presence of obstructive sleep apnea, so sleep patterns must be carefully monitored.

Laurence-Moon Syndrome and Biedl-Bardet Syndrome

Biedl-Bardet syndrome (OMIM #209900), associated with mutations on chromosome 16 (q21), is characterized by developmental delay, retinitis pigmentosa, polydactyly, and obesity. Laurence-Moon syndrome (OMIM #245800) is characterized by developmental delay, retinitis pigmentosa, delayed puberty, and spastic paraplegia. Both syndromes are associated with poor growth and obesity. They are inherited as autosomal recessive disorders. Study of large Canadian kindreds once again suggests combining the syndromes into one, as was done in the past. Biedl-Bardet syndrome is thought to be caused by a defect of the basal body of primary cilia resulting in cellular dysfunction.

Autosomal Chromosomal Disorders and Syndromes

Numerous other autosomal disorders and syndromes of dysmorphic children with or without developmental disorders are characterized by short stature. Often the key to diagnosis is the presence of several major or minor physical abnormalities that indicate the need for karyotype determination. Other abnormalities may include unusual body proportions, such as short extremities, leading to aberrant US:LS ratios, and arm spans quite discrepant from stature. Details of these syndromes can be found in the references listed at the end of the chapter.

Skeletal Dysplasias

There are more than 100 known types of genetic skeletal dysplasias (osteochondrodysplasias). Often they are noted at birth because of the presence of short limbs or trunk, but some are only diagnosed after a period of postnatal growth. The most common condition is autosomal dominant achondroplasia (OMIM #100800). This condition is characterized by short extremities in the proximal regions, a relatively large head with a prominent forehead due to frontal bossing and a depressed nasal bridge, and lumbar lordosis in later life. Adult height is decreased, with a mean of 132 cm for males and 123 cm for females. Intelligence is normal. Mutations of the tyrosine kinase domain of the *fibroblast growth factor receptor 3* (*FGFR3*) gene locus 4p16.3 (OMIM #134934) have been identified in this condition. Limb lengthening operations are used to increase stature in a few centers but the techniques are complex, and complications appear to be frequent.

Height, height velocity, weight, and BMI curves from birth to 16 years of age are available for achondroplasia. Children with achondroplasia who have received GH have in some instances demonstrated improved growth; however, atlanto-occipital dislocation is reported. The potential for abnormal brain growth and its relationship to aberrant skull shape mandates the caution that GH is not established therapy for this condition.

Hypochondroplasia (OMIM #146000) is manifested on a continuum from severe short-limbed dwarfism to apparent normal development until puberty, when there is an attenuated or absent pubertal growth spurt, leading to short adult stature. This disorder may be caused by an abnormal allele in the same gene causing achondroplasia (*FGFR3* at locus 4p16.3).

5. CHRONIC DISEASE

Severe chronic disease involving any organ system can cause poor growth in childhood and adolescence. In many cases, there are adequate physical findings by the time of consultation to permit diagnosis. In some cases, however—most notably celiac disease and regional enteritis—short stature and decreased growth may precede obvious signs of malnutrition or gastrointestinal disease. In some cases, growth is only delayed and may spontaneously improve. In others, growth can be increased by improved nutrition; patients with gastrointestinal disease, kidney disease, or cancer may benefit from nocturnal parenteral nutritional infusions. Cystic fibrosis combines several causes of growth failure: lung disease impairs oxygenation and predisposes to chronic infections, gastrointestinal disease decreases nutrient availability, and late-developing abnormalities of the endocrine pancreas cause diabetes mellitus. Children with cystic fibrosis experience decreased growth rates after 1 year of age following a normal birth size. The pubertal growth spurt is often decreased in magnitude and delayed in its timing; secondary sexual development may be delayed, especially in those with impaired pulmonary function. Study of growth in these patients allowed development of a cystic fibrosis specific growth chart and indicates that a reasonable outcome is an adult height in the 25th percentile. GH treatment in several studies demonstrated increased growth and weight gain in cystic fibrosis.

Children with congestive heart failure due to a variety of congenital heart diseases or acquired myocarditis grow poorly unless successfully treated with medications or surgery. Patients with cyanotic heart disease experience less deficits in growth.

Celiac disease is very common and may present initially with growth failure. Early diagnosis can be made by determination of tissue transglutaminase antibodies and IgA values while on a normal wheat-containing diet. However, a biopsy may still be required for diagnosis. On a gluten-free diet, patients experience catch-up growth. Adult height may still be impaired, depending on the duration of the period without treatment. Untreated patients with celiac disease have decreased serum IGF-I concentrations, presumably due to malnutrition, while IGF-I concentrations rise with dietary therapy. Thus, serum IGF-I in this condition, as in many with nutritional deficiencies, is not a reliable indicator of GH secretory status.

Crohn disease is associated with poor growth and decreased serum IGF-I concentrations. On an elemental diet, growth rate increases, and with glucocorticoid therapy (moderate doses), growth rate improves even though serum IGF-I decreases.

Patients with chronic hematologic diseases, such as sickle cell anemia or thalassemia, often have poor growth, delayed puberty, and short adult stature: iron deposition may itself cause endocrine complications. Juvenile rheumatoid arthritis may compromise growth before or after therapy with glucocorticoids. GH treatment is reported to increase the growth rate of these children, but it is too early to draw conclusions about the efficacy and safety of such therapy in juvenile rheumatoid arthritis. Hypophosphatemic vitamin D-resistant rickets usually leads to short adult stature, but treatment with 1,25-hydroxyvitamin D and oral phosphate in most cases will improve bone growth as well as increase adult stature. Chronic renal disease is known to interfere with growth, but increased growth rate occurs with improved nutrition and GH therapy which is approved for affected children.

Proximal or distal renal tubular acidosis (RTA) may both cause short stature. Proximal RTA demonstrates bicarbonate wasting at normal or low plasma bicarbonate concentrations; patients have hypokalemia, alkaline urine pH, severe bicarbonaturia, and later, acidemia. The condition may be inherited, sporadic, or secondary to many metabolic or medication-induced disorders. Distal RTA is caused by inability to acidify the urine; it may occur in sporadic or familial patterns or be acquired as a result of metabolic disorders or medication. Distal RTA is characterized by hypokalemia, hypercalciuria, and occasional hypocalcemia. The administration of bicarbonate is the primary therapy for proximal RTA, and proper treatment can substantially improve growth rate.

Obstructive sleep apnea is associated with poor growth. The amount of energy expended during sleep in children with sleep apnea appears to limit weight and length gain, a pattern which reverses with the resolution of the obstruction. Paradoxically, obstructive sleep apnea can be found with obesity that is more likely to be found with tall stature.

Hemoglobin, white blood cell count, erythrocyte sedimentation rate, serum carotene and folate levels, tissue transglutaminase antibodies, IgA values, plasma bicarbonate levels, and liver and kidney function should be assessed in short but otherwise apparently healthy children before endocrine screening tests are performed. Urinalysis should be done, with attention to specific gravity (to rule out diabetes insipidus) and ability to acidify urine (to evaluate possible RTA). All short girls without another diagnosis should undergo karyotype analysis to rule out Turner syndrome. A list of chronic diseases causing short stature is presented in Table 6–1.

6. MALNUTRITION

Malnutrition (other than that associated with chronic disease) is the most common cause of short stature worldwide and is the cause of much short stature in the developing world. Diagnosis in the developed world is based on historical and physical findings, particularly the dietary history. Food faddism and anorexia nervosa—as well as excessive voluntary dieting—can cause poor growth. Infection with parasites such as *Ascaris lumbricoides* or *Giardia lamblia* can decrease growth and is the cause of much short stature in the developing world.

Specific nutritional deficiencies can have particular effects on growth. For example, severe iron deficiency can cause a thin habitus as well as growth retardation. Zinc deficiency can cause anorexia, decreased growth, and delayed puberty, usually in the presence of chronic systemic disease or infection. Children with nutritional deficiencies characteristically demonstrate failure of weight gain before growth rate decreases, and weight for height decreases. This is in contrast to many endocrine causes of poor growth, where weight for height remains in the normal or high range. This simple rule often determines whether nutritional or endocrine evaluations are most appropriate. There are no simple laboratory tests for diagnosis of malnutrition. Serum IGF-I concentrations are low in malnutrition, as they are in GH deficiency. This distinction is important since misdiagnosing GH deficiency in the face of malnutrition would be tragic as well as costly.

7. MEDICATIONS

Children with hyperactivity disorders (or those incorrectly diagnosed as such) are frequently managed with chronic methylphenidate administration or similar medication. In larger doses, these agents can decrease weight gain—probably because of their effects on appetite—and they have been reported to lower growth rate, albeit inconsistently. These drugs must be used in moderation and only in children who definitely respond to them during careful evaluation and follow-up.

Exogenous glucocorticoids are a potent cause of poor growth (see discussed later), as are excessive endogenous glucocorticoids.

SHORT STATURE DUE TO ENDOCRINE DISORDERS

1. GROWTH HORMONE DEFICIENCY AND ITS VARIANTS

The incidence of GH deficiency is estimated to be between 1:4000 and 1:3500, so the disorder should not be considered rare. Using the conservative criteria of height (less than third percentile) and growth velocity (<5 cm/y for inclusion in the study), the incidence of endocrine disease in 114,881 Utah children who met these cutoff results was 5%, with a higher incidence in boys than girls by a ratio of more than 2.5:1. In this population, 48% of the children with Turner syndrome or GH deficiency were not diagnosed prior to the careful evaluation afforded by this study.

There may be abnormalities at various levels of the hypothalamic-pituitary, GH-IGF-I axis. Most patients with idiopathic GH deficiency apparently lack GHRH. One autopsied GH-deficient patient had an adequate number of pituitary somatotrophs that contained considerable GH stores. Thus, the pituitary gland produced GH, but it could not be released. Long-term treatment of such patients with GHRH can cause GH release and increase growth. Patients with pituitary tumors or those rare patients with congenital absence of the pituitary gland lack somatotrophs. Several kindreds have been described that lack various regions of the *GH* gene responsible for producing GH. Alternatively, gene defects responsible for the embryogenesis of the pituitary gland may cause multiple pituitary deficiencies. Absence of the *PIT1* gene encoding a pituitary-specific transcription factor causes deficient GH, TSH, and prolactin synthesis and secretion. Mutations of the prophet of PIT 1 (*PROP1*) gene cause deficiencies of GH, TSH, FSH, LH, and ACTH production.

Congenital Growth Hormone Deficiency

Congenital GH deficiency presents with slightly decreased birth length (–1 SD), but the growth rate decreases in some cases strikingly soon after birth. The disorder is identified by careful measurement in the first year and becomes more obvious by 1 to 2 years of age. Patients with classic GH deficiency have short stature, increased fat mass leading to a chubby or cherubic appearance with immature facial appearance, immature high-pitched voice, and delay in skeletal maturation. Less severe forms of partial GH deficiency are described with few abnormal characteristics apart from short stature and delayed bone age. GH-deficient patients lack the lipolytic effects of GH, partially accounting for the pudgy appearance. There is a higher incidence of hyperlipidemia with elevated total cholesterol and low-density lipoprotein (LDL) cholesterol in GH deficiency, and longitudinal studies demonstrate increases in high-density lipoprotein (HDL) cholesterol levels with GH treatment. Males with GH deficiency may have microphallus (penis <2 cm in length at birth), especially if the condition is accompanied by gonadotropin-releasing hormone (GnRH) deficiency (Figure 6–8). GH deficiency in the neonate or child can also lead to symptomatic hypoglycemia and seizures; if ACTH deficiency is also present, hypoglycemia is usually more severe. The differential diagnosis of neonatal hypoglycemia in a full-term infant who has not sustained birth trauma must include neonatal hypopituitarism. If microphallus (in a male subject), optic hypoplasia, or some other midline facial or central nervous system defect is noted, the diagnosis of congenital GH deficiency is more likely (see later). Congenital GH deficiency is also correlated with breech delivery. Intelligence is normal in GH deficiency unless repeated or severe hypoglycemia is present or a significant anatomic defect has compromised brain development. When thyrotropin-releasing hormone (TRH) deficiency is also present, there may be additional signs of hypothyroidism. Secondary or tertiary congenital hypothyroidism is not usually associated with physical findings of cretinism or developmental delay as is congenital primary hypothyroidism, but a few cases of isolated TRH deficiency and severe mental retardation have been reported.

Congenital GH deficiency may present with midline anatomic defects. Optic hypoplasia with visual defects ranging from nystagmus to blindness is found with variable hypothalamic endocrinopathies in 71.7% of one series: 64.1% of subjects had GH axis abnormalities, 48.5% hyperprolactinemia, 34.9% hypothyroidism,

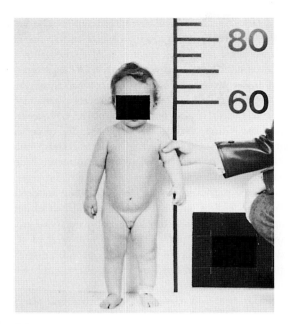

FIGURE 6–8 A 12-month-old boy with congenital hypopituitarism. He had hypoglycemic seizures at 12 hours of age. At 1 year, he had another hypoglycemic seizure (plasma glucose, 25 mg/dL) associated with an episode of otitis media, and it was noted that his penis was quite small. At 12 months, body length was 66.5 cm (−2 standard deviation [SD]) and weight was 8.5 kg [−3 SD]). The penis was less than 1.5 cm long, and both testes were descended (each 1 cm in diameter). Plasma GH did not rise above 1 ng/mL after arginine and levodopa testing (no insulin was given because of the history of hypoglycemia). LH rose very little after administration of GnRH (gonadorelin), 100 µg. Serum thyroxine was low (T$_4$, 6.6 µg/ dL; T$_4$ index, 1.5), and after administration of 200 µg of protirelin (TRH), serum TSH rose with a delayed peak characteristic of tertiary hypothyroidism. Plasma ACTH rose only to 53 pg/mL after metyrapone. Thus, the patient had multiple defects in the hypothalamic-pituitary axis including decreased secretion of GH, ACTH, and TSH probably due to deficient secretion of hypothalamic hormones. He was given six doses of 2000 units each of human chorionic gonadotropin (hCG) intramuscularly over 2 weeks, and plasma testosterone rose to 62 ng/dL, indicating normal testicular function. He was then treated with 25 mg of testosterone enanthate every month for 3 months, and his phallus enlarged to 3.5 × 1.2 cm without significant advancement of bone age. With hGH therapy (0.05 mg/kg intramuscularly every other day), he grew at a greater than normal rate for 12 months (catch-up growth), and growth then continued at a normal rate.

17.1% adrenal insufficiency, and 4.3% diabetes insipidus (DI) in this group of 47 subjects. About half of patients with optic hypoplasia have absence of the septum pellucidum on computed tomography (CT) or magnetic resonance imaging (MRI), leading to the diagnosis of septo-optic dysplasia. Septo-optic dysplasia is most often sporadic in occurrence. Affected individuals are reported with mutations of the *homeobox* gene expressed in ES cells (*HESX1*) (OMIM #601802) and septo-optic dysplasia (OMIM #182230). Cleft palate or other forms of oral dysraphism are associated with GH deficiency in about 7% of cases. Such children may need nutritional support to improve their growth. An unusual midline defect associated with GH deficiency is described in children with a single maxillary incisor.

Congenital absence of the pituitary gland, which occurs in an autosomal recessive pattern, leads to severe hypopituitarism with hypoglycemia. Affected patients have shallow development of or absence of the sella turcica. This defect is quite rare but clinically devastating if treatment is delayed. This is the most common MRI manifestation of PROP1 gene mutation (OMIM #601538).

Hereditary GH deficiency is described in several kindreds. Various genetic defects of the *GHN* gene (17q22-24) occur in affected families. Isolated type 1A GH deficiency (IGHDIA OMIM #262400) is inherited in an autosomal recessive pattern. Patients have deletions, frameshifts, and nonsense mutations in the *GH* gene. Unlike those with classic sporadic GH deficiency, some of these children are reported with significantly shortened birth lengths. Patients with absent or abnormal *GH* genes do initially respond to exogenous human GH (hGH) administration, but some soon develop high antibody titers that eliminate the effect of therapy. One reported kindred had a heterogeneous response: one sibling continued to grow and did not develop blocking antibodies, while the opposite effect occurred in two other siblings in the same family. Patients with high titers of blocking antibodies are reported to benefit from IGF-I therapy in place of GH therapy. Isolated GH deficiency (IGHD) type 1B (OMIM #612781) patients have autosomal recessive splice site mutations and incomplete GH deficiency. They are less severely affected. Type 2 (IGHD2) (OMIM #173100) patients have autosomal dominant GH deficiency due to splice site or missense mutations. Type 2 patients have X-linked GH deficiency often associated with hypogammaglobulinemia. A few patients are described with abnormalities of the *GHRH* gene, whereas others are described with mutant *GH* genes. Mutations in pituitary transcription factors can lead to various combinations of pituitary hormone deficiencies. Mutations in Pit1/POU1F1 (POU class 1 homeobox 1) (OMIM #173110) lead to GH, PRL, TSH deficiencies. Mutations in PROP 1 (Prophet of PIT1, paired-like homeodomain transcription factor) (OMIM #601538) leads to GH, PRL, TSH, LH, FSH, and sometimes ACTH deficiency. Mutations in HESX1 lead to GH, PRL, TSH, LH, FSH, ACTH, IGHD, and CPHD deficiencies.

Acquired Growth Hormone Deficiency

Onset of GH deficiency in late childhood or adolescence, particularly if accompanied by other pituitary hormone deficiencies, is ominous and may be due to a hypothalamic-pituitary tumor. The development of posterior pituitary deficiency in addition to anterior pituitary deficiency makes a tumor even more likely. The empty sella syndrome is more frequently associated with hypothalamic-pituitary abnormalities in childhood than in adulthood; thus, GH deficiency may be found in affected patients.

Some patients, chiefly boys with constitutional delay in growth and adolescence, may have transient GH deficiency on testing before the actual onset of puberty. When serum testosterone concentrations begin to increase in these patients, GH secretion and growth rate also increase. This transient state may incorrectly suggest bona fide GH deficiency but does not require therapy. A priming dose of estrogen is sometimes invoked to increase growth hormone secretion maximally so that bone fide GH deficiency is not diagnosed spuriously. Central nervous system conditions that cause acquired GH deficiency (eg, craniopharyngiomas, germinomas, gliomas, histiocytosis X) are described in Chapter 4. It is remarkable that after craniopharyngioma removal, some patients, mainly obese subjects, continue to grow quite well in spite of the absence of GH secretion. This persistent growth appears to be caused by hyperinsulinemia.

Cranial irradiation of the hypothalamic-pituitary region to treat CNS tumors or acute lymphoblastic leukemia may result in GH deficiency starting approximately 12 to 18 months later, owing to radiation-induced hypothalamic (or perhaps pituitary) damage. Higher doses of irradiation such as the 24-Gy regimen previously used for the treatment of central nervous system leukemia have greater effect (adult height may be as much as 1.7 SD below the mean) than the lower (eg, 18 Gy) regimens and higher doses are more likely to cause TSH, ACTH, and gonadotropin deficiency as well as hyperprolactinemia or even precocious puberty. Girls treated at an early age with this lower regimen still appear to be at risk of growth failure. All children must be carefully observed for growth failure after irradiation since growth failure may occur years later. If these patients receive spinal irradiation, upper body growth may also be impaired, causing a decreased US-LS ratio and a further tendency to short stature. Abdominal irradiation for Wilms tumor may also lead to decreased spinal growth (estimated loss of 10 cm height from megavoltage therapy at 1 year of age, and 7 cm from treatment at 5 years of age). Others receiving gonadal irradiation (or chemotherapy) have impaired gonadal function, lack onset or progression of puberty, and/or have diminished or absent pubertal growth spurt. Recent data suggests chemotherapy for acute lymphocytic leukemia without irradiation may also lead to GH deficiency, so follow-up of growth after treatment for cancer is always necessary.

CNS trauma is well established as a cause of hypopituitarism in adults. Cross sectional studies in children reveal both high and low rates of subsequent hypopitutirarism after head trauma but the rare prospective studies demonstrate lower risk in children than in adults.

Other Types of GH Dysfunction

Primary IGF-I deficiency is due to GH insensitivity (Laron syndrome and its variants (OMIM #262500). These disorders reflect GH receptor or postreceptor defects that are inherited in autosomal recessive fashion. The soluble GH-binding protein (GHBP) found in the circulation derives from the extracellular portion of the GH receptor, and since they derive from the same gene, circulating GHBP reflects the abundance of GH receptors. Patients with decreased or absent GH receptors have decreased serum GHBP levels, whereas those with postreceptor defects have normal GHBP concentrations. Affected children are found throughout the world, including Israel, where the syndrome was first

reported, and Ecuador, where several generations of a large kindred were studied in great detail. Defects in various kindreds include nonsense mutations, deletions, RNA processing defects, and translational stop codons. GH/JAK-STAT axis signal-transduction impairment leads to short stature when this intracellular system fails to activate in response to receptor occupancy by the GH ligand. Defects in the dimerization of the GH receptors also lead to short stature. Serum GH is elevated, due to decreased or absent IGF-I which results in lack of negative feedback inhibition. The condition does not respond to GH treatment. Patients are short at birth, confirming the importance of IGF-I in fetal growth (demonstrated previously in murine *IGF-I* gene knockout studies). About one-third have hypoglycemia, and half of boys have microphallus. Patients treated with recombinant IGF-I grow at an improved rate but do not respond quite as well to IGF-I as GH-deficient children do to GH treatment, indicating that GH may have a direct role in fostering growth above and beyond that conferred by IGF-I.

Other forms of GH resistance are described, but the majority of patients with disorders of the GH axis have abnormalities of GH secretion, not action. Very short, poorly growing children with delayed skeletal maturation, normal GH and IGF-I values, and no signs of organic disease have responded to GH therapy with increased growth rates equal to those of patients with bona fide GH deficiency. These patients may have a variation of constitutional delay in growth or genetic short stature, but a subtle abnormality of GH secretion or action is possible.

Pygmies (OMIM #265850) have normal serum GH, low IGF-I, and normal IGF-II concentrations. They have a congenital inability to produce IGF-I, which has greater importance in stimulating growth than IGF-II. Pygmy children are reported to lack a pubertal growth spurt, suggesting that IGF-I is essential to attain a normal peak growth velocity. Efe pygmies, the shortest of the pygmies, are significantly smaller at birth than neighboring Africans who are not pygmies, and their growth is slower throughout childhood, leading to statures displaced progressively below the mean. A few patients are reported with defects of the *IGF-I* gene or with deficiency of the IGF-I receptor and extreme short stature.

There are rare reports of IGF-I receptor (IGF-IR) defects (OMIM #147370) leading to short stature not responsive to IGF-I. Intrauterine growth deficiency is usually reported in these cases.

Why do certain normal children, perhaps within a short family, have stature significantly lower than the mean? There is no definite answer to this persistent question, but some patients have decreased serum GHBP concentration, which suggests a decrease in GH receptors in these children. A minority of short, poorly growing children have definable genetic abnormalities of their GH receptors. Short stature is the final common pathway of numerous biochemical abnormalities.

Adults who had GH deficiency in childhood or adolescence have decreased bone mass compared with normals even when bone mass is corrected for their smaller size. There is progressive bone loss in adults who are GH deficient even if bone density was improved with childhood therapy; GH is approved for adults with GH deficiency and can reverse this trend (see Chapter 4).

Diagnosis of GH Deficiency

Because basal values of serum GH are low in normal children and GH-deficient patients alike, the diagnosis of GH deficiency has classically rested on demonstration of an inadequate rise of serum GH after provocative stimuli or on some other measure of GH secretion. This process is complicated because different radioimmunoassay systems vary widely in their measurements of GH in the same blood sample (eg, a result on a single sample may be above 10 ng/mL in one assay but only 6 ng/mL in another). The physician must be familiar with the standards of the laboratory being used. Most insurance companies and state agencies accept inability of GH to rise above 10 ng/mL with stimulation as diagnostic of GH deficiency.

Another complicating factor is the state of pubertal development. Prepubertal children secrete less GH than pubertal subjects and, especially as they approach the onset of puberty, may have sufficiently reduced GH secretion to falsely suggest bona fide GH deficiency. This factor is sometimes addressed by administering a dose of estrogen to such subjects before testing. The very concept of GH testing provides a further complication. GH is released in episodic pulses. Although a patient who does not secrete GH in response to standard challenges is generally considered to be classically GH-deficient, a normal GH response to these tests may not rule out the efficacy of GH treatment. Testing should occur after an overnight fast; carbohydrate or fat ingestion suppresses GH response. Obesity suppresses GH secretion, and an overweight or obese child may falsely appear to have GH deficiency. Even within the normal range, variations of BMI affect peak GH after stimulation.

Because 10% or more of healthy children do not have an adequate rise in GH with one test of GH reserve, at least two methods of assessing GH reserve are necessary before the diagnosis of classic GH deficiency is assigned. Of course, if GH rises above 10 ng/mL in a single test, classic GH deficiency is eliminated. Serum GH values should rise after 10 minutes of vigorous exercise; this is used as a screening test. After an overnight fast, GH levels should rise in response to arginine infusion (0.5 g/kg body weight [up to 20 g] over 30 minutes), oral levodopa (125 mg for up to 15 kg body weight, 250 mg for up to 35 kg, or 500 mg for >35 kg), or clonidine (0.1 mg/m^2 orally). Side effects of levodopa include nausea; those of clonidine include some drop in blood pressure and drowsiness. Glucagon stimulation testing determines both GH and ACTH secretory ability.

GH levels also rise after acute hypoglycemia due to insulin administration; however, this test carries a risk of seizure if the blood glucose level drops excessively. An insulin tolerance test may be performed if a 10% to 25% dextrose infusion is available for emergency administration in the face of hypoglycemic coma or seizure and if the following conditions are satisfied: (1) an intravenous infusion line with heparin lock or low-rate saline infusion is available before the test begins, (2) the patient can be continuously observed by a physician, and (3) the patient has no history of hypoglycemic seizures. The patient must have a normal glucose concentration at the beginning of the test in the morning after an overnight fast (water intake is acceptable).

Regular insulin, 0.075 to 0.1 U/kg in saline, may be given as an intravenous bolus. In 20 to 40 minutes, a 50% drop in blood glucose will occur, and a rise in serum GH and cortisol and ACTH should follow. Serum glucose should be monitored, and an intravenous line must be maintained for emergency dextrose infusion in case the patient becomes unconscious or has a hypoglycemic seizure. If dextrose infusion is necessary, it is imperative that blood glucose not be raised far above the normal range, because hyperosmolality has been reported from overzealous glucose replacement; undiluted 50% dextrose should not be used (see Chapter 4).

A family of penta- and hexapeptides called GH-releasing peptides (GHRPs) stimulate GH secretion in normals and in GH-deficient subjects. GHRPs act via ghrelin receptors that are different from the GH-releasing factor (GHRF) receptors, and their effects are additive to that of GHRF. Ghrelin is a gastrointestinal-derived peptide that naturally binds to these receptors in the central nervous system, causing GH secretion, but it also stimulates appetite and is classified as an orexigenic agent. Recently, mutations in the GH secretagogue receptor (GHSR) were found in children with short stature; treatment with GH increases growth rate.

Patients who respond to the pharmacologic stimuli noted above, but not to physiologic stimuli such as exercise or sleep, were said to have neurosecretory dysfunction. These patients have decreased 24-hour secretion of GH (or integrated concentrations of GH) compared with healthy subjects, patterns similar to those observed in GH-deficient patients. It is not clear how frequently this condition is encountered.

This long discussion of the interpretation of GH after secretagogue testing brings into question the very standard for the diagnosis of GH deficiency. It is clear that pharmacologic testing cannot always determine which patients truly need GH therapy, and many authorities suggest that we abandon such dynamic testing in favor of measurements of IGF-I and IGFBP-3. This is the practice of the author whenever possible, although dynamic GH testing may still be required by a few insurance plans. Serum IGF-I and IGFBP-3 measurements are alternative methods for evaluating GH adequacy. Serum IGF-I values are low in most GH-deficient subjects, but, as noted above, some short patients with normal serum IGF-I concentrations may require GH treatment to improve growth rate. Moreover, starvation lowers IGF-I values in healthy children and incorrectly suggests GH deficiency. Children with psychosocial dwarfism—who need family therapy or foster home placement rather than GH therapy—have low GH and IGF-I concentrations and may falsely appear to have GH deficiency. Likewise, patients with constitutional delay in adolescence have low IGF-I values for chronologic age, but normal values for skeletal age, and may have temporarily decreased GH response to secretagogues. Thus, IGF-I determinations are not infallible in the diagnosis of GH deficiency. They must be interpreted with regard to nutrition, psychosocial status, and skeletal ages. IGFBP-3 is GH-dependent, and if its concentration is also low, it provides stronger evidence of GH deficiency than does the IGF-I determination alone.

The Growth Hormone Research Society produced criteria that attempt to deal with the diagnosis of GH deficiency in childhood in spite of the uncertainty of the methods. These criteria use clinical findings of various conditions associated with GH deficiency, the severity of short stature, and the degree and duration of decreased growth velocity to identify individuals that may have GH deficiency. The guidelines and diagnostic considerations in this chapter include most of the GH Society criteria. (See "Consensus guidelines" reference in the Short Stature section at the end of this chapter for details of the Growth Hormone Research Society statement.) A 3- to 6-month therapeutic trial of GH therapy may be necessary to determine growth response; if growth increases more than 2 cm/y, it is likely that the child will benefit from GH treatment, no matter what the tests originally showed.

Treatment of GH Deficiency

A. GH replacement   Before 1986, the only available method of treatment for GH deficiency was replacement therapy with hGH derived from cadaver donors. In 1985 and thereafter, Creutzfeldt-Jakob disease, a degenerative neurologic disease rare in patients so young, was diagnosed in some patients who had received natural hGH up to 10 to 15 years before. Because of the possibility that prions contaminating donor pituitary glands were transmitted to the GH-deficient patients, causing their deaths, natural GH from all sources was removed from distribution. Recombinant hGH now accounts for the world's current supply.

Commercial GH has the 191-amino acid natural sequence. GH is now available in virtually unlimited amounts, allowing innovative treatment regimens not previously possible owing to scarce supplies. The potential for abuse of GH in athletes or in children of normal size whose parents wish them to be taller than average, however, must now be addressed.

Growth disturbances due to disorders of GH release or action are shown in Table 6–2. GH-deficient children require biosynthetic

TABLE 6–2 Level of defect in growth.

Site of Defect	Clinical Condition
Hypothalamus	Idiopathic GH deficiency due to decreased GHRH secretion; hypothalamic tumors or congenital defects
Pituitary gland	Dysplasia, trauma, surgery, or tumor of the pituitary gland; defect in *GH* gene or in pituitary transcription factors
Sites of IGF production	Primary IGF1 deficiency: GH receptor defect (Laron dwarfism with high GH and low IGF concentrations)
	ALS deficiency
	Growth hormone/JAK-STAT axis signal-transduction defect
	Pygmies with normal GH, low IGF-1, and normal IGF-2 concentrations
Cartilage	Glucocorticoid-induced growth failure Resistance to IGF-1

somatropin (natural sequence GH) at a dose of 0.3 mg/kg/wk administered in one subcutaneous dose per day 6 or 7 times per week during the period of active growth before epiphyseal fusion. The increase in growth rate (Figures 6–9, 6–10, and 6–11) is most marked during the first year of therapy. Older children do not respond as well and may require larger doses. Higher doses, up to double the standard starting dose, are approved by the FDA for use in puberty, but there are varying reports of the effect of such higher doses on adult height as by far, most of the effect of GH on adult height is exerted in the years before puberty. GH does not increase growth rate without adequate nutrition and euthyroid status. During the roughly 50 years since the first use of GH in children, long-term effects are reported in several series. If only the children most recently treated with recombinant GH are considered, the mean adult height was 1.4 SD below the mean, a significant improvement over the –2.9 SD mean height at the start of therapy but not a true normalization of height in most patients. With earlier diagnosis and treatment, using new pubertal dosing schedules, adult height can reach genetic potential.

Monitoring of GH replacement is mainly accomplished by measuring growth rate and annually assessing bone age advancement. Serum IGF-I and IGFBP-3 will rise with successful therapy while GHBP will not change appreciably. Controlled clinical studies reported the utility of titrating the dose of GH to restore serum IGF-I to the high-normal range, monitoring serum IGF-I levels during clinical treatment. Serum bone-specific alkaline phosphatase rises with successful therapy. Urinary hydroxyproline, deoxypyridinoline, and galactosyl-hydroxylysine reflect growth rate and are used in clinical studies to reflect increased growth rate with therapy.

Antibodies to GH may be present in measurable quantities in the serum of children receiving GH. However, a high titer of blocking antibodies with significant binding capacity is rare except in patients with absence or abnormality of *GH* genes. Only a few patients are reported to have temporarily ceased growing because of antibody formation. GH exerts anti-insulin effects. Although clinical diabetes is not a likely result of GH therapy, the long-term effects of a small rise in glucose in an otherwise healthy child are unknown. If a tendency toward diabetes is already present, GH may cause the onset of clinical manifestations more quickly. Another potential risk is the rare tendency to develop slipped capital femoral epiphyses in children receiving GH therapy. Recent data have weakened the link between slipped capital femoral epiphyses and GH therapy, but the final import of the relationship is not yet clear. Slipped capital femoral epiphyses, if associated with endocrinopathies, are most common in treated hypothyroid patients (50% one series of 80 episodes of slipped capital femoral epiphyses), followed by treated GH-deficient patients (25% of the series). This condition may occur bilaterally, and prophylactic treatment of the nonaffected side is recommended by several authorities. Pseudotumor cerebri may rarely occur with GH therapy and is usually associated with severe headache and may be more common in obese individuals receiving GH treatment. It is reported to reverse after cessation of GH therapy, but if allowed to continue, it may impair vision and

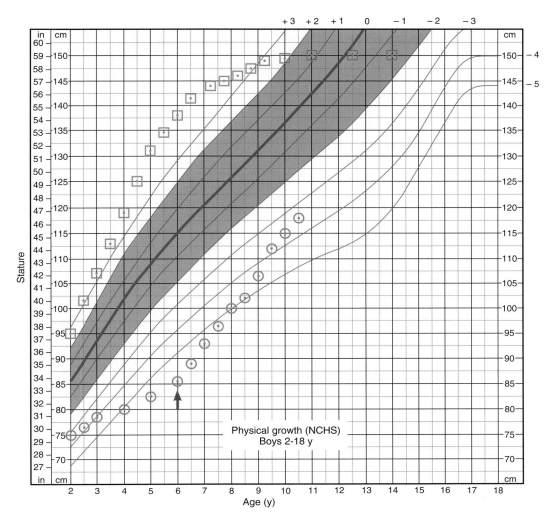

FIGURE 6–9 Examples of abnormal growth charts. Squares represent the growth pattern of a child (such as patient **A** in Figure 6–11) with precocious sexual development and early excessive growth leading to premature closure of the epiphyses and cessation of growth. Circles represent growth of a boy (such as patient **B** in Figure 6–11) with GH deficiency who showed progressively poorer growth until 6 years of age, when he was treated with hGH (arrow), after which catch-up growth occurred. The curves describe standard deviations from the mean.

cause severe complications. Organomegaly and skeletal changes like those found in acromegaly are other theoretical side effects of excessive GH therapy but do not occur with standard doses. Furthermore, a few cases of prepubertal gynecomastia are reported with GH therapy.

The discovery of leukemia in young adults previously treated with GH was worrisome, but no cause and effect relationship has been established, and GH treatment is not considered a cause of leukemia. GH does not increase the recurrence rate of tumors existing before therapy. Thus, patients with craniopharyngiomas, for example, may receive GH, if indicated, after the disease is clinically stable without significant worry that the GH will precipitate a recurrence. Clinicians usually wait 1 year after completion of tumor therapy before starting patients on GH therapy, but doing so is not a requirement. There are reports of a small increase in risk of colonic carcinoma decades after natural GH treatment in GH-deficient

children but no such information on long-term follow-up of children treated with recombinant derived GH is available.

GH deficiency is associated with an adverse lipid profile with elevated LDL cholesterol and decreased HDL cholesterol in addition to an increased BMI; GH-deficient adolescents treated with GH develop these findings within a few years after discontinuation of GH therapy. Low-dose GH therapy is now approved for use in adults with childhood-onset GH deficiency and is said to forestall these metabolic changes. Further, adult GH therapy maintains muscle strength and bone density in GH-deficient adults. One can, therefore, inform the parents of a child with GH deficiency that the patient may still benefit from GH therapy even after he or she stops growing, if profound GH deficiency remains after repeat testing.

GH has been combined with other substances to increase its impact on height. In patients who were diagnosed late, have

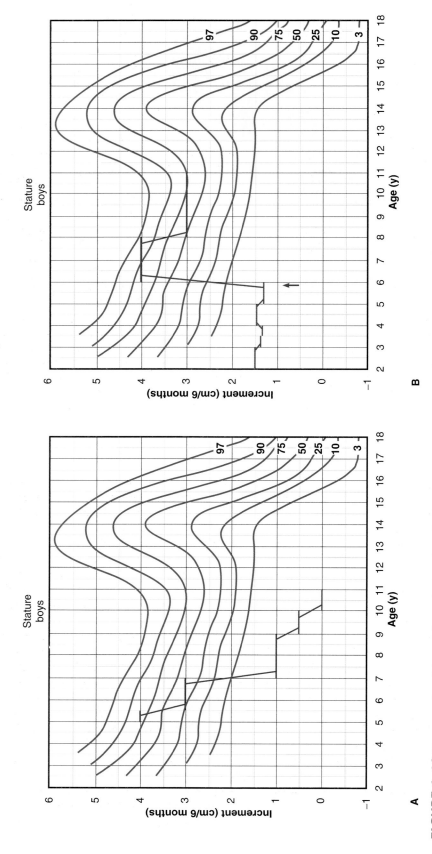

FIGURE 6–10 Two examples of abnormal growth plotted on a height velocity chart. **A.** The plot is taken from the data recorded as squares in Figure 6–9, describing a patient with precocious puberty such as patient **A** in Figure 6–11, with premature epiphysial closure, and cessation of growth. **B.** The plot is taken from the data recorded as circles in Figure 6–9, describing a patient with GH deficiency (such as patient **B** in Figure 6–11) who was treated with hGH (arrow) at age 6. Initial catch-up growth is noted for 2 years, with a lower (but normal) velocity of growth following. These charts display growth rate over 6 month growth intervals rather than 12-month intervals as shown on Figures 6–3 and 6–4.

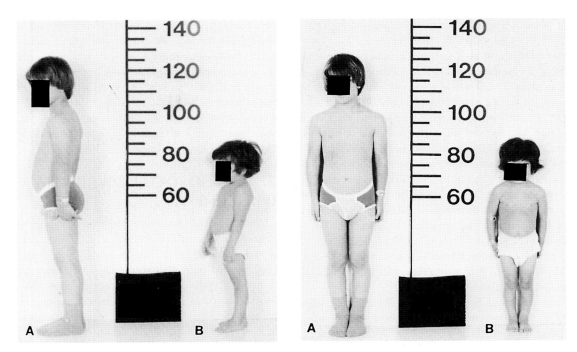

FIGURE 6–11 Two boys demonstrating extremes of growth. The boy at left in each photograph **(A)** has precocious puberty due to a central nervous system lesion. At 4½ years, he was 125.1 cm tall, which is 4.5 standard deviations (SDs) above the mean. (The mean height for a 4-year-old is 101.5 cm.) His testes measured 2 × 3.5 cm each, his penis 9.8 × 2.8 cm (all pubertal measurements). He was muscular and had acne and a deep voice. His bone age was 10 years, the testosterone level was 480 ng/dL, and the LH rose after 100 μg of GnRH (gonadorelin) to a pubertal response. His brain CT scan revealed a hamartoma of the tuber cinereum. The boy at right **(B)** at 6 years of age was 85 cm tall, which is more than 5 SD below the mean. He had the classic physical and historical characteristics of idiopathic GH deficiency, including early growth failure and a cherubic appearance. His plasma GH values were nondetectable and did not rise after provocative testing.

entered puberty, and appear to have limited time to respond to GH before epiphyseal fusion causes the cessation of growth, a GnRH agonist has been used to delay epiphyseal fusion in clinical trials with varying success, but this was not recommended by a consensus conference on the use of GnRH agonist therapy due to lack of strong evidence of effectiveness. While clinical trials continue, this off label use is not yet established as safe and effective. Aromatase inhibitors have been combined with GH in some studies and while this is not yet regular clinical practice, there appears to be an effect of decreasing bone age advancement while allowing increased growth and height obtained.

There are other conditions for which the FDA has approved the use of GH. GH therapy will increase adult height in Turner syndrome to an average of 5.1 cm if started early enough; the addition of low-dose oxandrolone is reported to further increase growth rate. Estrogen is used to promote feminization and maintain bone mineral density; the optimal time to initiate treatment with estrogen should be individualized based on bone age, height, and psychological factors. Usually estrogen is administered during the adolescent years in low doses and only after the normal age of onset of puberty is reached to preserve maximal adult height, although earlier initiation of therapy is gaining credence (see Chapter 15).

In the most successful series of children with SGA treated with GH, the agent increased adult height between 2.0 SD and 2.7 SD. Girls with Turner syndrome treated with GH reach adult height of more than 150 cm, an improvement from the average untreated height which is about 144 cm. When treatment starts at or before 4 years, an adult height is achieved in the normal range.

Treatment with GH is approved for chronic renal disease in childhood. GH increases growth rate above the untreated state without excessive advancement in bone age. Prader-Willi syndrome may also be treated with GH to increase growth rate and lean tissue mass and bone density. A recent study indicated that parental education exerted the most significant effect on body composition in these children. However, there are reports that patients with Prader-Willi syndrome have died of obstructive sleep apnea following GH treatment, demonstrating a need for sleep studies to exclude sleep apnea before initiating treatment and constant surveillance. The treatment of Noonan syndrome is described earlier. In general, males are more often treated with GH than females in the United States, but this is not the case in other developed countries.

The FDA has approved the use of GH in otherwise normal children, whose stature is below 2.25 standard deviations for age and who are predicted to fall short of reaching normal adult height

(<1 percentile of adult height). There may be pressure for treatment of children predicted to be taller than these guidelines from parents, but the FDA approval is for specific indications. While GH may increase the height of such severely affected children, it should not be used for a child whose predicted adult height is in the normal range. Treatment costs $30,000 to $40,000 per year or about $35,000 per cm gained. In the United States males are treated more often than females while the ratio is more equal in other countries, presumably due to social/cultural issues.

GHRH has been isolated, sequenced, and synthesized. It is available for use in diagnosis and treatment. GH-deficient patients demonstrate lower or absent GH secretion after administration of GHRH. However, episodic doses of GHRH can restore GH secretion, IGF-I production, and growth in children with idiopathic GH deficiency. The ability of GHRH administration to stimulate pituitary GH secretion further supports the concept that idiopathic GH deficiency is primarily a disease of the hypothalamus, not of the pituitary gland.

IGF-I is now produced by recombinant DNA technology. IGF-I is useful in the treatment of certain types of short stature, particularly Laron dwarfism (and perhaps for African pygmies, should treatment be desired) where neither GH nor any other treatment is effective. IGF-I has been studied clinically for more than 12 years. Side effects such as hypoglycemia (observed in 49% of treated subjects), injection site lipohypertrophy (32%), and tonsillar/adenoidal hypertrophy (22%) are common but not said to be severe. However, there is concern among some authorities as to the safety of this therapy.

B. Psychologic management and outcome   Research into the psychologic outcome of patients with short stature is flawed by lack of consistent methods of investigation and lack of controlled studies, but some results are of interest. Aromatase inhibitors have been combined with GH therapy in clinical studies to decrease the advancement of bone age and maximize adult height. This has not yet been introduced into common practice and is considered experimental.

Studies vary in their conclusions, as to whether short stature is harmful to a child's psychologic development or not, and whether, by inference, GH is helpful in improving the child's psychologic functioning. Children with GH deficiency are the most extensively studied; earlier investigations suggested that they have more passive personality traits than do healthy children, may have delayed emotional maturity, and suffer from infantilization from parents, teachers, and peers. Many of these children have been held back in school because of their size without regard to their academic abilities. Some patients retain a body image of short stature even after normal height has been achieved with treatment. More recent studies challenge these views and suggest that self-image in children with height below the fifth percentile, who do not have GH deficiency, is closely comparable to a population of children with normal height. These findings may not be representative of the patient population discussed above in that a normal ambulatory population of *short* children may differ from the selected group that seeks medical attention. The data suggest that short stature itself is not cause for grave

psychologic concern, and such concerns should not be used to justify GH therapy. We cannot avoid the fact that our *heightist* society values physical stature and equates it with the potential for success, a perception that is not lost on the children with short stature and their parents. A supportive environment in which they are not allowed to act younger than their age, nor to occupy a *privileged place* in the family is recommended for children with short stature. Psychologic help is indicated in severe cases of depression or maladjustment.

2. PSYCHOSOCIAL DWARFISM (FIGURE 6–12)

Children with psychosocial dwarfism present with poor growth, a *pot-bellied* and immature appearance. They often display bizarre eating and drinking habits. Parents may report that the affected child begs for food from neighbors, forages in garbage cans, and drinks from toilet bowls. As a rule, this tragic condition occurs in only one of several children in a family. Careful questioning and observation reveal a disordered family structure in which the child is either ignored or severely disciplined. Caloric deprivation or physical battering may or may not be a feature of the history. These children have functional hypopituitarism. Testing often reveals GH deficiency at first, but after the child is removed from the home, GH function quickly returns to normal. Diagnosis rests on improvement in behavior or catch-up growth in the hospital or in a foster home. Separation from the family is therapeutic, but the prognosis is guarded. Family psychotherapy may be beneficial, but long-term follow-up is lacking.

Growth disorder due to abnormal parent–child interaction in a younger infant is *maternal deprivation*. Caloric deprivation due to parental neglect may be of greater significance in this younger age group. Even in the absence of nutritional restriction or full-blown psychosocial dwarfism, constant negative interactions within a family may inhibit the growth of a child.

It is essential to consider family dynamics in the evaluation of a child with poor growth. It is not appropriate to recommend GH therapy for emotional disorders.

3. HYPOTHYROIDISM

Thyroid hormone deficiency decreases postnatal growth rate and skeletal development if onset is at or before birth. It leads to severe developmental delay unless treatment is rapidly provided after birth. Screening programs for the diagnosis of congenital hypothyroidism have been instituted all over the world. Early treatment following diagnosis in the neonatal period markedly reduces growth failure and has virtually eliminated mental retardation caused by this disorder. Indeed, early treatment of congenital hypothyroidism results in normal growth. Acquired hypothyroidism in older children (eg, due to lymphocytic thyroiditis) may lead to growth failure. Characteristics of hypothyroidism are decreased growth rate and short stature, retarded bone age, and an increased US-LS ratio for chronologic age due to poor growth of the extremities. Patients are apathetic and sluggish and have constipation, bradycardia, coarsening of features and hair, hoarseness, and delayed pubertal development if the condition is untreated.

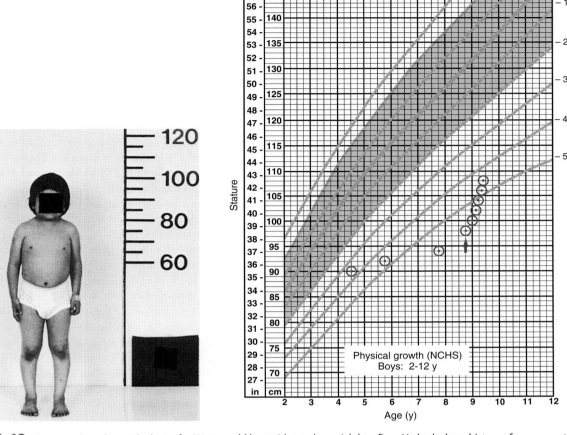

FIGURE 6-12 Photograph and growth chart of a 9½-year-old boy with psychosocial dwarfism. He had a long history of poor growth (<3 cm/y). The social history revealed that he was given less attention and punished more frequently than his seven siblings. He ate from garbage cans and begged for food, though he was not apparently deprived of food at home. When the photograph was taken, he was 99 cm tall (−7 standard deviation [SD]) and weighed 14.7 kg (−3 SD). His bone age was 5 years, with growth arrest lines visible. Serum thyroxine was 7.8 µg/dL. Peak serum GH varied from nondetectable to 8 ng/mL on different provocative tests between age 6 years and 8½ years. He was placed in a hospital chronic care facility (arrow) for a 6-month period and grew 9 cm, which projects to a yearly growth velocity of 18 cm. On repeat testing, the peak serum GH was 28 ng/mL.

Intelligence is unaffected in late-onset hypothyroidism, but the apathy and lethargy may make it seem otherwise. Although weight gain is possible with hypothyroidism, in contrast to common wisdom, it is not extreme.

The diagnosis of congenital hypothyroidism is usually made on the basis of neonatal screening studies. In this standard procedure, currently in use throughout the world, a sample of blood is taken from the heel or from the umbilical cord at birth and analyzed for total T_4 or TSH. A total T_4 of less than 6 µg/dL or a TSH more than 25 mU/L is usually indicative of congenital hypothyroidism, but values differ by state and laboratory. A low total T_4 alone may be associated with low circulating thyroxine-binding globulin (TBG), but the significantly elevated TSH is diagnostic of primary hypothyroidism. The diagnosis may be accompanied by radiologic evidence of retarded bone age or epiphyseal dysgenesis in severe congenital hypothyroidism.

In older children, serum TSH is the most reliable diagnostic test. Elevated TSH with decreased free T_4 may eliminate the potential confusion resulting from the use of total T_4, which may vary with the level of TBG or other thyroxine-binding proteins. A positive test for serum thyroglobulin antibodies or thyroperoxidase antibodies would lead to the diagnosis of autoimmune thyroid disease (Hashimoto thyroiditis) as an explanation for the development of hypothyroidism (see Chapter 7). If both FT_4 and TSH are low, the possibility of central hypothyroidism (pituitary or hypothalamic insufficiency) must be considered (this would not be determined in the newborn screening programs that use primarily TSH screening). This should lead to a search for other hypothalamic-pituitary endocrine deficiencies such as GH deficiency and central nervous system disease (see Chapter 4).

Treatment is accomplished by thyroxine replacement. The dose varies from a range of 10 to 15 µg/kg in infancy to 2 to 3 µg/kg in older children and teenagers. Suppression of TSH to normal values for age is a useful method for assessing the adequacy of replacement in acquired primary hypothyroidism. However, there are additional considerations in treatment of neonates, and consultation with a pediatric endocrinologist is essential in this age group to ensure optimal central nervous system development. Suppression of TSH is not necessarily appropriate in all affected newborns.

4. CUSHING SYNDROME

Excess glucocorticoids (either exogenous or endogenous) lead to decreased growth before obesity and other signs of Cushing syndrome develop. The underlying disease may be bilateral adrenal hyperplasia due to abnormal ACTH-cortisol regulation in Cushing disease, autonomous adrenal adenomas, or adrenal carcinoma. The appropriate diagnosis may be missed if urinary cortisol and 17-hydroxycorticosteroid determinations are not interpreted on the basis of the child's body size or if inappropriate doses of dexamethasone are used for testing (appropriate doses are 20 µg/kg/d for the low-dose and 80 µg/kg/d for the high-dose dexamethasone suppression test) (see Chapter 9). Furthermore, daily variations in cortisol production necessitate several urinary or plasma cortisol determinations before Cushing disease can be appropriately diagnosed or ruled out. The high-dose dexamethasone test was positive in 68% of a recent series of children with Cushing disease. The corticotropin-releasing hormone test was positive in 80% of affected patients, whereas MRI of the pituitary was positive in only 52%. Inferior petrosal sampling (see Chapters 4 and 9) was 100% accurate in the diagnosis of Cushing disease although technically difficult in children. The development of salivary cortisol assays makes the sampling of early morning cortisol after late-night dexamethasone doses an easier method to diagnose Cushing disease in children. Transsphenoidal microadenomectomy is the treatment of choice for Cushing disease.

Exogenous glucocorticoids used to treat asthma or even over-zealous use of topical corticosteroid ointments or creams may suppress growth. These iatrogenic causes of Cushing syndrome, if resolved early, may allow catch-up growth and so may not affect final height. Thus, an accurate history of prior medications is important in diagnosis. Treatment of the underlying disorder (eg, transsphenoidal microadenomectomy for Cushing disease) will restore growth rate to normal (catch-up growth may occur initially) if epiphyseal fusion has not occurred, but adult height will depend on the length of the period of growth suppression.

5. PSEUDOHYPOPARATHYROIDISM

Pseudohypoparathyroidism type 1A (OMIM #103580) is a rare disorder consisting of a characteristic phenotype and biochemical signs of hypoparathyroidism (low serum calcium and high serum phosphate) in its classic form. Phosphate is elevated in states of parathyroid hormone (PTH) deficiency, while phosphate is low in vitamin D deficiency. Circulating PTH levels are elevated, and target tissues fail to respond to exogenous PTH administration. Children with classic pseudohypoparathyroidism are short and overweight, with characteristic round facies and short fourth and fifth metacarpals. This constellation of physical findings is called Albright hereditary osteodystrophy, which may be expressed separately from the biochemical disorders (see later). Developmental

delay is common. The condition is due to heterozygous loss of function in the alpha subunit of the G_s protein transducer (*GNAS1* gene). When imprinted paternally, this results in a defect in the G-protein that couples PTH receptors to adenylyl cyclase. Thus, patients with pseudohypoparathyroidism type 1A have a blunted rise of urinary cAMP in response to administration of PTH. Remarkably, a defect occurs in the same regulatory protein system affected in McCune-Albright syndrome, in which hyperactive endocrine events result (see Chapters 1 and 8). A rarer variant of this disorder (pseudohypoparathyroidism type 1B; OMIM #603233) appears to be due to mutations in noncoding regions of the *GNAS1* gene. Treatment with high-dose vitamin D or 1,25-dihydroxyvitamin D (calcitriol) and exogenous calcium as well as phosphate-binding agents (if needed) will help correct the biochemical defects and control hypocalcemic seizures in patients with pseudohypoparathyroidism.

Two remarkable cousins are reported with pseudohypoparathyroidism and premature Leydig cell maturation, both due to abnormalities in the same G protein. The defective protein was shown to be inactive at normal body temperature, leading to defective PTH activity at the level of the kidney and bone. However, it was hyperactive at the cooler temperatures in the scrotum, leading to ligand-independent activation of Leydig cell function.

Children with the phenotype of Albright hereditary osteodystrophy but with normal circulating levels of calcium, phosphate, and PTH have pseudopseudohypoparathyroidism (OMIM #612463). They require no calcium or vitamin D therapy (see Chapter 8).

6. DISORDERS OF VITAMIN D METABOLISM

Short stature and poor growth are features of rickets in its obvious or more subtle forms. The cause may be vitamin D deficiency due to inadequate oral intake, fat malabsorption, inadequate sunlight exposure, anticonvulsant therapy, and/or renal or hepatic disease. Classic findings of vitamin D-deficient rickets include bowing of the legs, chest deformities (rachitic rosary), and characteristic radiographic findings of the extremities associated with decreased serum calcium and phosphate levels and elevated serum alkaline phosphatase levels. There are two forms of hereditary vitamin D-dependent rickets. Autosomal recessive type 1 hypophosphatemic rickets (OMIM #241520) involves a renal 25 OHD 1-hydroxylase deficiency, and type 2 (OMIM #613312) involves an absent or defective vitamin D receptor. However, the most common type of rickets in the United States is X-linked hypophosphatemic rickets, a dominant genetic disorder affecting renal reabsorption of phosphate. It is associated with short stature, severe and progressive bowing of the legs (but no changes in the wrists or chest), normal or slightly elevated serum calcium, very low serum phosphate, and urinary phosphate wasting. Short stature is linked with rickets in other renal disorders associated with renal phosphate wasting. Examples include Fanconi syndrome (including cystinosis and other inborn errors of metabolism) and renal tubular acidosis.

When treatment is effective in these disorders (eg, vitamin D for vitamin D deficiency or alkali therapy for appropriate types of RTA), growth rates will improve. Replacement of vitamin D and phosphate is appropriate therapy for vitamin D-resistant rickets. It improves the bowing of the legs and leads to improved growth, although there is a risk of nephrocalcinosis. This necessitates annual renal ultrasound examinations when patients are receiving vitamin D therapy.

In the Williams syndrome of elfin facies, supravalvular aortic stenosis, and mental retardation with gregarious personality, patients have SGA and greatly reduced height in childhood and as adults; this disorder may include infantile hypercalcemia but is no longer considered a disorder of vitamin D metabolism because a genetic defect in the *elastin* gene at 7q11.23 occurs in most affected patients (see Chapters 8 and 15).

7. DIABETES MELLITUS

Growth in type 1 diabetes mellitus depends on the efficacy of therapy. Well-controlled diabetes mellitus is compatible with normal growth, whereas poorly controlled diabetes often causes slow growth. Liver and spleen enlargement in a poorly controlled short diabetic child is known as Mauriac syndrome, rarely seen now owing to improved diabetic care. Another factor that may decrease growth rate in children with type 1 diabetes mellitus is the increased incidence of Hashimoto thyroiditis in this population. Yearly thyroid function screening is advisable, especially as the peripubertal period approaches. GH concentrations are higher in children with diabetes, and this factor may play a role in the development of diabetic complications. IGF-I concentrations tend to be normal or low, depending on glucose control, but judging from the elevated GH noted above, the stimulation of IGF-I production by GH appears to be partially blocked in these children.

8. DIABETES INSIPIDUS

Polyuria and polydipsia due to inadequate vasopressin (central or neurogenic diabetes insipidus) or inability of the kidney in the classic case to respond to vasopressin (nephrogenic diabetes insipidus) leads to poor caloric intake and decreased growth. With appropriate treatment (see Chapter 5), the growth rate should return to normal. Acquired neurogenic or central diabetes insipidus may herald a hypothalamic-pituitary tumor, and growth failure may be due to associated GH deficiency.

DIAGNOSIS OF SHORT STATURE (TABLE 6–3)

Evaluation of Short Stature

An initial decision must determine whether a child is pathologically short or simply distressed because height is not as close to the 50th percentile as desired by the patient or the parents. Performing unnecessary tests is expensive and may be a source of long-term concern to the parents—a concern that could be avoided by

TABLE 6–3 Basic diagnosis of short stature.

Medical History
Birth weight and gestational age
Prenatal substance abuse
Birth trauma or complications
Family heights
Age of puberty or menarche in family
Family history of or symptoms of chronic diseases
Dietary history

Physical Examination
Measured and charted height
Measured and charted weight and BMI
Signs of syndromes
Midline defects
Neurological examination
Findings of chronic disease

Laboratory Examination
Chemistry panel
   Electrolytes to rule out RTA
   Liver and kidney function to rule out chronic conditions
CBC to rule out anemia or hematological disease
Urinalysis to rule out RTA and renal disease
Free T_4 and TSH to rule out hypothyroidism
IGF-1 (Don't misinterpret low values in constitutional delay or malnutrition)
IGFBP-3 to confirm low IGF-1 in GH deficiency
Serum prolactin to evaluate potential hypothalamic/pituitary disease
Celiac panel
Karyotype in any girl without other diagnosis
Consider dexamethasone suppression in a short child who is gaining excessive weight (quite rare)

Radiographic Examination
Skeletal age to determine constitutional delay
Bone age determination will not make a diagnosis but may assist in making a diagnosis
Bone age determinations must be interpreted in terms of standard deviations from the mean
Bone age determinations must be read by an experienced evaluator
MRI with contrast is usually the best way to determine the presence of a CNS tumor

Growth Hormone Testing
Growth hormone testing is last and only performed if no other diagnosis is found
Never get basal serum GH unless you suspect gigantism!
Stimulated tests:
   L-Dopa
   Clonidine
   Arginine
   Glucagon
   Insulin-induced hypoglycemia (very dangerous)
   GHRH
   Growth hormone–releasing peptides (GRP)

appropriate reassurance. Alternatively, missing a diagnosis of pathologic poor growth may cause the patient to lose inches of final height or may allow progression of disease.

If a patient's stature, growth rate, or height adjusted for midparental height is sufficiently decreased to warrant evaluation, an orderly approach to diagnosis will eliminate unnecessary laboratory testing. The medical history will provide invaluable information. Birthweight and gestational age is used to determine whether the child is SGA or appropriate for gestational age (AGA), the intrauterine course and toxin exposure and the possibility of birth trauma. Evaluation for dietary abnormalities and for symptoms of any chronic disease is important since almost any systemic disease or nutritional compromise can decrease growth rate (see Table 6–1). Review of past growth charts is important, but in this modern era, children often change doctors frequently, and these data may not be available. Asking whether the child has changed clothing sizes or shoe sizes is useful in the absence of any other data that may allow determination of growth rate. Heights of parents and age of puberty of parents are recorded although usually only a mother will recall her age of menarche while the father will not remember anything about his pubertal development (unless the father continued to grow after he left high school which might indicate constitutional delay in puberty). The height of siblings and specifically their percentile of height and whether they entered puberty at an appropriate time is important. Chronic disease in the family is also found in the history. Evaluation of psychosocial factors affecting the family and the relationship of parents and child can be carried out during the history-taking encounter. Often the diagnosis can be made at this point.

It goes without stating that accurate measurement of growth is essential. The physical examination requires determination of height as described earlier, and comparison is carried out with any previous data available. Measurement of weight and the calculation of BMI is performed so that neither obesity nor malnutrition is missed. If past heights are not available, a history of lack of change in clothing and shoe sizes or failure to lengthen skirts or pants may reflect poor growth. Questions about how the child's stature compares with that of his or her peers and whether the child's height has always had the same relationship to that of classmates are useful. One of the most important features of the evaluation process is to determine height velocity and compare the child's growth rate with the normal growth rate for age. Adjustment for midparental height is calculated and nutritional status determined. Arm span, head circumference, and US-LS ratio are measured. Physical examination is directed to uncover signs of chronic disease or a midline defect of the central nervous system that may be related to hypothalamic pituitary dysfunction. Physical stigmas of syndromes or systemic diseases are evaluated. Neurologic examination is essential.

Any clues to a diagnosis in the history or physical examination should be pursued. However, if no historical or physical features lead to the etiology, laboratory examinations are performed. Complete blood count, urinalysis, and serum chemistry screening with electrolyte measurements may reveal anemia, abnormalities of hepatic or renal disease (including concentration defects), glucose intolerance, acidosis, calcium disorder, or other electrolyte disturbances. Age-adjusted values must be used, because, eg., the normal ranges of serum alkaline phosphatase and phosphorus values are higher in children than in adults. An elevated sedimentation rate, low serum carotene, or a positive antinuclear, antigliadin, antiendomysial, antireticulin, or antitissue transglutaminase antibody determination (with IgA determination) may indicate

connective tissue disease, Crohn disease, celiac disease, or malabsorption syndrome. Serum TSH and free T_4 are important measurements to exclude existing thyroid disease. Skeletal age evaluation does not alone provide a diagnosis; however, if the study shows delayed bone age, the possibility of constitutional delay in growth, hypothyroidism, or GH deficiency must be considered. The tests used for the diagnosis of GH deficiency are detailed above. If serum IGF-I is normal for age, classic GH deficiency or malnutrition is unlikely; if serum IGF-I is low, it must be considered in relation to skeletal age, nutritional status, and general health status before interpretation of the value can be made. Since IGF-I values are low under 2 or 3 years of age, the simultaneous measurement of IGFBP-3 is useful in infants. If either or both IGF-I and IGFBP-3 are low, the diagnosis may be GH deficiency if poor nutrition is ruled out. If GH deficiency or impairment is found or if there is another hypothalamic-pituitary defect, an MRI is indicated with particular attention to the hypothalamic-pituitary area to rule out a congenital defect or neoplasm in the area. Ectopic location of the posterior pituitary on MRI is relatively frequent in congenital GH deficiency, as is a decreased pituitary volume or apparent interruption of the pituitary stalk. Serum gonadotropin and sex steroid determinations are performed in pediatric assays if puberty is delayed (see Chapter 15). Serum prolactin may be elevated in the presence of a hypothalamic disorder.

Celiac disease is quite common as a cause of gastrointestinal distress and/or short stature. Serum IgA levels and antitissue transglutaminase antibody measurements are indicated in the evaluation of growth disorders. A karyotype is obtained in any short girl without another diagnosis to rule out Turner syndrome, especially if puberty is delayed or gonadotropins are elevated. If Turner syndrome is diagnosed, evaluation of thyroid function and determination of thyroid antibodies is also important.

Elevated urinary free cortisol (normal: <60 μg/m^2/24 h [<18.7 μmol/m^2/24 h]), elevated late night salivary cortisol, or abnormal dexamethasone suppression testing signifies Cushing syndrome.

If no diagnosis is apparent after all of the above have been considered and evaluated, more detailed procedures, such as provocative testing for GH deficiency, are indicated. It must be emphasized that a long and expensive evaluation is not necessary until it is demonstrated that psychologic or nutritional factors are not at fault. Likewise, if a healthy-appearing child presents with borderline short stature, normal growth rate, and short familial stature, a period of observation may be more appropriate than laboratory tests.

TALL STATURE DUE TO NONENDOCRINE CAUSES

1. CONSTITUTIONAL TALL STATURE

A subject who has been taller than his or her peers through most of childhood, is growing at a velocity within the normal range with a moderately advanced bone age, and has no signs of the disorders listed below may be considered to be constitutionally advanced. Predicted final height will usually be in the normal adult range for the family.

Obesity in an otherwise healthy child will often, especially in the presence of a melanocortin 4 receptor (MC4R) mutation, leads to moderate advancement of bone age, slightly increased growth rate, and tall stature in childhood. Puberty will begin in the early range of normal, and adult stature will conform to genetic influences. Thus, an obese child without endocrine disease should be tall; short stature and obesity are worrisome.

2. FAMILIAL/GENETIC TALL STATURE

Children with exceptionally tall parents have a genetic tendency to reach a height above the normal range. The child will be tall for age and will grow at a high normal rate. Bone age will be close to chronologic age, leading to a tall height prediction. Occasionally, children will be concerned about being too tall as adults. These worries are more common in girls and will often be of greater concern to the parents than to the patient. Adult height was limited in the past by promoting early epiphyseal closure with estrogen in girls or testosterone in boys, but such therapy is no longer considered appropriate. Testosterone therapy decreases HDL cholesterol levels. Acne fulminans may be caused by testosterone therapy and progression may occur, even after therapy has been withdrawn. Estrogen carries the theoretical risk of thrombosis, ovarian cysts, and galactorrhea, even if few of these complications are reported. High-dose estrogen therapy is estimated to decrease predicted final height by as much as 4.5 to 7 cm but only if started 3 to 4 years before epiphyseal fusion. Height-limiting therapy is extremely rare in the present era although, recently, long-acting somatostatin agonists have been used in an attempt to limit height. Counseling and reassurance are more appropriate.

3. SYNDROMES OF TALL STATURE

Cerebral Gigantism

The sporadic syndrome of rapid growth in infancy, prominent forehead, high-arched palate, sharp chin, and hypertelorism [Sotos syndrome (OMIM #117550)] is caused by mutation in the *nuclear receptor–binding SET domain protein 1* (*NSD1*) gene and is not associated with GH excess. Mentation is usually impaired. The growth rate decreases to normal in later childhood, but stature remains tall.

Marfan Syndrome

Marfan syndrome (OMIM #154700) is an autosomal dominant abnormality of connective tissue exhibiting variable penetrance. The disorder is due to mutation of the *fibrillin1* gene located on 15q21.1. This condition may be diagnosed by characteristic physical manifestations of tall stature, long thin fingers (arachnodactyly), hyperextension of joints, and superior lens subluxation. Pectus excavatum and scoliosis may be noted. Furthermore, aortic or mitral regurgitation or aortic root dilation may be present, and

aortic dissection or rupture may ultimately occur. In patients with this syndrome, arm span exceeds height, and the US-LS ratio is quite low owing to long legs. Aortic root ultrasound and slit lamp ophthalmologic examinations are indicated.

Homocystinuria

Patients with homocystinuria (OMIM #236200) have an autosomal recessive deficiency of cystathionine beta-synthase (gene locus 21q22.3) and phenotypes similar to those of patients with Marfan syndrome. Additional features of homocystinuria include developmental delay, increased incidence of seizures, osteoporosis, inferior lens dislocation, and increased urinary excretion of homocystine with increased plasma homocystine and methionine but low plasma cystine. Thromboembolic phenomena may precipitate a fatal complication. This disease is treated by restricting dietary methionine and, in responsive patients, administering pyridoxine.

Beckwith-Wiedemann Syndrome

Patients with Beckwith-Wiedemann syndrome (OMIM #130650) demonstrate macrosomia (birth weight >90th percentile) in 88% of cases, increased postnatal growth, omphalocele in 80%, macroglossia in 97%, and hypoglycemia due to the hyperinsulinism of pancreatic hyperplasia in 63%. Other reported features include fetal adrenocortical cytomegaly and large kidneys with medullary dysplasia. The majority of patients occur in a sporadic pattern due to a mutation at 11p15.5, but analysis of some pedigrees suggests the possibility of familial patterns. There is a risk of Wilms tumor, hepatoblastoma, adrenal carcinoma, and gonadoblastoma in this condition.

XYY Syndrome

Patients with one (47,XYY) or more (48,XYYY) extra Y chromosomes achieve greater than average adult heights. They have normal birth lengths but higher than normal growth rates. Excess GH secretion has not been documented (see Chapter 14).

Klinefelter Syndrome

Patients with Klinefelter syndrome (see Chapters 12 and 14) tend toward tall stature, but this is not a constant feature.

TALL STATURE DUE TO ENDOCRINE DISORDERS

1. PITUITARY GIGANTISM

Pituitary gigantism is caused by excess GH secretion before the age of epiphyseal fusion. The increased GH secretion may be due to somatotroph-secreting tumors or constitutive activation of GH secretion as is sometimes found in the McCune-Albright syndrome. Alternatively, it may result from excess secretion of GHRH. Patients—besides growing excessively rapidly—have coarse features, large hands and feet with thick fingers and toes, and often frontal bossing and large jaws.

Although this condition is quite rare, the findings appear similar to those observed in the more frequent acromegaly (which occurs with GH excess after epiphyseal fusion). Thus, glucose intolerance or frank diabetes mellitus, hypogonadism, and thyromegaly are predicted. Treatment is accomplished by surgery (the transsphenoidal approach is used if the tumor is small enough), radiation therapy, or by therapy with a somatostatin analog.

2. SEXUAL PRECOCITY

Early onset of estrogen or androgen secretion leads to abnormally increased height velocity. Because bone age is advanced, there is the paradox of the tall child who, because of early epiphyseal closure, is short as an adult. The conditions include complete and incomplete sexual precocity (including virilizing congenital adrenal hyperplasia) (see Chapter 14).

3. THYROTOXICOSIS

Excessive thyroid hormone, due to endogenous overproduction or overtreatment with exogenous thyroxine, leads to increased growth, advanced bone age, and, if occurring in early life, craniosynostosis. If the condition remains untreated, final height will be reduced.

4. INFANTS OF DIABETIC MOTHERS

Birth weight and size in infants of moderately diabetic mothers are quite high, although severely diabetic women who have poor control may have infants with IUGR due to placental vascular insufficiency. Severe hypoglycemia and hypocalcemia are evident in the infants soon after birth. The appearance and size of such infants is so striking that women have been diagnosed with gestational diabetes as a result of giving birth to affected infants. By 10 years of age, infants of diabetic mothers have an increased prevalence of obesity as well as insulin resistance and all of the comorbidities of the condition.

REFERENCES

Normal Growth

Himes JH. Minimum time intervals for serial measurements of growth in recumbent length or stature of individual children. *Acta Paediatr.* 1999;88:120. [PMID: 10102141]

Lofqvist C, Andersson E, Gelander L, Rosberg S, Blum WF, Albertsson Wikland K. Reference values for IGF-I throughout childhood and adolescence: a model that accounts simultaneously for the effect of gender, age, and puberty. *J Clin Endocrinol Metab.* 2001;86:5870. [PMID: 11739455]

Reiter EO, Rosenfeld RG. Normal and aberrant growth. In: Wilson JD, Foster DW, Kronenberg HM, Larsen PR, eds. *Williams Textbook of Endocrinology.* 11th ed. Philadelphia, PA: WB Saunders; 2007.

Silventoinen K, Haukka J, Dunkel L, Tynelius P, Rasmussen F. Genetics of pubertal timing and its associations with relative weight in childhood and adult height: the Swedish Young Male Twins Study. *Pediatrics.* 2008;121:e885. [PMID: 18381517]

Styne DM. Growth. In: *Handbook of Pediatric Endocrinology.* Philadelphia, PA: Lippincott Williams & Wilkins; 2004.

Towne B, Williams KD, Blangero J. Presentation, heritability, and genome-wide linkage analysis of the midchildhood growth spurt in healthy children from the Fels Longitudinal Study. *Hum Biol.* 2008;80:623. [PMID: 19728540]. http://www.cdc.gov/nchs/data/nhanes/growthcharts/set1/all.pdf.

Short Stature

Ahmad T, Garcia-Filion P, Borchert M, Kaufman F, Burkett L, Geffner M. Endocrinological and auxological abnormalities in young children with optic nerve hypoplasia: a prospective study. *J Pediatr.* 2006;148:78. [PMID: 16423602]

Albertsson-Wikland K, Aronson AS, Gustafsson J, et al. Dose-dependent effect of growth hormone on final height in children with short stature without growth hormone deficiency. *J Clin Endocrinol Metab.* 2008;93:4342. [PMID: 18728172]

Bullinger M, Kołtowska-Häggström M, Sandberg D, et al. Health-related quality of life of children and adolescents with growth hormone deficiency or idiopathic short stature—part 2: available results and future directions. *Horm Res.* 2009;72:74. [PMID: 19690424]

Chernausek SD, Backeljauw PF, Frane J, et al. Long-term treatment with recombinant insulin-like growth factor (IGF)-I in children with severe IGF-I deficiency due to growth hormone insensitivity. *J Clin Endocrinol Metab.* 2007;92:902. [PMID: 17192294]

Clayton PE, Cianfarani S, Czernichow P, Johannsson G, Rapaport R, Rogol A. Management of the child born small for gestational age through to adulthood: a consensus statement of the International Societies of Pediatric Endocrinology and the Growth Hormone Research Society. *J Clin Endocrinol Metab.* 2007;92:804. [PMID: 17200164]

Cohen P, Rogol AD, Deal CL, et al. Consensus statement on the diagnosis and treatment of children with idiopathic short stature: a summary of the Growth Hormone Research Society, the Lawson Wilkins Pediatric Endocrine Society, and the European Society for Paediatric Endocrinology Workshop. *J Clin Endocrinol Metab.* 2008;93:4210. [PMID: 18782877]

Collett-Solberg PF, Misra M. The role of recombinant human insulin-like growth factor-I in treating children with short stature. *J Clin Endocrinol Metab.* 2008;93:10. [PMID: 18165284]

Davenport ML, Crowe BJ, Travers SH, et al. Growth hormone treatment of early growth failure in toddlers with Turner syndrome: a randomized, controlled, multicenter trial. *J Clin Endocrinol Metab.* 2007;92:3406. [PMID: 17595258]

de Graaff LC, Argente J, Veenma DC, et al. Genetic screening of a Dutch population with isolated GH deficiency (IGHD). *Clin Endocrinol (Oxf).* 2009;70:742. [PMID: 18785993]

Donaldson MD, Gault EJ, Tan KW, Dunger DB. Optimising management in Turner syndrome: from infancy to adult transfer. *Arch Dis Child.* 2006;91:513. [PMID: 16714725]

GH Research Society. Consensus guidelines for the diagnosis and treatment of growth hormone (GH) deficiency in childhood and adolescence: summary statement of the GH Research Society. *J Clin Endocrinol Metab.* 2000;85:3990. [PMID: 11095419]

Gonc EN, Yordam N, Ozon A, Alikasifoglu A, Kandemir N. Endocrinological outcome of different treatment options in children with craniopharyngioma: a retrospective analysis of 66 cases. *Pediatr Neurosurg.* 2004;40:112. [PMID: 15367800]

Grote FK, van Dommelen P, Oostdijk W, et al. Developing evidence-based guidelines for referral for short stature. *Arch Dis Child.* 2008;93:212. [PMID: 17908714]

Hardin DS. GH improves growth and clinical status in children with cystic fibrosis—a review of published studies. *Eur J Endocrinol.* 2004;151(suppl 1): S81. [PMID: 15339250]

Huguenin M, Trivin C, Zerah M, Doz F, Brugieres L, Brauner R. Adult height after cranial irradiation for optic pathway tumors: relationship with neurofibromatosis. *J Pediatr.* 2003;142:699. [PMID: 12838200]

Keil MF, Stratakis CA. Pituitary tumors in childhood: update of diagnosis, treatment and molecular genetics. *Expert Rev Neurother.* 2008;8:563. [PMID: 18416659]

Kelly BP, Paterson WF, Donaldson MD. Final height outcome and value of height prediction in boys with constitutional delay in growth and adolescence treated with intramuscular testosterone 125 mg per month for 3 months. *Clin Endocrinol (Oxf).* 2003;58:267. [PMID: 12608930]

Laron Z. The essential role of IGF-I: lessons from the long-term study and treatment of children and adults with Laron syndrome. *J Clin Endocrinol Metab.* 1999;84:4397. [PMID: 10599694]

Leschek EW, Rose SR, Yanovski JA, et al. Effect of growth hormone treatment on adult height in peripubertal children with idiopathic short stature: a randomized, double-blind, placebo-controlled trial. *J Clin Endocrinol Metab.* 2004;89:3140. [PMID: 15240584]

Mauras N. Strategies for maximizing growth in puberty in children with short stature. *Endocrinol Metab Clin North Am.* 2009;38:613. [PMID: 19717007]

Mullis PE. Genetics of growth hormone deficiency. *Endocrinol Metab Clin North Am.* 2007;36:17. [PMID: 17336732]

Oberfield SE, Sklar CA. Endocrine sequelae in survivors of childhood cancer. *Adolesc Med.* 2002;13:161. [PMID: 11841962]

Phillip M, Lebenthal Y, Lebl J, et al. European multicentre study in children born small for gestational age with persistent short stature: comparison of continuous and discontinuous growth hormone treatment regimens. *Horm Res.* 2009;71:52. [PMID: 19039237]

Ranke MB, Schweizer R, Lindberg A, et al. Insulin-like growth factors as diagnostic tools in growth hormone deficiency during childhood and adolescence: the KIGS experience. *Horm Res.* 2004;62(suppl 1):17. [PMID: 15761228]

Saenger P, et al. Small for gestational age: short stature and beyond. *Endocr Rev.* 2007;28:219. [PMID: 17322454]

Simon D, Leger J, Carel JC. Optimal use of growth hormone therapy for maximizing adult height in children born small for gestational age. *Best Prac Res Clin Endocrinol Metab.* 2008;22:525. [PMID: 18538291]

Stanley TL, Levitsky LL, Grinspoon SK, Misra M. Effect of body mass index on peak growth hormone response to provocative testing in children with short stature. *J Clin Endocrinol Metab.* 2009;94:4875. [PMID: 19890023]

Styne DM, Grumbach MM, Kaplan SL, Wilson CB, Conte FA. Treatment of Cushing's disease in childhood and adolescence by transsphenoidal microadenomectomy. *N Engl J Med.* 1984;310:889. [PMID: 6321987]

Tanner JM, Davies PS. Clinical longitudinal standards for height and height velocity for North American children. *J Pediatr.* 1985;107:317. [PMID: 3875704]

van Dijk M, Bannink EM, van Pareren YK, Mulder PG, Hokken-Koelega AC. Risk factors for diabetes mellitus type 2 and metabolic syndrome are comparable for previously growth hormone-treated young adults born small for gestational age (SGA) and untreated short SGA controls. *J Clin Endocrinol Metab.* 2007;92:160. [PMID: 17062774]

Wickman S, Kajantie E, Dunkel L. Effects of suppression of estrogen action by the p450 aromatase inhibitor letrozole on bone mineral density and bone turnover in pubertal boys. *J Clin Endocrinol Metab.* 2003;88:3785. [PMID: 11888840]

Yanovski JA, Rose SR, Municchi G, et al. Treatment with a luteinizing hormone-releasing hormone agonist in adolescents with short stature. *N Engl J Med.* 2003;348:908. [PMID: 12621135]

Tall Stature

Eugster EA, Peskovitz OH. Gigantism. *J Clin Endocrinol Metab.* 1999;84:4379. [PMID: 10599691]

Leventopoulos G, Kitsiou-Tzeli S, Kritikos K, et al. A clinical study of Sotos syndrome patients with review of the literature. *Pediatr Neurol.* 2009;40:357. [PMID: 19380072]

Thomsett MJ. Referrals for tall stature in children: a 25-year personal experience. *J Paediatr Child Health.* 2009;45:58. [PMID: 19208068]

The Thyroid Gland

**David S. Cooper, MD, and
Paul W. Ladenson, MA (Oxon.), MD**

The thyroid gland is the body's largest single organ specialized for endocrine hormone production. Its function is to secrete an appropriate amount of the thyroid hormones, primarily 3,5,3',5'-l-tetraiodothyronine (thyroxine, T_4), and a lesser quantity of 3,5,3'-l-triiodothyronine (T_3), which arises mainly from the subsequent extrathyroidal deiodination of T_4. In target tissues, T_3 interacts with nuclear T_3 receptors that are, in turn, bound to special nucleotide sequences in the promoter regions of genes that are positively or negatively regulated by thyroid hormone. Among their life-sustaining actions, the thyroid hormones promote normal fetal and childhood growth and central nervous system development; regulate heart rate and myocardial contraction and relaxation; affect gastrointestinal motility and renal water clearance; and modulate the body's energy expenditure, heat generation, weight, and lipid metabolism. In addition, the thyroid contains parafollicular or C cells that produce calcitonin, a 32-amino-acid polypeptide that inhibits bone resorption, but has no apparent physiologic role in humans. However, calcitonin is clinically important as a tumor marker produced by medullary thyroid cancers that arise from these cells (Chapter 8).

EMBRYOLOGY, ANATOMY, AND HISTOLOGY

The thyroid gland originates in the embryo as a mesodermal invagination in the pharyngeal floor at the foramen cecum, from which it descends anterior to the trachea and bifurcates, forming two lateral lobes, each measuring approximately 4 cm in length, 2 cm in width, and 1 cm in thickness in adulthood. Ectopic thyroid tissue can be present anywhere along or beyond this thyroglossal duct, from the tongue base (lingual thyroid) to the mediastinum. The thyroglossal duct may also give rise to midline cysts lined with squamous epithelium, which can remain asymptomatic, or become infected or give rise to thyroid tumors. The caudal end of the thyroglossal duct forms the pyramidal lobe of the thyroid, which can become palpable in conditions causing diffuse thyroid inflammation or stimulation (Figure 7–1).

Upward growth of the thyroid gland is limited by the attachment of the sternothyroid muscle to the thyroid cartilage. However, posterior and downward growth is unimpeded, so that thyroid enlargement, or goiter, frequently extends posteriorly and inferiorly, even into the superior mediastinum (substernal goiter).

The thyroid gland has clinically important anatomical relationships to the recurrent laryngeal nerves, which course behind the gland, and two pairs of parathyroid glands that usually lie behind the upper and middle portions of the thyroid lobes. The thyroid is also draped around the trachea and the posterior margins of its lobes abut the esophagus. All of these structures can be compressed by gland enlargement, invaded by thyroid malignancies, or injured in the course of thyroid surgery (Figure 7–2). Because the posterior thyroid capsule is bound to the pretracheal fascia, the gland normally rises and falls with deglutition, facilitating its inspection and palpation.

The thyroid gland has a rich blood supply (Figure 7–3), which can be increased in hyperthyroidism, giving rise to an audible whooshing sound (bruit) or even a palpable vibration (thrill). Microscopically, thyrocytes form hollow spheres (follicles) that surround a central lumen containing an aggregation of iodinated thyroglobulin (colloid) that represents the gland's hormone stores (Figure 7–4).

PHYSIOLOGY

STRUCTURE AND SYNTHESIS OF THYROID HORMONES

The thyroid hormones are iodinated thyronines, which comprise of two tyrosine moieties joined by an ether linkage (Figure 7–5). The follicular cells of the thyroid gland are specialized in their ability to synthesize the large hormonal precursor protein thyroglobulin, concentrate iodide intracellularly from the circulation, and express a receptor that binds thyroid-stimulating hormone (thyrotropin, TSH), which promotes thyrocytes' growth and biosynthetic functions.

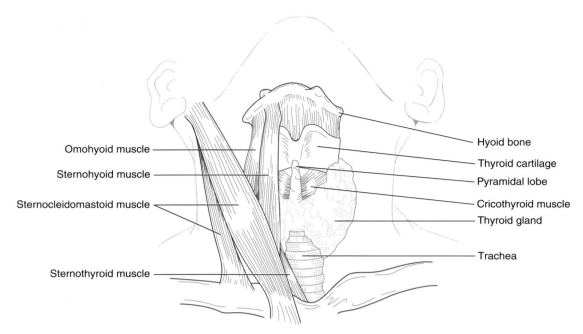

FIGURE 7–1 Gross anatomy of the human thyroid gland (anterior view).

IODINE METABOLISM

Iodine[1] is a key structural component of thyroid hormones. Consequently, it is an essential micronutrient consumed in food or water as iodide or iodate, which is converted to iodide in the stomach. The World Health Organization (WHO) recommends a daily dietary iodine intake of 150 μg for adults, 200 μg for pregnant and lactating women, and 50 to 250 μg for children. Because most iodide is excreted by the kidneys, urinary iodide excretion is an excellent index of dietary intake.

Over millennia, iodine has been leached from the soil in many mountainous and inland regions of the world. Consequently, according to WHO, dietary iodine deficiency, defined as a daily iodine intake less than 100 μg/d, affects an estimated two billion people, which is about one-third of the world's population. When iodide intake is less than 50 μg/d, a normal-sized thyroid cannot sustain adequate hormone production, with resulting gland enlargement (goiter) and, ultimately, hypothyroidism. The consequences of endemic dietary iodine deficiency are especially devastating for the developing fetus and children, who require thyroid hormone for normal neurologic development and growth. In the North American diet, iodine is principally derived from iodized salt, iodate preservatives in baked goods, dairy products containing traces of iodophore antibacterial agents used in milk collection, food coloring, and seafood.

Thyrocytes abundantly express the sodium-iodide symporter (Na-I⁻ symporter; NIS), which spans the cells' basal membranes and actively transports iodide from the blood. The thyroid gland concentrates and uses only a fraction of the iodide supplied to it for hormone synthesis, and the remainder returns to the extracellular fluid pool. Consequently, the normal fractional uptake of iodide, which can be quantified with a radioactive iodine tracer, is approximately 10% to 30% after 24 hours. Because of this active concentrating mechanism and the subsequent organification of intracellular iodide, the intrathyroidal pool of iodine is very large, 8 to 10 mg in the form of stored thyroid hormones and iodinated tyrosines. This iodine provides a buffer in the event of temporary dietary iodine deficiency.

THYROID HORMONE SYNTHESIS AND SECRETION

Synthesis of T_4 and T_3 by the thyroid gland involves six major steps: (1) active transport of iodide across the basement membrane into the thyroid cell (trapping); (2) oxidation of iodide and iodination of tyrosyl residues in thyroglobulin (organification); (3) linking pairs of iodotyrosine molecules within thyroglobulin to form the iodothyronines T_3 and T_4 (coupling); (4) pinocytosis and then proteolysis of thyroglobulin with release of free iodothyronines and iodotyrosines into the circulation; (5) deiodination of iodotyrosines within the thyroid cell, with conservation and reuse of the liberated iodide; and (6) intrathyroidal 5′-deiodination of T_4 to T_3.

Thyroid hormone synthesis requires that NIS, thyroglobulin, and the enzyme thyroid peroxidase (TPO) all be present, functional, and uninhibited. This process is summarized in Figures 7–6 and 7–7.

---

[1] In this chapter, the words "iodine," referring to the uncharged element, and "iodide," referring to its negatively charged anion form, are used interchangeably.

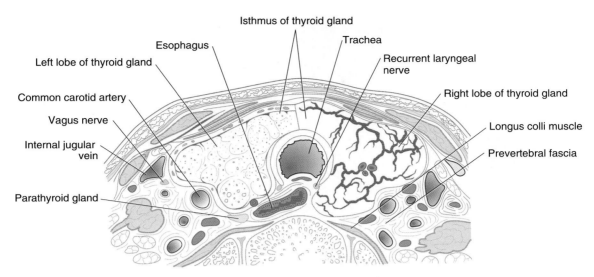

FIGURE 7–2 Cross-section of the neck at the level of T_1, showing thyroid relationships. (Reproduced, with permission, from Lindner HH. *Clinical Anatomy*. McGraw-Hill; 1989.)

Thyroglobulin

Thyroglobulin is a large glycoprotein molecule (MW 660,000 kD), composed of two subunits, each containing 5496 amino acids. Thyroglobulin includes approximately 140 tyrosyl residues, but only four tyrosyl sites are sterically oriented for effective hormonogenesis in each molecule. The iodine content of thyroglobulin can vary from 0.1% to 1% by weight. In thyroglobulin containing 0.5% iodine, for example, there are approximately three molecules of T_4 and one molecule of T_3.

The *thyroglobulin* gene, which resides on the long arm of chromosome 8, contains approximately 8500 nucleotides, which encode the prethyroglobulin protein monomer, including a

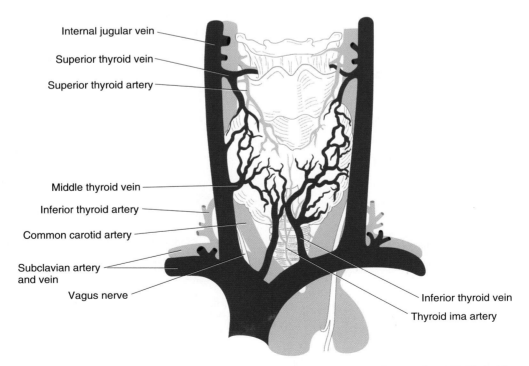

FIGURE 7–3 Arteries and veins related to the thyroid gland. (Reproduced, with permission, from Lindner HH. *Clinical Anatomy*. McGraw-Hill; 1989.)

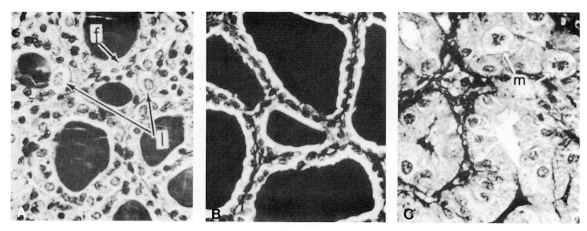

FIGURE 7–4 **A.** Normal rat thyroid. A single layer of cuboidal epithelial cells surrounds PAS-positive material in the follicular space (colloid). The larger, lighter-staining cells indicated by the arrows (I) are C cells that produce calcitonin. The follicular cells form an epithelial layer that surrounds the colloid (F). **B.** Inactive rat thyroid several weeks after hypophysectomy. The follicular lumens are larger and the follicular cells flatter. **C.** Rat thyroid under intensive TSH stimulation. The animal was fed an iodine-deficient diet and injected with propylthiouracil for several weeks. Little colloid is visible. The follicular cells are tall and columnar. Several mitoses (m) are visible. (Reproduced, with permission, from Halmi NS. In: Greep RO, Weiss L, eds. *Histology*. McGraw-Hill; 1973.)

19-amino acid signal peptide. TSH regulates expression of the *thyroglobulin* gene. After thyroglobulin mRNA is translated in the rough endoplasmic reticulum (RER), the protein is glycosylated during transport through the Golgi apparatus (see Figure 7–7), where thyroglobulin dimers are incorporated into exocytic vesicles. These vesicles then fuse with the cell's apical basement membrane, from which they are released into the follicular lumen. There, at the apical-colloid border, tyrosine residues in thyroglobulin are iodinated.

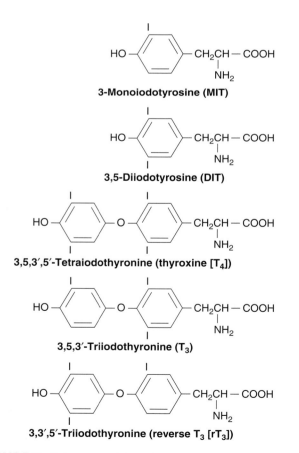

FIGURE 7–5 Structure of thyroid hormones and related compounds. (Reproduced, with permission, from Murray RK, et al. *Harper's Biochemistry*. 24th ed. McGraw-Hill; 1996.)

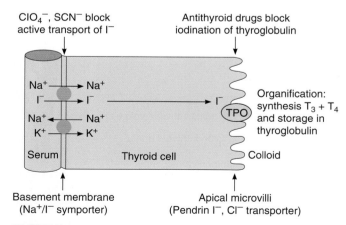

FIGURE 7–6 The iodide transporter in the thyroid cell. The large solid circle represents the Na$^+$/I$^-$ symporter actively transporting I$^-$ into the cell; the large blue circle represents Na$^+$-K$^+$ ATPase supplying the ion gradient which drives the reaction. I$^-$ is transported across the apical membrane by pendrin. Hormone synthesis takes place in the colloid at the colloid-apical membrane, catalyzed by thyroperoxidase (TPO).

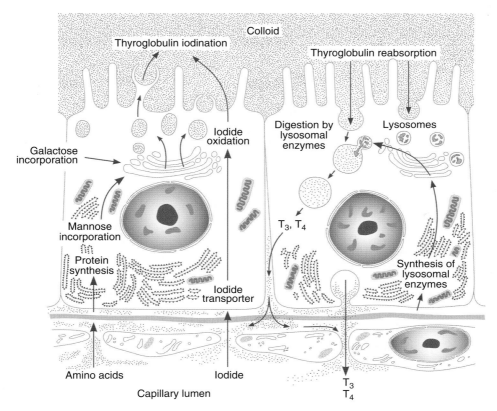

FIGURE 7–7 Processes of synthesis and iodination of thyroglobulin (left) and its reabsorption and digestion (right). These events occur in the same cell. (Reproduced, with permission, from Junqueira LC, Carneiro J, Kelley R. *Basic Histology*. 7th ed. McGraw-Hill; 1992.)

Iodide Transport

Iodide (I^-) is transported across thyrocytes' basal membrane by the NIS. Membrane-bound NIS, which derives its energy from a Na^+-K^+ ATPase, allows the human thyroid gland to maintain a concentration of free iodide 30 to 40 times higher than that in plasma. NIS action is stimulated physiologically by TSH and pathophysiologically by the TSH receptor–stimulating antibody of Graves disease. Although salivary, gastric, and breast tissues express NIS and concentrate iodide to a lesser extent than the thyroid, these other tissues do not organify or store iodide, and their NIS activities are not stimulated by TSH. Large amounts of iodide suppress both NIS activity and *NIS* gene expression, representing mechanisms of iodine autoregulation (see later). The perchlorate ion (ClO_4^-) competes with iodide for NIS; perchlorate has been used to treat hyperthyroidism and has the potential to be an environmental inhibitor of thyroid function. NIS can also concentrate pertechnetate (TcO_4^-) into thyroid cells, facilitating use of the radionuclide sodium pertechnetate ($Tc^{99m}O_4^-$) for visualization of the thyroid gland and quantification of its trapping activity.

At the thyrocyte's apical border, a second iodide transport protein, pendrin, transports iodide to the membrane–colloid interface, where it becomes a substrate for thyroid hormonogenesis (see Figures 7–6 and 7–7). Mutations in the *pendrin* (PDS or SLC26A4) gene impairing its function cause a syndrome of goiter and hearing loss acquired in infancy or early childhood (Pendred syndrome).

Thyroid Peroxidase

Thyroid peroxidase (TPO), a membrane-bound glycoprotein (MW 102 kD) containing a heme moiety, catalyzes both iodide oxidation and covalent linkage of iodine to the tyrosine residues of thyroglobulin. *TPO* gene expression is stimulated by TSH. After TPO is synthesized in the RER, it is inserted into the RER's cisternal membranes, from which it is transferred to the apical cell surface through Golgi elements and exocytic vesicles. Here, at the cell–colloid interface, TPO facilitates both iodination and coupling of the tyrosine residues within thyroglobulin.

Iodination of Thyroglobulin

Within the thyroid cell, at the apical–colloid interface, iodide is rapidly oxidized by locally produced hydrogen peroxide in a reaction catalyzed by TPO; the resulting active iodide intermediate is bound to tyrosyl residues in thyroglobulin. The required hydrogen peroxide is probably generated by an NADPH oxidase in the presence of calcium cations, a process that is also stimulated by TSH. TPO can also catalyze iodination of tyrosyl molecules in proteins other than thyroglobulin, such as albumin or thyroglobulin fragments; but no active hormones arise from these proteins.

Coupling of Iodotyrosyl Residues in Thyroglobulin

The coupling of iodotyrosyl residues in thyroglobulin is also catalyzed by TPO. This is believed to be an intramolecular process involving oxidation of two iodotyrosyl residues brought into proximity by the tertiary and quaternary structures of thyroglobulin, their linkage as a quinol ether intermediate, and splitting of the quinol ether to form an iodothyronine (Figure 7–8). Within the thyroglobulin molecule, two molecules of diiodotyrosine (DIT) couple to form T_4, and monoiodotyrosine (MIT) and DIT molecules couple to form T_3.

The thiocarbamide drugs, including methimazole, carbimazole, and propylthiouracil (PTU), are competitive inhibitors of TPO. Their resulting ability to block thyroid hormone synthesis (Figure 7–9) makes them useful in treatment of hyperthyroidism.

Proteolysis of Thyroglobulin and Thyroid Hormone Secretion

The processes of thyroglobulin proteolysis and secretion in thyroid hormonogenesis are illustrated in Figure 7–7. At the thyrocyte's apical membrane, colloid is engulfed in vesicles by pinocytosis and absorbed into the cell. Lysosomes containing proteolytic enzymes then fuse with the colloid vesicle. This releases T_4 and T_3, as well as inactive iodotyrosines, peptides, and individual amino acids. The biologically active thyroid hormones T_4 and T_3 enter the circulation; DIT and MIT are deiodinated and their iodide conserved. Thyroid hormone secretion is stimulated by TSH and inhibited by excess iodide (see later) and lithium. A small amount of intact thyroglobulin is normally released from thyroid cell and circulates in blood. The serum thyroglobulin concentration is markedly increased in a number of thyroid conditions, including thyroiditis, nodular goiter, and Graves disease. Because thyroglobulin is also synthesized by most malignancies arising from thyroid epithelium, such as papillary and follicular thyroid cancers, it is a useful circulating tumor marker.

Intrathyroidal Deiodination

MIT and DIT formed during the synthesis of thyroid hormone are deiodinated by intrathyroidal deiodinase, an NADPH-dependent flavoprotein found in mitochondria and microsomes that acts on the iodotyrosines MIT and DIT, but not on T_3 and T_4. Most of the iodide released is reused for hormone synthesis, and only a small amount normally leaks out of the thyroid gland (Figure 7–10).

The 5′-deiodinase that converts T_4 to T_3 in peripheral tissues is also found in the thyroid gland. When there is iodide deficiency and in various hyperthyroid states, the activity of this enzyme increases the amount of T_3 secreted by the gland, increasing metabolic efficiency of hormone synthesis.

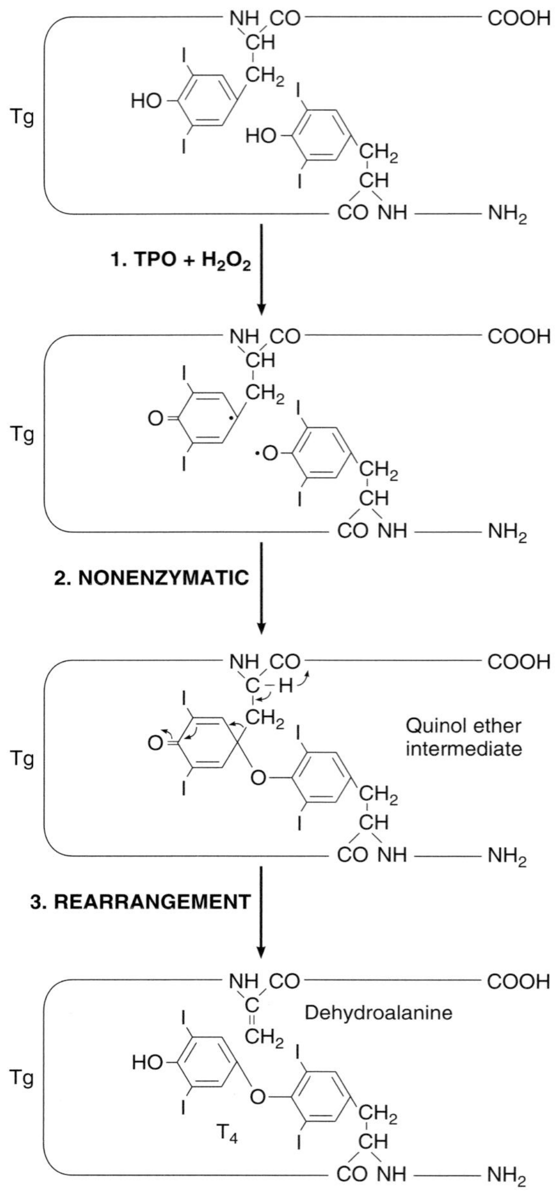

FIGURE 7–8 Hypothetical coupling scheme for intramolecular formation of T_4 within the thyroglobulin molecule. The major hormonogenic site at tyrosyl residue 5 is indicated. (Reproduced, with permission, from Taurog A. Thyroid hormone synthesis. Thyroid iodine metabolism. In Braverman LE, Utiger RD, eds. *Werner and Ingbar's The Thyroid.* 7th ed. Lippincott; 1996.)

ABNORMALITIES IN THYROID HORMONE SYNTHESIS AND RELEASE

Dietary Iodine Deficiency and Inherited Defects

A very low iodine diet and inherited defects in genes encoding the proteins required for thyroid hormone biosynthesis (dyshormonogenesis) can both result in insufficient hormone production. In

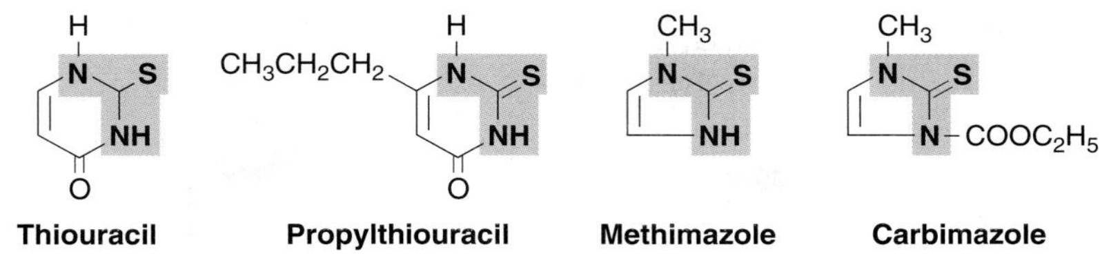

FIGURE 7–9 Thiocarbamide inhibitors of thyroidal iodide organification.

response to limited intrathyroidal iodine content or hormone production, the gland increases the ratios of MIT-to-DIT within thyroglobulin as well as the proportion of secreted T_3 relative to T_4. The hypothalamic-pituitary-thyroid axis also responds to thyroid hormone deficiency by increasing TSH secretion. Consequently, affected individuals typically present with thyroid gland enlargement (goiter), which may be sufficient to compensate for inefficient thyroid hormone production; but if not, they develop hypothyroidism. Severely affected neonates and infants can suffer the irreversible effects of thyroid hormone deficiency on development that result in cretinism. Specific inherited disorders are described in more detail in the section on nontoxic goiter, below.

Effects of Iodine Excess on Hormone Biosynthesis

Although iodide is an essential substrate for thyroid hormone production, excess iodide actually inhibits three steps in thyroid hormone production: iodide trapping, thyroglobulin iodination (the Wolff-Chaikoff effect), and thyroid hormone release from the gland. These inhibitory actions are transient, and the normal thyroid gland *escapes* after 10 to 14 days from these effects of excess iodide. These autoregulatory effects of iodide insulate physiologic thyroid function from short-term fluctuations in iodine intake.

These actions of excess iodide also have important clinical implications, sometimes causing iodine-induced thyroid dysfunction and permitting iodide treatment of certain thyroid conditions. If the thyroid is affected by autoimmune thyroiditis or certain inherited forms of dyshormonogenesis, it may be incapable of escaping from iodide-induced inhibition of gland function, and hypothyroidism can develop. Conversely, an iodide load can induce hyperthyroidism (Jod-Basedow effect[2]) in some patients with multinodular goiter, latent Graves disease, and rarely in individuals with thyroid glands that appear otherwise normal.

THYROID HORMONE TRANSPORT

Both thyroid hormones circulate in blood bound to plasma proteins; only 0.04% of T_4 and 0.4% of T_3 are unbound or free, and consequently, available for entry and action in target tissues (Figure 7–11). There are three major thyroid hormone transport proteins: thyroxine-binding globulin (TBG); transthyretin, formerly called thyroxine-binding prealbumin (TBPA), and albumin (Figure 7–12). The plasma protein binding permits blood delivery of the iodothyronines, which are otherwise poorly soluble in water. It also creates a large circulating thyroid hormone pool with a stable 7-day plasma half-life and ensures the homogeneous distribution of thyroid hormones in target tissues.

Thyroxine-Binding Globulin

Thyroxine-binding globulin (TBG) is a liver-derived glycoprotein member of the SERPIN family of serine antiproteases composed of a single 54-kDa polypeptide chain, to which are attached 4 carbohydrate chains normally containing approximately 10 sialic acid residues. Each TBG molecule has a single binding site for T_4 or T_3. The serum concentration of TBG is 15 to 30 μg/mL (280-560 nmol/L), and its high binding affinity for T_4 and T_3 allows it to carry about 70% of circulating thyroid hormones.

TBG and its binding of the thyroid hormones can be altered by congenital TBG derangements, certain physiologic and pathophysiologic circumstances, and several drugs. TBG deficiency occurs with a frequency of 1:5000 live births, with a number of variants described in several ethnic and racial groups. It is an X-linked recessive trait that, consequently, is much more commonly expressed in males. Despite low circulating total T_4 and T_3 levels in affected individuals, free hormone levels are normal, and these patients remain euthyroid. Congenital TBG deficiency is often associated with congenital corticosteroid-binding globulin deficiency (Chapter 9). Conversely, congenital TBG excess, which is rare, is characterized by elevated total T_4 and T_3 concentrations in blood, but normal free hormone levels and a euthyroid clinical state. Pregnancy, estrogen-secreting tumors, and estrogen therapy all increase the sialic acid content of the TBG molecule, resulting in decreased metabolic clearance and elevated serum TBG levels. TBG levels can decrease in major systemic illness, and due to cleavage by leukocyte proteases, its binding affinity for the thyroid hormones can also be reduced. Both effects lower the serum total thyroid hormone concentrations in sick patients (Table 7–1). Certain drugs can also decrease (androgenic steroids, glucocorticoids, danazol, L-asparaginase) or increase (estrogens, 5-fluourouracil) the plasma TBG concentration. Other drugs (eg, salicylates, high-dose phenytoin, and intravenous furosemide) can bind to TBG, displacing T_4 and T_3. In this circumstance, the hypothalamic-pituitary-thyroid axis (discussed later) preserves normal, free hormone concentrations

---

[2]Jod is German for iodine; Carl Adolph von Basedow was one of the first physicians to describe hyperthyroidism.

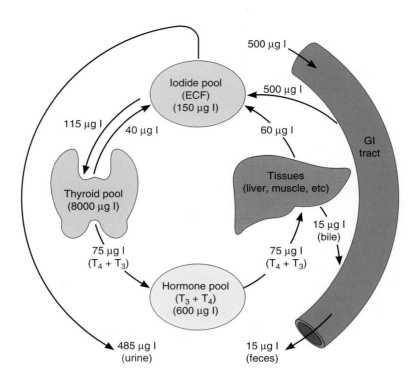

FIGURE 7–10 Iodine metabolism. The values indicated are representative of those that might be found in a healthy subject ingesting 500 μg of iodine a day. The actual iodine intake varies considerably among different individuals.

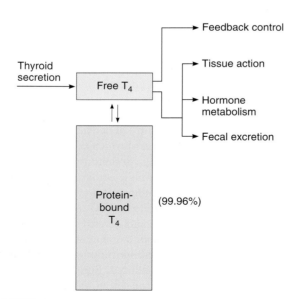

FIGURE 7–11 Representation of free T_4 (and free T_3) as the biologically active hormones at the level of the pituitary and the peripheral tissues. Most of the thyroid hormones circulating in plasma are protein-bound and have no biologic activity. This pool of bound hormone is in equilibrium with the free hormone pool. (Reproduced, with permission, from DeGroot LJ, Stanbury JB. *The Thyroid and Its Diseases.* 4th ed. Wiley; 1975.)

by lowering serum total thyroid hormone levels. Similarly, heparin stimulation of lipoprotein lipase releases free fatty acids that displace thyroid hormones from TBG. In vivo, this can result in lower total thyroid hormone concentrations, whereas in vitro (eg, in blood drawn through a heparin lock), heparin increases measured levels of free T_4 and T_3.

Transthyretin (Thyroxine-Binding Prealbumin)

Transthyretin, a 55-kDa globular polypeptide composed of four identical 127-amino acid subunits, binds 10% of circulating T_4. Its affinity for T_4 is 10-fold greater than for T_3. The dissociation of T_4 and T_3 from transthyretin is rapid, so that transthyretin is a source of readily available T_4. Increased affinity of transthyretin binding for T_4 can occur as a heritable condition. Affected individuals have an elevated total T_4 but a normal free T_4. Ectopic production of transthyretin, which has been reported to occur in patients with pancreatic and hepatic tumors, also causes euthyroid hyperthyroxinemia.

Albumin

Albumin binds to T_4 and T_3 with lesser affinity than TBG or transthyretin, but its high plasma concentration results in its

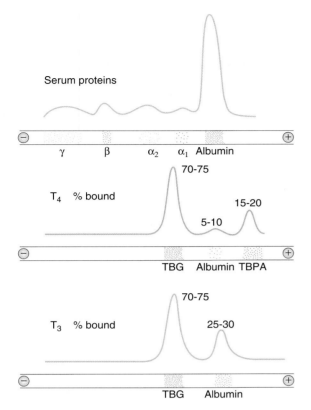

FIGURE 7–12 Diagrammatic representation of the distribution of radioactive T_4 and T_3 among serum thyroid hormone–binding proteins. **Top:** Paper electrophoretic pattern of serum proteins. **Middle:** Radioactive T_4 was added to serum and was then subjected to paper electrophoresis. The peaks represent the mobility of radioactive T_4 bound to different serum proteins. (TBG, thyroid hormone–binding globulin; TBPA, thyroxine-binding prealbumin.) **Bottom:** Radioactive T_3 was added to serum and subjected to paper electrophoresis. The peaks indicate the relative distribution of protein-bound radioactive T_3. The figures above each peak indicate the relative hormone distribution among the binding proteins in a normal adult. (Reproduced, with permission, from Rosenfield RL, et al. *Pediatric Nuclear Medicine.* James AE Jr, Wagner HN Jr, Cooke RE, ed. Saunders; 1974.)

TABLE 7–1 Causes of abnormal serum thyroxine determinations in euthyroid individuals.

Euthyroid Hyperthyroxinemia
↑ Plasma protein binding
  ↑ Thyroxine-binding globulin (TBG)
    Inherited
    Estrogen effect (pregnancy, estrogen therapy)
    Hepatitis
    Drugs: tamoxifen, 5-fluorouracil, clofibrate, methadone, heroin
  ↑ Transthyretin binding
    Inherited
    Paraneoplastic production by hepatic and pancreatic tumors
  ↑ Albumin binding
    Inherited (familial dysalbuminemic hyperthyroxinemia)
↓ T_4-to-T_3 conversion[a]
  Systemic illness
  Medications: amiodarone, radiocontrast agents, glucocor-ticoids, propranolol
Thyroxine therapy in hypothyroidism[a]
Generalized resistance to thyroid hormone[a]
Anti-T_4 antibody (assay interference)

Euthyroid Hypothyroxinemia
↓ Thyroxine-binding globulin
  ↓ TBG production
    Inherited
    Androgens
    Drugs: danazol, L-asparaginase
  ↑ TBG clearance
    Nephrotic syndrome
    Severe liver disease
    Protein-losing gastroenteropathy
Systemic illness[b]
Medications
    Exogenous thyromimetic compounds (T_3 [Cytomel])[b]
    Phenytoin and carbamazepine[b]
    Iodine deficiency (with normal serum T_3)[b]

[a]Both total and free T_4 elevated.
[b]Both total and free T_4 low.

transport of 15% of circulating T_4 and T_3. Rapid thyroid hormone dissociation rates from albumin make it a major source of free hormone to tissues. Hypoalbuminemia, as occurs in nephrosis or cirrhosis, is associated with a low total T_4 and T_3, but the free hormone levels are normal.

Familial dysalbuminemic hyperthyroxinemia is an autosomal dominant inherited disorder in which 25% of the albumin exhibits a higher than normal T_4-binding affinity. This results in an elevated total T_4 level but a normal free T_4 concentration and euthyroidism. In most affected kindreds, the T_3-binding affinity is normal. Because these albumin variants do not bind the thyroxine analogs used in many free T_4 immunoassays, they may falsely report elevation of the free T_4 in affected individuals.

METABOLISM OF THYROID HORMONES

The normal thyroid gland secretes about 100 nmol of T_4 and only 5 nmol of T_3 daily; less than 5 nmol of metabolically inactive reverse T_3 (rT_3) is produced (Figure 7–13). Most of the plasma pool of T_3 (80%) is derived from peripheral outer ring- or 5′-monodeiodination of T_4 in tissues outside of the thyroid gland, particularly the liver, kidney, and skeletal muscle (Table 7–2). Because T_3 has a higher binding affinity for the nuclear T_3 receptors that affect thyroid hormone action, this 5′-monodeiodination generates a more biologically active iodothyronine. On the other hand, deiodination of the *inner* ring of T_4 (5-deiodination) produces 3,3′,5′-triiodothyronine or reverse T_3 (rT_3), which is metabolically inert.

The three deiodinase enzymes that catalyze these reactions differ in tissue localization, substrate specificity, and physiologic and pathophysiologic modulation, as summarized in Table 7–2. Type 1 5′-deiodinase, the most abundant form, is found predominantly

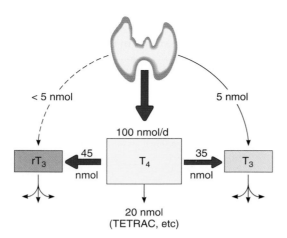

FIGURE 7–13 Major pathways of thyroxine metabolism in normal adult humans. Rates are expressed in nmol/24 h and are approximations based upon available data. 100 nmol of T_4 is equivalent to approximately 75 μg. (rT_3, reverse T_3; TETRAC, tetraiodothyroacetic acid.) (Reproduced, with permission, from Cavalieri RR, Rapoport B. Impaired peripheral conversion of thyroxine to triiodothyronine. *Ann Rev Med.* 1977;28:5765.)

in liver and kidney, and in lesser quantities in the thyroid gland, skeletal and heart muscle, and other tissues. The type 1 5'-deiodinase contains a selenocysteine moiety that is probably at the active deiodinating site. The major function of type 1 5'-deiodinase is to provide T_3 to the circulation. Its activity is increased in hyperthyroidism and decreased in hypothyroidism. This partially accounts for the relatively higher circulating T_3 levels compared to T_4 levels seen in hyperthyroid patients. The enzyme is inhibited by the thionamide antithyroid drug PTU, but not methimazole, and by the antiarrhythmic drug amiodarone and iodinated radiocontrast dyes, such as sodium ipodate. Dietary selenium deficiency can also impair T_4 to T_3 conversion.

Type 2 5'-deiodinase is predominantly expressed in the brain and pituitary gland, where it maintains a constant level of intracellular T_3 in the central nervous system. This deiodinase is very sensitive to circulating T_4, so a lower circulating T_4 rapidly increases enzyme concentration in brain and pituitary, by altering the rate of T_4 degradation and inactivation. In doing so, it maintains the level of intracellular T_3 and its neuronal cellular functions. Conversely, elevated plasma T_4 reduces the type 2 5'-deiodinase level, protecting brain cells from excessive T_3. Consequently, this deiodinase represents a mechanism by which the hypothalamus and pituitary can respond to the level of circulating T_4. rT_3 can also modify the activity of type 2 5'-deiodinase in the brain and the pituitary gland, and α-adrenergic compounds stimulate type 2 5'-deiodinase in brown fat, but the physiologic significance of these effects is not clear. Type 3 5-deiodinase is found in chorionic membranes of the placenta and glial cells in the central nervous system, where it inactivates T_4 by converting it to rT_3 and it inactivates T_3 by converting it to 3,3'-diiodothyronine (3,3'-T_2) (Figure 7–14). Type 3 deiodinase levels are elevated in hyperthyroidism and decreased in hypothyroidism and, therefore, may help insulate the fetus and the brain from T_4 excess or deficiency. Placental type 3 deiodinase accelerates thyroxine disposal in pregnant women, which partly explains the increased thyroxine dose requirements in treated hypothyroid women.

Overall, the functions of the deiodinases are physiologically important in three ways. First, they permit local tissue and cellular modulation of thyroid hormone actions. Second, they help the organism adapt to changing states, including iodine deficiency or chronic illness. Third, they regulate thyroid hormone actions in the early development of many vertebrates, including amphibia and mammals.

About 80% of T_4 is metabolized by deiodination, 35% to T_3 and 45% to rT_3 (see Figure 7–13). The remainder is inactivated mainly by glucuronidation in the liver and biliary secretion, and to a lesser extent, by sulfation in the liver or kidney. Other metabolic reactions include deamination of the alanine side chain, forming thyroacetic acid derivatives of low biologic activity; or decarboxylation or cleavage of the ether link, forming inactive compounds.

As a result of these metabolic pathways, approximately 10% of the total 1000 nmol extrathyroidal T_4 pool is cleared each day, and the plasma half-life of T_4 is 7 days. Due to T_3's lower binding affinity for plasma proteins, the turnover of its much smaller extrathyroidal pool is more rapid, with a plasma half-life of 1 day. The total body pool of rT_3 is about the same size as that of T_3, but rT_3 has an even more rapid turnover, with a plasma half-life of only 0.2 day.

TABLE 7–2   Iodothyronine deiodinase types and characteristics.

Deiodinase Type	D1	D2	D3
Substrates	$rT_3 > T_4 > T_3$	$T_4 > rT_3$	$T_3 > T_4$
Tissue distribution	Liver, kidney, skeletal muscle, thyroid	Brain, pituitary	Brain, placenta, fetal tissues
Function	Plasma T_3 production	Local T_3 production	T_3 degradation
PTU inhibition (IC50, μM)	5	> 1000	> 1000
Hypothyroidism	Decrease	Increase	Decrease
Hyperthyroidism	Increase	Decrease	Increase

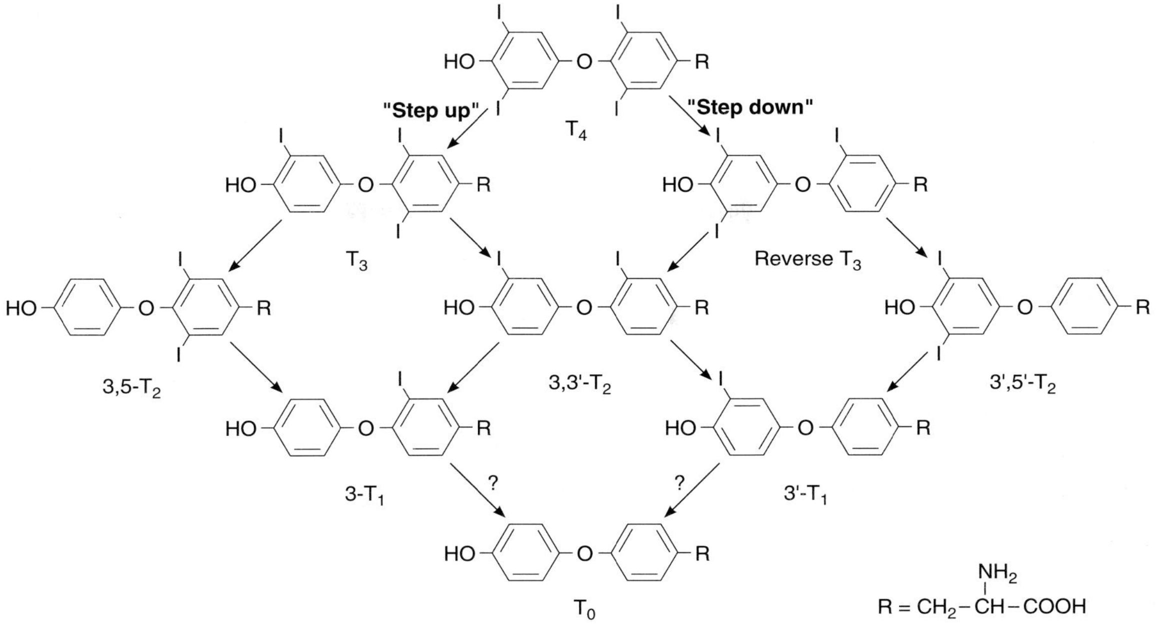

FIGURE 7–14 The deiodinative pathway of thyroxine metabolism. The monodeiodination of T_4 to T_3 represents a step-up in biologic potency, whereas the monodeiodination of T_4 to reverse T_3 has the opposite effect. Further deiodination of T_3 essentially abolishes hormonal activity.

CONTROL OF THYROID FUNCTION AND HORMONE ACTION

Growth and function of the thyroid gland are controlled by the hypothalamic-pituitary-thyroid axis (Figure 7–15) and, as previously discussed, by iodide through the elements of autoregulation. Hypothalamic thyrotropin-releasing hormone (TRH) stimulates thyrotrophic cells in the anterior pituitary to produce TSH, which in turn promotes thyroid gland growth and hormone secretion. In addition, deiodinases in the pituitary and peripheral tissues modulate thyroid hormone effects by their tissue-specific conversion of T_4 to the more active iodothyronine T_3. Finally, the molecular effects of T_3 in individual tissues are modulated by the subtype of T_3 receptor with which it interacts; the specific gene activation or repression response that it induces; and in a realm just now being revealed, the T_3 receptor's interaction with other ligands, closely related receptors (eg, retinoid X receptor; RXR), and coactivators and corepressors that interact with it in modulating gene expression.

Thyrotropin-Releasing Hormone

Thyrotropin-releasing hormone (TRH) is a tripeptide, pyroglutamyl-histidyl-proline amide (pyro-Glu-His-Pro-NH$_2$), synthesized by neurons in the supraoptic and supraventricular nuclei of the hypothalamus (Figure 7–16). TRH is stored in the median eminence of the hypothalamus and then transported via the pituitary portal venous system down the pituitary stalk to the anterior pituitary, where it controls synthesis and release of TSH. TRH is

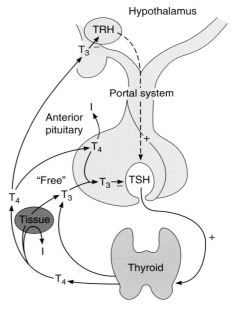

FIGURE 7–15 The hypothalamic-hypophysial-thyroidal axis. TRH produced in the hypothalamus reaches the thyrotrophs in the anterior pituitary by the hypothalamo-hypophysial portal system and stimulates the synthesis and release of TSH. In both the hypothalamus and the pituitary, it is primarily T_3 that inhibits TRH and TSH secretion, respectively. T_4 undergoes monodeiodination to T_3 in neural and pituitary as well as in peripheral tissues.

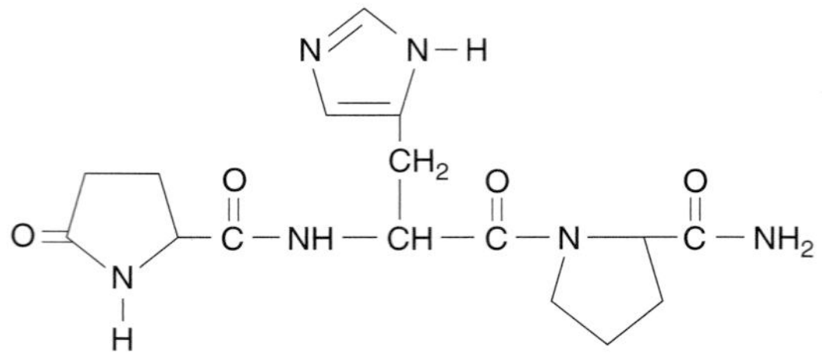

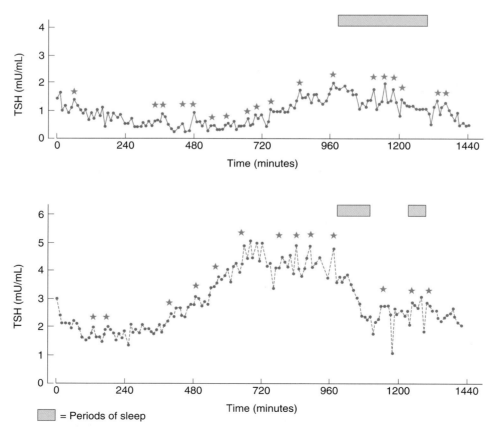

(pyro)Glu-His-Pro-(NH$_2$)

FIGURE 7–16 Chemical structure of thyrotropin-releasing hormone (TRH).

also found in other portions of the hypothalamus, brain, and spinal cord, where it may have distinct functions as a neurotransmitter. The pre-pro-*TRH* gene, which encodes a large molecule with five copies of the TRH progenitor sequence Glu-His-Pro-Gly, is located on chromosome 3. *TRH* gene expression is negatively regulated by thyroid hormone—both the T$_3$ delivered by the circulation and that arising from T$_4$ deiodination in peptidergic neurons themselves (see Table 7–2).

In the anterior pituitary, TRH binds to a specific membrane receptor located on TSH- and prolactin-secreting cells, stimulating

synthesis and release of their respective hormones. The TRH receptor is a member of the 7-transmembrane-spanning, G protein–coupled receptor family (Table 1–1; Figure 1–4). TRH binds to the receptor's third transmembrane helix, activating both its cyclic guanosine monophosphate-producing complex and the inositol 1,4,5-triphosphate (IP$_3$) signaling cascade that releases intracellular Ca^{2+} and generates 1,2-diacylglycerol, thereby activating protein kinase C. These pathways are responsible for stimulating TSH release. They coordinate transcription of the genes encoding the TSH subunits and posttranslational glycosylation of TSH, which is necessary for full biologic activity.

TRH-stimulated TSH secretion is pulsatile (Figure 7–17), with a mean TSH pulse amplitude of 0.6 mU/L every 2 hours. Normal individuals have a circadian rhythm in TSH release, with a peak circulating level between midnight and 4 AM, which is presumably controlled by a hypothalamic neuronal pulse generator driving TRH synthesis.

Thyroid hormones exert additional negative feedback on TSH production at the level of the pituitary by downregulating the number of TRH receptors on pituitary thyrotropes. Consequently, in patients with hyperthyroidism, both TSH pulses and its nocturnal surge are markedly suppressed; whereas in hypothyroid patients, the TSH pulse amplitude and nocturnal surge are much

= Periods of sleep

FIGURE 7–17 Serum TSH in two normal subjects demonstrating spontaneous pulses and the circadian rhythm of TSH secretion. (0 time is 0900; stars indicate significant pulses.) (Reproduced, with permission, from Greenspan SL, et al. Pulsatile secretion of TSH in man. *J Clin Endocrinol Metab.* 1986;63:664. Copyright 1986 by The Endocrine Society.)

greater. In experimental animals and newborn humans, exposure to cold temperature increases TRH and TSH secretion. Certain other hormones and drugs (eg, vasopressin and α-adrenergic agonists), stimulate TRH synthesis and release.

When synthetic TRH is administered intravenously to humans as a 200 to 500 μg bolus, it generates a prompt three- to fivefold rise in the serum TSH concentration, peaking at about 30 minutes and lasting for 2 to 3 hours (see Figure 4–14). In patients with primary hypothyroidism, in whom basal TSH is elevated, there is an exaggerated TSH response to exogenous TRH; and this response is suppressed in patients with hyperthyroidism, high-dose thyroxine therapy, and central hypothyroidism.

TRH is also found in the islet cells of the pancreas, gastrointestinal tract, placenta, heart, prostate, testes, and ovaries. TRH production in these peripheral tissues is not inhibited by T_3; the role of TRH in these tissues remains unknown.

Thyrotropin (Thyroid-Stimulating Hormone)

Thyroid-stimulating hormone (TSH) is 28-kD glycoprotein composed of α and β subunits that are noncovalently linked. The α subunit is common to the two other pituitary glycoproteins, follicle-stimulating hormone (FSH) and luteinizing hormone (LH), and the placental hormone human chorionic gonadotropin (hCG), whereas the β subunit is unique for each glycoprotein hormone, conferring specific binding properties and biologic activity. The genes for the TSH α and β subunits are located on chromosomes 6 and 1, respectively. The human α subunit has an apoprotein core of 92 amino acids and contains two oligosaccharide chains; the TSH β subunit has an apoprotein core of 112 amino acids and contains one oligosaccharide chain. The α and β subunit amino acid chains of TSH each form three loops that are intertwined into a cystine knot (Figure 7–18). Glycosylation takes place in the RER

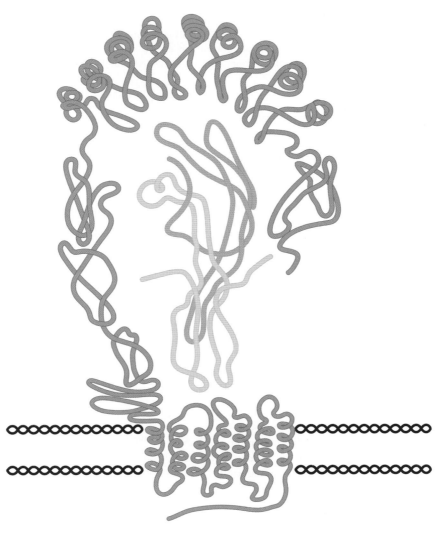

FIGURE 7–18 Schematic configuration of the TSH-TSHR complex. The central portion of the figure represents the ribbon-like structure of TSH within the TSH receptor. The dark blue line represents the β subunit and the light blue line the α subunit. See also Figure 7–19. (Reproduced, with permission, from Szkudlinski MW, et al. Thyroid-stimulating hormone and thyroid-stimulating hormone receptor structure-function relationships. *Physiol Rev.* 2002;82:473.)

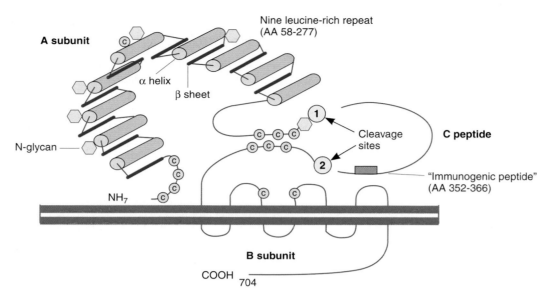

FIGURE 7–19 Schematic representation of the TSH receptor. The A subunit is the ligand-binding portion of the receptor and the B subunit is the activation portion. The ligands which bind to the receptor include TSH, TSH-stimulating antibody, and TSH-blocking antibody. There are two cleavage sites which allow breakage of the receptor and loss of the A subunit into the serum. (Reproduced, with permission, from Rapoport B, et al. The thyrotropin (TSH)-receptor: interaction with TSH and autoantibodies. *Endocr Rev.* 1998;19:673.)

and the Golgi, where glucose, mannose, and fucose residues and terminal sulfate or sialic acid residues are linked to the apoprotein core. These carbohydrate residues prolong its plasma half-life and enhance it ability to induce TSH receptor activation.

TSH controls thyroid cell growth and hormone production by binding to a specific TSH receptor, one of approximately 1000 located on the basolateral cell membrane of each thyroid cell. TSH binding activates both the cyclic adenosine monophosphate (cAMP) and the phosphoinositol pathways for signal transduction. The TSH receptor gene is located on chromosome 14; the product is a single-chain glycoprotein composed of 764 amino acids. The TSH receptor is a member of the 7-membrane spanning, G protein–coupled receptor family, with an ectodomain involved in ligand binding and an intramembrane and intracellular portion responsible for activation of the signaling pathways that promote thyroid cell growth and hormone synthesis and release (see Figure 7–19).

The TSH receptor is involved in the pathogenesis of numerous congenital and acquired forms of hypothyroidism and hyperthyroidism. Heritable defects resulting in impaired TSH synthesis or action have been described, including mutant genes for transcription factors required for pituitary thyrotrope differentiation (*POU1F1, PROP1, LHX3, HESX1*), TRH receptor, TSH β-chain, TSH receptor, and $G_{s\alpha}$, which transduces TSH receptor binding to adenylate cyclase activation. Acquired TSH receptor blocking antibodies can also cause hypothyroidism.

The most common TSH receptor–related disorder causing hyperthyroidism is Graves disease, in which autoantibodies bind and stimulate the TSH receptor. However, the TSH receptor is involved in the etiology of several other forms of hyperthyroidism. Germline mutations activating the TSH receptor can cause famil-

ial hyperthyroidism, and somatic activating mutations result in toxic adenomas. Other mutations can lead to aberrant TSH receptor activation by hCG, the placental glycoprotein hormone that is structurally similar to TSH, in familial gestational hyperthyroidism.

Effects of TSH on the Thyroid Cell

TSH has many actions on the thyroid cell. Most of its actions are mediated through the G protein-adenylyl cyclase-cAMP system, but activation of the phosphatidylinositol (PIP_3) system with a resulting increase in intracellular calcium is also involved. The major actions of TSH include the following:

A. Changes in thyroid cell morphology TSH rapidly induces pseudopods at the follicular cell-colloid border, accelerating thyroglobulin resorption. Colloid content is diminished as intracellular colloid droplets are formed and lysosome formation is stimulated, increasing thyroglobulin hydrolysis and thyroid hormone release.

B. Cell growth Individual thyroid cells increase in size; vascularity is increased; and, over a period of time, thyroid enlargement, or goiter, develops.

C. Iodine metabolism TSH stimulates all phases of iodide metabolism, from increased iodide uptake and transport to increased iodination of thyroglobulin and increased secretion of thyroid hormones and thyroglobulin itself. Increased NIS expression and the stimulation of cAMP production mediate increased iodide transport, and PIP_3 hydrolysis and increased intracellular

Ca^{2+} stimulate the iodination of thyroglobulin. The TSH effect on iodide transport across the cell is biphasic: initially, it is depressed (iodide efflux), and then, after a lag of several hours, iodide uptake is increased. The efflux of iodide may be due to the rapid increase in hydrolysis of thyroglobulin with release of hormone and leakage of iodide out of the gland. The TSH-mediated stimulation of thyrocyte iodine uptake and thyroglobulin secretion also occur after administration of recombinant TSH for radioiodine treatment and monitoring of patients with well-differentiated thyroid cancers.

D. Other effects of TSH   Other effects include increased transcription of the mRNAs for thyroglobulin and TPO; increased incorporation of iodide into MIT, DIT, T_3, and T_4; and increased lysosomal activity, with increased secretion of T_4 and T_3 from the gland. There is also increased activity of type 1 5'-deiodinase, which helps conserve intrathyroidal iodine.

TSH has additional effects on the thyroid gland, including stimulation of glucose uptake, oxygen consumption, and glucose oxidation. There is accelerated turnover of phospholipids and stimulation of synthesis of purine and pyrimidine precursors, with increased synthesis of DNA and RNA.

Serum TSH

Intact TSH and isolated α subunit are both present in circulating blood and detectable by immunoassay in concentrations that are normally 0.5 to 4.0 mU/L and 0.5 to 2 µg/L, respectively. The serum TSH level is increased in primary hypothyroidism and decreased in thyrotoxicosis, whether endogenous or from excessive oral intake of thyroid hormones. The plasma half-life of TSH is about 30 minutes, and the daily production rate is about 40 to 150 mU/d.

The glycoprotein α subunit is often disproportionately elevated in patients with TSH-secreting pituitary tumors (see later); it is also increased in normal postmenopausal women due to increased synthesis and secretion related to increased gonadotropin production.

Control of Pituitary TSH Secretion

Two major factors control synthesis and release of TSH: (1) T_3 level within thyrotrophic cells, which regulates mRNA expression, TSH translation, and the hormone's release; and (2) TRH, which controls posttranslational glycosylation and also release.

TSH synthesis and release are inhibited by high serum levels of T_4 and T_3 (hyperthyroidism) and stimulated by low levels of thyroid hormone (hypothyroidism). In addition, certain hormones and drugs inhibit TSH secretion. These include somatostatin, dopamine, dopamine agonists such as bromocriptine, and high doses of glucocorticoids. Severe disease may cause inhibition of TSH secretion, and there may be a rebound increase in TSH as the patient recovers. The magnitude of these effects varies; the drugs mentioned above usually only partially suppress serum TSH, but it remains detectable. In contrast, overt hyperthyroidism can suppress the TSH concentration to beneath the detection limits of even the most sensitive TSH immunoassays.

Tumors and other disorders of the hypothalamus or anterior pituitary gland can impair TRH and TSH secretion, respectively. Pituitary disorders causing hypothyroidism are termed *secondary*, whereas hypothalamic disease resulting in hypothyroidism is called *tertiary*. Differential diagnosis of these lesions is discussed later (see Thyroid Tests).

Other Thyroid Stimulators and Inhibitors

The thyroid follicle has a rich supply of capillaries that carry noradrenergic nerve fibers from the superior cervical ganglion and acetylcholine esterase-positive nerve fibers derived from the vagus nerve and thyroid ganglia. The parafollicular C cells secrete both calcitonin and calcitonin gene-related peptide (CGRP). In experimental animals, these and other neuropeptides modify thyroid blood flow and hormone secretion. In addition, growth factors such as insulin, insulin-like growth factor-1, insulin-like growth factor binding proteins, epidermal growth factor, transforming growth factor $\beta 1$, and fibroblast growth factors and their receptors, as well as autocrine factors such as prostaglandins and cytokines, modify thyroid cell growth and hormone production. However, it is not yet clear how clinically important these effects are.

Role of Pituitary and Peripheral Deiodinases

Pituitary type 2 5'-deiodinase converts T_4 to T_3 in the brain and pituitary, providing the main source of T_3 within thyrotropes. Its activity increases in hypothyroidism, initially maintaining a normal intracellular T_3 level in the cerebrum despite a falling plasma T_4 concentration. In hyperthyroidism, a decrease in its activity moderates exposure of pituitary and neural cells to thyroid hormone excess. In contrast, type 1 5'-deiodinase is decreased in hypothyroidism, conserving T_4, and increased in hyperthyroidism, accelerating T_4 metabolism but also leading to increased serum levels of T3 (see Table 7–2).

Thyroidal Autoregulation

Autoregulation may be defined as the capacity of the thyroid gland to modify its function to adapt to changes in the availability of iodine, independent of pituitary TSH. Thus, humans can maintain normal thyroid hormone secretion with iodide intakes varying from 50 µg to several milligrams per day. Some of the effects of iodide deficiency or excess are discussed earlier. The major adaptation to low iodide intake is the preferential synthesis of T_3 rather than T_4, increasing the metabolic effectiveness of the secreted hormone. Iodide excess, on the other hand, inhibits many thyroidal functions, including iodide transport, cAMP formation, hydrogen peroxide generation, and hormone synthesis and secretion. Some of these effects may be mediated by the formation of intrathyroidal iodinated fatty acids. The ability of the normal thyroid to *escape* from these inhibitory effects (Wolff-Chaikoff effect) allows the gland to continue to secrete hormone despite a high dietary iodide intake. It is important to note that this is different from the therapeutic effect of iodide in the treatment of

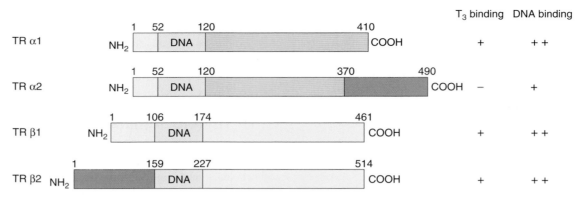

FIGURE 7–20 Deduced protein structure of the thyroid hormone receptor α and β gene products. The receptor protein has three domains: a DNA-binding domain with a high degree of similarity among the different types of receptors, a carboxyl terminal triiodothyronine (T_3)–binding domain, and an amino terminal domain that is not required for full function. The numbers above the structures represent amino acid numbers. The properties of the receptors with respect to their ability to bind T_3 and bind to a T_3-response element of DNA are shown on the right. Identical shading of receptor domains indicates identical amino acid sequences. (TR, thyroid hormone receptor.) (Reproduced, with permission, from Brent GA. The molecular basis of thyroid hormone action. *N Engl J Med.* 1994;331:847.)

Graves disease. Here, the high levels of iodide persistently inhibit thyroglobulin endocytosis and lysosomal activity, decreasing thyroid hormone release and lowering circulating hormone levels. In addition, pharmacologic amounts of iodide reduce the vascularity of the gland, which may be beneficial during thyroid surgery for Graves disease. However, this effect is also transient, lasting 10 to 14 days.

The Actions of Thyroid Hormones

1. THE THYROID HORMONE RECEPTORS AND MECHANISMS OF ACTION

The thyroid hormones exert their actions through two general mechanisms: (1) genomic actions effected through T_3 interactions with its nuclear receptors, regulating gene activity; and (2) nongenomic actions mediated by T_3 and T_4 interactions with certain enzymes (eg, calcium ATPase, adenylate cyclase, monomeric pyruvate kinase), glucose transporters, and mitochondrial proteins.

Thyroid hormones, that are unbound in plasma, are transported intracellularly, by either specific carriers including monocarboxylate transporter 8 (MCT8), MCT10, and organic anion transporting polypeptide (OATP1C1). OATP1C1 is expressed predominantly in brain capillaries and the choroid plexus, and transports T_4 preferentially, while MCT8 and MCT10 are expressed in many tissues and transport both T_4 and T_3. Thyroid hormones are transported through the cell membrane into the cytoplasm, and subsequently into the nucleus, where T_3 binds to its specific receptor. Clinical syndromes associated with mutations in these transporters have recently been recognized, such as the Allan-Herndon-Dudley syndrome in which affected male children develop mental retardation, myopathy, a movement disorder in association with elevated serum T_3 and low serum T_4 levels.

The T_3 nuclear receptor is member of a nuclear receptor superfamily that includes nuclear receptors for glucocorticoids,

mineralocorticoids, estrogens, progestins, vitamin D_3, and retinoids (see Figure 1–16). There are two thyroid hormone receptor (*TR*) genes in humans: *TRα* located on chromosome 17 and *TRβ* on chromosome 3. Each gene yields at least two differentially spliced products, TRα 1 and 2 and TRβ 1 and 2, although TRα 2 is believed to be biologically inactive (see Figure 7–20). Each of these receptors has a carboxyl terminal ligand-binding domain and a centrally located DNA-binding domain with two cysteine zinc fingers that facilitate their specific attachment to thyroid hormone response elements (TREs) in the promoters of target genes and regulate their transcription (see Figures 1–16 and 1–17). The concentration of these receptors in tissue varies among tissues and with their stage of development. For example, the brain contains predominantly TRα, the liver mostly TRβ, and cardiac muscle contains both. Point mutations in the ligand-binding domain of the *TRβ* gene have been shown to be responsible for the syndrome of generalized resistance to thyroid hormone (GRTH). The TRs bind to TREs, which are typically paired, specific oligonucleotide sequences (eg, AGGTCA) (Figure 7–21). The TRs can also function as heterodimers with receptors for other transcription factors, such as the retinoid X and retinoic acid receptors. TREs are generally located upstream of the transcription start site for the coding regions of thyroid hormone–responsive genes. In positively regulated genes, unbound TRs interact with corepressors (eg, nuclear receptor corepressor [NCoR] and silencing mediator for retinoic and thyroid hormone receptors [SMRT]) to repress basal transcription by recruiting histone deacetylases that alter the nearby chromatin structure. When TRs are bound by T_3, these corepressor complexes are released, and the T_3-bound TRs associate with coactivator complexes that promote local histone acetylation; they also associate with another protein complex (vitamin D receptor-interacting protein/TR-associated proteins) that recruits RNA polymerase II and starts gene transcription. Some genes are negatively regulated by T_3-bound TRs, such as pre-pro-*TRH* and *TSH-α* and -β subunit genes, but the

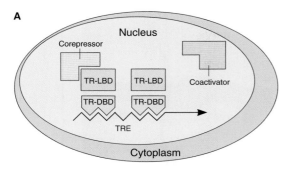

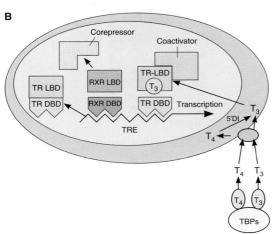

FIGURE 7–21 Model of the interaction of T_3 with the T_3 receptor. **Panel A, Inactive Phase:** The unliganded T_3 receptor dimer bound to the TRE along with corepressors acts as a suppressor of gene transcription. **Panel B, Active Phase:** T_3 and T_4 circulate bound to thyroid-binding proteins (TBPs). The free hormones are transported into the cell by a specific transport system. Within the cytoplasm, T_4 is converted to T_3 by 5′-deiodinase and T_3 moves into the nucleus. There it binds to the ligand-binding domain of the TR monomer. This promotes disruption of the TR homodimer and heterodimerization with RXR on the TRE, displacement of corepressors, and binding of coactivators. The TR-coactivator complex activates gene transcription, which leads to alteration in protein synthesis and cellular phenotype. (TR-LBD, T_3 receptor ligand-binding domain; TRDBD, T_3 receptor DNA–binding domain; RXR-LBD, retinoid X receptor ligand–binding domain; RXR-DBD, retinoid X receptor DNA–binding domain; TRE, thyroid hormone response element; TBPs, thyroxine-binding proteins; T_3, triiodothyronine; T_4, tetraiodothyronine, L-thyroxine; 5′DI, 5′-deiodinase.)

molecular mechanisms involved are currently less well understood. Thyroid hormone's actions to alter expression levels of specific mRNAs and their translated proteins generate a constellation of specific tissue responses (see Figure 7–21).

The nongenomic actions of thyroid hormones have long been suspected based on certain rapid tissue responses that take place before RNA transcription could occur and by recognition of T_3- and T_4-binding sites outside of the nucleus. For example, it has recently been shown that thyroid hormones bind the membrane protein integrin $\alpha V\beta3$, which is involved in thyroid

hormone–mediated activation of the MAP kinase cascade and stimulation of angiogenesis.

2. PHYSIOLOGIC EFFECTS OF THYROID HORMONES

The transcriptional effects of T_3 characteristically demonstrate a lag time of hours or days to achieve full effect. These genomic actions have a number of vital effects, including tissue growth, brain maturation, increased calorigenesis and oxygen consumption, as well as other specific effects on the heart, liver, kidneys, skeletal muscle, and skin. However, some actions of T_3 are believed not to be genomic, including its reduction of pituitary type 2 5′-deiodinase activity and the increased glucose and amino acid transport that it can induce in some tissues. Some specific effects of thyroid hormones are summarized below.

Effects on Fetal Development

Iodide concentration by thyroid tissue and pituitary TSH both appear in the human fetus at about 11 weeks' gestation. Because of the high placental content of type 3 5-deiodinase, most maternal T_3 and T_4 are inactivated, and very little free hormone reaches the fetal circulation. However, this small amount of free hormone from the mother may be important for early fetal brain development. After 15 to 18 weeks of gestation, the fetus is largely dependent on its own thyroidal secretion. Although some fetal growth occurs in the absence of fetal thyroid hormone secretion, brain development and skeletal maturation are markedly impaired if congenital hypothyroidism is undiagnosed and thyroid hormone therapy is not begun promptly after birth. Congenital hypothyroidism results in cretinism, the features of which include mental retardation and dwarfism.

Effects on Oxygen Consumption, Heat Production, and Free Radical Formation

T_3 increases O_2 consumption and heat production in part by stimulation of Na^+-K^+ ATPase in all tissues except the brain, spleen, and testis. This contributes to the increased basal metabolic rate (total somatic O_2 consumption at rest) and the increased sensitivity to heat in hyperthyroidism—and the opposite in hypothyroidism. Thyroid hormones stimulate mitochondriogenesis, augmenting the cell's oxidative capacity. They also induce changes in the mitochondrial inner membrane protein and lipid composition that increase oxidative metabolism by both genomic and nongenomic effects. The reduced efficiency of oxidative metabolism caused by thyroid hormone is also reflected in the increased futile cycling of intermediary carbohydrate metabolites.

Cardiovascular Effects (Figure 7–22)

T_3 stimulates transcription of sarcoplasmic reticulum Ca^{2+} ATPase, increasing the rate of myocardial diastolic relaxation. It also increases expression of the more rapidly contractile isoforms of myosin heavy chain, the α isoforms, which contributes to

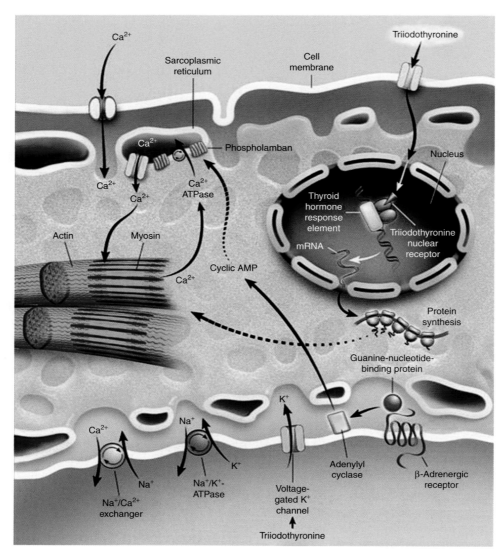

FIGURE 7-22 Sites of action of triiodothyronine on cardiac myocytes. Triiodothyronine enters the cell, possibly by a specific transport mechanism, and binds to nuclear triiodothyronine receptors. The complex then binds to thyroid hormone response elements of target genes and regulates transcription of these genes. Nonnuclear thyroid hormone effects on ion channels also occur. (Reproduced, with permission, from Klein I, Ojamaa K. Thyroid hormone and the cardiovascular system. *N Engl J Med.* 2001;344:501.)

enhanced systolic function. In myocardium, T$_3$ also alters expression of different isoforms of the Na$^+$-K$^+$ ATPase genes, increases expression of α-adrenergic receptors, and decreases the concentration of the inhibitory G protein Gi α. T$_3$ also increases the rates of both depolarization and repolarization of the sinoatrial node, increasing heart rate. Consequently, thyroid hormones have positive inotropic and chronotropic effects on the heart, which, along with the heightened adrenergic sensitivity (see later), accounts for the increased heart rate and contractility in hyperthyroidism and the reverse in hypothyroidism. Thyroid hormones also affect diastolic ventricular function, lower peripheral vascular resistance, and increase intravascular volume, which contributes further to the increase in cardiac output associated with thyroid hormone action.

Sympathetic Effects

Thyroid hormones increase the number of β-adrenergic receptors in heart and skeletal muscle, adipose tissue, and lymphocytes. They may also amplify catecholamine action at a postreceptor site. Many of the clinical manifestations of thyrotoxicosis appear to reflect increased sensitivity to catecholamines. Furthermore, therapy with β-adrenergic blocking agents is often helpful in controlling these sympathomimetic manifestations of thyroid hormone excess.

Pulmonary Effects

Thyroid hormones maintain ventilatory responses to hypoxia and hypercapnia in the brain stem respiratory center. Consequently, in patients with severe hypothyroidism, hypoventilation can occur.

Respiratory muscle functions are also regulated by thyroid hormone, and can be weakened in hyperthyroidism, leading to a sense of breathlessness.

Hematopoietic Effects

The increased cellular demand for O_2 in hyperthyroidism leads to increased production of erythropoietin and increased erythropoiesis. However, blood volume is usually not increased because of hemodilution and increased red cell turnover. Thyroid hormones increase the 2,3-diphosphoglycerate content of erythrocytes, allowing increased O_2 dissociation from hemoglobin and increasing O_2 availability to tissues. The reverse occurs in hypothyroidism.

Gastrointestinal Effects

Thyroid hormones promote gut motility, which can result in increased motility and hyperdefecation (ie, increased frequency of formed bowel movements) in hyperthyroidism. Conversely, slowed bowel transit and constipation occurs in hypothyroidism.

Skeletal Effects

Thyroid hormones stimulate bone turnover, increasing bone resorption and, to a lesser degree, bone formation. Consequently, hyperthyroidism can be associated with hypercalciuria, and less often, hypercalcemia. Furthermore, chronic thyroid hormone excess can cause clinically significant bone mineral loss.

Neuromuscular Effects

In hyperthyroidism, there is increased protein turnover and loss in skeletal muscle, which can lead to a characteristic proximal myopathy. There is also an increase in the speed of muscle contraction and relaxation, noted clinically as the hyperreflexia of hyperthyroidism and the delayed deep tendon reflex relaxation phase in hypothyroidism. A fine distal hand tremor is also typical in hyperthyroidism. As noted above, thyroid hormones are essential for normal development and function of the central nervous system, and failure of fetal thyroid function results in severe mental retardation. In the adult, hyperactivity in hyperthyroidism and sluggishness in hypothyroidism can be striking. Similarly, hyperthyroid patients can be anxious or agitated, while hypothyroidism is typically associated with a depressed mood.

Effects on Lipid and Carbohydrate Metabolism

Hyperthyroidism increases hepatic gluconeogenesis and glycogenolysis, as well as intestinal glucose absorption, and there may also be thyroid hormone–mediated decreases in insulin sensitivity. Thus, hyperthyroidism can worsen glycemic control in patients who also have diabetes mellitus. Cholesterol synthesis and degradation are both increased by thyroid hormones. The latter effect is due largely to an increase in hepatic low-density lipoprotein (LDL) receptor number, accelerating LDL clearance. Consequently,

total and LDL cholesterol levels are typically elevated in patients with hypothyroidism. Lipolysis is also increased, releasing fatty acids and glycerol into circulating plasma.

Endocrine Effects

Thyroid hormones alter the production, responsiveness, and metabolic clearance of a number of hormones. In hypothyroid children, impaired growth hormone release slows longitudinal growth. Hypothyroidism can cause delayed puberty by impairing gonadotropin-releasing hormone (GnRH) and gonadotropin secretion. Conversely, primary hypothyroidism can also cause precocious puberty, perhaps as an effect of very high TSH levels on gonadotropin receptors. In adults, hypothyroidism causes hyperprolactinemia in a minority of affected women. Menorrhagia (prolonged and heavier menses) and anovulation are common in hypothyroid women, the latter resulting in infertility. The responsiveness of the hypothalamic-pituitary-adrenal axis to stress is blunted in hypothyroid patients. A slowing of the cortisol metabolic clearance rate compensates for this in the hypothyroid state. Conversely, however, restoration of euthyroidism can rarely provoke adrenal insufficiency as cortisol metabolism is accelerated in patients with diminished cortisol reserve due to concomitant disease affecting the adrenal axis.

In hyperthyroidism, accelerated aromatization of androgens to estrogens and increased sex hormone–binding globulin levels contribute to the gynecomastia and elevated total testosterone levels seen in affected men. Hyperthyroidism can also impair normal GnRH and gonadotropin regulation of ovulation and menses, causing infertility and amenorrhea, respectively. All of the endocrine derangements occurring with thyroid dysfunction are reversed by appropriate treatment to restore euthyroidism.

PHYSIOLOGIC CHANGES IN THYROID FUNCTION

Thyroid Function in the Fetus

Before the fetus develops its own independent thyroid function, it depends on maternal thyroid hormones for early neural development. By the 11th week of gestation, however, the hypophysial portal system has developed, and measurable TSH and TRH are present. At about the same time, the fetal thyroid begins to trap iodine. The secretion of thyroid hormone probably begins in mid gestation (18-20 weeks). TSH increases rapidly to peak levels at 24 to 28 weeks, and T_4 levels peak at 35 to 40 weeks. T_3 levels remain low during gestation; T_4 is converted to rT_3 by type 3 5'-deiodinase during fetal development. At birth, there is a sudden marked rise in TSH stimulated by exposure to the colder extrauterine environment, with a rise in T_4, a rise in T_3, and a fall in rT_3. These parameters gradually stabilize over the first month of life.

Thyroid Function in Pregnancy

A number of thyroid parameters change during pregnancy. There is an increase in urinary iodide clearance; in areas of low dietary iodine intake, this can cause maternal goiter, or when severe, hypothyroidism. During pregnancy, there is a rise in TBG due to an estrogen-induced increase in hepatic glycosylation of TBG, prolonging its metabolic clearance rate. Consequently, serum total T_4, and to a lesser extent, total T_3 concentrations rise. Rising levels of hCG, which has weak TSH receptor agonist activity, contributes to minimal thyroid enlargement. Maternal hCG levels peak at approximately 12 weeks resulting in a transient high-normal or even modestly elevated serum-free T_4 level and a physiologic suppression of serum TSH to the low-normal or even subnormal range. Pathologically elevated hCG levels, found in women with a molar pregnancy or choriocarcinoma, can cause overt hyperthyroidism. Women with severe vomiting in pregnancy, called hyperemesis gravidarum, may also have higher levels of hCG, and can develop a transient gestational thyrotoxicosis. As noted earlier, placental type 3 deiodinase accelerates thyroxine clearance during pregnancy, which partly accounts for the increased thyroxine dose requirement in treated hypothyroid women, and occasionally causes mild hypothyroidism in women with autoimmune thyroiditis and decreased thyroid gland reserve.

Transplacental delivery of thyroid-related substances can have consequences for the fetus. Maternal iodide crossing the placenta is essential for fetal thyroid hormone production; however, large amounts of iodide can actually inhibit fetal thyroid function and cause a goiter substantial enough to obstruct delivery. In women with autoimmune thyroid disease, maternal immunoglobulins that stimulate or block the TSH receptor can cross the placenta and cause thyroid dysfunction in the fetus. The antithyroid drugs methimazole and PTU cross the placenta, and in large doses will impair fetal thyroid function (see Chapter 16).

Changes in Thyroid Function with Aging

T_4 turnover is highest in infants and children, and gradually falls to adult levels after puberty. The T_4 turnover rate is then stable until after age 60, when it again begins to decline. In the elderly, the metabolic clearance of T_4 can decrease by as much as 50%, necessitating a reduction in T_4 dose for treated patients.

TABLE 7–3 Conditions or factors associated with decreased conversion of T_4 or T_3.

1. Fetal life
2. Caloric restriction
3. Hepatic disease
4. Major systemic illness
5. Drugs:
    Propylthiouracil
    Glucocorticoids
    Propranolol (mild effect)
    Iodinated x-ray contrast agents (iopanoic acid, ipodate sodium)
    Amiodarone
6. Selenium deficiency

Effects of Acute and Chronic Illness on Thyroid Function (Euthyroid Sick Syndrome)

Acute or chronic illness has several striking effects on thyroid function and hormone economy. The most common and earliest effect is inhibition of T_4-to-T_3 conversion, with a resulting decrease in the circulating T_3 level. This change is accompanied by a rise in the serum reverse T_3 level, due to both its decreased conversion to $3,3'$-T_2 and some acceleration of its production from T_4. These changes occur physiologically in the fetus and pathologically in circumstances of caloric restriction, as in malnutrition, starvation, and anorexia nervosa, and in patients with a variety of acute or chronic systemic illnesses (Table 7–3). The pathogenesis of this *low T_3 syndrome* is thought to involve cytokines, such as tumor necrosis factor, secreted by inflammatory cells, which inhibit type 1 5'-deiodinase. Drugs can also inhibit type 1 5'-deiodinase and lower the serum T_3 levels in treated patients; these agents include corticosteroids, amiodarone, iodinated cholecystographic dyes, PTU, and high-dose propranolol. Initially, low serum T_3 levels are typically accompanied by total and free T_4 levels that are normal or, less commonly, slightly elevated (Figure 7–23). As illness becomes more severe, however, there is a

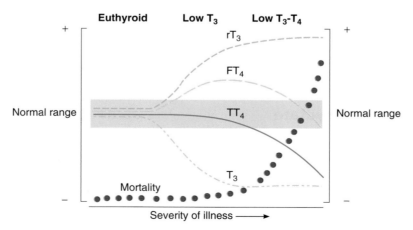

FIGURE 7–23 A schematic representation of the changes in serum thyroid hormone values with increasing severity of nonthyroidal illness. A rapidly rising mortality rate accompanies the fall in serum total T_4 (TT$_4$) and free T_4 (FT$_4$) values. (Reproduced, with permission, from Nicoloff JT. Abnormal measurements in nonendocrine illness. In: *Medicine for the Practicing Physician.* 2nd ed. Hurst JW, ed. Butterworth-Heinemann; 1991.)

decline in serum total and free T_4 as well. This hypothyroxinemia can have several causes. In certain illnesses (eg, nephrosis and severe liver disease), there can be a decline in the circulating TBG concentration. A rise in plasma free fatty acids can interfere with T_4 binding to TBG, liberating more free T_4 that, in turn, feeds back on the hypothalamus and pituitary to reduce TSH and establish a new equilibrium with a lower total T_4. TSH can also be suppressed by cytokines circulating in severely ill patients and by the dopamine or corticosteroids often used to treat critically ill patients. Finally, T_4 clearance is accelerated in illness. All of these factors can contribute to the lower serum levels of T_4 and free T_4, as measured by free hormone immunoassays and estimated T_3 resin-uptake procedures. However, the free T_4 level measured by equilibrium dialysis has been reported to be normal in most, but not all patients. This suggests that the low serum free T_4 levels reported by most commercially available free T_4 assays may be a measurement artifact that is unique to critically ill patients.

Two clinical questions arise in sick patients with this constellation of thyroid function test abnormalities. First, it can be challenging to distinguish the euthyroid sick syndrome from central hypothyroidism; in both conditions, the T_4 and TSH levels can be low. Clinical information can be helpful, including a history of known pituitary or thyroid disease, head trauma or surgery, or manifestations of other elements of hypopituitarism (eg, small testes in a man). Additional laboratory testing can sometimes be informative. The serum free T_4 level determined by equilibrium dialysis is typically normal in the euthyroid sick syndrome. In postmenopausal women, an elevated serum FSH attests to at least one intact pituitary function, although gonadotropin levels can be low in severe illness as well. Measurement of serum cortisol may be particularly helpful, because it should be normal or elevated in any patient with significant systemic illness. If it is normal or elevated, hypothalamic or pituitary disease is most unlikely. Sometimes, however, it is necessary to obtain emergent imaging of the hypothalamus or pituitary to resolve the question. These thyroid function test abnormalities normalize when the patient recovers. However, recovery can be accompanied by transient rebound elevation of the serum TSH that may be misinterpreted as hypothyroidism. In this setting, in the absence of clinically apparent hypothyroidism, it is best to avoid thyroid hormone therapy and to reevaluate a few weeks following recovery.

The second clinical question is whether the euthyroid sick syndrome itself should be treated with thyroid hormone. Certainly, many critically ill patients have clinical problems that are reminiscent of hypothyroidism, such as hypothermia, altered sensorium, ventilatory and myocardial dysfunction, and hyponatremia. It has been postulated that intracellular hypothyroidism may exist in these patients and that thyroid hormone therapy might be beneficial. Conversely, it has been proposed that these changes in thyroid status are, in fact, compensatory mechanisms for reducing rates of oxygen consumption and protein catabolism and that thyroid hormone therapy might actually be harmful. Furthermore, two randomized trials, small clinical series, and animal models of systemic illness all have failed to demonstrate any benefit of thyroid hormone therapy in this setting. Although the issue remains unresolved, current practice is generally to withhold thyroid hormone therapy unless there is convincing clinical and biochemical evidence of true hypothyroidism.

THYROID AUTOIMMUNITY

Autoimmunity is involved in the pathogenesis of many thyroid diseases, including hyperthyroid Graves disease, hypothyroidism with autoimmune or Hashimoto thyroiditis, silent and postpartum thyroiditis, and certain forms of neonatal thyroid dysfunction. Immunologic defense against foreign substances and neoplastic cells involves macrophages that ingest and digest the foreign material and present peptide fragments on the cell surface in association with a class II protein encoded by the HLA-DR region of the *MHC* gene complex. This complex is recognized by a T-cell receptor on a CD4 helper T cell, which stimulates the release of cytokines such as interleukin-2 (IL-2). These cytokines amplify the response by inducing T-cell activation and proliferation, induction of killer cell activity in CD8 suppressor cells, and stimulation of antibody formation against the foreign antigen by B lymphocytes. Eventually, the activation process is muted by the action of the CD8 suppressor cells (see Chapter 2).

Early observations suggested the possibility that immunologic reactions could affect the thyroid gland. Thyroiditis was induced by immunization of mice with thyroid tissue and Freund adjuvant. Thyroglobulin antibodies were identified in the sera from patients with thyroiditis, and a long-acting thyroid stimulator, later shown to be an antibody to the TSH receptor, was found in the sera of patients with Graves disease.

There are three major thyroidal autoantigens: thyroglobulin, TPO, and the TSH receptor. Circulating autoantibodies to these antigens are useful markers for thyroid autoimmunity, but T-cell-mediated immune mechanisms are central to the pathogenesis of thyroid diseases. Thyroid cells have the capacity to ingest antigen (eg, thyroglobulin) and, when stimulated by cytokines such as gamma interferon, express cell surface class II molecules (eg, HLA-DR4) that present these antigens to T lymphocytes. In addition to the antigen and the class II molecule, other factors such as costimulatory signals from antigen-presenting cells, are doubtless required to initiate autoimmune thyroid disease. One hypothesis is that the process is initiated or promoted by external antigens (eg, infectious agents) that lead to antibody and cellular immune responses through cross-reactivity. In addition, genetic factors clearly predispose individuals to thyroid autoimmunity. HLA typing in patients with Graves disease reveals a high frequency of HLA-B8 and HLA-DR3 in Caucasians, HLA-Bw46 and HLA-B5 in Chinese, and HLA-B17 in blacks. In Caucasians, atrophic thyroiditis has been associated with HLA-B8 and goitrous Hashimoto thyroiditis with HLA-DR5. It has been suggested that a genetically induced antigen-specific defect in suppressor T lymphocytes may be the basis for autoimmune thyroid disease.

The increased incidence of autoimmune thyroid disease in postpubertal and premenopausal women, as well as the occurrence of postpartum thyroiditis, implies a role for female sex hormones in the pathogenesis of autoimmune thyroid disease. A high iodine intake may result in more highly iodinated thyroglobulin that is more immunogenic and would favor the development of autoimmune thyroid disease. Therapeutic doses of lithium, used for the treatment of bipolar disorder, can interfere with suppressor cell function and may precipitate autoimmune thyroid disease.

TESTS OF THYROID FUNCTION

The high prevalence of thyroid dysfunction and neoplasia make testing for thyroid disease a daily necessity in virtually every field of medical practice—whether a pediatrician screening a neonate for congenital hypothyroidism, an internist considering possible thyroid dysfunction in a patient with nonspecific complaints, an obstetrician-gynecologist evaluating a woman with infertility, a surgeon assessing a thyroid nodule, or virtually any type of specialist considering thyroid disease as the potential cause for a complaint or test abnormality in the field of interest (eg, cardiologist, gastroenterologist, neurologist, psychiatrist, ophthalmologist).

Several levels of laboratory and radiologic investigation for thyroid diseases should be considered. First, it is common for clinicians with a relatively low index of suspicion for thyroid dysfunction in a particular patient to want to exclude its presence with greater certainty. For this purpose, a test with high sensitivity (ie, few false-negative results), wide availability, and low cost is most appropriate. The serum TSH concentration often plays this role in clinical consideration of hypothyroidism and hyperthyroidism. Second, when suspicion of thyroid disease is moderate to high, based on clinical or other routine laboratory results, testing with even greater sensitivity to detect rare thyroid disorders is required, as is a test that can begin to define the severity and underlying cause of thyroid dysfunction. For example, in a patient with hypothermia, confusion, periorbital edema, and hypercholesterolemia, measurement of both the serum TSH and free T_4 concentrations would permit exclusion of both primary and central forms of hypothyroidism; furthermore, if hypothyroidism is confirmed, the site of responsible disease would be implicated. Third, when thyroid dysfunction is clinically obvious or already biochemically confirmed by first-line testing, then more sophisticated studies are sometimes indicated to identify the underlying cause and plan appropriate therapy. For example, in a postpartum woman with thyrotoxicosis, an additional serum T_3, thyroid-stimulating immunoglobulin titer, and radionuclide thyroid uptake may be needed to differentiate Graves disease and postpartum thyroiditis—for which there are distinct therapeutic approaches.

TESTS OF THYROID HORMONES IN BLOOD

Serum TSH Measurement

Because thyroid dysfunction usually arises from primary disorders of the thyroid gland, serum TSH measurement is the most widely employed test to determine whether thyroid dysfunction exists. The sensitivity of the hypothalamic-pituitary-thyroid axis ensures that both primary hypothyroidism and thyrotoxicosis, due to

either primary thyroid disorders or exogenous thyroid hormones, are detected. Furthermore, even mild degrees of thyroid dysfunction, in which the serum thyroid hormone concentrations have fallen or risen significantly but remain within the broad reference range (ie, subclinical or mild thyroid dysfunction) are identified. The inverse logarithmic relationship between serum TSH and free T_4 concentration in various situations is shown in Figures 7–24A and 7–24B. TSH assays must be sensitive (ie, able to distinguish low from very low and undetectable TSH levels) to be used for diagnosis of thyrotoxicosis. A National Academy of Clinical Biochemistry guideline specifies that sensitivity, or lower limit of detection, for TSH assays should be less than 0.02 mU/L. It is better to assess and compare TSH assays by this quantitative criterion rather than marketing terms such as *third generation* or *ultrasensitive*.

There are, in general, two sorts of immunoassays used to measure TSH (and T_4 and T_3) in serum samples: immunometric assays (IMA) and radioimmunoassay (RIA). In an IMA or *sandwich assay*, an antibody—usually a mouse monoclonal antibody—directed against one epitope on the TSH molecule is fixed to a solid matrix, and a second monoclonal TSH antibody that binds another TSH epitope is labeled with a detectable marker, which can be a radioisotope, a colorimetrically quantifiable enzyme, or a fluorescent or chemiluminescent tag. In such IMAs, the concentration of TSH, which links the solid state and labeled antibodies, is proportionate to the intensity of signal emitted by the marker once unbound second antibody has been separated off. In contrast, in conventional RIAs, a small amount of a TSH tracer, to which a radioactive molecule has been linked, competes for binding to first antibody (eg, a rabbit antihuman TSH polyclonal antibody). Then antibody-bound TSH, both in the sample and the tracer, is separated from the free tracer in the supernatant using one of several techniques: a second antibody directed against the first (eg, goat antirabbit immunoglobulin antibody), polyethylene glycol, or staphylococcal protein A. In RIAs, the concentration of TSH in the sample is inversely proportionate to tracer activity. In general, TSH RIAs are less sensitive and less widely employed than IMAs.

There are infrequent but important limitations of the serum TSH assay alone for diagnosis of thyroid dysfunction when clinical suspicion of hypothyroidism is high and in certain other special circumstances (Table 7–4). First, central hypothyroidism can be overlooked. In patients with hypothyroidism due to a pituitary tumor, for example, the serum TSH is typically not elevated, but rather low or inappropriately normal. Consequently, simultaneous measurements of both the serum free T_4 and TSH would be required to further substantiate or exclude this diagnosis. Central hypothyroidism can also be confirmed by assessing the serum TSH response to an injection of TRH. To perform this test, serum samples for TSH are obtained before and 30 to 60 minutes after 200 μg of TRH is administered intravenously. The absence of a significant rise in serum TSH concentration (eg, to a peak value >7 mU/L) indicates pituitary or hypothalamic disease or suppression by exogenous thyroid hormone. A modest and delayed rise may be seen in patients with hypothalamic disease and tertiary hypothyroidism. Currently, TRH is not available in the

United States. Another cause of a misleadingly low serum TSH concentration is drug treatment with either high-dose corticosteroids or dopamine, both of which inhibit TSH secretion (see Table 7–4).

A second limitation of TSH testing alone is that there are other nonthyroidal causes of an elevated serum TSH concentration, as described in Table 7–4.

Serum T₄ and T₃ Measurements

The concentrations of total and free (unbound) T_4 and T_3 are measurable by a variety of automated assay techniques. Serum total thyroid hormone concentrations are widely available and accurate for assessment of most patients with overt thyroid dysfunction. However, a limitation of these assays is they can provide false-positive and false-negative results when changes in the concentration or binding affinity of the thyroid hormone–binding plasma proteins are altered. For example, a pregnant woman with an estrogen-induced increase in the concentration of TBG could

be misdiagnosed as being hyperthyroid if only a total T_4 assay was employed. Conversely, a pregnant patient with primary hypothyroidism might be overlooked if the elevated TBG concentration produced total T_4 within the reference range. Despite these reservations, diagnostic accuracy is high when total T_4 assay results are interpreted along with TSH assay findings.

These problems are circumvented by measuring the free thyroxine (FT_4) concentration by free T_4 IMAs or equilibrium dialysis or estimating it using the free thyroxine index (FT_4I), also called the **thyroid hormone–binding ratio** (THBR). Free T_4 assays employ strategies to measure only the unbound fraction of T_4 in serum samples. One approach is to employ a competing thyroxine analog tracer that binds to the assay antibody but not to plasma proteins. Such free T_4 assays are quite accurate in distinguishing straightforward TBG derangements from true FT_4 abnormalities. However, they may be influenced to some extent by variations in total T_4, and they can yield misleadingly high readings in dysalbuminemic hyperthyroxinemia. Because they are

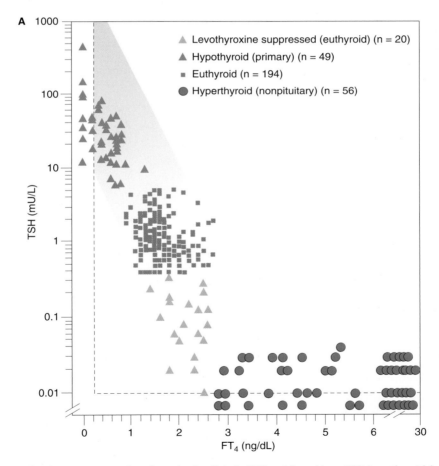

FIGURE 7–24 A. Relationship between serum-free thyroxine by dialysis (FT_4) ng/dL and $\log_{10}$ TSH in euthyroid, hyperthyroid, hypothyroid, and T_4-suppressed euthyroid individuals. Note that for each unit change in T_4 there is a logarithmic change in TSH. **B.** Relationship between FT_4 by dialysis and $\log_{10}$ TSH in normal subjects and subjects with various illnesses including primary hypothyroidism, central hypothyroidism and non–levothyroxine-suppressed TSH, levothyroxine-treated congenital hypothyroidism, TSH-secreting tumors, thyroid hormone resistance, non-thyroidal illness, and nonpituitary hyperthyroidism. (Reproduced, with permission, from Kaptein EM. Clinical applications of free thyroxine determinations. *Clin Lab Med*. 1993;13:654.)

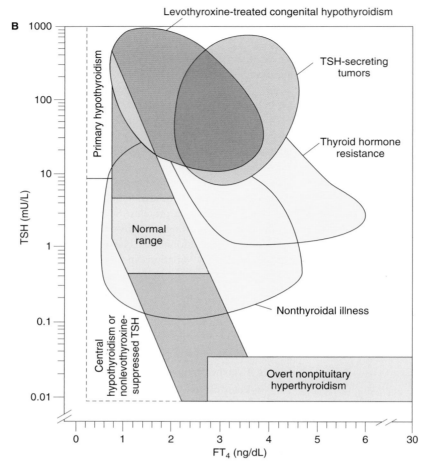

FIGURE 7–24   *(Continued)*

TABLE 7–4 Causes of inappropriate serum TSH concentration.[a]

Clinical hyperthyroidism
TSH-secreting pituitary adenoma
Isolated pituitary resistance to thyroid hormone
Clinical hypothyroidism
Central (pituitary or hypothalamic) hypothyroidism
Preceding TSH suppression (eg, recently treated hyperthyroidism)
Clinical euthyroidism
Systemic illnesses (↓ during acute phase, ↑ during recovery)
Generalized resistance to thyroid hormone (compensated)
Assay interference
Anti-TSH antibodies
Anti-mouse immunoglobulin antibodies
Drugs: dopamine, dobutamine, glucocorticoids

[a]"Inappropriate" refers to disruption of the usual reciprocal relationship between serum TSH and free thyroid hormone concentrations.

sufficiently accurate in most settings, automatable, and inexpensive, they are currently the most widely used method for free T_4 determination.

Equilibrium dialysis entails equilibrating a serum sample with buffer across a membrane with pores that permit passage only of unbound T_4; then the dialysate is assayed for its T_4 concentration, from which the serum concentration can be derived. Although equilibrium dialysis is considered the gold standard for free T_4 determination, it is cumbersome, relatively expensive, and not widely available. Consequently, it is not the optimal first-line method for free T_4 measurement, and it is best reserved for special circumstances.

Free T_4 estimation by free T_4 index entails measuring the total T_4 in a conventional IMA and then estimating the partition of a tracer iodothyronine between plasma proteins and a matrix with a virtually limitless binding capacity for small molecules (resin, charcoal, or talc). Radiolabeled T_3 is often the tracer employed, although T_4 tracer can be used as well. The free T_4 index is then calculated as the product of the total T_4 multiplied by the percentage of iodothyronine tracer taken up by the matrix, the so-called T_3 *uptake*. It is important to note that this refers to the T_3 tracer used in the assay, not the T_3 level in the serum sample.

When the free T_4 concentration alone is used to diagnose thyroid dysfunction, there are a number of conditions from which true hyperthyroidism or hypothyroidism must be distinguished. First, there are several conditions in which euthyroid individuals can develop hyperthyroxinemia (see Table 7–1). These include rare patients with nonthyroidal illnesses; unusual plasma-binding proteins abnormalities, such as familial dysalbuminemic hyperthyroxinemia (see later); and drugs that block T_4-to-T_3 conversion (eg, iodinated contrast media, amiodarone, glucocorticoids, and propranolol). In these conditions, true hyperthyroidism is excluded by the normal serum TSH level. Conversely, there are also conditions in which the serum-free thyroxine can be subnormal in euthyroid individuals. Antiepileptic drugs, such as phenytoin and carbamazepine, have multiple actions that lower total and free T_4 levels, including inhibition of TSH secretion and accelerating T_4 catabolism. However, the normal accompanying serum TSH and equilibrium dialysis T_4 levels implies that these patients are, in fact, euthyroid.

Total and free T_3 concentrations can also be quantitated in specific IMAs. Measurement of serum T_3 is used (1) to recognize patients who have T_3 toxicosis, a milder degree of hyperthyroidism in which the serum T_3 level is elevated with a normal serum T_4; (2) to fully define the severity of hyperthyroidism and monitor the response to therapy; and (3) to help in the differential diagnosis of patients with hyperthyroidism. Because T_3 is preferentially secreted in most patients with Graves disease, and some with toxic nodular goiter, the ratios of serum T_3:T_4 (expressed in ng/dL:μg/dL) are typically greater than 20 in patients with these conditions.

The serum T_3 concentration is not accurate for diagnosis of hypothyroidism because a normal T_3 level is often maintained in patients with mild to moderate primary hypothyroidism; TSH stimulation increases the relative secretion of T_3. Because T_3 is bound to TBG, the total serum T_3 concentration varies with the TBG level, although less than the serum total T_4 (Table 7–5). Serum-free T_3 can be measured by IMA or more precisely by equilibrium dialysis.

Reverse T_3 (rT_3) can be measured by RIA; its serum concentration in adults is about one-third of the total T_3 concentration. However, there is little or no clinical indication for rT_3 measurement. Previous claims that it is useful to differentiate hypothyroidism from the thyroid function test changes of nonthyroidal illness have not shown that rT_3 levels are sufficiently accurate for that purpose.

Thyroglobulin can be measured in serum by either IMA or RIA, which now have sensitivities as low as 0.1 ng/mL. There are two indications for thyroglobulin measurement: (1) detection of residual or recurrent epithelial thyroid cancers (papillary, follicular, and Hürthle cell carcinomas) after thyroidectomy (see section on Management of Thyroid Cancer); and (2) differentiation of thyrotoxicosis due to exogenous thyroid hormone, in which the thyroglobulin level is suppressed, from all forms of endogenous hyperthyroidism, including various forms of thyroiditis, in which it is elevated or normal.

There are several potential limitations of current thyroglobulin IMAs. The most important is interference caused by the presence of circulating antithyroglobulin antibodies. This typically leads to spuriously low values in thyroglobulin IMAs and elevated values in RIAs. Serum thyroglobulin determinations are not useful to differentiate malignant from benign thyroid nodules.

ASSESSMENT OF THYROID IODINE METABOLISM AND BIOSYNTHETIC ACTIVITY

Radionuclide uptake measurements can be useful to differentiate among the causes of thyrotoxicosis, particularly when used in conjunction with imaging. Radioiodine uptake determinations permit in vivo assessment of fractional iodine uptake and turnover by the thyroid gland. Iodine-123 is the ideal isotope for this purpose, with 13-hour half-life and emitting quantifiable 28-keV x-rays and 159-keV gamma photons but no tissue damage by beta particles. ^{123}I—or when it is unavailable, a low dose of ^{131}I—is given orally, and radioactivity over the thyroid is quantified with a scintillation counter at 4 or 6 hours and again at 24 hours (Figure 7–25). The fractional radioactive iodine uptake (RAIU) by

TABLE 7–5 Representative iodothyronine kinetic values in a euthyroid human.

	T_4	T_3	rT_3
Serum levels			
Total, μg/dL (nmol/L)	8 (103)	0.12 (1.84)	0.04 (0.51)
Free, ng/dL (pmol/L)	1.5 (19)	0.28 (4.3)	0.24 (3.69)
Body pool, μg (nmol)	800 (1023)	46 (70.7)	40 (61.5)
Distribution volume (L)	10	38	98
Metabolic clearance rate (MCR) (L/d)	1	22	90
Production (disposal) rate. MCR X serum concentration, μg/d (nmol/d)	80 (103)	26 (34)	36 (46)
Half-life in plasma (t1/2) (days)	7	1	0.2

(Note: T4 μg/dL × 12.87 = nmol/L; T3 μg/dL × 15.38 = nmol/L).

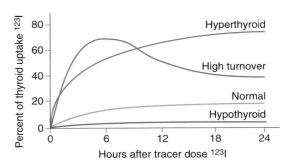

FIGURE 7–25 Typical curves of 24-hour radioiodine uptake in normal subjects and in patients with thyroid disease. A high-turnover curve may be seen in patients taking an iodine-deficient diet or with a defect in hormone synthesis.

the thyroid varies with recent dietary iodide intake. In countries with a relatively high iodide intake (eg, Chile, Brazil), the normal RAIU is 5% to 15% at 6 hours and 8% to 30% at 24 hours, whereas in areas of low iodide intake and endemic goiter (eg, some parts of Europe and sub-Saharan Africa), the 24-hour RAIU can be as high as 60% to 90%.

In hyperthyroid Graves disease, the 24-hour RAIU is markedly elevated (eg, 40%-95%), although if iodide turnover is very rapid, the 5-hour uptake may be even higher than the 24-hour uptake (Figure 7–25). Similarly, the 24-hour RAIU is increased to a lesser extent in toxic nodular goiter (eg, 30%-70%). Thyrotoxicosis with a low thyroidal RAIU occurs in patients with several conditions: (1) subacute and lymphocytic (postpartum, silent) thyroiditis with inflammatory release of preformed hormone causing spontaneously resolving thyrotoxicosis; (2) in iatrogenic or factitious thyrotoxicosis resulting from excessive thyroid hormone medication; and (3) following excess oral or intravenous iodide intake, as occurs, for example, with amiodarone therapy or after radiocontrast agents. There can also be low RAIU over the anterior neck when there is excessive thyroid hormone production elsewhere in the body, as occurs with ectopic thyroid tissue at the tongue base (lingual thyroid); in the mediastinum; with struma ovarii, an ovarian teratoma with functioning thyroid tissue; and with functioning metastases from thyroid carcinoma after total thyroidectomy.

The T_3 suppression test is a permutation of the RAIU that is rarely used to ascertain whether thyroid function is autonomous. When one gives T_3 to normal individuals (75-100 µg in divided doses daily for 5 days) it reduces the 24-hour RAIU by more than 50% from baseline. Failure of the radioiodine uptake to suppress indicates autonomous thyroid function, such as occurs in Graves disease or with an autonomously functioning thyroid nodule.

A rare use of RAIU is in determining whether a goitrous thyroid gland has an iodide organification defect. The perchlorate discharge test assesses efficiency of iodide organification by the gland. Perchlorate ($KClO_4$) acutely blocks the NIS, halting further influx of iodide into the gland and permitting leakage of trapped but nonorganified iodide out of the cell. Specifically, after

administering a radioiodine tracer dose and measuring an initial RAIU at 4 hours, 0.5 g $KClO_4$ is administered to block further radioiodine uptake. If a second RAIU 1 hour later shows that the measured RAIU has been diminished by 5% or more, this indicates an organification defect.

Positive perchlorate discharge tests are seen in some patients with congenital iodide organification defects, as well as in autoimmune thyroiditis, in Graves disease, especially after ^{131}I therapy, and in patients receiving antithyroid drug inhibitors of iodide organification. The perchlorate discharge test is rarely used clinically, and perchlorate is not available in the United States.

THYROID IMAGING

1. RADIONUCLIDE IMAGING

[123]I and technetium ^{99m}Tc pertechnetate ([99m]TcO_4) are useful for determining the functional activity and morphology of the thyroid gland. [123]I (200-300 µCi) is administered orally, and an image of the thyroid is obtained 8 to 24 hours later. [99m]TcO_4 (1-10 mCi), which is trapped by the NIS, but not organified and retained in the gland, is administered intravenously, and the scan image is obtained earlier than usual—at 30-60 minutes. Images can be obtained with either a rectilinear scanner or a gamma camera. The rectilinear scanner moves back and forth over the area of interest and produces a life-size picture, on which regions of interest, such as nodules, can be marked (Figure 7–26A). The gamma camera has a pinhole collimator, and the scan is obtained on a fluorescent screen and recorded on film or a computer monitor. The camera has greater resolution, but regions of interest must be identified with a radioactive marker for clinical correlation (Figure 7–26B).

Radionuclide scans provide information about the size and shape of the thyroid gland and the distribution of tracer activity within the gland. This is useful in differentiating among the causes of thyrotoxicosis; an enlarged gland with intense and homogenous concentration of tracer is typical of Graves disease. In contrast,

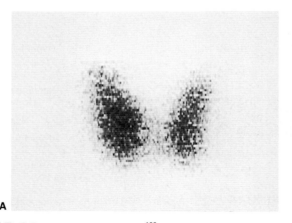

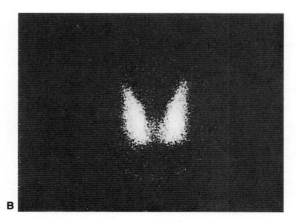

FIGURE 7–26 A. Rectilinear sodium ^{123}I scan performed 6 hours after the ingestion of 100 µCi of sodium [123]I. **B.** Scintiphoto (pinhole collimator) thyroid scan performed 6 hours after the ingestion of 100 µCi of sodium [123]I. (Both scans courtesy of Dr. R.R. Cavalieri.)

one or more discrete regions of tracer activity, especially corresponding to a palpable nodule or nodules, with suppression of extranodular tissue are characteristic of toxic nodular goiter.

Radionuclide imaging has a limited role in differentiation of benign from malignant thyroid nodules. When a patient with a thyroid nodule has a suppressed serum TSH concentration, a radionuclide scan is often appropriate to determine if the nodule is *hot* (ie, functioning with suppression of extranodular thyroid tissue). If this is the case, the nodule can generally be considered benign. Because both most benign and malignant thyroid nodules are *cold*, or hypofunctioning, documenting this is not particularly helpful, and cytologic evaluation must be performed in any case.

Radionuclide whole body scanning is useful in follow-up of patients with treated thyroid cancer and for confirmation that a mass on the tongue (lingual thyroid), in the midline of the neck (thyroglossal duct), or in the mediastinum (substernal goiter) represents ectopic thyroid tissue.

THYROID ULTRASONOGRAPHY AND OTHER IMAGING TECHNIQUES

The size of the thyroid gland and characteristics of nodular lesions within it are best ascertained by high-resolution ultrasonography (Figure 7–27). Sonography can differentiate solid nodules from cystic lesions and characterize complex cysts that have both solid and cystic components. Certain features of nodules are more common in malignant lesions (eg, irregular nodule capsule and microcalcifications), and other features are typical of benign lesions (eg, a *spongiform* appearance and cystic change), but none of these features can be considered definitive. Sonography can be used to serially monitor the size of thyroid nodules over time, to guide fine-needle aspiration of thyroid nodules, and to assess regional lymph nodes in thyroid cancer patients both preoperatively and in long-term follow-up.

Computed tomography (CT) and magnetic resonance imaging (MRI) are useful in patients with thyroid disease in special settings. They may be required to define the posterior cervical and substernal extent of large goiters, and whether there is tracheal deviation or compression. In thyroid cancer patients, they can be helpful in identifying metastatic disease outside of the neck (eg, in the lungs, liver). It should be remembered that administration of iodine-containing radiocontrast dye for CT imaging interferes with subsequent radioiodine imaging and therapy for up to several months. Positron emission tomography (PET) scanning has a role in localization of metastatic disease in treated thyroid cancer patients who have a serum thyroglobulin concentration greater than 10 ng/mL.

When any of the above-described techniques are used for other indications to image structures in the cervical region, thyroid nodules are commonly detected incidentally. Studies indicate that the prevalence of thyroid cancer in such thyroid incidentalomas is the same as in palpable nodules, so they should usually be biopsied if greater than 1.0 to 1.5 cm in diameter, and monitored by serial ultrasound if smaller. PET incidentalomas, in particular, should be thoroughly evaluated; as some studies have shown that as many as two-thirds of these hypermetabolic lesions have been found to be cancers.

THYROID BIOPSY

Fine-needle aspiration biopsy (FNAB) of a thyroid nodule is the best method for differentiating benign from malignant thyroid nodules and diffuse goiters. FNAB is a minor outpatient procedure performed in awake, nonfasting patients with appropriate aseptic technique; local anesthesia may or may not be required. The procedure is typically performed with a 27- or 25-gauge needle, which is inserted into the nodule or goiter, and moved in

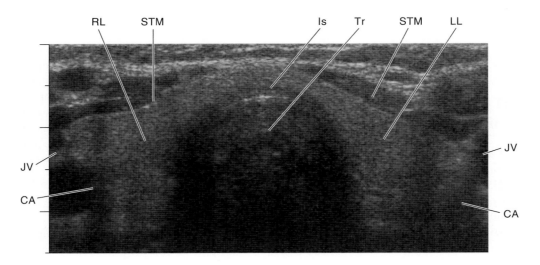

FIGURE 7–27 Ultrasound of the normal thyroid gland. (Tr, trachea; LL, left lobe of thyroid; RL, right lobe of thyroid; Is, isthmus; CA, carotid artery; JV, jugular vein; STM, sternothyroid muscle.) (Courtesy of Dr. R.A. Filly)

and out until a small amount of bloody material is seen in the hub of the needle. The aspirated material is then expressed onto a glass slide and prepared as a thin smear, which is either air-dried for immediate staining and preliminarily assessed, or placed in fixative for definitive staining and cytopathologic assessment. FNAB can also be useful to evacuate cystic lesions, although the fluid will recollect in one-half of these cysts.

Cytologic diagnosis of malignancy in thyroid nodules is highly accurate. The sensitivity (true-positive diagnoses divided by total number of nodules proven to be cancer by surgery) is 95% to 98%, and the specificity (true-negative results divided by total number of cases without disease) is also 95%.

TEST OF PERIPHERAL THYROID HORMONE ACTIONS

Theoretically, the most definitive test of thyroid function would be a method of quantifying thyroid hormone responses in peripheral tissues. In practice, however, these tests have limited accuracy because the response parameters may be imprecisely quantified (eg, ankle reflex relaxation time) or because they are also modulated by nonthyroidal factors (eg, serum cholesterol and echocardiographic systolic time intervals). Nonetheless, these techniques are useful in clinical research and in assessment of rare patients suspected of having resistance to thyroid hormone action.

Basal oxygen consumption reflects thyroid hormones' effects on oxygen consumption and calorigenesis in most body tissues, especially the liver. There is considerable overlap between the measured levels in hypothyroidism, euthyroidism, and hyperthyroidism. Echocardiography can be used to assess systolic and diastolic functions, both of which are altered with thyroid dysfunction; but this is exclusively a research technique.

Thyroid hormones influence the concentrations of a number of analytes in blood. For example, serum total and LDL cholesterol is usually elevated in hypothyroidism and lowered in hyperthyroidism. In hyperthyroidism, sex hormone–binding globulin, ferritin, and angiotensin-converting enzyme concentrations are often higher, as are markers of bone formation and degradation. However, none of these test results is sensitive or specific enough for routine diagnostic use.

MEASUREMENT OF THYROID AUTOANTIBODIES

Detection of thyroid autoantibodies can be helpful in establishing the diagnosis of autoimmune thyroid disease. To establish the diagnosis of autoimmune (Hashimoto) thyroiditis in a patient with diffuse goiter or hypothyroidism, serum anti-TPO or the less sensitive antithyroglobulin antibodies can be employed. An older test, antimicrosomal antibodies has intermediate sensitivity. Anti-TPO and antithyroglobulin antibodies can be measured by hemagglutination, enzyme-linked immunosorbent assay (ELISA), or RIA; RIA is more sensitive, precisely quantifiable, and generally preferred. Although these antibodies are most typical of autoimmune thyroiditis, they are also detected in significant proportions of patients with Graves disease. Due to their high prevalence in the population, especially in women, a positive result does not rule out presence of a second thyroid disorder (eg, cancer in an asymmetrical goiter).

TSH receptor stimulating, binding, and blocking antibodies can all be detected. Thyroid-stimulating immunoglobulin (TSI) is present in approximately 90% of patients with Graves disease and is almost never detected in unaffected patients or those with other autoimmune thyroid diseases. The test is performed by isolating the patient's immunoglobulins from a serum sample, exposing cultured thyroid cells to these antibodies, and then measuring their cAMP response in comparison with reference TSI and TSH standards. TSI testing is used in a few special settings: (1) pregnant women to define risk of subsequent neonatal hyperthyroidism in their fetus and neonate; (2) to differentiate Graves disease from postpartum thyroiditis in women who are breast feeding and cannot have a radionuclide thyroid uptake; and (3) to make the diagnosis of Graves disease in euthyroid patients with apparent thyroid-related ophthalmopathy. Some have advocated use of TSI to predict whether antithyroid drug-treated Graves patients will relapse when drug is later discontinued; however, its prognostic accuracy for this purpose is limited. TSH receptor–binding immunoglobulins can also be detected by in vitro demonstration that circulating immunoglobulins compete with radiolabeled TSH in binding to recombinant TSH receptors. It is a simpler and more sensitive alternative for the TSI indications described earlier, but does not distinguish between stimulating and blocking anti-TSH receptor antibodies. TSH receptor blocking antibodies have been implicated as the cause of hypothyroidism in a minority of hypothyroid patients in certain populations; they can also be transmitted transplacentally to the fetus and inhibit thyroid function during pregnancy and in the neonatal period.

DISORDERS OF THE THYROID

Patients with thyroid disease usually complain of one or more of the following: (1) thyroid enlargement, which may be diffuse or nodular; (2) symptoms of thyroid hormone deficiency, or hypothyroidism; (3) symptoms of thyroid hormone excess, or hyperthyroidism; or (4) complications of a specific form of hyperthyroidism—Graves disease—that may present with striking prominence of the eyes (exophthalmos) and, rarely, thickening of the skin over the lower legs (thyroid dermopathy or pretibial myxedema). Patients with thyroid nodules, whether benign or malignant, often have no symptoms, as do persons with mild perturbations of thyroid function.

History

The history should include evaluation of symptoms related to the above complaints, discussed in more detail later. Exposure to ionizing radiation in childhood has been associated with an increased incidence of thyroid disease, including cancer. Iodide ingestion in the form of amiodarone, an iodine-containing antiarrhythmic drug, or intravenous iodide-containing contrast media used in angiography or CT scanning may induce hypothyroidism or hyperthyroidism. Lithium carbonate, used in the treatment of bipolar disorder, can also induce hypothyroidism and goiter and possibly hyperthyroidism. Residence in an area of low dietary iodide is associated with iodine deficiency goiter (endemic goiter). Although dietary iodide is generally adequate in developed countries, there are still over 2 billion people with iodine-deficient diets in developing countries in Africa, Asia, South America, and inland mountainous areas in Europe. Finally, the family history should be explored with particular reference to goiter, hyperthyroidism, hypothyroidism, or thyroid cancer as well as immunologic disorders such as Type 1 diabetes, rheumatoid disease, pernicious anemia, alopecia, vitiligo, or myasthenia gravis, which may be associated with an increased incidence of autoimmune thyroid disease. Multiple endocrine neoplasia types 2A (Sipple syndrome) and 2B with medullary carcinoma of the thyroid gland are autosomal dominant conditions.

Physical Examination

Physical examination of the thyroid gland is illustrated in Figure 7–28. The thyroid is firmly attached to the anterior trachea midway between the sternal notch and the thyroid cartilage; it is often easy to see and to palpate. The patient should have a glass of water for comfortable swallowing. There are three maneuvers:

(1) With a good light coming from behind the examiner, the patient is instructed to swallow a sip of water. Observe the gland as it moves up and down. Enlargement and nodularity can often be noted.
(2) Palpate the gland anteriorly with swallowing. The thumb placed anteriorly along the trachea allows localization of the isthmus and connected lobes, as well as the pyramidal lobe, which extends superiorly from the isthmus and is often palpable in patients with autoimmune thyroid disease.
(3) Then, the examiner's right hand is placed on the patient's left shoulder, and the examiner's right thumb is used to palpate the left lobe, as the patient swallows. This permits a full appreciation of the size, texture, and contour of the lobe. Then, using the left hand, the right lobe can be palpated. The examiner's thumbs should be medial to the sternocleidomastoid muscles to avoid mistaking them for the thyroid lobes. Some experts recommend palpation from behind using three fingers to palpate each lobe while the patient swallows, but this technique has the disadvantage of not being able to see the gland during palpation.

Normally, the thyroid is just barely palpable, has a smooth surface, and has a soft to rubbery consistency. The palpable bulbous portion of each lobe of the normal thyroid gland measures about 2 cm in vertical dimension and about 1 cm in horizontal dimension above the isthmus. An enlarged thyroid gland is called a **goiter**. Generalized enlargement is termed **diffuse goiter**; irregular or lumpy enlargement is called **nodular goiter**. In Hashimoto thyroiditis, the gland is often symmetrically enlarged, firm, and has a bosselated (cobblestone) or finely nodular surface. In the atrophic form of Hashimoto thyroiditis, the gland may not be palpable at all. In patients with Graves disease, the gland is usually, but not always, symmetrically enlarged and smooth and rubbery in consistency. Multinodular goiters have one or more distinct nodules palpable, although both small and large and nodules are often not palpable because of their location or consistency. Tenderness of the gland should be noted. In patients with Graves disease, the presence of a bruit by auscultation should be sought, and a thrill may be palpated over the gland. Tracheal deviation by a goiter, cervical lymphadenopathy possibly related to thyroid cancer, and jugular venous distention and facial erythema from thoracic inlet obstruction by a large goiter should be noted as well. An outline of the gland can be traced on the skin of the neck and measured (Figure 7–28D). Nodules can be measured in a similar way. Thus, changes in the size of the gland or in nodules can easily be followed.

HYPOTHYROIDISM

Hypothyroidism is a clinical syndrome resulting from a deficiency of thyroid hormones, which in turn results in a generalized slowing down of metabolic processes. Hypothyroidism in infants and children results in marked slowing of growth and development, with serious permanent consequences, including mental retardation, when it occurs in infancy. Hypothyroidism with onset in adulthood causes a generalized decrease in metabolism, with slowed heart rate, diminished oxygen consumption, and deposition of glycosaminoglycans in intracellular spaces, particularly in skin and muscle, producing in extreme cases the clinical picture of **myxedema**. The symptoms and signs of hypothyroidism in adults are reversible with therapy.

Etiology and Incidence (Table 7–6)

Hypothyroidism may be classified as (1) primary (thyroid failure) (by far the most common), (2) secondary (due to pituitary TSH deficiency), or (3) tertiary (due to hypothalamic deficiency of TRH)—or may be due to (4) peripheral resistance to the action of thyroid hormones. Hypothyroidism can also be classified as goitrous or nongoitrous, but this classification is probably unsatisfactory, because Hashimoto thyroiditis (autoimmune thyroiditis) may produce hypothyroidism with or without goiter.

The incidence of various causes of hypothyroidism varies depending on geographic and environmental factors, such as dietary iodide and goitrogen intake, the genetic characteristics of the population, and the age distribution of the population (pediatric or adult). The causes of hypothyroidism, listed in approximate order of frequency in the United States, are presented in Table 7–6. Hashimoto thyroiditis is by far the most common cause of hypothyroidism in the developed world. In younger patients, it is more likely to be associated with goiter; in older patients, the gland may be totally destroyed by the immunologic process, and the only trace of the disease is a persistently positive test for TPO antibodies. Similarly, the end-stage of Graves disease may be hypothyroidism, occurring spontaneously or following destructive therapy with radioactive iodine or thyroidectomy.

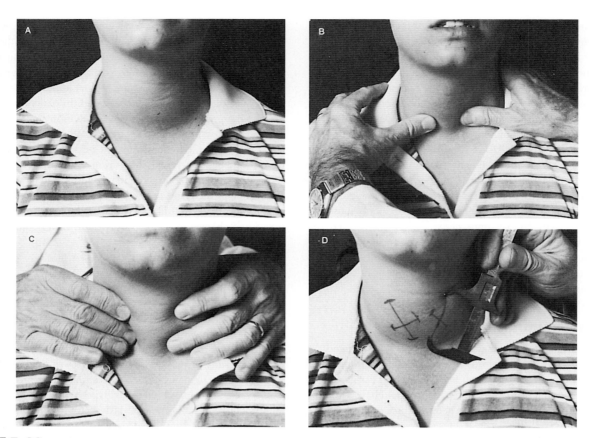

FIGURE 7–28 Examination of the thyroid gland. **A.** Observe the neck, especially as the patient swallows. **B.** Examine from the front, rotating the gland slightly with one thumb while palpating the other lobe with the other thumb. **C.** Examine from behind, using three fingers and the same technique. **D.** The size of each lobe or of thyroid nodules can be measured by first drawing an outline on the skin.

TABLE 7–6 Etiology of hypothyroidism.

Primary:
1. Hashimoto thyroiditis:
   a. With goiter
   b. "Idiopathic" thyroid atrophy, presumably end-stage autoimmune thyroid disease, following either Hashimoto thyroiditis or Graves disease
   c. Neonatal hypothyroidism due to placental transmission of TSH-R blocking antibodies
2. Radioactive iodine therapy for Graves disease
3. Subtotal thyroidectomy for Graves disease, nodular goiter, or thyroid cancer
4. Excessive iodide intake (kelp, radiocontrast dyes)
5. Subacute thyroiditis (usually transient)
6. Iodide deficiency (rare in North America)
7. Inborn errors of thyroid hormone synthesis
8. Drugs
   a. Lithium
   b. Interferon-alfa
   c. Amiodarone

Secondary: Hypopituitarism due to pituitary adenoma, pituitary ablative therapy, or pituitary destruction
Tertiary: Hypothalamic dysfunction (rare)
Peripheral resistance to the action of thyroid hormone

Thyroid glands involved in autoimmune disease are particularly susceptible to excessive iodide intake (eg, ingestion of kelp tablets, iodide-containing cough preparations, or the antiarrhythmic drug amiodarone) or intravenous administration of iodide-containing radiographic contrast media. Large amounts of iodide block thyroid hormone synthesis via the Wolff-Chaikoff effect (see earlier), producing iodine-induced hypothyroidism with goiter in the patient with an abnormal thyroid gland; the normal gland *escapes* from the Wolff-Chaikoff effect or iodide block, but for unclear reasons autoimmunity renders the gland more sensitive to the inhibitory effects of iodine. Hypothyroidism may occur during the late phase of subacute thyroiditis or silent thyroiditis; this is usually transient, but it may be permanent especially in silent thyroiditis, where permanent hypothyroidism occurs in about 25% of patients. Iodine deficiency is not a cause of hypothyroidism in the United States, but it is still frequently seen in developing countries, and is the most common cause of hypothyroidism world wide. Certain drugs can block hormone synthesis and produce hypothyroidism with goiter; at present, the most common pharmacologic causes of hypothyroidism (other than iodide) are lithium carbonate, used for the treatment of bipolar disease, and amiodarone. Chronic therapy of hyperthyroidism with the anti-thyroid drugs PTU and methimazole have the same effects. Interferon alfa, used to treat hepatitis C and other conditions, can cause altered immunity that can result in hypothyroidism due to Hashimoto thyroiditis. Inborn errors of thyroid hormone synthesis, called thyroid dyshormonogenesis, result from genetic deficiencies in enzymes necessary for hormone biosynthesis. These effects may be complete, resulting in a syndrome of severe congenital hypothyroidism (cretinism) with goiter; or partial, resulting in goiter with milder hypothyroidism. At least five separate biosynthetic abnormalities have been reported: (1) impaired transport of iodine; (2) deficient thyroid peroxidase with impaired oxidation of iodide to iodine and failure to incorporate iodine into thyroglobulin; (3) impaired coupling of iodinated tyrosines to triiodothyronine or tetraiodothyronine; (4) absence or deficiency of iodotyrosine deiodinase, so that iodine is not conserved within the gland; and (5) excessive production of metabolically inactive iodoprotein by the thyroid gland (see Figure 7–6). The latter may involve impaired or abnormal thyroglobulin synthesis.

Pituitary and hypothalamic deficiencies as causes of hypothyroidism are quite rare and are usually associated with other symptoms and signs of pituitary insufficiency (Chapter 4). Peripheral resistance to thyroid hormones is discussed later.

Pathogenesis

Thyroid hormone deficiency affects virtually every tissue in the body, so that the symptoms are multiple. Pathologically, the most characteristic finding is the accumulation of glycosaminoglycans—mostly hyaluronic acid—in interstitial tissues. Accumulation of this hydrophilic substance and increased capillary permeability to albumin account for the interstitial nonpitting edema that is particularly evident in the skin, heart muscle, and striated muscle. The accumulation is due not to excessive synthesis but to decreased metabolism of glycosaminoglycans.

Clinical Presentations and Findings

A. Newborn infants (cretinism)   The term cretinism was originally applied to infants born in areas of severe iodine deficiency with mental retardation, short stature, a characteristic puffy appearance of the face and hands, and (frequently) deaf mutism and neurologic signs of pyramidal and extrapyramidal tract abnormalities. In the United States, neonatal screening programs have revealed that in the Caucasian population the prevalence of sporadic neonatal hypothyroidism is 1:5000, whereas in the African American population the prevalence is only 1:32,000. In areas of iodine sufficiency, neonatal hypothyroidism typically results from failure of the thyroid to descend during embryonic development from its origin at the base of the tongue to its usual site in the lower anterior neck, resulting in an absent or *ectopic thyroid* gland that functions poorly. Placental transfer to the embryo of blocking anti-TSH receptor antibodies from a mother with Hashimoto thyroiditis may result in agenesis of the thyroid gland and athyreotic cretinism, but usually it only causes transient hypothyroidism. Inherited defects in thyroid hormone biosynthesis may also cause neonatal hypothyroidism and goiter. Other possible causes of neonatal hypothyroidism include exposure during pregnancy to iodides, antithyroid drugs given to the mother, or inadvertent administration of radioactive iodine for thyrotoxicosis or thyroid cancer.

The signs of hypothyroidism in newborns include respiratory difficulty, cyanosis, jaundice, poor feeding, hoarse cry, umbilical hernia, and marked retardation of bone maturation. The proximal tibial epiphysis and distal femoral epiphysis are present in almost all full-term infants with a body weight over 2500 g. Absence of these epiphyses strongly suggests hypothyroidism. The introduction of routine screening of newborns for TSH or T_4 in the developed world has been a major public health achievement, because early diagnosis can prevent permanent mental retardation. A drop of blood obtained by heel stick 24 to 48 hours after birth is placed on filter paper and sent to a central laboratory. A serum T_4 under 6 μg/dL or a serum TSH over 25 mU/L is suggestive of neonatal hypothyroidism. The diagnosis can then be confirmed by repeat testing and radiologic evidence of retarded bone age. Note that euthyroid infants born to hypothyroid mothers who have been inadequately treated with levothyroxine during pregnancy are not hypothyroid, but may have diminished intellectual potential later in childhood—emphasizing the importance of maintaining the mother in a euthyroid state throughout pregnancy.

B. Children and adolescents   Hypothyroidism in children and adolescents is characterized by retarded growth and short stature, the typical signs and symptoms of hypothyroidism seen in adults (see later), and variable but usually declining school performance. Precocious puberty may occur, and there may be enlargement of the sella turcica due to pituitary thyrotrope hyperplasia associated with augmented TSH production.

C. Adults   In adults, the common features of moderate to severe hypothyroidism include easy fatigability; cold sensitivity; weight gain (generally <10-20 lb); constipation; menstrual abnormalities, especially menorrhagia; and muscle cramps. Physical findings may include a cool, rough, dry skin; puffy face and hands; a hoarse, husky voice; and slow reflexes. Reduced conversion of carotene to vitamin A and increased blood levels of carotene may give the skin a yellowish color. However, many or all of the symptoms and signs are diminished or absent in patients with milder degrees of thyroid failure.

1. **Cardiovascular signs**—Hypothyroidism is manifested by impaired ventricular contraction, bradycardia, and increased peripheral resistance, resulting in diminished cardiac output. The electrocardiogram (ECG) may reveal low voltage of QRS complexes and P and T waves, with improvement in response to therapy. Cardiac enlargement may occur, due in part to interstitial edema, nonspecific myofibrillary swelling, and left ventricular dilation, as well as nonhemodynamically significant pericardial effusion (Figure 7–29). The degree of pericardial effusion can easily be determined by echocardiography. Although cardiac output is reduced, congestive heart failure and pulmonary edema are rarely noted. There is controversy about whether

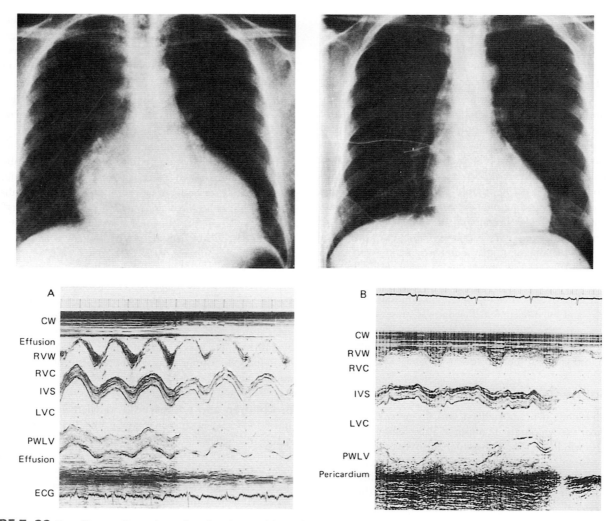

FIGURE 7–29 **Top.** Chest radiograph studies of patient with hypothyroid cardiomyopathy. **Left.** Before therapy, showing pronounced cardiomegaly. **Right.** Six months after institution of thyroxine therapy, the heart size has returned to normal. (Reproduced, with permission, from Reza MJ, Abbasi AS. Congestive cardiomyopathy in hypothyroidism. *West J Med*. 1975;123:228.)
Bottom. Echocardiogram of a 29-year-old woman with hypothyroidism **(A)** before and **(B)** after 2 months of therapy with levothyroxine sodium. Note disappearance of pericardial effusion following levothyroxine therapy. (CW, chest wall; RVW, right ventricular wall; RVC, right ventricular cavity; IVS, inter-ventricular septum; LVC, left ventricular cavity; PWLV, posterior wall left ventricle.)Reproduced, with permission, from Sokolow M, McIlroy MB. *Clinical Cardiology*. 4th ed. McGraw-Hill; 1986.

hypothyroidism induces coronary artery disease, but coronary artery disease is more common in patients with hypothyroidism, likely related to increased levels of total cholesterol, LDL cholesterol, and possibly other nontraditional atherogenic factors such as lipoprotein A and homocysteine. In patients with angina pectoris, hypothyroidism may protect the heart from ischemic stress, and replacement therapy may aggravate the angina by increasing myocardial oxygen consumption.

2. **Pulmonary function**—In the adult, hypothyroidism is characterized by shallow, slow respirations and impaired ventilatory responses to hypercapnia or hypoxia. Respiratory failure is a major problem in patients with myxedema coma (see later).

3. **Intestinal peristalsis**—Peristalsis is markedly slowed, resulting in chronic constipation and occasionally severe fecal impaction or ileus.

4. **Renal function**—Renal function is impaired, with decreased glomerular filtration rate and impaired ability to excrete a water load. This predisposes the hypothyroid patient to hyponatremia from water intoxication if excessive free water is administered.

5. **Anemia**—There are at least four mechanisms that may contribute to anemia in patients with hypothyroidism: (1) impaired hemoglobin synthesis as a result of thyroxine deficiency; (2) iron deficiency from increased iron loss with menorrhagia, as well as impaired intestinal absorption of iron; (3) folate deficiency from impaired intestinal absorption of folic acid; and (4) pernicious anemia, with vitamin B_{12}-deficient megaloblastic anemia. Pernicious anemia is often part of a cluster of autoimmune diseases, including hypothyroidism due to Hashimoto or autoimmune thyroiditis associated

with thyroid autoantibodies, pernicious anemia associated with parietal cell autoantibodies, diabetes mellitus associated with islet cell autoantibodies, and adrenal insufficiency associated with adrenal autoantibodies (Schmidt syndrome; see Chapter 2). These conditions are part of what has been termed the **polyglandular failure syndrome**.

6. **Neuromuscular system**—Many patients complain of symptoms referable to the neuromuscular system, including severe muscle cramps, paresthesias, and muscle weakness.

7. **Central nervous system**—Symptoms may include chronic fatigue, lethargy, and inability to concentrate. Patients with hypothyroidism are usually quite placid but can be severely depressed or even extremely agitated (myxedema madness).

8. **Reproductive system**—Hypothyroidism impairs the conversion of estrogen precursors to estrogens, resulting in altered FSH and LH secretion and in anovulatory cycles and infertility. This may be associated with menorrhagia, which may also be due, in part, to altered platelet function. Men may have decreased libido and erectile dysfunction.

Diagnosis

The combination of a low serum FT_4 and an elevated serum TSH is diagnostic of primary hypothyroidism (Figure 7–30). Serum T_3 levels are variable and may be within the normal range. Commonly, the serum FT_4 is normal or low-normal, and the serum TSH is elevated slightly, a situation termed **subclinical hypothyroidism**. This represents the mildest form of hypothyroidism and is a consequence of the very sensitive feedback relationship between the thyroid and the pituitary gland. In this situation, a small decrement in thyroid hormone output by the thyroid gland, in which serum T_4 levels are still within the normal range, results in a serum TSH level that is elevated, albeit usually less than 10 mU/L. Subclinical hypothyroidism is usually due to underlying Hashimoto thyroiditis, which can be confirmed by assessing anti-TPO antibody titers. In patients with secondary or central hypothyroidism, the serum FT_4 will be low and serum TSH will be low or normal, rather than elevated.

The patient may be taking thyroid hormone (T_4 tablets) when first seen. A palpable or enlarged thyroid gland and a positive test for thyroid autoantibodies would suggest underlying Hashimoto thyroiditis, in which case the medication should be continued. If antithyroid antibodies are absent and the indication for therapy is uncertain, the medication could be withdrawn for 6 weeks and determination made for FT_4 and TSH. The 6-week period of withdrawal is necessary because of the long half-life of T_4 (7 days) and to allow the pituitary gland to recover after a long period of suppression. The pattern of recovery of thyroid function after withdrawal of T_4 is noted in Figure 7–31. In hypothyroid individuals, serum TSH becomes elevated at 5 to 6 weeks and FT_4 remains subnormal, whereas both are normal after 6 weeks in euthyroid individuals.

The clinical picture of fully developed myxedema is usually quite clear, but the symptoms and signs of mild or subclinical hypothyroidism may be very subtle or absent. This has led to the recommendation by some professional organizations that screening for hypothyroidism be undertaken, especially in high-risk groups, such as older women where the prevalence is high (up to 20% in women >age 65), and in pregnant women, where untreated hypothyroidism may cause adverse outcomes in the child.

At times, patients with hypothyroidism present with unusual features: neurasthenia with symptoms of muscle cramps, paresthesias, and weakness; refractory anemia; disturbances in reproductive function, including infertility, delayed or precocious puberty, or menorrhagia; idiopathic edema or pleuropericardial effusions; retarded growth; obstipation; chronic rhinitis or hoarseness due to edema of nasal mucosa or vocal cords; and severe depression progressing to emotional instability or even frank paranoid psychosis. In the elderly, hypothyroidism may present with apathy and withdrawal, often attributed to senility (Chapter 23). In such cases, assessing thyroid function with serum FT_4 and TSH measurements confirms or rules out hypothyroidism as a contributing factor.

Complications

A. Myxedema coma   Myxedema coma, an extremely rare condition, is the end stage of untreated hypothyroidism (see also Chapter 24). It is characterized by progressive weakness, stupor, hypothermia, hypoventilation, hypoglycemia, and hyponatremia, and it may ultimately result in shock and death. It occurs most frequently in the winter in older female patients with underlying pulmonary and vascular disease, and the mortality rate may be greater than 50%.

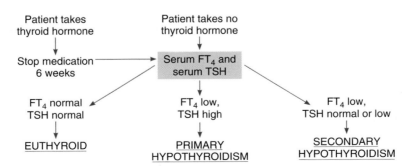

FIGURE 7–30 Diagnosis of hypothyroidism.

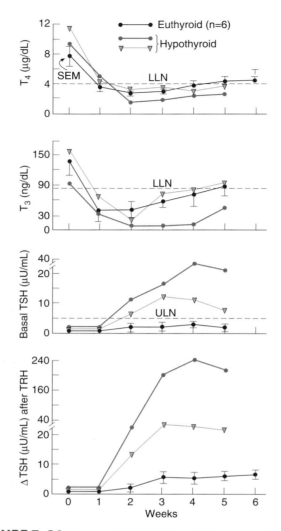

FIGURE 7–31 Changes in T_4, T_3, TSH, and TRH response following abrupt withdrawal of suppressive thyroxine therapy. Note that in euthyroid individuals, the T_4 may not return to normal until 6 weeks after withdrawal of therapy and that serum TSH is never elevated. In hypothyroid patients, TSH may be elevated as early as 2 weeks after withdrawal of therapy, and TRH response is exaggerated. (LLN, lower limit of normal; ULN, upper limit of normal). (Reproduced, with permission, from Wood LC. Controversial questions in thyroid disease. Workshop in the Thyroid, American Thyroid Association, Nov 1979, as adapted from Vagenakis AG, et al. Recovery of pituitary thyrotropic function after withdrawal of prolonged thyroid suppression therapy. *N Engl J Med*. 1975;293:681.)

The patient (or a family member if the patient is comatose) may recall previous thyroid disease, radioiodine or radiation therapy to the neck area, or thyroidectomy. The medical history is one of gradual onset of lethargy progressing to stupor or coma. Examination reveals bradycardia and marked hypothermia, with body temperature as low as 24°C (75°F). The patient is usually an obese elderly woman with yellowish skin, a hoarse voice, a large tongue, thin hair, puffy eyes, ileus, and slow reflexes. There may be signs of other illnesses such as pneumonia, myocardial

infarction, cerebral thrombosis, or gastrointestinal bleeding. Seizures, bleeding episodes, hypocalcemia, or hypercalcemia may occur. Laboratory clues to the diagnosis of myxedema coma include lactescent serum, high serum carotene, elevated serum cholesterol, and increased cerebrospinal fluid protein. Pleural, pericardial, or abdominal effusions with high protein content may be present. Serum tests reveal a low FT_4 and a markedly elevated TSH. Thyroid autoantibodies are usually strongly positive, indicating underlying Hashimoto thyroiditis. The ECG shows sinus bradycardia and low voltage. If laboratory studies are not immediately available, which is frequently the case, the diagnosis must be made clinically.

The pathophysiology of myxedema coma involves three major features: (1) CO_2 retention and hypoxia, (2) fluid and electrolyte imbalance, and (3) hypothermia. CO_2 retention and hypoxia are probably due in large part to a marked depression in the ventilatory responses to hypoxia and hypercapnia, although factors such as obesity, heart failure, ileus, immobilization, pneumonia, pleural or peritoneal effusions, central nervous system depression, and weak chest muscles may also contribute. Impairment of ventilatory drive is often severe, and assisted respiration is almost always necessary in patients with myxedema coma. Thyroid hormone therapy in patients with myxedema corrects the hypothermia and improves the ventilatory response to hypoxia. Water intoxication, due to reduced renal perfusion and impaired free water clearance, is the major fluid and electrolyte disturbance. This causes hyponatremia and is best managed by free water restriction. Hypothermia is frequently not recognized, because the ordinary clinical thermometer only goes down to about 34°C (93°F); a thermometer that registers a broader scale must be used to obtain accurate body temperature readings. Active rewarming of the body is contraindicated, because it may induce vasodilation and vascular collapse. A rise in body temperature is a useful indication of therapeutic effectiveness of T_4 therapy.

Disorders that may precipitate myxedema coma include heart failure, pneumonia, or administration of sedative or narcotic drugs to a patient with severe hypothyroidism. Adrenal insufficiency may occur occasionally in association with myxedema coma, either due to functional pituitary impairment or concurrent autoimmune adrenal insufficiency (Schmidt syndrome). Concomitant glucocorticoid therapy is recommended until normal adrenal function can be documented by laboratory testing. It is important to differentiate myxedema coma due to primary thyroid gland failure from that due to pituitary failure (central hypothyroidism). In the latter situation, glucocorticoid replacement is essential. Clinical clues to the presence of pituitary disease include the following: a history of amenorrhea or impotence, scanty pubic or axillary hair, and normal serum cholesterol and normal or low serum TSH levels. CT or MRI may reveal an enlarged sella turcica. The treatment of myxedema coma is discussed later.

B. Hypothyroidism and heart disease   In the past, treatment of patients with severe hypothyroidism and heart disease, particularly coronary artery disease, was very difficult, because levothyroxine replacement was sometimes associated with exacerbation of angina, heart failure, or myocardial infarction. Now that β-adrenergic blocking agents, coronary angioplasty, and coronary artery bypass surgery are available, hypothyroid patients with coronary artery disease can be treated medically or surgically first, and thyroxine replacement therapy is then better tolerated.

C. Hypothyroidism and neuropsychiatric disease

Hypothyroidism is often associated with depression, which may be quite severe. More rarely, severely hypothyroid patients may become confused, paranoid, or even manic (myxedema madness). Screening of psychiatric admissions with serum FT_4 and TSH is an efficient way to identify these patients, who frequently respond to T_4 therapy alone or in combination with psychopharmacologic agents. The effectiveness of T_4 therapy in depressed hypothyroid patients has given rise to the hypothesis that the addition of T_3 or T_4 to psychotherapeutic regimens for depression may be helpful in patients without demonstrable thyroid disease, but this concept has been difficult to prove.

Treatment

A. Treatment of hypothyroidism

Hypothyroidism is treated with T_4, which is available in pure form and is stable and inexpensive. Because T_4 is converted to T_3 in peripheral tissues, both hormones become available, even though only one is administered. Desiccated thyroid is now considered obsolete because it contains both T_4 and T_3, and triiodothyronine (as liothyronine) is unsatisfactory because of its rapid absorption, short half-life, and transient effects. The half-life of T_4 is about 7 days, so it needs to be given only once daily. It is well absorbed, and blood levels are easily monitored by following FT_4 and serum TSH levels. T_4 and T_3 levels are stable throughout the day, although there is a slight increase in free T_4 levels several hours after the medication is taken; this is not clinically significant.

B. Dosage of levothyroxine

Replacement doses of T_4 in adults range from 0.05 to 0.2 mg/d, with a mean of about 0.125 mg/d. The dose of T_4 varies according to the patient's age and body weight (Table 7–7). Because of more rapid T_4 metabolism, infants and young children require a surprisingly high dose of T_4 compared with adults. In adults, the mean replacement dose of T_4 is about 1.7 µg/kg/d, or about 0.8 µg/lb/d. In older adults,

the replacement dose is usually lower, about 1.6 µg/kg/d, or about 0.7 µg/lb/d. For TSH suppression in patients post-thyroidectomy for thyroid cancer, the average dose of T_4 is about 2.2 µg/kg/d (1 µg/lb/d). In most patients with hypothyroidism, one can begin treatment with the full estimated dose requirement. After 4 to 6 weeks, the final dose is adjusted based on the serum TSH level. The goal is to normalize the serum TSH, which is typically between 0.5 and 4 mU/L. In older patients or patients with underlying heart disease, it is best to start with a low dose of T_4 (eg, 0.025 mg daily) and increase the dose at 4- to 6-week intervals based on serum TSH measurements. Malabsorptive states or concurrent administration of soy products, aluminum hydroxide antacids, bile acid–binding resins such as cholestyramine and colestipol, calcium supplements, sucralfate, or iron compounds decrease T_4 absorption. In these patients, T_4 should be given before breakfast, when the stomach is empty, and the other compounds taken 4 hours later. Other drugs, such as the antiseizure medication carbamazepine, may increase thyroid hormone requirements by increasing T_4 metabolism. Proton pump inhibitors such as omeprazole may also impair T_4 absorption, possibly by decreasing gastric acid, but data on this point are conflicting. Estrogen replacement may increase T_4 requirements by increased binding of free T_4 to TBG, whereas androgen therapy has the opposite effect. T_4 has a sufficiently long half-life (7 days), so that if the patient is unable to take medications by mouth for a few days, omitting T_4 therapy will not be detrimental. If a hospitalized patient is being managed by sustained parenteral therapy, the parenteral dose of T_4 is about 75% to 80% of the usual oral dose.

C. Treatment of myxedema coma

Myxedema coma is an acute medical emergency and should be treated in the intensive care unit. Blood gases must be monitored regularly, and the patient usually requires intubation and mechanical ventilation. Associated illnesses such as infections or heart failure must be sought for and appropriately treated. Intravenous fluids should be administered with caution, and excessive free water intake must be avoided. Because patients with myxedema coma may absorb drugs poorly, it is imperative to give T_4 intravenously. These patients have marked total body depletion, and they should receive an initial loading dose of 300 to 400 µg of T_4 intravenously followed by 80% of the calculated full replacement dose intravenously daily. Management of patients with known or suspected heart disease is described later. If, after a few days, the clinical response has been suboptimal, some experts recommend adding intravenous T_3 to the regimen at a dose of 5 µg every 6 hours. The clinical guides to improvement are a rise in body temperature and the return of normal cerebral and respiratory function. The possibility of concomitant adrenal insufficiency (due to autoimmune adrenal disease or pituitary insufficiency) needs to be considered and ruled out with a cosyntropin stimulation test (see Chapter 9). Full adrenal support should then be administered (eg, hydrocortisone hemisuccinate) 100 mg intravenously, followed by 50 mg intravenously every 6 hours, tapering the dose over 7 days. Adrenal support can be withdrawn if the pretreatment plasma cortisol is 20 µg/dL or greater or if results of a cosyntropin stimulation test are within normal limits. When giving T_4 intravenously

TABLE 7–7 Replacement doses of levothyroxine.

Age	Dose of Levothyroxine (µg/kg/d)
0-6 mo	10-15
7-11 mo	6-8
1-5 y	5-6
6-10 y	4-5
11-20 y	1-3
Adult	1-2

Adapted and modified, with permission, from Foley TP Jr. Congenital hypothyroidism. In Braverman LE, Utiger RD: *Werner and Ingbar's The Thyroid.* 7th ed. Lippincott; 1996.

in large doses, there is an inherent risk of precipitating angina, heart failure, or arrhythmias in older patients with underlying coronary artery disease.

At one time, the mortality rate of myxedema coma was about 80%. The prognosis has been vastly improved as a result of recognition of the importance of mechanically assisted respiration and the use of intravenous T_4. At present, the outcome probably depends on how well the underlying comorbidities and consequences of severe hypothyroidism can be managed.

D. Myxedema with heart disease In older patients—particularly those with known cardiovascular disease—it is wise to start treatment slowly. T_4 is given in a dosage of 0.025 mg/d for 2 to 4 weeks, increasing by 0.025 mg every 2 to 4 weeks until a daily dose of 0.075 mg is reached. This dose is continued for about 6 weeks. Serum TSH is then measured and the dosage adjusted accordingly. It typically takes 2 to 4 months for a patient to come into equilibrium on full dosage. In some patients, the heart is very sensitive to the level of circulating T_4, and if angina pectoris or cardiac arrhythmia develops, it is essential to reduce the dose of T_4 immediately.

Adverse Effects of T_4 Therapy

There are no reported instances of allergy to pure T_4, although it is possible that a patient may develop an allergy to the coloring dye or some component of the tablet. The major toxic effects of T_4 overdosage are symptoms and signs of hyperthyroidism. Palpitations are the most common thyrotoxic cardiac symptom, and arrhythmias, particularly paroxysmal atrial tachycardia or fibrillation, may occur. Insomnia, tremor, restlessness, and excessive warmth may also be troublesome. Simply omitting the daily dose of T_4 for 3 days and then reducing the dosage will correct the problem.

Increased bone resorption and osteoporosis have been associated with long-standing hyperthyroidism and will also develop in postmenopausal women chronically overtreated with T_4. This can be prevented by regular monitoring and by maintaining normal serum TSH levels in patients receiving long-term replacement therapy. In patients receiving TSH-suppressive therapy for thyroid cancer, if serum FT_4 levels are kept in the upper range of normal—even if TSH is suppressed—the adverse effects of T_4 therapy on bone will be minimal (Chapter 23). In addition, concomitant administration of estrogen or bisphosphonates to postmenopausal women receiving high-dose T_4 therapy minimizes bone resorption.

Course and Prognosis

The course of untreated hypothyroidism is one of slow deterioration, potentially leading eventually to myxedema coma and death. With appropriate treatment, however, the long-term prognosis is excellent. Because of the long half-life (7 days) of T_4, it takes time to establish equilibrium on a fixed dose. Therefore, it is important to monitor the serum FT_4 and TSH every 4 to 6 weeks until equilibrium is reached. Thereafter, FT_4 and TSH can be monitored once in every 6 to 12 months. The dose of T_4 is increased by about

TABLE 7–8   Conditions associated with thyrotoxicosis.

1. Diffuse toxic goiter (Graves disease)
2. Toxic adenoma (Plummer disease)
3. Toxic multinodular goiter
4. Subacute thyroiditis
5. "Silent" thyroiditis
6. Thyrotoxicosis factitia
7. Rare forms of thyrotoxicosis: ovarian struma, metastatic thyroid carcinoma (follicular), hydatidiform mole, hamburger thyrotoxicosis TSH-secreting pituitary tumor, pituitary resistance to T_3 and T_4

50% in most women during pregnancy with the greatest dosage increases in those women with the least thyroid reserve (ie, in women who have had a thyroidectomy or who have received radioactive iodine therapy). Older patients metabolize T_4 more slowly, and the dose likely gradually decreases with age (see Chapter 23).

HYPERTHYROIDISM AND THYROTOXICOSIS

Thyrotoxicosis is the clinical syndrome that results when tissues are exposed to high levels of circulating thyroid hormones. It results in a generalized acceleration of metabolic processes. In most instances, thyrotoxicosis is due to hyperactivity of the thyroid gland, or hyperthyroidism. Occasionally, thyrotoxicosis may be due to other causes such as excessive ingestion of thyroid hormone or, very rarely, excessive secretion of thyroid hormones from an ovarian tumor (struma ovarii). The various forms of thyrotoxicosis are listed in Table 7–8. These syndromes will be discussed individually below.

1. DIFFUSE TOXIC GOITER (GRAVES DISEASE)

Graves disease is the most common form of thyrotoxicosis. Females are involved about five times more commonly than males. The disease may occur at any age, with a peak incidence in the 20- to 40-year age group (see section on Thyroid Autoimmunity, above). The syndrome consists of one or more of the following features: (1) thyrotoxicosis, (2) goiter, (3) ophthalmopathy (exophthalmos), and (4) dermopathy (pretibial myxedema).

Etiology

Graves disease is currently viewed as an autoimmune disease of unknown cause. There is a strong familial predisposition, in that about 15% of patients with Graves disease have a close relative with the same disorder, and about 50% of relatives of patients with Graves disease have circulating thyroid autoantibodies. There is a much higher concordance of Graves disease in monozygotic twins compared to dizygotic twins, but because the concordance rate in monozygotic twins is far less than 100%, there must be environmental factors that come into play as well. Proposed

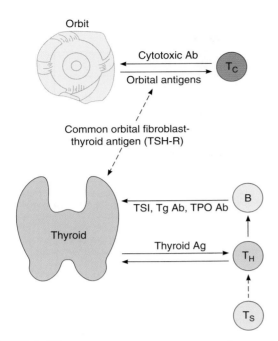

FIGURE 7–32 One theory of the pathogenesis of Graves disease. There is a defect in suppressor T lymphocytes (T$_s$) that allows helper T lymphocytes (T$_H$) to stimulate B lymphocytes (B) to synthesize thyroid auto-antibodies. The thyroid-stimulating immunoglobulin (TSI) is the driving force for thyrotoxicosis. The inflammatory process in the orbital muscles may be due to sensitization of cytotoxic T lymphocytes (T$_c$), or killer cells, to orbital antigens in association with cytotoxic antibodies. The thyroid and the eye are linked by a common antigen, the TSH-R, found in thyroid follicular cells and orbital fibroblasts. It is not yet clear what triggers this immunologic cascade. (Tg Ab, thyroglobulin antibody; TPO Ab, thyroperoxidase or microsomal antibody; Ag, antigen; Ab, antibody).

period; (2) iodide excess, particularly in geographic areas of iodide deficiency, where the lack of iodide may hold latent Graves disease in check; (3) interferon alfa, perhaps by modifying immune responsiveness; (4) viral or bacterial infections; and (5) psychological stress. The pathogenesis of ophthalmopathy may involve cytotoxic lymphocytes (killer cells) and cytotoxic antibodies sensitized to a common antigen such as the TSH receptor that is found in orbital fibroblasts, orbital muscle, and thyroid tissue (see Figure 7–32). Cytokines from these sensitized lymphocytes may cause activation and proliferation of orbital fibroblasts and preadipocytes, resulting in increased amounts of retro-orbital fat and glycosaminoglycans, as well as swollen extraocular muscles; this results in proptosis (protrusion) of the globes and diplopia, as well as redness, congestion, and conjunctival and periorbital edema (thyroid-associated ophthalmopathy or orbitopathy). For unclear reasons, smoking cigarettes is a potent risk factor for the development of thyroid-associated ophthalmopathy.

The pathogenesis of thyroid dermopathy (pretibial myxedema) (Figure 7–33) and the rare subperiosteal inflammation on the phalanges of the hands and feet (thyroid osteopathy or acropathy) (Figure 7–34) may also involve lymphocyte cytokine stimulation of fibroblasts in these locations. Many symptoms of thyrotoxicosis suggest a state of catecholamine excess, including tachycardia, tremor, sweating, lid lag, and stare. However, circulating levels of epinephrine and norepinephrine are normal or low; thus, in Graves disease, the body appears to have an increased sensitivity to

environmental triggers include stress, tobacco use, infection, and iodine exposure. The postpartum state, which may be associated with heightened immune function, also may trigger the development of Graves disease in genetically susceptible women.

Pathogenesis

In Graves disease, T lymphocytes become sensitized to antigens within the thyroid gland and stimulate B lymphocytes to synthesize antibodies to these antigens (see Chapter 2; see also the section on Thyroid Autoimmunity above and Figure 7–32). One such antibody is directed against the TSH receptor in the thyroid cell membrane, stimulating thyroid gland growth and function. The antibody is called a thyroid-stimulating antibody (TSAb), or thyroid-stimulating immunoglobulin (TSI). The presence of this circulating antibody is positively correlated with active disease and with relapse of the disease following therapy with antithyroid drugs. There is an underlying genetic predisposition, but it is not clear what triggers the initial onset of hyperthyroidism. Some factors that may incite the immune response of Graves disease are (1) pregnancy, particularly the postpartum

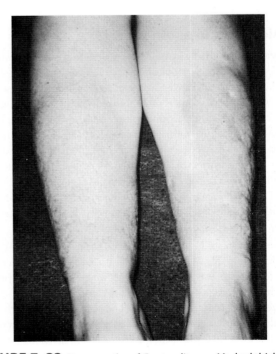

FIGURE 7–33 Dermopathy of Graves disease. Marked thickening of the skin is noted, usually over the pretibial area. Thickening occasionally extends downward over the ankle and the dorsal aspect of the foot but almost never above the knee.

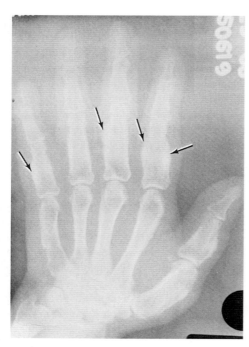

FIGURE 7–34 Radiograph of hand of a patient with thyroid osteopathy. Note marked periosteal thickening of the proximal phalanges.

TABLE 7–9 Classification of eye changes in Graves' disease.

Class	Definition
0	*No* signs or symptoms
1	*Only* signs, no symptoms. (signs limited to upper lid retraction, stare, lid lag)
2	*Soft* tissue involvement (symptoms and signs)
3	*Proptosis* (measured with Hertel exophthalmometer)[a]
4	*Extraocular* muscle involvement
5	*Corneal* involvement
6	*Sight* loss (optic nerve involvement)

[a]Upper limits of normal according to race: white, Asian, 20 mm; black, 22 mm. Increase in proptosis of 3-4 mm is mild involvement; 5-7 mm, moderate involvement; and over 8 mm, severe involvement. Other classes can be similarly graded as mild, moderate, or severe.

Reproduced, with permission, from Werner SC. Classification of the eye changes of Graves' disease. *J Clin Endocrinol Metab.* 1969; 29:782 and 1977;44:203.

catecholamines. This may be due in part to a thyroid hormone–mediated increase in membrane-bound β-adrenergic receptors in various tissues.

Clinical Features

A. Symptoms and signs   In younger individuals, common manifestations include palpitations, nervousness, easy fatigability, hyperkinesia, diarrhea, excessive sweating, intolerance to heat, and preference for cold. There is often marked weight loss without loss of appetite. Thyroid enlargement, thyrotoxic eye signs (see later), and mild tachycardia commonly occur. Muscle weakness and loss of muscle mass may be so severe that the patient cannot rise from a chair without assistance. In children, rapid growth with accelerated bone maturation occurs. In patients over age 60, cardiovascular and myopathic manifestations predominate; the most common presenting complaints are palpitations, dyspnea on exertion, tremor, nervousness, and weight loss (see Chapter 23).

The eye signs of Graves disease have been classified by Werner as set forth in Table 7–9. This classification is useful in describing the extent of the eye involvement. However, it is not helpful in following the progress of the illness, because one class does not necessarily progress into the next. The first letters of each class form the mnemonic *NO SPECS*. Class 1 involves retraction of the upper lids associated with active thyrotoxicosis and usually resolves spontaneously when the thyrotoxicosis is adequately controlled. Lid retraction can be seen in any form of thyrotoxicosis, because it is due to adrenergic stimulation of the upper eyelid. Classes 2 to 6 represent true infiltrative disease involving orbital muscles and

orbital tissues and are specific to Graves disease. Class 2 is characterized by soft tissue involvement with periorbital edema, congestion or redness of the conjunctiva, and edema of the conjunctiva (chemosis). Class 3 consists of proptosis as measured by the Hertel exophthalmometer. This instrument consists of two prisms with a scale mounted on a bar. The prisms are placed on the lateral orbital ridges, and the distance from the orbital ridge to the anterior cornea is measured on the scale (Figure 7–35). The upper limits of normal according to race are listed in the footnote to Table 7–9. Class 4 consists of extraocular muscle involvement, which typically is due to fibrosis and failure of muscle relaxation, limiting the function of the antagonist muscle. The inferior rectus is the muscle most commonly involved in the infiltrative process. By failing to relax normally, upward gaze limitation is the most common physical finding in patients with eye muscle involvement. The muscle next most commonly involved is the medial rectus, impairing lateral gaze. Class 5 is characterized by corneal involvement (keratitis) due to inability to close the eyes completely. Class 6 is a loss of vision from optic nerve involvement, likely due to ischemia of the nerve from compression of the surrounding enlarged extraocular muscles. As noted earlier, thyroid ophthalmopathy is due to infiltration of orbital fibroblasts and the extraocular muscles with lymphocytes and edema fluid due to an inflammatory reaction. The orbit is a cone enclosed by bone, and swelling of the extraocular muscles within this closed space causes proptosis of the globe and impaired muscle movement, resulting in diplopia. Ocular muscle enlargement can be demonstrated by orbital ultrasound, orbital CT scanning, or MRI (Figure 7–36).

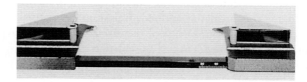

FIGURE 7–35 Hertel exophthalmometer.

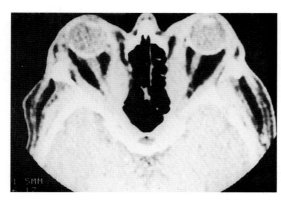

FIGURE 7–36 Orbital CT scan in a patient with severe ophthalmopathy and visual failure. Note the marked enlargement of extraocular muscles posteriorly, with compression of the optic nerve at the apex of the orbital cone.

Although only about one-third of patients have eye involvement clinically, enlarged muscles can be detected by imaging in over 90% of patients.

Thyroid dermopathy consists of thickening of the skin, particularly over the lower tibia, due to accumulation of glycosaminoglycans (see Figure 7–33). It is relatively rare, occurring in about 2% to 3% of patients with Graves disease. It is usually associated with significant ophthalmopathy and with a very high serum titer of TSAb. The skin is markedly thickened with a *peau d'orange* surface, and cannot be picked up between the fingers. Sometimes the dermopathy involves the entire lower leg and may extend onto the feet. Finally, bony involvement (osteopathy or thyroid acropachy), with subperiosteal bone formation and swelling, is particularly evident in the metacarpal bones (see Figure 7–34) and as clubbing of the digits. This too is a relatively rare finding. A more common finding in Graves disease is separation of the fingernails from their beds (onycholysis or Plummer nails), likely caused by rapid growth of the nails (Figure 7–37).

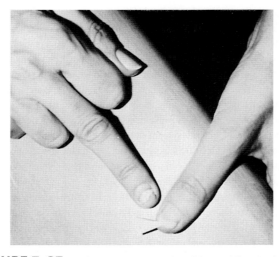

FIGURE 7–37 Onycholysis (separation of the nail from its bed) in Graves disease usually resolves spontaneously as the patient improves.

B. Laboratory findings The laboratory findings in hyperthyroidism are summarized in Figure 7–38. The combination of an elevated FT_4 and a suppressed TSH makes the diagnosis of hyperthyroidism. Approximately 5% of patients have normal FT_4 levels but elevated serum T_3 levels, a situation termed **T_3 thyrotoxicosis**. Also, very mild Graves disease may result in FT_4 and T_3 serum levels that are within the range of normal but are high enough to lead to suppressed serum TSH levels, a situation termed **subclinical hyperthyroidism**. If both FT_4 and TSH are elevated, and the RAIU is also elevated, consider a TSH-secreting pituitary tumor or generalized or pituitary-resistance syndromes. Patients who are severely ill may have low serum TSH levels but also have low serum FT_4 and T_3 levels (the so-called *sick euthyroid syndrome*).

In the condition called **familial dysalbuminemic hyperthyroxinemia**, an abnormal albumin is present in serum that preferentially binds T_4 but not T_3. This results in elevation of serum T_4 and FT_4I, and often the free T_4 when measured by usual clinical analogue free T_4 assays, but free T_4 is usually normal by equilibrium dialysis methods, as are serum T_3 and TSH. It is important to differentiate this euthyroid state from true hyperthyroidism. In addition to the absence of clinical features of hyperthyroidism, a normal serum T_3 and a normal TSH level rule out hyperthyroidism.

If eye signs are present, the diagnosis of Graves disease can be made without further tests. If eye signs are absent and the patient is hyperthyroid with or without a goiter, a RAIU test should be done. An elevated uptake is typical of Graves disease. In contrast, a low uptake is seen in patients with several forms of spontaneously resolving hyperthyroidism, as in subacute thyroiditis or *silent thyroiditis* also termed **postpartum thyroiditis**, (see discussed later). A low radioiodine uptake is also found in patients who are iodine-loaded or who are taking T_4 therapy—or, rarely, in association with a struma ovarii, where ectopic thyroid tissue is located within an ovarian teratoma. Thyroid autoantibodies—to thyroglobulin and TPO—are usually present in the serum in both Graves disease and *silent thyroiditis*, a variant of Hashimoto thyroiditis, but TSAb is relatively specific for Graves disease. This may be a useful diagnostic test in the patient who presents with unilateral or bilateral exophthalmos without obvious signs or laboratory manifestations of Graves disease (so called "euthyroid Graves disease"). The ^{123}I or technetium scan is useful to evaluate the size of the gland as well as the presence of hot or cold nodules. CT and MRI scans of the orbits reveal extraocular muscle enlargement in most patients with Graves disease even when there is no clinical evidence of ophthalmopathy. In patients with clinical ophthalmopathy, orbital muscle enlargement may be striking (see Figure 7–36).

Other Presentations

Graves disease occasionally presents in an unusual or atypical fashion, in which case the diagnosis may not be obvious. Marked muscle atrophy may suggest severe myopathy that must be differentiated from a primary neuromuscular disorder. *Thyrotoxic periodic paralysis* usually occurs in Asian males and presents with a sudden attack of flaccid paralysis and hypokalemia due to a shift

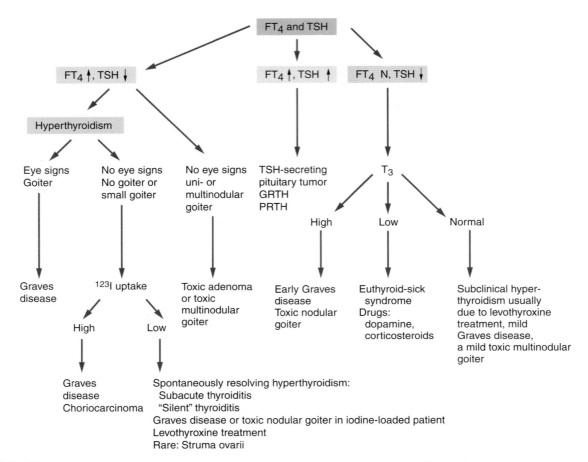

FIGURE 7–38 Laboratory tests useful in the differential diagnosis of hyperthyroidism (see text for details).

of K^+ intracellularly. The paralysis usually subsides spontaneously and can be prevented by K^+ supplementation and β-adrenergic blockade. The illness is cured by appropriate treatment of the thyrotoxicosis (see Chapter 24). Patients with thyrocardiac disease, especially those over age 60, present primarily with symptoms of heart involvement—especially refractory atrial fibrillation insensitive to digoxin—or with high-output heart failure. About 50% of these patients have no evidence of underlying heart disease, and cardiac problems are cured by treatment of the thyrotoxicosis. Some older patients present with weight loss, small goiter, slow atrial fibrillation, and severe depression, with none of the clinical features of increased catecholamine reactivity. These placid patients have apathetic thyrotoxicosis. Finally, some young women may present with amenorrhea or infertility as the primary symptom. In all of these instances, the diagnosis of hyperthyroidism can usually be made on the basis of the clinical and laboratory studies described earlier.

Complications

Thyrotoxic crisis (thyroid storm) is the acute exacerbation of all of the symptoms and signs of thyrotoxicosis, often presenting as a syndrome that may be of life-threatening severity (see Chapter 24).

Occasionally, thyroid storm may be mild and present simply as an unexplained febrile reaction after thyroid surgery in a patient who has been inadequately prepared. More commonly, it occurs in a more severe form after surgery, radioactive iodine therapy, or parturition in a patient with inadequately controlled thyrotoxicosis—or during a severe, stressful illness or disorder such as uncontrolled diabetes, trauma, acute infection, severe drug reaction, or myocardial infarction. The clinical manifestations of thyroid storm are marked hypermetabolism and excessive adrenergic response. Fever ranges from 38°C to 41°C and is associated with flushing and sweating. There is marked tachycardia, often with atrial fibrillation and high pulse pressure; occasionally heart failure occurs. Central nervous system symptoms include marked agitation, restlessness, delirium, and coma. Gastrointestinal symptoms include nausea, vomiting, diarrhea, and jaundice. A fatal outcome is associated with heart failure and shock.

At one time it was thought that thyroid storm was due to sudden release or dumping of stored T_4 and T_3 from the thyrotoxic gland. Careful studies have revealed, however, that the serum levels of T_4 and T_3 in patients with thyroid storm are not necessarily higher than in thyrotoxic patients without this condition. There is no evidence that thyroid storm is due to excessive production of T_3. Also, in thyrotoxicosis, the number of adrenergic-binding sites for catecholamines increases, so that heart and nerve tissues have increased sensitivity to circulating catecholamines. In addition, there is decreased binding to TBG, with further elevation of free T_3 and T_4. One theory is that in this setting, with increased binding sites available for catecholamines, an acute illness, infection, or surgical stress triggers an outpouring of catecholamines which, in association with high levels of free T_4 and T_3, precipitates the acute problem.

The most striking clinical diagnostic feature of thyrotoxic crisis is hyperpyrexia out of proportion to other findings. Laboratory findings include elevated serum T_4, FT_4, and T_3 as well as a suppressed TSH (see Chapter 24).

Treatment of Graves Disease

Although autoimmune mechanisms are responsible for the syndrome of Graves disease, management has been largely directed toward controlling the hyperthyroidism. Three good methods are available: (1) antithyroid drug therapy, (2) surgery, and (3) radioactive iodine therapy.

A. Antithyroid drug therapy (Figure 7–9) The antithyroid drugs methimazole, carbimazole, and PTU act by inhibiting TPO-mediated iodination of thyroglobulin to form T_4 and T_3 within the thyroid gland. PTU but not methimazole blocks peripheral T_4 to T_3 conversion; however, this effect is not generally considered to be clinically important except possibly in patients with severe thyrotoxicosis or thyroid storm. Carbimazole, used in the United Kingdom and parts of the British Commonwealth, is a derivative of methimazole that is rapidly metabolized to methimazole. Additionally, each of these drugs may have immunosuppressive effects that may be responsible for the remission from the disease that some patients have after 1 to 2 years of treatment. In general, antithyroid drug therapy as a first-line therapy is most useful in young patients with small glands and mild disease. The drug is given for 1 to 2 years and then it is tapered or discontinued to see whether the patient has achieved a remission. Remissions, defined as normal thyroid function for 1 year following discontinuation of the antithyroid drug, occur in 20% to 50% of patients but may not be lifelong. Antithyroid drug therapy is generally started with larger doses. When the patient becomes biochemically euthyroid after 4 to 12 weeks, maintenance therapy may be achieved with a lower dose. Because of the potential for severe and potentially fatal hepatotoxicity with PTU, methimazole is the antithyroid drug of choice in most patients. Methimazole has a longer duration of action and single daily dosing leads to improved compliance. A typical regimen starts with a 10 to 20-mg dose of methimazole each morning for 1 to 2 months; this dose would then be reduced to 5 to 10 mg each morning for maintenance therapy. PTU could be considered in patients with mild allergic reactions to methimazole, and is preferred in pregnant women in the first trimester because of rare teratogenic effects of methimazole in the fetus. A common regimen consists of giving PTU, 100 mg every 8 hours initially, and then in 4 to 8 weeks, reducing the dose to 50 to 200 mg once or twice daily. The laboratory tests of most value in early monitoring the course of therapy

are serum FT_4 and T_3. TSH levels often remain suppressed for many weeks or even months, and hence are not a reliable index of thyroid function early in the course of treatment.

An alternative method of therapy utilizes the concept of a total block of thyroid activity. The patient is treated with methimazole until euthyroid (about 3-6 months), but instead of continuing to taper the dose of antithyroid drug, at this point T_4 is added in a dose of about 0.1 mg/d. The patient then continues to receive the combination of antithyroid drug and T_4 (0.1 mg/d) for another 12 to 24 months. At the end of this time or when the size of the gland has returned to normal, the drugs are discontinued. This combined therapy prevents the development of hypothyroidism due to excessive doses of antithyroid drugs, but the frequency of relapse is about the same as after treatment with antithyroid drugs alone. It is more expensive, because two drugs are needed, and there may be a greater frequency of side effects. Consequently, this strategy is not recommended for most patients.

1. **Duration of therapy and other factors related to remissions**—The duration of therapy with antithyroid drugs in Graves disease is usually 12 to 24 months; some patients prefer to be treated, if necessary, for prolonged periods of time (eg, decades) but this is not typical. A sustained remission is most likely in the following circumstances: (1) if the thyroid gland returns to normal size, (2) if the disease can be controlled with a relatively small dose of antithyroid drugs, and (3) if TSAbs are no longer detectable in the serum at the end of the course of therapy.

2. **Reactions to antithyroid drugs**—Allergic reactions to antithyroid drugs can be minor, especially a rash (about 5% of patients) or major, especially agranulocytosis (about 0.5% of patients). The rash can often be managed by administering antihistamines, and unless it is severe, it is not an indication for discontinuing the medication. Agranulocytosis requires immediate cessation of antithyroid drug therapy, institution of appropriate antibiotic therapy, and shifting to an alternative therapy, usually radioactive iodine. Agranulocytosis is usually heralded by a severe sore throat and fever. Thus, all patients receiving antithyroid drugs are instructed that if sore throat or fever develops, they should stop the drug, contact their physician, and obtain a white blood cell and differential count. If the white blood cell count is normal, the antithyroid drug can be resumed. Cholestatic jaundice with methimazole, hepatocellular toxicity and vasculitis with PTU, and acute arthritis with either drug are serious but rare side effects that also require cessation of drug therapy. As noted earlier, the severity of hepatotoxicity from PTU has led to the warning by the FDA that PTU be used only in special circumstances: in patients who are allergic to methimazole who are not candidates for radioiodine or surgery and in the first trimester of pregnancy. PTU may also be preferred in patients with thyroid storm, where the inhibition of T_4 to T_3 conversion may be clinically important.

B. Radioactive iodine therapy In the United States, sodium iodide ^{131}I is the preferred treatment for most patients over age 21. In many patients without underlying heart disease, radioactive iodine may be given immediately in a dosage of 80 to 200 μCi/g of thyroid weight estimated on the basis of physical examination. The dosage is corrected for iodine uptake according to the following formula:

$$\text{Dose} = \frac{80-200 \text{microcuries}}{\text{Estimated gram thyroid tissue}}$$
$$\times \frac{\text{Estimated gram thyroid tissue}}{\text{fractional 24-hour radioiodine uptake}}$$

Following the administration of radioactive iodine, which typically is given orally as a single capsule, the gland will shrink, and the patient will usually become euthyroid over a period of 2 to 6 months.

In elderly patients and in those with underlying heart disease or other medical problems, severe thyrotoxicosis, or large glands (>100 g), it is desirable to achieve a euthyroid state prior to ^{131}I therapy, because there may be occasional exacerbations of thyroid function in the weeks following radioiodine therapy. For this purpose, patients usually are treated with methimazole until they are euthyroid, medication is then stopped for 3 to 7 days, and the radioiodine therapy is given. Methimazole (or PTU) pretreatment have been associated with a diminished effectiveness of radioiodine therapy, which can be overcome by modestly increasing the dose of radioactive iodine.

Hypothyroidism is the almost inevitable complication of radioactive iodine therapy, ultimately developing in more than 80% of patients who are adequately treated. Hypothyroidism usually occurs in the first 6 to 12 months after therapy and is the best assurance that the patient will not have a recurrence of hyperthyroidism. Serum FT_4 and TSH levels should be followed every 6 to 8 weeks, and when hypothyroidism develops, prompt replacement therapy with T_4, 0.05 to 0.2 mg daily, is instituted. Long-term follow-up studies have shown that radioiodine therapy does not cause infertility, birth defects, or cancer later in life. Severe Graves eye disease is a relative contraindication to radioiodine therapy; several prospective studies have shown that radioiodine can exacerbate eye problems when they are severe at baseline. Patients with severe underlying hyperthyroidism and those patients who smoke cigarettes are particularly prone to an exacerbation following radioiodine treatment. However, potential worsening can be prevented by the administration of prednisone 30 to 60 mg daily for 1 to 2 months following the radioiodine treatment. Prednisone is typically used in patients with moderate to severe Graves eye disease, especially in those who smoke cigarettes.

Hypothyroidism may also occur as a late development after an earlier course of antithyroid drug therapy for Graves disease; in such patients, *burned-out* Graves disease is likely the end result of autoimmune thyroid destruction. Accordingly, all patients with Graves disease who have not become hypothyroid require lifetime follow-up to be certain that they remain euthyroid.

C. Surgical treatment   Total or near-total thyroidectomy is the treatment of choice for patients with very large glands or multinodular goiters, for patients with a concomitant suspicious or malignant thyroid nodule, for patients who are allergic to or noncompliant with antithyroid drugs, for patients who refuse radioactive iodine, and for pregnant women with severe Graves disease who are allergic or develop reactions to antithyroid drugs.

The patient is prepared with antithyroid drugs until euthyroid (about 6 weeks). In addition, starting 2 weeks before the day of operation, the patient may be given saturated solution of potassium iodide, five drops twice daily. This regimen is thought to diminish the vascularity of the gland and thereby decrease intraoperative blood loss.

An experienced surgeon is required and total thyroidectomy is recommended, because if too much thyroid tissue is left behind, the disease may recur. Hypoparathyroidism and recurrent laryngeal nerve injury occur as complications of surgery in about 1% of cases, with lower rates in the hands of *high volume* surgeons.

D. Other medical measures   During the acute phase of thyrotoxicosis, β-adrenergic blocking agents are extremely helpful. Propranolol, 10 to 40 mg every 6 hours, or longer acting betablockers such as Inderal LA, nadolol, atenolol, or metoprolol control many adrenergic symptoms, tachycardia, hypertension, and atrial fibrillation. The drug is gradually withdrawn as serum FT_4 and T_3 levels return to normal. Adequate nutrition and rest are both essential. The oral cholecystographic dyes, sodium ipodate and iopanoic acid (no longer available in the United States), have been shown to inhibit both thyroid hormone synthesis and release as well as peripheral conversion of T_4 to T_3. In a dosage of 1 g daily, these drugs may help to rapidly restore the euthyroid state in very ill patients. They leave the gland saturated with iodide, so they should not be used immediately before ^{131}I therapy. Cholestyramine, 4 g orally three times daily, lowers serum T_4 by binding it in the gut, and may be useful in severely hyperthyroid patients.

Choice of Therapy

The choice of therapy varies with the nature and severity of the illness and prevailing customs. For example, in the United States, radioiodine therapy has been the preferred treatment for the average patient, whereas in Europe and Asia, primary antithyroid drug therapy is preferred. In general, antithyroid drugs are a reasonable initial therapy for children and adolescents and in adults with mild disease and small goiters. In all other patients, radioiodine is the treatment of choice. Nowadays, the role of surgery is limited to noncompliant patients who refuse radioiodine, patients with large goiters, and other unusual circumstances noted earlier.

Treatment of Complications

A. Thyrotoxic crisis   Thyrotoxic crisis (thyroid storm) requires vigorous management. Propranolol, 1 to 2 mg slowly intravenously every 5 to 10 minutes for a total of 10 mg, or 40 to 80 mg every 6 hours orally, is helpful in controlling arrhythmias. Large doses of propranolol also have the ability to block T_4 to T_3 conversion. Esmolol, a very rapidly acting beta blocker, is given at a dose of 250 to 500 mg/kg/min as a loading dose followed by 50 μg/kg/min with cardiac monitoring. In the presence of severe heart failure or asthma and arrhythmia, where beta blockers may be contraindicated, cautious intravenous administration of verapamil in a dose of 5 to 10 mg may be effective. Hormone synthesis is blocked by the administration of PTU, 250 mg every 6 hours. In thyroid storm, PTU may be preferable to methimazole because PTU blocks T_4 to T_3 conversion. If the patient is unable to take medication by mouth, methimazole in a dose of 60 mg every 24 hours or PTU, 400 mg every 6 hours, can be given by rectal suppository or enema.[3] After administration of an antithyroid drug, hormone release is retarded by the oral administration of a saturated solution of potassium iodide, 10 drops twice daily. As noted above, the oral cholecystographic agents, sodium ipodate (Oragrafin) or iopanoic acid (Telepaque), provide a source of iodine and potently block T_4 to T_3 conversion, but these drugs are not available currently in the United States. The administration of hydrocortisone hemisuccinate, or its equivalent, 50 mg intravenously every 6 hours, is usually recommended, but its role in thyroid storm management is uncertain. Supportive therapy includes a cooling blanket and acetaminophen to help control fever. Aspirin is contraindicated because of its tendency to bind to TBG and displace T_4, rendering more T_4 available in the free state. Proper fluid, electrolyte, and nutritional support are important. For sedation, phenobarbital may be useful because it accelerates the peripheral metabolism and inactivation of T_4 and T_3. Oxygen, diuretics, and digoxin are indicated for heart failure and/or atrial fibrillation. Finally, it is essential to treat the underlying disease process that may have precipitated the acute exacerbation. As an extreme measure (rarely needed) to control thyrotoxic crisis, plasmapheresis or peritoneal dialysis may be used to remove high levels of circulating free thyroid hormones (see Chapter 24).

B. Ophthalmopathy For mild disease, keeping the patient's head elevated at night and the administration of diuretics may help diminish periorbital edema. As noted above, prednisone begun immediately after radioiodine in a dose of 30 to 60 mg/d, reducing the dose by 10 mg every 2 weeks, protects against exacerbation of ophthalmopathy following ^{131}I therapy. Management of severe ophthalmopathy due to Graves disease involves close cooperation between the endocrinologist and the ophthalmologist. For severe acute inflammatory reactions, a short course of high-dose corticosteroid therapy is frequently effective (eg, prednisone, 100 mg daily orally in divided doses for 7-14 days, then every other day in gradually diminishing dosage for 6-12 weeks). Alternatively, pulse therapy with high doses of intravenous methylprednisolone can be used. If corticosteroid therapy is not effective or if there is recurrence after the drug is tapered, external x-ray therapy to the retrobulbar area may be helpful. The dose is usually 2000 cGy in 10 fractions given over a period of 2 weeks. The lens and anterior chamber structures must be shielded.

In very severe cases where vision is threatened, orbital decompression can be used. One operation involves a transantral approach through the maxillary sinus, removing the floor and the lateral walls of the orbit. In the alternative anterior approach, the orbit is entered under the globe, and portions of the floor and the walls of the orbit are removed. Both approaches are effective, and exophthalmos can be reduced by 5 to 7 mm in each eye by these techniques. After the acute process has subsided, the patient is frequently left with double vision or lid abnormalities owing to muscle fibrosis and contracture or the postoperative position of the globe. These problems can be corrected by cosmetic lid surgery or eye muscle surgery.

C. Thyrotoxicosis and pregnancy Thyrotoxicosis during pregnancy presents a special problem. It is unusual, affecting approximately 0.1% of pregnancies. It is important to recall that serum TSH levels may be subnormal at the end of the first trimester in up to 20% of normal women. This is due to the effects of serum hCG, the levels of which normally peak at the end of the first trimester; hCG activates the TSH receptor. This is a transient phenomenon and is physiologic, not pathologic. Hyperemesis gravidarum may cause mild hyperthyroidism (so-called *gestational thyrotoxicosis*), which is likely due to extremely high serum levels of hCG, present in this condition, that stimulates the TSH receptor. However, no treatment is indicated, because the hyperthyroid state resolves when the hyperemesis resolves, usually by midgestation.

In pregnant patients with Graves disease, the patient is treated with antithyroid drugs throughout most of the pregnancy, postponing the decision regarding long-term management until after delivery. Radioactive iodine is absolutely contraindicated because it crosses the placenta freely and may injure the fetal thyroid. The dosage of antithyroid drugs must be kept to the minimum necessary to control symptoms, because both PTU and methimazole cross the placenta and may affect the function of the fetal thyroid gland. PTU is preferred over methimazole because methimazole has rare teratogenic effects (aplasia cutis and methimazole embryopathy [choanal atresia, tracheoesophageal fistulae, and other defects]). Current recommendations advise limiting PTU use to the first trimester, and then switching to methimazole. However, methimazole can be used when PTU allergy or a poor clinical response to PTU is present. If the disease can be controlled by initial doses of PTU of 250 mg/d (in divided doses) or less and maintenance doses of 25 to 100 mg/d, the likelihood of fetal hypothyroidism is extremely small. The FT_4I or FT_4 should be maintained in the upper range of normal for nonpregnant women by appropriately reducing the antithyroid drug dosage. In a significant minority of patients, the drug can be discontinued in the latter part of pregnancy because of spontaneous disappearance of TSAb. Serum levels of TSAb should be measured in the third trimester; high titers can be associated with neonatal Graves disease (see later). Breastfeeding is permissible with either antithyroid drug, because the low levels found in breast milk do not affect thyroid function in the neonate.

Graves disease may occur in the newborn infant (*neonatal Graves disease*) due to transplacental passage of TSAb. Although

---

[3]**Preparation of rectal methimazole:** Dissolve 1200 mg methimazole in 12 mL of water to which a mixture of two drops of Span 80 in 52 mL of cocoa butter warmed to 37°C has been added. Stir the mixture to form a water-oil emulsion, pour into 2.6 mL suppository molds, and cool. Each suppository supplies approximately 60 mg methimazole-absorbed dose (Nabil et al, 1982).
Preparation of rectal PTU: Dissolve 400 mg PTU in 60 mL of Fleet Mineral Oil for the first dose and then dissolve 400 mg PTU in 60 mL of Fleet Phospho-Soda for subsequent enemas.

most infants with this rare syndrome are born to mothers with active Graves disease, it occasionally can occur in infants born to hypothyroid mothers who have been treated for Graves disease with radioiodine in the past but who still retain circulating TSAb. The disease may not be evident at birth, because the antithyroid drugs used to treat the mother can cross the placenta and affect the infant's thyroid as well. The child is born small, with weak muscles, tachycardia, fever, and frequently with distress or neonatal jaundice. Examination reveals an enlarged thyroid gland and occasionally prominent, puffy eyes. The heart rate is rapid, temperature is elevated, and heart failure may ensue. Laboratory studies reveal an elevated FT_4I or FT_4, a markedly elevated T_3, and usually a low TSH—in contrast to normal infants, who have elevated TSH at birth. Bone age may be accelerated. TSAb is usually found in the serum of both the infant and the mother. The pathogenesis of this syndrome is thought to involve transplacental transfer of TSAb from mother to fetus, with subsequent development of thyrotoxicosis. The disease is self-limited and subsides over a period of 4 to 12 weeks, coinciding with the fall in the child's serum TSAb levels. Therapy for the infant includes PTU in a dose of 5 to 10 mg/kg/d (in divided doses at 8-hour intervals); Lugol solution, one drop (8 mg potassium iodide) every 8 hours; and propranolol, 2 mg/kg/d in divided doses. In addition, adequate nutrition, antibiotics for infection if present, sedatives if necessary, and supportive therapy are indicated. If the child is very thyrotoxic, corticosteroid therapy (prednisone, 2 mg/kg/d) partially blocks conversion of T_4 to T_3 and may be helpful in the acute phase. The above medications are gradually reduced as the child improves and can usually be discontinued by 6 to 12 weeks.

Maternal sera may also contain TSAb that functions as blocking antibodies that can cross the placenta to produce transient hypothyroidism in the infant. This condition may need to be treated with T_4 supplementation for a short time.

Course and Prognosis

In general, the course of Graves disease treated with antithyroid drugs is one of remissions and exacerbations over a protracted period of time, unless the gland is destroyed by surgery or radioactive iodine. Although some patients may remain euthyroid for long periods after antithyroid drug treatment, at least 25% eventually develop hypothyroidism. Lifetime follow-up is therefore indicated for all patients with Graves disease.

2. OTHER FORMS OF THYROTOXICOSIS

Toxic Adenoma

A functioning adenoma hypersecreting T_3 and T_4 causes hyperthyroidism. These lesions start out as a small autonomously functioning nodule that slowly increases in size to produce excessive quantities of thyroid hormones. This gradually suppresses endogenous TSH secretion, which results in reduced function of the contralateral lobe of the gland (Figure 7–39). The typical patient is an older individual (usually >40) who has noted recent growth of a long-standing thyroid nodule. Symptoms of weight loss, weakness, shortness of breath, palpitations, tachycardia, and

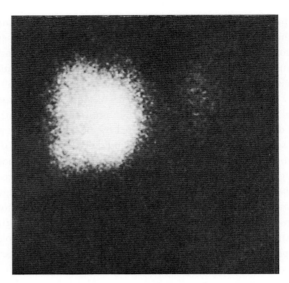

FIGURE 7–39 Solitary toxic nodule as it appears on ^{99m}Tc pertechnetate scan. Note suppression of contralateral lobe (left) by toxic nodule (right).

heat intolerance are noted. Infiltrative ophthalmopathy is never present.

Physical examination reveals a definite nodule on one side, with very little thyroid tissue on the other side. Laboratory studies usually reveal suppressed TSH and elevation in serum T_3 levels, often with only borderline elevation of FT_4 levels. A radionuclide scan reveals that the nodule is hot, with diminished or absent function of the contralateral lobe. Toxic adenomas are usually benign follicular adenomas and almost never malignant.

Treatment with radioactive iodine is generally effective and is attractive because the contralateral lobe can be spared the destructive effects of the radiation, and the patient should therefore remain euthyroid. Radioiodine therapy in doses of 20 to 30 mCi is usually required to destroy the benign neoplasm. If antithyroid drugs are used to pretreat the patient, it is important that the serum TSH remain low, so that the contralateral lobe will not be stimulated to take up the radioiodine. Surgery is an option, if the nodule is very large and causing obstructive symptoms such as dysphagia, neck pressure, or difficulty breathing. Antithyroid drugs may be used to normalize thyroid function prior to radioiodine or surgery but are not a good long-term solution, because, unlike the situation with Graves disease, remissions do not occur.

Toxic Multinodular Goiter (Plummer Disease)

This disorder usually occurs in older patients with long-standing euthyroid multinodular goiter. The patient presents with tachycardia, heart failure, or arrhythmia and sometimes weight loss, nervousness, weakness, tremors, and sweats. Physical examination reveals a multinodular goiter that may be small or quite large and may even extend substernally. Laboratory studies reveal a suppressed TSH and elevation in serum T_3 levels, with less striking elevation of serum T_4. Radioiodine scan reveals multiple

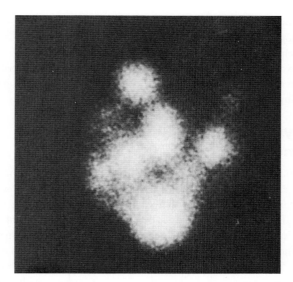

FIGURE 7–40 Toxic multinodular goiter as it appears on ^{99m}Tc pertechnetate scan. Note multiple functioning thyroid nodules. (Courtesy of Dr. J.M. Lowenstein.)

functioning nodules in the gland or occasionally an irregular, patchy distribution of radioactive iodine (Figure 7–40).

Hyperthyroidism in patients with long-standing multinodular goiters can be precipitated by the administration of pharmacologic doses of iodide-containing drugs (called the Jod-Basedow phenomenon or iodide-induced hyperthyroidism). The pathophysiology of iodine-induced hyperthyroidism is unknown but likely involves the inability of some thyroid nodules to adapt to an iodide load, with resulting excess hormone production. This is one mechanism for the development of hyperthyroidism after administration of the iodine-containing antiarrhythmic drug amiodarone (see later).

The management of toxic nodular goiter may be difficult, because patients are often elderly with other comorbidities. Control of the hyperthyroid state with antithyroid drugs followed by radioiodine is the therapy of choice. If the goiter is very large, thyroidectomy can be contemplated if the patient is a good surgical candidate.

Amiodarone-Induced Thyrotoxicosis

Amiodarone is an antiarrhythmic drug that contains 37.3% iodine by weight. In the body, it is stored in fat, myocardium, liver, and lung and has a half-life of about 50 days. In the United States, about 2% of patients treated with amiodarone develop amiodarone-induced thyrotoxicosis. In some patients, the thyrotoxicosis is due to the excess iodine; in others, it is due to an amiodarone-induced thyroiditis, with inflammation and release of stored hormone into the bloodstream as the result of thyroidal inflammation. Thyroid ultrasound with Doppler examination of the thyroid circulation may be helpful in differentiating the two syndromes: the thyroidal blood flow is increased in iodide-induced hyperthyroidism and diminished in thyroiditis. Treatment is often

difficult. Iodide-induced thyrotoxicosis can be controlled with methimazole, 40 to 60 mg/d, and β-adrenergic blockade. Although potassium perchlorate (250 mg every 6 hours) could be added to block further iodide uptake, long-term, high-dose treatment with this agent has been associated with aplastic anemia and requires careful monitoring. Also, this drug is no longer available in the United States. The drug-induced thyroiditis responds to prednisone therapy, which may need to be continued for several months. Some patients have what appears to be a mixed form of disease and respond to a combination of antithyroid drugs and prednisone. Total thyroidectomy is curative and may be needed in patients who are nonresponsive to pharmacologic therapy. Of course, surgery is feasible only if the patient can withstand the stress of surgery (see Chapter 24).

Subacute and Silent Thyroiditis

These entities will be discussed in a separate section, but it should be mentioned here that thyroiditis, either subacute or silent, may present with symptoms of mild to severe thyrotoxicosis following an acute release of T_4 and T_3 into the circulation. These illnesses can be differentiated from other forms of thyrotoxicosis in that the RAIU is markedly suppressed and the symptoms usually subside spontaneously over a period of weeks or months.

Thyrotoxicosis Factitia

This is a psychoneurotic disturbance in which the patient surreptitiously ingests excessive amounts of T_4 or thyroid hormone preparations, usually for purposes of weight control. The individual, usually a woman, is often someone connected with the health-care field who can easily obtain thyroid medication. Features of thyrotoxicosis, including weight loss, nervousness, palpitation, tachycardia, and tremor, may be present, but goiter and eye signs are absent. Characteristically, TSH is suppressed, serum FT_4 and T_3 levels are elevated, serum thyroglobulin is low, and RAIU is nil. Management requires careful discussion of the hazards of long-term thyroid hormone therapy, particularly cardiovascular damage, muscle wasting, and osteoporosis. Formal psychotherapy may be necessary.

Rare Forms of Thyrotoxicosis

A. Struma ovarii In this syndrome, a teratoma of the ovary contains thyroid tissue that becomes hyperactive. Mild features of thyrotoxicosis result, such as weight loss and tachycardia, but there is no evidence of goiter or eye signs. Serum FT_4 and T_3 are mildly elevated, serum TSH is suppressed, and RAIU over the neck is low. Total body scan reveals uptake of radioiodine in the pelvis, rather than in the neck. The disease is curable by removal of the teratoma.

B. Thyroid carcinoma Follicular carcinoma of the thyroid may concentrate radioactive iodine, but only rarely does it retain the ability to convert this iodide into active hormone. Only a few cases of metastatic thyroid cancer are described in which patients have presented with hyperthyroidism. The clinical picture consists of weakness, weight loss, palpitations, and a thyroid nodule but no ophthalmopathy. Body scan with ^{131}I reveals areas of uptake usually distant from the thyroid (eg, bone or lung). Treatment with large doses of radioactive iodine may destroy the metastatic deposits and treat the hyperthyroidism.

C. Hydatidiform mole and choriocarcinoma

Hydatidiform moles and choriocarcinomas produce high levels of chorionic gonadotropin, which has intrinsic TSH-like activity. This may induce thyroid hyperplasia, increased radioiodine uptake, suppressed TSH, and mild elevation of serum T_4 and T_3 levels. It is rarely associated with overt thyrotoxicosis and is curable by removal of the mole or treatment of the tumor.

D. Hamburger thyrotoxicosis

In the 1970s an epidemic of thyrotoxicosis in the midwestern United States was traced to hamburger made from *neck trim*, the strap muscles from the necks of slaughtered cattle that contained beef thyroid tissue. The United States Department of Agriculture has now prohibited the use of this material for human consumption.

E. Syndrome of inappropriate TSH secretion

A group of patients have been reported with elevated serum FT_4 concentrations in association with elevated or inappropriately normal serum immunoreactive TSH levels. This has been called the **syndrome of inappropriate TSH secretion**. Two conditions may explain this unusual combination of laboratory values: (1) TSH-secreting pituitary adenoma, and (2) non-neoplastic pituitary hypersecretion of TSH.

Patients with TSH-secreting pituitary adenomas usually present with mild thyrotoxicosis and goiter and may have a concurrent pituitary hormonal deficiency, such as central hypogonadism causing amenorrhea or impotence. Rarely, a TSH-secreting tumor may cosecrete other pituitary hormones such as growth hormone or prolactin. There are no eye signs of Graves disease. Laboratory evaluation reveals elevated FT_4 and T_3, whereas serum TSH, usually undetectable in Graves disease, is within the normal range or even elevated. The TSH α subunit secretion from these tumors is markedly elevated; a molar ratio of α subunit:TSH greater than 5.7 is usually diagnostic of the presence of a TSH-secreting pituitary adenoma.[4]

In addition, the increased serum TSH is not suppressible with high doses of exogenous thyroid hormones. Visual field examination may reveal a bitemporal defect, and CT or MRI of the sella usually reveals a pituitary tumor. Management usually involves control of the thyrotoxicosis with antithyroid drugs and removal of the pituitary tumor via transsphenoidal hypophysectomy. These tumors are often quite aggressive and may extend widely out of the sella. If the tumor cannot be completely removed, it may be necessary to treat residual tumor with radiation therapy and to control

thyrotoxicosis with radioactive iodine. Long-acting somatostatin analog (octreotide) suppresses TSH secretion in many of these patients and may even inhibit tumor growth in some.

Non-neoplastic pituitary hypersecretion of TSH is essentially a form of tissue resistance to T_3 and T_4. This is discussed in the following section.

Thyroid Hormone Resistance Syndromes

Two forms of resistance to thyroid hormones are recognized: (1) generalized resistance to thyroid hormones (GRTH), (2) selective pituitary resistance to thyroid hormones (PRTH).

GRTH was first described in 1967 as a familial syndrome of deaf mutism, stippled epiphyses, goiter, and abnormally high thyroid hormone levels with normal TSH. The clinical presentation in more than 500 cases that have been reported has been variable; although most patients are clinically euthyroid, some present with goiter, stunted growth, delayed maturation, attention deficits, hyperactivity disorders, and resting tachycardia. Seventy-five percent of reported cases are familial. Inheritance is autosomal dominant. Laboratory tests reveal elevated T_4, FT_4, T_3, and normal or elevated TSH. Dynamic tests to distinguish generalized resistance to thyroid hormones from TSH-secreting adenomas usually reveal a fall in TSH with T_3 administration, and a molar ratio of α subunit-TSH of less than 1. In addition, in patients with GRTH, pituitary MRI fails to demonstrate a pituitary tumor. Molecular studies have revealed point mutations in the carboxyl terminal ligand-binding portion of the human *TR*β, which produces a defective TR that fails to bind T_3 but retains the ability to bind to DNA. In addition, the mutant TR occupies the TRE as an inactive dimer or heterodimer, perhaps inducing sustained gene repression (see Figures 7–20 and 7–21). Individual point mutations in different families may account in part for the differences in clinical expression of the syndrome. Furthermore, identification of the mutation in affected individuals may allow the use of molecular screening methods for the diagnosis of the syndrome in some families.

In most patients with GRTH, the increased levels of T_3 and T_4 compensate in part for the receptor defect, and treatment is not necessary. In fact, some patients are erroneously thought to have Graves disease and undergo inappropriate therapy with radioiodine or surgery. In some children, administration of thyroid hormones may be necessary to correct defects in growth or mental development.

Selective PRTH is less common and usually presents with symptoms of mild hyperthyroidism, goiter, elevated serum T_4 and T_3, and normal or elevated serum TSH. It is currently thought that selective PRTH is not a distinct syndrome, but rather the result of the poor sensitivity and specificity of the signs and symptoms of hyperthyroidism, and the fact that thyroid hormone resistance is not necessarily complete and may vary from tissue to tissue. In fact, identical mutations in the TRβ receptor have been found in patients with both variants of thyroid hormone resistance. If the hyperthyroid state is causing significant symptoms, therapy with beta-blocking drugs, antithyroid drugs, or radioactive iodine could be considered.

[4]The α subunit-TSH molar ratio is calculated as follows: (α subunit in μg/L divided by TSH in mU/L) × 10. Normal range (for a patient with normal TSH and gonadotrophins) is less than 1.

TSH Receptor **Gene Mutations**

Mutations in the *TSH receptor* (*TSH-R*) gene can produce a variety of clinical syndromes. Somatic mutations in the seven-transmembrane loop of the TSH-R may activate the receptor, producing solitary or multiple hyperfunctioning adenomas, whereas germline mutations may result in congenital hyperthyroidism in the newborn that can mimic neonatal Graves disease. Mutations in the extracellular amino terminal portion of the TSH-R produce resistance to TSH with uncompensated or compensated hypothyroidism. Some patients may have normal serum FT_4 and T_3 levels and normal growth and development but persistently elevated serum TSH. Others may be severely hypothyroid (cretinoid), with low FT_4 levels, elevated TSH, and no response to exogenous TSH. In this group, the defect may be in the coupling of TSH-R and the G_s protein necessary for activation of adenylyl cyclase.

NONTOXIC GOITER

Etiology

Nontoxic goiter (ie, goiter not associated with hyperthyroidism) can be diffuse or nodular. In some circumstances, it results from TSH stimulation, which in turn results from inadequate thyroid hormone synthesis. Some goiters are due to mutations in genes involved in thyroid growth and/or thyroid function. In many patients, however, the cause of the goiter is obscure, because serum TSH levels are normal. Worldwide, iodine deficiency remains the most common cause of nontoxic goiter or *endemic goiter*. With the widespread use of iodized salt and the introduction of iodides into fertilizers, animal feeds, and food preservatives, iodide deficiency in developed countries has become relatively rare, and it probably does not exist in the United States. However, there are large areas such as central Africa, the mountainous areas of central Asia, the Andes of central South America, parts of central Europe, and Indonesia (particularly New Guinea), where iodine intake is still markedly deficient. Optimal iodine requirements for adults are in the range of 150 to 300 μg/d. In endemic goiter areas, the daily intake (and urinary excretion) of iodine falls below 50 μg/d; in areas where iodine is extremely scarce, excretion falls below 20 μg/d. It is in these areas that 90% of the population has goiters, and 5% to 15% of infants are born with myxedematous or neurologic changes of cretinism. The variability in the extent of goiter in these areas may be related to the presence of other, unidentified goitrogens such as goitrin, an organic compound found in certain roots and seeds; and cyanogenic glycosides, found in cassava and cabbage, that release thiocyanate that can exacerbate the effects of iodide deficiency. In addition, compounds such as phenols, phthalates, pyridines, and polyaromatic hydrocarbons found in industrial waste water are weakly goitrogenic.

The most common cause of thyroid enlargement in developed countries is chronic thyroiditis (Hashimoto thyroiditis; see later). The cause of goiter not due to autoimmune thyroid disease or iodine sufficiency is uncertain. In some patients, mild defects in thyroid hormone synthesis (dyshormonogenesis) (discussed above in the section on Hypothyroidism) may result in goiter with relatively normal thyroid function. Finally, thyroid enlargement can be due to gene mutations producing a benign lesion, such as adenoma, or to a malignant one, such as carcinoma.

Pathogenesis

The development of nontoxic goiter in patients with dyshormonogenesis or severe iodine deficiency involves impaired hormone synthesis and, secondarily, an increase in TSH secretion. TSH induces diffuse thyroid hyperplasia, followed by focal hyperplasia with necrosis and hemorrhage, and finally the development of new areas of focal hyperplasia. Focal or nodular hyperplasia usually involves a clone of cells that may or may not be able to concentrate iodine or synthesize thyroglobulin. Thus, the nodules vary from hot nodules that can concentrate iodine to cold ones that cannot, and from colloid nodules that can synthesize thyroglobulin to microfollicular ones that cannot. Initially, the hyperplasia is TSH dependent, but later the nodules become TSH independent, or autonomous. Thus, a diffuse nontoxic TSH-dependent goiter may progress over an extended period of time to become a toxic multinodular TSH-independent goiter.

The mechanism for the development of autonomous growth and function of thyroid nodules may involve mutations that activate the G_s protein in the cell membrane. Mutations of this gene, called the *gsp* oncogene, have been found in a high proportion of nodules from patients with multinodular goiter. Chronic activation of the G_s protein results in thyroid cell proliferation and hyperfunction even when TSH is suppressed.

In iodine-sufficient parts of the world such as the United States, euthyroid nontoxic goiter is a very common problem affecting up to 15% of women. The cause of goiter in the absence of iodine deficiency, autoimmunity, or obvious biosynthetic defects is unknown. In some kindreds with euthyroid multinodular goiter, mutations in the *thyroglobulin* gene have been identified, suggesting the presence of subclinical or mild defects in thyroid hormone synthesis that do not cause overt hypothyroidism or even elevation in serum TSH levels.

Clinical Features

A. Symptoms and signs Patients with nontoxic goiter usually present with thyroid enlargement, which, as noted above, may be diffuse or multinodular. The gland may be relatively firm but is often soft or rubbery in consistency. Over a period of time, the gland may become progressively larger, so that in long-standing cases, huge goiters may develop and extend substernally to the level of the aortic arch. Facial flushing and dilation of cervical veins on lifting the arms over the head is a positive **Pemberton sign** and indicates obstruction to jugular venous flow (Figure 7–41). The patient may complain of pressure symptoms in the neck, particularly on moving the head upward or downward, and of difficulty in swallowing. Vocal cord paralysis due to recurrent laryngeal nerve involvement is rare. The vast majority of patients are euthyroid. Thyroid enlargement probably represents compensated hypothyroidism.

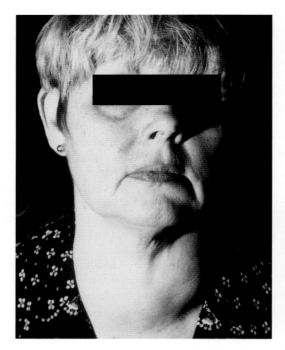
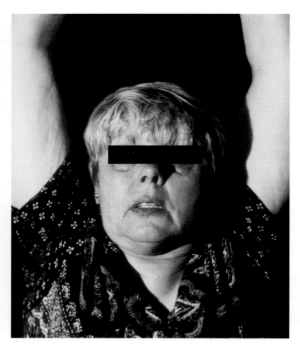
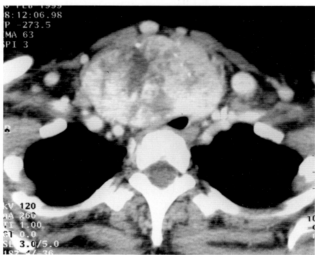

FIGURE 7–41 Pemberton sign (facial plethora) when the arms are raised above the head due to obstruction of jugular venous flow as the thyroid is forced downward into the sternal notch. This patient has a large goiter shown on an MRI. (Reproduced, with permission, from Basaria S, Salvatori R. Pemberton sign. *N Engl J Med.* 2004;350:1338.)

B. Laboratory findings   Laboratory studies reveal a normal FT_4 and, usually, normal levels of TSH. The increased mass of thyroid tissue may compensate for inefficient synthesis of hormone. RAIU may be high, normal, or low, depending on the iodide pool and the serum TSH level.

C. Imaging studies   Isotope scanning usually reveals a patchy uptake, frequently with focal areas of increased uptake corresponding to hot nodules and areas of decreased uptake corresponding to cold nodules. RAIU of the hot nodules may not be suppressible

following administration of thyroid hormones such as liothyronine. Thyroid ultrasound is a simple way to follow the growth of the goiter and in addition may reveal cystic changes and coarse calcifications in one or more of the nodules, representing previous hemorrhage and necrosis.

Differential Diagnosis

The major problem in differential diagnosis is to rule out cancer. This will be discussed in the section on thyroid carcinoma.

Treatment

With the exception of those due to neoplasm, the current management of nontoxic goiters consists simply of observation, without any specific therapy. Nontoxic goiters are very slow growing and usually never cause compressive symptoms or thyroid dysfunction. Thyroid hormone suppression therapy rarely results in clinically significant decrements in goiter size. Also, long-standing goiters may have areas of necrosis, hemorrhage, and scarring as well as autonomously functioning nodules that will not regress on T_4 therapy. Furthermore, to suppress the serum TSH level, doses of T_4 are required that could cause harm, especially in elderly patients who are at risk of developing atrial fibrillation and osteoporosis. Also, many nontoxic goiters have areas of autonomy within them that do not depend on TSH for function, and therefore, will not decrease in size and may contribute to the iatrogenic hyperthyroidism.

Surgery is indicated for goiters that continue to grow or that produce obstructive symptoms. Substernal extension of a goiter is not, in and of itself, an indication for surgical removal. The gross appearance of a multinodular goiter at the time of surgery is presented in Figure 7–42. Note that the left lobe of the gland extends downward from the middle of the thyroid cartilage to just above the clavicle. The pressure of this enlargement has caused deviation of the trachea to the right. The surface of the gland is irregular, with many large and small nodules. Although multinodular goiters are rarely malignant, the size of the mass with resulting pressure symptoms may require subtotal thyroidectomy.

If the patient is not a suitable candidate for surgery, radioiodine ablation of functioning thyroid tissue may provide palliative relief of obstructive symptoms. An adequate dose of radioiodine reduces the size of the goiter about 30% to 50% and usually alleviates obstructive symptoms.

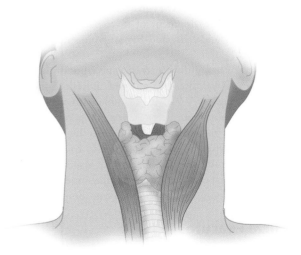

FIGURE 7–42 Multinodular goiter at the time of surgery. The asymmetric enlargement and the nodularity are apparent, as is the rightward deviation of the trachea resulting from marked enlargement of the lobe.

Course and Prognosis

Patients with nontoxic goiter should avoid pharmacologic doses of iodides, which may induce either hyperthyroidism or, in the presence of thyroidal autoimmunity, hypothyroidism. Occasionally, single adenomas or several adenomas become hyperfunctional, producing a toxic nodular goiter (discussed earlier). Nontoxic goiter is often familial and other members of the family should be examined and observed for the possible development of goiter.

THYROIDITIS

1. SUBACUTE THYROIDITIS

Subacute thyroiditis (De Quervain thyroiditis or granulomatous thyroiditis) is an acute inflammatory disorder of the thyroid gland most likely due to viral infection. A number of viruses, including mumps virus, coxsackievirus, and adenoviruses, have been implicated, either by finding the virus in biopsy specimens taken from the gland or by demonstration of rising titers of viral antibodies in the blood during the course of the infection. Pathologic examination reveals moderate thyroid enlargement and a mild inflammatory reaction involving the capsule. Histologic features include destruction of thyroid parenchyma and the presence of many large phagocytic cells, including giant cells. Subacute thyroiditis is more common in the summer months, in women, and in individuals who are HLA-Bw35 positive.

Clinical Features

A. Symptoms and signs Subacute thyroiditis usually presents with fever, malaise, and soreness in the anterior neck, which may extend up to the angle of the jaw or toward the ear lobes on one or both sides of the neck. Initially, the patient may have symptoms of hyperthyroidism, with palpitations, nervousness, and sweats. There is no ophthalmopathy. On physical examination, the gland is exquisitely tender, so that the patient objects to pressure on it. There are no signs of local redness or heat suggestive of abscess formation. Clinical signs of thyrotoxicosis, including tachycardia, tremor, and hyperreflexia, may be present.

B. Laboratory findings Laboratory studies vary with the course of the disease (Figure 7–43). Initially, FT_4 and T_3 are elevated, whereas serum TSH and RAIU are extremely low. Because the thyroid hormone levels in the blood are a reflection of leakage of glandular hormonal stores, serum FT_4 levels are elevated disproportionately to serum T_3 levels. The erythrocyte sedimentation rate is markedly elevated, sometimes greater than 100 mm/h by the Westergren scale. Thyroid autoantibodies are usually not detectable in serum. As the disease progresses, FT_4 and T_3 drop, TSH rises, and symptoms of hypothyroidism may be noted. Later, RAIU rises, reflecting recovery of the gland from the acute insult.

Differential Diagnosis

Subacute thyroiditis can be differentiated from other viral illnesses by the involvement of the thyroid gland. It is differentiated from

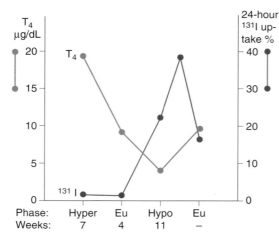

FIGURE 7–43 Changes in serum T₄ and radioactive iodine uptake in patients with subacute, silent, and postpartum thyroiditis. In the initial phase, serum T₄ is elevated and the patient may have symptoms of thyrotoxicosis, but radioactive iodine uptake is markedly suppressed. The illness may pass through phases of euthyroidism and hypothyroidism before remission. (Data adapted, with permission, from Woolf PD, Daly R. Thyrotoxicosis with painless thyroiditis. *Am J Med.* 1976;60:73.)

Graves disease by the presence of thyroidal pain, low RAIU associated with elevated serum T₃ and FT₄ and suppressed serum TSH, and by the absence of thyroid antibodies.

Treatment

In many cases, only symptomatic treatment is necessary (eg, aspirin or other nonsteroidal anti-inflammatory drugs). In severe cases or in patients who do not respond to nonsteroidal agents, a glucocorticoid such as prednisone, 20 mg three times daily for 7 to 10 days, may be necessary to reduce the inflammation. β-Adrenergic–blocking agents can be employed during the hyperthyroid phase to treat bothersome symptoms of hyperthyroidism.

T₄, 0.1 to 0.15 mg once daily, may be indicated during the hypothyroid phase of the illness if hypothyroid symptoms are present. T₄ therapy may also prevent exacerbations of inflammation due to elevated TSH levels.

Course and Prognosis

Subacute thyroiditis usually resolves completely and spontaneously over weeks or months. Occasionally, the disease may begin to resolve and then suddenly become worse, sometimes involving first one lobe of the thyroid gland and then the other (migrating or *creeping* thyroiditis). Exacerbations may occur when the FT₄ levels have fallen, the TSH level has risen, and the gland is starting to recover function. Rarely, the course may extend over several years, with repeated bouts of inflammatory disease. Ninety percent of patients recover without any sequelae. In about 10% of patients, permanent hypothyroidism ensues, and long-term T₄ therapy is necessary.

2. CHRONIC THYROIDITIS

Chronic thyroiditis (Hashimoto thyroiditis, lymphocytic thyroiditis) is the most common cause of hypothyroidism and goiter in the United States. It is certainly the major cause of goiter in children and young adults and is the cause of *idiopathic myxedema*, which represents an end stage of Hashimoto thyroiditis, with total destruction of the gland. **Riedel thyroiditis** may be a very rare variant of Hashimoto thyroiditis, with extensive fibrosis extending outside the gland and involving overlying muscle and surrounding tissues. Riedel struma (struma is an old term for the thyroid) presents as a stony-hard mass that must be differentiated from thyroid cancer. It is also associated with fibrosis in other parts of the body including the mediastinum and retroperitoneum.

Etiology and Pathogenesis

Hashimoto thyroiditis is an immunologic disorder in which lymphocytes become sensitized to thyroidal antigens and autoantibodies are formed that react with these antigens (see thyroid autoimmunity, above). In Hashimoto thyroiditis, the three most important thyroid autoantibodies are thyroglobulin antibody, TPO Ab, and TSH-R–blocking antibody. During the early phases of Hashimoto thyroiditis, thyroglobulin antibody is markedly elevated, and TPO Ab is slightly elevated. Later, thyroglobulin antibody may disappear, but TPO Ab is present for many years. Blocking antibodies may be found in patients with atrophic thyroiditis and myxedema and, rarely, in mothers giving birth to infants with no detectable thyroid tissue (**athyreotic cretins**). The pathology of Hashimoto thyroiditis involves a heavy infiltration of lymphocytes totally destroying normal thyroidal architecture. Lymphoid follicles and germinal centers may be formed. The follicular epithelial cells are frequently enlarged and contain an eosinophilic cytoplasm laden with mitochondria (Hürthle cells). Destruction of the gland results in a fall in serum T₃ and FT₄ and a rise in TSH. Initially, TSH may maintain adequate hormonal synthesis by the development of thyroid enlargement or goiter, but often the gland fails, and hypothyroidism with or without goiter ensues.

Hashimoto thyroiditis is part of a spectrum of thyroid diseases that includes Graves disease at one end and idiopathic myxedema at the other (Figure 7–44). It is familial and may be associated with other autoimmune diseases, including pernicious anemia, adrenocortical insufficiency, idiopathic hypoparathyroidism, myasthenia gravis, and vitiligo. *Schmidt syndrome* consists of Hashimoto thyroiditis, idiopathic adrenal insufficiency, and, commonly, type 1 diabetes mellitus. This phenomenon has also been called the autoimmune polyglandular syndrome (see Chapter 2).

Clinical Features

A. Symptoms and signs Hashimoto thyroiditis usually presents with goiter in a patient who is euthyroid or has mild hypothyroidism. The female:male sex distribution is about 4:1. The process is painless, and the patient may be unaware of the goiter unless it becomes very large. Older patients may present

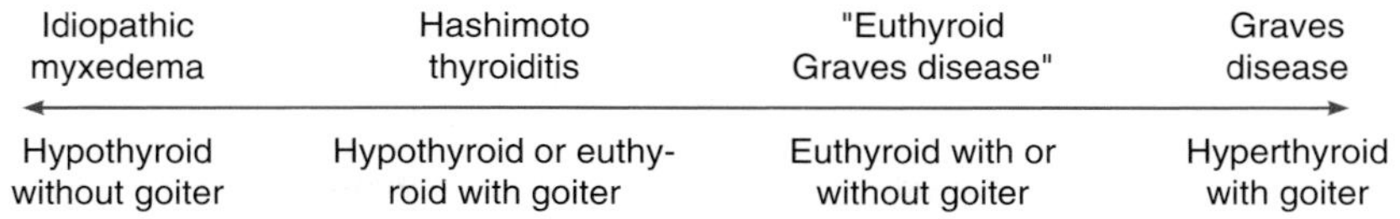

Idiopathic myxedema	Hashimoto thyroiditis	"Euthyroid Graves disease"	Graves disease
Hypothyroid without goiter	Hypothyroid or euthyroid with goiter	Euthyroid with or without goiter	Hyperthyroid with goiter

FIGURE 7–44 Spectrum of autoimmune disease of the thyroid gland. The clinical manifestations of autoimmune disease of the thyroid gland range from idiopathic myxedema, through nontoxic goiter, to diffuse toxic goiter, or Graves disease. Progression of autoimmune disease from one form to another in the same patient can occasionally occur.

with severe hypothyroidism with only a small, firm atrophic thyroid gland (idiopathic myxedema).

B. Laboratory findings   There are multiple defects in iodine metabolism. Peroxidase activity is decreased, so that organification of iodine is impaired. This can be demonstrated by a positive perchlorate discharge test. RAIU may be high, normal, or low. Circulating thyroid hormone levels are usually normal or low, and if low, TSH will be elevated.

The most striking laboratory finding is the high titer of autoantibodies to thyroidal antigens in the serum. Serum tests for either thyroglobulin antibody or TPO Ab are positive in most patients with Hashimoto thyroiditis. Another diagnostic test that may be helpful is FNAB, which reveals lymphocytic infiltration as well as the presence of Hürthle cells.

Differential Diagnosis

Hashimoto thyroiditis can be differentiated from other causes of nontoxic goiter by serum antibody studies and, if necessary, by FNAB.

Complications and Sequelae

The major complication of Hashimoto thyroiditis is progressive hypothyroidism. Most patients with Hashimoto thyroiditis initially have a small goiter and subclinical hypothyroidism, which is defined as normal serum levels of FT_4 and T_3, but mildly elevated serum TSH levels, usually less than 10 mU/L. This is in contrast to overt hypothyroidism, in which FT_4 levels are subnormal. Whether subclinical hypothyroidism is a significant health problem that warrants therapy is a matter of debate. Some patients may have mild symptoms of hypothyroidism as well as increased lipid levels and other risk factors for atherosclerotic cardiovascular disease. There may be progression to overt hypothyroidism over time, especially if serum levels of antithyroid antibodies are high. On the other hand, most patients are asymptomatic, especially when TSH serum levels are less than 10 mU/L, and the link between atherosclerosis is still controversial.

One variant of Hashimoto thyroiditis has been termed **silent or painless thyroiditis**. It has a predilection for occurring in the postpartum period, developing in about 5% of postpartum women. In this setting it is called **postpartum thyroiditis**. Most patients have symptoms and signs of mild hyperthyroidism that may be difficult to distinguish from mild Graves disease. There are no eye findings, and unlike subacute thyroiditis, the thyroid is not tender to palpation. The serum FT_4 is elevated out of proportion to the serum T_3, typical of most forms of thyroiditis, when there is leakage of stored hormone into the bloodstream. The erythrocyte sedimentation rate is normal, which distinguishes it from subacute thyroiditis, and TPO Ab titers are elevated. Importantly, the 24-hour RAIU is low, rather than elevated, which readily distinguishes this condition from postpartum Graves disease. Silent thyroiditis evolves with a triphasic course, similar to what is seen in subacute thyroiditis, with the hyperthyroid phase lasting 1 to 3 months, followed by a hypothyroid phase lasting several months as well. In postpartum thyroiditis, the hyperthyroid phase generally begins 3 to 4 months after delivery. Although recovery is the rule, about 25% of patients have permanent mild or subclinical hypothyroidism, which can progress with time to overt hypothyroidism. Long-term follow-up is required because permanent hypothyroidism can eventually develop in patients after many years. Also, recurrent episodes of silent thyroiditis can occur, and postpartum thyroiditis often develops following subsequent pregnancies.

Rarely, a patient with Hashimoto thyroiditis may develop lymphoma of the thyroid gland. Although the etiology of thyroid lymphoma is unknown, Hashimoto thyroiditis is a definite risk factor. It is possible that thyroid lymphoma may be the result of the expansion of an abnormal clone of an immortalized population of intrathyroidal lymphocytes. Thyroid lymphoma is characterized by rapid growth of the gland despite continued T_4 therapy; the diagnosis of lymphoma can be made by FNAB and immunocytochemical analysis, looking for a monoclonal population of lymphocytes, but sometimes requires surgical biopsy (see later).

Whether adenocarcinoma of the thyroid gland occurs more frequently in patients with Hashimoto thyroiditis is controversial, but the two diseases—chronic thyroiditis and carcinoma—can coexist in the same gland. Recent studies have shown that the presence of thyroid cancer in thyroid nodules is more frequent in patients whose serum TSH is higher, even when it is within the normal range. Cancer must be suspected when a solitary nodule or thyroid mass grows or fails to regress while the patient is receiving doses of T_4 that normalize or suppress the serum TSH. FNAB is critical in the differential diagnosis in this situation.

Treatment

The indications for treatment of Hashimoto thyroiditis are goiter or overt hypothyroidism; a patient with a positive thyroid antibody test alone does not require therapy. Surgery is rarely indicated for Hashimoto thyroiditis but occasionally is performed if a goiter does not regress and continues to cause compressive symptoms. The treatment of subclinical hypothyroidism is a matter of debate but is often instituted because of (1) mild symptoms; (2) dyslipidemia which could be ameliorated by T_4 therapy; and (3) positive antithyroid antibody titers, which predicts a higher chance of progression to overt hypothyroidism over time. Sufficient T_4 is given to normalize TSH and allow regression of the goiter.

The treatment of silent or postpartum thyroiditis varies with the patient's thyroid status. During the hyperthyroid phase, β-adrenergic–blocking drugs can be used to treat the symptoms of tremor, palpitations, and nervousness. T_4 can be used in the hypothyroid phase, but it is usually not needed, because symptoms are usually mild.

Course and Prognosis

Without treatment, Hashimoto thyroiditis usually progresses from goiter and subclinical hypothyroidism to overt hypothyroidism over many years. In severe cases, myxedema and myxedema coma may be the end result of untreated disease. With T_4 therapy, the goiter usually resolves, although not necessarily completely, and hypothyroid symptoms are reversed.

Because Hashimoto thyroiditis may be part of a syndrome of multiple autoimmune diseases (see Chapter 2), the patient should be monitored for other autoimmune diseases such as pernicious anemia, adrenal insufficiency, and type 1 diabetes mellitus. Patients with Hashimoto thyroiditis may also develop true Graves disease, occasionally with severe ophthalmopathy or dermopathy (see Figure 7–44). The chronic thyroiditis may blunt the severity of the thyrotoxicosis, so that the patient may present with eye or skin complications of Graves disease without marked thyrotoxicosis, a syndrome often called **euthyroid Graves disease**. The ophthalmopathy and dermopathy are treated as if thyrotoxic Graves disease were present.

3. OTHER FORMS OF THYROIDITIS

The thyroid gland may be subject to acute abscess formation in patients with septicemia or acute infective endocarditis or from local extension of a pharyngeal infection. Immunocompromised hosts may develop opportunistic thyroidal infections, with involvement of organisms such as aspergillus, mycobacteria, and pneumocystis. Abscesses cause symptoms of pyogenic infection, with local pain and tenderness, swelling, and warmth and redness of the overlying skin. Needle aspiration confirms the diagnosis and identifies the organism. Treatment includes antibiotic therapy and occasionally incision and drainage. A thyroglossal duct cyst may become infected and present as acute suppurative thyroiditis. This too responds to antibiotic therapy and occasionally incision and drainage.

EFFECTS OF IONIZING RADIATION ON THE THYROID GLAND

Ionizing radiation can induce both acute and chronic thyroiditis. Thyroiditis may occur acutely in patients treated with large doses of radioiodine and may be associated with release of thyroid hormones and an acute thyrotoxic crisis. Such an occurrence is extremely rare, however, and pretreatment with antithyroid drugs to bring the patient to a euthyroid state prior to ^{131}I therapy should prevent this complication. Radioiodine therapy, which exposes the thyroid to a dosage of around 10,000 rads (cGy), is not associated with the development of thyroid cancer, presumably because the thyroid gland is largely destroyed by high doses of radiation. Thus, although the incidence of postradiation hypothyroidism is high, the incidence of thyroid cancer is extremely low.

External radiation was used many years ago for the treatment of respiratory problems in the newborn, thought to be due to thymic hyperplasia, and for the treatment of benign conditions such as severe acne and chronic tonsillitis or adenoiditis. This treatment has been associated with the later development of nodular goiter, hypothyroidism, or thyroid cancer. Fortunately, such therapy has not been used since the early 1960s. In addition, high doses of therapeutic radiation in children with Hodgkin disease or other cancers have also been associated with the development of thyroid cancer later in life. Almost all radiation-related thyroid cancers have been of the papillary type. In some parts of the world, radiation exposure from fallout from atomic bomb testing or a nuclear reactor accident has been associated with nodular thyroid disease and thyroid cancer. Although the overall frequency of thyroid carcinoma in irradiated patients is low, data from several large series suggest that the incidence of cancer in a patient who presents with a solitary cold nodule of the thyroid gland and a history of therapeutic radiation of the head, neck, or chest is about 50%.

The most recent episode of large-scale radiation-induced thyroid neoplasia was the Chernobyl disaster in April, 1986, at which time huge amounts of radioactive material, especially radioiodine, were released. As early as 4 years later, a striking increase in the incidence of thyroid nodules and thyroid cancer was noted in children in Gomel, an area in the Republic of Belarus that is close to Chernobyl and was heavily contaminated by the accident. A high proportion of the cancers arose in very young children and developed after a very short latency period. The sex distribution was equal. Most of the cancers have been papillary carcinomas and have been more aggressive than typical papillary cancer, with intraglandular, capsular, local, and lymph node invasion.

Patients who have been exposed to ionizing radiation should be followed carefully for life. Annual studies should include physical examination of the neck for goiter or nodules and FT_4 or TSH determinations to rule out hypothyroidism. Periodic thyroid ultrasound may detect nodules that are not palpable. If a nodule is found and is greater than 1 cm in diameter, FNAB should be performed. If the nodule is malignant, the patient should have total thyroidectomy. If it is benign, follow-up with periodic thyroid ultrasound is recommended. If the nodule enlarges, repeat biopsy or surgery should be considered.

THYROID NODULES AND THYROID CANCER

Thyroid nodules are extremely common, particularly among women. The prevalence of palpable thyroid nodules in the United States

TABLE 7–10 Etiology of benign thyroid nodules.

1. Focal thyroiditis
2. Dominant nodule in a multinodular goiter
3. Benign adenomas:
   a. Follicular
   b. Hürthle cell
4. Thyroid, parathyroid, or thyroglossal cysts
5. Agenesis of a thyroid lobe
6. Postsurgical remnant hyperplasia
7. Postradioiodine remnant hyperplasia
8. Rare: teratoma, lipoma, hemangioma

has been estimated to be about 4% of the adult population, with a female-male ratio of 4:1. In young children, the prevalence is less than 1%; in persons aged 11 to 18 years, about 1.5%; and in persons over age 60, about 5%. In contrast to the relatively low prevalence of palpable nodules, thyroid nodules are detected on thyroid ultrasound in up to 50% of healthy individuals, especially middle-aged and older women.

Although thyroid nodules are common, thyroid cancer is a relatively rare condition, with an annual incidence of approximately 8.7 per 100,000 population. In 2009, there are expected to be approximately 37,000 new cases in the United States. Thus, the vast majority (95%) of thyroid nodules are benign, and it is important to identify those that are likely to be malignant in the most rational and cost-effective manner. In 95% of cases, thyroid cancer presents as a nodule or lump in the thyroid. Occasionally, especially in children, enlarged cervical lymph nodes are the first sign of the disease, although on careful examination a small thyroid nodule can often be felt. Rarely, distant metastasis in lung or bone is the first sign of thyroid cancer.

1. BENIGN THYROID NODULES

Etiology

Benign conditions that can produce nodularity in the thyroid gland are listed in Table 7–10. They include focal areas of chronic thyroiditis; colloid-filled or hyperplastic cellular nodules within a multinodular goiter; a cyst involving thyroid tissue; rarely parathyroid tissue or thyroglossal duct remnants; and agenesis of one lobe of the thyroid, with hypertrophy of the other lobe presenting as a mass in the neck and mimicking a nodule. It is usually the left lobe of the thyroid that fails to develop, and the hypertrophy occurs in the right lobe. Finally, benign areas of hyperplasia and neoplasms in the thyroid, including follicular adenomas and Hürthle cell adenomas (also called oxyphil adenomas) present as thyroid nodules. Rare benign thyroidal lesions include teratomas, lipomas, and hemangiomas.

Differentiation of Benign and Malignant Lesions

Risk factors that predispose to benign or malignant disease are set forth in Table 7–11 and discussed below.

A. History A family history of goiter suggests benign disease, as does residence in an area of endemic goiter. However, a family history of papillary or medullary carcinoma or a history of recent thyroid growth, hoarseness, dysphagia, or obstruction suggests cancer, as does exposure to ionizing radiation, as discussed earlier.

B. Clinical features Clinical features associated with a lower risk of thyroid cancer include middle age, female sex, a soft

TABLE 7–11 Risk factors useful in distinguishing benign from malignant thyroid lesions.

	More Likely Benign	More Likely Malignant
History	Family history of benign goiter Residence in endemic goiter area	Family history of medullary cancer of thyroid Previous therapeutic irradiation of head or neck Recent growth of nodule Hoarseness, dysphagia, or obstruction
Physical characteristics	Older woman Soft nodule Multinodular goiter	Child, young adult, male Solitary, firm nodule clearly different from rest of gland (dominant nodule) Vocal cord paralysis, firm lymph nodes, distant metastases
Serum factors	High titer of thyroid autoantibodies	Elevated serum calcitonin
Scanning techniques		
^{123}I or ^{99m}TcO$_4$	Hot nodule	Cold nodule
Sonogram	Cyst (pure)	Solid or complex
Biopsy (needle)	Benign appearance on cytologic examination	Malignant or suggestion of malignancy
Levothyroxine therapy (TSH suppression for 3-6 mo)	Regression	No regression

thyroid nodule on physical examination, and the presence of a multinodular goiter. Individuals at higher risk of thyroid cancer include children, young adults, and older males. A solitary firm or dominant nodule that is clearly different from the rest of the gland signifies an increased risk of malignancy. Vocal cord paralysis, enlarged cervical lymph nodes, and suspected metastases are strongly suggestive of malignancy.

C. Serum factors   A serum TSH level should be the initial laboratory study in the evaluation of a thyroid nodule. If the serum TSH level is normal, which is the case for most patients, no further blood tests are needed. If the serum TSH is below normal, a radionuclide thyroid scan should be considered to see whether the nodule is hot or autonomously functioning (see later). A high normal or elevated serum TSH has been associated with modestly higher risk of thyroid cancer. In the presence of a firm thyroid gland or other clinical features of Hashimoto thyroiditis (eg, positive family history of hypothyroidism), serum antithyroid antibodies should be assessed. A high titer of thyroid autoantibodies in serum suggests chronic thyroiditis as the cause of thyroid enlargement and nodules, but does not rule out an associated malignancy. Measurement of serum calcitonin is not routinely advised. However, an elevated serum calcitonin in patients with a family history of medullary carcinoma strongly suggests the presence of medullary thyroid cancer. Elevated serum thyroglobulin following total thyroidectomy for papillary or follicular thyroid cancer usually indicates residual or metastatic disease, but serum thyroglobulin is not helpful in determining the nature of a thyroid nodule.

D. Imaging studies   Thyroid ultrasound has become an important tool in the confirmation and differential diagnosis of thyroid nodules. Ultrasound is used to confirm that a cervical mass is within the thyroid; measure a nodule's size precisely; detect other nonpalpable nodules elsewhere in the gland; and distinguish cystic from solid lesions, as a small pure cyst is almost never malignant. Cystic lesions that have internal septa or solid lesions on ultrasound may be benign or malignant. Certain ultrasound characteristics can suggest that a nodule is more likely to be malignant, including microcalcifications, irregular borders, and high internal blood flow on Doppler imaging. Other ultrasound characteristics, such as the so-called *comet tail* artifact due to the presence of colloid within the nodule favor a benign nodule.

In patients with low serum TSH levels, radionuclide thyroid scanning with ^{123}Iodine or ^{99m}Technetium pertechnetate can be used to identify a hot or cold nodule (ie, a nodule that takes up more or less radioactive iodine than surrounding tissue). Hot nodules are almost never malignant, and although 5% to 10% of cold nodules may be malignant, 90% to 95% of cold nodules are benign (Figure 7–45).

E. Needle biopsy   Fine-needle aspiration biopsy (FNAB) of thyroid nodules to obtain cytological material for pathological examination is the principal test to distinguish benign from malignant lesions. The technique of FNAB is relatively simple, safe, reliable, and well tolerated. FNAB is now generally performed under sonographic guidance and definitely should be done so if the nodule is nonpalpable, difficult to localize by palpation, or is cystic. FNAB separates thyroid nodules into three groups:

1. Cytologically benign thyroid nodules (70%-80% of all biopsy specimens), which exclude cancer with a negative predictive value of 95%-98%.
2. Cytologically malignant thyroid nodules (3%-5% of all biopsy specimens), which have a positive predictive value for cancer of 95% for all types of thyroid malignancies.
3. Cytologically indeterminate or suspicious thyroid nodules (10%-15% of all biopsy specimens), among which 15% ultimately prove to be malignant and 85% benign.

There are several subcategories of cytologically indeterminate lesions, including suspicions for malignancy (60%-75% risk of cancer) and follicular neoplasm (15%-30% risk of cancer). In the

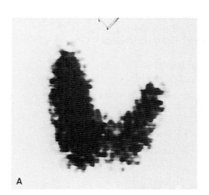
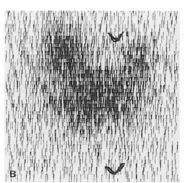
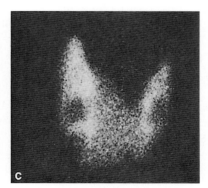

FIGURE 7–45 Demonstration of resolution obtained utilizing different scanning techniques: **A.** ^{123}I scintiscan with rectilinear scanner. **B.** Fluorescent scan with rectilinear scanner. **C.** ^{99m}Tc pertechnetate scan with the pinhole collimated gamma camera. Note the presence of two cold nodules, one in each lobe of the thyroid, easily detected in **C** but not clearly delineated in the other two scans. The lesion in the right lobe was palpable, about 1 cm in diameter, and was shown to be follicular carcinoma on needle biopsy. The lesion in the left lobe was either a metastatic tumor or a second primary follicular carcinoma. (Courtesy of Dr. M.D. Okerlund.)

future, assessment of genetic and molecular markers of malignancy (eg, BRAF mutational analysis, galectin-3 immunostaining) in FNAB specimens may assist in distinguishing benign from malignant indeterminate nodules. These markers of malignancy, and others, are currently being studied to see whether they may provide increased sensitivity and specificity for predicting malignancy in suspicious nodules, beyond what can be ascertained by traditional cytopathology.

Management of Thyroid Nodules

A decision tree for management of a thyroid nodule is presented in Figure 7–46. A patient with a thyroid nodule should have a serum TSH performed. If TSH is low, thyroid scanning should be done to avoid performing FNAB in a patient with a hot nodule. If the serum TSH is normal or elevated, ultrasound should be performed to document the presence of the nodule and to see whether other nodules are present. If one or more nodules are confirmed, FNAB should be performed on those nodules that are larger than 1.0 to 1.5 cm or that have suspicious ultrasound characteristics. If the nodule is cytologically malignant, the patient is generally referred for thyroid surgery unless there are other serious medical problems associated with high operative risk and/or a prognosis much graver than thyroid cancer. If the nodule is cytologically benign and neither local compressive symptoms nor hyperthyroidism are present, only reassessment of nodule size in 6 to 12 months by physical examination and/or ultrasound is required. If the nodule grows, defined as an increase of 20% or more in two of three dimensions, repeat FNAB and cytological examination are indicated to verify the benign diagnosis.

In patients with cytologically indeterminate nodules, those with lesions categorized as suspicious for malignancy are generally best referred for surgery. In those with a cytological follicular neoplasm, a radionuclide scan may be obtained. If the scan reveals the nodule to be hot (ie, functioning and suppressing the remainder of the gland), the patient can be observed to detect future overt hyperthyroidism. If the lesion is cold and >2 cm in diameter, has suspicious ultrasound features, or is present in a younger patient, surgery is usually preferable. On the other hand, if the nodule is <1 cm in diameter, soft, or present in an older patient, observation with serial sonography and surgery only if the lesion grows is an alternative.

2. THYROID CANCER

Pathology

The types and approximate frequency of malignant thyroid tumors are listed in Table 7–12.

A. Papillary carcinoma   Papillary carcinoma of the thyroid gland typically presents as a nodule that is firm and solid on thyroid ultrasound, sometimes with internal calcifications. In multinodular goiter, the cancer is usually a dominant nodule—larger, firmer, and/or with ultrasound characteristics more suspicious than other nodules in the gland. About 10% of papillary carcinomas, especially in children, present with enlarged cervical nodes. Careful examination then often also reveals a nodule in the thyroid. Sometimes, there is hemorrhage, necrosis, and cyst formation in the malignant nodule, but on thyroid ultrasound of these lesions, a defined solid component is an indication for FNAB of this nodule component. Finally, papillary carcinoma may be found incidentally as a microscopic focus of cancer in a gland removed for other reasons, such as another indeterminate nodule, multinodular goiter, or Graves disease. Microscopically, papillary cancer typically consists of single layers of thyroid cells arranged in vascular stalks, with papillary projections extending into microscopic cystlike spaces. The nuclei of the cells are large and pale and frequently contain clear, glassy intranuclear inclusion bodies. About 40% of papillary carcinomas form laminated calcified spheres—often at the tip of a papillary projection—called psammoma bodies. Most papillary thyroid cancers grow slowly and

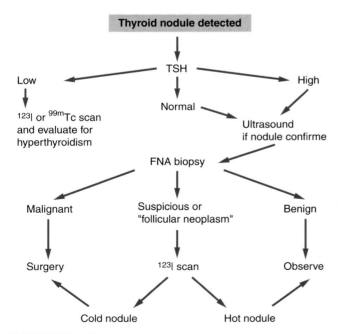

FIGURE 7–46 Decision matrix for workup of a thyroid nodule (see text for details). (FNAB, fine-needle aspiration biopsy.)

TABLE 7–12 Approximate frequency of malignant thyroid tumors.

Papillary carcinoma (including mixed papillary and follicular)	80%
Follicular carcinoma (including Hürthle cell carcinoma)	10%
Medullary carcinoma	5%
Undifferentiated (anaplastic) carcinomas	3%
Miscellaneous (including lymphoma, fibrosarcoma, squamous cell carcinoma, malignant hemangioendothelioma, teratomas, and metastatic carcinomas)	1%

remain confined to the thyroid gland and local lymph nodes. However, these cancers can exhibit intraglandular metastasis and lymph node spread. In some children with papillary thyroid cancer, there are extensive lymph node and pulmonary micrometastases. In older patients, papillary cancer can be aggressive and invade locally into adjacent muscles, nerves, and trachea. In later stages, these tumors may spread to the lung, bone, brain, and other organs. Death is usually due to local disease, with invasion of deep tissues in the neck; less commonly, death may be due to extensive distant metastases. In some older patients, a long-standing, slowly growing papillary carcinoma begins to grow rapidly and converts to undifferentiated or anaplastic carcinoma.

Most papillary carcinomas secrete thyroglobulin, which can be used as a marker for recurrence or metastasis of the cancer. Some papillary cancers concentrate radioiodine, albeit less efficiently than normal thyroid tissue. In such patients, radioiodine is an effective tool for identification and treatment of extrathyroidal disease.

B. Follicular carcinoma   Follicular carcinoma is characterized histologically by the presence of small follicles with poor colloid formation. Follicular carcinoma is distinguished from benign follicular adenoma microscopically by the presence of the capsule and/or vascular invasion within the tumor capsule. When only the capsule is involved, follicular cancer is categorized as minimally invasive, a tumor that typically has an indolent course similar to low-grade papillary cancers. When capsular blood vessels are also invaded, follicular cancers are categorized as invasive and have the potential for distant metastatic spread to bone, lung, and other sites. These tumors often retain the ability to concentrate radioactive iodine, form thyroglobulin, and, rarely, synthesize T_3 and T_4. This may render these tumors responsive to radioactive iodine therapy. When death occurs, it is attributable to local extension or distant metastases with extensive involvement of bone, lungs, and viscera.

A variant of follicular carcinoma is the **Hürthle cell or oxyphil cell carcinoma,** characterized by large individual cells with pink-staining cytoplasm filled with mitochondria. They behave like follicular cancer except that they rarely take up radioiodine.

C. Medullary carcinoma   Medullary thyroid cancer is a disease of the C cells (parafollicular cells) derived from the ultimobranchial body. These cells are capable of secreting calcitonin, carcinoembryonic antigen (CEA), histaminase, prostaglandins, serotonin, and other peptides (see Chapters 8 and 22). Microscopically, these tumors consist of sheets of cells separated by a pink-staining substance that stains with Congo red, typical of amyloid.

Medullary thyroid carcinoma is typically more aggressive than papillary or follicular carcinoma, extending locally to cervical lymph nodes and into surrounding tissues. It may also invade lymphatics and blood vessels and metastasize to lungs, liver, and other viscera. The calcitonin and CEA secreted by the tumor are clinically useful markers for diagnosis and follow-up.

Eighty percent of medullary carcinomas are sporadic, and the remainder are familial. There are three familial patterns: (1) familial medullary cancer without associated endocrine disease; (2) multiple endocrine neoplasia 2A (MEN 2A), consisting of medullary thyroid carcinoma, pheochromocytoma, and hyperparathyroidism; and (3) MEN 2B, consisting of medullary thyroid cancer, pheochromocytoma, multiple mucosal neuromas, as well as intestinal ganglioneuromatosis simulating Hirschsprung disease. There is also a variant of MEN 2A with cutaneous lichen amyloidosis, a pruritic skin lesion located on the upper back. These familial syndromes are due to *ret* protooncogene mutations, most commonly in exons 10, 11, or 16 (see later and Chapter 22).

If medullary thyroid cancer is diagnosed by FNAB or at surgery, it is essential that the patient be screened for one of the familial medullary thyroid carcinoma syndromes by DNA analysis for mutations in the *ret* protooncogene. If screening is negative, the tumor is almost certainly sporadic, and no investigation of family members is required. If a mutation is found, family members should then be screened.

D. Undifferentiated (anaplastic) carcinoma   Undifferentiated thyroid gland cancer include small cell, giant cell, and spindle cell carcinomas. They usually occur in older patients, who often have a long history of goiter with sudden gland enlargement over weeks or months, causing pain, dysphagia, hoarseness, and/or dyspnea. Death from aggressive local extension and metastatic disease typically occurs within 6 to 36 months. These tumors are very resistant to all currently available therapies.

E. Miscellaneous types

1. **Lymphoma**—Thyroid lymphoma may develop as part of a generalized lymphoma or may be primary in the thyroid gland. Primary thyroid lymphoma usually develops in patients with long-standing Hashimoto thyroiditis. It may be difficult to distinguish from chronic thyroiditis histologically. There is a monoclonal lymphocyte population with invasion of thyroid follicles and blood vessel walls. If there is no systemic involvement, the tumor may respond dramatically to combined radiation and chemotherapy.

2. **Cancer metastatic to the thyroid**—Systemic cancers can metastasize to the thyroid gland. Common primary cancers responsible for these metastases include breast, kidney, lung carcinomas, and malignant melanoma. The primary site of involvement is usually obvious. Occasionally, the diagnosis is made by biopsy of an enlarging cold thyroid nodule. The prognosis is that of the primary tumor.

F. Molecular biology of thyroid neoplasms   Extensive studies have revealed frequent gene mutations in both benign and malignant thyroid neoplasms (Figure 7–47). Activating mutations in the *gsp* oncogene, encoding Gsα or the TSH receptor in thyroid cells have been associated with increased growth and function in benign hot or toxic thyroid nodules. Activating mutations of the *ras* oncogene and loss of function of *PTEN* a tumor suppressor gene, are common in benign follicular adenomas. Progression to follicular carcinoma may occur after another genetic event involving a chromosomal translocation forming a fusion gene between the thyroid transcription factor *PAX8* gene and the *PPARγ* gene (*PAX8-PPARγ*). Further loss of the suppressor gene *P53* may allow

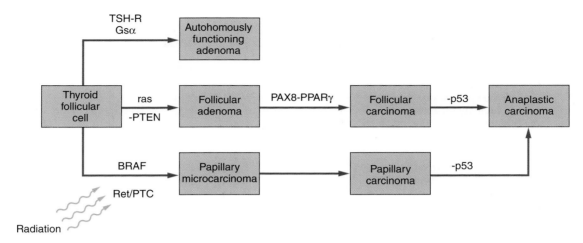

FIGURE 7–47 Molecular defects associated with development and progression of human thyroid neoplasms. The hypothetical role of specific mutational events in thyroid tumorigenesis is inferred from their prevalence in the various thyroid tumor phenotypes (see text for details). (Adapted, with permission, from Fagin JA. Genetic basis of endocrine disease 3: molecular defects in thyroid gland neoplasia. *J Clin Endocrinol Metab.* 1992;75:1398.)

progression to an anaplastic carcinoma. Papillary cancer is likely caused by mutations in genes in the MAP kinase–signaling pathway, especially *BRAF*. Another common finding in papillary thyroid cancers, especially after radiation exposure, are gene rearrangements in which a portion of the *RET* gene, a receptor tyrosine kinase not normally expressed in the thyroid, is linked to a portion of one of several unrelated genes at its 5′ end, producing a constitutively active chimeric RET receptor. Subsequent loss of *P53* suppressor gene may allow progression to anaplastic carcinoma. As noted above, activating mutations of the *RET* protooncogene on chromosome 10 have been shown to be associated with MEN 2A, MEN 2B, and familial medullary thyroid cancer. About 85% to 90% of the mutations found in MEN 2A and familial medullary thyroid cancer occur in exons 10 and 11, whereas about 95% of the mutations associated with MEN 2B are found in codon 918 in exon 16 of the *RET* oncogene. These mutations can be demonstrated in DNA from peripheral white blood cells utilizing the polymerase chain reaction and DNA sequencing. In patients with MEN 2 or familial medullary thyroid cancer who do not demonstrate a mutation in *RET*, family unit linkage analysis may be used to identify gene carriers. Thus, families can be screened for the carrier state, and early diagnosis and treatment can be instituted (Figure 7–48). Somatic mutations in the *ret* oncogene occur in about 30% of sporadic medullary thyroid cancer cells, but this does not occur in white blood cells and does not represent a germline mutation (see also Chapter 22).

Management of Thyroid Cancer (Figure 7–49)

A. Papillary and follicular carcinoma: treatment Because both papillary and follicular cancers arise from thyroid epithelial cells and sometimes respond to TSH and concentrate iodine, they are grouped together as **differentiated thyroid cancers.** These patients may be classified loosely into low-risk and high-risk groups. The low-risk group includes patients under age 45 with primary lesions under 2 cm and no evidence of intra- or extraglandular spread. For these patients, total thyroidectomy is generally recommended, although lobectomy is probably adequate therapy for small (<1 cm) tumors. All other patients should be considered high-risk, and for these, total thyroidectomy and—if there is preoperative evidence of lymphatic spread—central compartment neck dissection are indicated. In the absence of evidence of lymphatic spread, prophylactic neck dissection may not be necessary, but can be considered for larger tumors (>4 cm).

For many low-risk patients and all high-risk patients, postoperative radioiodine ablation of residual thyroid remnant is recommended to decrease the likelihood of recurrent disease. To achieve maximal uptake of radioiodine into the remnant, an elevated serum TSH level is required. This can be achieved using injections of recombinant human TSH (rhTSH) given to patients in the euthyroid state. Alternatively, TSH stimulation can be achieved by withdrawing the patient from thyroxine therapy, which causes transient clinical hypothyroidism. If the latter method is employed, T_3 is often prescribed temporarily at a dose of 25 to 50 μg daily in divided doses for 2 to 4 weeks; the medication is then stopped for 2 weeks, and, because of its 1-day half-life, patients quickly become hypothyroid prior to radioiodine therapy. In general, rhTSH is preferred, since clinical hypothyroidism is avoided and whole body radiation exposure is lower as the radioiodine is cleared from the body more rapidly because renal function is preserved. Regardless of how the patient achieves an elevated serum TSH level, a low-iodine diet is prescribed for 1 to 2 weeks to enhance uptake of the radioisotope. Following either rhTSH stimulation or thyroid hormone withdrawal, the serum thyroglobulin level is determined, and the patient is scanned 24 to

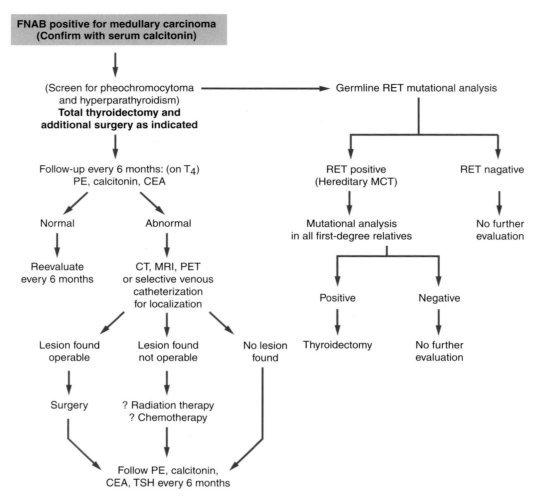

FNAB positive for medullary carcinoma
(Confirm with serum calcitonin)

(Screen for pheochromocytoma and hyperparathyroidism)
Total thyroidectomy and additional surgery as indicated

Germline RET mutational analysis

Follow-up every 6 months: (on T$_4$) PE, calcitonin, CEA

Normal → Reevaluate every 6 months

Abnormal → CT, MRI, PET or selective venous catheterization for localization

Lesion found operable → Surgery

Lesion found not operable → ? Radiation therapy ? Chemotherapy

No lesion found

RET positive (Hereditary MCT) → Mutational analysis in all first-degree relatives

RET nagative → No further evaluation

Positive → Thyroidectomy

Negative → No further evaluation

Follow PE, calcitonin, CEA, TSH every 6 months

FIGURE 7–48 Decision matrix for the management of medullary thyroid carcinoma (see text for details). (FNAB, fine-needle aspiration biopsy; PE, physical examination.)

72 hours after a low dose of radioiodine (ie, 1-4 mCi of ^{131}I or 1-2 mCi ^{123}I). If there is evidence of residual radioactive iodine uptake in the neck or elsewhere, or if there is a rise in serum thyroglobulin to detectable levels, radioactive iodine (^{131}I) is administered in a dose of 30 to 200 mCi, depending on the size and invasiveness of the primary tumor. A whole body radioiodine scan is then repeated 4 to 7 days later (called a **posttherapy scan**) to be sure no additional areas of radioiodine uptake are revealed. Nine to 12 months later, rhTSH is administered or thyroid hormone therapy is withdrawn, and a radioiodine scan and serum thyroglobulin are repeated to document ablation of all functioning thyroid tissue. An undetectable serum thyroglobulin level at a time when the serum TSH is elevated is the most sensitive evidence that all thyroid tissue has been eradicated. Indeed, a repeat whole body radioiodine scan may not be needed in low-risk patients. For the first year, patients are typically maintained on doses of T$_4$ that are adequate to suppress serum TSH to levels that are less than 0.1 mU/L. Once it has been established that the patient is free of disease, the dose of T$_4$ can be increased to allow the serum TSH to rise into the low-normal range (0.3-2 mU/L).

rhTSH, rather than thyroid hormone withdrawal, is usually employed for follow-up evaluations. When using rhTSH, the patient continues to take his T$_4$, avoiding the adverse effects of hypothyroidism. If the patient's TSH-stimulated serum thyroglobulin is less than 1 ng/mL and the whole body radioiodine scan, if obtained, is negative, the patient is likely free of disease. On the other hand, if the serum thyroglobulin concentration rises above 2 ng/mL and/or if the radioiodine scan is positive, the patient is likely to have either persistent thyroid remnant tissue or residual thyroid cancer. Neck sonography, CT, or MRI should be considered in this circumstance to look for evidence of residual thyroid cancer. If disease is localized anatomically and proven to be thyroid cancer, additional surgery may be warranted. If the stimulated thyroglobulin is greater than 20 ng/mL and other anatomic imaging studies are negative, some experts recommend empiric radioiodine therapy because of the high suspicion of residual disease that might then be visualized on the posttreatment scan.

Follow-up at intervals of 6 to 12 months should include careful examination of the neck, sometimes including neck ultrasound, looking for recurrent masses, which typically develop in ipsilateral cervical nodes. If an abnormal lymph node is discovered, FNAB is

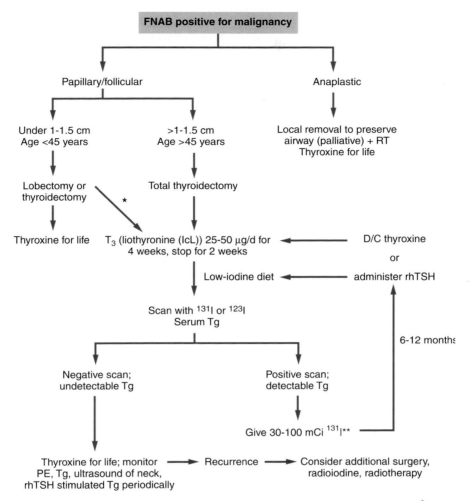

FIGURE 7–49 Decision matrix for the management of papillary, follicular, or anaplastic thyroid carcinoma. *Some experts recommend radioiodine therapy following total thyroidectomy for tumors >1.0 cm and for multifocal disease. **Some patients have a negative scan but detectable serum Tg and require further evaluation. See text for details. (FNAB, fine-needle aspiration biopsy; PE, physical examination; RT, radiotherapy; rhTSH, recombinant human TSH [Thyrogen]; Tg, thyroglobulin.)

indicated to confirm or rule out cancer. The patient's serum TSH should be checked to be certain it is adequately suppressed. The serum thyroglobulin should be periodically assessed to be certain it is undetectable. A rise in serum thyroglobulin to detectable levels while TSH is suppressed suggests tumor recurrence, and imaging studies such as neck ultrasound, CT, and MRI are necessary. PET scanning may also be useful to localize residual disease, especially in patients with very high serum thyroglobulin levels (>50 ng/mL) when conventional imaging studies have been unrevealing.

Thyroglobulin autoantibodies present in 20% of patients interfere with accurate measurement of thyroglobulin in radioimmunometric assays which are used in the majority of commercial laboratories and hospitals, causing falsely low values. Patients with thyroglobulin autoantibodies must be followed with periodic imaging studies, such as thyroid ultrasound or CT scan.

The patient with a rising thyroglobulin and a negative ^{131}I scan presents a common and difficult problem. Serial anatomic imaging, especially with cervical sonography, can sometimes identify the site

of residual cervical disease. Administration of large empiric ^{131}I doses has not been shown to be of significant benefit. For patients with noniodine-avid metastatic disease that is progressive, recent studies have shown that several kinase–inhibiting drugs, including sorafenib and sunitinib, can be effective in halting further tumor growth for 1 to 2 years. The kinases involved include the vascular endothelial growth factor receptor family (VEGF), RET, and BRAF. For patients with bone or brain metastases, combined external radiation and ^{131}I therapy may be effective.

B. Differentiated thyroid cancer: course and prognosis

Staging of cancer usually relies on the tumor-nodes-metastases (TNM) system for staging thyroid cancer (Table 7–13). Papillary and follicular thyroid carcinomas are grouped together, and staging is related to the age of the patient at the time of diagnosis. The cause-specific 5-year mortality rates are for stage 1, 0%; stage 2, 1%; stage 3, 5%; and stage 4, 77%. The TNM system may underestimate the risk of recurrence and death in younger patients with

TABLE 7–13 Tumor (T), lymph node (N), and distant metastasis (M) classification and staging of thyroid cancer.

DEFINITION of TNM

Primary Tumor (T)

All categories may be subdivided: (s) solitary tumor and (m) multifocal tumor (the largest determines the classification).

TX	Primary tumor cannot be assessed
T0	No evidence of primary tumor
T1	Tumor 2 cm or less in greatest dimension limited to the thyroid
T1a	Tumor 1 cm or less, limited to the thyroid
T1b	Tumor more than 1 cm but not more than 2 cm in greatest dimension, limited to the thyroid
T2	Tumor more than 2 cm but not more than 4 cm in greatest dimension, limited to the thyroid
T3	Tumor more than 4 cm in greatest dimension limited to the thyroid, or any tumor with minimal extrathyroid extension (e.g., extension to sternothyroid muscle or perithyroid soft tissues)
T4a	Moderately advanced disease. Tumor of any size extending beyond the thyroid capsule to invade subcutaneous soft tissues, larynx, trachea, esophagus, or recurrent laryngeal nerve
T4b	Very advanced disease. Tumor invades prevertebral fascia or encases carotid artery or mediastinal vessels

All anaplastic carcinomas are considered T4 tumors

T4a	Intrathyroidal anaplastic carcinoma
T4b	Anaplastic carcinoma with gross extrathyroid extension

Regional Lymph Nodes (N)

Regional lymph nodes are the central compartment, lateral cervical, and upper mediastinal lymph nodes.

NX	Regional lymph nodes cannot be assessed.
N0	No regional lymph node metastasis
N1	Regional lymph node metastasis
N1a	Metastasis to Level VI (pretracheal, paratracheal, and prelaryngeal/Delphian lymph nodes)
N1b	Metastasis to unilateral, bilateral, or contralateral cervical (Levels I, II, III, IV or V) or retropharyngeal or superior mediastinal lymph nodes (Level VII)

Distant Metastasis (M)

M0	No distant metastasis (no pathologic M0; use clinical M to complete stage group)
M1	Distant metastasis

STAGE GROUPING

Separate stage groupings are recommended for papillary or follicular, medullary, and anaplastic (undifferentiated) carcinoma.

Clinical — Papillary or Follicular (Differentiated) Under 45 y

	T	N	M
Stage I	Any T	Any N	M0
Stage II	Any T	Any N	M1

Pathologic — Papillary or Follicular (Differentiated)

	T	N	M
Stage I	Any T	Any N	M0
Stage II	Any T	Any N	M1

Clinical — Papillary or Follicular (Differentiated) 45 y and Older

	T	N	M
Stage I	T1	N0	M0
Stage II	T2	N0	M0
Stage III	T3	N0	M0
	T1	N1a	M0
	T2	N1a	M0
	T3	N1a	M0
Stage IVA	T4a	N0	M0
	T4a	N1a	M0
	T1	N1b	M0
	T2	N1b	M0
	T3	N1b	M0
	T4a	N1b	M0
Stage IVB	T4b	Any N	M0
Stage IVC	Any T	Any N	M1

Pathologic — Papillary or Follicular (Differentiated) 45 y and Older

	T	N	M
Stage I	T1	N0	M0
Stage II	T2	N0	M0
Stage III	T3	N0	M0
	T1	N1a	M0
	T2	N1a	M0
	T3	N1a	M0
Stage IVA	T4a	N0	M0
	T4a	N1a	M0
	T1	N1b	M0
	T2	N1b	M0
	T3	N1b	M0
	T4a	N1b	M0
Stage IVB	T4b	Any N	M0
Stage IVC	Any T	Any N	M1

Clinical — Medullary Carcinoma

	T	N	M
Stage I	T1	N0	M0
Stage II	T2	N0	M0
	T3	N0	M0
Stage III	T1	N1a	M0
	T2	N1a	M0
	T3	N1a	M0
Stage IVA	T4a	N0	M0
	T4a	N1a	M0
	T1	N1b	M0
	T2	N1b	M0
	T3	N1b	M0
	T4a	N1b	M0
Stage IVB	T4b	Any N	M0
Stage IVC	Any T	Any N	M1

Pathologic — Medullary Carcinoma (All age groups)

	T	N	M
Stage I	T1	N0	M0
Stage II	T2	N0	M0
	T3	N0	M0
Stage III	T1	N1a	M0
	T2	N1a	M0
	T3	N1a	M0
Stage IVA	T4a	N0	M0
	T4a	N1a	M0
	T1	N1b	M0
	T2	N1b	M0
	T3	N1b	M0
	T4a	N1b	M0
Stage IVB	T4b	Any N	M0
Stage IVC	Any T	Any N	M1

Clinical — Anaplastic Carcinoma

All anaplastic carcinomas are considered Stage IV

	T	N	M
Stage IVA	T4a	Any N	M0
Stage IVB	T4b	Any N	M0
Stage IVC	Any T	Any N	M1

Pathologic — Anaplastic Carcinoma

All anaplastic carcinomas are considered Stage IV

	T	N	M
Stage IVA	T4a	Any N	M0
Stage IVB	T4b	Any N	M0
Stage IVC	Any T	Any N	M1

Reproduced with permission from: Edge SB et al. *AJCC Cancer Staging Manual.* 7th ed. New York: Springer; 2010.

aggressive disease. An optimal outcome is also dependent on adequate therapy. There has been controversy over the extent of initial surgery for papillary and follicular thyroid cancer. As noted above, lesions under 1 cm with no evidence of local or distant metastases (T1, N0, M0) can probably be treated with lobectomy alone. However, in all other groups, total thyroidectomy and modified regional neck dissection (if gross evidence of spread is noted at the time of surgery) is indicated for two reasons: (1) it removes all local disease, and (2) it sets the stage for ^{131}I therapy and follow-up utilizing serum thyroglobulin measurements. Total or near-total thyroidectomy must be performed by an experienced thyroid surgeon to minimize the complications of surgery. The improvement in outcome following total thyroidectomy is presented in Figure 7–50.

A second factor in survival is the use of radioiodine for ablation of residual thyroid tissue after thyroidectomy and the treatment of residual or recurrent disease. Low doses of 30 to 50 mCi ^{131}I are used to ablate residual thyroid tissue, but larger doses of 100 to 200 mCi are necessary for the treatment of invasive or metastatic disease. Acute adverse effects of the larger doses include radiation sickness, sialadenitis, gastritis, and transient oligospermia. Cumulative doses of ^{131}I above 500 mCi may be associated with transient infertility in females and azoospermia in males, pancytopenia in about 4% of patients, and leukemia in about 0.3%. Radiation pneumonitis may occur in patients with diffuse pulmonary metastases, but this is minimized by utilization of high-dose treatment no more than once a year. The effectiveness of ^{131}I therapy in reducing cancer mortality is presented in Figure 7–51.

A third factor in survival is the adequate use of TSH suppression therapy. T_4 in a dose of 2.2 μg/kg/d (1 μg/lb/d) usually suppresses TSH to 0.1 mU/L or less, which removes a major growth factor for papillary or follicular thyroid cancer (see Figure 7–51). However, high-dose T_4 therapy is not without risk: there may be angina, tachycardia, or heart failure in older patients or tachycardia and nervousness in younger patients. In addition, there is an increased risk of osteoporosis in postmenopausal women. Estrogen or bisphosphonate therapy may prevent bone loss in these patients, but the treatment program must be individualized.

C. Medullary carcinoma   Early and adequate initial thyroidectomy and cervical node dissection is the best therapy for medullary cancer. Once the disease has metastasized, it is very difficult to control, though the more favorable tumor types often progress very slowly. Patients with medullary cancer should be followed postoperatively with periodic measurement of serum markers (eg, calcitonin and CEA) that indicate residual disease. Family members of patients with an *RET* oncogene mutation should be screened for the mutation as noted above (Figure 7–48). If a patient has a persistently elevated serum calcitonin concentration after total thyroidectomy and regional node dissection, neck ultrasound, CT, MRI, and/or selective venous catheterization and sampling for serum calcitonin may reveal the location of the metastases. Metastatic foci of medullary cancer may also be revealed by PET, indium-labeled somatostatin (octreotide), or sestamibi scans. If these studies fail to localize the lesion (as is often the case), the patient must be followed until the metastatic lesions become evident by physical examination or imaging studies. External x-ray therapy may be useful in the treatment of some metastatic lesions. Chemotherapy with tyrosine kinase inhibitors,

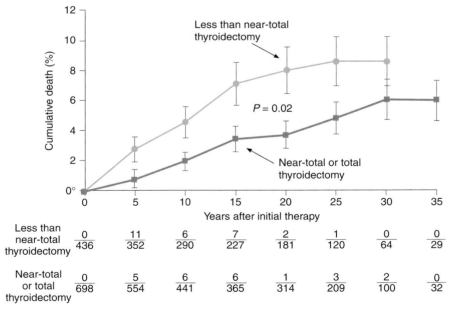

FIGURE 7–50 Improved survival in patients with papillary or follicular thyroid carcinoma following total or near-total thyroidectomy compared to less than near-total thyroidectomy. (Reproduced, with permission, from Mazzaferri EL, Jhiang SM. Long term impact of initial surgical and medical therapy on papillary and follicular thyroid cancer. *Am J Med.* 1994;97:418.)

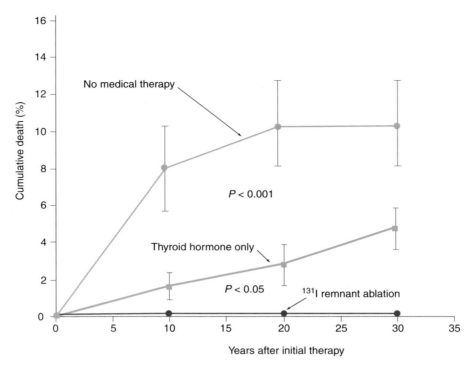

FIGURE 7–51 Cancer death rates after thyroid remnant ablation, thyroid hormone therapy alone, or no postoperative medical therapy. (Modified and reproduced, with permission, from Mazzaferri EL. Thyroid remnant ^{131}I ablation for papillary and follicular thyroid carcinoma. *Thyroid.* 1997;7:265.)

especially the experimental *RET* inhibitor vandetanib (ZD 6474), has recently been shown to be highly effective in preventing disease progression in many patients with medullary cancer. Metastatic medullary cancer cannot be treated with ^{131}I, and TSH-suppressive doses of T_4 are not required.

Medullary thyroid cancer is most aggressive in patients with MEN 2B, less aggressive in the sporadic type, and least aggressive in MEN 2A and familial medullary thyroid cancer.

D. Anaplastic carcinoma   Anaplastic carcinoma of the thyroid has a very poor prognosis. Treatment consists of minimal surgery to biopsy the tumor and establish the diagnosis, and sometimes to debulk the tumor and prevent tracheal compression. Standard treatment incorporates combined radiotherapy and chemotherapy with doxorubicin, which is sometimes combined with other agents (see Figure 7–49). Occasionally, patients have prolonged survival, but most succumb to their disease within 1 year.

REFERENCES

Anatomy

Gillam MP, Kopp P. Genetic regulation of thyroid development. *Curr Opin Pediatr.* 2001;13:358. [PMID: 11717563]

Hegedus L. Thyroid ultrasound. *Endocrinol Metab Clin North Am.* 2001;30:339. [PMID: 11444166]

Monfared A, Gorti G, Kim D. Microsurgical anatomy of the laryngeal nerves as related to thyroid surgery. *Laryngoscope.* 2002;112:386. [PMID: 11889402]

Physiology

Baxter JD, Dillmann WH, Wes BL, et al. Selective modulation of thyroid hormone receptor action. *J Steroid Biochem Mol Biol.* 2001;76:31. [PMID: 11384861]

Bianco AC, Salvatore D, Gereben B, Berry MJ, Larsen PR. Biochemistry, cellular and molecular biology, and physiological roles of the iodothyronine selenodeiodinases. *Endocr Rev.* 2002;23:38. [PMID: 11844744]

Chiamolera MI, Wondisford FE. Minireview: thyrotropin-releasing hormone and the thyroid hormone feedback mechanism. *Endocrinology.* 2009;150:1091. [PMID: 19179434]

Davies TF, Ando T, Lin RY, Tomer Y, Latif R. Thyrotropin receptor-associated diseases: from adenomata to Graves disease. *J Clin Invest.* 2005;115:1972. [PMID: 16075037]

Dunn JT, Dunn AD. Update on intrathyroidal iodine metabolism. *Thyroid.* 2001;11:407. [PMID: 11396699]

Gershengorn MC, Osman R. Minireview: insights into G protein-coupled receptor function. *Endocrinology.* 2001;142:2. [PMID: 11145559]

Glinoer D. Pregnancy and iodine. *Thyroid.* 2001;11:471. [PMID: 11396705]

Heuer H, Visser TJ. Pathophysiological importance of thyroid hormone transporters. *Endocrinology.* 2009;150:1078. [PMID: 19179441]

Klein I, Danzi S. Thyroid disease and the heart. *Circulation.* 2007;116:1725. [PMID: 17923583]

Kohn LD, Suzuki K, Nakazato M, Royaux IE, Green ED. Effects of thyroglobulin and pendrin on iodide flux through the thyrocyte. *Trends Endocrinol Metab.* 2001;12:10. [PMID: 11137035]

Kopp P. The TSH receptor and its role in thyroid disease. *Cell Mol Life Sci.* 2001;58:1301. [PMID: 11577986]

Marino M, McCluskey RT. Role of thyroglobulin endocytic pathways in the control of thyroid hormone release. *Am J Physiol Cell Physiol.* 2000;279:C1295. [PMID: 11029276]

Rose SR. Disorders of thyrotropin synthesis, secretion, and function. *Curr Opin Pediatr.* 2000;12:375. [PMID: 10943820]

Schussler GC. The thyroxine-binding proteins. *Thyroid*. 2000;10:141. [PMID: 10718550]

Shen DH, Kloos RT, Mazzaferri EL, Jhian SM. Sodium iodide symporter in health and disease. *Thyroid*. 2001;11:415. [PMID: 11396700]

St Germain DL, Galton VA, Hernandez A. Minireview: defining the roles of the iodothyronine deiodinases: current concepts and challenges. *Endocrinology*. 2009;150:1097. [PMID: 19179439]

Szkudlinski MW, Fremont V, Ronin C, Weintraub BD. Thyroid-stimulating hormone and thyroid-stimulating hormone receptor structure-function relationships. *Physiol Rev*. 2002;82:473. [PMID: 11917095]

Wonerow P, Neumann S, Gudermann T, Paschke R. Thyrotropin receptor mutations as a tool to understand thyrotropin receptor action. *J Mol Med*. 2001;79:707. [PMID: 11862314]

Wrutniak-Cabello C, et al. Thyroid hormone action in mitochondria. *J Mol Endocrinol*. 2001;26:67. [PMID: 11174855]

Wu Y, Koenig RJ. Gene regulation by thyroid hormone. *Trends Endocrinol Metab*. 2000;11:207. [PMID: 10878749]

Yen PM. Physiological and molecular basis of thyroid hormone action. *Physiol Rev*. 2001;81:1097. [PMID: 11427693]

Zhang J, Lazar MA. The mechanism of action of thyroid hormones. *Annu Rev Physiol*. 2000;62:439. [PMID: 10845098]

Zimmermann MB. Iodine deficiency. *Endocr Rev*. 2009;30:376. [PMID: 19460960]

Tests of Thyroid Function

Adler SM, Wartofsky L. The nonthyroidal illness syndrome. *Endocrinol Metab Clin North Am*. 2007;36:657. [PMID: 17673123]

Dayan CM. Interpretation of thyroid function tests. *Lancet*. 2001;357:619. [PMID: 11558500]

Glinoer D. The regulation of thyroid function during normal pregnancy: importance of the iodine nutrition status. *Best Pract Res Clin Endocrinol Metab*. 2004;18(2):133. [PMID: 15157832]

Hollowell JG, Staehling NW, Flanders WD, et al. Serum TSH, T(4), and thyroid antibodies in the United States population (1988 to 1994): National Health and Nutrition Examination Survey (NHANES III). *J Clin Endocrinol Metab*. 2002;87:489. [PMID: 11836274]

Klein I. Clinical, metabolic, and organ specific indices of thyroid function. *Endocrinol Metab Clin North Am*. 2001;30:415. [PMID: 11444169]

Nayar R, Frost AR. Thyroid aspiration cytology: a "cell pattern" approach to interpretation. *Semin Diagn Pathol*. 2001;18:81. [PMID: 11403258]

Raymond J, LaFranchi SH. Fetal and neonatal thyroid function: review and summary of significant new findings. *Curr Opin Endocrinol Diabetes Obes*. 2010;17(1):1. [PMID: 19901830]

Ross DS. Serum thyroid-stimulating hormone measurement for assessment of thyroid function and disease. *Endocrinol Metab Clin North Am*. 2001;30:24. [PMID: 11444162]

Hypothyroidism

Cappola AR, Ladenson PW. Hypothyroidism and atherosclerosis. *J Clin Endocrinol Metab*. 2003;88(6):2438. [PMID: 12788839]

Cooper DS. Clinical practice. Subclinical hypothyroidism. *N Engl J Med*. 2001;345:260. [PMID: 11474665]

Glinoer D. Potential consequences of maternal hypothyroidism on the offspring: evidence and implications. *Horm Res*. 2001;55:109. [PMID: 11549871]

Haddow JE, Palomaki GE, Allan WC, et al. Maternal thyroid deficiency during pregnancy and subsequent neuropsychological development of the child. *N Engl J Med*. 1999;341:549. [PMID: 1041459]

Kopp P. Pendred's syndrome and genetic defects in thyroid hormone synthesis. *Rev Endocr Metab Disord*. 2000;1:109. [PMID: 11704986]

McDermott MT. Hypothyroidism. *Ann Intern Med*. 2009;151:61. [PMID: 19949140]

Wiersinga WM. Thyroid hormone replacement therapy. *Horm Res*. 2001;56 (suppl 1):74. [PMID: 11786691]

Hyperthyroidism

Alsanea O, Clark OH. Treatment of Graves' disease: the advantages of surgery. *Endocrinol Metab Clin North Am*. 2000;29: 321. [PMID:10874532]

Bahn RS. Graves' ophthalmopathy. *N Engl J Med*. 2010;362:726. [PMID: 20181974]

Bartalena L, Tanda ML. Clinical practice. Graves' ophthalmopathy. *N Engl J Med*. 2009;360:994. [PMID: 19264688]

Brent GA. Clinical practice. Graves' disease. *N Engl J Med*. 2008;358:2594. [PMID: 18550875]

Cooper DS. Antithyroid drugs. *N Engl J Med*. 2005;352:905. [PMID: 15745981]

Fadel BM, Ellahham S, Ringel MD, Lindsay J Jr, Wartofsky L, Burman KD. Hyperthyroid heart disease. *Clin Cardiol*. 2000;23:402. [PMID: 10875028]

Fontanilla JC, Schneider AB, Sarne DH. The use of oral radiographic contrast agents in the management of hyperthyroidism. *Thyroid*. 2001;11:561. [PMID: 11442003]

Gough SC. The genetics of Graves' disease. *Endocrinol Metab Clin North Am*. 2000;29:255. [PMID: 10874528]

Heufelder AE. Pathogenesis of ophthalmopathy in autoimmune thyroid disease. *Rev Endocr Metab Disord*. 2000;1:87. [PMID: 11704996]

Kraiem Z, Newfield RS. Graves' disease in childhood. *J Pediatr Endocrinol Metab*. 2001;229:43. [PMID: 11308041]

Kung AW. Clinical review: thyrotoxic periodic paralysis: a diagnostic challenge. *J Clin Endocrinol Metab*. 2006;91(7):2490. [PMID: 16608889]

Nabil N, Miner DJ, Amatruda JM. Methimazole: an alternative route of administration. *J Clin Endocrinol Metab*. 1982;54:180. [PMID: 7054215]

Pauwels EK, Smit JW, Slats A, Bourguignon M, Overbeek F. Health effects of therapeutic use of 131I in hyperthyroidism. *Q J Nucl Med*. 2000;44:333. [PMID: 11302261]

Rapoport B, McLachlan SM. The thyrotropin receptor in Graves' disease. *Thyroid*. 2007;17:911. [PMID: 17822379]

Stanbury JB, Ermans AE, Bourdoux P, et al. Iodine-induced hyperthyroidism: occurrence and epidemiology. *Thyroid*. 1998;8:83. [PMID: 9492158]

Volpe R. The immunomodulatory effects of anti-thyroid drugs are mediated via actions on thyroid cells, affecting thyrocyte-immunocyte signalling: a review. *Curr Pharm Des*. 2001;7:451. [PMID: 11281852]

Thyroid Hormone Resistance

Agrawal NK, Goyal R, Rastogi A, Naik D, Singh SK. Thyroid hormone resistance. *Postgrad Med J*. 2008;84(995):473. [PMID: 18940949]

Refetoff S. Resistance to thyroid hormone. *Clin Lab Med*. 1993;13:563. [PMID: 8222575]

Syndrome of Inappropriate TSH Secretion

Beck-Peccoz P, Persani L, Mannavola D, Campi I. Pituitary tumours: TSH-secreting adenomas. *Best Pract Res Clin Endocrinol Metab*. 2009;23:597-606. [PMID: 19945025]

Sanno N, Teramoto A, Osamura RY. Thyrotropin-secreting pituitary adenomas. Clinical and biological heterogeneity and current treatment. *J Neurooncol*. 2001;54:179. [PMID: 11761434]

Multinodular Goiter

Bononi M, de Cesare A, Atella F, et al. Surgical treatment of multinodular goiter: incidence of lesions of the recurrent nerves after total thyroidectomy. *Int Surg*. 2000;85:190. [PMID: 11324993]

Derwahl M, Studer H. Nodular goiter and goiter nodules: where iodine deficiency falls short of explaining the facts. *Exp Clin Endocrinol Diabetes*. 2001;109:250. [PMID: 11507648]

Freitas JE. Therapeutic options in the management of toxic and nontoxic nodular goiter. *Semin Nucl Med*. 2000;30:88. [PMID: 10787189]

Hashmi SM, Premachandra DJ, Bennett AM, Parry W. Management of retrosternal goitres: results of early surgical intervention to prevent airway morbidity, and a review of the English literature. *J Laryngol Otol*. 2006;120(8):644. [PMID: 16884549]

Thyroiditis

Barbesino G, Chiovato L. The genetics of Hashimoto's disease. *Endocrinol Metab Clin North Am*. 2000;29:357. [PMID: 10874534]

Fatourechi V, Aniszewski JP, Fatourechi GZ, Atkinson EJ, Jacobsen SJ. Clinical features and outcome of subacute thyroiditis in an incidence cohort: Olmsted County, Minnesota. *J Clin Endocrinol Metab.* 2003;88:2100. [PMID: 12727961]

McLachlan SM, Rapoport B. Autoimmune response to the thyroid in humans: thyroid peroxidase—the common autoantigenic denominator. *Int Rev Immunol.* 2000;19:587. [PMID: 11129117]

Michels AW, Eisenbarth GS. Immunologic endocrine disorders. *J Allergy Clin Immunol.* 2010;125:S226. [PMID: 20176260]

Muller AF, Drexhage HA, Berghout A. Postpartum thyroiditis and autoimmune thyroiditis in women of childbearing age: recent insights and consequences for antenatal and postnatal care. *Endocr Rev.* 2001; 22:605. [PMID: 11588143]

Interferon-Induced Thyroiditis

Tomer Y, Menconi F. Interfereon induced thyroiditis. *Best Pract Res Clin Endocrinol Metab.* 2009;23:703. [PMID: 19942147]

Radiation Exposure

Gilbert ES, Land CE, Simon SL. Health effects from fallout. *Health Phys.* 2002;82:726. [PMID: 12003021]

Inskip PD. Thyroid cancer after radiotherapy for childhood cancer. *Med Pediatr Oncol.* 2001;36:568. [PMID: 11340614]

Rubino C, Cailleux AF, De Vathaire F, Schlumberger M. Thyroid cancer after radiation exposure. *Eur J Cancer.* 2002;38:645. [PMID: 11916545]

Williams D. Radiation carcinogenesis: lessons from Chernobyl. *Oncogene.* 2008;27(suppl 2):S9. [PMID: 19956182]

Thyroid Nodules and Thyroid Cancer

Alsanea O, Clark OH. Familial thyroid cancer. *Curr Opin Oncol.* 2001;13:44. [PMID: 11148685]

Cibas ES, Ali SZ. The Bethesda System for Reporting Thyroid Cytopathology. *Thyroid.* 2009;19:1159. [PMID: 19846805]

Cooper DS, Doherty GM, Haugen BR, et al. Revised American Thyroid Association management guidelines for patients with thyroid nodules and differentiated thyroid cancer. *Thyroid.* 2009;19:1167. [PMID: 19860577]

Csako G, Csako G, Byrd D, Wesley RA, et al. Assessing the effects of thyroid suppression on benign solitary thyroid nodules. A model for using quantitative research synthesis. *Medicine. (Baltimore)* 2000;79:9. [PMID: 10670406]

Giuffrida D, Gharib H. Anaplastic thyroid carcinoma: current diagnosis and treatment. *Ann Oncol.* 2000;11:1083. [PMID: 11061600]

Haugen BR, Pacini F, Reiners C, et al. A comparison of recombinant thyrotropin and thyroid hormone withdrawal for the detection of thyroid remnant or cancer. *J Clin Endocrinol Metab.* 1999;84:3877. [PMID: 10566623]

Kato MA, Fahey TJ, 3rd. Molecular markers in thyroid cancer diagnostics. *Surg Clin North Am.* 2009;89:1139. [PMID: 19836489]

Kloos RT, Eng C, Evans DB, et al. Medullary thyroid cancer: management guidelines of the American Thyroid Association. *Thyroid.* 2009;19:565. [PMID: 19469690]

Krohn K, Paschke R. Somatic mutations in thyroid nodular disease. *Mol Genet Metab.* 2002;75:202. [PMID: 11914031]

Leenhardt L, Aurengo A. Post-Chernobyl thyroid carcinoma in children. *Baillieres Best Pract Res Clin Endocrinol Metab.* 2000;14:667. [PMID: 11289741]

Lind P, Kumnig G, Matschnig S, et al. The role of F-18FDG PET in thyroid cancer. *Acta Med Austriaca.* 2000;27:38. [PMID: 10812462]

Pacini F, Ladenson PW, Schlumberger M, et al. Radioiodine ablation of thyroid remnants after preparation with recombinant human thyrotropin in differentiated thyroid carcinoma: results of an international, randomized, controlled study. *J Clin Endocrinol Metab.* 2006;91:926. [PMID: 16384850]

Ringel MD. Molecular diagnostic tests in the diagnosis and management of thyroid carcinoma. *Rev Endocr Metab Disord.* 2000;1:173. [PMID: 11705003]

Robbins RJ, Larson SM. The value of positron emission tomography (PET) in the management of patients with thyroid cancer. *Best Pract Res Clin Endocrinol Metab.* 2008;22:1047. [PMID: 19041831]

Ruben Harach H. Familial nonmedullary thyroid neoplasia. *Endocr Pathol.* 2001;12:97. [PMID: 11579685]

Schlumberger M, Sherman SI. Clinical trials for progressive differentiated thyroid cancer: patient selection, study design, and recent advances. *Thyroid.* 2009;19:1393. [PMID: 20001721]

Weiss RE, Lado-Abeal J. Thyroid nodules: diagnosis and therapy. *Curr Opin Oncol.* 2002;14:46. [PMID: 11790980]

Wiersinga WM. Thyroid cancer in children and adolescents—consequences in later life. *J Pediatr Endocrinol Metab.* 2001;14(suppl 5):1289. [PMID: 11964025]

Metabolic Bone Disease

Dolores Shoback, MD, Deborah Sellmeyer, MD, and Daniel D. Bikle, MD, PhD

ACTH	Adrenocorticotropin		MEPE	Matrix extracellular phosphoglycoprotein
ADHR	Autosomal dominant hypophosphatemic rickets		NALP5	NACHT leucine-rich-repeat protein 5
			OPG	Osteoprotegerin
AHO	Albright hereditary osteodystrophy		PHP	Pseudohypoparathyroidism
AIRE	Autoimmune regulator		PIP$_2$	Phosphatidylinositol 4,5-bisphosphate
BMD	Bone mineral density		PPHP	Pseudo pseudohypoparathyroidism
CaSR	Extracellular calcium-sensing receptor		PTH	Parathyroid hormone
CGRP	Calcitonin gene–related peptide		PTHrP	Parathyroid hormone–related protein
DBP	Vitamin D–binding protein		RANK	Receptor activator of nuclear factor kappa B
DXA	Dual-energy x-ray absorptiometry		RANKL	Receptor activator of nuclear factor kappa-B ligand
FBHH	Familial benign hypocalciuric hypercalcemia		RAR	Retinoic acid receptor
FGF23	Fibroblast-derived growth factor 23		RBP	Retinol-binding protein
GALNT3	UDP-N-acetyl-α-D-galactosamine transferase		RXR	Retinoid X receptor
HPT-JT	Hyperparathyroidism-jaw tumor		SERMs	Selective estrogen response modulators
HT	Hormone therapy		sFRP	Secreted frizzled related protein
ICMA	Immunochemiluminescent assay		TNF	Tumor necrosis factor
IFN	Interferon		TPN	Total parenteral nutrition
IGF	Insulin-like growth factor		TRP	Tubular reabsorption of phosphate
IL	Interleukin		VDR	Vitamin D receptor
IP$_3$	Inositol 1,4,5-triphosphate		VDRE	Vitamin D response element
IRMA	Immunoradiometric assay		VIP	Vasoactive intestinal polypeptide
LDL	Low-density lipoprotein		WHI	Women's Health Initiative
MCT	Medullary carcinoma of thyroid		WHO	World Health Organization
MEN	Multiple endocrine neoplasia		XLH	X-linked hypophosphatemia

CELLULAR AND EXTRACELLULAR CALCIUM METABOLISM

The calcium ion plays a critical role in intracellular and extracellular events in human physiology. Extracellular calcium levels in humans are tightly regulated within a narrow physiologic range to provide for proper functioning of many tissues: excitation-contraction coupling in the heart and other muscles, synaptic transmission and other functions of the nervous system, platelet aggregation, coagulation, and secretion of hormones and other regulators by exocytosis. The level of intracellular calcium is also tightly controlled, at levels about 10,000-fold lower than extracellular calcium, in order for calcium to serve as an intracellular second messenger in the regulation of cell division, muscle contractility, cell motility, membrane trafficking, and secretion.

TABLE 8–1   Calcium concentrations in body fluids.

Total serum calcium	8.5-10.5 mg/dL (2.1-2.6 mmol/L)
Ionized calcium	4.4-5.2 mg/dL (1.1-1.3 mmol/L)
Protein-bound calcium	4.0-4.6 mg/dL (0.9-1.1 mmol/L)
Complexed calcium	0.7 mg/dL (0.18 mmol/L)
Intracellular free calcium	0.00018 mmol/L (180 nmol/L)

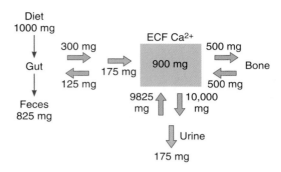

FIGURE 8–1   Calcium fluxes in a normal individual in a state of zero external mineral balance. The blue arrows denote unidirectional calcium fluxes; the pink arrows denote net fluxes. (Reproduced, with permission, from Felig P, et al, ed. *Endocrinology and Metabolism*. 2nd ed. McGraw-Hill; 1987.)

It is the concentration of ionized calcium ($[Ca^{2+}]$) that is regulated in the extracellular fluid. The ionized calcium concentration averages 1.25 ± 0.07 mmol/L (Table 8–1). However, only about 50% of the total calcium in serum and other extracellular fluids is present in the ionized form. The remainder is bound to albumin (about 40%) or complexed with anions such as phosphate and citrate (about 10%). The protein-bound and complexed fractions of serum calcium are metabolically inert and are not regulated by hormones; only the ionized $[Ca^{2+}]$ serves a regulatory role, and only this fraction is itself regulated by the calciotropic hormones parathyroid hormone (PTH) and 1,25 dihydroxyvitamin D [$1,25(OH)_2D$]. Large increases in the serum concentrations of phosphate or citrate can, however, by mass action, markedly increase the complexed fraction of calcium. For example, massive transfusions of blood, in which citrate is used as an anticoagulant, can reduce the ionized $[Ca^{2+}]$ enough to produce tetany. In addition, because calcium and phosphate circulate at concentrations close to saturation, a substantial rise in the serum concentration of either calcium or phosphate can lead to the precipitation of calcium phosphate salts in tissues. This is a source of major clinical problems in patients with severe hypercalcemia (eg, malignant tumors) and in those with severe hyperphosphatemia (eg, in renal failure or rhabdomyolysis).

What is remarkable about calcium metabolism is that the serum-ionized $[Ca^{2+}]$, which represents a tiny fraction of the total body calcium, can be so tightly regulated in the face of the rapid fluxes of calcium through body compartments that take place during the course of calcium metabolism (Figure 8–1). The total calcium in extracellular fluid amounts to about 1% of total body calcium, with most of the remainder sequestered in bone. Yet from the extracellular fluid compartment, which contains about 900 mg of calcium, 10,000 mg/d is filtered at the glomerulus and 500 mg/d is added to a labile pool in bone; and to the extracellular fluid compartment are added about 200 mg absorbed from the diet, 9800 mg reabsorbed by the renal tubule, and 500 mg from bone.

The challenge of calcium homeostasis, then, is to maintain a constant level of ionized $[Ca^{2+}]$ in the extracellular fluid, simultaneously providing adequate amounts of calcium to cells, to bone, and for renal excretion—and all the while compensating, on an hourly basis, for changes in daily intake of calcium, bone metabolism, and renal function. It is scarcely surprising that this homeostatic task requires two hormones, PTH and $1,25(OH)_2D$, or that the secretion of each hormone is exquisitely sensitive to small changes in the serum calcium, or that each hormone is able to

regulate calcium exchange across all three interfaces of the extracellular fluid: the gut, the bone, and the renal tubule. We will reexamine the integrated roles of PTH and $1,25(OH)_2D$ in calcium homeostasis after their actions and secretory control have been described.

The challenge of the cellular calcium economy is to maintain a cytosolic $[Ca^{2+}]$, or $[Ca^{2+}]_i$, of about 100 nmol/L, about 10,000-fold less than what is present outside cells (~1.0 mmol/L), providing for rapid fluxes through the intracellular compartment as required for regulation while maintaining a large gradient across the cell membrane. The calcium gradient across the cell membrane is maintained by ATP-dependent calcium pumps, Na^+-Ca^{2+} exchangers, and the storage of calcium within intracellular sites. Calcium can enter cells through several types of calcium channels, some of which are voltage operated or receptor operated, to provide for rapid influx in response to depolarization or receptor stimulation. The cell also maintains large stores of calcium in microsomal and mitochondrial pools and in some cells the Golgi apparatus. Calcium can be released from microsomal stores rapidly by cellular signals such as 1,4,5-inositol trisphosphate (IP_3). Reuptake mechanisms are also present, so that cytosolic calcium transients can be rapidly terminated by returning calcium to storage pools or pumping it across the plasma membrane.

PARATHYROID HORMONE

Anatomy and Embryology of the Parathyroid Glands

PTH is secreted from four glands located adjacent to the thyroid gland in the neck. The glands weigh an average of 40 mg each. The two superior glands are usually found near the posterior aspect of the thyroid capsule; the inferior glands are most often located near the inferior thyroid margin. However, the exact location of the glands is variable, and 12% to 15% of normal persons have a fifth parathyroid gland. The parathyroid glands arise from the third and fourth branchial pouches. The inferior glands are actually those derived from the third branchial pouches. Beginning cephalad to the other pair, they migrate further caudad, and one of them sometimes follows the thymus gland into the superior mediastinum. The small size of the parathyroids and the vagaries of their location and number make parathyroid surgery a challenging enterprise for all but the expert surgeon.

The parathyroid glands are composed of epithelial cells and stromal fat. The predominant epithelial cell is the **chief cell**. The chief cell is distinguished by its clear cytoplasm from the **oxyphil cell**, which is slightly larger and has eosinophilic granular cytoplasm. Both cell types contain PTH, and it is not known whether their secretory regulation differs in any fundamental way.

Secretion of Parathyroid Hormone

To regulate the extracellular calcium concentration [Ca^{2+}], PTH is under tight control by the serum calcium concentration. Thus, the negative feedback relationship of PTH with serum [Ca^{2+}] is steeply sigmoidal, with the steep portion of the curve corresponding exactly to the normal range of serum calcium—precisely the relationship to create a high "gain" controller and ensure maintenance of the normal serum-ionized [Ca^{2+}] by PTH (Figure 8–2).

To sense the ionized [Ca^{2+}] and thereby regulate the secretion of PTH, the parathyroid cell relies on relatively high levels of expression of the extracellular calcium-sensing receptor (CaSR). CaSR is a 120-kDa G protein–coupled receptor belonging to family C of this superfamily (see Chapter 1). The CaSR has sequence

homologies to the metabotropic glutamate receptors of the central nervous system, the type B gamma-aminobutyric acid receptor, and a large family of pheromone receptors. The large extracellular domain of the CaSR mediates the sensing of calcium and other ions. Like other G protein–coupled receptors, the CaSR has seven membrane-spanning domains. The intracellular loops that connect these domains are directly involved in coupling the receptor to G proteins.

Shortly after the identification of the CaSR, it was shown that mutations in this receptor were responsible for familial benign hypocalciuric hypercalcemia (FBHH), a disorder of calcium sensing by the parathyroid glands and kidney. The CaSR is not unique to the parathyroid. CaSRs are widely distributed in the brain, skin, growth plate, intestine, stomach, C cells, and other tissues. This receptor regulates the responses to calcium in thyroid C cells, which secrete calcitonin in response to high extracellular [Ca^{2+}], and in the distal nephron of the kidney, where the receptor regulates calcium excretion. The function of CaSRs in many other sites is still unclear.

The primary cellular signal by which an increased extracellular [Ca^{2+}] inhibits the secretion of PTH appears to be an increase in [Ca^{2+}]$_i$. The CaSR is directly coupled by G$_q$ to the enzyme phospholipase C, which hydrolyzes the phospholipid phosphatidylinositol 4,5-bisphosphate (PIP$_2$) to liberate the intracellular messengers IP$_3$ and diacylglycerol (see Chapter 1). IP$_3$ binds to a receptor in endoplasmic reticulum that releases calcium from membrane stores. The release of stored calcium raises the [Ca^{2+}]$_i$ rapidly and is followed by a sustained influx of extracellular calcium, through channels that produce a rise and sustained plateau in [Ca^{2+}]$_i$. Increased [Ca^{2+}]$_i$ may be sufficient for inhibition of PTH release, but it is unclear whether calcium release from intracellular stores or sustained calcium influx from the cell exterior is more important. The other product of phospholipase C action is the lipid diacylglycerol, an activator of the calcium- and phospholipid-sensitive protein kinases in the protein kinase C family. The effects of protein kinase C isoenzymes on the release of PTH from the gland are complex. CaSRs also couple to the inhibition of cyclic adenosine-3',5'-monophosphate (cAMP) generation, which also may play a role in setting the response of parathyroid cells to ambient calcium levels.

The initial effect of high extracellular calcium is to inhibit the secretion of preformed PTH from storage granules in the gland by blocking the fusion of storage granules with the cell membrane and release of their contents. In most cells, stimulation of exocytosis (*stimulus-secretion coupling*) is a calcium-requiring process, which is inhibited by depletion of extracellular calcium. The parathyroid cell is necessarily an exception to this rule, because this cell must increase secretion of PTH when the ionized [Ca^{2+}] is low. In the parathyroids, intracellular magnesium may serve the role in stimulus-secretion coupling that calcium does in other cells. As discussed later in the section on hypoparathyroidism, depletion of magnesium stores can paralyze the secretion of PTH, leading to reversible hypoparathyroidism.

Besides calcium, there are several regulators of PTH secretion. Hypermagnesemia inhibits PTH, and during the treatment of premature labor with infusions of magnesium sulfate, reductions

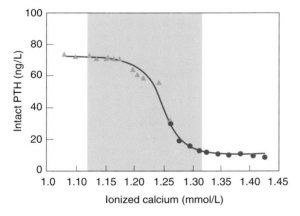

FIGURE 8-2 The relationship between the serum-ionized calcium level and the simultaneous serum concentration of intact PTH in normal humans. The serum calcium concentration was altered by the infusion of calcium (closed circles) or citrate (closed triangles). Parathyroid sensitivity to changes in serum calcium is maximal within the normal range (the shaded area). Low concentrations of PTH persist in the face of hypercalcemia. (Modified from Conlin PR, et al. Hysteresis in the relationship between serum ionized calcium and intact parathyroid hormone during recovery from induced hyper- and hypocalcemia in normal humans. *J Clin Endocrinol Metab.* 1989;69:593. By permission of the *Journal of Clinical Endocrinology and Metabolism.*)

in PTH levels and occasionally hypocalcemia are observed. Conversely, moderate hypomagnesemia can stimulate PTH secretion, even though prolonged depletion of magnesium will paralyze it. On a molar basis, magnesium is less potent in controlling secretion than calcium. Catecholamines, acting through β-adrenergic receptors and cAMP, stimulate the secretion of PTH. This effect does not appear to be clinically significant. The hypercalcemia sometimes observed in patients with pheochromocytoma usually has another basis—secretion of parathyroid hormone–related protein (PTHrP) by the tumor.

Not only do changes in serum calcium regulate the secretion of PTH—they also regulate the synthesis of PTH at the level of stabilizing preproPTH mRNA levels. It is estimated that glandular stores of PTH are sufficient to maintain maximal rates of secretion for no more than 1.5 hours, so increased synthesis is required to meet sustained hypocalcemic challenges.

Transcription of the *PTH* gene is also regulated by vitamin D: high levels of 1,25(OH)$_2$D inhibit *PTH* gene transcription. This is one of many ways that the calciotropic hormones cooperatively regulate calcium homeostasis, and it has therapeutic implications. Vitamin D analogs are used to treat secondary hyperparathyroidism in dialysis patients with renal osteodystrophy.

Synthesis and Processing of Parathyroid Hormone

PTH is an 84-amino-acid peptide with a molecular weight of 9300. Its gene is located on chromosome 11. The gene encodes a precursor called preproPTH with a 29-amino-acid extension added at the amino terminus of the mature PTH peptide (Figure 8–3). This extension includes a 23-amino-acid signal sequence (the *pre* sequence) and a 6-residue prohormone sequence. The signal sequence in preproPTH functions precisely as it does in most other secreted protein molecules, to allow recognition of the peptide by a signal recognition particle, which binds to nascent peptide chains as they emerge from the ribosome and guides them to the endoplasmic reticulum, where they are inserted through the membrane into the lumen (Figure 8–4).

In the lumen of the endoplasmic reticulum, a signal peptidase cleaves the signal sequence from preproPTH to leave proPTH, which exits the endoplasmic reticulum and travels to the Golgi apparatus, where the *pro* sequence is cleaved from PTH by an enzyme called furin. Whereas preproPTH is evanescent, proPTH has a life span of about 15 minutes. The processing of proPTH is quite efficient, and proPTH, unlike other prohormones

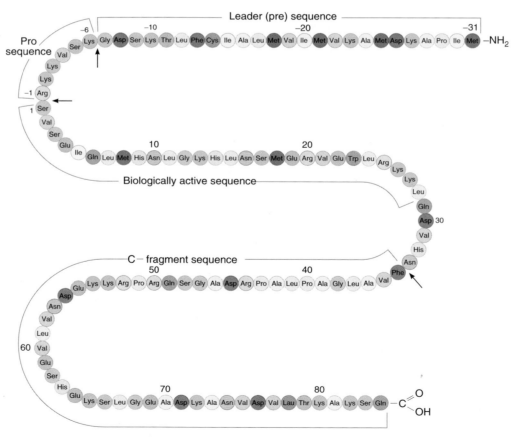

FIGURE 8–3 Primary structure of human preproparathyroid hormone. The arrows indicate sites of specific cleavages which occur in the sequence of biosynthesis and peripheral metabolism of the hormone. The biologically active sequence is enclosed in the center of the molecule. (Reproduced, with permission, from Felig P, Baxter JD, Frohman LA, ed. *Endocrinology and Metabolism*. 3rd ed. McGraw-Hill; 1995.)

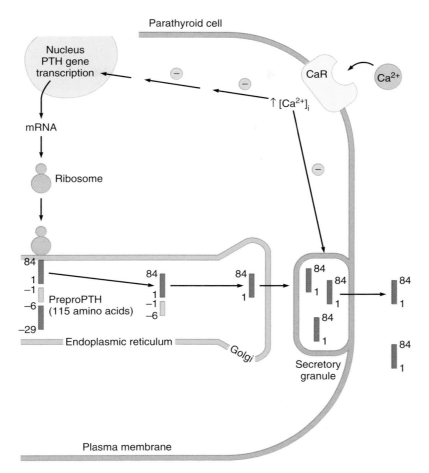

FIGURE 8–4 Biosynthetic events in the production of PTH within the parathyroid cell. *PreproPTH* gene is transcribed to its mRNA, which is translated on the ribosomes to preproPTH(amino acids −29 to +84). The presequence is removed within the endoplasmic reticulum, yielding proPTH(−6 to +84). Mature PTH(1-84) released from the Golgi is packaged in secretory granules and released into the circulation in the presence of hypocalcemia. The CaSR, or CaR, senses changes in extracellular calcium that affect both the release of PTH and the transcription of the *preproPTH* gene. (Reproduced, with permission, from McPhee SJ, et al, ed. *Pathophysiology of Disease: An Introduction to Clinical Medicine.* Originally published by Appleton & Lange. Copyright 1995 by The McGraw-Hill Companies, Inc.)

(eg, proinsulin), is not secreted. As it leaves the Golgi apparatus, PTH is repackaged into dense neuroendocrine-type secretory granules, where it is stored to await secretion.

Clearance and Metabolism of PTH

PTH secreted by the gland has a circulating half-life of 2 to 4 minutes. Intact PTH(1-84) is predominantly cleared in the liver and kidney. There, PTH is cleaved at the 33 to 34 and 36 to 37 positions to produce an amino terminal fragment and a carboxyl terminal fragment. Amino terminal fragments of PTH do not circulate to the same extent as carboxyl terminal fragments. The latter are cleared from blood by renal filtration, and they accumulate in chronic renal failure. Although the classic activities of PTH are encoded in the amino terminal portion of the molecule, mid region and carboxyl terminal fragments of the hormone may not be metabolically inert. Recent evidence suggests that they may have their own receptors and biologic actions.

Assays of PTH

Current assays of intact PTH(1-84) employ two-site immunoradiometric assay (IRMA) or immunochemiluminescent assay (ICMA) techniques, in which the normal range for PTH is approximately 10 to 60 pg/mL (1-6 pmol/L). By utilizing antibodies to two determinants, one near the amino terminal end of the PTH molecule and the other near the carboxyl terminal end of PTH, these assays are designed to measure the intact, biologically active hormone species (Figure 8–5). In practice, such assays have sufficient sensitivity and specificity to detect not only increased levels of PTH in patients with hyperparathyroid disorders but also suppressed levels of PTH in patients with nonparathyroid hypercalcemia. The ability to detect suppression of PTH makes these assays powerful tools for the differential diagnosis of hypercalcemia. If hypercalcemia results from a form of hyperparathyroidism, then the serum PTH level will be high; if hypercalcemia has a *nonparathyroid* basis, then PTH will be suppressed.

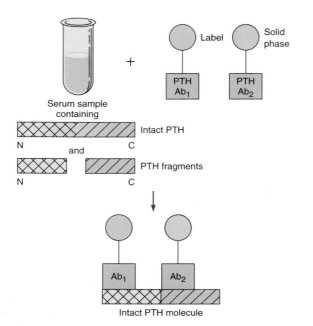

FIGURE 8–5 Schematic representation of the principle of the two-site assay for intact PTH. The label may be a luminescent probe or ^{125}I in the immunochemiluminescent or immunoradiometric assay, respectively. Two different region-specific antibodies are used (Ab$_1$ and Ab$_2$). Only the hormone species containing both immunodeterminants is counted in the assay. Most recent whole or intact PTH immunoassays employ an Ab$_1$ directed against extreme N-terminal PTH epitopes as shown. (Reproduced and modified, with permission, from McPhee SJ, et al, ed. *Pathophysiology of Disease: An Introduction to Clinical Medicine.* Originally published by Appleton & Lange. Copyright 1995 by The McGraw-Hill Companies, Inc.)

Recently, intact PTH assays have been further refined so that the amino-terminal antibody recognizes only the most amino terminal residues of PTH (essentially amino acids 1-6). This improvement was made because it became clear that antibodies used in first-generation, two-site intact PTH assays were detecting species of PTH that were not PTH (1-84). There are non-PTH(1-84) amino-terminally truncated PTH fragments generated in vivo by peripheral metabolism that can accumulate in patients with chronic renal failure. About 50% of circulating PTH in patients with renal failure consists of large fragments of non-(1-84)PTH. Assays specific for full-length PTH, in which the amino terminal antibodies truly detect residues at the extreme N-terminus of the molecule (residues 1-6), are designated as *whole, bioactive,* or *intact* PTH.

Biologic Effects of PTH

The central function of PTH is to regulate ionized $[Ca^{2+}]$ levels by concerted effects on three principal target organs: bone, intestinal mucosa, and kidney. The effect of PTH on intestinal calcium absorption is indirect, resulting from increased renal production of the intestinally active vitamin D metabolite $1,25(OH)_2D$. By its integrated effects on the kidney, gut, and bone, PTH acts to increase the inflow of calcium into the extracellular fluid and thus defend against hypocalcemia. Removal of the parathyroid glands results in profound hypocalcemia and ultimately in tetany and death.

In the kidney, PTH has direct effects on the tubular reabsorption of calcium, phosphate, and bicarbonate. Although the bulk of calcium is resorbed from tubule fluid together with sodium in the proximal convoluted tubule, the fine tuning of calcium excretion occurs in the distal nephron. There, PTH markedly increases the reabsorption of calcium, predominantly in the distal convoluted tubule. Although calcium is actively transported against an electrochemical gradient, the precise nature of the calcium transport process that is regulated by PTH is controversial. However, from a physiologic standpoint, the ability to limit renal losses of calcium is one important means by which PTH defends the serum calcium level.

PTH inhibits the reabsorption of phosphate in the renal proximal tubule. In this nephron segment, phosphate is transported across the apical membrane of the tubule cell by specific sodium-phosphate cotransporters, with phosphate influx driven by the energy of the sodium gradient. PTH inhibits sodium-phosphate reabsorption by reducing the rate of insertion of transporters from a sequestered cytoplasmic pool into the apical membrane. The phosphaturic effect of PTH is profound. It is best quantified by calculating the tubular reabsorption of phosphate (TRP) from the clearances of phosphate and creatinine (TRP = $1 - C_P/C_{creat}$, normal range 80%-97%), or by calculating the renal phosphate threshold (TmP/GFR) from a standard nomogram. Because it is primarily the renal phosphate threshold that sets the level of serum phosphate, the phosphaturic effect of PTH is mirrored in the serum phosphorus level (eg, hypophosphatemia in hyperparathyroidism). Hyperparathyroid states may also be characterized by impaired bicarbonate reabsorption and a mild hyperchloremic metabolic acidosis, because of inhibition of Na^+-H^+ antiporter activity by PTH.

Although the hypocalciuric effect of PTH is readily understood as part of the concerted actions of the hormone to defend the serum $[Ca^{2+}]$, the utility of the phosphaturic effect of PTH is less obvious. One consideration is that the phosphaturic effect tends to prevent an increase in serum phosphate, which would otherwise result from the obligatory release of phosphate with calcium during bone resorption and would tend to dampen the homeostatic increase in serum calcium by complexing calcium in blood. An example is renal osteodystrophy. When phosphate clearance is impaired by renal failure, the hypocalcemic effect of phosphate released during bone remodeling is an important contributor to progressive secondary hyperparathyroidism as part of a positive feedback loop—the more that bone resorption is stimulated and phosphate released, the more hyperparathyroidism is induced.

Mechanism of Action of Parathyroid Hormone

There are two mammalian receptors for PTH. The first receptor to be identified recognizes PTH and PTHrP and is designated the PTH/PTHrP receptor, or the PTH-1 receptor (PTH-1R). The

PTH-2R is activated by PTH only. These receptors also differ in their tissue distribution. The PTH-1R in kidney and bone is an 80,000-MW glycoprotein and member of the G protein receptor superfamily. It has the canonical architecture of such receptors, with a large first extracellular domain, seven consecutive membrane-spanning domains, and a cytoplasmic tail (see Chapter 1). PTH binds to sites in the large extracellular domain of the receptor. The hormone-bound form of the receptor then activates associated G proteins via several determinants in the intracellular loops. PTH receptors are closely related to a small subfamily of peptide hormone receptors, which includes those for secretin, vasoactive intestinal polypeptide (VIP), adrenocorticotropin (ACTH), and calcitonin.

PTH itself has a close structural resemblance to a sister protein, PTHrP, and also resembles the peptides secretin, VIP, calcitonin, and ACTH. As noted above, the receptors for these related ligands are themselves members of a special family. These peptide hormones are characterized by an amino terminal alpha helical domain, thought to be directly involved in receptor activation, and an adjacent alpha helical domain that seems to be the primary receptor-binding domain. In the case of PTH, residues 1 to 6 are required for activation of the receptor; truncated analogs without these residues (eg, PTH[7-34]) can bind the receptor but cannot efficiently activate it and thus serve as competitive antagonists of PTH action. The primary receptor-binding domain consists of PTH(18-34). Although the intact form of PTH is an 84-amino-acid peptide, PTH(35-84) does not seem to have any important role in binding to the bone-kidney receptor. However, a separate PTH(35-84) receptor may exist; the carboxyl terminal PTH receptor could mediate an entirely different set of actions of PTH.

The PTH-1 receptor binds PTH and PTHrP with equal affinity. Physiologic activation of the receptor by binding of either PTH or PTHrP induces the active, GTP-bound state of two receptor-associated G proteins. G_s couples the receptor to the effector adenylyl cyclase and thereby to the generation of cAMP as a cellular second messenger. G_q couples the receptor to a separate effector system, phospholipase C, and thereby to an increase in $[Ca^{2+}]_i$ and to activation of protein kinase C (see Chapter 1). Although it is not clear which of the cellular messengers, cAMP, intracellular calcium, or diacylglycerol is responsible for each of the various cellular effects of PTH, there is evidence from an experiment of nature that cAMP is the intracellular second messenger for maintaining calcium homeostasis and renal phosphate excretion. The experiment is pseudohypoparathyroidism (PHP), in which null mutations in one allele of the stimulatory G protein subunit G_s alpha (GNAS1) cause hypocalcemia and unresponsiveness of renal phosphate excretion to PTH.

PTHrP

When secreted in abundance by malignant tumors, PTHrP produces severe hypercalcemia by activating the PTH-1 receptor. However, the physiologic roles of PTHrP are quite different from those of PTH. PTHrP is produced in many fetal and adult tissues. Based on gene knockout experiments and overexpression of PTHrP in individual tissues, we now know that PTHrP is required for normal development as a regulator of the proliferation and mineralization of chondrocytes and as a regulator of placental calcium transport. In postnatal life, PTHrP also appears to regulate epithelial-mesenchymal interactions that are critical for development of the mammary gland, skin, and hair follicle. In most physiologic circumstances, PTHrP carries out local rather than systemic actions. PTHrP is discussed fully in Chapter 21.

CALCITONIN

Calcitonin (CT) is a 32-amino-acid peptide whose principal function is to inhibit osteoclast-mediated bone resorption. CT is secreted by parafollicular C cells of the thyroid. These are neuroendocrine cells derived from the ultimobranchial body, which fuses with the posterior lobes of the thyroid to become the C cell mass (about 0.1% of the thyroid gland).

The secretion of CT is under the control of the ionized $[Ca^{2+}]$. The C cell uses the same CaSR as the parathyroid cell to sense changes in the ambient ionized $[Ca^{2+}]$. In contrast to parathyroid cells, C cells increase secretion of CT in response to hypercalcemia and shut off hormone secretion during hypocalcemia.

CT is a member of the *CT* gene–related peptide (CGRP) superfamily that includes: CT, CGRP, CT-receptor–stimulating peptide (CRSP), adrenomedullin, and amylin. CT and CGRP are encoded by one gene, and the respective peptides are generated from alternative splicing of primary RNA transcripts in a tissue-selective manner with CT made predominantly in the thyroid C cells. The genomic structure of the *CT/CGRP/CRSP* gene family is shown in Figure 8–6. In humans, there are two genes (*CALCA* and *CALCB*) that encode CGRPs and CT and one pseudogene

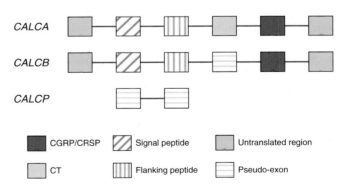

FIGURE 8–6 Genomic structure of the human calcitonin (CT)/calcitonin gene–related peptide (CGRP)/CT-receptor–stimulating peptide (CRSP) family of genes which includes CALCA and CALCB and the pseudogene CALCP. Alternative splicing generates the two gene products (CT in the thyroid C cells and CGRP in the nervous system) with well-defined functions in humans. Straight lines indicate the introns while the coding sequences are shown by specifically designated boxes. (Reproduced and modified, with permission from Katafuchi T, et al. Calcitonin receptor-stimulating peptide: its evolutionary and functional relationship with calcitonin/calcitonin gene-related peptide based on gene structure. *Peptides.* 2009;30:1753.)

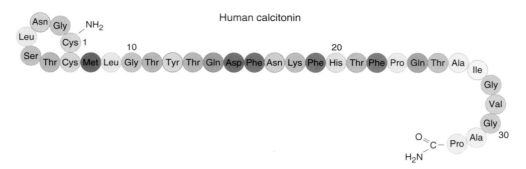

FIGURE 8–7 Amino acid sequence of human calcitonin, demonstrating its biochemical features, including an amino terminal disulfide bridge and carboxyl terminal prolinamide. (Reproduced, with permission, from McPhee SJ, et al, ed. *Pathophysiology of Disease: An Introduction to Clinical Medicine.* Originally published by Appleton & Lange. Copyright 1995 by The McGraw-Hill Companies, Inc.)

(CALCP). Transcription of CALCA produces CT and CGRP in a tissue-specific manner by alternative splicing. The *CALCB* gene has a coding CGRP-beta exon and an exon that codes for CT but in which there is an in-frame stop codon. Thus, CALCB generates only CGRP-beta. In the thyroid C cell, mature CT (Figure 8–7) is incorporated within a 141-amino-acid precursor. In neurons of the central nervous system, CGRP is produced from a 128-amino-acid precursor. CGRP is a 37-amino-acid peptide with considerable homology to CT. The amino termini of both peptides incorporate a seven-member disulfide-bonded ring (see Figure 8–7). Acting through its own receptor, CGRP is among the most potent vasodilator substances known. When administered intravenously, CT produces a rapid and dramatic decline in levels of serum calcium and phosphate, primarily through actions on bone. The major effect of the hormone is to inhibit osteoclastic bone resorption. After exposure to CT, the morphology of the osteoclast changes rapidly. Within minutes, the cell withdraws its processes, shrinks in size, and retracts the ruffled border, the organelle of bone resorption, from the bone surface. Osteoclasts and cells of the proximal renal tubule express CT receptors. Like the PTH receptor, this is a G protein–coupled receptor with seven membrane-spanning regions that is coupled by G_s alpha to adenylyl cyclase and thereby to the generation of cAMP in target cells. CT also has renal effects. In the kidney, CT inhibits the reabsorption of phosphate, thus promoting renal phosphate excretion. CT also induces a mild natriuresis and increases the renal excretion of calcium. The renal effects of CT are not essential for its acute effect on serum calcium levels, which results from blockade of bone resorption.

Although its secretory control by calcium and its antiresorptive actions enable CT to counter PTH in the control of calcium homeostasis, thus engendering bihormonal regulation, it is actually unlikely that CT plays an essential physiologic role in humans and other terrestrial animals. This is supported by two lines of evidence. First, removal of the thyroid gland—the major if not the only source of CT in mammals—has no perceptible impact on calcium handling or bone metabolism in postnatal life. Second, secretion of extremely high CT levels by medullary carcinoma of the thyroid (MCT), a malignancy of the C cell, likewise has no

apparent effect on mineral homeostasis. Thus, in humans, CT is a hormone in search of a function. It plays a much more obvious homeostatic role in saltwater fish, in which the major challenge is maintenance of blood calcium levels in the sea, where the ambient calcium concentration of sea water is very high.

CT is of clinical interest for two reasons. First, CT is important as a tumor marker in MCT. Second, CT has therapeutic uses as an inhibitor of osteoclastic bone resorption. CT can be administered either parenterally or as a nasal spray and is used in the treatment of Paget disease of bone, hypercalcemia, and osteoporosis.

VITAMIN D

Nomenclature

The term vitamin D (calciferol) refers to two secosteroids: vitamin D_2 (ergocalciferol) and vitamin D_3 (cholecalciferol) (Figure 8–8). Both are produced by photolysis from naturally occurring sterol precursors. Vitamin D_2 is the principal form of vitamin D available for pharmaceutical purposes other than as dietary supplements (Table 8–2). Vitamin D_3 is produced from 7-dehydrocholesterol, a precursor of cholesterol found in high concentration in the skin. Although vitamin D_2 is metabolized somewhat differently than vitamin D_3, the active metabolites of vitamin D_2 and vitamin D_3 have equivalent biologic activity so the term vitamin D, unless otherwise qualified, will be understood here to denote both. Vitamins D_2 and D_3 differ in their side chains: vitamin D_2 has a methyl group at C24 and a double bond at C22 to C23. These features alter the metabolism of vitamin D_2 compared with vitamin D_3; however, both are converted to 25-hydroxyvitamin D (25[OH]D) and 1,25-dihydroxyvitamin D (1,25[OH]$_2$D).

In the process of forming vitamins D_2 and D_3, the B ring of the sterol precursor is cleaved, and the A ring is rotated around the C5 to C6 double bond so that the 3β-hydroxyl group is positioned below the plane of the A ring. By convention, this hydroxyl group retains its designation as 3β, and the one position above the plane of the A ring is designated 1α. Hydroxylations in the side chain can lead to stereoisomers

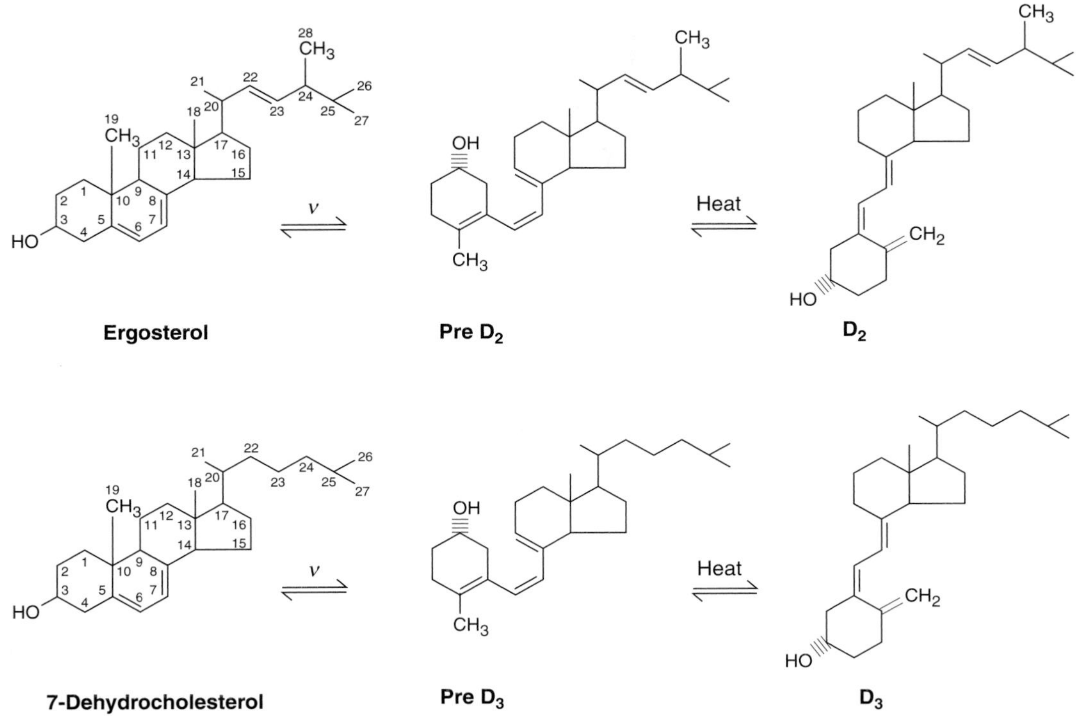

FIGURE 8–8 The photolysis of ergosterol and 7-dehydrocholesterol to vitamin D_2 (ergocalciferol) and vitamin D_3 (cholecalciferol), respectively. An intermediate is formed after photolysis, which undergoes a thermal-activated isomerization to the final form of vitamin D. The rotation of the A-ring puts the 3-beta-hydroxyl group into a different orientation with respect to the plane of the A-ring during production of vitamin D.

designated R and S. The natural position for the C24 hydroxyl group is R. Both the R and the S positions can be hydroxylated at C25 in the formation of 25,26(OH)$_2$D.

Because vitamin D can be formed in vivo (in the epidermis) in the presence of adequate amounts of ultraviolet light, it is more properly considered a hormone (or prohormone) than a vitamin. To be biologically active, vitamin D must be metabolized further. The liver is the major but not the only organ that can metabolize vitamin D to its principal circulating form, 25(OH)D. The

kidney and other tissues metabolize 25(OH)D to a variety of other metabolites, the most important of which are 1,25(OH)$_2$D and, perhaps, 24,25(OH)$_2$D. A large number of other metabolites have been identified, but their physiologic roles are unclear. They may represent products destined only for elimination. Normal circulating levels of the principal metabolites are listed in Table 8–3. The recommended daily allowance for vitamin D in adults is 400 units (1 unit = 0.025 μg vitamin D), although recent data indicate that is inadequate especially in older individuals.

TABLE 8–2 Commonly used vitamin D metabolites and analogs.

	Cholecalciferol, Ergocalciferol	Paricalcitol	Doxercalciferol	Calcitriol
Abbreviation	D_3, D_2	19-nor calcitriol	1αOHD$_2$	1,25(OH)$_2$D
Physiologic dose	2.5-10 ug (1 ug = 40 units)		1-5 ug	0.25-0.5 ug
Pharmacologic dose	0.625-5 mg	1-4 μg po 2.5 μg/mL IV	20-200 ug	1-3 ug
Duration of action	1-3 mo	Hours to days	Hours to days	Hours to days
Clinical applications	Vitamin D deficiency Vitamin D malabsorption Hypoparathyroidism	Secondary hyperparathyroidism of chronic renal failure	Secondary hyperparathyroidism of chronic renal failure	Secondary hyperparathyroidism of chronic renal failure Hypoparathyroidism Hypophosphatemic rickets Acute hypocalcemia Vitamin D-dependent rickets types I and II

TABLE 8–3 **Vitamin D and its metabolites.**

Name	Abbreviation	Generic Name	Serum Concentration[a]

Vitamin D
  Vitamin D_3
  Vitamin D_2
	D
	D_3
	D_2
		Calciferol
		Cholecalciferol
		Ergocalciferol
			1.6 ± 0.4 ng/mL

25-Hydroxyvitamin D	25(OH)D	Calcifediol	26.5 ± 5.3 ng/mL
1,25-Dihydroxyvitamin D	$1,25(OH)_2D$	Calcitriol	34.1 ± 0.4 pg/mL
24,25-Dihydroxyvitamin D	$24,25(OH)_2D$		1.3 ± 0.4 ng/mL
25,26-Dihydroxyvitamin D	$25,26(OH)_2D$		0.5 ± 0.1 ng/mL

[a]Values differ somewhat from laboratory to laboratory depending on the methodology used, sunlight exposure, and dietary intake of vitamin D in the population study. Children tend to have higher $1,25(OH)_2D$ levels than do adults.

Data from Lambert PW et al. In: Bikle D, ed. *Assay of Calcium Regulating Hormones.* Springer; 1983.

Cutaneous Synthesis of Vitamin D

Vitamin D_3 is formed in the skin from 7-dehydrocholesterol, which is distributed throughout the epidermis and dermis but has its highest concentration in the lower layers of the epidermis, the stratum spinosum, and stratum basale. These epidermal layers also account for the highest production of vitamin D. The cleavage of the B ring of 7-dehydrocholesterol to form previtamin D_3 (see Figure 8–8) requires ultraviolet light with a spectrum of 280 to 320 nm (UVB). Following cleavage of the B ring, the previtamin D_3 undergoes thermal isomerization to vitamin D_3 but also to the biologically inactive compounds lumisterol and tachysterol. Formation of pre-D_3 is rapid and reaches a maximum within hours during exposure to solar or ultraviolet irradiation. The degree of epidermal pigmentation, the age of the skin, and the intensity of exposure all affect the time required to reach the maximum pre-D_3 concentration but do not alter that maximum. Continued ultraviolet light exposure then results in continued formation of the inactive compounds from pre-D_3. The formation of lumisterol is reversible, so lumisterol can be converted back to pre-D_3 as pre-D_3 levels fall. Short exposure to sunlight causes prolonged release of vitamin D_3 from the exposed skin because of the slow conversion of pre-D_3 to vitamin D_3 and the conversion of lumisterol to pre-D_3. Prolonged exposure to sunlight does not produce toxic quantities of vitamin D_3 because of the photoconversion of pre-D_3 to lumisterol and tachysterol.

Vitamin D_3 transport from the skin into the circulation has not been thoroughly studied. Vitamin D_3 is carried in the bloodstream primarily bound to vitamin D–binding protein (DBP), an α-globulin produced in the liver. DBP has a lower affinity for vitamin D_3 than other vitamin D metabolites such as 25(OH)D and $24,25(OH)_2D$. 7-Dehydrocholesterol, pre-D_3, lumisterol, and tachysterol bind to DBP even less well. Therefore, vitamin D_3 could be selectively removed from skin by the gradient established by selective binding to DBP. Because the deepest levels of the epidermis make the most vitamin D_3 when the skin is irradiated, the distance over which vitamin D_3 must diffuse to reach the circulation is short. However, simple diffusion is an unlikely means for so hydrophobic a molecule to enter the bloodstream. Epidermal lipoproteins may play a role in transport, but this remains to be established.

Dietary Sources and Intestinal Absorption

Dietary sources of vitamin D are clinically important because exposure to ultraviolet light may not be sufficient to maintain adequate production of vitamin D in the skin. The farther away from the equator one lives, the shorter the period of the year during which the intensity of sunlight is sufficient to produce vitamin D_3. Most milk products in the United States are supplemented with vitamin D. Unfortified milk products contain little or no vitamin D. Although plants and mushrooms contain ergosterol, their content of vitamin D_2 is limited unless they are irradiated with ultraviolet light during processing. Vitamin D is found in moderate to high concentrations in fish oils and fish liver and in lesser concentrations in eggs. Vitamin D is absorbed from the diet in the small intestine with the help of bile salts. Drugs that bind bile salts such as colestipol and various malabsorption syndromes reduce vitamin D absorption. Most of the vitamin D passes into the lymph in chylomicrons, but a significant amount is absorbed directly into the portal system. The presence of fat in the lumen decreases vitamin D absorption. 25(OH)D and calcitriol are preferentially absorbed into the portal system and are less influenced by the amount of fat in the lumen. Biliary conjugates of the vitamin D metabolites have been identified, and an enterohepatic circulation of these metabolites has been established. Vitamin D is taken up rapidly by the liver and is metabolized to 25(OH)D. 25(OH)D is also transported in the blood bound to DBP. Little vitamin D is stored in the liver. Excess vitamin D is stored in adipose tissue and muscle.

Binding Proteins for Vitamin D Metabolites

As noted above, vitamin D metabolites are transported in the blood bound principally to DBP (85%) and albumin (15%). DBP binds 25(OH)D and $24,25(OH)_2D$ with approximately 30 times greater affinity than it binds $1,25(OH)_2D$ and vitamin D. DBP circulates at a concentration (5×10^{-6} mol/L) approximately

50 times greater than the total concentrations of the vitamin D metabolites. DBP levels are reduced in liver disease and in the nephrotic syndrome and increased during pregnancy and with estrogen administration, but are not altered by states of vitamin D deficiency or excess. The high affinity of DBP for the vitamin D metabolites and the large excess-binding capacity maintain the free and presumed biologically active concentrations of the vitamin D metabolites at very low levels—approximately 0.03% and 0.4% of the total 25(OH)D and 1,25(OH)$_2$D levels, respectively. Liver disease reduces the total level of the vitamin D metabolites commensurate with the reduction in DBP and albumin levels, but the free concentrations of the vitamin D metabolites remain normal in most subjects. This fact must be borne in mind when evaluating a patient with liver disease to determine whether such a patient is truly vitamin D deficient. Pregnancy, on the other hand, increases both the free and total concentrations by increasing DBP levels, altering the binding of the metabolites to DBP, and increasing the production of 1,25(OH)$_2$D. The binding of the vitamin D metabolites to DBP appears to occur at the same site, and saturation of this site by one metabolite can displace the other metabolites. This is an important consideration in vitamin D toxicity because the very high levels of 25(OH)D that characterize this condition displace the often normal levels of 1,25(OH)$_2$D, leading to elevated free and biologically active concentrations of 1,25(OH)$_2$D. This phenomenon at least partially explains the hypercalcemia and hypercalciuria that mark vitamin D intoxication even in patients with normal total 1,25(OH)$_2$D levels.

At present, it is not clear whether DBP functions just to maintain a circulating reservoir of vitamin D metabolites or whether DBP participates in transporting the vitamin D metabolites to their target tissues. A different set of proteins related to heat shock proteins are found within the cell that bind the vitamin D metabolites and appear to facilitate their further metabolism. These proteins are distinct from DBP and the nuclear hormone receptors for calcitriol, which will be discussed subsequently.

Metabolism

The conversion of vitamin D to 25(OH)D occurs principally in the liver (Figure 8–9). Both mitochondria and microsomes have the capacity to produce 25(OH)D but with different kinetics and with different enzymes. The mitochondrial enzyme has been identified as the 5βcholestane-3α,7α,12α-triol-27(26)-hydroxylase (CYP27A1), a cytochrome P450 mixed-function oxidase, and its cDNA has been isolated. A number of microsomal P450 enzymes have been shown to have 25-hydroxylase activity with variable preference for D$_2$ or D$_3$ and their 1-hydroxylated metabolites. The microsomal 25-hydroxylase that has received the most attention is CYP2R1. Like the mitochondrial enzyme, these are not specific

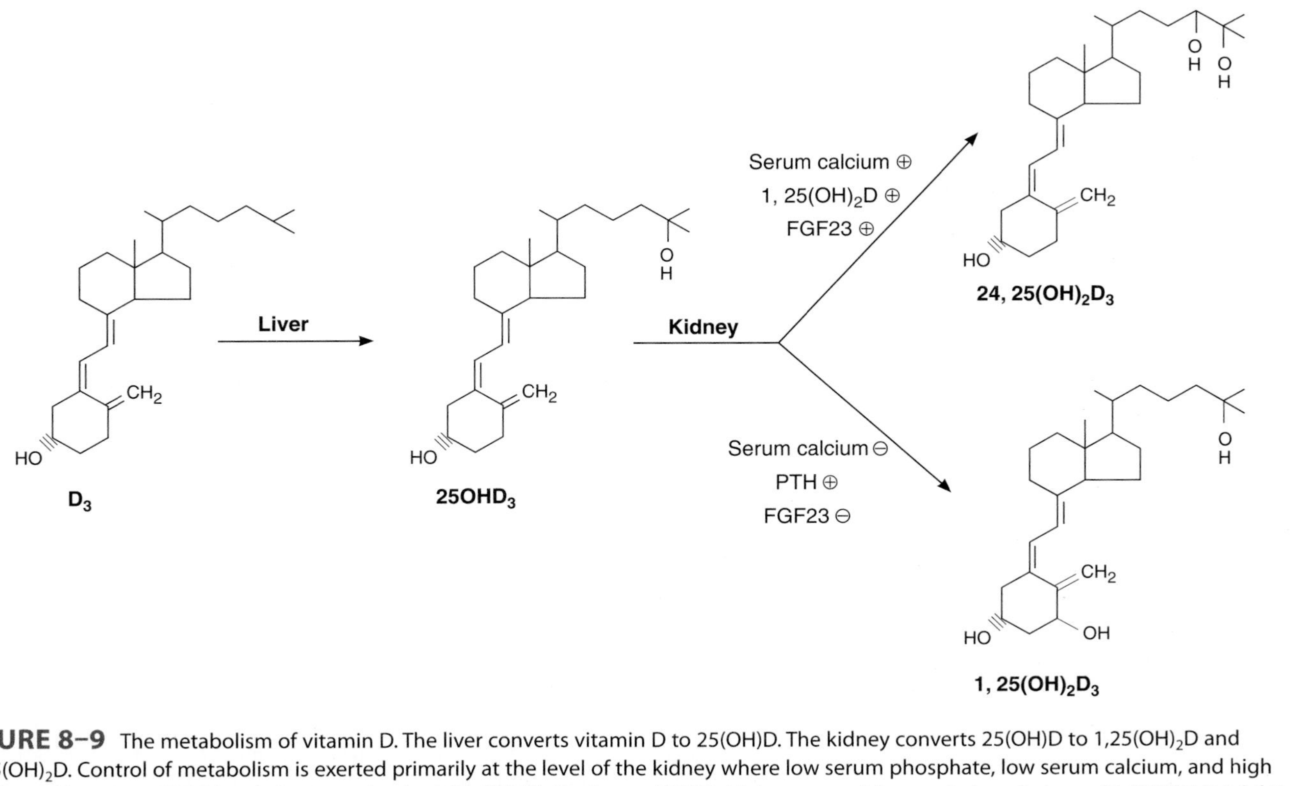

FIGURE 8–9 The metabolism of vitamin D. The liver converts vitamin D to 25(OH)D. The kidney converts 25(OH)D to 1,25(OH)$_2$D and 24,25(OH)$_2$D. Control of metabolism is exerted primarily at the level of the kidney where low serum phosphate, low serum calcium, and high parathyroid hormone (PTH) levels favor production of 1,25(OH)$_2$D whereas FGF23; high serum calcium and phosphate, and 1,25(OH)$_2$D inhibit 1,25(OH)$_2$D production while increasing 24,25(OH)$_2$D production. Plus (+) and minus (–) signs denote the stimulatory and inhibitory enzymatic reactions, respectively, driving the metabolic steps indicated.

for vitamin D. Regulation of 25(OH)D production is difficult to demonstrate. Drugs such as phenytoin and phenobarbital reduce serum 25(OH)D levels, primarily by increased catabolism of 25(OH)D and vitamin D. Liver disease leads to reduced total (but not necessarily free) serum 25(OH)D levels, primarily because of reduced DBP and albumin synthesis and not reduced synthesis of 25(OH)D. Vitamin D deficiency is marked by low blood levels of 25(OH)D, primarily because of lack of substrate for the 25-hydroxylase. Vitamin D intoxication, on the other hand, leads to increased levels of 25(OH)D because of the lack of feedback inhibition on the 25-hydroxylases.

Control of vitamin D metabolism is exerted principally in the kidney (see Figure 8–9). 1,25(OH)$_2$D and 24,25(OH)$_2$D are produced by cytochrome mixed-function oxidases in mitochondria of the proximal tubules. cDNAs encoding these enzymes have both been identified and show substantial homology to each other and to the mitochondrial 25-hydroxylase (CYP27A1). Their homology to other mitochondrial steroid hydroxylases is considerable but not as high. Although the 24-hydroxylase is widely distributed, the 1-hydroxylase is more limited, being found primarily in the epidermis, placenta, bone, macrophages, and prostate in addition to kidney, although low levels of expression have been observed in a number of other tissues such as breast, lung, testes, T and B lymphocytes, dendritic cells, heart, and brain.

The kidney remains the principal source of circulating 1,25(OH)$_2$D. Production of 1,25(OH)$_2$D in the kidney is stimulated by PTH and insulin-like growth factor-1 (IGF-1) and is inhibited by fibroblast-derived growth factor 23 (FGF23) and high blood levels of calcium and phosphate. Production of FGF23, a recently identified cytokine, occurs primarily in bone and is regulated by the levels of serum phosphate and 1,25(OH)$_2$D (Figure 8–10). FGF23 inhibits 1,25(OH)$_2$D production, blocks renal phosphate reabsorption, and acts to lower serum phosphate (see Figure 8–10 and Chapter 21).

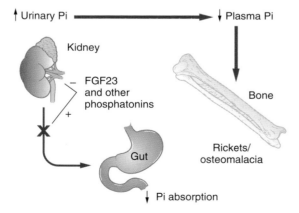

FIGURE 8–10 Regulation of phosphate homeostasis and 1,25(OH)$_2$D production by FGF23 and other phosphatonins. FGF23 decreases phosphate reabsorption by the kidney and lowers plasma phosphate levels. FGF23 also blocks 1,25(OH)$_2$D synthesis by the kidney, which reduces intestinal calcium and phosphate absorption. Excessive FGF23 production and/or action result in abnormal bone matrix mineralization, causing rickets or osteomalacia.

Calcium and phosphate also have both direct and indirect effects on 1,25(OH)$_2$D production. In addition to direct actions on 1-hydroxylase to reduce its activity, calcium inhibits PTH secretion by the parathyroid glands, and this lowers 1,25(OH)$_2$D production. Phosphate inhibits the production of growth hormone by the pituitary gland, leading to decreased IGF-1 generation, and stimulates FGF23 production, each step contributing to the indirect inhibition of 1,25(OH)$_2$D production by phosphate.

1,25(OH)$_2$D inhibits its own synthesis and stimulates the production of 24,25(OH)$_2$D and 1,24,25(OH)$_3$D by the 24-hydroxylase, which are the initial products of both 25(OH)D and 1,25(OH)$_2$D catabolism, respectively. Other hormones such as prolactin and CT may regulate 1,25(OH)$_2$D production, but their roles under normal physiologic conditions in humans have not been demonstrated.

Extrarenal production of 1,25(OH)$_2$D is regulated in a cell-specific fashion. Cytokines such as γ-interferon (γ-IFN) and tumor necrosis factor-α (TNF-α) stimulate 1,25(OH)$_2$D production by macrophages and keratinocytes. 1,25(OH)$_2$D and calcium have minimal effects on 1,25(OH)$_2$D production by these cells. This is important in understanding the pathophysiology of hypercalcemia and the increased 1,25(OH)$_2$D levels in patients with sarcoidosis, lymphomas, and other granulomatous diseases.

Mechanisms of Action

The main function of vitamin D metabolites is the regulation of calcium and phosphate homeostasis, which occurs in conjunction with PTH. The gut, kidney, and bone are the principal target tissues for this regulation. The major pathologic complication of vitamin D deficiency is rickets (in children with open epiphyses) or osteomalacia (in adults), which results mainly from the deficiency of calcium and phosphate required for bone mineralization. 1,25(OH)$_2$D is the most biologically active, if not the only vitamin D metabolite involved in maintaining calcium and phosphate homeostasis.

Most of the cellular processes regulated by 1,25(OH)$_2$D involve the nuclear vitamin D receptor (VDR), a 50-kDa protein related by structural and functional homology to a large class of nuclear hormone receptors including the steroid hormone receptors, thyroid hormone receptors (TRs), retinoic acid and retinoid X receptors (RARs, RXRs), and endogenous metabolite receptors, including peroxisome proliferation activator receptors (PPARs), liver X receptors (LXRs), and farnesoid X receptors (FXRs) (see Chapter 1). These receptors are transcription factors. The VDR, as is the case with TRs, RARs, PPARs, LXRs, and FXRs, generally acts by forming heterodimers with RXRs. The VDR–RXR complex then binds to specific regions within the regulatory portions of the genes whose expression is controlled by 1,25(OH)$_2$D (Figure 8–11). The regulatory regions are called vitamin D response elements (VDREs) and are generally composed of two stretches of six nucleotides (each called a half-site) with a specific and nearly identical sequence separated by three nucleotides with a less specific sequence (a direct repeat with three base-pair separation; DR3). Numerous exceptions to this rule can be found such as a VDR–RAR complex binding to a DR6 (direct repeat with six

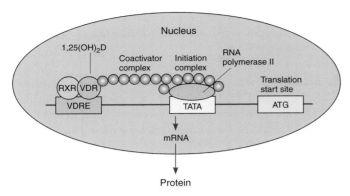

FIGURE 8–11 1,25(OH)$_2$D-initiated gene transcription. 1,25(OH)$_2$D enters the target cell and binds to its receptor, VDR. The VDR then heterodimerizes with the retinoid X receptor, RXR. This increases the affinity of the VDR–RXR complex for the vitamin D response element (VDRE), a specific sequence of nucleotides in the promoter region of a vitamin D responsive gene. Binding of the VDR–RXR complex to the VDRE attracts a complex of proteins termed coactivators to the VDR–RXR complex, some of which open up the gene for transcription by acetylating the histones and other proteins which communicate with and activate the RNA polymerase II complex. Transcription of the gene is initiated to produce the corresponding mRNA, which leaves the nucleus for the cytoplasm to be translated to the corresponding protein.

base-pair separation) or inverted palindromes (repeat elements going in opposite directions) with various degrees of spacing (eg, IP9). Other nuclear hormone receptors bind to similar elements but with different spacing or orientation of the half-sites. The binding of the VDR–RXR complex to the VDRE then attracts a number of other proteins called coactivators, which may function to open up the gene for transcription by acetylating the histones covering the gene or by bridging the gap between the VDRE and the initiation complex containing the RNA polymerase to signal the beginning of transcription. Not all actions of 1,25(OH)$_2$D, however, can be explained by changes in gene expression. VDR in the membrane and a membrane-bound protein called the 1,25D$_3$-membrane–associated rapid response steroid binding protein (1,25D$_3$-MARRS) may mediate the rapid effects of 1,25(OH)$_2$D on calcium influx and protein kinase C activity observed in a number of tissues, effects too rapid to be explained by genomic activity.

A. Intestinal calcium transport   Intestinal calcium transport is the best-understood target tissue response of 1,25(OH)$_2$D. Calcium transport through the intestinal epithelium proceeds by at least three distinct steps: (1) entrance into the cell from the lumen across the brush border membrane down a steep electrochemical gradient; (2) passage through the cytosol, probably within subcellular organelles such as mitochondria and endosomes; and (3) removal from the cell against a steep electrochemical gradient at the basolateral membrane. Each of these steps is regulated by 1,25(OH)$_2$D. At the brush border, 1,25(OH)$_2$D induces a change in the binding of calmodulin to brush border

myosin 1, a unique form of myosin found only in the intestine, where it resides primarily in the microvillus bound to actin and to the plasma membrane. The calmodulin-myosin 1 complex may provide the mechanism for removing calcium from the brush border after it crosses the membrane into the cell. Changes in the phospholipid composition of the brush border may explain the increased flux of calcium across this membrane after calcitriol administration. None of these changes requires new protein synthesis. However, evidence now indicates that a calcium channel, the transient receptor potential cation channel 6 (TRPV6) in the brush border membrane is induced by 1,25(OH)$_2$D and is likely the major mechanism by which calcium enters the intestinal epithelial cell. The transport of calcium through the cytosol requires a vitamin D-inducible protein called calbindin. Calbindin exists either in a 28-kDa or 9-kDa form, depending on the species and tissue. Calbindin has a high affinity for calcium. If its synthesis is blocked, the calcium content of the cytosol and mitochondria increases, and efficiency of transport is reduced. At the basolateral membrane, calcium is removed from the cell by an ATP-driven pump, the Ca^{2+}-ATPase (PMCA1b), a protein also induced by 1,25(OH)$_2$D. Recent studies, however, in which calbindin or TRPV6 expression is deleted show surprisingly little impact on intestinal calcium transport (calbindin knockout) or only a partial reduction (TRPV6 knockout) suggesting that there is more to learn about the mechanisms governing intestinal calcium transport. Nevertheless in mice in which the VDR is rendered nonfunctional (VDR knockout), intestinal calcium transport is markedly impaired, indicating the importance of VDR function—presumably via regulation of gene expression—in governing intestinal calcium transport.

B. Actions of vitamin D in bone   The critical role of 1,25(OH)$_2$D in regulating bone formation and resorption is evidenced by the development of rickets in children who are vitamin D-deficient, have inactivating mutations in CYP27B1 (the 1-hydroxylase) (pseudovitamin D-deficient rickets), or lack a functioning VDR (hereditary 1,25[OH]$_2$D-resistant rickets). The histologic and radiologic appearance of bone in these genetic conditions is quite similar to that in patients with severe vitamin D deficiency.

Patients with inactivating mutations in the *1-hydroxylase* gene can be treated successfully with calcitriol (but not with vitamin D), whereas those with mutations in the VDR are resistant to calcitriol as well as to vitamin D. These experiments of nature, however, do not exclude the possibility that other vitamin D metabolites, in combination with 1,25(OH)$_2$D, are essential for normal bone metabolism.

In vitamin D deficiency, all vitamin D metabolites are reduced, but 25(OH)D and 24,25(OH)$_2$D tend to be reduced out of proportion to 1,25(OH)$_2$D, which may be maintained in the low normal range despite clear abnormalities in bone mineralization. Thus, it is reasonable to ask whether 1,25(OH)$_2$D is the only vitamin D metabolite of consequence for the regulation of skeletal homeostasis. In fact, a number of studies point to unique actions of 24,25(OH)$_2$D that cannot be replicated by 1,25(OH)$_2$D, especially in cartilage, although this remains controversial. Studies in mice, in which the *24-hydroxylase* gene has been inactivated (knocked out), support the concept that 24,25(OH)$_2$D has a role in bone formation that is not replaced by 1,25(OH)$_2$D. At least some of the skeletal abnormalities in 24-hydroxylase–null animals may be explained by their inability to regulate 1,25(OH)$_2$D levels. Nevertheless, the need for more than just 1,25(OH)$_2$D is an important concept in the treatment of vitamin D deficiency; this is best done with vitamin D or 25(OH)D rather than calcitriol alone, because vitamin D serves as a precursor for both 1,25(OH)$_2$D and 24,25(OH)$_2$D.

The mechanisms by which 1,25(OH)$_2$D regulates skeletal homeostasis remain uncertain. Provision of adequate calcium and phosphate for mineralization is clearly important. The rickets present in patients with defective VDRs can be cured with calcium and phosphate infusions. Similarly, in mice in which the VDR is rendered nonfunctional (knocked out), rickets is prevented with diets high in calcium and phosphate. Thus, even though the osteoblast, the cell responsible for forming new bone, contains a VDR and the transcription of a number of proteins in bone is regulated by 1,25(OH)$_2$D, it is not clear how essential the direct actions of 1,25(OH)$_2$D on bone are for bone formation and mineralization. Thus, the bone is a good example of a tissue in which 1,25(OH)$_2$D and calcium work together, such that limited quantities of one may be compensated for by increased amounts of the other.

In organ cultures of bone, the best established action of 1,25(OH)$_2$D is to stimulate bone resorption. This is accompanied by an increase in osteoclast number and activity and decreased collagen synthesis. The increase in osteoclast number and activity is now known to be mediated by the production in osteoblasts of a membrane-bound protein called receptor activator of NF-kappa B ligand (RANKL), which acts on its receptor (RANK) in osteoclasts and their precursors to stimulate osteoclast differentiation and activity (see later). 1,25(OH)$_2$D is one of several hormones (PTH and selected cytokines are others) that stimulate RANKL production. Vitamin D deficiency does not decrease bone resorption, probably because PTH levels are elevated. High levels of PTH could, therefore, compensate for the lack of 1,25(OH)$_2$D at the level of RANKL production. The presence of partial skeletal resistance to PTH in patients with vitamin D deficiency may be explained by this mechanism.

1,25(OH)$_2$D also promotes the differentiation of osteoblasts. This action is less well-delineated than the promotion of osteoclast differentiation. Osteoblasts pass through a well-defined sequence of biochemical processes as they differentiate from proliferating osteoprogenitor cells to cells capable of producing and mineralizing matrix. The effect of 1,25(OH)$_2$D on the osteoblast depends on the stage of differentiation at which the 1,25(OH)$_2$D is administered. Early in the differentiation process, in cells characterized as immature osteoblast-like cells, 1,25(OH)$_2$D stimulates collagen production and alkaline phosphatase activity. These functions are inhibited in more mature osteoblasts. On the other hand, osteocalcin production is stimulated by 1,25(OH)$_2$D only in mature osteoblasts. Experiments in vivo demonstrating that excessive 1,25(OH)$_2$D can inhibit normal bone mineralization—leading to the paradoxical appearance of osteomalacia—can be understood in the context of these differential effects of 1,25(OH)$_2$D on the osteoblast as it differentiates. Excess 1,25(OH)$_2$D can disrupt the differentiation pathway.

C. Actions of vitamin D in kidney   The kidney expresses VDRs, and 1,25(OH)$_2$D stimulates the expression of calbindin, TRPV5 (the renal homolog of the intestinal TRPV6), and Ca^{2+}-ATPase (PMCA) in the distal tubule as well as 24,25(OH)$_2$D production in the proximal tubule. However, the role of 1,25(OH)$_2$D in regulating calcium and phosphate transport across the renal epithelium remains controversial. 25(OH)D may be more important than 1,25(OH)$_2$D in acutely stimulating calcium and phosphate reabsorption by the kidney tubules. In vivo studies are complicated by the effect of 1,25(OH)$_2$D on other hormones, particularly PTH, which appears to be more important than the vitamin D metabolites in regulating calcium and phosphate handling by the kidney.

D. Actions of vitamin D in other tissues   An exciting observation is that VDRs are found in a large number of tissues beyond the classic target tissues—gut, bone, and kidney—and these tissues respond to 1,25(OH)$_2$D. Furthermore, many of these tissues contain CYP27B1 (the 1-hydroxylase) and so are capable of producing their own 1,25(OH)$_2$D from circulating 25(OH)D. These tissues include elements of the hematopoietic and immune systems; cardiac, skeletal, and smooth muscle; and brain, liver, breast, endothelium, skin (keratinocytes, melanocytes, and fibroblasts), and endocrine glands (pituitary, parathyroid, pancreatic islets [B cells], adrenal cortex and medulla, thyroid, ovary, and testis). Furthermore, malignancies developing in these tissues often contain VDRs and respond to the antiproliferative actions of 1,25(OH)$_2$D.

The responses of these tissues to 1,25(OH)$_2$D are as varied as the tissues themselves. 1,25(OH)$_2$D regulates hormone production and secretion, including stimulation of insulin secretion from the pancreas and prolactin from the pituitary, but inhibiting PTH secretion from the parathyroid gland, renin secretion from the kidney, and atrial naturetic peptides from the heart. 1,25(OH)$_2$D enables the innate immune system by inducing antimicrobial peptides such as cathelidicin but suppresses the adaptive immune response by blocking the maturation of dendritic cells and shifting the balance of T-helper cell differentiation from Th1 and Th17 to Th2 and Treg. Myocardial contractility and vascular tone are modulated by 1,25(OH)$_2$D. 1,25(OH)$_2$D reduces the rate of proliferation of many cell lines, including normal keratinocytes, fibroblasts, lymphocytes, and thymocytes as well as abnormal cells of mammary, skeletal, intestinal, lymphatic, and myeloid origin. Differentiation of numerous normal cell types, including keratinocytes, lymphocytes, hematopoietic cells, intestinal epithelial cells, osteoblasts, and osteoclasts as well as abnormal cells of the same lineage is enhanced by 1,25(OH)$_2$D. Thus, the potential for manipulating a vast array of physiologic and pathologic processes with calcitriol and its analogs is enormous. This promise is starting to be realized in that vitamin D analogs are being used to treat psoriasis, uremic hyperparathyroidism, and osteoporosis.

Epidemiologic and animal studies indicate a role for vitamin D in the prevention and treatment of both type 1 and type 2 diabetes mellitus, autoimmune diseases such as multiple sclerosis and inflammatory bowel disease, and infections such as tuberculosis. Trials of vitamin D analogs in the treatment of a variety of cancers are also being conducted. Thus, although regulation of bone mineral homeostasis remains the major physiologic function of vitamin D and its metabolites, clinical applications for these compounds and their analogs are being found outside the classic target tissues.

HOW VITAMIN D AND PTH CONTROL MINERAL HOMEOSTASIS

Consider a person who switches from a high normal to a low normal intake of calcium and phosphate—from 1200 mg/d to 300 mg/d of calcium (the equivalent of leaving three glasses of milk out of the daily diet). The net absorption of calcium falls sharply, causing a transient decrease in the serum calcium level. The homeostatic response to this transient hypocalcemia is led by an increase in PTH, which stimulates the release of calcium and phosphate from bone and the retention of calcium by the kidney. The phosphaturic effect of PTH allows elimination of phosphate, which is resorbed from bone together with calcium. In addition, the increase in PTH, along with the fall in serum calcium and serum phosphate, activates renal $1,25(OH)_2D$ synthesis. In turn, $1,25(OH)_2D$ increases the fractional absorption of calcium and further increases bone resorption. External calcium balance is thus restored by increased fractional absorption of calcium and increased bone resorption at the expense of higher steady state levels of PTH and $1,25(OH)_2D$.

MEDULLARY CARCINOMA OF THE THYROID

MCT, a neoplasm of thyroidal C cells, accounts for 5% to 10% of all thyroid malignancies. Approximately 75% of MCTs are sporadic. The remainder is familial and associated with one of three heritable syndromes: familial isolated MCT; multiple endocrine neoplasia 2A (MEN 2A), consisting of MCT, pheochromocytoma, and primary hyperparathyroidism; or multiple endocrine neoplasia 2B (MEN 2B), consisting of MCT, pheochromocytoma, multiple mucosal neuromas, and, rarely, primary hyperparathyroidism (Table 8–4). The MEN syndromes are more extensively discussed in Chapter 22.

Understanding the pathogenesis of MCT has been greatly enhanced by the identification of causative mutations in the *RET* proto-oncogene located on chromosome 10q11.2. The *RET* gene encodes a membrane tyrosine kinase receptor whose ligands belong to the glial cell line-derived neurotrophic factor (GDNF) family. This receptor is expressed developmentally in migrating neural crest cells that give rise to hormone-secreting neuroendocrine

TABLE 8–4 Clinical presentations resulting from RET mutations.

Disorder	Characteristic Components
MEN 2A	MCT, pheochromocytoma, primary hyper-parathyroidism
MEN 2A with lichen amyloidosis	MEN 2A + pruritic lesions of upper back
Familial MCT	MCT
MEN 2A or Familial MCT and Hirschsprung disease	MCT, Hirschsprung disease
MEN 2B	MCT, pheochromocytoma, marfanoid habitus, intestinal and mucosal ganglioneuromatosis

Modified from Brandi ML, et al. Guidelines for diagnosis and therapy of MEN type 1 and type 2. *J Clin Endocrinol Metab.* 2001;86:5658 and Sakorafas GH, et al. The genetic basis of hereditary medullary thyroid cancer: clinical implications for the surgeon with a particular emphasis on the role of prophylactic thyroidectomy. *Endo Rel Cancer.* 2008;15:871.

cells (eg, C cells and adrenal medullary cells) and to the parasympathetic and sympathetic ganglia of the peripheral nervous system. Remarkably, different mutations in *RET* can produce five distinct diseases (see Table 8–4). Inheritance of certain activating mutations is responsible for MEN 2A and familial MCT. Inheritance of a different set of activating mutations causes MEN 2B. In over half of sporadic MCTs, the tumor has a clonal somatic mutation (present in the tumor but not in genomic DNA), which is identical to one of the mutations that is responsible for the familial forms of MCT. These somatic mutations clearly play a causative role in sporadic MCT. Mutations in the *RET* gene can also produce Hirschsprung disease, a congenital absence of the enteric parasympathetic ganglia, that can lead to a disturbance in intestinal motility, resulting in megacolon.

MCT is usually located in the middle or upper portions of the thyroid lobes. It is typically unilateral in sporadic cases but often multicentric and bilateral in familial forms of the disease. The natural history of MCT is variable. Sporadic tumors may be quite aggressive or very indolent; the mean 5-year survival rate is about 50%. The behavior of familial forms varies among syndromes. MEN 2B has the most aggressive form of MCT, with a 2-year survival of about 50%; MEN 2A has a course similar to that of sporadic forms of this tumor, and familial MCT has the most indolent course of all MCT. The natural history of the tumor in familial MCT, MEN 2A, and MEN 2B syndromes has been dramatically impacted by early prophylactic total thyroidectomy that is now advised in most carriers of disease-causing RET mutations. MCT may spread to regional lymph nodes or undergo hematogenous spread to the lungs and other viscera. When metastatic, this tumor is sometimes associated with a chronic diarrhea syndrome. The pathogenesis of the diarrhea is unclear. In addition to CT, these tumors secrete a variety of other bioactive products, including prostaglandins, serotonin, histamine, and peptide hormones (ACTH, somatostatin, corticotropin-releasing hormone). In some cases, the associated diarrhea responds dramatically to treatment with long-acting somatostatin analog such as octreotide, which blocks secretion of these bioactive products.

CT is a tumor marker for MCT. It is most sensitive for this purpose when secretion is stimulated with provocative agents. The standard provocative tests use pentagastrin (0.5 ug/kg intravenously over 5 seconds) or a rapid infusion of calcium gluconate (2 mg calcium/kg over 1 minute). Blood samples are obtained at baseline and 1, 2, and 5 minutes after the stimulus. For maximal sensitivity, both tests are usually combined, with the calcium infusion immediately followed by administration of pentagastrin. Although basal CT levels are often normal in early tumors, CT levels may be many times higher than normal in patients with disseminated MCT. Despite this, the patients are uniformly normocalcemic. Although tumors secrete larger molecular weight forms of CT with decreased biologic activity, monomeric CT levels are often high as well. *RET* oncogene analysis has replaced provocative testing in most cases, although basal CT levels are still used to follow disease burden postoperatively and during chemotherapy trials.

Members of families carrying *RET* mutations must be screened for MCT and, if positive, for the associated tumors that occur in MEN 2A and MEN 2B (see Table 8–4 and Chapter 22). In the case of MCT, the presence of the *RET* mutation in an individual generally leads to the recommendation for a total thyroidectomy prior to the development of frank malignancy or abnormal CT levels. It is recommended in a kindred with a known *RET* mutation that children be screened at birth for the carrier state. Total thyroidectomy with or without central compartment lymph node dissection can be performed in mutation carriers, and further testing can be discontinued in genetically normal family members. The timing of prophylactic thyroidectomy in carriers of *RET* mutations, however, depends on the genotype present (ie, codon mutated in *RET*) (Table 8–5). As supported by the genotype-phenotype correlations in these diseases, surgery is recommended in certain high-risk cases before 1 year of age, in cases of intermediate risk before 5 years of age, and in lower-risk patients later in childhood usually by 10 years of age. Because a limited number of mutations in *RET* cause more than 95% of hereditary MCT and up to 25% of sporadic disease, it is possible to screen the majority of patients using commercial reference laboratories.

Apparent sporadic MCT also calls for genetic testing and family studies. Up to 25% of new cases of MCT may actually be probands of families who harbor one of the familial syndromes. It has been noted in some kindreds after careful and lengthy follow-up that some individuals develop pheochromocytomas or primary hyperparathyroidism. Therefore, patients with apparent familial MCT should be followed indefinitely for one of these components of MEN 2A. Screening of family members can be accomplished by genetic testing, once the index case is identified. Identification of a mutation that is present only in tumor tissue would establish the mutation as somatic and the tumor as a sporadic one. Identification of the same *RET* mutation in tumor and genomic DNA would make

TABLE 8-5   RET mutations: their frequency and age at which surgery is recommended in gene carriers based on level of risk of MCT.

Codon	Frequency (Percent of Total)
MEN 2A[a]	
634	87
620	6
618	3
611	2
609	<1
MEN 2B[b]	
918	94
883	5
804	<1
Familial MCT[c]	
618	30
634	26
620	21
768	8
609	4
804	3
790, 791, 891	Uncertain

[a]Surgery recommended before 5 years of age.

[b]Surgery recommended in the first year of life.

[c]Recommendations for surgery by some experts at 5 years of age and by others before 10 years of age.

Reproduced, with permission, from Sakorafas GH, et al. The genetic basis of hereditary medullary thyroid cancer: clinical implications for the surgeon, with a particular emphasis on the role of prophylactic thyroidectomy. *Endo Rel Cancer.* 2008;15:871.

the diagnosis of a familial form of the disorder and would mandate careful screening of the family.

HYPERCALCEMIA

Clinical Features

A number of symptoms and signs accompany hypercalcemia. They include central nervous system effects such as lethargy, depression, psychosis, ataxia, stupor, and coma; neuromuscular effects such as weakness, proximal myopathy, and hypertonia; cardiovascular effects such as hypertension, bradycardia (and eventually asystole), and a shortened QT interval; renal effects such as stones, decreased glomerular filtration, polyuria, hyperchloremic acidosis, and nephrocalcinosis; gastrointestinal effects such as nausea, vomiting, constipation, and anorexia; eye findings such as band keratopathy; and systemic metastatic calcification. Primary hyperparathyroidism, one of the most common etiologies for hypercalcemia, has the mnemonic for recalling its signs and symptoms as *stones, bones, abdominal groans, and psychic moans* (Figure 8–12).

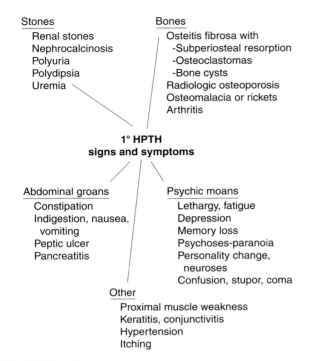

FIGURE 8–12 Signs and symptoms of primary hyperparathyroidism.

Mechanisms

Although many disorders are associated with hypercalcemia (Table 8–6), they produce it by a limited number of mechanisms: (1) increased bone resorption, (2) increased gastrointestinal absorption of calcium, or (3) decreased renal excretion of calcium. Although any of these mechanisms can be involved in a given patient, the common feature of virtually all hypercalcemic disorders is accelerated bone resorption. The only hypercalcemic disorder in which bone resorption does not play a part is the milk-alkali syndrome.

The central feature of the defense against hypercalcemia is suppression of PTH secretion. This reduces bone resorption, renal production of $1,25(OH)_2D$, and, thereby, intestinal calcium absorption and increases urinary calcium losses. The kidney plays a key role in the adaptive response to hypercalcemia as the only route of net calcium elimination. The level of renal calcium excretion is markedly increased by the combined effects of an increased filtered load of calcium and the suppression of PTH. However, the patient who relies on the kidneys to excrete an increased calcium load is in precarious balance. Glomerular filtration is impaired by hypercalcemia; the urinary concentrating ability is diminished, predisposing to dehydration; poor mentation may interfere with access to fluids; and nausea and vomiting may further predispose to dehydration and renal azotemia. Renal insufficiency, in turn, compromises calcium clearance, leading to a downward spiral (Figure 8–13). Thus, once established, many hypercalcemic states are self-perpetuating or aggravated through the *vicious cycle of hypercalcemia*. The only alternative to the renal route for elimination of calcium from the extracellular fluid is deposition of

TABLE 8–6 Causes of hypercalcemia.

Primary hyperparathyroidism
Sporadic
Associated with MEN 1 or MEN 2A
Familial
Postrenal transplantation
Variant forms of hyperparathyroidism
Familial benign hypocalciuric hypercalcemia
Lithium therapy
Tertiary hyperparathyroidism in chronic renal failure
Malignancies
Humoral hypercalcemia of malignancy
Caused by PTHrP (solid tumors, adult T-cell leukemia syndrome)
Caused by $1,25(OH)_2D$ (lymphomas)
Caused by ectopic secretion of PTH (rare)
Local osteolytic hypercalcemia (multiple myeloma, leukemia, lymphoma)
Sarcoidosis or other granulomatous diseases
Endocrinopathies
Thyrotoxicosis
Adrenal insufficiency
Pheochromocytoma
VIPoma
Drug induced
Vitamin A intoxication
Vitamin D intoxication
Thiazide diuretics
Lithium
Milk-alkali syndrome
Estrogens, androgens, tamoxifen (in breast carcinoma)
Immobilization
Acute renal failure
Idiopathic hypercalcemia of infancy
ICU hypercalcemia
Serum protein disorders

calcium phosphate and other salts in bone and soft tissues. Soft tissue calcification is observed with massive calcium loads, with massive phosphate loads (as in tumor lysis syndrome, crush injuries and compartment syndromes), and when renal function is markedly impaired and the calcium-phosphate product rises.

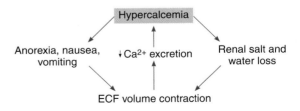

FIGURE 8–13 Vicious cycle of hypercalcemia. Once established, hypercalcemia can be maintained or aggravated as depicted. (Reproduced, with permission, from Felig P, Baxter JD, Frohman LA, ed. *Endocrinology and Metabolism*. 3rd ed. McGraw-Hill; 1995.)

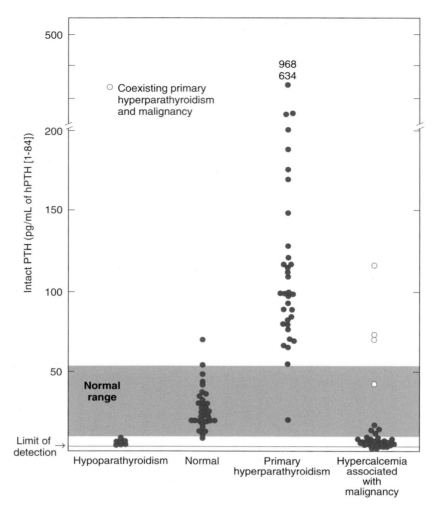

FIGURE 8–14 Clinical utility of immunoradiometric assay for intact PTH. (Reproduced, with permission, from Endres DB, et al. Measurement of parathyroid hormone. *Endocrinol Metab Clin North Am.* 1989;18:611.)

Differential Diagnosis

As a practical matter, the categories for differential diagnosis are primary hyperparathyroidism and *everything else* (see Table 8–6). Hyperparathyroidism is by far the most common cause of hypercalcemia and has distinctive pathophysiologic features. Thus, the first step in the differential diagnosis is determination of intact PTH (Figure 8–14). If the PTH level is high, and thus inappropriate for hypercalcemia, little further workup is required except to consider the variant forms of hyperparathyroidism that are discussed later. If the PTH level is suppressed, then a search for other entities must be conducted. Most other entities in Table 8–6 are readily diagnosed by their distinctive features, as discussed later.

DISORDERS CAUSING HYPERCALCEMIA

1. PRIMARY HYPERPARATHYROIDISM

Primary hyperparathyroidism results from the excessive secretion of PTH and typically produces frank hypercalcemia. With the

advent of multiphasic screening of serum chemistries, we have come to recognize that primary hyperparathyroidism is a common and usually asymptomatic disorder. Its incidence is approximately 42 per 100,000, and its prevalence is up to 4 per 1000 in women over age 60. Primary hyperparathyroidism is approximately 2 to 3 times more common in women than in men.

Etiology and Pathogenesis

Primary hyperparathyroidism is caused by a single parathyroid adenoma in about 80% of cases and by primary hyperplasia of the parathyroids in 10% to 15%. Parathyroid carcinoma is a rare cause of hyperparathyroidism, accounting for 1% to 2% of cases. Parathyroid carcinoma is often recognizable preoperatively because it presents with severe hypercalcemia or a palpable neck mass.

Sporadic parathyroid adenomas have a clonal origin, indicating that they can be traced back to an oncogenic mutation in a single progenitor cell. A few of these genetic alterations have been identified and/or assigned to chromosomal loci. About 25% of sporadic parathyroid adenomas have chromosomal deletions involving chromosome 11q12-13 that are thought to eliminate the putative tumor suppressor gene *MENIN*. As reviewed later and in Chapter 22, loss of the functioning menin protein, a tumor suppressor, is the cause of parathyroid, pituitary, and pancreatic tumors in the MEN 1 syndrome. An additional 40% of parathyroid adenomas display allelic loss on chromosome 1p (1p32pter).

Another important locus on chromosome 11 that has been implicated in approximately 4% of sporadic parathyroid adenomas involves the *cyclin D1* gene. In the initial elucidation of this pathogenic mechanism, a chromosomal rearrangement was found in a parathyroid tumor. Breakage and then inversion of a piece of chromosome 11 led to the expression of cyclin D1, a cell-cycle regulatory protein, under the control of the PTH promoter. As expected, this promoter is highly active in parathyroid cells, resulting in marked overexpression of cyclin D1 in these tumor cells. Cyclin D1 is normally expressed at high levels in the G_1 phase of the cell cycle and permits entry of cells into the mitotic phase of the cycle. Thus, a parathyroid-specific disorder of cell-cycle regulation leads to abnormal cell proliferation and ultimately excessive PTH production.

Parathyroid hyperplasia accounts for 12% to 15% of cases of primary hyperparathyroidism and is the pathologic basis for these inherited conditions: MEN 1, MEN 2A, the hyperparathyroidism-jaw tumor (HPT-JT) syndromes, and isolated familial hyperparathyroidism. In all of these instances four or fewer glands may be involved at the time of presentation. Inheritance of all of these conditions is autosomal dominant.

Parathyroid hyperplasia was traditionally viewed as an example of true hyperplasia, a polyclonal expansion of cell mass. This occurs in other endocrine tissues when a trophic hormone present in excess (eg, ACTH excess) induces bilateral adrenal hyperplasia. Molecular analysis, however, has revised this view. Parathyroid hyperplasia appears to share similar pathogenic mechanisms with parathyroid adenomas. The MEN 1 syndrome illustrates this. MEN 1 is due to the inherited inactivation of one allele of the *MENIN* gene, which encodes a tumor suppressor. Acquired postnatal somatic mutations in the remaining *MENIN* gene result in loss of the other allele's function. This leads to tumors in those endocrine tissues in which the gene is expressed. In this view, multicentric somatic mutations would account for the occurrence of four-gland hyperparathyroidism.

Kindreds with a presentation like MEN 1 but without mutations in *MENIN* have been investigated for germline mutations in cyclin-dependent kinase inhibitors (CDKIs) of which there are seven known genes. In an analysis of 196 consecutive cases of MEN 1 or other tumor states without germline mutations in *MENIN*, one laboratory found seven probable pathologic mutations in these genes. Three of the seven mutations were in *p27* with the remainder in three other CDKIs (*p15, p18,* and *p27*). These mutations are thought to be disease causing because abnormalities in CDKI–protein interaction were uncovered in the majority of these mutations tested. The CDKIs negatively control the cell cycle through interaction with and inhibition of cyclins D, E, and A. The germline mutations in these kindreds would, therefore, involve loss of function in known inhibitors of cell growth and cell cycle activity.

In MEN 2A, the occurrence of parathyroid hyperplasia is also a consequence of expression of activating mutations of the *RET* gene in the four glands. These and other studies clearly indicate that parathyroid hyperplasia is typically monoclonal in its origin, implying that cell hyperproliferation arose from a single progenitor cell in each gland.

In addition to hyperparathyroidism, as one part of classical MEN 1, it is now clear that a subset of cases of familial isolated hyperparathyroidism is due to germline mutations in the *MENIN* gene. This observation established the concept that isolated familial hyperparathyroidism can be an allelic variant of the MEN 1 syndrome. The variation from MEN 1 lies in the absence of tumors in the other endocrine glands.

Other cases of familial isolated hyperparathyroidism are explained, albeit rarely, by mutations in the gene that causes the HPT-JT syndrome (see later). Additional families with isolated hyperparathyroidism have, as yet, no identified mutations.

In contrast to MEN 1 and MEN 2A, both benign and malignant parathyroid tumors occur in the HPT-JT syndrome. This is an autosomal dominant disorder that includes primary hyperparathyroidism (90%), jaw tumors (ossifying fibromas of the mandible or maxilla) (30%), renal cysts (10%), and less frequently renal hamartomas and Wilms tumor. Linkage analysis originally determined the locus for this syndrome, which had been designated as *hyperparathyroidism 2 or HRPT2* to be at 1q24-q32. Inactivating mutations in *HRPT2* gene, encoding the protein parafibromin, have been identified in HPT-JT kindreds. Mutations in the *HRPT2* gene inactivate parafibromin. This protein like menin normally functions as a tumor suppressor. Its function(s) in parathyroid cells have not yet been elucidated.

Inactivating mutations in the *HRPT2* gene have also been identified in kindreds with isolated familial hyperparathyroidism. Both single- and multiple-gland disease have been noted. It was further noted that approximately 15% of affected individuals with HPT-JT syndrome develop parathyroid cancer, instead of adenomas or hyperplasia, suggesting that reduced parafibromin function also contributes to a malignant phenotype. Several groups have shown that a large percentage (~70%) of patients with sporadic parathyroid cancer harbor somatic mutations in the *HRPT2* gene. Surprisingly, approximately 30% of individuals with isolated parathyroid cancer have also been found to have germline mutations in *HRPT2* without the other manifestations of the HPT-JT syndrome. It is now thought that the majority of sporadically occurring parathyroid cancers are due to somatic mutations in the coding region of the *HRPT2* gene. It is anticipated that mutations in the noncoding regulatory regions of this gene may explain additional cases. A pathologic study of more than 50 cases of parathyroid cancer indicates that the loss of parafibromin immunoreactivity is a specific and key feature of malignancy with a sensitivity of 96% (CI, 85%-99%) and specificity of 99% (CI, 92%-100%).

Clinical Features

A. Symptoms and signs The typical clinical presentation of primary hyperparathyroidism has evolved considerably over the past few decades. As the disease continues to be detected primarily by multiphasic screening that includes determination of serum calcium levels, there has been a marked reduction in the frequency of the classic signs and symptoms of primary hyperparathyroidism. Renal disease (stones, decreased renal function, and occasionally nephrocalcinosis) and the classic hyperparathyroid bone disease osteitis fibrosa cystica are decidedly rare today. In fact, about 85% of patients presenting today have neither bone nor renal manifestations of hyperparathyroidism and are regarded as asymptomatic or at most minimally symptomatic. At the same time, we have begun to recognize more subtle manifestations of hyperparathyroidism. This has presented a number of questions about the role of parathyroid surgery in primary hyperparathyroidism, which are discussed later (see Treatment).

1. **Hyperparathyroid bone disease**—The classic bone disease of hyperparathyroidism is osteitis fibrosa cystica. Formerly common, this disorder now occurs in less than 10% of patients. Clinically, osteitis fibrosa cystica causes bone pain and sometimes pathologic fractures. The most common laboratory finding is an elevation of the alkaline phosphatase level, reflecting high bone turnover. Histologically, there is an increase in the number of bone-resorbing osteoclasts, marrow fibrosis, and cystic lesions that may contain fibrous tissue (brown tumors). The most sensitive and specific radiologic finding of osteitis fibrosa cystica is subperiosteal resorption of cortical bone, best seen in high-resolution films of the phalanges (Figure 8–15A). A similar process in the skull leads to a salt-and-pepper appearance (Figure 8–15B). Bone cysts or brown tumors may present as osteolytic lesions. Dental films may disclose loss of the lamina dura of the teeth, but this is a nonspecific finding also seen in periodontal disease.

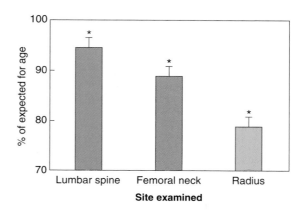

FIGURE 8–16 Bone mineral density at several sites in primary hyperparathyroidism shown as the percentage of expected for age. (Reproduced, with permission, from Silverberg SJ, et al. Nephrolithiasis and bone involvement in primary hyperparathyroidism. *Am J Med.* 1990;89:327.)

The other important skeletal consequence of hyperparathyroidism is osteoporosis. Unlike other osteoporotic disorders, hyperparathyroidism often results in the preferential loss of cortical bone (Figure 8–16). In general, both the mass and mechanical strength of trabecular bone are relatively maintained in mild primary hyperparathyroidism. Patients who are followed medically with this disease generally do not experience progressive bone loss for as long as 8 years after diagnosis (Figure 8–17). This may be due to the fact that mild PTH excess has an anabolic effect on the skeleton to maintain or even increase bone mass. Although osteoporosis, defined by bone mineral density (BMD) T-scores by dual-energy x-ray

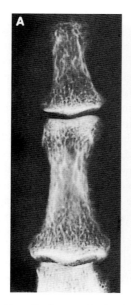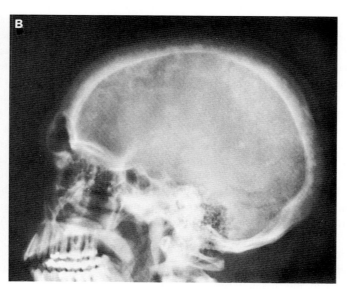

FIGURE 8–15 **A**: Magnified x-ray of index finger on fine-grain industrial film showing classic subperiosteal resorption in a patient with severe primary hyperparathyroidism. Note the left (radial) surface of the distal phalanx, where the cortex is almost completely resorbed, leaving only fine wisps of cortical bone. **B**: Skull x-ray from a patient with severe secondary hyperparathyroidism due to end-stage renal disease. Extensive areas of demineralization alternate with areas of increased bone density, resulting in the "salt and pepper" skull x-ray. (Both films courtesy of Dr. Harry Genant.)

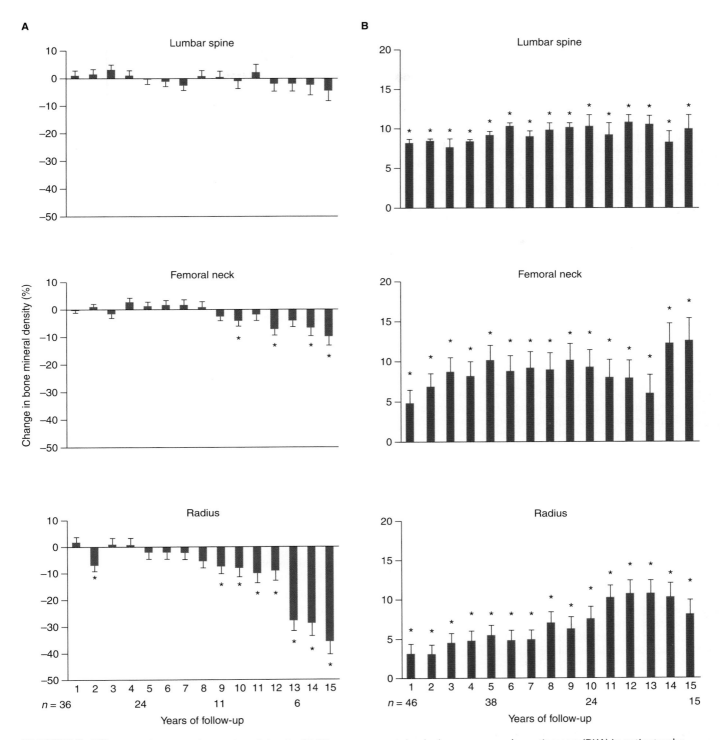

FIGURE 8-17 Mean changes in bone mineral density (BMD) measurements by dual-energy x-ray absorptiometry (DXA) in patients who underwent parathyroidectomy compared with medical follow-up during a 15-year observational study. BMD changes are reported compared with baseline and were statistically different from baseline as shown (*$P < .05$, **$P < .01$, ***$P < 0.001$). The number of patients whose measurements are included are shown underneath each time point. Either just before (distal 1/3 radius) or after 10 years of conservative follow-up (femoral neck) BMD measurements began to fall significantly, while lumbar spine BMD remained unchanged (**Panel A**). Patients who underwent parathyroidectomy demonstrated improved BMD which persisted during 15 years of follow-up (**Panel B**). (Reproduced and modified, with permission, from Rubin MR, et al. The natural history of primary hyperparathyroidism with or without parathyroid surgery after 15 years. *J Clin Endocrinol Metab*. 2008;93:3462. Copyright 2008 by The Endocrine Society. All rights reserved.)

absorptiometry (DXA) of –2.5 or lower, is generally considered to be an indication for surgical treatment of primary hyperparathyroidism, the impact of low bone mass on morbidity is difficult to corroborate clinically (see Treatment of Hypercalcemia).

2. **Hyperparathyroid kidney disease**—Once common in primary hyperparathyroidism, kidney stones now occur in 10% to 20% of cases depending on the series. These are usually calcium oxalate stones. From the perspective of a stone clinic, only about 7% of calcium stone formers prove to have primary hyperparathyroidism. They are difficult to manage medically, and stones constitute one of the agreed indications for parathyroidectomy. Clinically evident nephrocalcinosis rarely occurs, but a gradual loss of renal function is not uncommon. Renal function is stabilized after a successful parathyroidectomy, and otherwise unexplained renal insufficiency (defined as an estimated glomerular filtration rate [eGFR] <60 mL/min) in the setting of primary hyperparathyroidism is also considered to be an indication for surgery because of the risk of progression. Chronic hypercalcemia can also compromise the renal concentrating ability, giving rise to polydipsia and polyuria.

3. **Nonspecific features of primary hyperparathyroidism**—Although stupor and coma occur in severe hypercalcemia, the degree to which milder impairments of central nervous system function affect the typical patient with primary hyperparathyroidism is unclear. Lethargy, fatigue, depression, difficulty in concentrating, and personality changes may occur; however, some patients appear to benefit from parathyroidectomy. Frank psychosis also responds to surgery on occasion. Muscle weakness with characteristic electromyographic changes is also seen, and there is evidence from controlled clinical trials that surgery can improve muscle strength. A number of studies have examined quality of life (QOL) and psychological function in patients with primary hyperparathyroidism pre- and post-parathyroid surgery, compared to a medically followed group. Results vary as to whether QOL improves with surgery. It was formerly thought that the incidence of hypertension was increased in primary hyperparathyroidism, but more recent evidence suggests that it is probably no greater than in age-matched controls, and parathyroidectomy appears to be of no benefit. Dyspepsia, nausea, and constipation all occur, probably as a consequence of hypercalcemia, but there is probably no increase in the incidence of peptic ulcer disease. The articular manifestations of primary hyperparathyroidism include chondrocalcinosis in up to 5% of patients. Acute attacks of pseudogout, however, are less frequent.

B. Laboratory findings   Hypercalcemia is virtually universal in primary hyperparathyroidism, although the serum calcium sometimes fluctuates into the upper normal range. In patients with subtle hyperparathyroidism, repeated serum calcium measurements over a period of time may be required to establish the pattern of intermittent hypercalcemia. Both total and ionized calcium are elevated, and in most clinical instances there is no advantage to measuring the ionized calcium level. Patients with normocalcemic primary hyperparathyroidism, in whom subtle vitamin D deficiency and malabsorption have been eliminated, are being recognized more frequently. In patients with primary hyperparathyroidism, the serum phosphorus level is low-normal (<3.5 mg/dL) or low (<2.5 mg/dL) because of the phosphaturic effect of PTH. A mild hyperchloremic metabolic acidosis may also manifest itself.

The diagnosis of primary hyperparathyroidism in a hypercalcemic patient can be made by determining the intact PTH level. As shown in Figure 8–14, an elevated or even upper-normal level of PTH is clearly inappropriate in a hypercalcemic patient and establishes the diagnosis of hyperparathyroidism or one of its variants—FBHH or lithium-induced hypercalcemia. The reliability of the two-site intact PTH assay allows for the definitive diagnosis of primary hyperparathyroidism. In a patient with a high PTH level, there is no need to screen for such disorders as metastatic cancer or sarcoidosis. Determinations of BMD, renal function, and a plain abdominal radiograph for renal stones are often obtained for clinical decision-making reasons. A determination of urinary calcium concentration and urinary creatinine excretion should always be obtained to exclude FBHH.

Treatment

The definitive treatment of primary hyperparathyroidism is parathyroidectomy. The surgical strategy (ie, minimally invasive vs bilateral neck exploration) depends on the ability of localizing studies such as sestamibi scanning to identify one clearly abnormal gland and the availability of intraoperative PTH determinations to verify that the disease-producing lesion has been removed during surgery. If multiple enlarged glands are suspected, the likely diagnosis is parathyroid hyperplasia or double adenoma. In patients with hyperplasia, the preferred operation is a 3½ gland parathyroidectomy, leaving a remnant sufficient to prevent hypocalcemia. Double parathyroid adenomas are both removed in affected patients. The pathologist is of little help in distinguishing among normal tissue, parathyroid adenoma, and parathyroid hyperplasia: these in essence are surgical diagnoses, based on the size and appearance of the glands. The recurrence rate of hypercalcemia is high in patients who have parathyroid hyperplasia—particularly in those with MEN 1 or allelic variants of MEN 1 or the HPT-JT syndromes, because of the inherited propensity for tumor growth. In such cases, the parathyroid remnant can be removed from the neck and implanted in pieces in forearm muscles to allow for easy subsequent removal of some parathyroid tissue if hypercalcemia recurs.

In experienced hands, the cure rate for a single parathyroid adenoma is more than 95%. The success rate in primary parathyroid hyperplasia is somewhat lower, because of missed glands and recurrent hyperparathyroidism in patients with MEN syndromes. There is a 20% incidence of persistent or recurrent hypercalcemia. However, parathyroidectomy is difficult surgery: the normal parathyroid gland weighs only about 40 mg and may be located throughout the neck or upper mediastinum. It is mandatory in this situation not only to locate a parathyroid adenoma, but also to find the other gland or glands and determine whether or not they are normal in size. Complications of surgery include damage to the recurrent laryngeal nerve, which passes close to the posterior thyroid capsule, and inadvertent removal or devitalization of all parathyroid tissue, producing permanent hypoparathyroidism. In skilled hands, the incidence of these complications is less than 1%.

It is critical that parathyroid surgery be performed by someone with specialized skill and experience (see Chapter 26).

Localization studies of the parathyroid glands in patients with primary hyperparathyroidism and intraoperative PTH testing are critical components in the contemporary surgical management of patients presenting for minimally invasive surgical procedures. If localizing studies clearly indicate a single abnormal gland and if intraoperative PTH testing is available, surgical management generally consists of unilateral exploration with the removal of the single abnormal gland. Localization studies continue to be essential in the management of patients with recurrent or persistent hyperparathyroidism. The most successful procedures are ^{99m}Tc-sestamibi scanning, computed tomography, magnetic resonance imaging, and ultrasound. Individually, each has a sensitivity of 60% to 80% in experienced hands. Used in combination, they are successful in at least 80% of reoperated cases. Invasive studies, such as angiography and venous sampling, are reserved for the most difficult cases.

There is no definitive medical therapy for primary hyperparathyroidism. In postmenopausal women, estrogen therapy in high doses (1.25 mg of conjugated estrogens or 30-50 μg of ethinyl estradiol) produces an average decrease of 0.5 to 1 mg/dL in the serum calcium and an increase in BMD. The effects of estrogen are on the skeletal responses to PTH. PTH levels do not fall. Small series of patients provide experience with oral bisphosphonates (eg, alendronate) and the selective estrogen response modulator (SERM) raloxifene in these patients. Treatment with alendronate for 1 or 2 years reduces biochemical markers of bone turnover and improves BMD by DXA, especially in the spine and also in the femoral neck, compared to baseline values prior to treatment. Studies have shown that raloxifene, administered over several weeks, to postmenopausal women with mild primary hyperparathyroidism also reduces bone turnover markers significantly. Neither alendronate nor raloxifene have significant and or persistent effects on serum calcium or intact PTH levels, nor is either agent approved for treatment of primary hyperparathyroidism by the U.S. Food and Drug Administration (FDA). Calcimimetic agents that activate the parathyroid CaSR, currently under investigation, may offer an alternative to surgery. The calcimimetic cinacalcet is FDA-approved for the management of secondary hyperparathyroidism in patients on dialysis (see later). In small clinical trials, cinacalcet was shown to normalize serum [Ca^{2+}] and raise serum phosphate with modest lowering of PTH levels in patients with mild asymptomatic primary hyperparathyroidism for up to 5 years of therapy. No significant changes in BMD by DXA were seen. This therapy, therefore, is most effective at controlling hypercalcemia in these patients.

The relatively asymptomatic status of most patients with primary hyperparathyroidism today presents a dilemma. Which of them should be subjected to surgery? To answer this question definitively, it is necessary to know more about the natural history of untreated primary hyperparathyroidism. Most observational studies lack long-term follow-up and appropriate control groups. However, one observational study of 15 years duration showed modest increases in serum [Ca^{2+}] (after 10 years) and slow but consistent downward trends in BMD at cortical sites (femoral neck and distal radius) (after 8-10 years of follow-up) (see Figure 8–17A). This study has challenged the skeletal safety of long-term observation of otherwise asymptomatic patients. On the other hand, surgery is usually curative. In experienced hands, surgery has a low morbidity rate. Although parathyroid surgery has a substantial initial cost, over the long term, the cost-benefit ratio may be favorable when compared with a lifetime of medical follow-up. Moreover, there is a marked improvement in BMD after surgery (see Figure 8–17B), with sustained increases over 15 years postoperatively. Consensus Development Conferences or International Workshops in 1990, 2002, and 2008 examined evidence and published recommendations for surgery in mild asymptomatic primary hyperparathyroidism and for conservative management. Current recommendations are for surgery (1) if the serum calcium is greater than 1 mg/dL above the upper limits of normal; (2) if there had been a previous episode of life-threatening hypercalcemia; (3) if the eGFR is <60 mL/min; (4) if a kidney stone is present; (5) if the BMD by DXA at the lumbar spine, hip, or distal radius is substantially reduced (≥2.5 SD below peak bone mass; T-score ≤–2.5); (6) if the patient is young (<50 years of age); or (7) if long-term medical surveillance is not desired or possible. Patients with a coexisting illness complicating the management of hypercalcemia should also be referred for surgery.

The expert panel also considered neuropsychiatric dysfunction, impending onset of menopause, older age and functional status, biochemical markers of bone turnover, and nonclassical symptoms of primary hyperparathyroidism (eg, gastrointestinal and cardiovascular manifestations) in their recommendations. The participants thought that there was sufficient uncertainty regarding these factors that firm recommendations for surgical referral based on these factors alone was not warranted. This panel agreed, however, that these clinical issues should be carefully considered in making decisions regarding surgery and/or long-term follow-up in individual patients.

Variants of Primary Hyperparathyroidism

A. Familial benign hypocalciuric hypercalcemia

Inherited as an autosomal dominant trait, this disorder is responsible for lifelong asymptomatic hypercalcemia, first detectable in cord blood. Hypercalcemia is usually mild (10.5-12 mg/dL [2.7-3 mmol/L]) and is often accompanied by mild hypophosphatemia and hypermagnesemia. The PTH level is normal or slightly elevated, indicating that this is a PTH-dependent form of hypercalcemia. The parathyroid glands are normal in size or slightly enlarged. The most notable laboratory feature of the disorder is hypocalciuria. The urinary calcium level is usually less than 50 mg/24 h, and the calcium/creatinine clearance ratio is less than 0.01 and calculated as follows:

$$\frac{\text{Urine calcium} \times \text{Serum creatinine}}{\text{Serum calcium} \times \text{Urine creatinine}}$$

Hypocalciuria is an intrinsic renal trait; it persists even in patients who have undergone total parathyroidectomy and become hypocalcemic.

Because FBHH is asymptomatic and benign, the most important role of diagnosis is to distinguish it from primary hyperparathyroidism and avoid an unnecessary parathyroidectomy. If subtotal parathyroidectomy is performed, the serum calcium invariably returns shortly to preoperative levels; these persons resist attempts to lower the serum calcium while functioning parathyroid tissue remains. Unfortunate patients with this condition who have undergone total parathyroidectomy are rendered hypoparathyroid and are dependent on calcium and vitamin D supplementation.

The diagnosis must be considered in patients with asymptomatic mild hypercalcemia who are relatively hypocalciuric. However, an unequivocal diagnosis cannot be made biochemically because the serum and urinary calcium and PTH levels all overlap with typical primary hyperparathyroidism. Family screening or sequencing of the *CaSR* gene in an affected individual is necessary to make the diagnosis and can be obtained commercially. The penetrance of the phenotype is essentially 100%, and affected family members are hypercalcemic throughout life, so if the proband has the disorder, each first-degree relative who is screened has a 50% chance of being hypercalcemic.

Most cases of FBHH are caused by loss-of-function mutations in the CaSR. Loss of the functional output of one CaSR allele shifts the set point for inhibition of PTH release to the right, producing hypercalcemia. The same receptor is expressed in the kidney, where it regulates renal calcium excretion. A variety of point mutations in different exons of the CaSR produce the phenotype. Acquired hypocalciuric hypercalcemia has been described in association with antibodies that interact with the parathyroid CaSRs and block the ability of high $[Ca^{2+}]$ to suppress PTH.

A child of two parents with FBHH may inherit a mutant allele from each parent, producing **neonatal severe hypercalcemia,** a life-threatening disorder in which failure to sense extracellular calcium causes severe hyperparathyroidism, requiring total parathyroidectomy soon after birth.

B. MEN syndromes   As noted above, primary hyperparathyroidism is a feature of both MEN 1 and MEN 2A (see also Chapter 22). The penetrance of primary hyperparathyroidism in MEN 1 is over 90% by age 40. Patients with the MEN 1 syndrome inherit a loss-of-function germline mutation in the tumor suppressor gene *MENIN* on chromosome 11q12-13. Menin is a nuclear protein that appears to interact with JunD, a member of the AP1 family of transcription factors. A mutation during mitosis of a parathyroid cell that resulted in loss of function in the remaining allele in that cell would abrogate the cell's growth control mechanism and permit clonal expansion of its progeny ultimately to generate the parathyroid tumor. A similar mechanism appears also to operate in a small fraction of sporadic parathyroid adenomas with 11q12-13 deletions.

The penetrance of primary hyperparathyroidism in MEN 2A is about 30%. As discussed in the above section on MCT, the disorder is caused by activating mutations in the *RET* gene, a tyrosine kinase growth factor receptor. Evidently, the *RET* gene product is less important for growth of the parathyroids than for

thyroid C cells, because the penetrance of primary hyperparathyroidism is fairly low and because (in MEN 2B) a separate class of activating *RET* mutations produces MCT and pheochromocytoma and very rarely primary hyperparathyroidism. The treatment for parathyroid hyperplasia in MEN 1 or MEN 2 is subtotal parathyroidectomy. The recurrence rate is higher than in sporadic parathyroid hyperplasia and may approach 50% in MEN 1.

C. Lithium therapy   Both in patients and in isolated parathyroid cells, exposure to extracellular lithium shifts the set point for inhibition of PTH secretion to the right. Clinically, this results in hypercalcemia and a detectable or elevated level of PTH. Lithium treatment also produces hypocalciuria and is thus a virtual phenocopy of FBHH. Most patients with therapeutic lithium levels for bipolar affective disorder have a slight increase in the serum calcium level, and up to 10% become mildly hypercalcemic, with PTH levels that are high normal or slightly elevated. Lithium treatment can also unmask underlying primary hyperparathyroidism. It is difficult to diagnose primary hyperparathyroidism in a lithium-treated patient, particularly when temporary cessation of lithium therapy is difficult. However, the likelihood of underlying primary hyperparathyroidism is high when the serum calcium is greater than 11.5 mg/dL, and the decision to undertake surgery must be based on clinical criteria. Unfortunately, surgical cure of hyperparathyroidism rarely ameliorates the underlying psychiatric condition.

2. MALIGNANCY-ASSOCIATED HYPERCALCEMIA

Malignancy-associated hypercalcemia is the second most common form of hypercalcemia, with an incidence of 15 cases per 100,000 per year—about one-half the incidence of primary hyperparathyroidism. It is, however, much less prevalent than primary hyperparathyroidism, because most patients have a very limited survival. Nonetheless, malignancy-associated hypercalcemia is the most common cause of hypercalcemia in hospitalized patients. The clinical features and pathogenesis of malignancy-associated hypercalcemia are presented in Chapter 21. The treatment of nonparathyroid hypercalcemia is presented later.

3. SARCOIDOSIS AND OTHER GRANULOMATOUS DISORDERS

Hypercalcemia is seen in up to 10% of subjects with sarcoidosis. A higher percentage has hypercalciuria. This is due to inappropriately elevated $1,25(OH)_2D$ levels and abnormal vitamin D metabolism. Lymphoid tissue and pulmonary macrophages from affected individuals contain 25(OH)D 1-hydroxylase activity that is not seen in normal individuals. The 1-hydroxylase enzyme, responsible for the overproduction of $1,25(OH)_2D$ in sarcoidosis, is the same as that in the kidney (CYP27B1). 1-Hydroxylase activity in these cells is not readily inhibited by calcium or $1,25(OH)_2D$, indicating a lack of feedback inhibition. Macrophages expressing the 1-hydroxylase in these patients do not express a normally functioning 24-hydroxylase so that the catabolism and clearance of $1,25(OH)_2D$ in these cells are lacking. This makes these subjects vulnerable to hypercalcemia or hypercalciuria during periods of increased vitamin D production (eg, summertime with increased sunlight exposure). γ-IFN stimulates 1-hydroxylase activity in these cells, which makes such subjects more vulnerable to altered calcium homeostasis when their disease is active. Glucocorticoids, on the other hand, suppress the inflammation, and subsequently 1-hydroxylase activity, and antagonize 1,25(OH)$_2$D action, providing effective treatment for both the disease and this complication of it.

Other granulomatous diseases are associated with abnormal vitamin D metabolism, resulting in hypercalcemia and/or hypercalciuria. These disorders include tuberculosis, berylliosis, disseminated coccidioidomycosis, histoplasmosis, leprosy, and pulmonary eosinophilic granulomatosis. Furthermore, a substantial number of subjects with Hodgkin or non-Hodgkin lymphomas develop hypercalcemia associated with inappropriately elevated 1,25(OH)$_2$D levels. Although most such patients are normocalcemic on presentation, they may be hypercalciuric, and this should be evaluated as part of the workup. Hypercalcemia and hypercalciuria may not become apparent until situations such as increased sunlight exposure or vitamin D and calcium ingestion are experienced. Thus, one should remain alert to this complication even when the initial evaluation of serum calcium is within normal limits.

4. ENDOCRINOPATHIES

Thyrotoxicosis

Mild hypercalcemia is found in about 10% of patients with thyrotoxicosis. The PTH level is suppressed, and the serum phosphate is in the upper normal range. The serum alkaline phosphatase and biochemical markers of bone turnover may be mildly increased. Significant hypercalcemia may develop in patients with thyrotoxicosis, particularly if it is severe and if patients are temporarily immobilized. Thyroid hormone has direct bone-resorbing properties causing a high turnover state, which often eventually progresses to mild osteoporosis.

Adrenal Insufficiency

Hypercalcemia can be a feature of acute adrenal crisis and responds rapidly to glucocorticoid therapy. Animal studies suggest that hemoconcentration is a critical factor. In experimental adrenal insufficiency, ionized [Ca^{2+}] is normal.

5. ENDOCRINE TUMORS

Hypercalcemia in patients with pheochromocytoma is most often a manifestation of the MEN 2A syndrome, but hypercalcemia is found occasionally in uncomplicated pheochromocytoma, where it appears to result from secretion of PTHrP by the tumor. About 40% of tumors secreting VIP (VIPomas) are associated with hypercalcemia. The cause is unknown. It is known, however, that high levels of VIP may activate PTH/PTHrP receptors.

6. THIAZIDE DIURETICS

The administration of thiazides and related diuretics such as chlorthalidone, metolazone, and indapamide can produce an increase in the serum calcium that is not fully accounted for by hemoconcentration. Hypercalcemia is mild and usually transient, lasting for days or weeks, but occasionally it persists. Thiazide administration can also exacerbate the effects of underlying primary hyperparathyroidism; in fact, thiazide administration was formerly used as a provocative test for hyperparathyroidism in patients with borderline hypercalcemia. Most patients with persistent hypercalcemia while receiving thiazides prove to have primary hyperparathyroidism.

7. VITAMIN D AND VITAMIN A

Hypervitaminosis D

Hypercalcemia may occur in individuals ingesting large doses of vitamin D either therapeutically or accidentally (eg, irregularities in milk product supplementation with vitamin D have been reported). The initial signs and symptoms of vitamin D intoxication include weakness, lethargy, headaches, nausea, and polyuria and are attributable to hypercalcemia and hypercalciuria. Ectopic calcification may occur, particularly in the kidneys, resulting in nephrolithiasis or nephrocalcinosis; other sites include blood vessels, heart, lungs, and skin. Infants appear to be quite susceptible to vitamin D intoxication and may develop disseminated atherosclerosis, supravalvular aortic stenosis, and renal acidosis.

Hypervitaminosis D is readily diagnosed by the very high serum levels of 25(OH)D, because the conversion of vitamin D to 25(OH)D is not tightly regulated. In contrast, 1,25(OH)$_2$D levels are often normal, but not suppressed. This reflects the expected feedback regulation of 1,25(OH)$_2$D production by the elevated calcium and reduced PTH levels. Levels of free 1,25(OH)$_2$D when measured have been found to be increased. This is in part caused by the high levels of 25(OH)D that displace 1,25(OH)$_2$D from DBP, raising the ratio of free:total 1,25(OH)$_2$D. The elevated free concentration of 1,25(OH)$_2$D, plus the intrinsic biologic effects of the elevated 25(OH)D concentration, combine to increase intestinal calcium absorption and bone resorption. The hypercalciuria, which is invariably seen, may lead to dehydration and coma as a result of hyposthenuria, prerenal azotemia, and worsening hypercalcemia due, in part, to decreased renal clearance.

The dose of vitamin D required to induce toxicity varies among patients, reflecting differences in absorption, storage, and subsequent metabolism of the vitamin as well as in target tissue response to the active metabolites. For example, an elderly patient is likely to have reduced intestinal calcium transport and renal production of 1,25(OH)$_2$D. Such an individual may be able to tolerate 50,000 to 100,000 units of vitamin D daily (although these levels far exceed daily requirements). However, patients with unsuspected hyperparathyroidism receiving such doses for the treatment of osteoporosis are more likely to experience hypercalcemia. Treatment consists of withdrawing the vitamin D, rehydration, reducing calcium intake, and administering glucocorticoids, which antagonize the ability of 1,25(OH)$_2$D to stimulate intestinal calcium absorption. Excess vitamin D is slowly cleared from the body (weeks to months), so treatment is prolonged.

Hypervitaminosis A

Excessive ingestion of vitamin A, usually from self-medication with vitamin A preparations, causes a number of abnormalities, including gingivitis, cheilitis, erythema, desquamation, and hair loss. Bone resorption is increased, leading to osteoporosis and fractures, hypercalcemia, and hyperostosis. Excess vitamin A causes hepatosplenomegaly with hypertrophy of fat storage cells, fibrosis, and sclerosis of central veins. Many of these effects can be attributed to the effects of vitamin A on cellular membranes. Under normal circumstances, such effects are prevented because vitamin A is bound to retinol-binding protein (RBP), and its release from the liver is regulated. In vitamin A toxicity, however, these protective mechanisms are overcome, and retinol and its retinyl esters appear in blood unbound to RBP. The mechanism by which vitamin A stimulates bone resorption is not clear.

8. MILK-ALKALI SYNDROME

The ingestion of large quantities of calcium together with an absorbable alkali can produce hypercalcemia with alkalosis, renal impairment, and often nephrocalcinosis. The syndrome was more common when absorbable antacids were the standard treatment for peptic ulcer disease, but it is still seen occasionally. This is the only recognized example of pure absorptive hypercalcemia. The details of its pathogenesis are poorly understood.

9. MISCELLANEOUS CONDITIONS

Immobilization

In immobilized patients there is a marked increase in bone resorption, which often produces hypercalciuria and occasionally hypercalcemia, mainly in individuals with a preexisting high bone turnover state, such as adolescents and patients with thyrotoxicosis or Paget disease. Intact PTH and PTHrP levels are suppressed. The disorder remits with the restoration of activity. If acute treatment is required, bisphosphonates appear to be the treatment of choice.

Acute Renal Failure

Hypercalcemia is often seen when renal failure is precipitated by rhabdomyolysis and usually occurs during the early recovery stage, presumably as calcium deposits are mobilized from damaged muscle tissue. It typically resolves over a few weeks.

TREATMENT OF HYPERCALCEMIA

Initial management of hypercalcemia consists of assessing the hydration state of the patient and rehydrating as necessary with saline. The first goal is to restore renal function, which is often impaired in hypercalcemia because of reduced glomerular filtration and dehydration. Hypercalcemia impairs the urinary concentrating ability, leading to polyuria, and at the same time impairs the sensorium, diminishing the sense of thirst. Once renal function is restored, excretion of calcium can be further enhanced by inducing a saline diuresis. Because most of the filtered calcium is reabsorbed by bulk flow in the proximal tubule along with sodium chloride, a saline diuresis markedly increases calcium excretion. However, a vigorous saline diuresis also induces substantial urinary losses of potassium and magnesium, and these must be monitored and replaced as necessary.

After these initial steps, attention should be given to finding a suitable chronic therapy. It is important to start chronic therapy soon after hospitalization, because several of the most useful agents take up to 5 days to have their full effect. Intravenous bisphosphonates (pamidronate or zoledronic acid) are the first choice for most patients. Bisphosphonates act by inhibiting osteoclastic bone resorption. The initial dose of pamidronate is 60 to 90 mg by intravenous infusion over 1 hour, and the dose of zoledronic acid is 4 mg infused over 15 minutes. In two large trials, 88% and 70% of patients with malignancy-associated hypercalcemia normalized their serum calcium values after infusions of zoledronic acid (4 mg) and pamidronate (90 mg), respectively. Zoledronic acid produced a longer duration of response when treating hypercalcemia of malignancy—32 days versus 18 days for pamidronate. The nadir of serum calcium does not occur until 4 to 5 days after administration of either agent. Retreatment with either agent can be conducted after recurrence of hypercalcemia. Transient fever and myalgia occur in between 10 and 20% of patients who undergo intravenous bisphosphonate therapy. Increases in serum creatinine of ≥ 0.5 mg/dL occur in about 15% of patients. Intravenous bisphosphonates should be used cautiously (if at all) and at reduced doses when the baseline serum creatinine exceeds 2.5 mg/dL.

In patients with severe hypercalcemia and in those with renal insufficiency that is refractory to rehydration, it may be necessary to use an alternative second-line antiresorptive agent for a few days while awaiting the full therapeutic effect of intravenous bisphosphonates. For this purpose, synthetic salmon CT may be administered at a dose of 4 to 8 IU/kg subcutaneously every 12 hours. This is a useful adjunct acutely, but most patients become totally refractory to CT within days to weeks, so it is not suitable for chronic use.

The use of an antiresorptive agent together with saline diuresis provides for a two-pronged approach to hypercalcemia. Other agents besides bisphosphonates may be considered (eg, plicamycin or gallium nitrate), but their toxicity and lack of superior efficacy discourage their use. Both agents act to inhibit osteoclastic bone resorption.

Glucocorticoid administration is first-line treatment for hypercalcemia in patients with multiple myeloma, lymphoma, sarcoidosis, or intoxication with vitamin D or vitamin A. Glucocorticoids are also beneficial in some patients with breast carcinoma. However, they are of little use in most other patients with solid tumors and hypercalcemia.

HYPOCALCEMIA

Classification

Both PTH and $1,25(OH)_2D$ maintain a normal serum calcium and are thus central to the defense against hypocalcemia.

TABLE 8–7 Causes of hypocalcemia.

Hypoparathyroidism
Surgical
Idiopathic
Neonatal
Familial
Autoimmune
Deposition of metals (iron, copper, aluminum)
Postradiation
Infiltrative
Functional (in hypomagnesemia)

Resistance to PTH action
Pseudohypoparathyroidism
Renal insufficiency
Medications that block osteoclastic bone resorption
    Plicamycin
    Calcitonin
    Bisphosphonates

Failure to produce 1,25(OH)$_2$D normally
Vitamin D deficiency
Hereditary vitamin D-dependent rickets, type 1 (renal 25-OH-vitamin D 1alpha-hydroxylase deficiency)

Resistance to 1,25(OH)$_2$D action
Hereditary vitamin D-dependent rickets, type 2 (defective VDR)

Acute complexation or deposition of calcium
Acute hyperphosphatemia
    Crush injury with myonecrosis
    Rapid tumor lysis
    Parenteral phosphate administration
    Excessive enteral phosphate
    Oral (phosphate-containing antacids)
    Phosphate-containing enemas
Acute pancreatitis
Citrated blood transfusion
Rapid, excessive skeletal mineralization
    Hungry bones syndrome
    Osteoblastic metastasis
    Vitamin D therapy for vitamin D deficiency

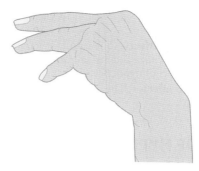

FIGURE 8–18 Position of fingers in carpal spasm due to hypocalcemic tetany. (Reproduced, with permission, from Ganong WF. *Review of Medical Physiology*. 16th ed. Originally published by Appleton & Lange. Copyright 1993 by The McGraw-Hill Companies, Inc.)

Hypocalcemic disorders are best understood as failures of the adaptive response. Thus, chronic hypocalcemia can result from a failure to secrete PTH, altered responsiveness to PTH, a deficiency of vitamin D, or a resistance to vitamin D (Table 8–7). Acute hypocalcemia is most often the consequence of an overwhelming challenge to the adaptive response such as rhabdomyolysis, in which a flood of phosphate from injured skeletal muscle inundates the extracellular fluid.

Clinical Features

Most of the symptoms and signs of hypocalcemia occur because of increased neuromuscular excitability (tetany, paresthesias, seizures, organic brain syndrome) or because of deposition of calcium in soft tissues (cataract, calcification of basal ganglia).

A. Neuromuscular manifestations Clinically, the hallmark of severe hypocalcemia is tetany. Tetany is a state of spontaneous tonic muscular contraction. Overt tetany is often heralded by tingling paresthesias in the fingers and around the mouth, but

the classic muscular component of tetany is carpopedal spasm. This begins with adduction of the thumb, followed by flexion of the metacarpophalangeal joints, extension of the interphalangeal joints, and flexion of the wrists to produce the *main d'accoucheur* posture (Figure 8–18). These involuntary muscle contractions are painful. Although the hands are most typically involved, tetany can involve other muscle groups, including life-threatening spasm of laryngeal muscles. Electromyographically, tetany is typified by repetitive motor neuron action potentials, usually grouped as doublets. Tetany is not specific for hypocalcemia. It also occurs with hypomagnesemia and metabolic alkalosis, and the most common cause of tetany is respiratory alkalosis from hyperventilation.

Lesser degrees of neuromuscular excitability (eg, serum [Ca] 7.5-8.5 mg/dL) produce latent tetany, which can be elicited by testing for Chvostek and Trousseau signs. Chvostek sign is elicited by tapping the facial nerve about 2 cm anterior to the earlobe, just below the zygoma. The response is a contraction of facial muscles ranging from twitching of the angle of the mouth to hemifacial contractions. The specificity of the test is low; about 25% of normal individuals have a mild Chvostek sign. Trousseau sign is elicited by inflating a blood pressure cuff to about 20 mm Hg above systolic pressure for 3 minutes. A positive response is carpal spasm. Trousseau sign is more specific than Chvostek, but 1% to 4% of normal individuals have positive Trousseau signs.

Hypocalcemia predisposes to focal or generalized seizures. Other central nervous system effects of hypocalcemia include pseudotumor cerebri, papilledema, confusion, lassitude, and organic brain syndrome. Twenty percent of children with chronic hypocalcemia develop mental retardation. The basal ganglia are often calcified in patients with long-standing hypoparathyroidism or PHP. This is usually asymptomatic but can produce a variety of movement disorders.

B. Other manifestations of hypocalcemia

1. **Cardiac effects**—Repolarization is delayed, with prolongation of the QT interval. Excitation-contraction coupling may be impaired, and refractory congestive heart failure is sometimes

observed, particularly in patients with underlying cardiac disease.

2. **Ophthalmologic effects**—Subcapsular cataract is common in chronic hypocalcemia, and its severity is correlated with the duration and level of hypocalcemia.

3. **Dermatologic effects**—The skin is often dry and flaky and the nails brittle.

CAUSES OF HYPOCALCEMIA

1. HYPOPARATHYROIDISM

Hypoparathyroidism may be surgical, autoimmune, familial, or idiopathic. The signs and symptoms are those of chronic hypocalcemia. Biochemically, the hallmarks of hypoparathyroidism are hypocalcemia, hyperphosphatemia (because the phosphaturic effect of PTH is lost), and an inappropriately low or undetectable PTH level.

Surgical Hypoparathyroidism

The most common cause of hypoparathyroidism is surgery on the neck, with removal or destruction of the parathyroid glands. The operations most often associated with hypoparathyroidism are cancer surgery, total thyroidectomy, and parathyroidectomy, but the skill and experience of the surgeon are more important predictors than the nature of the operation. Tetany ensues 1 or 2 days postoperatively, but about half of patients with postoperative tetany recover sufficiently so they do not require long-term replacement therapy. In these cases, a devitalized parathyroid remnant has recovered its blood supply and resumes secretion of PTH. In some patients, hypocalcemia may not become evident until years after the procedure. Surgical hypoparathyroidism is the presumptive diagnosis for hypocalcemia in any patient with a surgical scar on the neck.

In patients with severe hyperparathyroid bone disease preoperatively, a syndrome of postoperative hypocalcemia can follow successful parathyroidectomy. This is the **hungry bones syndrome**, which results from avid uptake of calcium and phosphate by the bones. The parathyroids, although intact, cannot compensate. The syndrome is usually seen in patients with an elevated preoperative serum alkaline phosphatase and/or severe uremic secondary hyperparathyroidism. It can usually be distinguished from surgical hypoparathyroidism by the serum phosphorus, which is low in the hungry bones syndrome, because of skeletal avidity for phosphate, and high in hypoparathyroidism, and by the serum PTH, which becomes appropriately elevated in the hungry bones syndrome.

Idiopathic Hypoparathyroidism

Acquired hypoparathyroidism is sometimes seen in the setting of polyglandular endocrinopathies. Most commonly, it is associated with primary adrenal insufficiency and mucocutaneous candidiasis in the syndrome of *autoimmune polyglandular syndrome type 1 (APS1)* (see Chapter 3). The typical age at onset of hypoparathyroidism is 5 to 9 years. A similar form of hypoparathyroidism can

occur as an isolated finding. The age at onset of idiopathic hypoparathyroidism is 2 to 10 years, and there is a preponderance of female cases. Circulating parathyroid antibodies are common in both APS1 and in isolated hypoparathyroidism. Many patients have antibodies that recognize the CaSR. Many patients with autoimmune hypoparathyroidism have antibodies reactive with NALP5 (NACHT leucine-rich-repeat protein 5), an intracellular signaling molecule expressed in the parathyroid. The pathogenetic role of any of these antibodies is not yet clarified. APS1 is an autosomal recessive disorder in which mutations are found in the *AIRE* (autoimmune regulator) protein. AIRE is a transcription factor involved in negative selection in the thymus and periphery.

Another form of autoimmune hypoparathyroidism has been reported in patients with autoantibodies to the CaSR that functionally activate it and suppress PTH secretion. These rare cases have been detected along with other autoimmune disorders such as Addison disease and Hashimoto thyroiditis.

Familial Hypoparathyroidism

Hypoparathyroidism is an uncommon disorder and presents in familial forms transmitted as either autosomal dominant or recessive traits. Autosomal recessive hypoparathyroidism occurs in families with *PTH* gene mutations that interfere with the normal processing of PTH. Another autosomal recessive form of this disease is due to a deletion of the 5′ sequence of the gene encoding the transcription factor *glial cell missing 2*, which is necessary for parathyroid gland development. Hypoparathyroidism is evident in the newborn period because of parathyroid gland agenesis.

Autosomal dominant hypoparathyroidism can be due to point mutations in the *CaSR* gene, which render the protein constitutively active. This property enables the receptor to mediate suppression of PTH secretion at normal and even subnormal serum calcium levels. Several families with different mutations have been described; affected individuals typically have mild hypoparathyroidism (mildly reduced serum $[Ca^{2+}]$ and PTH levels). These patients also demonstrate marked hypercalciuria due to CaSR mutations in their kidneys. The set point for calcium-induced suppression of PTH secretion in these patients is shifted to the left as is the effect of serum $[Ca^{2+}]$ on renal calcium excretion. Thus, this syndrome is the mirror image of FBHH. Therapy is often not necessary and risks precipitating even greater degrees of hypercalciuria, nephrocalcinosis, and renal stones.

Other Causes of Hypoparathyroidism

Neonatal hypoparathyroidism can be part of the **DiGeorge syndrome** (dysmorphic facies, cardiac defects, immune deficiency, and hypoparathyroidism) due to a microdeletion (or other genetic abnormalities) on chromosome 22q11.2; the **HDR syndrome** (hypoparathyroidism, sensorineural deafness, and renal anomalies) due to mutations in or deletion of an allele of the GATA3 transcription factor; and other rare conditions. Transfusion-dependent individuals with thalassemia or red cell aplasia who survive into the third decade of life are susceptible to

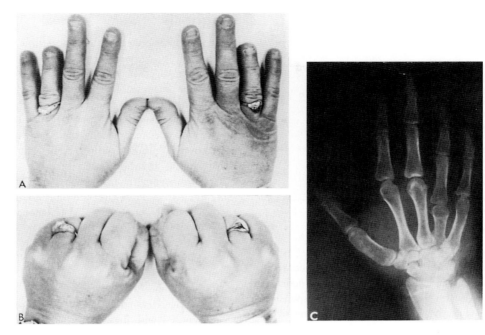

FIGURE 8–19 Hands of a patient with pseudohypoparathyroidism. **A**: Note the short fourth fingers. **B**: Note the "absent" fourth knuckle. **C**: Film shows the short fourth metacarpal. (Reproduced, with permission, from Potts JT. Pseudohypoparathyroidism: clinical features; signs and symptoms; diagnosis and differential diagnosis. In: Stanbury JB, Wyngaarden JB, Fredrickson DS, eds. *The Metabolic Basis of Inherited Disease.* 4th ed. McGraw-Hill; 1978.)

hypoparathyroidism as the result of iron deposition in the parathyroid glands. Copper deposition can cause hypoparathyroidism in Wilson disease. Infiltration with metastatic carcinoma is a very rare cause of hypoparathyroidism.

Severe magnesium depletion temporarily paralyzes the parathyroid glands, preventing secretion of PTH. Magnesium depletion also blunts the actions of PTH on target organs (kidney and bone) to counteract the hypocalcemia. This is seen with magnesium losses due to gastrointestinal and renal disorders and alcoholism. The syndrome responds immediately to infusion of magnesium. As discussed above in the section on regulation of PTH secretion, magnesium is probably required for effective stimulus-secretion coupling in the parathyroids.

2. PSEUDOHYPOPARATHYROIDISM

PHP is a genetic disorder of target-organ unresponsiveness to PTH. Biochemically, it mimics hormone-deficient forms of hypoparathyroidism, with hypocalcemia and hyperphosphatemia, but the PTH level is elevated, and there is a markedly blunted response to the administration of PTH (see Diagnosis, later).

Clinical Features

Two distinct forms of PHP are recognized. PHP type IB is a disorder of isolated resistance to PTH, which presents with the biochemical features of hypocalcemia, hyperphosphatemia, and secondary hyperparathyroidism. PHP type IA has, in addition to these biochemical features, a characteristic somatic phenotype known as **Albright hereditary osteodystrophy (AHO).** This consists of short stature, round face, short neck, obesity, brachydactyly (short digits), shortened metatarsals, subcutaneous ossifications, and often reduced intelligence. Because of shortening of the metacarpal bones—most often the fourth and fifth metacarpals—affected digits have a dimple, instead of a knuckle, when a fist is made (Figure 8–19). Primary hypothyroidism is frequently seen. Less commonly, these patients have abnormalities of reproductive function—oligomenorrhea in females and infertility in males due to primary hypogonadism. Interestingly, certain individuals in families with PHP inherit the somatic phenotype of AHO without any disorder of calcium metabolism; this state, which mimics PHP, is called **pseudo-PHP** or **PPHP**.

Pathophysiology

PHP type IA is caused by the loss of function of one allele (haploinsufficiency) of the gene encoding the stimulatory G protein alpha subunit, (G_s alpha or GNAS). This abnormality is predicted to produce only 50% of the normal levels of the alpha subunit of the heterotrimeric G_s, which couples the PTH receptor to adenylyl cyclase. Patients with PHP type IA have a markedly blunted response of urinary cAMP to administration of PTH. Because G_s also couples many other receptors to adenylyl cyclase, the expected result of this mutation would be a generalized disorder of hormonal unresponsiveness. The presence of primary hypothyroidism and primary hypogonadism in these patients indicates that resistance to TSH, LH, and FSH occurs fairly commonly. Responsiveness to other hormones (eg, ACTH, glucagon) is fairly

TABLE 8–8 Features of pseudohypoparathyroidism.

	PHP 1A	PPHP[a]	PHP 1B
Hypocalcemia	Yes	No	Yes
Response to PTH	No	Yes	No
Albright hereditary osteodystrophy	Yes	Yes	No
GNAS coding region mutation	Yes	Yes	No
GNAS regulatory region mutation or deletion	No	No	Yes
Generalized target organ unresponsiveness	Yes	No	No

[a]Pseudopseudohypoparathyroidism.

normal. Thus, a 50% loss of the G$_s$ alpha protein produces resistance to some hormones but not others. G$_s$ alpha is also deficient in individuals with PPHP, who have AHO but normal responsiveness to PTH. Thus, a mutation in the *G$_s$ alpha* gene invariably produces AHO but only sometimes produces resistance to PTH, suggesting that the occurrence of a metabolic phenotype is determined by other factors described below (Table 8–8).

In PHP type IB, there is resistance to PTH but no somatic phenotype (ie, AHO), and levels of G$_s$ alpha protein in red blood cell or fibroblast membranes are normal. The disorder, however, is also linked to the GNAS locus, but it does not involve mutations in the coding region of GNAS. Instead epigenetic defects in GNAS are present that cause the differentially methylated region at exon A/B to lose its imprinting. Most cases demonstrate a maternally derived 3-kb deletion of DNA sequences located more than 200 kb centromeric of the GNAS locus at the STX16 locus. Other deletions remove this entire differentially methylated region—a key regulator of the levels of GNAS transcription. Transcription directed by this (unmethylated) promoter does not produce appropriate levels of G$_s$ alpha protein in the renal cortex where this biallelic promoter activity is important. Thus, abnormal methylation of GNAS regulatory sequences plays a key role in the pathogenesis of PHP1B.

Genetics

PHP type IA is inherited as an autosomal dominant trait. Individuals who have acquired the trait from their fathers almost always present with PPHP and lack hormone resistance. When the mutant allele is derived from the mother, PHP with hormone resistance is always present. This pattern of inheritance is due to genomic imprinting of the GNAS1 locus. In the kidney cortex, the maternal allele is preferentially expressed and the paternal allele is silenced. Thus, if the mutant GNAS1 allele is maternally derived, the resulting offspring will have PHP; if the mutant GNAS1 allele is paternally derived (and therefore silenced), the resulting offspring will have PPHP. Tissue-specific imprinting of the *GNAS1* gene, therefore, determines the expression of hormone resistance in the kidney and thyroid. The expression of AHO does not depend on imprinting mechanisms and occurs in PHP type IA and PPHP.

Diagnosis

Several disorders present with hypocalcemia and secondary hyperparathyroidism (eg, vitamin D deficiency), but when these features occur together with hyperphosphatemia or AHO, this suggests the diagnosis of PHP. To confirm that resistance to PTH is present, the patient can be challenged with PTH (the Ellsworth-Howard test). For this purpose, synthetic human PTH(1-34) (teriparatide acetate, 3 IU/kg body weight) is infused intravenously over 10 minutes during a water diuresis, and urine is collected during the hour preceding the infusion, during the half-hour following the infusion, 30 to 60 minutes after the infusion, and 1 to 2 hours after the infusion and assayed for cAMP and creatinine. Data are expressed as nanomoles of cAMP per liter of glomerular filtrate, based on creatinine measurements. Normally, there is an increase in urinary cAMP of more than 300 nmol/L glomerular filtrate after administration of PTH. The use of the urinary phosphate response as a gauge of PTH responsiveness is much less reliable. For practical purposes, hypocalcemia, hyperphosphatemia, elevated PTH levels, and normal levels of vitamin D metabolites (with or without AHO) confirm the presence of resistance to PTH.

3. VITAMIN D DEFICIENCY

Pathogenesis

Vitamin D deficiency results from one or more factors: inadequate sunlight exposure, inadequate nutrition, or malabsorption. In addition, drugs that activate the catabolism of vitamin D and its metabolites, such as phenytoin and phenobarbital, can precipitate vitamin D deficiency in subjects with marginal vitamin D status. Although the human skin is capable of producing sufficient amounts of vitamin D if exposed to sunlight of adequate intensity, institutionalized patients frequently do not get adequate exposure. Furthermore, the fear of skin cancer has led many to avoid sunlight exposure or to apply protective agents that block the ultraviolet portion of sunlight from reaching the lower reaches of the epidermis where most of the vitamin D is produced. Heavily pigmented and elderly individuals have less efficient production of vitamin D for a given exposure to ultraviolet irradiation. Serum levels of 25(OH)D are used to indicate vitamin D status. Although there is no consensus on what level of 25(OH)D constitutes sufficiency, 30 ng/mL has become the preferred target in North America. With that standard, a large portion of the population is vitamin D insufficient. A recent NHANES survey found that in the population over age 60, 67% of Caucasians, 82% of Hispanics, and 88% of African Americans had 25(OH)D levels below 30 ng/mL. Studies of hospitalized patients or those in nursing homes show almost universal vitamin D insufficiency if not frank deficiency. The intensity of sunlight is an important factor that limits effective vitamin D production as a function of season (summer > winter) and latitude (less intense the higher the latitude). The supplementation of milk has reduced the incidence of vitamin D deficiency in the United States, but most countries do not follow this practice. Even in the United States, severe vitamin D deficiency and rickets may occur in children of vegetarian mothers who avoid milk products (and presumably have reduced vitamin D stores) and in children who are not weaned to vitamin D-supplemented milk by age 2. Breast milk contains little vitamin D, although vitamin D content can be increased by supplementing the mother. Adults who avoid milk as well as sunlight are likewise at risk. Individuals with a variety of small bowel, pancreatic, and biliary tract disease and those after partial gastrectomy or intestinal bypass surgery have reduced capacity to absorb the vitamin D from the diet.

Clinical Features

The clinical features of individuals with severe vitamin D deficiency will be discussed more thoroughly in the section on "Osteomalacia and Rickets." Severe vitamin D deficiency should be suspected in individuals complaining of lethargy, proximal muscle weakness, and bone pain who have frankly low or low normal serum calcium and phosphate and low urine calcium on routine biochemical evaluation. A low serum 25(OH)D level is diagnostic in this setting. $1,25(OH)_2D$ levels are often normal and reflect the increased 1-hydroxylase activity in these subjects that is responding appropriately to the increased PTH levels as well as the low serum calcium and phosphate levels. However, there is increasing awareness that less severe degrees of vitamin D deficiency may not present with obvious musculoskeletal signs and symptoms. These individuals may be more susceptible to conditions such as hyperparathyroidism, osteoporosis, increased risk of falls and fractures, but also increased infections, hypertension, increased cardiovascular disease, diabetes mellitus, and various malignancies. Solid data from large-scale randomized placebo controlled clinical trials demonstrating cause and effect for vitamin D deficiency and many of these disorders are lacking, although animal studies and a large body of epidemiologic evidence and case control studies point in this direction.

Treatment

The goal in treating severe vitamin D deficiency manifesting as rickets or osteomalacia is to normalize the clinical, biochemical, and radiologic abnormalities without producing hypercalcemia, hyperphosphatemia, hypercalciuria, nephrolithiasis, or ectopic calcification. To realize this goal, patients must be followed carefully. As the bone lesions heal or the underlying disease improves, the dosage of vitamin D, calcium, or phosphate needs to be adjusted to avoid such complications. With the appreciation that most individuals have a less severe form of vitamin D deficiency and do not have obvious signs or symptoms associated with rickets or osteomalacia, the goal of treatment is to achieve a level of 25(OH)D that existing data indicate will reduce the predisposition of such individuals to the numerous diseases associated with vitamin D deficiency. Correction of vitamin D deficiency can usually be achieved by the weekly administration of 50,000 IU ergocalciferol for 6 to 8 weeks followed by replacement doses of 800 to 2000 IU/d based on maintenance of adequate serum 25(OH)D levels. Patients with malabsorption may respond to larger amounts of vitamin D (25,000-100,000 IU/d or one to three times per week). 25(OH)D (50-100 µg/d) is better absorbed than

vitamin D and may be used if malabsorption of vitamin D is a limiting factor, but is not readily available in the United States. Calcitriol $(1,25(OH)_2D)$ and its analogs are not appropriate therapy for patients with vitamin D deficiency because of the likely requirement for vitamin D metabolites other than $1,25(OH)_2D$ and the advantage of providing adequate substrate (25(OH)D) for tissues capable of producing their own $1,25(OH)_2D$ as the need arises (eg, as in the immune response). The exception to this rule is in patients with renal failure incapable of producing adequate $1,25(OH)_2D$. Vitamin D therapy should be supplemented with 1 to 3 g of elemental calcium per day. Care must be taken in managing patients with vitamin D deficiency who also have elevated PTH levels, because long-standing vitamin D deficiency may produce a degree of autonomy in the parathyroid glands such that rapid replacement with calcium and vitamin D could result in hypercalcemia or hypercalciuria. A listing of available vitamin D metabolites and analogs with their main indications for clinical use is presented in Table 8–2.

4. PSEUDOVITAMIN D DEFICIENCY

Pseudovitamin D deficiency is a rare autosomal recessive disease in which rickets is accompanied by low levels of $1,25(OH)_2D$ but normal levels of 25(OH)D. The disease is due to mutations in the *25(OH)D 1-hydroxylase* gene (*CYP27B1*) that render it nonfunctional. Both alleles need to be defective in order for the disease to be manifest. Although affected patients do not respond to doses of vitamin D that are effective in subjects with vitamin D deficiency, they can respond to pharmacologic doses of vitamin D and to physiologic doses of calcitriol, which is the preferred treatment.

5. HEREDITARY VITAMIN D–RESISTANT RICKETS

Hereditary vitamin D–resistant rickets is a rare autosomal recessive disease that presents in childhood with rickets similar to that seen in patients with vitamin D deficiency. Many of these patients also have alopecia, which is not characteristic of vitamin D deficiency or pseudovitamin D deficiency. The biochemical changes are similar to those reported in subjects with vitamin D deficiency except that the $1,25(OH)_2D$ levels are generally very high. The disease is caused by inactivating mutations in the *VDR* gene. The location of the mutation can affect the severity of the disease. In particular, mutations in the DNA-binding domain (exons 2, 3) that prevent DNA binding and mutations in the ligand-binding domain (exons 5-7) that prevent $1,25(OH)_2D$ binding lead to a more. The latter mutations may alter but not inhibit DNA/ligand binding. These patients are treated with large doses of calcitriol and dietary calcium and may show partial or complete remission as they grow older. An animal model of this disease (inactivation or knockout of both VDR alleles) demonstrates that the bone disease can be corrected with high dietary intake of calcium and phosphate, although the alopecia is not altered. This disease points to a role for the VDR in epidermis and hair development that is independent of its activity in the intestine and bone.

6. OTHER HYPOCALCEMIC DISORDERS

Hypoalbuminemia produces a low total serum $[Ca^{2+}]$ because of a reduction in the bound fraction of calcium, but the ionized $[Ca^{2+}]$ is normal. The ionized $[Ca^{2+}]$ can be determined directly, or the effect of hypoalbuminemia can be roughly corrected for by using the following formula:

Corrected serum calcium = Measured serum calcium + (0.8)
(4 − Measured serum albumin)

Thus, in a patient with a serum $[Ca^{2+}]$ of 7.8 mg/dL and a serum albumin of 2 g/dL, the corrected serum $[Ca^{2+}]$ is 7.8 + (0.8) (4 − 2) = 9.4 mg/dL.

Several disorders produce acute hypocalcemia even if homeostatic mechanisms are intact, simply because they overwhelm these mechanisms. Acute hyperphosphatemia resulting from rhabdomyolysis or tumor lysis, often in the setting of renal insufficiency, may produce severe symptomatic hypocalcemia. Transfusion of large volumes of cit-rated blood causes acute hypocalcemia by complexation of calcium as calcium citrate. In this instance, total calcium may be normal, but the ionized fraction is reduced. In acute pancreatitis, hypocalcemia is an ominous prognostic sign. The mechanism of hypocalcemia is sequestration of calcium by saponification with fatty acids, which are produced in the retroperitoneum by the action of pancreatic lipases. Skeletal mineralization, when very rapid, can cause hypocalcemia. This is seen in the **hungry bones syndrome**, which was discussed above in the section on surgical hypoparathyroidism, and occasionally with widespread osteoblastic metastases from prostatic carcinoma.

TREATMENT OF HYPOCALCEMIA

Acute Hypocalcemia

Patients with tetany should receive intravenous calcium as calcium chloride (272 mg calcium/10 mL), calcium gluconate (90 mg calcium/10 mL), or calcium gluceptate (90 mg calcium/10 mL). Approximately 200 mg of elemental calcium can be given over several minutes. The patient must be observed for stridor and the airway secured if necessary. Oral calcium and a rapidly acting preparation of vitamin D should be started. If necessary, calcium can be infused in doses of 400 to 1000 mg/24 h until oral therapy has taken effect. Intravenous calcium is irritating to the veins and is best infused into a large vein or through a central venous catheter.

Chronic Hypocalcemia

The objective of chronic therapy is to keep the patient free of symptoms and to maintain a serum $[Ca^{2+}]$ of approximately 8.5 to 9.0 mg/dL. With lower serum $[Ca^{2+}]$, the patient may not only experience symptoms but may be predisposed over time to cataract formation if the phosphate level is also high. With serum calcium concentrations in the upper normal range, there may be marked hypercalciuria, which occurs because the hypocalciuric effect of PTH has been lost. This may predispose to nephrolithiasis,

nephrocalcinosis, and chronic renal insufficiency. In addition, the patient with borderline elevated calcium is at increased risk of overshooting the therapeutic goal and may develop symptomatic hypercalcemia.

The mainstays of treatment are calcium and a form of vitamin D. Oral calcium can be given in a dose of 1.5 to 3 g of elemental calcium or more per day. These large doses of calcium reduce the doses of vitamin D that are needed and allow for rapid normalization of serum calcium if vitamin D intoxication subsequently occurs. Numerous preparations of calcium are available. A short-acting preparation of vitamin D (calcitriol) and the very long-acting preparations such as vitamin D_2 (ergocalciferol) are available (see Table 8–2). By far the most inexpensive regimens are those that use ergocalciferol. In addition to economy, they have the advantage of rather easy maintenance in most patients. The disadvantage is that ergocalciferol can slowly accumulate and produce prolonged vitamin D intoxication. Caution must be exercised in the introduction of other drugs that influence calcium metabolism. For example, thiazide diuretics have a hypocalciuric effect. By reducing urinary calcium excretion in treated patients, whose other adaptive mechanisms such as the modulation of PTH secretion by calcium, are nonoperative and who are thus absolutely dependent on renal excretion of calcium to maintain the serum calcium level, thiazides may produce significant hypercalcemia. In a similar way, intercurrent illnesses that compromise renal function (and therefore calcium excretion) may produce dangerous hypercalcemia in the patient who is maintained on large doses of vitamin D. Short-acting preparations are less prone to some of these effects but may require more frequent titration and are much more expensive than vitamin D_2.

BONE ANATOMY AND REMODELING

FUNCTIONS OF BONE

Bone has four major functions.

(1) It provides rigid support to extremities and body cavities containing vital organs. In diseases in which the skeleton is weakened or defective, erect posture may be impossible and vital organ function may be compromised. An example is the cardiopulmonary dysfunction that occurs in patients with severe kyphosis due to vertebral collapse.
(2) Bones are crucial to locomotion in that they provide efficient levers and sites of attachment for muscles. With bony deformity, these levers become defective, and severe abnormalities of gait develop.
(3) Bone provides a large reservoir of ions, such as calcium, phosphate, magnesium, and sodium that are critical for life and can be mobilized when the external environment fails to provide them.
(4) Bone houses the hematopoietic elements. There is increasing evidence of a trophic relationship between the stromal cells in bone and the hematopoietic elements.

STRUCTURE OF BONE

The material properties of normal bone strike an ideal balance between rigidity and elasticity. Bone is rigid enough to provide structural stability and resist applied forces but not overly mineralized and brittle, which would result in an increased tendency to fracture. Bone must also be light enough to be moved by muscle contractions. Cortical bone, composed of densely packed layers of mineralized collagen, provides rigidity and is the major component of tubular bones (Figure 8–20). Trabecular (cancellous) bone is spongy in cross-section, provides strength and elasticity, and constitutes the major portion of the axial skeleton. Disorders in which cortical bone is defective or reduced in mass lead to fractures of the long bones. Disorders in which trabecular bone is defective or scanty, in contrast, lead preferentially to vertebral fractures. Fractures of long bones may also occur because normal trabecular bone reinforcement is lost.

Two-thirds of the weight of bone is due to mineral; the remainder is due to water and type I collagen. Minor organic components such as proteoglycans, lipids, acidic proteins containing gamma-carboxyglutamic acid, osteonectin, osteopontin, and growth factors comprise the remainder.

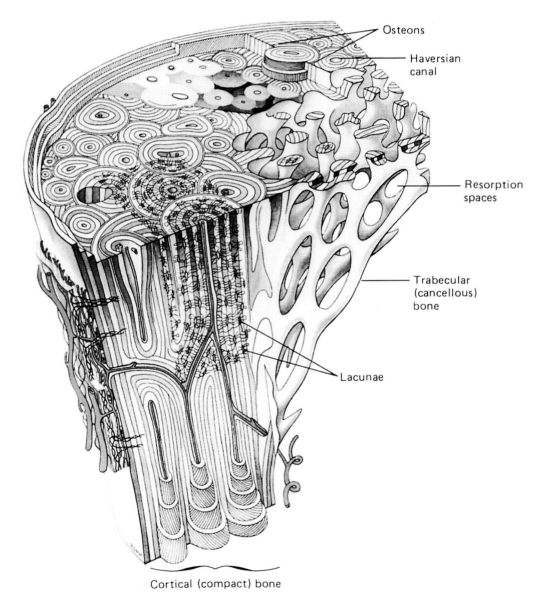

FIGURE 8–20 Diagram showing features of the microstructure of mature bone seen in both transverse (top) and longitudinal section. Areas of cortical (compact) and trabecular (cancellous) bone are included. (Reproduced, with permission, from Warwick R, Williams PL, eds. *Gray's Anatomy*. 35th ed. Longman; 1973.)

Bone Mineral

The mineral of bone is present in two forms. The major form consists of hydroxyapatite in crystals of varying maturity. The remainder is amorphous calcium phosphate, which lacks a coherent x-ray diffraction pattern, has a lower calcium-to-phosphate ratio than pure hydroxyapatite, occurs in regions of active bone formation, and is present in larger quantities in young bone.

Bone Cells

Bone is composed of three types of cells: the osteoblast, the osteocyte, and the osteoclast.

A. Osteoblast   The osteoblast is the principal bone-forming cell. It arises from a pool of mesenchymal stem cells in the bone marrow, which as they differentiate, acquire a set of characteristics, including expression of PTH and vitamin D receptors; surface expression of the ectoenzyme alkaline phosphatase; and expression of bone matrix protein genes—type I collagen, osteocalcin, osteopontin, and others. Differentiated osteoblasts are directed to the bone surface, where they line regions of new bone formation, laying down bone matrix (osteoid) in orderly lamellae and inducing its mineralization (Figure 8–21). In the mineralization process, hydroxyapatite crystals are deposited on the collagen layers to produce lamellar bone. Mineralization requires an adequate supply of extracellular calcium and phosphate as well as alkaline phosphatase, which is secreted in large amounts by active osteoblasts. The fate of senescent osteoblasts is not well defined. Some probably become flattened, inactive lining cells on trabecular bone

surfaces, some are buried in cortical bone as osteocytes, and others undergo apoptosis.

B. Osteocyte   Osteoblasts that remain within cortical bone during the remodeling process become osteocytes. Protein synthetic activity decreases markedly, and the cells develop multiple processes (canaliculi) that reach out through lacunae in bone tissue to communicate with nutrient capillaries, with processes of other osteocytes within a unit of bone (osteon), and also with the cell processes of surface osteoblasts (see Figure 8–20). The physiologic functions of osteocytes are poorly understood. They are believed to (1) act as a cellular syncytium that permits the translocation of mineral in and out of regions of bone removed from surfaces, and (2) serve as the sensors of mechanical loading by providing key signals that trigger bone modeling and remodeling.

C. Osteoclast   The osteoclast is a multinucleated giant cell that is specialized for resorption of bone. Osteoclasts are terminally differentiated cells that arise from hematopoietic precursors in the monocyte lineage and do not divide. Osteoblasts stimulate both osteoclast formation and activation via the cell surface molecule *RANKL*. RANKL stimulates its cognate ligand RANK on the surface of osteoclast precursors and mature osteoclasts (Figure 8–22). Osteoblasts also elaborate macrophage colony stimulating factor-1 (M-CSF), which potentiates the effects of RANKL on osteoclastogenesis. In addition, osteoblasts and other cells produce a decoy receptor, *osteoprotegerin (OPG)*, which binds to RANKL and blocks its actions. PTH and $1,25(OH)_2D$ both increase RANKL expression by osteoblasts, as do cytokines such as

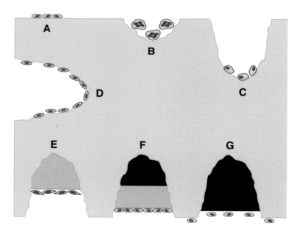

FIGURE 8–21   The remodeling cycle. **A:** Resting trabecular surface. **B:** Multinucleated osteoclasts dig a cavity of approximately 20 microns. **C:** Completion of resorption to 60 microns by mononuclear phagocytes. **D:** Recruitment of osteoblast precursors to the base of the resorption cavity. **E:** Secretion of new matrix (gray shading) by osteoblasts. **F:** Continued secretion of matrix, with initiation of calcification (black areas). **G:** Completion of mineralization of new matrix. Bone has returned to quiescent state, but a small deficit in bone mass persists.

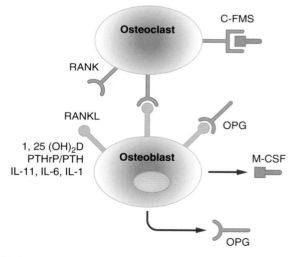

FIGURE 8–22   Regulation of osteoclast formation and activation by the osteoblast. The osteoblast stimulates osteoclast formation and activation via the interaction of RANKL on the osteoblast with RANK on the osteoclast. M-CSF secreted by the osteoblast enhances the process via its receptor on the osteoclast C-FMS, whereas OPG, also secreted by the osteoblast, blocks the process by blocking RANKL. RANKL expression is stimulated by $1,25(OH)_2D$ and PTHrP/PTH as well as by the cytokines IL-1, IL-6, and IL-11.

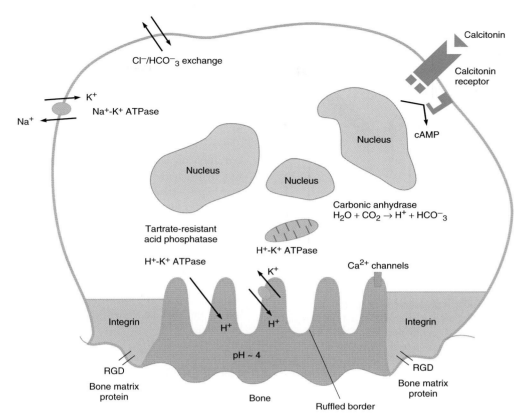

FIGURE 8–23 Osteoclast-mediated bone resorption. The osteoclast attaches to the bone surface via integrin-mediated binding to bone matrix bone proteins. When enough integrin binding has occurred, the osteoclast is anchored and a sealed space is formed. The repeatedly folded plasma membrane creates a ruffled border. Secreted into the sealed space are acid and enzymes forming an extracellular lysosome. (Reproduced, with permission, from Felig P, Baxter JD, Frohman LA, ed. *Endocrinology and Metabolism*. 3rd ed. McGraw-Hill; 1995.)

IL-1, IL-6, and IL-11. TNF potentiates the ability of RANKL to stimulate osteoclastogenesis, whereas IFN-gamma blocks this process by direct effects on the osteoclast.

To resorb bone, the motile osteoclast alights on a bone surface and seals off an area by forming an adhesive ring. Having isolated an area of bone surface, the osteoclast develops above the surface an elaborately invaginated plasma membrane structure called the **ruffled border** (Figure 8–23). The ruffled border is a distinctive organelle, but it acts essentially as a huge lysosome that dissolves bone mineral by secreting acid onto the isolated bone surface and simultaneously breaks down bone matrix by secretion of proteases, in particular cathepsin K. The collagen breakdown products from bone resorption can be assayed in serum and urine as measures of bone resorption rates (*N*- and *C*-telopeptides). Bone resorption can be controlled in two ways: by regulating the formation of osteoclasts via changes in cell numbers or by regulating the activity of mature osteoclasts. The mature osteoclast has receptors for CT but does not appear to have PTH or vitamin D receptors.

BONE REMODELING

Bone remodeling is a continuous process of breakdown and renewal that occurs throughout life. During childhood and adolescence, remodeling proceeds at a vigorous rate but is quantitatively overwhelmed by the concomitant occurrence of bone modeling and linear growth. Once peak bone mass has been established, remodeling supervenes as the common mechanism by which bone mass is modified for the remainder of a person's life. Each remodeling event is carried out by individual "bone remodeling units" on bone surfaces throughout the skeleton (see Figure 8–21). Normally, about 90% of these surfaces lie dormant, covered by a thin layer of lining cells. Following physical or biochemical signals, precursor cells from the bone marrow migrate to specific loci on the bone surface, where they fuse into multinucleated bone-resorbing cells known as osteoclasts that then excavate a resorption cavity into the bone.

Cortical bone is remodeled from within by cutting cones, groups of osteoclasts that cut tunnels through the compact bone (Figure 8–24). They are followed by trailing osteoblasts that line the tunnels with a cylinder of new bone, progressively narrowing the tunnels until all that remains are the tiny haversian canals by which the cells left behind as resident osteocytes are fed. The packet of new bone formed by a single cutting cone is called an osteon (see Figure 8–20).

By contrast, trabecular resorption creates scalloped areas of the bone surface called Howship lacunae. Two to three months after initiation, the resorption phase reaches completion, having created

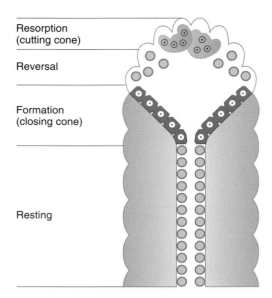

FIGURE 8–24 Schematic representation of the four principal stages involved in the formation of a new basic structural unit in cortical bone. (Reproduced, with permission, from Felig P, Baxter JD, Frohman LA, ed. *Endocrinology and Metabolism*. 3rd ed. McGraw-Hill; 1995.)

a cavity about 60 um deep. This is accompanied by ingress from marrow stroma into the base of the resorption cavity of precursors for bone-forming osteoblasts. These cells develop an osteoblastic phenotype, expressing characteristic bone-specific proteins such as alkaline phosphatase, osteopontin, and osteocalcin, and begin to replace the resorbed bone by elaborating new bone matrix. Once the newly formed osteoid reaches a thickness of about 20 um, mineralization begins. Completion of a full remodeling cycle normally lasts about 6 months (see Figure 8–21).

Bone remodeling does not absolutely require systemic hormones except to maintain intestinal absorption of minerals by 1,25(OH)$_2$D and thus ensure an adequate supply of calcium and phosphate. For example, bone is normal, aside from being in a state of low turnover, in patients with hypoparathyroidism. However, systemic hormones use the "bone pool" as a source of minerals for regulation of extracellular calcium homeostasis. When they do, the coupling mechanism ensures that bone is replenished. For example, when bone resorption is activated by PTH to provide calcium to correct hypocalcemia, bone formation also increases, tending to replenish lost bone. Although the role of the osteoblast in regulating osteoclast activity is reasonably well understood, the mechanism by which osteoblasts are recruited to sites of bone resorption is not. One possibility is that bone resorption releases IGF-1 from the bone matrix, and IGF-1 then stimulates osteoblast proliferation and differentiation. However, it is also becoming clear that the osteoclast itself can regulate osteoblast differentiation through bidirectional signaling molecules of the ephrin/Eph family.

If the replacement of resorbed bone matched the amount that was removed, remodeling would lead to no net change in bone mass. However, small deficits in bone mass persist on completion

of each cycle, reflecting inefficiency in remodeling dynamics. Consequently, lifelong accumulation of remodeling deficits underlies the well-documented phenomenon of age-related bone loss, a process that begins shortly after growth stops. Alterations in remodeling activity represent the final pathway through which diverse stimuli, such as dietary insufficiency, hormones, and drugs affect bone balance. A change in whole body remodeling rate can be brought about through distinct perturbations in remodeling dynamics. Changes in the hormonal milieu often increase the activation of remodeling units. Examples include hyperthyroidism, hyperparathyroidism, and hypervitaminosis D. Other factors may impair osteoblastic functional adequacy, such as high doses of glucocorticoids or ethanol. Yet other perturbations, such as estrogen or androgen deficiency, may augment osteoclastic resorptive capacity. At any given time, a transient deficit in bone exists called the **remodeling space** representing sites of bone resorption that have not yet filled in. In response to any stimulus that alters the birth rate of new remodeling units, the remodeling space either increases or decreases accordingly until a new steady state is established, and this adjustment is seen as an increase or decrease in bone mass.

OSTEOPOROSIS

Osteoporosis is a condition of low bone mass and microarchitectural disruption that results in fractures with minimal trauma. The term **primary osteoporosis** denotes reduced bone mass and fractures in postmenopausal women (postmenopausal osteoporosis) or in older men and women due to age-related factors. The term **secondary osteoporosis** refers to bone loss resulting from specific clinical disorders, such as thyrotoxicosis or hyperadrenocorticism (Table 8–9). There is overlap in these designations; for example, many postmenopausal women with low bone mass have vitamin D insufficiency or deficiency which could be considered a secondary cause of osteoporosis.

Osteoporotic fractures are a major public health problem for older women and men in Western society. Half the men and women over age 55 have low bone mass or osteoporosis, placing them at increased risk of fracture. At any age, women experience twice as many osteoporosis-related fractures as men, reflecting gender-related differences in skeletal properties as well as the almost universal loss of bone at menopause. However, the number of osteoporotic fractures in older men is not trivial (Figure 8–25). One white woman in six suffers a hip fracture; mortality after hip fracture is as high as 20% in the first year. One-third of hip fractures occur in men and have been associated with an even higher mortality rate than in women. Billions of dollars are spent annually for acute hospital care of hip fracture alone. The consequences of vertebral deformity are also significant and include chronic pain, inability to conduct daily activities, depression, increased mortality, and high risk of additional vertebral fractures.

Typically, fractures attributed to bone fragility are those due to trauma equal to or less than a fall from a standing position. Common sites of fragility-related fractures include the vertebral bodies, distal forearm, and proximal femur, but because the

TABLE 8–9 Causes of secondary osteoporosis.

Endocrinopathies
  Thyrotoxicosis
  Hyperprolactinemia
  Primary hyperparathyroidism
  Acromegaly
  Hypogonadism
  Glucocorticoid excess

Gastrointestinal/nutritional
  Vitamin D deficiency
  Chronic liver disease
  Celiac sprue
  Malabsorption

Medications
  Glucocorticoids
  Androgen deprivation therapy with gonadotropin-releasing
  hormone agonists
  Certain anticonvulsants
  Excess thyroid hormone replacement

Other
  Alcoholism
  Osteogenesis imperfecta
  Rheumatoid arthritis
  Multiple myeloma
  Chronic obstructive pulmonary disease
  Idiopathic hypercalciuria

TABLE 8–10 Risk factors for fractures.

Advanced age

Postmenopausal fracture

First-degree relative with a fracture

Current tobacco use

Low body weight

Inability to rise without using arms

Lifelong low calcium intake

Vitamin D deficiency

Inactivity/bed rest

Early estrogen loss

Low testosterone in men

Dementia

Alcoholism

Impaired vision

History of falls

Low bone mineral density

skeletons of patients with osteoporosis are diffusely fragile, other sites, such as ribs and long bones, also fracture with high frequency. Vertebral compression fractures are the most common fragility-related fractures. Pain sufficient to require medical attention occurs in approximately one-third of vertebral fractures, the majority being detected only when height loss or spinal deformity (kyphosis) occurs. However, even asymptomatic vertebral fractures confer an increased risk of future vertebral fractures and mortality. Thus, incidentally detected vertebral fractures have the same clinical significance as a clinical vertebral fracture. Furthermore, even fractures that appear to be due to trauma portend an increased future fracture risk. Both skeletal and extraskeletal factors determine fracture risk (Table 8–10).

Gain, Maintenance, and Loss of Bone

The amount of bone mineral present at any time in adult life represents that which has been gained at skeletal maturity (peak bone mass) minus that which has been subsequently lost. Bone acquisition is completed in the late teenage years and early twenties in girls and by the second decade in boys. Heredity accounts for most of the variance in bone acquisition. African American adolescent girls have greater calcium retention on a fixed calcium intake compared to Caucasian adolescent girls, potentially explaining at least part of the racial differences in bone mass. Specific genes implicated in bone acquisition include those affecting body size, hormone responsiveness, and bone-specific proteins such as type 1 collagen and transforming growth factor beta.

Recent evidence indicates that the *Wnt pathway* plays a central role in determining bone mass. The low-density lipoprotein (LDL) receptor-like protein 5 (LRP5) along with the frizzled protein serves as coreceptor for members of the Wnt family of ligands. Activation of Wnt and its downstream signaling pathways mediates increased osteoblastic activity (gene expression, cell proliferation). Mutations that render LRP5 constitutively active are associated with high bone mass, and autosomal recessive inactivating mutations in LRP5 play a causative role in the osteoporosis-pseudoglioma syndrome. These mutations lead to accelerated bone loss and fractures as well as blindness. These two disorders of bone mass have firmly established Wnts, LRP5, and frizzled as essential molecules in osteoblast-mediated bone formation.

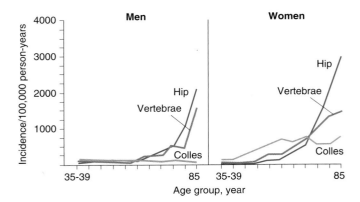

FIGURE 8–25 Incidence rates for the three common osteoporotic fractures (Colles, hip, and vertebral) in men and women, plotted as a function of age at the time of the fracture. (Reproduced, with permission, from Cooper C, Melton LJ, III. Epidemiology of osteoporosis. *Trend Endocrinol Metab.* 1992;314:224.)

Other factors contributing to the acquisition of peak bone mass include circulating gonadal steroids, physical activity, and nutrient intake. In adolescents, calcium retention is maximal at a calcium intake of 1300 mg/d; this is the current recommended intake for individuals aged 9 to 18 years. Adolescence is a critical time for the skeleton; bone gained during adolescence accounts for about 60% of final adult bone mass. Assuming adequate exposure to key nutrients, physical activity, and reproductive hormones, adolescent growth supports acquisition of the maximum bone mass permitted by the genetic endowment. Estradiol plays a decisive role in the initiation of adolescent growth and bone acquisition. Rare examples have been reported of young men bearing mutations in the estradiol receptor or in aromatase, the enzyme that converts androgen to estrogen. Although these men had normal or increased circulating concentrations of testosterone, estradiol was either absent or totally ineffective. In all cases, severe deficits in BMD were observed, and these patients had not undergone the anticipated acceleration in linear growth at the time of puberty. In the patients with aromatase deficiency, substantial gains in bone were observed shortly after initiating estrogen therapy.

Adolescent bone acquisition falters in the face of inadequacies in diet, physical activity, or reproductive function, resulting in a lower peak bone mass and less reserve to accommodate future losses. Recent trends in habitual physical activity and calcium intake for North American teenagers, particularly girls, offer little encouragement in this regard. A list of representative conditions often associated with reduced peak bone mass acquisition is presented in Table 8–11.

TABLE 8–11 Examples of disorders associated with reduced peak bone mass.

Anorexia nervosa
Ankylosing spondylitis
Childhood immobilization (therapeutic bed rest)
Cystic fibrosis
Delayed puberty
Exercise-associated amenorrhea
Galactosemia
Intestinal or renal disease
Marfan syndrome
Osteogenesis imperfecta

Once peak bone mass is achieved, bone mass remains fairly stable until the late third or early fourth decades (Figure 8–26). Successful bone maintenance requires continued attention to the same factors that influenced bone acquisition: diet, physical activity, and sex hormone status. Maintenance of bone requires sufficiency in all areas, and deficiency in one is not compensated by the others. For example, amenorrheic athletes lose bone despite frequent high-intensity physical activity and supplemental calcium intake. Successful bone maintenance is also jeopardized by known toxic exposures such as smoking, alcohol excess, and immobility as well as by systemic illnesses and many medications.

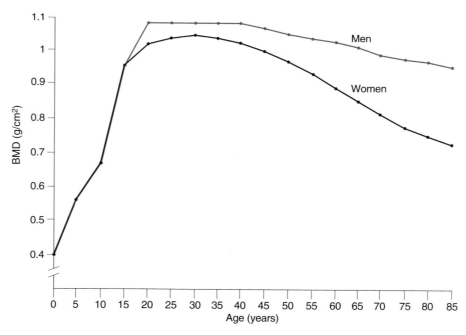

FIGURE 8–26 Mean bone mineral density by DXA in white males (upper curve) and females (lower curve) aged 5 to 85 years. (The data are from Southard RN, et al. Bone mass in healthy children: measurement with quantitative DXA. *Radiology.* 1991;179:735; and from Kelly TL. Bone mineral reference databases for American men and women. *J Bone Miner Res.* 1990;5(suppl 2):702. Courtesy of Hologic, Inc.)

Bone Loss Associated with Estrogen Deficiency

Estrogen deprivation promotes bone remodeling by releasing constraints on the production and activity of cytokines, particularly IL-6, which stimulates the proliferation of osteoclast precursors. Estradiol suppresses IL-6 secretion by marrow stromal osteoblastic cells, and treatment of mice with neutralizing IL-6 antibodies suppresses osteoclast production after oophorectomy. Estradiol directly suppresses IL-6 production in human osteoblasts, and *IL-6* gene knockout prevents bone loss in oophorectomized mice. Thus, a strong case implicates IL-6 as a critical molecule by which osteoblasts signal increased bone remodeling and suggests that this link is a major site for estrogen action in bone. Subsidiary roles for IL-1 and IL-11 have also been described. As discussed above, the RANK-RANKL-OPG system acts as a bone regulatory system through which osteoblast signals stimulate the production of osteoclasts. With estrogen deficiency, OPG secretion is low, permitting a robust response of osteoclast precursors to RANKL. With estrogen sufficiency, increased local concentrations of OPG bind to RANKL, reduce osteoclast production, and thereby decrease bone turnover.

With accelerated bone turnover, delivery of calcium from bone to the circulation increases, and the resultant subtle increase in plasma calcium concentration suppresses the secretion of PTH, thereby enhancing calciuria, suppressing renal production of $1,25(OH)_2D$, and reducing intestinal calcium absorption efficiency. At menopause, loss of endogenous estrogen promotes an increase in daily calcium loss from 20 mg to about 60 mg, reflecting a relative increase in bone resorption over formation activity. Although small, this magnitude of change in mineral balance accounts, after a decade, for about 13% of an original whole body calcium mass of 1000 g, equivalent to a standard deviation in BMD, and leads to a two- to threefold increase in the risk of fracture (see Figure 8–26). In the 5 years after menopause, women not on estrogen can lose as much as 5% to 8% of bone mass. To accommodate menopausal changes in calcium economy by dietary means alone, a rise in daily calcium intake from 1000 mg to about 1500 mg would be necessary. Increased calcium intake can slow but usually does not entirely prevent the bone loss that occurs with menopause.

Bone Loss in Later Life

Progressive deficits in renal and intestinal function impair whole body calcium economy during normal human aging. These deficits include progressive inefficiency of vitamin D production by the skin as well as declining ability to convert $25(OH)D$ to $1,25(OH)_2D$ in the kidney. Consequently, intestinal calcium absorption becomes less efficient, leading to modest reductions in plasma ionized calcium activity and compensatory hypersecretion of PTH. PTH maintains blood calcium concentrations by activating new bone remodeling units, although as a result of its inherent inefficiency, increased bone remodeling leads to accelerated bone loss. Little can be done to counteract remodeling inefficiency, but the impact of these physiologic deficits can be minimized by suppressing the stimulus for PTH secretion by consuming adequate amounts of dietary calcium (about 1500 mg/d) and vitamin D (at least 800-1200 units/d).

Diagnosis of Osteoporosis

The diagnosis of osteoporosis may be obvious in patients who have sustained fragility fractures (Figure 8–27), but noninvasive

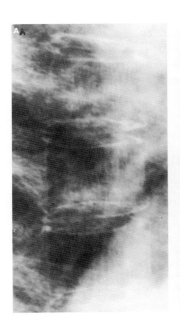
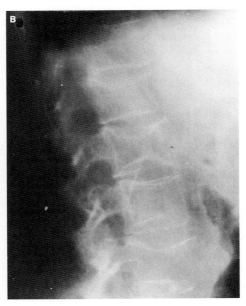

FIGURE 8–27 A: Magnified x-rays of thoracic vertebrae from a woman with osteoporosis. Note the relative prominence of vertical trabeculae and the absence of horizontal trabeculae. **B:** Lateral x-ray of the lumbar spine of a woman with postmenopausal osteoporosis. Note the increased density of the superior and inferior cortical margins of vertebrae, the marked demineralization of vertebral bodies, and the central compression of articular surfaces of vertebral bodies by intervertebral disks. (Courtesy of Dr. G. Gordan.)

methods to estimate BMD are required to identify high-risk patients who have not yet sustained a fracture. Due to the significant consequences of fractures, diagnosis prior to fracture is essential. Several techniques have been developed for this purpose, but DXA offers the most precise measurements at multiple skeletal sites for the least amount of radiation exposure. Current guidelines recommend that all women over the age of 65 years be screened for osteoporosis using bone densitometry. Under age 65, the National Osteoporosis Foundation (NOF) guidelines recommend that screening start after menopause in women with risk factors for fracture. NOF recommends screening men over 70 and targeted screening of men between age 50 and 70 if there is a risk factor for bone loss and or fracture. There are no routine screening recommendations for younger individuals. Younger men and women should have bone density testing as clinically indicated (eg, clinical evidence of bone fragility). Assessment of skeletal health should be based on age-matched normative data (Z-scores). Although there are no formal guidelines and a paucity of long-term data, most experts consider a BMD more than two standard deviations below the age-matched normal reference population (a Z score of −2 or lower) to indicate low BMD in a young person. However, BMD in younger individuals must be interpreted in light of the clinical situation and other risk factors for fracture.

BMD is a highly significant predictor of fracture risk. For each standard deviation BMD below the average BMD of individuals at the age of peak bone mass, fracture risk approximately doubles. Site-specific measurements best predict fracture risk at that site (ie, hip BMD best predicts hip fracture), but a measurement at any site predicts overall fracture risk. Based on data from Caucasian postmenopausal women and originally intended to be used as an epidemiologic tool, a World Health Organization (WHO) panel in 1994 offered an absolute standard for categorization of BMD. By this criterion, BMD values 2.5 or more SD below the average value for a person at the age of peak bone mass (a T-score of −2.5 or below) are categorized as **osteoporosis.** BMD values between −1.0 and −2.5 SD below the standard (T-score between −1 and −2.5) are categorized as low bone density or **osteopenia.**

While not their original intended purpose, these T-score cut points became integrated into clinical practice and have been used to place individuals with low BMD into diagnostic categories. Problematically, there are no risk thresholds at these values and an individual with a T-score of −2.4 and an individual with a T-score of −2.5 have nearly identical fracture risk, but one is considered to have osteoporosis and one is not. Additionally, two individuals with the same T-score value can have very different fracture risk. A woman in her fifties with no personal or family history of fracture but a femoral neck T-score of −2.5 has a 10-year risk of fracture of less than 10%. However, an 80-year-old woman whose mother had a hip fracture and who has a personal history of fracture but the same femoral neck T-score of −2.5 has a 10-year risk of fracture of more than 50%. It has long been recognized that the combination of risk factors for fracture and BMD can improve fracture risk prediction. An approach to formally estimating individual fracture risk from

femoral neck bone density and risk factors for fracture was developed by the WHO and became available in 2008 at the website http://www.shef.ac.uk/FRAX/index.htm. While still undergoing revisions and improvements, the FRAX tool has greatly improved the clinician's ability to estimate fracture risk for an individual patient. The levels of risk at which treatment should be initiated are country specific and being revised, but a cost-effectiveness analysis in the United States suggests that individuals with a 10-year probability of major osteoporotic fracture of 20% or of hip fracture of 3% should be considered for treatment. Limitations of this fracture prediction model include that it only incorporates BMD by DXA at the hip, many risk factors are not available in the model, and there is no way to incorporate the effect of prior treatment on fracture risk.

TREATMENT OF OSTEOPOROSIS

Drugs used for prevention and treatment of osteoporosis act either by decreasing the rate of bone resorption, thereby slowing the rate of bone loss, or by increasing bone formation (Table 8–12). Because of the coupled nature of bone resorption and formation, agents that decrease bone resorption ultimately decrease the rate of bone formation. Thus, increases in BMD, representing a reduction of the remodeling space to a new steady-state level, are commonly observed during the first year or two of therapy, after which BMD increases slowly and may even reach a plateau. It is not uncommon for there to be minimal changes in BMD observed with treatment in clinical practice. Analysis of data from the Fracture Intervention Trial demonstrated that women in the alendronate treatment group whose bone density did not increase during treatment still benefited with rates of fracture reduction similar to the women whose BMD measurably increased. Thus, women on treatment with stable BMD should not be considered treatment failures based on a perceived lack of response.

TABLE 8–12   Pharmacologic approaches to osteoporosis.

Antiresorptive agents
Calcium
Vitamin D and calcitriol
Estrogen
SERMs
Calcitonin
Bisphosphonates
RANK-ligand inhibition
Bone-forming agents
Fluoride[a]
Androgens[a]
Parathyroid hormone
Strontium ranelate[a]

[a]Not approved in the United States.

TABLE 8–13 Current daily recommendations for adequate intake of calcium and food sources of calcium.

Children/adolescents	
Age 1-3	500 mg
Age 4-8	800 mg
Ages 9-18	1300 mg
Adults	
Age 19-50	1000 mg
Age >51	1200 mg
Food sources of calcium	
Dairy-free diet	300 mg
Milk (8 oz)	300 mg
Calcium set tofu (1/2 cup)	400 mg
Cheese (1 oz)	250 mg
Yogurt (1 cup)	300 mg
Cooked greens (1 cup)	100 mg
Fortified foods	Varies

Specific Antiresorptive Agents

A. Calcium In the seventh decade and beyond, supplemental calcium and vitamin D therapy suppresses bone turnover, increases bone mass, and has been shown in clinical trials to decrease fracture incidence. Studies confirming the clinical efficacy of various pharmacologic agents to increase BMD or decrease fracture have been performed in the setting of calcium and vitamin D sufficiency. Thus, adequate intake of calcium and vitamin D should be considered a basic approach for prevention and treatment of osteoporosis in all patients (Table 8–13).

The current recommended intake of calcium is 1300 mg/d for adolescents, 1000 mg/d for adults up to age 50, and 1200 mg/d for adults over age 50 years. Intakes of 1500 mg/d for individuals with or at risk of developing osteoporosis are recommended by some authors. A dairy-free diet contains approximately 250 mg/d of calcium. Achieving the recommended calcium intake goals by food alone typically requires consumption of three to four servings per day of dairy foods or calcium-fortified foods. Patients who are unable to increase dietary calcium by diet alone may choose from many palatable, low-cost calcium preparations, the most frequently prescribed being the carbonate salt. Others include the lactate, gluconate, and citrate salts and hydroxyapatite. Absorption of most commonly prescribed calcium products is similar. For many patients, cost and palatability outweigh modest differences in absorption. Calcium carbonate requires an acid environment for optimal absorption. For older individuals who may have hypo- or achlorhydria, taking calcium carbonate tablets with meals generally provides adequate acidity for this requirement. To maximize absorption, calcium should be taken in doses of 500 mg or less at a time and spread throughout the day. Calcium can interfere with the absorption of iron and L-thyroxine and should be ingested separately from these medications.

B. Vitamin D and calcitriol In recent years, it has become necessary to reassess our concepts of vitamin D sufficiency (see also Vitamin D earlier). Although circulating 25(OH)D concentrations above 10 ng/mL appear adequate for preventing histologic evidence of osteomalacia, a strong case can now be made that values below 25 to 30 ng/mL are associated with hypersecretion of PTH, proximal muscle weakness predisposing to falls, and increased bone turnover. In some regions of the United States, healthy adults show average 25(OH)D concentrations of 30 ng/mL or above, but in others, such as New England or in states farther north than Missouri, the ultraviolet component of sunlight fails to contain sufficient amounts, at the critical region of approximately 270 to 310 nm, to support cutaneous vitamin D synthesis. In those areas, vitamin D insufficiency is very common, particularly in frail, homebound, or hospitalized patients. Vitamin D supplementation in individuals with marginal or deficient vitamin D status improves intestinal calcium absorption, suppresses PTH and bone remodeling, increases bone mass, and, in doses of 800 IU/d or greater, reduces fracture risk.

The use of potent vitamin D analogs or metabolites—such as calcitriol—to treat osteoporosis is an intervention distinct from ensuring vitamin D nutritional adequacy. In the treatment of osteoporosis, the rationale is to exploit the ability of these compounds to interact with the VDR in parathyroid cells to suppress PTH secretion directly and reduce bone turnover. Clinical experience with calcitriol remains mixed. Higher doses impose an added risk of hypercalciuria and hypercalcemia.

C. Estrogen Conjugated equine estrogens at a dose of 0.625 mg/d increase BMD about 5% and 2.5% at the lumbar spine and proximal femur respectively, and reduce the risk of hip and vertebral fractures by 35% to 40%. Both oral and transdermal estrogen offers protection against bone loss. Cessation of estrogen administration leads to rapid bone loss, and protection against fracture dissipates within a few years of stopping even after prolonged treatment.

Data from the Women's Health Initiative (WHI) released since 2002 underscore the lack of cardiovascular disease prevention in estrogen-treated postmenopausal woman and the small but statistically significant increases in breast cancer and venous thromboembolic phenomena that occur with estrogen and progesterone therapy (hormone therapy; HT) in postmenopausal women. The WHI has led to a marked change in prescribing of HT for postmenopausal women such that only patients suffering from significant vasomotor effects of estrogen deficiency and early in menopause are currently prescribed HT and for the shortest possible time. Reduced BMD is not considered an indication for HT, because effective alternative therapies for skeletal preservation exist. In older women who also receive adequate calcium supplementation, 0.3 mg of conjugated estrogens produces similar gains in bone density, but this dose has not been tested for antifracture effects. In the relatively small randomized trials in which lower doses of estrogen have been studied, increases in vascular events or breast cancer have not been seen. Interest remains in whether there might be a low dose of estrogen at which the skeletal benefits could be achieved without incurring the adverse vascular and malignant consequences. It is unclear whether a trial of sufficient size to address this question is feasible at the present time.

D. Selective estrogen response modulators The past decade has witnessed the design and development of several molecules that act as estrogens on some tissues but antiestrogens on others. The only currently approved SERM, raloxifene, is an estrogen agonist at bone and liver, that promotes conservation of BMD and lowering of LDL cholesterol concentrations, but it is inert at the endometrium and a potent antiestrogen at the breast. Raloxifene has been shown to decrease the vertebral fracture incidence in older osteoporotic women and has received FDA approval for both prevention and treatment of osteoporosis in postmenopausal women.

E. Calcitonin The role of endogenous calcitonin in calcium metabolism is unclear. However, given as a pharmacologic agent, calcitonin inhibits osteoclastic bone resorption. Originally available only as an injectable form, calcitonin is now also available as a nasal spray, and both formulations are approved for postmenopausal osteoporosis treatment. CT nasal spray (200 IU/d) increases BMD by 2% to 3% and reduces vertebral fractures by about 35%. CT has not been shown to reduce hip or nonspine fractures in randomized trials; however, a meta-analysis of 14 CT trials suggested a significant reduction in both vertebral and nonvertebral fractures with CT therapy. CT may provide some analgesic benefit in women with acute or painful vertebral fractures, possibly through central nervous system effects. Side-effects of nasal spray CT appear mild and include rhinitis. The nasal spray daily dose should be alternated between nostrils. Injectable CT has additional side-effects of flushing, nausea, and local injection reactions, making the nasal option the preferred form of administration.

F. Bisphosphonates Bisphosphonates bind avidly to the hydroxyapatite crystals in bone, particularly at sites of active remodeling. The currently approved amino bisphosphonates interfere with protein prenylation in the osteoclast, impairing osteoclast-mediated bone resorption as well as enhancing osteoclast apoptosis. Four bisphosphonates, alendronate, risedronate, ibandronate, and zoledronic acid are FDA-approved for prevention and treatment of osteoporosis. Three of them, alendronate, risedronate, and zoledronic acid are approved for treatment of glucocorticoid-induced osteoporosis in men and women and for the treatment of osteoporosis in men.

All the approved bisphosphonates have been shown to reduce vertebral fractures by approximately 50% to 60%. Alendronate, risedronate, and zoledronic acid have also been shown to reduce the risk of nonvertebral fractures. In clinical trials, hip fractures were reduced by 51% after treatment with alendronate, 30% after treatment with risedronate, and 41% after annual infusions of zoledronic acid for 3 years. Head-to-head comparisons, however, have not been performed. Treatment of individuals (men and women) who have had a hip fracture with zoledronic acid has also been shown to reduce subsequent fractures and decrease mortality

in individuals. Ibandronate has not been shown to reduce the risk of nonvertebral fractures except in the post hoc analysis of women with T-scores less than -3. The fracture trials for all the bisphosphonates were conducted using daily dosing, except for zoledronic acid which was given as a 5 mg annual intravenous dose. Based on equivalent effects on BMD to daily dosing, alendronate and risedronate are approved for weekly dosing, and risedronate and ibandronate are approved for monthly dosing. Ibandronate is also approved for quarterly intravenous dosing.

Oral bisphosphonate absorption is very low, less than 1% of the administered dose. Consequently, patients must take these medications on first arising in the morning, on an empty stomach, with at least 8 oz of water, remain upright to ensure passage of the pill into the stomach, and ingest nothing else for 30 minutes for alendronate and risedronate, and 60 minutes for ibandronate. Side-effects from the oral bisphosphonates are primarily upper gastrointestinal, most notably esophageal irritation if the pill does not clear the esophagus. Hence the requirement to administer with sufficient water and remain upright after dosing. None of the bisphosphonates are recommended for use in patients with significant renal impairment (creatinine clearance <35 mL/min).

Intravenous therapy can be given conveniently for zoledronic acid (5 mg annually) and ibandronate (3 mg quarterly).

Osteonecrosis of the jaw has been reported in patients taking bisphosphonates, and a warning regarding this possible adverse effect was recently added to all bisphosphonate labeling. The vast majority of cases have occurred after dental work in patients with malignancies on intravenous bisphosphonates at more frequent intervals and at much higher doses of drug than the annual infusions for patients with osteoporosis. Several cases, however, have been reported in patients with osteoporosis. Estimates of the incidence of this complication related to bisphosphonate treatment in benign conditions vary widely, but appear to be approximately 1/50,000 patient years. Rates are significantly higher in malignant conditions such as multiple myeloma or breast cancer. Osteonecrosis of the jaw is a difficult disorder to treat, and additional oral procedures including biopsy of the affected site may worsen the condition. Suspected cases should be referred to an experienced dental professional.

Other bisphosphonate related side-effects include bone pain and, for the intravenous agents, an acute phase reaction temporally related to dosing and typically limited to the patient's first dose.

G. Rank-L inhibition Denosumab, a human monoclonal IgG2 antibody to RANK-L, has been shown to reduce spine fractures by 68%, hip fractures by 40%, and nonvertebral fractures by 20% in postmenopausal women with low bone density (T-score <−2.5 and >−4.0) aged 60 to 90 years. In the pivotal trial establishing this antifracture efficacy, 60 mg denosumab was administered subcutaneously every 6 months for 3 years. Denosumab has been approved by the FDA for the treatment of patients with severe osteoporosis at high risk for fracture. Adverse events include eczema and cellulitis. Another clinical trial in men with prostate cancer undergoing androgen deprivation therapy has shown substantial increases in BMD and reduced risk of vertebral fractures in these men. At present, the FDA has not given formal approval to the use of denosumab in these high-risk men.

Bone-Forming Agents

A. Parathyroid hormone

Fractures, skeletal deformity, and bone pain are well-described manifestations of bone disease associated with severe primary hyperparathyroidism. It may seem counterintuitive, therefore, to suggest that administration of PTH to individuals with low BMD may not only improve BMD but also reduce the risk of fractures. Yet, that is what experience over the past two decades indicates. The decisive element apparently that determines the effects of PTH to be destructive or therapeutic is whether PTH concentrations in blood are elevated constantly or only intermittently. In severe hyperparathyroidism, PTH concentrations remain high, varying little throughout the day. In most cases of mild hyperparathyroidism seen today, PTH concentrations are lower, sometimes even within the normal range. In such patients, normal and even increased lumbar spine BMD measurements are commonly observed. Administration of PTH as daily pulse injections has been shown to increase BMD in both animals and humans. Abundant evidence now indicates that PTH is truly an osteotropic agent, and several groups have shown increases in vertebral BMD of patients with osteoporosis. In a large clinical trial conducted in postmenopausal women with osteoporosis, recombinant human PTH(1-34)(rhPTH[1-34]), given in daily subcutaneous doses for approximately 21 months, reduced the incidence of vertebral fractures by more than 60% and that of nonvertebral fractures by 50%. During the course of this trial, a long-term carcinogenicity study showed that rats given near-lifetime daily injections of rhPTH(1-34) showed a dose-related incidence of osteosarcoma. Clinical studies with this agent were immediately suspended, pending a thorough review of all relevant information by an independent group of cancer biologists, who concluded that the rat osteosarcoma finding was not likely to predict a relationship to osteosarcoma in humans. Consequently, human trials with rhPTH(1-34) were resumed. rhPTH(1-34) or teriparatide was approved by the FDA for use in both men and postmenopausal women with osteoporosis who are at high risk for fractures as well as in glucocorticoid-induced osteoporosis. Therapeutic use is limited to 2 years and is recommended for individuals who have had a fracture related to osteoporosis, who have multiple risk factors for fracture, or who cannot use other osteoporosis treatments. Side-effects include hypercalcemia, hypercalciuria, and bone pain. Teriparatide is contraindicated for patients with conditions placing them at increased risk for osteosarcoma such as Paget disease of bone, unexplained elevations of alkaline phosphatase, open epiphyses, or patients who have received radiation therapy involving the skeleton. Over 430,000 patients have received teriparatide therapy, and there have been two reported cases of possible osteosarcoma; this approximates the background risk of osteosarcoma in the general population. After cessation of PTH therapy, bone loss resumes, and all bone gained may be lost over 1 to 2 years. It is strongly recommended that PTH therapy be followed with a bisphosphonate, thus maintaining the gain in BMD achieved with PTH administration. Given

the potency of bisphosphonates like alendronate and zoledronic acid, it is not recommended that patients treated with these agents receive teriparatide therapy concomitantly.

B. Androgen

Testosterone increases bone mass in hypogonadal men. Androgens also improve bone mass in osteoporotic women, but therapy is frequently limited by virilizing side-effects. Nandrolone decanoate, 50 mg intramuscularly every 3 weeks, and the androgenic progestin norethisterone acetate increased BMD in osteoporotic women without bothersome side-effects. Fracture data do not yet permit a conclusion about the clinical utility of these agents.

Nonpharmacologic Aspects of Osteoporosis Management

Much of the day-to-day management of osteoporotic patients involves issues that are not specific for bone. These include depression therapy as appropriate, pain control, maintaining nutritional status, exercise, fall prevention, and assisting the patient to organize activities of daily living.

Minimal attention has been devoted to the role of exercise for patients with established osteoporosis. Patients and physicians often show reluctance to participate in exercise because of concerns for additional injury. However, activity avoidance aggravates bone loss and places the skeleton in even greater jeopardy, whereas improving muscle strength, particularly of the back extensor groups, constitutes a powerful means for reducing pain and increasing functional capacity. Even the most frail individuals can successfully implement exercise regimens with the assistance of a trained physical therapist.

Exercise regimens that include a component of weight bearing and/or resistance exercise have been shown to increase BMD approximately 1% per year in randomized trials. If exercise is discontinued, these gains in BMD are lost.

Because the great majority of hip fractures are the immediate result of a fall, strategies aimed at reduction of falls are of critical importance. Muscle weakness is an important predictor of fall risk, and decreased muscle mass and strength are consequences of normal human aging. Resistance exercise (ie, weight training) promotes muscle strength even in very old men and women, and evidence suggests that increased lower extremity strength may reduce falls risk by improving postural stability. Thus, a widely disseminated program of leg-strengthening exercise could lower the risk of falling and reduce hip fracture incidence even if no changes in BMD are achieved.

Several additional measures may lower the risk of fracture for osteoporotic patients. Proper footwear and installation of safety features around the home may minimize the risk of falling. Such features include bathroom safety rails and night lights, rails and lighting for stairways, and elimination of floor clutter. Canes and other walking aids should be recommended to patients with an unsteady gait. Physicians may need to overcome substantial patient resistance, but these aids can be lifesaving. Visual acuity should be maximized and visual impairments corrected to the extent possible. Corsets and other support garments stabilize posture and relieve strain on paraspinous muscles. Metal braces may be indicated at times, but they are expensive, poorly accepted by most patients, and frequently end up unused. Attention should be given to other comorbid conditions that may affect fracture risk such as pain and depression and the effects of medications that may cause diminished alertness and responsiveness by causing sedation or orthostatic hypotension.

GLUCOCORTICOID-INDUCED OSTEOPOROSIS

In children, chronic exposure to glucocorticoids impairs skeletal growth. Glucocorticoid-induced deficits in childhood bone mass reflect failure of normal skeletal acquisition occasionally compounded by bone loss. In adults, initiation of glucocorticoid therapy leads to rapid bone loss, resulting in significant BMD deficits within even a few months with a greater impact on trabecular than cortical bone. The magnitude of bone loss can be large, typically approaching 40% reduction of the initial BMD. Approximately half of long-term glucocorticoid-treated patients suffer a fracture. Skeletal fragility is not the only risk factor for fracture in steroid-treated patients, because glucocorticoids (and the illnesses for which they are prescribed) are also associated with muscle weakness, which itself creates instability and increases the risk of falling.

Glucocorticoid-induced bone loss generally follows sustained administration of systemic doses greater than 5 mg/d of prednisone or its equivalent. Short, infrequent courses of glucocorticoids, such as for poison oak dermatitis, do not appear to have long-term skeletal consequences. Used according to manufacturer recommendations, most steroid inhalers available in the United States also appear to be without skeletal consequence, because systemic absorption of glucocorticoids is minimal. However, excessive use of standard preparations may achieve systemic concentrations, adequate to suppress the hypothalamic-pituitary axis and predictably lead to loss of bone mass. Patients receiving maintenance hydrocortisone dosages (eg, 20 mg/d) for adrenocortical insufficiency do not generally have an increased skeletal risk. However, based on accurate measurements of steroid production rates in normal humans, maintenance doses of hydrocortisone are now estimated to be lower (ie, 15 mg/d) than have traditionally been recommended (about 30 mg/d). Patients who continue to be treated according to older recommendations may be at risk of excessive bone loss.

Pathophysiology

Glucocorticoids affect mineral balance through alterations in renal, intestinal, and skeletal function.

A. Renal calcium losses   Within a few days after initiating therapy, direct inhibition of renal tubular calcium reabsorption leads to hypercalciuria, which is magnified by excessive dietary sodium intake and attenuated by thiazide diuretics.

B. Intestinal calcium losses   Glucocorticoids, given in high doses for several weeks, inhibit intestinal calcium absorption, lowering plasma ionized $[Ca^{2+}]$. This is thought to stimulate compensatory hypersecretion of PTH, which restores ionized $[Ca^{2+}]$ by increasing the efficiency of renal calcium reabsorption and by activating bone turnover to increase delivery of calcium to the circulation from bone. However, it has never been shown consistently that plasma PTH concentrations are actually elevated in steroid-treated patients. Evidence suggests that PTH action in bone and kidney may be enhanced even if there are minimal or no increases in detectable PTH. PTH may contribute to the pathophysiology of bone loss in glucocorticoid-treated patients. Consistent effects of glucocorticoids on the production, clearance, and circulating concentrations of vitamin D metabolites have not been demonstrable, so it appears that the intestinal actions of glucocorticoids are independent of the vitamin D system.

C. Skeletal losses   Glucocorticoids affect the skeleton by multiple mechanisms. There is evidence for direct stimulation of bone resorption via increased RANK-L expression and decreased OPG production. Glucocorticoids also inhibit osteoblastic maturation and activity. Recent information indicates that glucocorticoids shift multipotent stem cell maturation away from osteoblastic lineage toward other cell lines, particularly adipocytes. Glucocorticoids also promote apoptosis in osteoblasts and osteocytes. In patients chronically treated with glucocorticoids, bone formation is suppressed. High-dose glucocorticoid administration also suppresses gonadotropin secretion and creates a hypogonadal state in both men and women. Thus, a component of the bone loss in some steroid-treated patients is likely to be related to loss of gonadal function.

Prevention and Treatment of Glucocorticoid-Related Osteoporosis

A. Reduction of steroid dose   Prevention of bone loss remains the approach most likely to give a favorable outcome. The most important aspect of a preventive strategy is to limit exposure to glucocorticoids and to find alternative treatments if possible. Opportunities should be sought for initiating dose reduction or switching to nonsystemic forms of steroid administration. Unfortunately, the use of alternate-day steroids, which is known to protect growth in steroid-treated children, appears not to offer skeletal protection to adults. The possibility that a bone-sparing glucocorticoid might be developed has been under consideration for many years, but no such agent is currently available. In patients who require immunosuppression following organ transplantation, the use of cyclosporine and tacrolimus has permitted reductions in glucocorticoid use. However, these newer drugs also have been associated with lower BMD; whether long-term therapy will have less negative skeletal effects than glucocorticoids is not established.

B. Calcium and vitamin D   Providing supplemental calcium and vitamin D to glucocorticoid-treated patients normalizes plasma-ionized $[Ca^{2+}]$, suppresses PTH secretion, and reduces bone remodeling, thereby reducing the number of active remodeling units at a given time. So long as the patient continues to take glucocorticoids, however, suppression of osteoblast function does not reverse. Patients should receive 1200 mg/d of supplemental calcium on the condition that such supplementation does not result in hypercalciuria. Vitamin D dosing should be targeted to maintain values at or above the current target of 30 ng/mL. However, periodic surveillance of glucocorticoid-treated patients for urinary calcium excretion is warranted, because they are at higher risk of developing kidney stones as a consequence of hypercalciuria.

C. Physical activity Skeletal immobilization precipitates bone loss, so inactivity must be avoided in steroid-treated patients. Some conditions such as polymyalgia rheumatica respond exuberantly to steroid therapy, giving patients a rapid and complete recovery of function. These patients may have little difficulty maintaining a vigorous schedule of weight-bearing activities during treatment. Patients with other conditions may not regain full mobility and may have residual functional disabilities. It is particularly important that such patients receive physical therapy or other appropriate support for maintaining and restoring functional capacity.

D. Hormone therapy In some rheumatologic conditions (eg, systemic lupus erythematosus), estrogens have traditionally been avoided. If there are no contraindications to estrogen administration, HT will counteract the negative skeletal consequences of pituitary-gonadal suppression. Evaluation of gonadal hormone status should be considered in all glucocorticoid-treated patients and estrogen or testosterone therapy utilized where appropriate.

Pharmacologic Therapy of Glucocorticoid-Related Osteoporosis

Alendronate, risedronate, zoledronic acid, and teriparatide have been shown to increase BMD and decrease the risk of new vertebral fractures by up to 70% in patients on glucocorticoid therapy.

Because the bone loss associated with glucocorticoid therapy has a very rapid onset and occurs in approximately 50% of treated patients, it is prudent to assess BMD prior to initiating therapy and consider starting a bisphosphonate along with the glucocorticoids in patients whose BMD is already low. Patients with normal BMD may be followed by repeating the BMD at a shorter interval than is typically done with osteoporosis, namely, in 6 to 9 months. If significant bone loss is evident, a bisphosphonate or teriparatide may then be started. All patients should receive appropriate calcium and vitamin D and other risk factors for fracture addressed.

OSTEOMALACIA AND RICKETS

Osteomalacia and rickets are caused by the abnormal mineralization of bone and cartilage. Osteomalacia is a bone defect occurring after the epiphyseal plates have closed (ie, in adults). Rickets occur

in growing bone (ie, in children). Abnormal mineralization in growing bone affects the transformation of cartilage into bone at the zone of provisional calcification. As a result, an enormous profusion of disorganized, nonmineralized, degenerating cartilage appears in this region, leading to widening of the epiphyseal plate (observed radiologically as a widened radiolucent zone) with flaring or cupping and irregularity of the epiphyseal-metaphyseal junctions. This latter problem gives rise to the clinically obvious beaded swellings along the costochondral junctions known as the **rachitic rosary** and the swelling at the ends of the long bones. Growth is retarded by the failure to make new bone. Once bone growth has ceased (ie, after closure of the epiphyseal plates), the clinical evidence for defective mineralization becomes more subtle, and special diagnostic procedures may be required for its detection.

Pathogenesis

The best-known cause of abnormal bone mineralization is vitamin D deficiency (see discussed earlier). Vitamin D, through its biologically active metabolites, ensures that the calcium and phosphate concentrations in the extracellular milieu are adequate for mineralization. Vitamin D may also permit osteoblasts to produce a bone matrix that can be mineralized and then allows them to mineralize that matrix normally. Phosphate deficiency can also cause defective mineralization, as in diseases in which phosphate is lost in the urine or poorly absorbed in the intestine. Phosphate deficiency may act independently or in conjunction with other predisposing abnormalities, because most hypophosphatemic disorders associated with osteomalacia or rickets also affect the vitamin D endocrine system. Dietary calcium deficiency has been shown to lead to rickets in children in the absence of vitamin D deficiency and may contribute to the osteomalacia of elderly adults who are also susceptible to vitamin D deficiency.

Osteomalacia or rickets may develop despite adequate levels of calcium, phosphate, and vitamin D if the bone matrix cannot undergo normal mineralization as a result of enzyme deficiencies, such as decreased alkaline phosphatase in patients with hypophosphatasia, or in the presence of inhibitors of mineralization, such as aluminum, fluoride, or etidronate. Table 8–14 lists diseases associated with osteomalacia or rickets according to their presumed mechanism. Several diseases appear under several headings, indicating that they contribute to bone disease by several mechanisms.

Diagnosis

The following discussion refers primarily to vitamin D deficiency. In children, the presentation of rickets is generally obvious from a combination of clinical and radiologic evidence. The diagnostic challenge is to determine the cause. In adults, the clinical, radiologic, and biochemical evidence of osteomalacia is often subtle. In situations in which osteomalacia should be suspected such as malnutrition or malabsorption, BMD is strikingly low, and the clinician must decide whether to obtain a bone biopsy for histomorphometric examination. This decision rests on the

TABLE 8–14   Causes of osteomalacia.

Disorders of the vitamin D endocrine system
  Decreased bioavailability
    Insufficient sunlight exposure
    Nutritional vitamin D deficiency
    Nephrotic syndrome (urinary loss)
    Malabsorption (fecal loss)
      Billroth type II gastrectomy
      Sprue
      Regional enteritis
      Jejunoileal bypass
      Pancreatic insufficiency
      Cholestatic disorders
      Cholestyramine
  Abnormal metabolism
    Liver disease
    Chronic renal failure
    Vitamin D-dependent rickets type I
    Tumoral hypophosphatemic osteomalacia
    X-linked hypophosphatemia
    Chronic acidosis
    Anticonvulsants
  Abnormal target tissue response
    Vitamin D-dependent rickets type II
    Gastrointestinal disorders

Disorders of phosphate homeostasis
  Decreased intestinal absorption
    Malnutrition
    Malabsorption
    Antacids containing aluminum hydroxide
  Increased renal loss
    X-linked hypophosphatemic rickets
    Tumoral hypophosphatemic osteomalacia
    De Toni-Debré-Fanconi syndrome

Calcium deficiency

Primary disorders of bone matrix
  Hypophosphatasia
  Fibrogenesis imperfecta ossium
  Axial osteomalacia

Inhibitors of mineralization
  Aluminum
    Chronic renal failure
    Total parenteral nutrition
  Etidronate
  Fluoride

availability of resources to obtain and examine the biopsy specimen, the index of suspicion coupled with the lack of certainty from other diagnostic procedures, and the degree to which the therapeutic approach will be altered by the additional information. In many cases, a therapeutic trial of vitamin D supplements suffices to establish the diagnosis without the need for bone biopsy.

Clinical Features

A. Symptoms and signs   The clinical presentation of rickets depends on the age of the patient and, to some extent, the cause of the syndrome. The affected infant or young child may be apathetic, listless, weak, hypotonic, and growing poorly. A soft, somewhat misshapen head, with widened sutures and frontal bossing,

may be observed. Eruption of teeth may be delayed, and teeth that do appear may be pitted and poorly mineralized. The enlargement and cupping of the costochondral junctions produce the *rachitic rosary* on the thorax. The tug of the diaphragm against the softened lower ribs may produce an indentation at the point of insertion of the diaphragm (Harrison groove). Muscle hypotonia can result in a pronounced potbelly and a waddling gait. The limbs may become bowed, and joints may swell because of flaring at the ends of the long bones (including phalanges and metacarpals) (Figure 8–28). Pathologic fractures may occur in patients with florid rickets. After the epiphyses have closed, the clinical signs of rickets or osteomalacia are subtle and cannot be relied on to make the diagnosis. Patients with severe osteomalacia complain of bone pain and proximal muscle weakness. Difficulty climbing stairs or rising from chairs may be reported and should be looked for. Such individuals may have a history of fractures and be diagnosed as having osteoporosis.

B. Laboratory findings

1. **Biochemistry**—Vitamin D deficiency results in decreased intestinal absorption of calcium and phosphate. In conjunction with the resulting secondary hyperparathyroidism, vitamin D deficiency leads to an increase in bone resorption, increased excretion of urinary phosphate, and increased renal tubular reabsorption of calcium. The net result tends to be low-normal

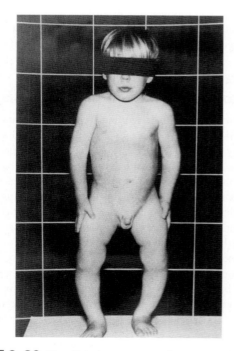

FIGURE 8–28 The clinical appearance of a young child with rickets. The most striking abnormalities are the bowing of the legs and protuberant abdomen. Flaring of the ends of the long bones can also be appreciated. (Photograph courtesy of Dr. Sara Arnaud.)

serum calcium, low serum phosphate, elevated serum alkaline phosphatase, increased PTH, decreased urinary calcium, and increased urinary phosphate levels. Finding a low 25(OH)D level, in combination with these other biochemical alterations, strengthens the diagnosis of vitamin D deficiency. The $1,25(OH)_2D$ level may be normal, making this determination less useful for the diagnosis of osteomalacia. Both 25(OH)D and $1,25(OH)_2D$ levels may be reduced in patients with liver disease or nephrotic syndrome because the binding proteins for the vitamin D metabolites are low secondary to decreased production (liver disease) or increased renal losses (nephrotic syndrome; see later). Such individuals may have normal free concentrations of these metabolites and so are not vitamin D deficient. Other factors, such as age and diet, must be considered. For example, serum phosphate values are normally lower in adults than in children. Dietary history is important, because urinary phosphate excretion and, to a lesser extent, urinary calcium excretion reflect dietary phosphate and calcium content. Because phosphate excretion depends on the filtered load (the product of the glomerular filtration rate and plasma phosphate concentration), urinary phosphate levels may be reduced despite the presence of hyperparathyroidism, when serum phosphate levels are particularly low. Expressions of renal phosphate clearance that account for these variables (eg, renal threshold for phosphate, or T_mP/GFR) are a better indicator of renal phosphate handling than is total phosphate excretion. The T_mP/GFR can be calculated from a nomogram using measurements of a fasting serum and urine phosphate concentration.

2. **Histologic examination**—Transcortical bone biopsy is the definitive means of making the diagnosis of osteomalacia. A rib or the iliac crest is the site at which biopsy is usually performed. To assess osteoid content and mineral appositional rate, the bone biopsy specimen is processed without decalcification. This requires special equipment. In osteomalacia, bone is mineralized poorly and slowly, resulting in wide osteoid seams (>12 μm) and a large fraction of bone covered by unmineralized osteoid. States of high bone turnover (increased bone formation and resorption), such as hyperparathyroidism, can also cause wide osteoid seams and an increased osteoid surface, producing a superficial resemblance to osteomalacia. Therefore, the rate of bone turnover should be determined by labeling bone with tetracycline, which provides a fluorescent marker of the calcification front. When two doses of tetracycline are given at different times, the distance between the two labels divided by the time interval between the two doses equals the mineral appositional rate. The normal appositional rate is approximately 0.74 um/d. Mineralization lag time—the time required for newly formed osteoid to be mineralized—can be calculated by dividing osteoid seam width by the appositional rate corrected by the linear extent of mineralization of the calcification front (a measure of the bone surface that is undergoing active mineralization as measured by tetracycline incorporation). Mineralization lag time is normally about 20 to 25 days. Bone formation rate is calculated as the product of the appositional rate times the linear extent of mineralization of the calcification front. Depressed appositional rate, increased mineralization lag time, and reduced bone formation rate clearly distinguish osteomalacia from high-turnover states such as hyperparathyroidism. Low-turnover states, as can be seen in various forms of osteoporosis, also have low appositional and bone formation rates, but these conditions are distinguished from osteomalacia by normal or reduced osteoid surface and volume.

C. Imaging studies The radiologic features of rickets can be quite striking, especially in the young child. In growing bone, the radiolucent epiphyses are wide and flared, with irregular epiphyseal-metaphyseal junctions. Long bones may be bowed. The cortices of the long bones are often indistinct. Occasionally, evidence of secondary hyperparathyroidism—subperiosteal resorption in the phalanges and metacarpals and erosion of the distal ends of the clavicles—is observed. Pseudofractures (also known as looser zones or milkman fractures) are an uncommon but nearly pathognomonic feature of rickets and osteomalacia (Figure 8–29). These radiolucent lines are most often found along the concave side of the femoral neck, pubic rami, ribs, clavicles, and lateral aspects of the scapulae. Pseudofractures may result from unhealed microfractures at points of stress or at the entry point of blood vessels into bone. They may progress to complete fractures that go unrecognized and thus lead to substantial deformity and disability. BMD is not a reliable indicator of osteomalacia, because BMD can be decreased in patients with vitamin D deficiency or increased in patients with chronic renal failure. In adults with normal renal function, radiologic evidence of a mineralization defect is often subtle and not readily distinguished from osteoporosis, with which it often coexists.

Treatment

The treatment of vitamin D deficiency is covered under that heading. The treatment of other diseases causing rickets or osteomalacia is found below under the specific disease headings.

NEPHROTIC SYNDROME

Nephrotic syndrome may lead to osteomalacia because of losses of vitamin D metabolites in the urine. Vitamin D metabolites are tightly bound to DBP, an α-globulin, and less tightly bound to

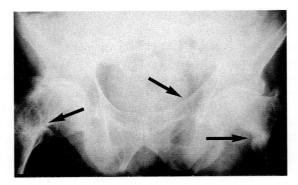

FIGURE 8–29 X-ray of the pelvis of an elderly woman with osteomalacia. Note marked bowing of both femoral necks, with pseudofractures of the medial aspect of the femoral necks and the superior aspect of the left pubic ramus (arrows). (Photograph courtesy of Dr. Harry Genant.)

albumin as described earlier. Patients with the nephrotic syndrome may lose large amounts of DBP and albumin in their urine and so deplete their vitamin D stores. Such patients can have very low levels of vitamin D metabolites in their serum, although the free concentrations are less affected. Thus, the measurement of total 25(OH)D or 1,25(OH)$_2$D may be misleading with respect to the severity of the vitamin D deficiency. Although bone disease has been recognized as a complication of the nephrotic syndrome, the prevalence of osteomalacia in this population is unknown. If vitamin D deficiency is suspected, treatment with vitamin D is indicated with the proviso that normal total levels of 25(OH)D and 1,25(OH)$_2$D are not the goal. Blood levels of calcium, phosphate, and PTH are a more reliable guide to treatment.

HEPATIC OSTEODYSTROPHY

Hepatic osteodystrophy is the bone disease associated with liver disease. In the United States, patients with severe liver disease generally have osteoporosis, not osteomalacia. Both osteomalacia and osteoporosis are found in patients with liver disease in Great Britain, where vitamin D deficiency is more common. Although the liver is the site of the first step in the bioactivation of vitamin D—the conversion of vitamin D to 25(OH)D—this process is not tightly controlled, and until the liver disease is severe it is not rate limiting. Neither cholestatic nor parenchymal liver disease has much effect on 25(OH)D production until the late stages of liver failure. The low levels of 25(OH)D and 1,25(OH)$_2$D associated with liver disease can usually be attributed to the reduced production of DBP and albumin, poor nutrition, or malabsorption rather than a deficiency in the vitamin D 25-hydroxylase. As in patients with the nephrotic syndrome, the low total levels of the vitamin D metabolites may be misleading, as they reflect a reduction in DBP and albumin rather than a reduction in the free concentrations of these metabolites.

DRUG-INDUCED OSTEOMALACIA

Phenytoin and phenobarbital are anticonvulsants that induce drug-metabolizing enzymes in the liver that alter the hepatic metabolism of vitamin D and its metabolites. This action is not limited to anticonvulsants; the antituberculosis drug rifampin has been reported to do likewise. This effect may account for the lower circulating levels of 25(OH)D found in patients treated with such drugs. Levels of 1,25(OH)$_2$D are less affected. Chronic anticonvulsant or antituberculosis therapy does not appear to lead to clinically significant bone disease except in subjects with other predisposing factors such as inadequate sunlight exposure (institutionalized patients) and poor nutrition. Children may be more vulnerable than adults. In animal studies, phenytoin has been noted to exert a direct inhibitory effect on bone mineralization, but the relevance of this observation to the human use of this drug is uncertain. The decrease in 25(OH)D levels in patients taking these drugs can be readily reversed with supplemental vitamin D administration.

HYPOPHOSPHATEMIC DISORDERS

Chronic hypophosphatemia may lead to rickets or osteomalacia independently of other predisposing abnormalities. The principal diseases in which hypophosphatemia is associated with osteomalacia or rickets, however, also include other abnormalities that can interfere with bone mineralization. Chronic phosphate depletion is caused by dietary deficiency (as in strict vegetarians), decreased intestinal absorption, or increased renal clearance (renal wasting). Acute hypophosphatemia can result from movement of phosphate into cells (eg, after infusion of insulin and glucose), but this condition is transient and does not result in bone disease.

Seventy to ninety percent of dietary phosphate is absorbed under normal conditions in the jejunum. This process is not tightly regulated, although 1,25(OH)$_2$D stimulates phosphate absorption, a factor that needs to be considered when calcitriol is being used to treat other conditions. Meat and dairy products are the principal dietary sources of phosphate. The incidence of osteomalacia in vegetarians who avoid all meat and dairy products is unknown, but its occurrence has been reported. Intrinsic small bowel disease and small bowel surgery interfere with phosphate absorption and, if coupled with diarrhea or steatorrhea, can result in phosphate depletion. A number of antacids (eg, Mylanta, Maalox, Basaljel, and Amphojel) contain aluminum hydroxide, which binds phosphate and prevents its absorption. Patients who ingest large amounts of these antacids may become phosphate depleted. When this occurs in the setting of renal failure, reductions in serum phosphate plus aluminum intoxication in these individuals, who also have reduced 1,25(OH)$_2$D production, can produce profound osteomalacia. Eighty-five to ninety percent of the phosphate filtered by the glomerulus is reabsorbed, primarily in the proximal tubule. This process is regulated by PTH which reduces renal tubular phosphate reabsorption. It is also probably regulated by various vitamin D metabolites that appear to increase renal tubular phosphate reabsorption, and importantly by FGF23, which blocks the insertion of sodium phosphate cotransporters into and increases their internalization from the luminal membrane of renal proximal tubular cells. Many diseases that affect renal handling of phosphate are associated with osteomalacia—especially those also associated with abnormalities in vitamin D metabolism and in FGF23 production and or clearance, as discussed later (see also Chapter 21).

Treatment of phosphate deficiency is generally geared to correction of the primary problem. Oral preparations of phosphate (and the amounts required to provide 1 g of elemental phosphorus) include Fleet Phospho-soda (6.12 mL) and Neutra-Phos (300 mL). These preparations are usually given in amounts that provide 1 to 3 g of phosphorus daily in divided doses, although diarrhea may limit the dose. Careful attention to both serum calcium and serum phosphate concentrations is required to avoid hypocalcemia, ectopic calcification, or secondary hyperparathyroidism.

X-Linked and Autosomal Dominant Hypophosphatemia

X-linked hypophosphatemia (XLH), formerly called vitamin D-resistant rickets, is characterized by renal phosphate wasting, hypophosphatemia, and decreased $1,25(OH)_2D$ production relative to the degree of hypophosphatemia. Clinical presentation is variable, but children often present with florid rickets. This X-linked dominant disorder generally affects males more severely than females. A similar but genetically distinct syndrome, autosomal dominant hypophosphatemic rickets (ADHR), is less common, affects females to the same extent as males, and may present later in life (second to fourth decades). Animal studies have indicated that the cause of the renal phosphate wasting in XLH is humoral rather than a structural defect in the phosphate transporter itself. Recent evidence strongly suggests that this humoral factor is FGF23, although other candidates have been proposed. Circulating FGF23 appears to be responsible for both the reduction in phosphate reabsorption in the renal proximal tubule and the blunted response of the proximal tubule to the ensuing hypophosphatemia with respect to $1,25(OH)_2D$ production. The gene responsible for XLH has been identified and is called *PHEX*. It shares structural homology with a number of endopeptidase genes and it is located on the X chromosome. As is implicit in this ambiguous name, the role of *PHEX* in renal phosphate transport is not clear. The prevailing hypothesis is that *PHEX* indirectly leads to the cleavage and subsequent inactivation of FGF23, thus relieving the inhibition of phosphate reabsorption and $1,25(OH)_2$ production.

ADHR is due to a mutation in FGF23 that renders it resistant to cleavage. Recent evidence suggests that the defects in XLH and ADHR may not be restricted to the proximal renal tubule but may affect osteoblast function as well, a cell in which *PHEX* is expressed. With the recent cloning of *PHEX* and FGF23, our understanding of these diseases should rapidly increase.

Treatment of XLH and ADHR generally requires a combination of phosphate (1-4 g/d in divided doses) combined with calcitriol (1-3 μg/d) as tolerated. Vitamin D is less effective than calcitriol and should not be used for this condition. Appropriate therapy heals the rachitic lesions and increases growth velocity. A frequent complication of these diseases, however, is the development of hyperparathyroidism, which may become autonomous and require parathyroidectomy. It is unclear whether the hyperparathyroidism is a complication of therapy or intrinsic to the disease process itself. Treatment with phosphate and calcitriol may also lead to ectopic calcification, including nephrocalcinosis. Thus, these patients need to be followed closely.

Tumor-Induced Osteomalacia

The association of osteomalacia and hypophosphatemia with tumors, primarily of mesenchymal origin, has been recognized for half a century (see Chapter 21). The cause of this syndrome has until recently remained obscure. Removal of the tumors, which are often small and difficult to find, cures the disease. Although most implicated tumors are mesenchymal, including fibromas and osteoblastomas, other tumors, including breast, prostate, and lung carcinomas; multiple myeloma; and chronic lymphocytic leukemia have been associated with this syndrome. The patient generally presents with bone pain, muscle weakness, and osteomalacia. Symptoms may occur for years before the diagnosis is made. Renal phosphate wasting, hypophosphatemia, and normal serum calcium and 25(OH)D levels but inappropriately low $1,25(OH)_2D$ levels characterize the disease. Thus, it resembles XLH or ADHR. Tumor extracts contain molecules that inhibit renal phosphate transport and $1,25(OH)_2D$ production, suggesting that a phosphate-regulating substance or **phosphatonin** is involved. Thus, it was of great interest to observe that many of these tumors overproduce FGF23 and that production by the tumor of FGF23 can explain the metabolic abnormalities associated with the hypophosphatemic syndrome (see Figure 8–10). Other tumor products such as MEPE (matrix extracellular phosphoglycoprotein) and sFRP4 (secreted frizzled related protein 4) have also been implicated. The best treatment is removal of the tumor, but this is not always possible. Phosphate and calcitriol have been the mainstays of treatment but with limited success. Patients should be dosed to tolerance as in XLH and ADHR.

Fibrous Dysplasia

Fibrous dysplasia results from activating mutations in the *GNAS* gene, which encodes Gs alpha. Fibrous dysplasia of bone is a component of the McCune-Albright syndrome. The bony lesions in this disorder overproduce FGF23 which like tumor-induced osteomalacia, described above, leads to hypophosphatemia, osteomalacia, and inappropriately normal $1,25(OH)_2D$. These lesions can be mono-ostotic or polyostotic, with the extent of bone involved correlating with the degree of FGF23 hypersecretion, and hence the hypophosphatemia observed.

De Toni-Debré-Fanconi Syndrome and Hereditary Hypophosphatemic Rickets with Hypercalciuria

The De Toni-Debré-Fanconi syndrome includes a heterogeneous group of disorders affecting the proximal tubule and leading to phosphaturia and hypophosphatemia, aminoaciduria, glycosuria, bicarbonaturia, and proximal renal tubular acidosis. Not all features must be present to make the diagnosis. Damage to the renal proximal tubule secondary to genetic or environmental causes is the underlying cause. This syndrome may be divided into two types depending on whether vitamin D metabolism is also abnormal. In the more common type I, $1,25(OH)_2D$ production is reduced relative to the degree of hypophosphatemia. In type II, $1,25(OH)_2D$ production is appropriately elevated in response to the hypophosphatemia, and this leads to hypercalciuria. The reason that $1,25(OH)_2D$ production is reduced in type I, despite the hypophosphatemia, is unclear but may suggest damage to the mitochondria where the 1-hydroxylase is located.

The type II Fanconi syndrome shares the principal features of hereditary hypophosphatemic rickets with hypercalciuria (HHRH).

This rare disorder results from mutations in *SLC34A3*, the gene that encodes the type IIc sodium phosphate cotransporter (NaPiIIc), leading to loss of function of this transporter. Mutations in NaPiIIa, the other major renal sodium phosphate cotransporter, produces a similar picture. The key difference between HHRH and ADHR or XLH is that FGF23 is not elevated—so 1-hydroxylase activity is not suppressed. Thus, the hypophosphatemia leads to increased 1,25(OH)$_2$D production, increased intestinal calcium absorption, and hypercalciuria. HHRH is heterogeneous in clinical presentation, but in severely affected individuals, it begins in childhood with bone pain and skeletal deformities. The syndrome is characterized by renal phosphate wasting and hypophosphatemia, hypercalciuria and normal serum calcium, and elevated 1,25(OH)$_2$D levels. The osteomalacia associated with these renal phosphate-wasting syndromes is probably the result of the hypophosphatemia, with contributions from the acidosis and decreased 1,25(OH)$_2$D levels in the type I syndrome.

The ideal treatment is correction of the underlying defect, which may or may not be identified and/or reversible. Otherwise, treatment includes phosphate supplementation in all cases, correction of the acidosis, and 1,25(OH)$_2$D replacement in the type I syndrome, but not in HHRH as this will aggravate the hypercalciuria.

CALCIUM DEFICIENCY

Calcium deficiency may contribute to the mineralization defect that complicates gastrointestinal disease and proximal tubular disorders, but it is less well established as a cause of osteomalacia than is vitamin D or phosphate deficiency. In carefully performed studies of children who ingested a very low-calcium diet in Africa, there was clinical, biochemical, and histologic evidence of osteomalacia. The serum phosphate and 25(OH)D and 1,25(OH)$_2$D levels were normal; serum alkaline phosphatase levels were elevated; and serum and urine calcium levels were low. Because intestinal absorption of calcium decreases with age, the daily requirement for calcium increases from approximately 800 mg in young adults to 1400 mg in the elderly. Calcium deficiency can result not only from inadequate dietary intake but also from excessive fecal and urinary losses. Except in cases in which a renal leak of calcium plays an important role in the etiology of calcium deficiency (certain forms of idiopathic hypercalciuria or following glucocorticoid therapy for inflammatory diseases), urinary calcium excretion provides a useful means to determine the appropriate level of oral calcium replacement. Because of its low cost and high percentage of elemental calcium, calcium carbonate is the treatment of choice.

PRIMARY DISORDERS OF THE BONE MATRIX

Several diseases lead to abnormalities in bone mineralization because of intrinsic defects in the matrix or in the osteoblast producing that matrix. With the exception of osteogenesis imperfecta, these tend to be rare. Examples are listed below.

OSTEOGENESIS IMPERFECTA

Osteogenesis imperfecta is a heritable disorder of connective tissue due to a qualitative or quantitative abnormality in type I collagen, the most abundant collagen in bone. The disease is typically transmitted in an autosomal dominant mode, although autosomal recessive inheritance has also been described. Clinical expression is highly variable, depending on the location and type of mutation observed. Although skeletal deformity and fracture are the hallmarks of this disease, other tissues are often affected, including the teeth, skin, ligaments, and scleras. Routine biochemical studies of bone and mineral metabolism are generally normal; however, elevated serum alkaline phosphatase and increased excretion of biochemical markers of bone turnover and calcium are often found. Bone histology shows abundant disorganized, poorly mineralized matrix but with a high rate of bone turnover as reflected by increased tetracycline labeling.

Treatment is supportive and includes orthopedic, rehabilitative, and dental intervention as appropriate. Bisphosphonates have recently been shown to be of value in children to prevent fractures and reduce bone pain and skeletal morbidity.

Hypophosphatasia

Hypophosphatasia, transmitted in an autosomal recessive or dominant pattern, has considerable variability in clinical expression ranging from a severe form of rickets in children to a predisposition to fractures in adults. The biochemical hallmarks are low serum and tissue levels of alkaline phosphatase (liver-bone-kidney but not intestine-placenta) and increased urinary levels of phosphoethanolamine. Serum calcium and phosphate levels may be high, and many patients have hypercalciuria. Levels of vitamin D metabolites and PTH are generally normal. In some families, a mutation in the *alkaline phosphatase* gene has been identified. Radiologic examination shows osteopenia, with the frequent occurrence of stress fractures and chondrocalcinosis. Bone biopsy specimens show osteomalacia. It is not clear why these patients develop osteomalacia or rickets. Skeletal alkaline phosphatase cleaves pyrophosphate, an inhibitor of bone mineralization. Thus, patients deficient in alkaline phosphatase may be unable to hydrolyze this inhibitor and so develop a mineralization defect.

There is no established medical therapy. Use of vitamin D or its metabolites may further increase the already elevated serum calcium and phosphate and should not be used.

Fibrogenesis Imperfecta Ossium

Fibrogenesis imperfecta ossium is a rare, painful disorder that affects middle-aged subjects in what appears to be a sporadic fashion. Serum alkaline phosphatase activity is increased. The bones have a dense, amorphous mottled appearance radiologically and a disorganized arrangement of collagen with decreased birefringence histologically when viewed with polarized light microscopy. Presumably, the disorganized collagen matrix retards normal bone mineralization. There is no specific therapy.

Axial Osteomalacia

This rare disease involves only the axial skeleton and affects mostly middle-aged or elderly males. Most cases are sporadic. It is not particularly painful. Alkaline phosphatase activity may be increased, but calcium, phosphate, and vitamin D metabolite levels are normal. Histologically, the bone shows increased osteoid and reduced tetracycline incorporation. The reason for the mineralization disorder is uncertain. No effective medical therapy has been established.

INHIBITORS OF MINERALIZATION

Several drugs are known to cause osteomalacia or rickets by inhibiting mineralization. However, the mechanisms by which this occurs are not fully understood.

Aluminum

Aluminum-induced bone disease is found primarily in patients with renal failure on chronic hemodialysis and in patients being treated with total parenteral nutrition (TPN). With the recognition of this complication and the switch to deionized water for dialysis, decreased use of aluminum-containing antacids, and the use of purified amino acids rather than casein hydrolysates (which contained large amounts of aluminum) for TPN, the incidence and prevalence of this complication have been markedly reduced. The problem, however, still exists. As described under renal osteodystrophy, the bone disease is osteomalacia and can be severe and painful. Aluminum deposits in the mineralization front and appears to inhibit the mineralization process. Removal of the aluminum with deferoxamine chelation therapy is the treatment of choice.

Fluoride

Fluoride is a potent stimulator of bone formation. If administered at high doses with inadequate calcium supplementation, the bone formed as a result is poorly mineralized. The mechanisms underlying the effects of fluoride on osteoblast function and bone mineralization remain unclear.

PAGET DISEASE OF BONE (OSTEITIS DEFORMANS)

Paget disease is a focal disorder of bone remodeling that leads to greatly accelerated rates of bone turnover, disruption of the normal architecture of bone, and sometimes to gross deformities of bone. As a focal disorder it is not, strictly speaking, a metabolic bone disease. Paget disease is prevalent in northern Europe, particularly in England and Germany. It is also common in the United States but is unusual in Africa and Asia.

Etiology

It has long been thought that Paget disease, with its late onset and spotty involvement of the skeleton, might be due to a chronic slow virus infection of bone. Inclusion bodies that resemble paramyxovirus inclusions have been identified in pagetic osteoclasts, and the presence of measles virus transcripts has been detected by molecular techniques. However, considerably more work would be required to prove the infectious etiology of Paget disease. There are also familial clusters of the disease, with up to 20% of patients in some studies having afflicted first-degree relatives so a heterogeneity of pathogenetic mechanisms is likely (see later).

Pathology

At the microscopic level, the disorder is characterized by highly vascular and cellular bone, consistent with its high metabolic activity. The osteoclasts are sometimes huge and bizarre, with up to 100 nuclei per cell. Because pagetic osteoclasts initiate the bone remodeling cycle in a chaotic fashion, the end result of remodeling is a mosaic pattern of lamellar bone. Paget disease (and other high turnover states) can also produce woven bone—bone that is laid down rapidly and in a disorganized fashion, without the normal lamellar architecture.

Pathogenesis

Abnormal osteoclastic bone resorption is the probable initiating event in Paget disease. Not only are the osteoclasts very abnormal histologically and prone to unruly behavior, but some forms of the disease are marked by an early resorptive phase in which pure osteolysis occurs without an osteoblastic response. Additionally, Paget disease responds dramatically to inhibitors of osteoclastic bone resorption.

The rate of bone resorption is often increased by as much as 10- to 20-fold, and this is reflected in biochemical indices of bone resorption. Over the skeleton as a whole, osteoblastic new bone formation responds appropriately to this challenge. Even though local disparities in remodeling may result in areas with the radiographic appearance of osteolysis or dense new bone, there is a close relationship between biochemical markers of bone resorption (eg, N-telopeptide, C-telopeptide, deoxypyridinoline) and formation (eg, alkaline phosphatase, osteocalcin). Because this tight coupling is maintained in Paget disease, in the face of enormously increased skeletal turnover rates, systemic mineral homeostasis is usually unperturbed.

Genetic Forms

Approximately 20% of patients with Paget disease have a positive family history. This interesting observation plus the uncertain viral etiology has led several groups to determine the genetic loci responsible for the disease. These studies plus work done to unravel the molecular defects in patients with rare but clear disorders of accelerated and unregulated bone remodeling have shed light on molecular pathways that may be important in sporadic Paget disease.

Mutations in RANK and OPG are important in the pathogenesis of high bone remodeling states. Whyte and colleagues investigated two unrelated Navajo patients with autosomal recessive juvenile Paget disease in whom they found approximately 100-kb deletions of the gene encoding TNFRSF11B or OPG on chromosome 8q24.2. In two other clinical disorders of high bone remodeling designated as familial expansile osteolysis and expansile skeletal hyperphosphatasia, tandem duplications are present within the signal peptide of RANK, leading to a gain-of-function in the activity of RANK. This is predicted to enhance osteoclastogenesis.

Familial Paget disease is not, however, generally explained by abnormalities in *RANK* or *OPG* genes. In contrast, several groups have uncovered mutations in SQSTM1 or sequestosome 1 (also known as p62) in multiple kindreds with Paget disease. SQSTM1 is a ubiquitin-binding protein involved in signaling pathways for IL-1, TNF, and RANKL—all molecules important in the production and function of osteoclasts. A variety of different SQSTM1 mutations are thought to explain approximately 30% of cases of familial Paget disease. The identification of additional candidate genes is in progress.

Clinical Features

A. Symptoms and signs   Typical Paget disease may affect any of the bones, but the most common sites are the sacrum and spine (50% of patients), femur (46%), skull (28%), and pelvis (22%). The clinical features of Paget disease are pain, fractures, deformity, and manifestations of the neurologic, rheumatologic, or metabolic complications of the disease. However, at least two-thirds of patients are asymptomatic. Thus, Paget disease is often discovered as an incidental radiologic finding or during the investigation of an elevated alkaline phosphatase level. On physical examination, enlargement of the skull, frontal bossing, or deafness may be evident. Involvement of the weight-bearing long bones of the lower extremity often results in bowing. The femur and tibia bow anteriorly and laterally, but the fibula is almost never affected. Cutaneous erythema and warmth, as well as bone tenderness, may be evident over affected areas of the skeleton, reflecting greatly increased blood flow through pagetic bone. The findings of pain, warmth, and erythema led to the appellation osteitis deformans, although Paget disease is not truly an inflammatory disorder. The most common fractures in Paget disease are vertebral crush fractures and incomplete *fissure* fractures through the cortex, usually on the convex surface of the tibia or femur. Affected bones may fracture completely; when they do, healing is usually rapid and complete—the increased metabolic activity of pagetic bone seems to favor fracture healing.

B. Laboratory findings   The serum alkaline phosphatase activity is usually increased, sometimes to very high levels. Levels of biochemical markers of bone turnover are often high, but it is not clear that their determination offers any special advantage over that of serum alkaline phosphatase activity. The serum calcium and phosphate concentrations and the urinary calcium excretion are normal, although if a patient sustains a fracture and becomes immobilized, hypercalciuria and hypercalcemia may occur.

C. Imaging studies   The early stages of Paget disease are often osteolytic. Examples are erosion of the temporal bone of the skull, osteoporosis circumscripta, and pagetic lesions in the extremities, which begin in the metaphysis and migrate down the shaft as a V-shaped resorptive front (Figure 8–30). Over years or even decades, the typical mixed picture of late Paget disease evolves. Trabeculae are thickened and coarse. The bone may be enlarged or bowed. In the pelvis, the iliopectineal line or pelvic brim is often thickened (Figure 8–31). In the spine, osteoblastic lesions of the vertebral bodies may present a *picture-frame* appearance or a homogeneously increased density, the *ivory vertebra*. Associated osteoarthritis may present with narrowing of the joint space (see Figure 8–31). Osteosarcoma may present with cortical destruction or a soft tissue mass (see Figure 8–31). Radionuclide bone scanning with technetium-labeled bisphosphonates or other bone-seeking agents is uniformly positive in active Paget disease and is useful for surveying the skeleton when a focus of Paget disease has been found radiographically (Figure 8–32) or the disease is suspected.

Complications

Complications of Paget disease may be neurologic, otologic, rheumatologic, neoplastic, or cardiac (Table 8–15).

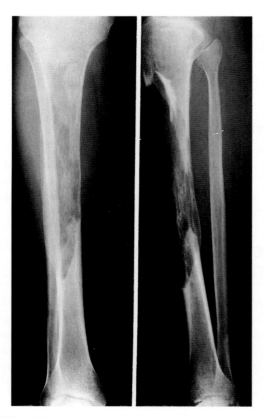

FIGURE 8–30 Lytic Paget disease in the tibia before (**left**) and after (**right**) immobilization in a cast. The lytic area has a flame- or V-shaped leading edge (**left**). (Reproduced, with permission, from Strewler GJ. Paget's disease of bone. *West J Med*. 1984;140:763.)

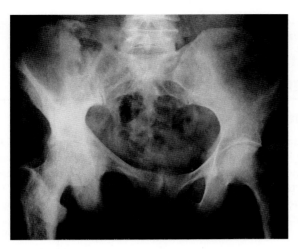

FIGURE 8–31 Paget disease of the right femur and pelvis. The right femur displays cortical thickening and coarse trabeculation. The right ischium is enlarged, with sclerosis of ischial and pubic rami and the right ilium. Two complications of Paget disease are present. There is concentric bilateral narrowing of the hip joint space, signifying osteoarthritis. The destructive lesion interrupting the cortex of the right ilium is an osteosarcoma. (Reproduced, with permission, from Strewler GJ. Paget disease of bone. *West J Med.* 1984;140:763.)

TABLE 8–15   Complications of Paget disease.

Rheumatologic
Osteoarthritis
Gout
Calcific periarthritis
Neurologic/Otologic
Basilar impression
Hydrocephalus (rare)
Cranial nerve dysfunction (especially deafness)
Spinal cord and root compression
Peripheral nerve entrapment (carpal and tarsal tunnel syndromes)
Metabolic
Immobilization hypercalciuria-hypercalcemia
Urolithiasis
Neoplastic
Sarcoma
Giant cell tumor

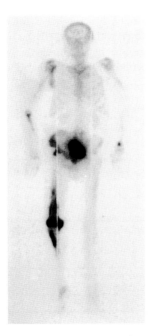

FIGURE 8–32 Bone scan of a patient with Paget disease of the pelvis, right femur, and acetabulum. Note localization of bone-seeking isotope (^{99m}Tc-labeled bisphosphonate) in these areas.

A. Neurologic/Otologic   The brain, spinal cord, and peripheral nerves are all at risk. Sensorineural deafness occurs in up to 50% of patients in whom the skull is involved, and compression of the other cranial nerves can also occur. At the base of the skull, Paget disease can produce platybasia and basilar impression of the

brain stem, with symptoms of brain stem compression, obstructive hydrocephalus, or vertebrobasilar insufficiency. Spinal stenosis is common in vertebral Paget disease, in part because the pagetic vertebra can be enlarged, and may extend posteriorly when collapse occurs, but spinal stenosis responds well to medical treatment of the disease.

B. Rheumatologic   Osteoarthritis is common in Paget disease. It may be an unrelated finding in elderly patients with the disorder, or it may result directly from pagetic deformities and their effects on wear and tear in the joints. Arthritis presents a conundrum to the clinician attempting to relieve pain, as it may be difficult to determine whether the pain originates in pagetic bone or in the nearby joint. An association of osteitis deformans and gout was first noted by James Paget himself, and asymptomatic hyperuricemia is also common.

C. Neoplastic   The most dreaded complication of Paget disease is development of a sarcoma. The tumor arises in pagetic bone, typically in individuals with polyostotic involvement, and may present with soft tissue swelling, increased pain, or a rapidly increasing alkaline phosphatase. Osteosarcoma, chondrosarcoma, and giant cell tumors all occur in Paget disease, with a combined incidence of about 1%. Because osteosarcoma is otherwise uncommon in the elderly, fully 30% of elderly patients with osteosarcoma have underlying Paget disease.

D. Cardiac   High-output congestive heart failure occurs rarely and is due to markedly increased blood flow to bone, usually in patients with more than 50% involvement of the skeleton.

Treatment

In a patient known to have Paget disease, bone pain that is unresponsive to nonsteroidal anti-inflammatory agents deserves a trial of specific therapy. As noted earlier, it may not be easy to differentiate pagetic bone pain from that due to osteoarthritis. The other indications for treatment of Paget disease are controversial. Treatment has been advocated for neurologic compression syndromes, as preparation for surgery, and to prevent deformities. Neurologic deficits often respond to medical treatment, and a trial of treatment is often warranted. Pretreatment for 2 to 3 months before orthopedic surgery prevents excessive bleeding and postoperative hypercalcemia, but satisfactory bone healing usually occurs without medical treatment. Paget disease is sometimes treated in the hope of arresting the progress of deformities (eg, bowing of the extremities and resultant osteoarthritis), but it is not certain whether medical treatment can achieve this aim or whether it will arrest the progression of deafness in patients with skull involvement.

Two classes of agents are used in the treatment of Paget disease: bisphosphonates and CT. Both inhibit osteoclastic bone resorption.

A. Bisphosphonates   The oral bisphosphonates (alendronate and risedronate) are commonly used in the treatment of Paget disease. Alendronate is administered at a dose of 40 mg daily for 6 months. On average, alkaline phosphatase activity is suppressed by about 80% using such treatment. Biochemical remissions are often prolonged for more than 1 year, after the drug is stopped. The main side-effect is gastrointestinal upset, requiring discontinuation of therapy in about 6% of patients. Risedronate, given at a dosage of 30 mg/d for 2 months, is also highly efficacious in lowering and even normalizing alkaline phosphatase activity and reducing bone pain. For patients with gastrointestinal intolerance to oral bisphosphonates or more severe bony involvement, it may be more convenient or appropriate to administer intravenous bisphosphonates. If the disease is highly active and surgery is planned in the immediate future, intravenous therapy is generally preferred. Pamidronate, an aminobisphosphonate closely related to alendronate, has been used for this purpose. Intravenous infusions of pamidronate (60 or 90 mg) produce a high remission rate and a durable response. More recently, intravenous zoledronic acid (5 mg) has been shown to be efficacious, in terms of both the strength and duration of alkaline phosphatase suppression, in patients with Paget disease. The principal side-effect observed with intravenous aminobisphosphonate administration is an acute-phase response, including fever and myalgias, that occurs in about 10% of patients and may last for several days after a dose. A very small percentage of patients receiving multiple and typically high doses of intravenous bisphosphonates can develop osteonecrosis of the jaw.

B. Calcitonin   Salmon CT is administered initially at a dosage of 50 to 100 IU daily until symptoms are improved; thereafter, many patients can be maintained on 50 units three times a week. Improvement in pain is usually evident within 2 to 6 weeks. On average, the alkaline phosphatase falls by 50% within 3 to 6 months. Many patients have a sustained response to treatment extending over years, and biochemical parameters are often suppressed for 6 months to 1 year after treatment is discontinued. Up to 20% of patients receiving chronic CT treatment develop late resistance to CT, which may be antibody-

mediated. Data on the use of nasal spray CT's efficacy in Paget disease are limited.

RENAL OSTEODYSTROPHY

Pathogenesis

Metabolism of 25(OH)D to 1,25(OH)$_2$D and 24,25(OH)$_2$D in the kidney is tightly regulated. Renal disease results in reduced circulating levels of both of these metabolites. With the reduction in 1,25(OH)$_2$D levels, intestinal calcium absorption falls, and bone resorption appears to become less sensitive to PTH—a result that leads to hypocalcemia. Phosphate excretion by the diseased kidney is decreased, resulting in hyperphosphatemia, which amplifies the fall in serum calcium and independently increases PTH secretion. The fall in serum calcium combined with the low levels of 1,25(OH)$_2$D, which is an inhibitor of PTH secretion, and the hyperphosphatemia result in hyperparathyroidism (Figure 8–33). The parathyroid glands, under chronic proliferative stimulation in uremic individuals, can develop clonal expansion of cells that harbor mutations in known parathyroid growth-promoting genes. This can result in nodular hyperplasia. In addition, the expression of both VDRs and CaSRs is often depressed in tissues from individuals with chronic secondary hyperparathyroidism. Both calcium, likely acting via CaSRs, and 1,25(OH)$_2$D, acting via VDRs, exert inhibitory effects on parathyroid cell growth. Furthermore, the hyperphosphatemia of uremia stimulates FGF23 production by bone, and this can further inhibit 1,25(OH)$_2$D production.

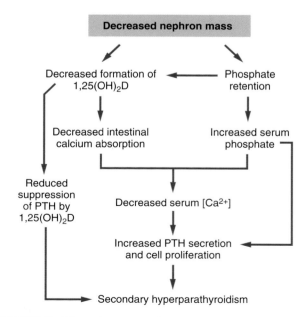

FIGURE 8–33 Pathogenesis of renal secondary hyperparathyroidism.

The net effect of deficient 1,25(OH)$_2$D and 24,25(OH)$_2$D and excess PTH and FGF23 on bone in uremia is complex. Patients may have osteitis fibrosa (reflecting excessive PTH), osteomalacia (in part reflecting decreased vitamin D metabolites and high FGF23 which have complex effects on bone mineralization), or a combination of the two. One particularly debilitating form of renal osteodystrophy is now found in an increasing percentage of patients on hemodialysis in whom only osteomalacia occurs. Rarely now, some patients have increased aluminum content in their bones, particularly in the region where mineralization is occurring (calcification front), and this appears to inhibit mineralization. More commonly, however, these patients do not have aluminum excess or increased osteoid but have low bone turnover, a state termed **adynamic bone disease**. These patients are particularly prone to develop symptoms of bone pain, fractures, and muscle weakness, and are particularly sensitive to developing hypercalcemia when treated with calcitriol despite the relatively low levels of PTH.

Clinical Features

Most patients with renal osteodystrophy have osteitis fibrosa alone or in combination with osteomalacia. If not well controlled, these patients will have a low serum level of calcium and high serum levels of phosphorus, alkaline phosphatase, and PTH. A few patients develop severe secondary hyperparathyroidism in which the PTH level increases dramatically and stays elevated even with restoration of the serum calcium to normal. Such patients are prone to developing hypercalcemia with the usual replacement doses of calcium (sometimes referred to as tertiary hyperparathyroidism). Another subset of patients with renal osteodystrophy present with relatively normal levels of PTH and alkaline phosphatase. Their serum calcium levels are often elevated after treatment with small doses of calcitriol. These patients generally have adynamic bone disease on bone biopsy and may suffer from aluminum intoxication (see discussed earlier).

Treatment

Patients with renal osteodystrophy generally respond to calcitriol (0.5-1 μg/d) or one of the vitamin D analogs paricalcitol (19-nor-1-alpha, 25[OH]$_2$D$_2$) or doxercalciferol (1αOHD$_2$), calcium supplementation (1-3 g/d), and phosphate restriction. Vitamin D supplementation is also recommended to ensure adequate 25(OH)D levels (30 ng/mL). Because of the concern about aluminum intoxication, sevelamer (Renagel) and other nonaluminum phosphate binders have replaced aluminum hydroxide to reduce intestinal phosphate absorption. To minimize the calcium-phosphate product, absorbable calcium-containing salts are used only at low doses to maintain sufficient calcium intake and not to act as a phosphate binder. The goal is to maintain normal serum levels of calcium, phosphate, and alkaline phosphatase. This regimen treats osteitis fibrosa more effectively than osteomalacia.

To prevent the development of adynamic bone disease, intact PTH levels higher than the upper limit of normal in standard intact PTH assays are allowed. The optimal intact PTH level for preserving skeletal integrity in end-stage renal disease and in patients on dialysis is uncertain. Newer or so-called *biointact* or *whole* PTH assays give a better reflection of the levels of the full-length PTH(1-84) molecule in these settings (described earlier). As previously noted, aluminum toxicity is associated with low-turnover bone disease rarely now. In the absence of aluminum toxicity, the etiology of uremic adynamic bone disease is unknown.

Patients with aluminum intoxication are very sensitive to and respond poorly to calcitriol and calcium, with rapid onset of hypercalcemia and little improvement in their bone disease. These patients may respond to chelation therapy with deferoxamine, a drug also used for iron chelation.

Severe secondary hyperparathyroidism is difficult to manage. These patients are prone to the development of hypercalcemia with calcium supplementation. Intravenous doses of calcitriol with hemodialysis may preferentially inhibit PTH secretion with less effect on raising serum calcium. Several analogs of calcitriol with less hypercalcemic potential than calcitriol itself have recently been approved for the management of such patients, as has the calcimimetic cinacalcet. Cinacalcet inhibits PTH secretion by activating the CaSR on parathyroid cells. Calcimimetic therapy has the distinct advantage of lowering PTH and presumably bone turnover, and thereby serum phosphate, calcium, and their product unlike the vitamin D analogs which tend to raise serum calcium and phosphate. Cinacalcet has contributed substantially to the management of uremic secondary hyperparathyroidism, although its major side effect, nausea and vomiting, limits its use in some patients.

HEREDITARY FORMS OF HYPERPHOSPHATEMIA

Tumoral Calcinosis

Mutations in genes leading to reduced FGF23 production, secretion, or action have recently been described which result in hyperphosphatemia and increased 1,25(OH)2D production. FGF23 requires glycosylation for its export from the cell where it is produced. Although FGF23 utilizes FGF receptors in common with many other members of the FGF family (FGFR 1 and 3), it also requires a coreceptor alpha klotho, to activate FGF23-mediated signaling in target cells. Inactivating mutations in FGF23 itself, the enzyme that glycosylates FGF23 which is necessary for secretion, **GALNT3** (UDP-*N*-acetyl-α-D-galactosamine transferase), and alpha klotho all lead to hyperphosphatemia and increased 1,25(OH)2D levels, although serum calcium levels are generally normal. Urinary phosphate reabsorption is increased. These findings are the opposite of those of familial hypophosphatemic disorders described earlier. As a result of the increased calcium-phosphate product, ectopic calcification occurs, generally around joints and soft tissues. Dentition may be affected in some individuals. Treatment involves the use of phosphate binders in an effort to reduce the serum phosphate levels and reduce the painful and sometimes disfiguring ectopic calcifications which can become very large.

REFERENCES

Parathyroid Hormone, Parathyroid Hormone–Related Peptide, and Their Receptors

Gensure RC, Gardella TJ, Juppner H. Parathyroid hormone and parathyroid hormone-related peptide, and their receptors. *Biochem Biophys Res Commun.* 2005;328:666. [PMID: 15694400]

Murray TM, Rao LG, Divieti P, Bringhurst FR. Parathyroid hormone secretion and action: evidence for discrete receptors for the carboxyl-terminal region and related biological actions of carboxyl-terminal ligands. *Endocr Rev.* 2005;26:78. [PMID: 15689574]

Calcitonin

Findlay DM, Sexton PM. Calcitonin. *Growth Factors.* 2004;22:217. [PMID: 15621724]

Katafuchi T, Yasue H, Osaki T, Minamino N: Calcitonin receptor-stimulating peptide: its evolutionary and functional relationship with calcitonin/calcitonin-gene related peptide based on gene structure. *Peptides.* 2009;30:1753. [PMID: 19540291]

Naot D, Cornish J. The role of peptides and receptors of the calcitonin family in the regulation of bone metabolism. *Bone.* 2008;43:813. [PMID: 18687416]

Vitamin D

Bikle DD. Nonclassic actions of vitamin D. *J Clin Endocrinol Metab.* 2009;94:26. [PMID: 18854395]

Bikle DD. Extrarenal synthesis of 1,25-dihydroxyvitamin D and its health implications. *Clin Rev Bone Miner Metab.* 2009;7:114.

Bouillon R, Carmeliet G, Verlinden L, et al. Vitamin D and human health: lessons from vitamin D receptor null mice. *Endo Rev.* 2008;29:726. [PMID: 18694980]

Christakos S, Dhawan P, Benn B, et al. Vitamin D: molecular mechanism of action. *Ann NY Acad Sci.* 2007;1116:340. [PMID: 18083936]

Dawson-Hughes B. Serum 25-hydroxyvitamin D and functional outcomes in the elderly. *Am J Clin Nutr.* 2008;88:537S. [PMID: 18689397]

Holick MF. Vitamin D deficiency. *N Engl J Med.* 2007;357:266. [PMID: 17634462]

Khanal RC, Nemere I. Regulation of intestinal calcium transport. *Ann Rev Nutr.* 2008;28:179. [PMID: 18598134]

Medullary Thyroid Carcinoma

Costante G, Durante C, Francis Z, Schlumberger M, Filetti S. Determination of calcitonin levels in C-cell disease: clinical interest and potential pitfalls. *Nat Clin Pract Endo Metab.* 2009;5:35. [PMID: 19079202]

Frank-Raue K, Rondot S, Raue F. Molecular genetics and phenomics of RET mutations: impact on prognosis of MTC. *Mol Cell Endocrinol.* 2010;322:2. [PMID: 20083156]

Moo-Young TA, Traugott AL, Moley JF. Sporadic and familial medullary thyroid carcinoma: state of the art. *Surg Clin North Am.* 2009;89:1193. [PMID: 19836492]

Raue F, Frank-Raue K. Update multiple endocrine neoplasia type 2. *Fam Cancer.* Epub 20 Jan 2010. [PMID: 20087666]

Sakorafas GH, Friess H, Peros G. The genetic basis of hereditary medullary thyroid cancer: clinical implications for the surgeon, with a particular emphasis on the role of prophylactic thyroidectomy. *Endo Rel Canc.* 2008;15:871. [PMID: 19015274]

Tuttle RM, Ball DW, Byrd D, et al. Medullary carcinoma. *J Natl Compr Canc Netw.* 2010;8:512. [PMID: 20495082]

Hypercalcemic Disorders

Agarwal SK, Mateo CM, Marx SJ. Rare germline mutations in cyclin-dependent kinase inhibitor genes in multiple endocrine neoplasia type 1 and related states. *J Clin Endocrinol Metab.* 2009;94:1826. [PMID: 19141585]

Bilezikian JP, Potts JT Jr., Fuleihan G, et al. Guidelines for management of asymptomatic primary hyperparathyroidism: summary statement from the Third International Workshop. *J Clin Endocrinol Metab.* 2009;94:335. [PMID: 19193908]

Conron M, Young C, Beynon HL. Calcium metabolism in sarcoidosis and its clinical implications. *Rheumatology (Oxford).* 2000;39:707. [PMID: 10908687]

Eastell R, Arnold A, Brandi ML, Diagnosis of asymptomatic primary hyperparathyroidism: proceedings of the Third International Workshop. *J Clin Endocrinol Metab.* 2009;94:340. [PMID: 19193909]

Egbuna OI, Brown EM. Hypercalcaemic and hypocalcaemic conditions due to calcium-sensing receptor mutations. *Best Pract Res Clin Rheum.* 2008;22:129. [PMID: 18328986]

Fraser WD. Hyperparathyroidism. *Lancet.* 2009;374:145. [PMID: 19595349]

Iqbal AA, Burgess EH, Gallina DL, Nanes MS, Cook CB. Hypercalcemia in hyperthyroidism: patterns of serum calcium, parathyroid hormone, and 1,25-dihydroxyvitamin D3 levels during management of thyrotoxicosis. *Endocr Pract.* 2003;9:517. [PMID: 14715479]

Jacobs TP, Bilezikian JP. Clinical review: rare causes of hypercalcemia. *J Clin Endocrinol Metab.* 2005;90:6316. [PMID: 16131579]

Khan A, Grey A, Shoback D. Medical management of asymptomatic primary hyperparathyroidism: proceedings of the Third International Workshop. *J Clin Endocrinol Metab.* 2009;94:373. [PMID: 19193912]

Marcocci C, Cetani F, Rubin MR, Silverberg SJ, Pinchera A, Bilezikian JP. Parathyroid carcinoma. *J Bone Min Res.* 2008;23:1869. [PMID: 19016595]

Marcocci C, Chanson P, Shoback D, et al. Cinacalcet reduces serum calcium concentrations in patients with intractable primary hyperparathyroidism. *J Clin Endocrinol Metab.* 2009;94:2766. [PMID: 19470620]

Marx SJ. Molecular genetics of multiple endocrine neoplasia types 1 and 2. *Nat Rev Cancer.* 2005;5:367. [PMID: 15864278]

Peacock M, Bolognese MA, Borofsky M, et al. Cinacalcet treatment of primary hyperparathyroidism: biochemical and bone densitometric outcomes in a five-year study. *J Clin Endocrinol Metab.* 2009;94:4860. [PMID: 19837909]

Ralston SH, Coleman R, Fraser WD, et al. Medical management of hypercalcemia. *Calcif Tissue Int.* 2004;74:1. [PMID: 14523593]

Rubin MR, Bilezikian JP, McMahon DJ, et al. The natural history of primary hyperparathyroidism with or without parathyroid surgery after 15 years. *J Clin Endocrinol Metab.* 2008;93:3462. [PMID: 18544625]

Saunders Y, Ross JR, Broadley KE, Edmonds PM, Patel S; Steering Group. Systematic review of bisphosphonates for hypercalcaemia of malignancy. *Palliat Med.* 2004;18:418. [PMID: 15332420]

Shepard MM, Smith JW, 3rd. Hypercalcemia. *Am J Med Sci.* 2007;334:381. [PMID: 18004092]

Stewart AF. Clinical practice. Hypercalcemia associated with cancer. *N Engl J Med.* 2005;352:373. [PMID: 15673803]

Udelsman R, Pasieka JL, Sturgeon C, Young JE, Clark OH. Surgery for asymptomatic primary hyperparathyroidism: proceedings of the Third International Workshop. *J Clin Endocrinol Metab.* 2009;94:366. [PMID: 19193911]

Hypocalcemic Disorders

Alimohammadi M, Björklund P, Hallgren A, et al. Autoimmune polyendocrine syndrome type 1 and NALP5, a parathyroid autoantigen. *N Engl J Med.* 2008;358:1018. [PMID: 18322283]

Bhattacharyya A, et al. Hungry bone syndrome—revisited. *J R Coll Phys Edinb.* 2002;32:83.

Brown EM. Anti-parathyroid and anti-calcium sensing receptor antibodies in autoimmune hypoparathyroidism. *Endocrinol Metab Clin N Am.* 2009;38:437. [PMID: 19328421]

Cooper MS, Gittoes NJL. Diagnosis and management of hypocalcemia. *BMJ.* 2008;336;1298. [PMID: 18535072]

Husebye ES, Perheentupa J, Rautemaa R, Kämpe O. Clinical manifestations and management of patients with autoimmune polyendocrine syndrome type I. *J Intern Med.* 2009;265:514. [PMID: 19382991]

Kobrysnki LJ, Sullivan KE. Velocardiofacial syndrome, DiGeorge syndrome: the chromosome 22q11.2 deletion syndromes. *Lancet*. 2007;370:1443. [PMID: 17950858]

Mannstadt M, Bertrand G, Muresan M, et al. Dominant-negative GCMB mutations cause an autosomal dominant form of hypoparathyroidism. *J Clin Endocrinol Metab*. 2008;93:3568. [PMID: 18583467]

Mantovani G, Spada A. Mutations in Gs alpha gene causing hormone resistance. *Best Pract Res Clin Endocrinol Metabol*. 2006;20:501. [PMID: 17161328]

Plagge A, Kelsey G, Germain-Lee EL. Physiological functions of the imprinted Gnas locus and its protein variants G{alpha}s and XL{alpha}s in human and mouse. *J Endocrinol*. 2008;196:193. [PMID: 18252944]

Shoback D. Hypoparathyroidism. *N Engl J Med*. 2008;358:391. [PMID: 18650515]

Zahirieh A, Nesbit MA, Ali A, et al. Functional analysis of a novel GATA3 mutation in a family with the hypoparathyroidism, deafness, and renal dysplasia syndrome. *J Clin Endocrinol Metab*. 2005;90:2445. [PMID: 15705923]

Bone Anatomy and Remodeling

Almeida M, Han L, Martin-Millan M, et al. Skeletal involution by age-associated oxidative stress and its acceleration by loss of sex steroids. *J Biol Chem*. 2007;282:27285. [PMID: 17623659]

Fukumoto S, Martin TJ. Bone as an endocrine organ. *Trends Endo Metab*. 2009:20:230. [PMID: 19546009]

Henriksen K, Neutzsky-Wulff AV, Bonewald LF, Karsdal MA. Local communication on and within bone controls bone remodeling. *Bone*. 2009;44:1026. [PMID: 19345750]

Kearns AE, Khosla S, Kostenuik PJ. Receptor activator of nuclear factor kappaB ligand and osteoprotegerin regulation of bone remodeling in health and disease. *Endo Rev*. 2008;29:155. [PMID: 18057140]

Matsuo K, Irie N. Osteoclast-osteoblast communication. *Arch Biochem Biophys*. 2008;473:201. [PMID: 18406338]

Quarles LD. Endocrine function of bone in mineral metabolism regulation. *J Clin Invest*. 2008;118:3820. [PMID: 19033649]

Teitelbaum SL. Osteoclasts: what do they do and how do they do it? *Am J Pathol*. 2007;170:427. [PMID: 17255310]

Yadav VK, Ryu JH, Suda N, et al. Lrp5 controls bone formation by inhibiting serotonin synthesis in the duodenum. *Cell*. 2008;135:825. [PMID: 19041748]

Yadav VK, Oury F, Suda N, et al. A serotonin-dependent mechanism explains the leptin regulation of bone mass, appetite, and energy expenditure. *Cell*. 2009;138:976. [PMID: 19737523]

Osteoporosis

Anderson GL, Limacher M, Assaf AR, et al. Effects of conjugated equine estrogen in postmenopausal women with hysterectomy: the Women's Health Initiative randomized controlled trial. *JAMA*. 2004;291:1701. [PMID: 15082697]

Bischoff-Ferrari HA, Giovannucci E, Willett WC, Dietrich T, Dawson-Hughes B, et al. Estimation of optimal serum concentrations of 25-hydroxyvitamin D for multiple health outcomes. *Am J Clin Nutr*. 2006;84:18. [PMID: 16825677]

Cadarette SM, Katz JN, Brookhart MA, Stürmer T, Stedman MR, Solomon DH. Relative effectiveness of osteoporosis drugs for preventing nonvertebral fracture. *Ann Int Med*. 2008;148:637. [PMID: 18458276]

Canalis E, Giustina A, Bilezikian JP. Mechanism of anabolic therapies for osteoporosis. *N Engl J Med*. 2007;357:905. [PMID: 17761594]

Center JR, Bliuc D, Nguyen TV, Eisman JA. Risk of subsequent fracture after low-trauma fracture in men and women. *JAMA*. 2007;297:387. [PMID: 17244835]

Cummings SR, San Martin J, McClung MR, et al. Denosumab for prevention of fracture in postmenopausal women with osteoporosis. *N Engl J Med*. 2009;361:756. [PMID: 19671655]

Dawson-Hughes B, Tosteson AN, Melton LJ 3rd, et al. Implications of absolute fracture risk assessment for osteoporosis practice guidelines in the USA. *Osteo Int*. 2008;19:449. [PMID: 18292975]

deKam D, Smulders E, Weerdesteyn V, Smits-Engelsman BC. Exercise interventions to reduce fall-related fractures and their risk factors in individuals with low bone density: a systematic review of randomized controlled trials. *Osteoporos Int*. 2009;20:2111. [PMID: 19421702]

Ebeling PR. Clinical practice. Osteoporosis in men. *N Engl J Med*. 2008;358:1474. [PMID: 18385499]

Hofbauer LC, Rauner M. Minireview: live and let die: molecular effects of glucocorticoids on bone cells. *Mol Endocrinol*. 2009;23:1525. [PMID: 19477950]

Kanis JA, Oden A, Johnell O, et al. The use of clinical risk factors enhances the performance of BMD in the prediction of hip and osteoporotic fractures in men and women. *Osteo Int*. 2007:18:1033. [PMID: 17323110]

Khosla S, Burr D, Cauley J, et al. Bisphosphonate-associated osteonecrosis of the jaw: report of a Task Force of the American Society for Bone and Mineral Research. *J Bone Min Res*. 2007;22:1479. [PMID: 176663640]

Khosla S, Westendorf JJ, Oursler MJ. Building bone to reverse osteoporosis and repair fractures. *J Clin Invest*. 2008;118:421. [PMID: 18246192]

Liu H, Paige NM, Goldzweig CL, et al. Screening for osteoporosis in men: a systematic review for an American College of Physicians guideline. *Ann Int Med*. 2008;148:685. [PMID: 18458282]

MacLean C, Newberry S, Maglione M, et al. Systematic review: comparative effectiveness of treatment to prevent fractures in men and women with low bone density or osteoporosis. *Ann Int Med*. 2008;148:197. [PMID: 18087050]

National Osteoporosis Foundation. *Clinician's Guide to Prevention and Treatment of Osteoporosis*. Washington, DC: National Osteoporosis Foundation. www. nof.org.

Pleiner-Duxneuner J, Zwettler E, Paschalis E, Roschger P, Nell-Duxneuner V, Klaushofer K. Treatment of osteoporosis with parathyroid hormone and teriparatide. *Calcif Tiss Int*. 2009;84:159. [PMID: 19189037]

Qaseem A, Snow V, Shekelle P, et al. Screening for osteoporosis in men: a Clinical Practice Guideline from the American College of Physicians. *Ann Int Med*. 2008;148:680. [PMID: 18458281]

Richards JB, Kavvoura FK, Rivadeneira F, et al. Genetic factors for osteoporosis. Collaborative meta-analysis: associations of 150 candidate genes with osteoporosis and osteoporotic fracture. *Ann Int Med*. 2009;151:528. [PMID: 19841454]

Rossouw JE, Anderson GL, Prentice RL, et al. Risks and benefits of estrogen plus progestin in healthy postmenopausal women: principal results from the Women's Health Initiative randomized controlled trial. *JAMA*. 2002;288:321. [PMID: 12117397]

Russell RG, Watts NB, Ebetino FH, Rogers MJ. Mechanisms of action of bisphosphonates: similarities and differences and their potential influence on clinical efficacy. *Osteo Int*. 2008;19:733. [PMID: 18214569]

Sambrook P, Cooper C. Osteoporosis. *Lancet*. 2006;367:2010. [PMID: 16782492]

Smith MR, Egerdie B, Hernández Toriz N, et al. Denosumab in men receiving androgen-deprivation therapy for prostate cancer. *N Engl J Med*. 2009;361:745. [PMID: 19671656]

Styrkarsdottir U, Halldorsson BV, Gretarsdottir S, et al. Multiple genetic loci for bone mineral density and fractures. *N Engl J Med*. 2008;358:2355. [PMID: 18445777]

Tang BMP, Eslick GD, Nowson C, Smith C, Bensoussan A. Use of calcium or calcium in combination with vitamin D supplementation to prevent fractures and bone loss in people aged 50 years and older: a meta-analysis. *Lancet*. 2007;370:657. [PMID: 17720017]

Tosteson ANA, Melton LJ 3rd, Dawson-Hughes B, et al. Cost-effective osteoporosis treatment thresholds: the United States perspective. *Osteo Int*. 2008;19:437. [PMID: 18292976]

Osteomalacia, Rickets, and Hypophosphatemia

De Prisco C, Levine SN. Metabolic bone disease after gastric bypass surgery for obesity. *Am J Med Sci*. 2005;329:57. [PMID: 15711420]

Feng JQ, Ward LM, Liu S, et al. Loss of DMP1 causes rickets and osteomalacia and identifies a role for osteocytes in mineral metabolism. *Nat Gen*. 2006;38:1310. [PMID: 17033621]

Ichikawa S, Sorenson AH, Imel EA, Friedman NE, Gertner JM, Econs MJ. Intronic deletions in the SLC34A3 gene cause hereditary hypophosphatemic rickets with hypercalciuria. *J Clin Endocrinol Metab*. 2006;91:4022. [PMID: 16849419]

Jonsson KB, Zahradnik R, Larsson T. Fibroblast growth factor 23 in oncogenic osteomalacia and X linked hypophosphatemia. *N Engl J Med*. 2003;348:1656. [PMID: 12711740]

Lawson J. Drug-induced metabolic bone disorders. *Semin Musculoskelet Radiol.* 2002;6:285. [PMID: 12541185]

Levine BS, Kleeman CR, Felsenfeld AJ. The journey from vitamin D-resistant rickets to the regulation of renal phosphate transport. *Clin J Am Soc Nephrol.* 2009;4:1866. [PMID: 19808223]

Tiosano D, Hochberg Z. Hypophosphatemia: the common denominator of all rickets. *J Bone Miner Metab.* 2009;27:392. [PMID: 195044043]

Ward LM. Renal phosphate-wasting disorders in childhood. *Pediatr Endocrinol Rev.* 2005;2(suppl 3):342. [PMID: 16456503]

FGF23 and Alpha Klotho

Fukomoto S, Yamashita T. FGF23 is a hormone regulating phosphate metabolism—unique biological characteristics of FGF23. *Bone.* 2007;40:1190. [PMID: 17276744]

Garringer HJ, Malekpour M, Esteghamat F, et al. Molecular genetic and biochemical analyses of FGF23 mutations in familial tumoral calcinosis. *Am J Physiol Endocrinol Metab.* 2008;295:E929. [PMID: 18682534]

Ichikawa S, Sorenson AH, Austin AM, et al. Ablation of the Galnt3 gene leads to low circulating intact fibroblast growth factor 23 (Fgf23) concentrations and hyperphosphatemia despite increased Fgf23 expression. *Endocrinology.* 2009;150:2543. [PMID: 19213845]

Kuro-OM. Overview of the FGF23-klotho axis. *Pediatr Nephrol.* 2010;25:583. [PMID: 19626341]

Ramon I, Kleynen P, Body JJ, Karmali R, et al. Fibroblast growth factor 23 and its role in phosphate homeostasis. *Eur J Endocrinol.* 2010;162:1. [PMID: 19776202]

Strom TM, Juppner H. PHEX, FGF23, DMP1 and beyond. *Curr Opin Nephrol Hypertens.* 2008;17:357. [PMID: 18660670]

Urakawa I, Yamazaki Y, Shimada T, et al. Klotho converts canonical FGF receptor into a specific receptor for FGF23. *Nature.* 2006;444:770. [PMID: 17086194]

Paget Disease

Daroszewska A, Ralston SH. Mechanisms of disease: genetics of Paget's disease of bone and related disorders. *Nat Clin Pract Rheum.* 2006;2:270. [PMID: 16932700]

Hosking D, Lyles K, Brown JP, et al. Long-term control of bone turnover in Paget's disease with zoledronic acid and risedronate. *J Bone Min Res.* 2007;22:142. [PMID: 1703222148]

Langston AL, Campbell MK, Fraser WD, et al. Randomized trial of intensive bisphosphonate treatment versus symptomatic management in Paget's disease of bone. *J Bone Min Res.* 2010;25:20. [PMID: 19580357]

Ralston SH, Langston, Reid IR. Pathogenesis and management of Paget's disease of bone. *Lancet.* 2008;372:155. [PMID: 18620951]

Reid IR, Miller P, Lyles K, et al. Comparison of a single infusion of zoledronic acid with risedronate for Paget's disease. *N Engl J Med.* 2006;353:898. [PMID: 16135834]

Singer FR. Paget disease: when to treat and when not to treat. *Nat Rev Rheum.* 2009;5:483. [PMID: 19652650]

Whyte MP. Paget's disease of bone. *N Engl J Med.* 2006;355:593. [PMID: 16899779]

Renal Osteodystrophy

Block GA, Martin KJ, de Francisco AL, et al. Cinacalcet for secondary hyperparathyroidism in patients receiving hemodialysis. *N Engl J Med.* 2004;350:1516. [PMID: 15071126]

Bover J, Canal C, Marco H, Fernandez-Llama P, Bosch RJ, Ballarín J. Diagnostic procedures and rationale for specific therapies in chronic kidney disease-mineral and bone disorders. *Contrib Nephrol.* 2008;161:222. [PMID: 18451681]

Cunningham J. New vitamin D analogues for osteodystrophy in chronic kidney disease. *Pediatr Nephrol.* 2004;19:705. [PMID: 15141342]

de Francisco AL. Secondary hyperparathyroidism: review of the disease and its treatment. *Clin Ther.* 2004;26:1976. [PMID: 15823762]

Gutierrez OM, Mannstadt M, Isakova T, et al. Fibroblast growth factor 23 and mortality among patients undergoing hemodialysis. *N Engl J Med.* 2008;359:584. [PMID: 18687639]

Hruska KA, Mathew S, Lund R, Qiu P, Pratt R. Hyperphosphatemia of chronic kidney disease. *Kidney Int.* 2008;74:148. [PMID: 18449174]

Martin KJ, Akhtar I, Gonzalez EA. Parathyroid hormone: new assays, new receptors. *Semin Nephrol.* 2004;24:3. [PMID: 14730504]

Navneethan SD, Palmer SC, Craig JC, Elder GJ, Strippoli GF. Benefits and harms of phosphate binders in CKD: a systematic review of randomized controlled trials. *Am J Kid Dis.* 2009;54:619. [PMID: 19692157]

Ott SM. Bone histomorphometry in renal osteodystrophy. *Semin Nephrol.* 2009;29:122. [PMID: 19371803]

Tentori F, Blayney MJ, Albert JM, et al. Mortality risk for dialysis patients with different levels of serum calcium, phosphorus, and PTH: the Dialysis Outcomes and Practice Patterns Study (DOPPS). *Am J Kidney Dis.* 2008;52:519. [PMID: 18514987]

Glucocorticoids and Adrenal Androgens

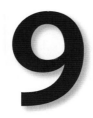

Ty B. Carroll, MD, David C. Aron, MD, MS, James W. Findling, MD, and J. Blake Tyrrell, MD

ACTH	Adrenocorticotropic hormone		**HPLC**	High-performance liquid chromatography
ADH	Antidiuretic hormone (vasopressin)		**IL**	Interleukin
APS	Autoimmune polyglandular syndrome		**IPSS**	Inferior petrosal sinus sampling
AVP	Arginine vasopressin		**IRMA**	Immunoradiometric assay
CBG	Corticosteroid-binding globulin		**LH**	Luteinizing hormone
CRH	Corticotropin-releasing hormone		**LPH**	Lipotropin
DAX1	Dosage-sensitive sex reversal-adrenal hypoplasia gene product		**PMN**	Polymorphonuclear neutrophil
DHEA	Dehydroepiandrosterone		**PRA**	Plasma renin activity
DOC	Deoxycorticosterone		**PRL**	Prolactin
GH	Growth hormone		**PTH**	Parathyroid hormone
GIP	Glucose-dependent insulinotropic peptide/Gastrointestinal inhibitory polypeptide		**SF-1**	Steroidogenic factor-1a
			SHBG	Sex hormone–binding globulin
GnRH	Gonadotropin-releasing hormone		**StAR**	Steroidogenic acute regulatory protein
HLA	Human leukocyte antigen		**TRH**	Thyrotropin-releasing hormone
HPA	Hypothalamic-pituitary-adrenal		**TSH**	Thyroid-stimulating hormone (thyrotropin)
			VLCFA	Very long chain fatty acid

The adrenal cortex produces many steroid hormones of which the most important are cortisol, aldosterone, and the adrenal androgens. Disorders of the adrenal glands lead to classic endocrinopathies such as Cushing syndrome, Addison disease, hyperaldosteronism, and the syndromes of congenital adrenal hyperplasia. This chapter describes the physiology and disorders of the glucocorticoids and the adrenal androgens. Disorders of aldosterone secretion are discussed in Chapter 10 and congenital defects in adrenal hormone biosynthesis in Chapters 10 and 14. Hirsutism and virilization (which reflect excess androgen action) are discussed in Chapter 13.

Advances in diagnostic procedures have simplified the evaluation of adrenocortical disorders; in particular, the assay of plasma glucocorticoids, androgens, and adrenocorticotropin (ACTH) has allowed more rapid and precise diagnosis. In addition, advances in surgical and medical treatment have improved the outlook for patients with these disorders.

EMBRYOLOGY AND ANATOMY

Embryology

The adrenal cortex is of mesodermal origin and derives from a single cell lineage characterized by expression of certain transcription factors such as steroidogenic factor-1 (SF-1). At 2 months' gestation, the cortex, already identifiable as a separate organ, is composed of a fetal zone and a definitive zone similar to the adult adrenal cortex. The adrenal cortex then increases rapidly in size; at mid gestation, it is considerably larger than the kidney and much larger than the adult gland in relation to total body mass. The fetal zone makes up the bulk of the weight of the adrenal cortex at this time. Several genes encoding transcription factors are important in adrenal development and differentiation. These include SF-1 and the product of the dosage-sensitive sex reversal–adrenal hypoplasia gene (*DAX1*), among others; mutations of the *DAX1* gene are associated with congenital adrenal hypoplasia.

The fetal adrenal is under the control of ACTH by mid pregnancy, but the fetal zone is deficient in the activity of 3β-hydroxysteroid dehydrogenase (see section on biosynthesis of cortisol and adrenal androgens, later) and thus produces mainly dehydroepiandrosterone (DHEA) and DHEA sulfate, which serve as precursors of maternal-placental estrogen production after conversion in the liver to 16α-hydroxylated derivatives. The definitive zone synthesizes a number of steroids and is the major site of fetal cortisol synthesis. Mutations of the ACTH- or *melanocortin-2 receptor* gene are associated with familial glucocorticoid deficiency.

Anatomy

The anatomic relationship of the fetal and definitive zones is maintained until birth, at which time the fetal zone gradually disappears, with a consequent decrease in adrenocortical weight in the 3 months following delivery. During the next 3 years, the adult adrenal cortex develops from cells of the outer layer of the cortex and differentiates into the three adult zones: glomerulosa, fasciculata, and reticularis–adrenal zonation.

The adult adrenal glands, with a combined weight of 8 to 10 g, lie in the retroperitoneum above or medial to the upper poles of the kidneys (Figure 9–1). A fibrous capsule surrounds the gland; the cortex comprises 90% of the adrenal weight, the inner medulla is about 10%.

The adrenal cortex is richly vascularized and receives its main arterial supply from branches of the inferior phrenic artery, the renal arteries, and the aorta. These small arteries form an arterial plexus beneath the capsule and then enter a sinusoidal system that penetrates the cortex and medulla, draining into a single central vein in each gland. The right adrenal vein drains directly into the posterior aspect of the vena cava; the left adrenal vein enters the left renal vein. These anatomic features account for the fact that it is relatively easier to catheterize the left adrenal vein than it is to catheterize the right adrenal vein.

Microscopic Anatomy

Histologically, the adult cortex is composed of three zones: an outer zona glomerulosa, a zona fasciculata, and an inner zona reticularis (Figure 9–2). However, the inner two zones appear to function as a unit (see later). The zona glomerulosa, which produces aldosterone and constitutes about 15% of adult cortical volume, is deficient in 17α-hydroxylase activity and thus cannot produce cortisol or androgens (see later and Chapter 10). The zona glomerulosa lacks a well-defined structure, and the small lipid-poor cells are scattered beneath the adrenal capsule. The zona fasciculata is the thickest layer of the adrenal cortex, making up about 75% of the cortex, and produces cortisol and androgens. The cells of the zona fasciculata are larger and contain more lipid and thus are termed **clear cells**. These cells extend in columns from the narrow zona reticularis to either the zona glomerulosa or to the capsule. The inner zona reticularis surrounds the medulla and also produces cortisol and androgens. The compact cells of this narrow zone lack significant lipid content but do contain lipofuscin granules. The zonae fasciculata and reticularis are regulated by ACTH; excess or deficiency of this hormone alters their

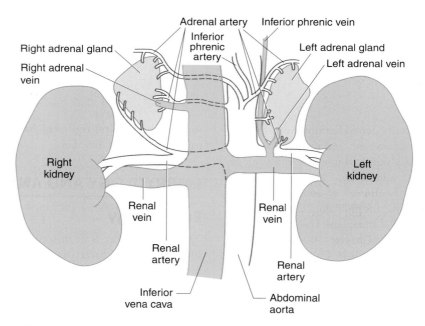

FIGURE 9–1 Location and blood supply of the adrenal glands (schematic). (Reproduced, with permission, from Miller WL, Tyrrell JB. The adrenal cortex. In: Felig P, et al, eds. *Endocrinology and Metabolism*. 4th ed. McGraw-Hill; 2002.)

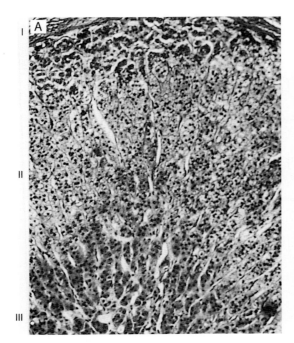

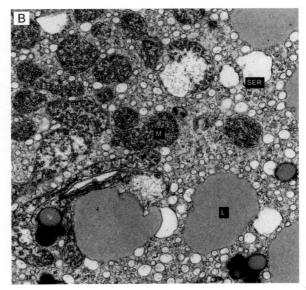

FIGURE 9–2 Photomicrograph of the adrenal cortex (H&E stain). **A.** A low-power general view. I, the glomerulosa; II, the fasciculata; III, the reticularis. (Reproduced, with permission, from Junqueira LC, Carneiro J. *Basic Histology.* 7th ed. McGraw-Hill; 1992.)
B. Electron micrograph of a normal adrenocortical steroid-producing cell (L, lipid vacuole; M, large mitochondria with tubular cristae; SER, smooth endoplasmic reticulum). (Courtesy of Dr. Medhat O. Hasan, Pathology Department, Louis Stokes Cleveland Department of Veterans Affairs Medical Center.)

structure and function. Thus, both zones atrophy when ACTH is deficient; when ACTH is present in excess, hyperplasia and hypertrophy of these zones occur. In addition, chronic stimulation with ACTH leads to a gradual depletion of the lipid from the clear cells of the zona fasciculata at the junction of the two zones; these cells thus attain the characteristic appearance of the compact reticularis cells. With chronic excessive stimulation, the compact reticularis cells extend outward and may reach the outer capsule. It is postulated that the zona fasciculata cells can respond acutely to ACTH stimulation with increased cortisol production, whereas the reticularis cells maintain basal glucocorticoid secretion and that induced by prolonged ACTH stimulation.

BIOSYNTHESIS OF CORTISOL AND ADRENAL ANDROGENS

Steroidogenesis

The major hormones secreted by the adrenal cortex are cortisol, the androgens, and aldosterone. The carbon atoms in the steroid molecule are numbered as shown in Figure 9–3, and the major biosynthetic pathways and hormonal intermediates are illustrated in Figures 9–4 and 9–5.

The scheme of adrenal steroidogenic synthesis has been clarified by analysis of the steroidogenic enzymes. Most of these enzymes belong to the family of cytochrome P450 oxygenases (see Table 9–1 for current and historical nomenclature conventions). In mitochondria, the *CYP11A* gene, located on chromosome 15, encodes

C_{21} steroid (progesterone)

C_{19} steroid (dehydroepiandrosterone)

FIGURE 9–3 Structure of adrenocortical steroids. The letters in the formula for progesterone identify the A, B, C, and D rings; the numbers show the positions in the basic C_{21} steroid structure. The angular methyl groups (positions 18 and 19) are usually indicated simply by straight lines, as in the lower formula. Dehydroepiandrosterone is a 17-ketosteroid formed by cleavage of the side chain of the C_{21} steroid 17-hydroxypregnenolone and its replacement by an O atom. (Reproduced, with permission, from Ganong WF. *Review of Medical Physiology.* 14th ed. McGraw-Hill; 1989.)

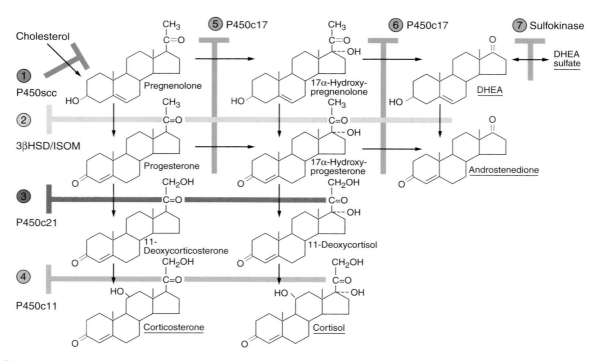

FIGURE 9–4 Steroid biosynthesis in the zona fasciculata and zona reticularis of the adrenal cortex. The major secretory products are underlined. The enzymes for the reactions are numbered on the left and at the top of the chart, with the steps catalyzed shown by the shaded bars. ① P450scc, cholesterol 20,22-hydroxylase:20,22 desmolase activity; ② 3βHSD/ISOM, 3-hydroxysteroid dehydrogenase; δ^5-oxosteroid isomerase activity; ③ P450c21, 21α-hydroxylase activity; ④ P450c11, 11β-hydroxylase activity; ⑤ P450c17, 17α-hydroxylase activity; ⑥ P450c17, 17,20-lyase/desmolase activity; ⑦ sulfokinase. (Modified and reproduced, with permission, from Ganong WF. *Review of Medical Physiology.* 16th ed. McGraw-Hill; 1993.)

P450scc, the enzyme responsible for cholesterol side chain cleavage. *CYP11B1*, a gene located on chromosome 8, encodes P450c11, another mitochondrial enzyme, which mediates 11β-hydroxylation in the zona reticularis and zona fasciculata. This reaction converts 11-deoxycortisol to cortisol and 11-deoxycorticosterone (11-DOC) to corticosterone. In the zona glomerulosa, *CYP11B2*, also located on chromosome 8, encodes the enzyme P450aldo, also known as aldosterone synthase. P450aldo mediates 11β-hydroxylation, 18-hydroxylation, and 18-oxidation to convert 11-DOC to corticosterone, 18-hydroxycorticosterone, and aldosterone, respectively. In the endoplasmic reticulum, gene *CYP17*, located on chromosome 10, encodes a single enzyme, P450c17, which mediates both 17α-hydroxylase activity and 17,20-lyase activity, and the gene *CYP21A2* encodes the enzyme P450c21, which mediates 21-hydroxylation of both progesterone and 17-hydroxyprogesterone. The 3β-hydroxysteroid dehydrogenase: Δ^{5,4}-isomerase activities are mediated by a single non-P450 microsomal enzyme (see Figure 9–4).

A. Zones and steroidogenesis   Because of enzymatic differences between the zona glomerulosa and the inner two zones, the adrenal cortex functions as two separate units, with differing regulation and secretory products. Thus, the zona glomerulosa, which produces aldosterone, lacks 17α-hydroxylase activity and cannot synthesize 17α-hydroxypregnenolone and 17α-hydroxyprogesterone, which are the precursors of cortisol and the adrenal androgens. The synthesis of aldosterone by this zone is primarily regulated by the renin-angiotensin system and by potassium (see Chapter 10).

The zona fasciculata and zona reticularis (see Figure 9–4) produce cortisol, androgens, and small amounts of estrogens. These zones, primarily regulated by ACTH, do not express the gene *CYP11B2* (encoding P450aldo) and therefore cannot convert 11-DOC to aldosterone (see Chapter 10).

B. Cholesterol uptake and synthesis   Synthesis of cortisol and the androgens by the zonae fasciculata and reticularis begins with cholesterol, as does the synthesis of all steroid hormones. Plasma lipoproteins are the major source of adrenal cholesterol, although synthesis within the gland from acetate also occurs. Low-density lipoprotein accounts for about 80% of cholesterol delivered to the adrenal gland. A small pool of free cholesterol within the adrenal is available for rapid synthesis of steroids when the adrenal is stimulated. When stimulation occurs, there is also increased hydrolysis of stored cholesteryl esters to free cholesterol, increased uptake from plasma lipoproteins, and increased cholesterol synthesis within the gland. The acute response to a steroidogenic stimulus is mediated by the steroidogenic acute regulatory protein (StAR). This mitochondrial phosphoprotein enhances cholesterol transport from the outer to the inner mitochondrial membrane. Mutations in the *StAR* gene result in congenital lipoid adrenal hyperplasia with severe cortisol and aldosterone deficiencies at birth.

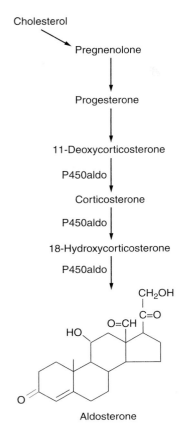

Cholesterol

Pregnenolone

Progesterone

11-Deoxycorticosterone

P450aldo

Corticosterone

P450aldo

18-Hydroxycorticosterone

P450aldo

Aldosterone

FIGURE 9–5 Steroid biosynthesis in the zona glomerulosa. The steps from cholesterol to 11-deoxycorticosterone are the same as in the zona fasciculata and zona reticularis. However, the zona glomerulosa lacks 17α-hydroxylase activity and thus cannot produce cortisol. Only the zona glomerulosa can convert corticosterone to 18-hydroxycorticosterone and aldosterone. The single enzyme P450aldo catalyzes the conversion of 11-deoxycorticosterone to corticosterone to 18-hydroxycorticosterone to aldosterone. (Modified and reproduced, with permission, from Ganong WF. *Review of Medical Physiology*. 16th ed. McGraw-Hill; 1993.)

C. Cholesterol metabolism The conversion of cholesterol to pregnenolone is the rate-limiting step in adrenal steroidogenesis and the major site of ACTH action in the adrenal. This step occurs in the mitochondria and involves two hydroxylations and then the side chain cleavage of cholesterol. A single enzyme, CYP11A, mediates this process; each step requires molecular oxygen and a pair of electrons. The latter are donated by NADPH to adrenodoxin reductase (ferredoxin reductase), a flavoprotein, and then to adrenodoxin, an iron-sulfur protein, and finally to CYP11A. Both adrenodoxin reductase and adrenodoxin are also involved in the action of CYP11B1 (see earlier). Electron transport to microsomal cytochrome P450 involves P450 reductase, a flavoprotein distinct from adrenodoxin reductase. Pregnenolone is then transported outside the mitochondria before further steroid synthesis occurs.

D. Synthesis of cortisol Cortisol synthesis proceeds by 17α-hydroxylation of pregnenolone by CYP17 within the smooth endoplasmic reticulum to form 17α-hydroxypregnenolone. This steroid is then converted to 17α-hydroxyprogesterone after conversion of its 5,6 double bond to a 4,5 double bond by the 3β-hydroxysteroid dehydrogenase: $\Delta^{5,4}$-oxosteroid isomerase enzyme complex, which is also located within the smooth endoplasmic reticulum. An alternative but apparently less important pathway in the zonae fasciculata and reticularis is from pregnenolone to progesterone to 17α-hydroxyprogesterone (see Figure 9–4).

The next step, which is again microsomal, involves the 21-hydroxylation by CYP21A2 of 17α-hydroxyprogesterone to form 11-deoxycortisol; this compound is further hydroxylated within mitochondria by 11β-hydroxylation (CYP11B1) to form cortisol. The zona fasciculata and zona reticularis also produce 11-DOC, 18-hydroxydeoxycorticosterone, and corticosterone. However, as noted above, the absence of the mitochondrial enzyme CYP11B2 prevents production of aldosterone by these zones of the adrenal cortex (Figure 9–5). Cortisol secretion under basal (ie, non-stressed) conditions ranges from 8 to 25 mg/d (22-69 μmol/d), with a mean of about 9.2 mg/d (25 μmol/d)—rates lower than most previous calculations.

E. Synthesis of androgens The production of adrenal androgens from pregnenolone and progesterone requires prior 17α-hydroxylation (CYP17) and thus does not occur in the zona glomerulosa. The major quantitative production of androgens is by conversion of 17α-hydroxypregnenolone to the 19-carbon compounds (C-19 steroids) DHEA and its sulfate conjugate DHEA sulfate. Thus, 17α-hydroxypregnenolone undergoes removal of its two-carbon side chain at the C_{17} position by microsomal 17,20-desmolase (CYP17), yielding DHEA with a keto group at C_{17}. DHEA is then converted to DHEA sulfate by a reversible adrenal sulfokinase. The other major adrenal androgen, androstenedione, is produced mostly from DHEA, mediated by CYP17, and possibly from 17α-hydroxyprogesterone, also by CYP17. Androstenedione can be converted to testosterone, although adrenal secretion of this hormone is minimal. The adrenal androgens, DHEA, DHEA sulfate, and androstenedione, have minimal intrinsic androgenic activity, and they contribute to androgenicity by their peripheral conversion to the more potent androgens testosterone and dihydrotestosterone. Although DHEA and DHEA sulfate are secreted in greater quantities, androstenedione is qualitatively more important, because it is more readily converted peripherally to testosterone (see Chapter 12). Of note, recent studies have identified de novo synthesis of some steroid hormones in nerve and cardiac tissues, where they appear to act as paracrine or autocrine factors. Steroidogenic enzymes (eg, 3β-hydroxysteroid dehydrogenase and aromatase) are expressed in many tissues.

Regulation of Secretion

A. Secretion of CRH and ACTH ACTH is the trophic hormone of the zonae fasciculata and reticularis and the major regulator of cortisol and adrenal androgen production, although other factors produced within the adrenal, including neurotransmitters, neuropeptides, and nitric oxide also play a role. ACTH in turn is regulated by the hypothalamus and central nervous system via neurotransmitters and corticotropin-releasing hormone (CRH)

TABLE 9–1 The main components of the steroidogenic pathway.

Enzyme	Gene	Chromosomal Location	Enzyme Activity (or Activities)	Subcellular Localization	Characteristic Features of Normal Tissue-Specific Expression
Steroidogenic acute regulatory protein (StAR)	StAR	8p11.2	Activation of peripheral type benzodiazepine receptor	Outer mitochondrial membrane	All steroid hormone–producing cells except the placenta, Schwann cells, and the brain
Peripheral type benzodiazepine receptor	PDA	22q13.31	Regulated cholesterol channel	Forms channel at the contact sites between the outer and inner mitochondrial membranes	All steroid hormone–producing cells
P450scc	CYP11A	15q23-24	Cholesterol-20,22-desmolase	Matrix side of inner mitochondrial membrane	All steroid hormone–producing cells
3β-Hydroxysteroid dehydro genase (HSD)/isomerase	3β-Hydroxysteroid dehydrogenase type I	1p13, the HSD3B1 and HSD3B2 loci are located 1-2 cm from the centromeric marker D1Z5	3β-Hydroxysteroid dehydrogenase	Smooth endoplasmic reticulum	Expressed in syncytiotrophoblast cells, sebaceous glands
	3β-Hydroxysteroid dehydrogenase type II				Expressed in the definitive adrenal cortex and the gonads. Absent from the fetal zone of the adrenal cortex
P450c21	CYP21B	6p21.3 (close to HLA locus)	21-hydroxylase	Smooth endoplasmic reticulum	Only in adrenal cortex (all zones); low levels in fetal zone
	CYP21A	6p21.3 (close to HLA locus)	Pseudogene	N/A	N/A
P450c11	CYP11B1	8q21-22	11β-hydroxylase	Matrix side of inner mitochondrial membrane	Only expressed in zona fasciculata and zona reticularis of the adrenal cortex; low levels in fetal zone
P450aldo	CYP11B2	8q24.3	Aldosterone synthase: 11β-hydroxylase, 18-hydroxylase, 18-oxidase	Matrix side of inner mitochondrial membrane	Only expressed in the zona glomerulosa of the adrenal cortex; low levels in fetal zone
P450c17	CYP17	10q24-25	17α-hydroxylase, 17,20-lyase	Smooth endoplasmic reticulum	Absent from the zona glomerulosa in adults, the placenta, and the definitive zone of fetal adrenal cortex until the third trimester
P450arom	CYP19	15q	Aromatase	Smooth endoplasmic reticulum	Expressed in numerous tissues including gonads, brain, adrenal, adipose tissue, and bone

Modified from Kacsoh B. *Endocrine Physiology.* McGraw-Hill; 2000.

and arginine vasopressin (AVP). The neuroendocrine control of CRH and ACTH secretion involves three mechanisms (see later and Chapter 4).

B. ACTH effects on the adrenal cortex   ACTH administration leads to the rapid synthesis and secretion of steroids; plasma levels of these hormones rise within minutes. ACTH increases RNA, DNA, and protein synthesis. Chronic stimulation leads to adrenocortical hyperplasia and hypertrophy; conversely, ACTH deficiency results in decreased steroidogenesis and is accompanied by adrenocortical atrophy, decreased gland weight, and decreased protein and nucleic acid content.

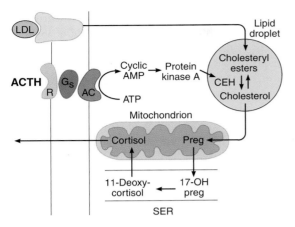

FIGURE 9–6 Mechanism of action of ACTH on cortisol-secreting cells in the inner two zones of the adrenal cortex. When ACTH binds to its receptor (R), adenylyl cyclase (AC) is activated via G_s. The resulting increase in cAMP activates protein kinase A, and the kinase phosphorylates cholesteryl ester hydrolase (CEH), increasing its activity. Consequently, more free cholesterol is formed and converted to pregnenolone in the mitochondria. Note that in the subsequent steps in steroid biosynthesis, products are shuttled between the mitochondria and the smooth endoplasmic reticulum (SER). (Reproduced, with permission, from Ganong WF. *Review of Medical Physiology.*16th ed. McGraw-Hill; 1993.)

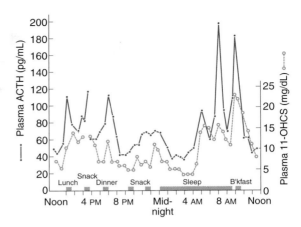

FIGURE 9–7 Fluctuations in plasma ACTH and glucocorticoids (11-OHCS) throughout the day. Note the greater ACTH and glucocorticoid rises in the morning before awakening. (Reproduced, with permission, from Krieger DT, et al. Characterization of the normal temporal pattern of corticosteroid levels. *J Clin Endocrinol Metab.* 1971;32:266.)

C. ACTH and steroidogenesis   ACTH binds to high-affinity plasma membrane receptors, thereby activating adenylyl cyclase and increasing cyclic adenosine monophosphate, which in turn activates intracellular phosphoprotein kinases (Figure 9–6), including StAR. ACTH action results in increased free cholesterol formation as a consequence of increased cholesterol esterase activity and decreased cholesteryl ester synthetase as well as increased lipoprotein uptake by the adrenal cortex. This process stimulates the rate-limiting step—cholesterol delivery to the side chain cleavage enzyme (P450scc or CYP11A1) for conversion to Δ^5-pregnenolone, thereby initiating steroidogenesis.

D. Neuroendocrine control   Cortisol secretion is closely regulated by ACTH, and plasma cortisol levels parallel those of ACTH (Figure 9–7). There are three mechanisms of neuroendocrine control: (1) episodic secretion and the circadian rhythm of ACTH, (2) stress responsiveness of the hypothalamic-pituitary-adrenal (HPA) axis, and (3) feedback inhibition by cortisol of ACTH secretion.

1. **Circadian rhythm**—Circadian rhythm is superimposed on episodic secretion; it is the result of central nervous system events that regulate both the number and magnitude of CRH and ACTH secretory episodes. Cortisol secretion is low in the late evening and continues to decline in the first several hours of sleep, at which time plasma cortisol levels may be undetectable. During the third and fifth hours of sleep there is an increase in secretion; but the major secretory episodes begin in the sixth to eighth hours of sleep

(see Figure 9–7) and then begin to decline as wakefulness occurs. About half of the total daily cortisol output is secreted during this period. Cortisol secretion then gradually declines during the day, with fewer secretory episodes of decreased magnitude; however, there is increased cortisol secretion in response to eating and exercise.

Although this general pattern is consistent, there is considerable intra- and interindividual variability, and the circadian rhythm may be altered by changes in sleep pattern, light-dark exposure, and feeding times. The rhythm is also changed by (1) physical stresses such as major illness, surgery, trauma, or starvation; (2) psychologic stress, including severe anxiety, endogenous depression, and the manic phase of manic-depressive psychosis; (3) central nervous system and pituitary disorders; (4) Cushing syndrome; (5) liver disease and other conditions that affect cortisol metabolism; (6) chronic renal failure; and (7) alcoholism. Cyproheptadine inhibits the circadian rhythm, possibly by its antiserotonergic effects, whereas other drugs usually have no effect.

2. **Stress responsiveness**—Plasma ACTH and cortisol secretion are also characteristically responsive to physical stress. Thus, plasma ACTH and cortisol are secreted within minutes following the onset of stresses such as surgery and hypoglycemia, and these responses abolish circadian periodicity if the stress is prolonged. Stress responses originate in the central nervous system and increase hypothalamic CRH and thus pituitary ACTH secretion. Stress responsiveness of plasma ACTH and cortisol is abolished by prior high-dose glucocorticoid administration and in spontaneous Cushing syndrome; conversely, the responsiveness of ACTH secretion is enhanced following adrenalectomy. Regulation of the HPA axis is linked to that of the immune system. For example, interleukin-1 (IL-1) stimulates ACTH secretion, and cortisol inhibits IL-1 synthesis.

3. **Feedback inhibition**—The third major regulator of ACTH and cortisol secretion is that of feedback inhibition by glucocorticoids of CRH, ACTH, and cortisol secretion. Glucocorticoid feedback inhibition occurs at both the pituitary and hypothalamus and involves two distinct mechanisms—fast and delayed feedback inhibition.

Fast feedback inhibition of ACTH secretion is rate-dependent; that is, it depends on the rate of increase of the glucocorticoid but not the dose administered. This phase is rapid (within minutes) and transient (lasting <10 minutes), suggesting mediation by a noncytosolic glucocorticoid receptor mechanism. **Delayed feedback inhibition** is both time- and dose-dependent. With continued glucocorticoid administration, ACTH levels continue to decrease and become unresponsive to stimulation, ultimately resulting in suppression of CRH and ACTH release and atrophy of the zonae fasciculata and reticularis. The suppressed HPA axis fails to respond to stress and stimulation. Delayed feedback appears to act via the classic glucocorticoid receptor mechanism (see later).

E. ACTH effects on regulation of androgen production

Adrenal androgen production in adults is also regulated by ACTH; both DHEA and androstenedione exhibit circadian periodicity in concert with ACTH and cortisol. In addition, plasma concentrations of DHEA and androstenedione increase rapidly with ACTH administration and are suppressed by glucocorticoid administration. DHEA sulfate, because of its slow metabolic clearance rate, does not exhibit a diurnal rhythm. The existence of a separate anterior pituitary hormone that regulates adrenal androgen secretion has long been postulated but not yet proved.

CIRCULATION OF CORTISOL AND ADRENAL ANDROGENS

Cortisol and the adrenal androgens circulate bound to plasma proteins. The plasma half-life of cortisol (60-90 minutes) is determined by the extent of plasma binding and by the rate of metabolic inactivation.

Plasma-Binding Proteins

Cortisol and adrenal androgens are secreted in an unbound state; however, these hormones bind to plasma proteins on entering the circulation. Cortisol binds mainly to corticosteroid-binding globulin (CBG, transcortin) and to a lesser extent to albumin, whereas the androgens bind chiefly to albumin. Bound steroids are biologically inactive; the unbound or free fraction is active. The plasma proteins may provide a pool of circulating cortisol by delaying metabolic clearance, thus preventing more marked fluctuations of plasma-free cortisol levels during episodic secretion by the gland. Because there are no binding proteins in saliva, salivary cortisol reflects free cortisol.

Free and Bound Cortisol

Under basal conditions, about 10% of the circulating cortisol is free, about 75% is bound to CBG, and the remainder is bound to albumin. The plasma free cortisol level is approximately 1 μg/dL, and it is this biologically active cortisol that is regulated by ACTH.

A. Corticosteroid-binding globulin

Corticosteroid-binding globulin (CBG) has a molecular weight of about 50,000, is produced by the liver, and binds cortisol with high affinity. The CBG in plasma has a cortisol-binding capacity of about 25 μg/dL. When total plasma cortisol concentrations rise above this level, the free concentration rapidly increases and exceeds its usual fraction of 10% of the total cortisol. Other endogenous steroids usually do not appreciably affect cortisol binding to CBG; an exception is in late pregnancy, when progesterone may occupy about 25% of the binding sites on CBG. Synthetic steroids do not bind significantly to CBG—with the exception of prednisolone. CBG levels are increased in high-estrogen states (pregnancy; estrogen or oral contraceptive use), hyperthyroidism, diabetes, certain hematologic disorders, and on a genetic basis. CBG concentrations are decreased in familial CBG deficiency, hypothyroidism, and protein deficiency states such as severe liver disease or nephrotic syndrome.

B. Albumin

Albumin has a much greater capacity for cortisol binding but a lower affinity. It normally binds about 15% of the circulating cortisol, and this proportion increases when the total cortisol concentration exceeds the CBG-binding capacity. Synthetic glucocorticoids are extensively bound to albumin (eg, about 75% of dexamethasone in plasma is bound to albumin).

C. Androgen binding

Androstenedione, DHEA, and DHEA sulfate circulate weakly bound to albumin. However, testosterone is bound extensively to a specific globulin, sex hormone–binding globulin (SHBG) (see Chapter 12).

METABOLISM OF CORTISOL AND ADRENAL ANDROGENS

The metabolism of these steroids renders them inactive and increases their water solubility, as does their subsequent conjugation with glucuronide or sulfate groups. These inactive conjugated metabolites are more readily excreted by the kidney. The liver is the major site of steroid catabolism and conjugation, and 90% of these metabolized steroids are excreted by the kidney.

Conversion and Excretion of Cortisol

Cortisol is modified extensively before excretion in urine; less than 1% of secreted cortisol appears in the urine unchanged.

A. Hepatic conversion

Hepatic metabolism of cortisol involves a number of metabolic conversions of which the most important (quantitatively) is the irreversible inactivation of the steroid by Δ^4-reductases, which reduce the 4,5 double bond of the A ring. Dihydrocortisol, the product of this reaction, is then converted to tetrahydrocortisol by a 3-hydroxysteroid dehydrogenase. Cortisol is also converted extensively by 11β-hydroxysteroid dehydrogenase to the biologically inactive cortisone, which is then metabolized by the enzymes described above to yield tetrahydrocortisone. Tetrahydrocortisol and tetrahydrocortisone can be further altered to form the cortoic acids. These conversions result in the excretion of approximately equal amounts of cortisol and cortisone metabolites. Cortisol and cortisone are also metabolized to the cortols and cortolones and to a lesser extent by other pathways (eg, to 6β-hydroxycortisol).

B. Hepatic conjugation More than 95% of cortisol and cortisone metabolites are conjugated by the liver and then reenter the circulation to be excreted in the urine. Conjugation is mainly with glucuronic acid at the 3α-hydroxyl position.

C. Variations in clearance and metabolism The metabolism of cortisol is altered by a number of circumstances. It is decreased in infants and in the elderly. It is impaired in chronic liver disease, leading to decreased renal excretion of cortisol metabolites; however, the plasma cortisol level remains normal. Hypothyroidism decreases both metabolism and excretion; conversely, hyperthyroidism accelerates these processes. Cortisol clearance may be reduced in starvation and anorexia nervosa and is also decreased in pregnancy because of the elevated CBG levels. The metabolism of cortisol to 6β-hydroxycortisol is increased in the neonate, in pregnancy, with estrogen therapy, and in patients with liver disease or severe chronic illness. Cortisol metabolism by this pathway is also increased by drugs that induce hepatic microsomal enzymes, including barbiturates, phenytoin, mitotane, aminoglutethimide, and rifampin. These alterations generally are of minor physiologic importance as the free cortisol levels remain relatively stable in these conditions. However, they result in decreased excretion of the urinary metabolites of cortisol measured as 17-hydroxycorticosteroids. These conditions and drugs have a greater influence on the metabolism of synthetic glucocorticoids and may result in inadequate plasma levels of the administered glucocorticoid because of rapid clearance and metabolism.

D. Cortisol-cortisone shunt Aldosterone is the principal mineralocorticoid controlling sodium and potassium exchange in the distal nephron. Mineralocorticoid receptors in the kidney are responsible for this effect, and the sensitivities of both the glucocorticoid receptor and the mineralocorticoid receptor for cortisol in vitro are similar. Small changes in aldosterone affect sodium and potassium exchange in the kidney, whereas free and biologically active cortisol does not, yet cortisol circulates in much higher concentrations. This apparent paradox is explained by an intracellular enzyme—11β-hydroxysteroid dehydrogenase type 2 (11β-HSD2)—that metabolizes cortisol to the inactive cortisone and protects the mineralocorticoid receptor from cortisol binding (Figure 9–8). However, when circulating cortisol is extremely high

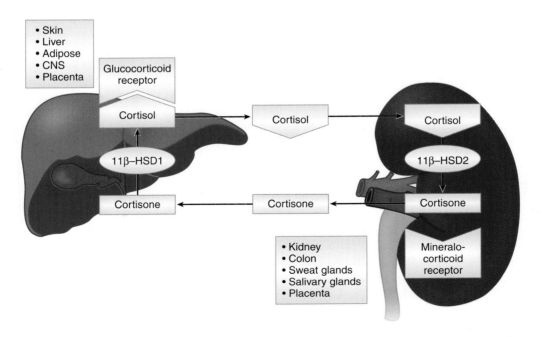

FIGURE 9–8 Cortisol-cortisone shunt. Contrasting functions of the isozymes of 11β-HSD. 11β-HSD2 is an exclusive 11β-dehydrogenase that acts in classical aldosterone target tissues to exclude cortisol from otherwise nonselective mineralocorticoid receptors. Inactivation of cortisol also occurs in placenta. 11β-HSD1 is a predominant 11β-reductase in vivo that acts in many tissues to increase local intracellular glucocorticoid concentrations and thereby maintain adequate exposure of relatively low affinity glucocorticoid receptors to their ligand.

(as in severe Cushing syndrome), this prereceptor metabolism of cortisol is overwhelmed and the mineralocorticoid receptor is activated by cortisol, resulting in volume expansion, hypertension, and hypokalemia. The active ingredient of licorice (glycyrrhizic acid) actually inhibits 11β-HSD2 and gives cortisol free access to the unprotected mineralocorticoid receptor in the kidney, causing hypokalemia and hypertension. In addition, some tissues can actually convert the inactive cortisone to cortisol with the isoform called 11β-hydroxysteroid dehydrogenase type 1 (11β-HSD1). The skin expresses this enzyme, explaining why cortisone cream can be effective. More importantly, the liver expresses 11β-HSD1 and can activate cortisone to cortisol, thereby completing the cortisol-cortisone shunt such that the kidney inactivates cortisol to cortisone and the liver can reactivate cortisone to cortisol. The expression of 11β-HSD1 in adipose tissue may contribute to abdominal obesity seen in metabolic syndrome without biochemical hypercortisolism.

Conversion and Excretion of Adrenal Androgens

Adrenal androgen metabolism results either in degradation and inactivation or the peripheral conversion of these weak androgens to their more potent derivatives testosterone and dihydrotestosterone. DHEA is readily converted within the adrenal to DHEA sulfate, the adrenal androgen secreted in greatest amount. DHEA secreted by the gland is also converted to DHEA sulfate by the liver and kidney, or it may be converted to Δ^4-androstenedione. DHEA sulfate may be excreted without further metabolism; however, both it and DHEA are also metabolized to 7α- and 16α-hydroxylated derivatives and by 17β reduction to Δ^5-androstenediol and its sulfate. Androstenedione is converted either to testosterone or by reduction of its 4,5 double bond to etiocholanolone or androsterone, which may be further converted by 17α reduction to etiocholanediol and androstanediol, respectively. Testosterone is converted to dihydrotestosterone in androgen-sensitive tissues by 5β reduction, and it, in turn, is mainly metabolized by 3α reduction to androstanediol. The metabolites of these androgens are conjugated either as glucuronides or sulfates and excreted in the urine.

BIOLOGIC EFFECTS OF ADRENAL STEROIDS

Glucocorticoids

Although glucocorticoids were originally so called because of their influence on glucose metabolism, they are currently defined as steroids that exert their effects by binding to specific cytosolic receptors that mediate the actions of these hormones. These glucocorticoid receptors are present in virtually all tissues, and glucocorticoid-receptor interaction is responsible for most of the known effects of these steroids. Alterations in the structure of the glucocorticoids have led to the development of synthetic compounds with greater glucocorticoid activity. The increased activity

of these compounds is due to increased affinity for the glucocorticoid receptors and delayed plasma clearance, which increases tissue exposure. In addition, many of these synthetic glucocorticoids have negligible mineralocorticoid effects and thus do not result in sodium retention, hypertension, and hypokalemia. This section describes the molecular mechanisms of glucocorticoid action and the effects on individual metabolic functions and tissues (Table 9–2).

Molecular Mechanisms

Glucocorticoid action is initiated by entry of the steroid into the cell and binding to the cytosolic glucocorticoid–receptor proteins (see Figures 1–13, 1–14, and 1–15). The most abundant cytoplasmic glucocorticoid–receptor complex includes two subunits of the 90-kDa heat shock protein (hsp) 90. After binding, the hsp90 subunits dissociate and activated hormone–receptor complexes enter the nucleus and interact with nuclear chromatin acceptor sites. The DNA-binding domain of the receptor is a cysteine-rich region which, when it chelates zinc, assumes a conformation called a **zinc finger**. The receptor–glucocorticoid complex acts via two mechanisms: (1) binding to specific sites in nuclear DNA, the glucocorticoid regulatory elements; and (2) interactions with other transcription factors such as nuclear factor κB, an important regulator of cytokine genes. These result in altered expression of specific genes and the transcription of specific mRNAs. The resulting proteins elicit the glucocorticoid response, which may be inhibitory or stimulatory depending on the specific gene and tissue affected. Although glucocorticoid receptors are similar in many tissues, the proteins synthesized in response to glucocorticoids vary widely and are the result of expression of specific genes in different cell types. The mechanisms underlying this specific regulation are unknown. Analyses of cloned complementary DNAs for human glucocorticoid receptors have revealed marked structural and amino acid sequence homology between glucocorticoid receptors and receptors for other steroid hormones (eg, mineralocorticoids, estrogen, progesterone) as well as for thyroid hormone and the oncogene v-erb-A. Although the steroid-binding domain of the glucocorticoid receptor confers specificity for glucocorticoid binding, glucocorticoids such as cortisol and corticosterone bind to the mineralocorticoid receptor with an affinity equal to that of aldosterone. Mineralocorticoid receptor specificity is maintained by the expression of 11β-HSD in classic mineralocorticoid-sensitive tissues—the cortisol-cortisone shunt (see earlier).

Although glucocorticoid–receptor complexes and their subsequent regulation of gene expression are responsible for most glucocorticoid effects, other effects may occur through plasma membrane receptors.

Glucocorticoid Agonists and Antagonists

The study of glucocorticoid receptors has led to the definition of glucocorticoid agonists and antagonists. These studies have also identified a number of steroids with mixed effects termed partial agonists, partial antagonists, or partial agonist–partial antagonists. In addition, novel glucocorticoid receptor ligands are being

TABLE 9–2 The main targets and actions of glucocorticoids and the consequences of Cushing disease and Addison disease.

Target System	Specific Target	Physiologic Function	Cushing Disease	Addison Disease
Intermediary metabolism	Liver	Increased expression of gluconeogenic enzymes, phosphoenolpyruvate carboxykinase, glucose-6-phosphatase, and fructose-2,6-bisphosphatase	Increased hepatic glucose output; together with insulin, increased hepatic glycogen stores	Diminished hepatic glucose output and glycogen stores
	Adipose tissue	Permissive for lipolytic signals (catecholamines, GH) leading to elevated plasma FFA to fuel gluconeogenesis	Overall effect (together with insulin): central obesity (truncal obesity, moon facies, and buffalo hump)	Decreased adiposity and decreased lipolysis
	Skeletal muscle	Degradation of fibrillar muscle proteins by activating the ubiquitin pathway, thereby providing amino acid substrates for gluconeogenesis	Muscle weakness and wasting mainly in proximal muscles; increased urinary nitrogen excretion (urea from amino acids)	Muscle weakness, decreased muscle glycogen stores; decreased urinary nitrogen excretion
	Plasma glucose	Maintains plasma glucose during fasting (antihypoglycemic action); increases plasma glucose during stress (hyperglycemic action)	Impaired glucose tolerance, insulin-resistant diabetes mellitus; increased plasma glucose is due to decreased peripheral glucose utilization and increased hepatic glucose output	Hypoglycemia, increased insulin sensitivity
Calcium homeostasis	Kidney	Decreased reabsorption of calcium	Hypercalciuria without hypercalcemia leading to secondary hyperparathyroidism	Retardation of bone growth mainly through decreased GH; hypercalcemia possible
	Bone, cartilage	Inhibition of collagen synthesis and bone deposition	Retardation of bone growth and bone age by direct action and by decreasing GH; osteoporosis in adults	
	Gastrointestinal tract	Inhibition of calcium, magnesium, and phosphate absorption by antagonizing calcitriol actions		
Other endocrine systems	Hypothalamus, pituitary	Decreases endogenous opioid production; depresses gonadotroph responsiveness to GnRH; stimulates *GH* gene expression by the pituitary; inhibits GH secretion via the hypothalamus	Scanty menses due to suppressed gonadotroph sensitivity to GnRH; suppressed GH secretion by hypothalamic action; minimal suppression of the TRH-TSH axis	Scanty menses by upregulated CRH-endogenous opioid pathway-mediated suppression of GnRH; suppressed GH secretion; hypothyroidism (if present) is due to autoimmune mechanism
	Pancreas	Inhibits insulin secretion by decreasing the efficacy of cytoplasmic Ca^{2+} on the exocytotic process	Absolute hyperinsulinemia with relative hypoinsulinemia (lower plasma insulin than expected for the degree of hyperglycemia)	Absolute hypoinsulinemia with relative hyperinsulinemia
	Adrenal medulla	Increases PNMT expression and activity (epinephrine synthesis)	Increased responses to sympathoadrenal activation	Decreased responses to sympathoadrenal activation
	Carrier proteins (CBG, SHBG, TBG)	Decreases all major hormone-binding proteins	Decrease in total T_4, free T_4 remains normal	
Immune system	Thymus, lymphocytes	Causes age-related involution of the thymus; induces thymic atrophy	Immunocompromised state; lymphocytopenia	Relative lymphocytosis in peripheral blood
	Monocytes	Inhibits monocyte proliferation and antigen presentation; decreased production of IL-1, IL-6, and TNFα	Monocytopenia in peripheral blood	Monocytosis in peripheral blood
	Granulocytes	Demargination of neutrophils by suppressing the expression of adhesion molecules	Peripheral blood: granulocytosis, eosinopenia	Peripheral blood: granulocytopenia, eosinophilia

(Continued)

TABLE 9–2 The main targets and actions of glucocorticoids and the consequences of Cushing disease and Addison disease. (*Continued*)

Target System	Specific Target	Physiologic Function	Cushing Disease	Addison Disease
	Inflammatory response	Inhibition of inflammation by inhibiting PLA_2, thereby inhibiting production of leukotrienes and prostaglandins; suppresses COX-2 expression		
	Erythrocytes	No significant effect	Increased hemoglobin and hematocrit are due to ACTH-mediated overproduction of androgens	Anemia is more pronounced in women and is due to loss of adrenal androgens; anemia may be related to direct autoimmune targeting of gastric parietal cells
Skin and connective tissue		Antiproliferative for fibroblasts and keratinocytes	Easy bruisability due to dermal atrophy; striae or sites of increased tension, especially sites of adipose tissue accumulation; poor wound healing; hirsutism and acne are due to ACTH-mediated increase of adrenal androgens; hyperpigmentation is a direct effect of ACTH on melanocortin 1 receptors	Darkening of the skin is due to ACTH-mediated stimulation of epidermal melanocortin 1 receptors; vitiligo may occur due to direct autoimmune destruction of melanocytes in circumscribed areas
Breast	Mammary epithelium	Mandatory requirement for lactation	Cushing disease may be associated with galactorrhea	Addison disease is not associated with galactorrhea
Lung	Type II alveolar cell	Stimulation of surfactant production		
Cardiovascular system	Heart	Increased contractility	Hypertension	Lower peripheral resistance; hypertension with further postural decrease in blood pressure (orthostatic hypotension); low-voltage ECG
	Vasculature	Increased vascular reactivity to vasoconstrictors (catecholamines, angiotensin II)		
Na^+, K^+, and ECF volume	Kidney	Increased GFR and nonphysiologic actions on mineralocorticoid receptors	Hypokalemic alkalosis, increased ECF volume due to mineralocorticoid activity (increased DOC, saturation of type 2 11β-hydroxysteroid dehydrogenase by high levels of cortisol)	Hyponatremia, hyperkalemic acidosis, and decreased ECF volume are mainly due to loss of mineralocorticoid activity
	Posterior pituitary		Hyponatremia due to SIADH	Increased ADH mainly via hypovolemia-related baroreceptor mechanism
Psychiatric parameters of CNS function	Mood	Eucortisolemia maintains emotional balance	Initially, euphoria; long-term, depression, psychosis	Depression
	Appetite	Increases appetite	Hyperphagia	Decreased appetite in spite of improved taste and smell
	Sleep	Suppression of REM sleep	Sleep disturbances	
	Memory	Sensitizes hippocampal glutamate receptors, induces atrophy of dendrites	Impaired memory, bilateral hippocampal atrophy	
	Eye	Increasing intraocular pressure	Cataract formation; increased intraocular pressure	Decreased intraocular pressure

Modified from Kacsoh B. *Endocrine Physiology*. McGraw-Hill; 2000.

developed that have more selectivity in terms of receptor binding or transcription of specific genes.

A. Agonists In humans, cortisol, synthetic glucocorticoids (eg, prednisolone, dexamethasone), corticosterone, and aldosterone are glucocorticoid agonists. The synthetic glucocorticoids have substantially higher affinity for the glucocorticoid receptor, and these have greater glucocorticoid activity than cortisol when present in equimolar concentrations. Corticosterone and aldosterone have substantial affinity for the glucocorticoid receptor; however, their plasma concentrations are normally much lower than that of cortisol, and thus these steroids do not have significant physiologic glucocorticoid effects.

B. Antagonists Glucocorticoid antagonists bind to the glucocorticoid receptors but do not elicit the nuclear events required to cause a glucocorticoid response. These steroids compete with agonist steroids such as cortisol for the receptors and thus inhibit agonist responses. Other steroids have partial agonist activity when present alone (ie, they elicit a partial glucocorticoid response). However, in sufficient concentration, they compete with agonist steroids for the receptors and thus competitively inhibit agonist responses; that is, these partial agonists may function as partial antagonists in the presence of more active glucocorticoids. Steroids such as progesterone, 11-deoxycortisol, DOC, testosterone, and 17β-estradiol have antagonist or partial agonist-partial antagonist effects; however, the physiologic role of these hormones in glucocorticoid action is probably negligible, because they circulate in low concentrations. The antiprogestational agent mifepristone has substantial glucocorticoid antagonist properties and has been used to block glucocorticoid action in patients with Cushing syndrome.

Intermediary Metabolism (Table 9–2)

Glucocorticoids in general inhibit DNA synthesis. In addition, in most tissues they inhibit RNA and protein synthesis and accelerate protein catabolism. These actions provide substrate for intermediary metabolism; however, accelerated catabolism also accounts for the deleterious effects of glucocorticoids on muscle, bone, connective tissue, and lymphatic tissues. In contrast, RNA and protein synthesis in liver is stimulated.

A. Hepatic glucose metabolism Glucocorticoids increase hepatic gluconeogenesis by stimulating the gluconeogenic enzymes phosphoenolpyruvate carboxykinase and glucose-6-phosphatase. They have a permissive effect in that they increase hepatic responsiveness to the gluconeogenic hormone glucagon, and they also increase the release of substrates for gluconeogenesis from peripheral tissues, particularly muscle. This latter effect may be enhanced by the glucocorticoid-induced reduction in peripheral amino acid uptake and protein synthesis. Glucocorticoids also increase glycerol and free fatty acid release by lipolysis and increase muscle lactate release. They enhance hepatic glycogen synthesis and storage by stimulating glycogen synthetase activity and to a lesser extent by inhibiting glycogen breakdown. These effects are insulin dependent.

B. Peripheral glucose metabolism Glucocorticoids also alter carbohydrate metabolism by inhibiting peripheral glucose uptake in muscle and adipose tissue. This effect and the others described earlier may result in increased insulin secretion in states of chronic glucocorticoid excess.

C. Effects on adipose tissue In adipose tissue, the predominant effect is increased lipolysis with release of glycerol and free fatty acids. This is partially due to direct stimulation of lipolysis by glucocorticoids, but it is also contributed to by decreased glucose uptake and enhancement by glucocorticoids of the effects of lipolytic hormones. Although glucocorticoids are lipolytic, increased fat deposition is a classic manifestation of glucocorticoid excess. This paradox may be explained by the increased appetite caused by high levels of these steroids and by the lipogenic effects of the hyperinsulinemia that occurs in this state. The reason for abnormal fat deposition and distribution in states of cortisol excess is unknown. In these instances, fat is classically deposited centrally in the face, cervical area, trunk, and abdomen; the extremities are usually spared.

D. Summary The effects of the glucocorticoids on intermediary metabolism can be summarized as follows:

(1) Effects are minimal in the fed state. However, during fasting, glucocorticoids contribute to the maintenance of plasma glucose levels by increasing gluconeogenesis and decreasing uptake of glucose by adipose tissue.

(2) Hepatic glucose production is enhanced, as is hepatic RNA and protein synthesis.

(3) The effects on muscle are catabolic (ie, decreased glucose uptake and metabolism, decreased protein synthesis, and increased release of amino acids). This provides amino acid substrates for gluconeogenesis in the liver.

(4) In adipose tissue, lipolysis is stimulated. This increases fatty acid delivery to the liver where their metabolism provides energy to support gluconeogenesis.

(5) In glucocorticoid deficiency, hypoglycemia may result, whereas in states of glucocorticoid excess there may be hyperglycemia, hyperinsulinemia, muscle wasting, and weight gain with abnormal fat distribution.

Effects on Other Tissues and Functions (Table 9–2)

A. Connective tissue Glucocorticoids in excess inhibit fibroblasts, lead to loss of collagen and connective tissue, and thus result in thinning of the skin, easy bruising, stria formation, and poor wound healing.

B. Bone The physiologic role of glucocorticoids in bone metabolism and calcium homeostasis is unknown; however, in excess, they have major deleterious effects. Glucocorticoids directly inhibit bone formation by decreasing cell proliferation and the synthesis of RNA, protein, collagen, and hyaluronate. Initially, supraphysiologic doses of glucocorticoids also stimulate bone resorption, at least in part via interference of the receptor activator of nuclear factor kappa B (RANK)-ligand/RANK/osteo-protegerin pathway. This leads to osteolysis and increased biochemical markers of bone turnover. In addition, glucocorticoids may potentiate the proresorptive actions of parathyroid hormone (PTH) and 1,25-dihydroxycholecalciferol (1,25[OH]$_2$D$_3$) on bone, and this may further contribute to net bone resorption. Chronically, however, the key effect to promote bone loss is due to the detrimental impact on bone formation (see Chapter 8).

C. Calcium metabolism Glucocorticoids also have other major effects on mineral homeostasis. They markedly reduce intestinal calcium absorption, which tends to lower serum calcium. This theoretically promotes a state of secondary hyperparathyroidism to maintain the serum calcium within the normal range. In reality, however, chronic elevations in intact PTH levels have been difficult to demonstrate consistently in patients on glucocorticoid therapy. The mechanism of decreased intestinal calcium absorption is thought to result from antagonism of 1,25(OH)$_2$D action in the intestine. It is not due to decreased synthesis or decreased serum levels of the active vitamin D metabolites; in fact, 1,25(OH)$_2$D levels are normal or even increased in the presence of glucocorticoid excess. Increased 1,25(OH)$_2$D synthesis in this setting may result from decreased serum phosphorus levels (see later), increased PTH secretion, direct stimulation by glucocorticoids of renal 1α-hydroxylase, and or reduced target cell (intestine) responsiveness. Glucocorticoids increase urinary calcium excretion, and hypercalciuria is a frequent feature of cortisol excess. They also reduce the tubular reabsorption of phosphate, leading to phosphaturia and decreased serum phosphorus concentrations.

Thus, glucocorticoids in excess result in negative calcium balance, with decreased calcium absorption and increased urinary calcium excretion. Serum calcium levels are maintained, but at the expense of net bone resorption. Decreased bone formation and increased resorption ultimately result in the disabling osteoporosis that is often a major complication of spontaneous and iatrogenic glucocorticoid excess (see Chapter 8).

D. Growth and development Glucocorticoids accelerate the development of a number of systems and organs in fetal and differentiating tissues, although the mechanisms are unclear. As discussed above, glucocorticoids are generally inhibitory, and these stimulatory effects may be due to glucocorticoid interactions with other growth factors. Examples of these development-promoting effects are increased surfactant production in the fetal lung and the accelerated development of hepatic and gastrointestinal enzyme systems.

Glucocorticoids in excess inhibit growth in children, and this adverse effect is a major complication of therapy. This may be a direct effect on bone cells, although decreased growth hormone (GH) secretion and insulin-like growth factor I generation also contribute (see Chapter 6).

E. Blood cells and immunologic function

1. **Erythrocytes**—Glucocorticoids have little effect on erythropoiesis and hemoglobin concentration. Although mild polycythemia and anemia may be seen in Cushing syndrome and Addison disease, respectively, these alterations are more likely to be secondary to altered androgen metabolism.

2. **Leukocytes**—Glucocorticoids influence both leukocyte movement and function. Thus, glucocorticoid administration increases the number of intravascular polymorphonuclear neutrophils/leukocytes (PMNs) by increasing PMN release from bone marrow, by increasing the circulating half-life of PMNs, and by decreasing PMN movement out of the vascular compartment. Glucocorticoid administration reduces the number of circulating lymphocytes, monocytes, and eosinophils, mainly by increasing their movement out of the circulation. The converse (ie, neutropenia, lymphocytosis, monocytosis, and eosinophilia) is seen in adrenal insufficiency. Glucocorticoids also decrease the migration of inflammatory cells (PMNs, monocytes, and lymphocytes) to sites of injury, and this is probably a major mechanism of the anti-inflammatory actions and increased susceptibility to infection that occur following chronic administration. Glucocorticoids also decrease lymphocyte production and the mediator and effector functions of these cells.

3. **Immunologic effects**—Glucocorticoids influence multiple aspects of immunologic and inflammatory responsiveness, including the mobilization and function of leukocytes, as discussed earlier. They inhibit phospholipase A$_2$, a key enzyme in the synthesis of prostaglandins. This inhibition is mediated by a class of peptides called lipocortins or annexins. They also impair the release of effector substances such as the lymphokine IL-1, antigen processing, antibody production and clearance, and other specific bone marrow–derived and thymus-derived lymphocyte functions. The immune system, in turn, affects the HPA axis; IL-1 stimulates the secretion of CRH and ACTH. Although traditionally used as anti-inflammatory and/or immunosuppressive agents, glucocorticoids, especially at lower doses, also have stimulatory and permissive effects on the inflammatory response to injury.

F. Cardiovascular function Glucocorticoids may increase cardiac output, and they also increase peripheral vascular tone, possibly by augmenting the effects of other vasoconstrictors (eg, the catecholamines). Glucocorticoids also regulate expression of adrenergic receptors. Thus, refractory shock may occur when the glucocorticoid-deficient individual is subjected to stress. Glucocorticoids in excess may cause hypertension independently of their mineralocorticoid effects. Although the incidence and the precise cause of this problem are unclear, it is likely that the mechanism involves the renin-angiotensin system; glucocorticoids regulate renin substrate, angiotensinogen, the precursor of angiotensin I.

G. Renal function These steroids affect water and electrolyte balance by actions mediated either by mineralocorticoid receptors (sodium retention, hypokalemia, and hypertension) or via glucocorticoid receptors (increased glomerular filtration rate due to increased cardiac output or due to direct renal effects on salt and water retention). Thus, corticosteroids such as betamethasone or dexamethasone, which have little mineralocorticoid activity, increase sodium and water excretion. Glucocorticoid-deficient subjects have decreased glomerular filtration rates and are unable to excrete a water load. This may be further aggravated by increased ADH secretion, which may occur in glucocorticoid deficiency.

H. Central nervous system function Glucocorticoids readily enter the brain, and although their physiologic role in central nervous system function is unknown, their excess or deficiency may profoundly alter behavior and cognitive function.

1. **Excessive glucocorticoids**—In excess, the glucocorticoids initially cause euphoria; however, with prolonged exposure, a variety of psychologic abnormalities occur, including irritability, emotional lability, and depression. Hyperkinetic or manic behavior is less common; overt psychoses occur in a small number of patients, particularly those with underlying bipolar disorder. Many patients also note impairment in cognitive functions, most commonly memory and concentration. Other central effects include increased appetite, decreased libido, and insomnia, with decreased rapid eye movement sleep and increased stage II sleep.
2. **Decreased glucocorticoids**—Patients with Addison disease are apathetic and depressed and tend to be irritable, negativistic, and reclusive. They have decreased appetite but increased sensitivity of taste and smell mechanisms.

I. Effects on other hormones

1. **Thyroid function**—Glucocorticoids in excess affect thyroid function. Thyroid-stimulating hormone (TSH) synthesis and release are inhibited by glucocorticoids, and TSH responsiveness to thyrotropin-releasing hormone (TRH) is frequently subnormal. Although basal levels are usually normal, the TSH concentration may be acutely low in patients treated with moderate- to high-dose glucocorticoids. Serum total thyroxine (T_4) concentrations are usually low normal because of a decrease in thyroxine-binding globulin, but free T_4 levels are normal. Total and free T_3 (triiodothyronine) concentrations may be low, because glucocorticoid excess decreases the conversion of T_4 to T_3 and increases conversion to reverse T_3. Despite these alterations, manifestations of hypothyroidism are not apparent.
2. **Gonadal function**—Glucocorticoids also affect gonadotropin and gonadal function. In males, they inhibit gonadotropin secretion, as evidenced by decreased responsiveness to administered gonadotropin-releasing hormone (GnRH) and subnormal plasma testosterone concentrations. In females, glucocorticoids also suppress luteinizing hormone (LH) responsiveness to GnRH, resulting in suppression of estrogens and progestins with inhibition of ovulation and amenorrhea.

J. Miscellaneous effects

1. **Peptic ulcer**—The role of steroid excess in the production or reactivation of peptic ulcer disease is controversial. However, there appears to be a modest independent effect of glucocorticoids to promote peptic ulcer disease (relative risk about 1.4), and when this effect is combined with that of nonsteroidal anti-inflammatory drugs there is a synergistic interaction that considerably increases the risk.
2. **Ophthalmologic effects**—Intraocular pressure varies with the level of circulating glucocorticoids and parallels the circadian variation of plasma cortisol levels. In addition, glucocorticoids in excess increase intraocular pressure in patients with open-angle glaucoma. Glucocorticoid therapy may also cause cata-

ract formation. Central serous chorioretinopathy, an accumulation of subretinal detachment, may also complicate endogenous or exogenous glucocorticoid excess.

ADRENAL ANDROGENS

The direct biologic activity of the adrenal androgens (androstenedione, DHEA, and DHEA sulfate) is minimal, and they function primarily as precursors for peripheral conversion to the active androgenic hormones, testosterone and dihydrotestosterone. Thus, DHEA sulfate secreted by the adrenal androgens undergoes limited conversion to DHEA; this peripherally converted DHEA and that secreted by the adrenal cortex can be further converted in peripheral tissues to androstenedione, the immediate precursor of the active androgens.

The actions of testosterone and dihydrotestosterone are described in Chapter 12. This section will deal only with the adrenal contribution to androgenicity.

Effects in Males

In males with normal gonadal function, the conversion of adrenal androstenedione to testosterone accounts for less than 5% of the production rate of this hormone, and thus the physiologic effect is negligible. In adult males, excessive adrenal androgen secretion has no clinical consequences; however, in boys, it causes premature penile enlargement and early development of secondary sexual characteristics.

Effects in Females

In females, the adrenal substantially contributes to total androgen production by the peripheral conversion of androstenedione to testosterone. In the follicular phase of the menstrual cycle, adrenal precursors account for two-thirds of testosterone production and one-half of dihydrotestosterone production. During midcycle, the ovarian contribution increases, and the adrenal precursors account for only 40% of testosterone production.

In females, abnormal adrenal function as seen in Cushing syndrome, adrenal carcinoma, and congenital adrenal hyperplasia results in excessive secretion of adrenal androgens, and their peripheral conversion to testosterone results in androgen excess, manifested by acne, hirsutism, and virilization.

LABORATORY EVALUATION

Cortisol and the adrenal androgens are measured by specific plasma assays. Certain urinary assays, particularly measurement of 24-hour urine free cortisol, are also useful. In addition, plasma concentrations of ACTH can be determined. The assays for plasma steroids commonly used measure the total hormone concentrations and are therefore influenced by alterations in plasma-binding proteins. Furthermore, because ACTH and the plasma concentrations of the adrenal hormones fluctuate markedly (see Figure 9–7), single plasma measurements are frequently unreliable.

Thus, plasma levels must be interpreted cautiously, and more specific diagnostic information is usually obtained by performing appropriate dynamic tests (stimulation and suppression) or other tests that reflect cortisol secretory rate.

Plasma ACTH

A. Methods of measurement   Plasma ACTH measurements are extremely useful in the diagnosis of pituitary-adrenal dysfunction. The normal range for a plasma ACTH, using a sensitive immunoradiometric assay (IRMA) or immunochemiluminometric assay (ICMA), is 9 to 52 pg/mL (2-11.1 pmol/L).

B. Interpretation   Plasma ACTH levels are most useful in differentiating pituitary causes from adrenal causes of adrenal dysfunction as follows:

(1) In adrenal insufficiency due to primary adrenal disease, plasma ACTH levels are elevated. Conversely, in pituitary ACTH deficiency and secondary hypoadrenalism, plasma ACTH levels are inappropriately normal or less than 10 pg/mL (2.2 pmol/L).

(2) In Cushing syndrome due to primary glucocorticoid-secreting adrenal tumors, plasma ACTH is suppressed, and a level less than 5 pg/mL (1.1 pmol/L) is diagnostic. In patients with Cushing disease (pituitary ACTH hypersecretion), plasma ACTH levels are inappropriately normal or elevated.

(3) Plasma ACTH levels are usually markedly elevated in the ectopic ACTH syndrome, but there is a considerable amount of overlap with levels seen in Cushing disease. In addition, values lower than expected may be observed rarely in ectopic ACTH syndrome when the two-site immunoradiometric assay (IRMA) is used; this assay may not detect high-molecular-weight precursors of ACTH that can be produced in ectopic ACTH syndrome.

(4) Plasma ACTH levels are also elevated in patients with the common forms of congenital adrenal hyperplasia and are useful in the diagnosis and management of these disorders (see Chapters 10 and 14).

Plasma Cortisol

A. Methods of measurement   The most common methods of measurement of plasma cortisol are radioimmunoassay, enzyme-linked immunosorbent assay (ELISA), high-performance liquid chromatography (HPLC), and liquid chromatography tandem mass spectroscopy (LC/MS/MS). These methods measure total cortisol (both bound and free) in plasma. Most commonly used drugs and medications do not interfere with this assay. In contrast to radioimmunoassays, HPLC and LC/MS/MS do not demonstrate cross-reactivity with synthetic glucocorticoids.

B. Interpretation   The diagnostic utility of single plasma cortisol concentrations is limited by the episodic nature of cortisol secretion and its appropriate elevations during stress. As explained below, more information is obtained by dynamic testing of the HPA axis.

1. **Normal values**—Normal plasma cortisol levels vary with the method used and time of day the sample is obtained. With

radioimmunoassay, levels at 8 AM range from 3 to 20 μg/dL (80-550 nmol/L) and average 10 to 12 μg/dL (275.9-331.1 nmol/L). Values obtained later in the day are lower and at 4 PM are approximately half of morning values. At 10 PM to 2 AM, the plasma cortisol concentrations by these methods are usually less than 3 μg/dL (80 nmol/L).

2. **Levels during stress**—Cortisol secretion increases in patients who are acutely ill, during surgery, and following trauma. Plasma concentrations may reach greater than 40 to 60 μg/dL (1100-1655 nmol/L).

3. **High-estrogen states**—The total plasma cortisol concentration is also elevated with increased CBG-binding capacity, which occurs most commonly when circulating estrogen levels are high (eg, during pregnancy and when exogenous estrogens or oral contraceptives are being used). In these situations, plasma cortisol may reach levels two to three times normal.

4. **Other conditions**—CBG levels may be increased or decreased in other situations, as discussed above in the sections on circulation and metabolism. Total plasma cortisol concentrations may also be increased in severe anxiety, endogenous depression, starvation, anorexia nervosa, alcoholism, and chronic kidney disease.

Salivary Cortisol

Cortisol in the saliva is in equilibrium with the free and biologically active cortisol in the blood. Salivary cortisol concentrations are not affected by changes in serum cortisol–binding proteins, by salivary flow or composition, and they are stable at room temperature for many days. Measurements of salivary cortisol can be obtained from late-night, ambulatory saliva samples, which are used as a means of establishing the presence or absence of Cushing syndrome. Salivary cortisol may also be used to obtain accurate free cortisol levels in patients with abnormal serum-binding proteins.

A. Methods of measurement   Saliva can easily be sampled at home by the patient using a variety of techniques, including the use of a commercially available sampling device or by passive drooling. The same methods that are employed to measure plasma cortisol, radioimmunoassay, ELISA, HPLC, and LC/MS/MS, are used to measure salivary cortisol concentrations.

B. Interpretation

1. **Normal values**—Reference ranges for late-night salivary cortisol concentrations are dependent on the assays employed, but with radioimmunoassay and ELISA, the normal salivary cortisol level at midnight is generally less than 0.15 μg/dL (4 nmol/L).

2. **Diagnostic utility**—As with single plasma cortisol measurements, randomly obtained salivary cortisol concentrations are of limited use. However, plasma and salivary cortisol in normal individuals reach a nadir from 10 PM to 2 AM. Patients with Cushing syndrome do not reach a normal nadir at this time, and several studies have shown that elevated late-night time salivary cortisol is a sensitive and specific diagnostic test for Cushing syndrome.

Plasma Free Cortisol

This assay measures the free or biologically active fraction of plasma cortisol and, thus, is not influenced by alterations in corticosteroid-binding globulin and serum albumin. The best current method involves equilibrium dialysis to separate bound and free hormone followed by measurement of the free fraction by radioimmunoassay. In patients with normal serum albumin and CBG, the free cortisol correlates well with total cortisol levels; however, in patients with disturbances in plasma-binding proteins this correlation is lost.

Although this assay is not in common use, it is of importance in the assessment of adrenal function in patients with critical illness. In these patients the measurement of total plasma cortisol and its response to ACTH has overestimated the number of patients with adrenal insufficiency especially in the most severely ill patients who frequently have hypoalbuminemia and subnormal corticosteroid-binding globulin levels.

Urinary Corticosteroids

A. Free cortisol

1. **Methods of measurement**—The assay of unbound cortisol excreted in the urine is an excellent method for the diagnosis of Cushing syndrome. Normally, less than 1% of the secreted cortisol is excreted unchanged in the urine. However, in states of excess secretion, the binding capacity of CBG is exceeded, and plasma free cortisol therefore increases, as does its urinary excretion. Urine free cortisol is measured in a 24-hour urine collection by HPLC, radioimmunoassay, and by LC/MS/MS.

2. **Normal values**—HPLC and LC/MS/MS provide the most specific measurement of cortisol and are the current procedures of choice. The normal range for urine free cortisol assayed by HPLC or LC/MS/MS is 5 to 50 μg/24 h (14-135 nmol/24 h).

3. **Diagnostic utility**—This method is particularly useful in differentiating simple obesity from Cushing syndrome, because urine free cortisol levels are not elevated in obesity, as are the urinary 17-hydroxycorticosteroids (see later). The levels may be elevated in the same conditions that increase plasma cortisol (see earlier), including a slight elevation during pregnancy. This test is not useful in adrenal insufficiency, because it lacks sensitivity at low levels and because low cortisol excretion is often found in normal persons.

B. 17-Hydroxycorticosteroids

These urinary steroids are largely of historical interest and should not be measured at present because of the greater utility of plasma cortisol and urine free cortisol measurements.

Dexamethasone Suppression Tests

A. Low-Dose test

This procedure is used to establish the presence of Cushing syndrome regardless of its cause. Dexamethasone, a potent glucocorticoid, normally suppresses pituitary ACTH release with a resulting fall in plasma and urine cortisol, thus assessing feedback inhibition of the HPA axis. In Cushing syndrome, this mechanism is abnormal, and steroid secretion fails to be suppressed in the normal way. Dexamethasone in the doses used does not interfere with the measurement of plasma and urinary cortisol.

The overnight 1-mg dexamethasone suppression test is commonly used as a screening test for Cushing syndrome. Dexamethasone, 1 mg orally, is given as a single dose at 11:00 PM, and the following morning a plasma sample is obtained for cortisol determination. Cushing syndrome is probably excluded if the serum or plasma cortisol level is less than 1.8 μg/dL (50 nmol/L). Utilizing this criterion leads to very high sensitivity but also has an increased false-positive rate and results in a specificity of 80% to 90%.

Eighty to ninety-nine percent of patients with Cushing syndrome have abnormal responses. False-negative results are more common in mild hypercortisolism and may also occur in patients in whom dexamethasone metabolism is abnormally slow, because plasma levels of dexamethasone in these patients are higher than normally achieved and result in apparently normal suppression of cortisol. Simultaneous measurement of plasma dexamethasone and cortisol levels identifies these patients.

False-positive results occur in hospitalized and chronically ill patients. Acute illness, depression, anxiety, alcoholism, high-estrogen states, and uremia may also cause false-positive results. Patients taking phenytoin, barbiturates, and other inducers of hepatic microsomal enzymes may have accelerated metabolism of dexamethasone and thus fail to achieve adequate plasma levels to suppress ACTH.

B. High-dose tests

High-dose dexamethasone suppression testing has historically been used to differentiate Cushing disease (pituitary ACTH hypersecretion) from ectopic ACTH and adrenal tumors. This rationale has been based on the fact that in some patients with Cushing disease, the HPA axis is suppressible with supraphysiologic doses of glucocorticoids, whereas cortisol secretion is autonomous in patients with adrenal tumors and in most patients with the ectopic ACTH syndrome. Unfortunately, exceptions to these rules are so common that high-dose dexamethasone suppression testing must be interpreted with extreme caution.

1. **Overnight high-dose dexamethasone suppression test**—After a baseline morning cortisol specimen is obtained, a single dose of dexamethasone, 8 mg orally, is administered at 11:00 PM and plasma cortisol is measured at 8:00 AM the following morning. Generally, patients with Cushing disease suppress plasma cortisol level to less than 50% of baseline values—in contrast to patients with the ectopic ACTH syndrome, who fail to suppress to this level. Patients with cortisol-producing adrenal tumors also fail to suppress: their cortisol secretion is autonomous, and ACTH secretion is already suppressed by the high endogenous levels of cortisol.

2. **Two-day high-dose dexamethasone suppression test**—This test is performed by administering dexamethasone, 2 mg orally every 6 hours for 2 days. Twenty-four-hour urine samples are collected before and on the second day of dexamethasone administration. Patients with Cushing disease have a reduction of urine cortisol excretion to less than 50% of baseline values, whereas those with adrenal tumors or the ectopic ACTH syndrome usually have little or no reduction in urinary cortisol excretion. However, some patients with an ectopic ACTH-secreting neoplasm suppress steroid secretion with high doses of dexamethasone, and some patients with pituitary

ACTH-dependent Cushing syndrome fail to suppress to these levels. The diagnostic sensitivity, specificity, and accuracy of the high-dose dexamethasone suppression test are only about 80%. Better specificity and accuracy can be achieved by utilizing different criteria. However, it has become increasingly clear that high-dose dexamethasone suppression testing, regardless of the criteria employed, cannot distinguish pituitary from nonpituitary ACTH hypersecretion with certainty. Currently, the only biochemical test with a high enough diagnostic accuracy to distinguish between these causes is inferior petrosal sinus ACTH sampling.

Pituitary-Adrenal Reserve

These tests are used to evaluate the ability of the HPA axis to respond to stress. ACTH administration directly stimulates adrenal secretion; metyrapone inhibits cortisol synthesis, thereby stimulating pituitary ACTH secretion; and insulin-induced hypoglycemia stimulates ACTH release by increasing CRH secretion. More recently, CRH has been utilized to directly stimulate pituitary corticotrophs to release ACTH. The relative utility of these procedures is discussed below in the section on adrenocortical insufficiency and also in Chapter 4.

A. ACTH stimulation testing

1. **Procedure and normal values—High-dose ACTH stimulation test.** The rapid ACTH stimulation test measures the acute adrenal response to ACTH and is used to diagnose both primary and secondary adrenal insufficiency. A synthetic human α^{1-24}-ACTH called tetracosactin or cosyntropin is used. Fasting is not required, and the test may be performed at any time of the day. A baseline cortisol sample is obtained; cosyntropin is administered in a dose of 250 μg intramuscularly or intravenously; and additional samples for plasma cortisol are obtained at 30 or 60 minutes following the injection. Because the peak concentration of ACTH with this test achieves a pharmacologic level exceeding 10,000 pg/mL, this study assesses maximal adrenocortical capacity. The peak cortisol response, 30 to 60 minutes later, should exceed 18 to 20 μg/dL (>497-552 nmol/L). The 30-minute peak cortisol response to ACTH is constant and is unrelated to the basal cortisol level. In fact, there is no difference in the peak cortisol level at 30 minutes regardless of whether 250 μg, 5 μg, or even 1 μg of ACTH is administered. Early studies of the salivary or plasma free cortisol response to ACTH suggest that this method may be useful in patients with abnormal levels of cortisol-binding proteins.

   Low-dose ACTH stimulation test. Since the standard or high-dose test may be normal in patients with partial secondary adrenal insufficiency, a low-dose (1 μg) ACTH stimulation test was developed. Although some studies reported increased sensitivity and specificity, two meta-analyses did not establish a distinct advantage for the low-dose test.

   To perform the low-dose test appropriately it must be undertaken in the morning and the ACTH must be given intravenously. In addition, technical limitations are significant (ie, ACTH is available only in 250-μg vials, it is unstable in solution, and adheres to glass and plastic syringes and IV tubing). Thus, there are serious issues as to the accuracy of the dose of ACTH during reconstitution, dilution, and IV injection. For these reasons, the low-dose ACTH stimulation test is not practical for routine clinical practice.

2. **Subnormal responses**—If the cortisol response to the rapid ACTH stimulation test is inadequate, adrenal insufficiency is present. In primary adrenal insufficiency, destruction of cortical cells reduces cortisol secretion and increases pituitary ACTH secretion. Therefore, the adrenal is already maximally stimulated, and there is no further increase in cortisol secretion when exogenous ACTH is given; that is, there is decreased adrenal reserve. In secondary adrenal insufficiency due to ACTH deficiency, there is atrophy of the zonae fasciculata and reticularis, and the adrenal thus is either hyporesponsive or unresponsive to acute stimulation with exogenous ACTH. In either primary or secondary types, a subnormal response to the rapid ACTH stimulation test accurately predicts deficient responsiveness of the axis to insulin hypoglycemia, metyrapone, and surgical stress.

3. **Normal responses**—A normal response to the rapid ACTH stimulation test excludes both primary adrenal insufficiency (by directly assessing adrenal reserve) and overt secondary adrenal insufficiency with adrenal atrophy. However, a normal response does not rule out partial ACTH deficiency (decreased pituitary reserve) in patients whose basal ACTH secretion is sufficient to prevent adrenocortical atrophy and patients with recently developed secondary adrenal insufficiency who have not yet undergone adrenal atrophy. These patients may be unable to further increase ACTH secretion and thus may have subnormal pituitary ACTH responsiveness to stress or hypoglycemia. In such patients, further testing with metyrapone, hypoglycemia, or CRH may be indicated. For further discussion, see the section on diagnosis of adrenocortical insufficiency.

B. Metyrapone testing

Metyrapone testing has been used to diagnose adrenal insufficiency and to assess pituitary-adrenal reserve. The test procedures are detailed in Chapter 4. Metyrapone blocks cortisol synthesis by inhibiting the 11β-hydroxylase enzyme that converts 11-deoxycortisol to cortisol. This stimulates ACTH secretion, which in turn increases the secretion and plasma levels of 11-deoxycortisol. The overnight metyrapone test is most commonly used and is best suited to patients with suspected pituitary ACTH deficiency; patients with suspected primary adrenal failure are usually evaluated with the rapid ACTH stimulation test as described earlier and discussed in the section on diagnosis of adrenocortical insufficiency. The normal response to the overnight metyrapone test is a plasma 11-deoxycortisol level greater than 7 ng/dL (0.2 nmol/L) and a plasma ACTH level greater than 100 pg/mL (22 pmol/L) and indicates both normal ACTH secretion and adrenal function. A subnormal response establishes adrenocortical insufficiency. A normal response to metyrapone accurately predicts normal stress responsiveness of the hypothalamic-pituitary axis and correlates well with responsiveness to insulin-induced hypoglycemia. Metyrapone is only available directly from the manufacturer.

C. Insulin-induced hypoglycemia testing

The details of this procedure are described in Chapter 4. Hypoglycemia induces a central nervous system stress response, increases CRH release, and in this way increases ACTH and cortisol secretion. It therefore measures the integrity of the axis and its ability to respond to stress. The normal plasma cortisol response is an increment greater than 8 μg/dL (220 nmol/L) and a peak level greater than 18 to 20 μg/dL (497-552 nmol/L). The plasma ACTH response to hypoglycemia is usually greater than 100 pg/mL (22 pmol/L). A normal plasma cortisol response to hypoglycemia excludes adrenal insufficiency and decreased pituitary reserve. Thus, patients with normal responses do not require cortisol therapy during illness or surgery.

D. CRH testing   The procedure for CRH testing is described in Chapter 4. ACTH responses are exaggerated in patients with primary adrenal failure and absent in patients with hypopituitarism. Delayed responses may occur in patients with hypothalamic disorders. CRH testing has also been used to differentiate among the causes of Cushing syndrome (see later).

Androgens

Androgen excess is usually evaluated by the measurement of basal levels of these hormones, because suppression and stimulation tests are not as useful as in disorders affecting glucocorticoids. Assays are available for total plasma levels of DHEA, DHEA sulfate, androstenedione, testosterone, and dihydrotestosterone. Plasma-free testosterone (ie, testosterone not bound to SHBG) can be measured and is a more direct measure of circulating biologically active testosterone than the total plasma level, but commercially available methods vary widely in their accuracy (see Chapter 12).

DISORDERS OF ADRENOCORTICAL INSUFFICIENCY

Deficient adrenal production of glucocorticoids or mineralocorticoids results in adrenocortical insufficiency, which is either the consequence of destruction or dysfunction of the cortex (primary adrenocortical insufficiency, or Addison disease) or secondary to deficient pituitary ACTH secretion (secondary adrenocortical insufficiency). Glucocorticoid therapy is the most common cause of secondary adrenocortical insufficiency.

PRIMARY ADRENOCORTICAL INSUFFICIENCY (ADDISON DISEASE)

Etiology and Pathology (Figure 9–9)

The etiology of primary adrenocortical insufficiency has changed over time. Prior to 1920, tuberculosis was the major cause of adrenocortical insufficiency. Since 1950, autoimmune adrenalitis with adrenal atrophy has accounted for about 80% of cases. It is associated with a high incidence of other immunologic and autoimmune endocrine disorders (see later). Causes of primary adrenal insufficiency are listed in Table 9–3. Primary adrenocortical insufficiency, or Addison disease, is rare, with a reported prevalence of 35 to 140 per million population. When part of the polyglandular system, it is more common in females, with a female-male ratio of

approximately 2:1. Addison disease is usually diagnosed in the third to fifth decades.

A. Autoimmune adrenocortical insufficiency   Pathologically, the adrenals are small and atrophic, and the capsule is thickened. The adrenal medulla is preserved, although cortical cells are largely absent, show degenerative changes, and are surrounded by a fibrous stroma and the characteristic lymphocytic infiltrates.

Autoimmune Addison disease is frequently accompanied by other immune disorders. There are two different syndromes in which autoimmune adrenal insufficiency may occur. The best characterized one is known as autoimmune polyendocrinopathy-candidiasis-ectodermal dystrophy syndrome (APCED), or autoimmune polyglandular syndrome type 1 (APS-1). This is an autosomal recessive disorder that usually presents in childhood and is accompanied by hypoparathyroidism, adrenal failure, and mucocutaneous candidiasis. APS-1 results in most cases from a mutation of the autoimmune regulator gene (*AIRE*), which is located on chromosome 21q22.3. These patients have a defect in T-cell–mediated immunity, especially toward the candidal antigens. APS-1 has no relationship to human leukocyte antigen (HLA) and is often associated with hepatitis, dystrophy of dental enamel and nails, alopecia, vitiligo, and keratopathy and may be accompanied by hypofunction of the gonads, thyroid, pancreatic B cell, and gastric parietal cells. Autoantibodies against the cholesterol side chain cleavage enzyme (P450scc, CYP11A1) and others have been described in patients with this disorder.

The more common presentation of autoimmune adrenocortical insufficiency is associated with HLA-related disorders including type 1 diabetes mellitus and autoimmune thyroid disease. Other less common related disorders include alopecia areata, vitiligo, primary hypogonadism, pernicious anemia, and celiac disease. This disorder is often referred to as APS type 2. The genetic susceptibility to this disorder is linked to HLA-DR3 or DR4 (or both). These patients have antiadrenal cytoplasmic antibodies that may be important in the pathogenesis of this disorder, and autoantibodies directed against 21α-hydroxylase (P450c21, CYP21A2) have been identified (see Chapter 2).

B. Adrenal hemorrhage   Bilateral adrenal hemorrhage is a rare cause of adrenal insufficiency. The diagnosis is usually made in critically ill patients in whom a computed tomography (CT) scan of the abdomen is performed. Bilateral adrenal enlargement is found, leading to an assessment of adrenocortical function. Anatomic factors predispose the adrenal glands to hemorrhage. The adrenal glands have a rich arterial blood supply, but they are drained by a single vein. Adrenal vein thrombosis may occur during periods of stasis or turbulence, thereby increasing adrenal vein pressure and resulting in a *vascular dam*. This causes hemorrhage into the gland and is followed by adrenocortical insufficiency.

Most patients with adrenal hemorrhage have been taking anticoagulant therapy for an underlying coagulopathy or are predisposed to thrombosis. Heparin-induced thrombocytopenia syndrome may be accompanied by adrenal vein thrombosis and

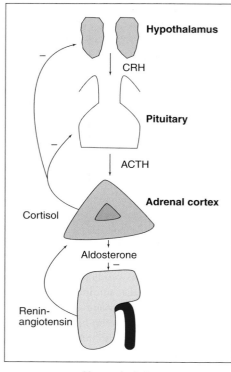

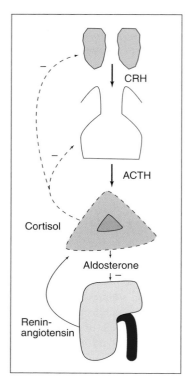

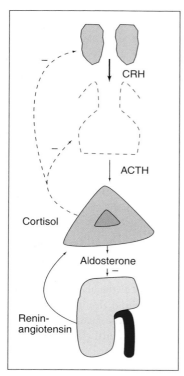

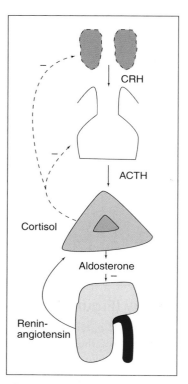

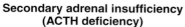

FIGURE 9–9 Hypothalamic-pituitary axis in adrenal insufficiency of different causes. These panels illustrate hormone secretion in the normal state (upper left), primary adrenal insufficiency (upper right), secondary adrenal insufficiency—ACTH deficiency (lower left), and tertiary adrenal insufficiency—CRH deficiency (lower right). Renin-angiotensin system is also illustrated. In contrast to normal secretion and hormone levels, decreased hormonal secretion is indicated by a dotted line and increased secretion by a dark solid line.

TABLE 9-3   Causes of primary adrenocortical insufficiency.

Autoimmune
Metastatic malignancy or lymphoma
Adrenal hemorrhage
Infectious
   Tuberculosis, CMV, fungi (histoplasmosis, coccidioidomycosis), HIV
Adrenoleukodystrophy
Infiltrative disorders
   Amyloidosis, hemochromatosis
Congenital adrenal hyperplasia
Familial glucocorticoid deficiency and hypoplasia
Drugs
   Ketoconazole, metyrapone, aminoglutethimide, trilostane,
   mitotane, etomidate

hemorrhage. The primary antiphospholipid antibody syndrome (lupus anticoagulant) has emerged as one of the more common causes of adrenal hemorrhage.

C. Infections   Although tuberculosis is a common cause of primary adrenal insufficiency in the rest of the world, it is a rare cause of this problem in the United States. Clinically significant adrenal insufficiency appears to occur in only about 5% of patients with disseminated tuberculosis. With the use of antituberculous chemotherapy, it may even be reversible if detected in early stages. It is important to recognize that rifampin may accelerate the metabolic clearance of cortisol, thereby increasing the replacement dose needed in these patients. Most if not all systemic fungal infections can involve and destroy the adrenal cortex. Tuberculosis and fungal infections are associated with enlarged adrenals that may show calcifications. Of note, the azole antifungal agents, such as ketoconazole, inhibit adrenal cytochrome P450 steroidogenic enzymes that are essential for cortisol biosynthesis. Thus, azole antifungal treatment, especially with ketoconazole, in patients with marginal adrenocortical reserve due to fungal disease may precipitate adrenal crisis.

HIV/AIDS has been associated with pathologic involvement of the adrenal gland. Although adrenal necrosis is commonly seen in postmortem examination of patients with AIDS, primary adrenal insufficiency appears to complicate only a few patients with this disorder. Primary adrenal insufficiency in AIDS is usually caused by opportunistic infections such as fungal infection, cytomegalovirus, and mycobacterium avium complex. Adrenocortical insufficiency usually occurs as a late manifestation in AIDS patients with very low CD4 counts (see Chapter 25).

D. Adrenoleukodystrophy   X-linked adrenoleukodystrophy is an important cause of adrenal insufficiency in men. This disorder represents two distinct entities that may cause malfunction of the adrenal cortex and demyelination in the central nervous system. These disorders are characterized by abnormally high levels of very long chain fatty acids (VLCFAs) due to their defective beta oxidation within peroxisomes. The abnormal accumulation of VLCFAs in the brain, adrenal cortex, testes, and liver result in the clinical manifestations of this disorder.

Adrenoleukodystrophy has an incidence of approximately one in 25,000 and is an X-linked disorder (chromosome Xq28) with incomplete penetrance. Molecular analysis is available clinically and can be used both in family screening and in prenatal evaluation. Two clinical phenotypes have been described. Cerebral adrenoleukodystrophy usually presents in childhood, and its neurologic symptoms include cognitive dysfunction, behavioral problems, emotional lability, and visual and gait disturbances. It may progress to dementia. Because 30% of these patients develop adrenal insufficiency before the onset of neurologic symptoms, a young man with primary adrenal insufficiency should always be screened for adrenoleukodystrophy. A clinically milder phenotype, adrenomyeloneuropathy, usually presents in the second to fourth decades of life. Spinal cord and peripheral nerve demyelination occur over years and may result in loss of ambulation, cognitive dysfunction, urinary retention, and impotence. Once again, adrenal insufficiency may occur before the onset of neurologic symptoms.

The diagnosis of adrenoleukodystrophy can be confirmed by demonstration of the defect in fatty acid metabolism with the abnormal accumulation of saturated VLCFAs, especially C26:0 fatty acid.

E. Metastatic adrenal disease   The adrenal glands are common sites of metastasis for lung, gastrointestinal, breast, and renal neoplasia. Bilateral adrenal involvement is present in approximately 50% of patients; however, adrenal insufficiency does not occur with unilateral metastatic disease. Even with bilateral involvement adrenal insufficiency appears to be uncommon. Despite being uncommon, patients with bilateral disease should be evaluated for adrenal insufficiency and then followed as adrenal insufficiency is a potentially life threating condition. In addition, non-Hodgkin and Hodgkin lymphoma may present with involvement of the adrenal glands with bilateral adrenal enlargement and primary adrenal insufficiency.

F. Familial glucocorticoid deficiency and congenital adrenal hypoplasia   Familial glucocorticoid deficiency is a rare disorder in which there is hereditary adrenocortical unresponsiveness to ACTH. This leads to adrenal insufficiency with subnormal glucocorticoid and adrenal androgen secretion as well as elevated plasma ACTH levels. As a rule, aldosterone secretion is preserved. At least two distinct types of this disorder have been described. One type is associated with mutations in the ACTH receptor on the cells of the adrenal cortex. Another type is often associated with achalasia and alacrima (Allgrove syndrome; triple A syndrome) and progressive neurologic impairment, but no mutations in the ACTH receptor have been seen in these patients. The responsible gene is on chromosome 12 (12q13) and encodes a protein belonging to the WD repeat proteins. Its function remains unknown. Congenital adrenal hypoplasia is a developmental abnormality usually presenting in the neonatal period. X-linked forms associated with mutations of DAX1 and autosomal recessive forms have been reported.

G. Cortisol resistance   Primary cortisol resistance is an unusual disorder representing target cell resistance to cortisol due to either qualitative or quantitative abnormalities of the glucocorticoid receptor. This disorder is characterized by hypercortisolism without clinical manifestations of glucocorticoid excess. Pituitary resistance to cortisol results in hypersecretion of ACTH, which stimulates the adrenal gland to produce excessive amounts of cortisol, mineralocorticoids, and adrenal androgens. The increased production of cortisol and these nonglucocorticoid adrenal steroids may cause hypertension, hypokalemia, virilization, and sexual precocity. Because cortisol is essential for life, this disorder actually represents partial rather than complete resistance.

H. Drug-induced adrenal insufficiency   Drugs associated with primary adrenal insufficiency include the azole antifungal agents, the anesthetic agent etomidate, the antiparasitic agent suramin as well as the steroid synthesis inhibitors aminoglutethimide, metyrapone, and mitotane. Mifepristone is a progesterone antagonist that also antagonizes the glucocorticoid receptor and may cause adrenal insufficiency if given in a sufficient dose. Megestrol acetate, a synthetic progesterone derivative used to stimulate appetite, binds to the glucocorticoid receptor and suppresses the HPA axis leading to adrenal insufficiency after withdrawal of therapy. Opioid narcotics cause a transient suppression of the HPA axis and can lead to suppression of plasma cortisol levels. Additionally, the use of protease inhibitors with exogenous glucocorticoids (from oral, injectable, inhaled, or even optic routes) can cause secondary adrenal insufficiency after cessation of glucocorticoid use.

I. Cortisol in critical illness   In 2002 it was reported that 77% of 299 patients with severe sepsis had plasma cortisol increments of less than 9 μg/dL to standard ACTH-stimulation testing. These patients were classified as having *relative adrenal insufficiency* (also termed *partial adrenal insufficiency* or *decreased adrenal reserve*) and randomized to therapy with hydrocortisone and fludrocortisones with a modest survival benefit. The study led to a widespread recommendation that all severely ill patients with sepsis be tested with ACTH and treated with corticosteroids. However, the study was compromised by two major issues. First, 30% of the patients classified as relatively adrenal insufficient had received etomidate (a drug which causes adrenal insufficiency) within 12 hours of enrollment. Second, the authors did not recognize that total plasma cortisol levels and their response to ACTH are lowered in severely ill patients who frequently have hypoalbuminemia and low corticosteroid-binding globulin levels. Subsequent studies have shown that both plasma free cortisol and salivary cortisol are appropriately elevated and respond normally to ACTH in patients with sepsis. In addition, several studies have shown no survival benefit following corticosteroid therapy. Thus, there is no convincing evidence that adrenal insufficiency is frequent in critically ill patients.

Pathophysiology

Loss of more than 90% of both adrenal cortices results in the clinical manifestations of adrenocortical insufficiency. Gradual destruction, such as occurs in the idiopathic and invasive forms of the disease, leads to chronic adrenocortical insufficiency. However,

more rapid destruction occurs in many cases; about 25% of patients are in crisis or impending crisis at the time of diagnosis. With gradual adrenocortical destruction, the initial phase is that of decreased adrenal reserve; that is, basal steroid secretion is normal, but secretion does not increase in response to stress. Thus, acute adrenal crisis can be precipitated by the stresses of surgery, trauma, or infection, which require increased corticosteroid secretion. With further loss of cortical tissue, even basal secretion of glucocorticoids becomes deficient, leading to the manifestations of chronic adrenocortical insufficiency. Mineralocorticoid deficiency may occur early or late in the course. Destruction of the adrenals by hemorrhage results in sudden loss of both glucocorticoid and mineralocorticoid secretion, accompanied by acute adrenal crisis.

With decreasing cortisol secretion, plasma levels of ACTH are increased because of decreased negative feedback inhibition of their secretion. In fact, an elevation of plasma ACTH may be the earliest and most sensitive indication of suboptimal adrenocortical reserve.

Clinical Features

A. Symptoms and signs   Cortisol deficiency causes weakness, fatigue, anorexia, nausea and vomiting, hypotension, hyponatremia, and hypoglycemia. Mineralocorticoid deficiency produces renal sodium wasting and potassium retention and can lead to severe dehydration, hypotension, hyponatremia, hyperkalemia, and acidosis.

1. Chronic primary adrenocortical insufficiency—The chief symptoms (Table 9–4) are hyperpigmentation, weakness and fatigue, weight loss, anorexia, and gastrointestinal disturbances.

Hyperpigmentation is the classic physical finding, and its presence in association with the above manifestations should suggest primary adrenocortical insufficiency. Generalized hyperpigmentation of the skin and mucous membranes is one of the earliest manifestations of Addison disease. It is increased in sun-exposed areas and accentuated over pressure areas such as the knuckles, toes, elbows, and knees. It is accompanied by increased numbers of black or dark-brown freckles. The classic hyperpigmentation of the buccal mucosa and gums is preceded by generalized hyperpigmentation of the skin; adrenal insufficiency should also be suspected when there is increased pigmentation of the palmar creases, nail beds, nipples, areolae,

TABLE 9–4 Clinical features of primary adrenocortical insufficiency.

	Percent
Weakness, fatigue, anorexia, weight loss	100
Hyperpigmentation	92
Hypotension	88
Gastrointestinal disturbances	56
Salt craving	19
Postural symptoms	12

Reproduced, with permission, from Baxter JD, Tyrrell JB. In: Felig P, Baxter JD, Frohman LA, eds. *Endocrinology and Metabolism*. 3rd ed. McGraw-Hill; 1995.

and perivaginal and perianal mucosa. Scars that have formed after the onset of ACTH excess become hyperpigmented, whereas older ones do not.

General weakness, fatigue and malaise, anorexia, and weight loss are invariable features of the disorder. Weight loss may reach 15 kg with progressive adrenal failure. Gastrointestinal disturbances, especially nausea and vomiting, occur in most patients; diarrhea is less frequent. An increase in gastrointestinal symptoms during an acute adrenal crisis may confuse the diagnosis by suggesting a primary intra-abdominal process.

Hypotension is present in about 90% of patients and is accompanied by orthostatic symptoms and occasionally syncope. In more severe chronic cases and in acute crises, recumbent hypotension or shock is almost invariably present. Vitiligo occurs in 4% to 17% of patients with autoimmune Addison disease but is rare in Addison disease due to other causes. Salt craving occurs in about 20% of patients.

Severe hypoglycemia may occur in children. This finding is unusual in adults but may be provoked by fasting, fever, infection, or nausea and vomiting, especially in acute adrenal crisis. Hypoglycemia occurs more commonly in secondary adrenal insufficiency.

Amenorrhea is common in Addison disease. It may be due to weight loss and chronic illness or to primary ovarian failure. Loss of axillary and pubic hair may occur in women as a result of decreased secretion of adrenal androgens.

Partial adrenal insufficiency may have subtle clinical manifestations. Adrenal insufficiency should be considered in the differential diagnosis of unexplained weight loss and in patients with hypotension and fever.

2. **Acute adrenal crisis**—Acute adrenal crisis represents a state of acute adrenocortical insufficiency and occurs in patients with Addison disease who are exposed to the stress of infection, trauma, surgery, or dehydration due to salt deprivation, vomiting, or diarrhea.

The symptoms are listed in Table 9–5. Anorexia and nausea and vomiting increase and worsen the volume depletion and dehydration. Hypovolemic shock frequently occurs, and adrenal insufficiency should be considered in any patient with unexplained vascular collapse. Abdominal pain may occur and mimic an acute abdominal emergency. Weakness, apathy, and confusion are common. Fever is also common and may be due to infection or to hypoadrenalism per se. Hyperpigmentation is present unless the onset of adrenal insufficiency is rapid and should suggest the diagnosis.

Additional findings that suggest the diagnosis are hyponatremia, hyperkalemia, lymphocytosis, eosinophilia, and hypoglycemia.

Shock and coma may rapidly lead to death in untreated patients (see Chapter 24).

TABLE 9–5 Clinical features of acute adrenal crisis.

Hypotension and shock
Fever
Dehydration, volume depletion
Nausea, vomiting, anorexia
Weakness, apathy, depressed mentation
Hypoglycemia

TABLE 9–6 Clinical features of adrenal hemorrhage.

	Percent
General features	
Hypotension and shock	74
Fever	59
Nausea and vomiting	46
Confusion, disorientation	41
Tachycardia	28
Cyanosis or lividity	28
Local features	
Abdominal, flank, or back pain	77
Abdominal or flank tenderness	38
Abdominal distention	28
Abdominal rigidity	20
Chest pain	13
Rebound tenderness	5

Reproduced, with permission, from Baxter JD, Tyrrell JB. In: Felig P, Baxter JD, Frohman LA, eds. *Endocrinology and Metabolism.* 3rd ed. McGraw-Hill; 1995.

3. **Acute adrenal hemorrhage (Table 9–6)**—Bilateral adrenal hemorrhage and acute adrenal destruction in an already compromised patient with major medical illness follow a progressively deteriorating course. The usual manifestations are abdominal, flank, or back pain and abdominal tenderness. Abdominal distention, rigidity, and rebound tenderness are less frequent. Hypotension, shock, fever, nausea and vomiting, confusion, and disorientation are common; tachycardia and cyanosis are less frequent.

With progression, severe hypotension, volume depletion, dehydration, hyperpyrexia, cyanosis, coma, and death ensue.

The diagnosis of acute adrenal hemorrhage should be considered in the deteriorating patient with unexplained abdominal or flank pain, vascular collapse, hyperpyrexia, or hypoglycemia, particularly in the setting of an underlying coagulopathy.

B. Laboratory and electrocardiographic findings and imaging studies

1. **Gradual adrenal destruction**—Hyponatremia and hyperkalemia are classic manifestations of the glucocorticoid and mineralocorticoid deficiency of primary adrenal insufficiency and should suggest the diagnosis. Hematologic manifestations include normocytic, normochromic anemia, neutropenia, eosinophilia, and a relative lymphocytosis. Azotemia with increased concentrations of blood urea nitrogen and serum creatinine is due to volume depletion and dehydration. Mild acidosis is frequently present. Hypercalcemia of mild to moderate degree occurs in about 6% of patients.

Abdominal radiographs reveal adrenal calcification in half the patients with tuberculous Addison disease and in some patients with other invasive or hemorrhagic causes of adrenal insufficiency. CT is a more sensitive detector of adrenal calcification and adrenal enlargement. Bilateral adrenal enlargement in association with adrenal insufficiency may be seen with tuberculosis, fungal infections, cytomegalovirus, malignant and nonmalignant infiltrative diseases, and adrenal hemorrhage.

Electrocardiographic features are low voltage, a vertical QRS axis, and nonspecific ST-T wave abnormalities secondary to abnormal electrolytes.

2. Acute adrenal hemorrhage—Hyponatremia and hyperkalemia occur in only a small number of cases, but azotemia is a usual finding. Increased circulating eosinophils may suggest the diagnosis. The diagnosis is frequently established only when imaging studies reveal bilateral adrenal enlargement.

SECONDARY ADRENOCORTICAL INSUFFICIENCY

Etiology

Secondary adrenocortical insufficiency due to ACTH deficiency is most commonly a result of exogenous glucocorticoid therapy. Pituitary or hypothalamic tumors are the most common causes of naturally occurring pituitary ACTH hyposecretion. These and other less common causes are reviewed in Chapter 4.

Pathophysiology

ACTH deficiency is the primary event and leads to decreased cortisol and adrenal androgen secretion. Aldosterone secretion remains normal except in a few cases. In the early stages, basal ACTH and cortisol levels may be normal; however, ACTH reserve is impaired, and ACTH and cortisol responses to stress are, therefore, subnormal. With further loss of basal ACTH secretion, there is atrophy of the zonae fasciculata and reticularis of the adrenal cortex; and, therefore, basal cortisol secretion is decreased. At this stage, the entire pituitary adrenal axis is impaired; that is, there is not only decreased ACTH responsiveness to stress but also decreased adrenal responsiveness to acute stimulation with exogenous ACTH.

The manifestations of glucocorticoid deficiency are similar to those described for primary adrenocortical insufficiency. However, because aldosterone secretion by the zona glomerulosa is usually preserved, the manifestations of mineralocorticoid deficiency are absent.

Clinical Features

A. Symptoms and signs   Secondary adrenal insufficiency is usually chronic, and the manifestations may be nonspecific. However, acute crisis can occur in undiagnosed patients or in corticosteroid-treated patients who do not receive increased steroid dosage during periods of stress.

The clinical features of secondary adrenal insufficiency differ from those of primary adrenocortical insufficiency in that pituitary secretion of ACTH is deficient and hyperpigmentation is, therefore, not present. In addition, mineralocorticoid secretion is usually normal. Thus, the clinical features of ACTH and glucocorticoid deficiency are nonspecific.

Volume depletion, dehydration, and hyperkalemia are usually absent. Hypotension is usually not present except in acute presentations. Hyponatremia may occur, as a result of water retention and inability to excrete a water load, but is not accompanied by hyperkalemia. Prominent features are weakness, lethargy, easy fatigability, anorexia, nausea, and occasionally vomiting. Arthralgias

and myalgias also occur. Hypoglycemia is occasionally the presenting feature. Acute decompensation with severe hypotension or shock unresponsive to vasopressors may occur.

B. Associated features   Patients with secondary adrenal insufficiency commonly have additional features that suggest the diagnosis. A history of glucocorticoid therapy, or if this is not available, the presence of cushingoid features suggests prior glucocorticoid use. Hypothalamic or pituitary tumors leading to ACTH deficiency usually cause loss of other pituitary hormones (hypogonadism and hypothyroidism). Hypersecretion of GH or prolactin (PRL) from a pituitary adenoma may be present.

C. Laboratory findings   Findings on routine laboratory examination consist of normochromic, normocytic anemia, neutropenia, lymphocytosis, and eosinophilia. Hyponatremia is not uncommon and may be the presenting laboratory abnormality. Hyponatremia is due to the lack of glucocorticoid-negative feedback on AVP as well as the reduction in glomerular filtration associated with hypocortisolism. Serum potassium, creatinine, and bicarbonate and blood urea nitrogen are usually normal; plasma glucose may be low, although severe hypoglycemia is unusual.

DIAGNOSIS OF ADRENOCORTICAL INSUFFICIENCY

Although the diagnosis of adrenal insufficiency should be confirmed by assessment of the pituitary adrenal axis, therapy should not be delayed, and the patient should not be subjected to procedures that may increase volume loss and dehydration and further contribute to hypotension. If the patient is acutely ill, therapy should be instituted and the diagnosis established when the patient is stable.

Diagnostic Tests

Because basal levels of adrenocortical steroids in either urine or plasma may be normal in partial adrenal insufficiency, tests of adrenocortical reserve are necessary to establish the diagnosis (Figure 9–10). These tests are described in the section on laboratory evaluation and in Chapter 4.

Rapid ACTH Stimulation Test

The rapid ACTH stimulation test assesses adrenal reserve and is the initial procedure in the assessment of possible adrenal insufficiency, either primary or secondary. As previously discussed, the low-dose ACTH (1-μg cosyntropin) stimulation test has been suggested to represent a more physiologic stimulus to the adrenal cortex; however, many experienced clinicians continue to employ the standard 250-μg cosyntropin dose.

Subnormal responses to exogenous ACTH administration are an indication of decreased adrenal reserve and establish the diagnosis of adrenocortical insufficiency. Further diagnostic procedures

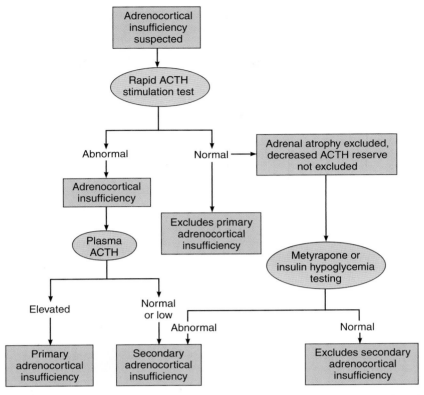

FIGURE 9–10 Evaluation of suspected primary or secondary adrenocortical insufficiency. Boxes enclose clinical decisions, and circles enclose diagnostic tests. (Redrawn and reproduced, with permission, from Miller WL, Tyrrell JB. The adrenal cortex. In: Felig P, et al, eds. *Endocrinology and Metabolism.* McGraw-Hill; 1995.)

are not required, because subnormal responses to the rapid ACTH stimulation test indicate lack of responsiveness to metyrapone, insulin-induced hypoglycemia, or stress. However, this test does not permit differentiation of primary and secondary causes. This is best accomplished by measurement of basal plasma ACTH levels, as discussed later.

A normal response to the rapid ACTH stimulation test excludes primary adrenal failure, because a normal cortisol response indicates normal cortical function. However, normal responsiveness does not exclude partial secondary adrenocortical insufficiency in those few patients with decreased pituitary reserve and decreased stress responsiveness of the HPA axis who maintain sufficient basal ACTH secretion to prevent adrenocortical atrophy. If this situation is suspected clinically, pituitary ACTH responsiveness may be tested directly with metyrapone or insulin-induced hypoglycemia (see section "Laboratory Evaluation" and below).

Plasma ACTH Levels

If adrenal insufficiency is present, plasma ACTH levels are used to differentiate primary and secondary forms. In patients with primary adrenal insufficiency, plasma ACTH levels exceed the upper limit of the normal range (>52 pg/mL [11 pmol/L]) and usually exceed 200 pg/mL (44 pmol/L). Plasma ACTH

concentrations are inappropriately normal or less than 10 pg/mL (2.2 pmol/L) in patients with secondary adrenal insufficiency (Figure 9–11). However, basal ACTH levels must always be interpreted in light of the clinical situation, especially because of the episodic nature of ACTH secretion and its short plasma half-life. For example, ACTH levels frequently exceed the normal range during the recovery of the HPA axis from secondary adrenal insufficiency and may be confused with levels seen in primary adrenal insufficiency. Patients with primary adrenal insufficiency consistently have elevated ACTH levels. In fact, the ACTH concentration is elevated early in the course of adrenal insufficiency even before a significant reduction in the basal cortisol level or its response to exogenous ACTH occurs. Therefore, plasma ACTH measurements serve as a valuable screening study for primary adrenal insufficiency.

Partial ACTH Deficiency

When partial ACTH deficiency and decreased pituitary reserve are suspected despite normal responsiveness to the rapid ACTH stimulation test, the following procedures may be used for more direct assessment of hypothalamic-pituitary function.

A. Methods of testing The overnight metyrapone test is used in patients with suspected hypothalamic or pituitary disorders when

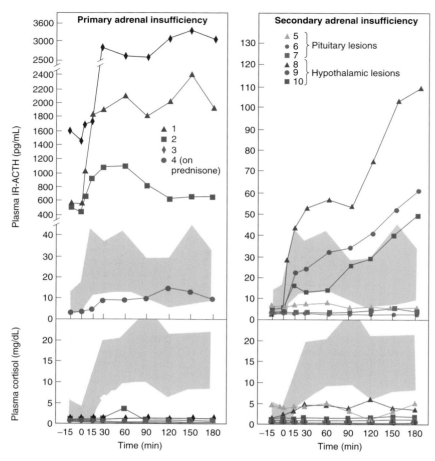

FIGURE 9–11 Plasma ACTH (top) and cortisol (bottom) responses to CRH in subjects with primary adrenal insufficiency (left) or secondary adrenal insufficiency (right). Patients with hypothalamic lesions had clearly distinct ACTH responses to CRH, different from those in three patients with pituitary adrenal insufficiency. **Shaded area:** Absolute range from 15 normal subjects. (IR-ACTH, ACTH by IRMA.) (Reproduced, with permission, from Schulte HM, et al. The corticotropin-releasing hormone stimulation test: a possible aid in the evaluation of patients with adrenal insufficiency. *J Clin Endocrinol Metab.* 1984;58:1064.)

hypoglycemia is contraindicated and in those with prior glucocorticoid therapy. Insulin-induced hypoglycemia is used in patients with suspected hypothalamic or pituitary tumors, because both ACTH and GH responsiveness can be assessed (see Chapter 4).

B. Interpretation   A normal response to either metyrapone or hypoglycemia excludes secondary adrenocortical insufficiency (see section "Laboratory Evaluation"). Subnormal responses, even in the presence of a normal response to ACTH administration, establish the diagnosis of secondary adrenal insufficiency.

TREATMENT OF ADRENOCORTICAL INSUFFICIENCY

The aim of treatment of adrenocortical insufficiency is to produce levels of glucocorticoids and mineralocorticoids equivalent to those achieved in an individual with normal HPA function under similar circumstances.

Acute Addisonian Crisis (Table 9–7)

Treatment for acute Addisonian crisis should be instituted as soon as the diagnosis is suspected. Therapy includes administration of glucocorticoids; correction of dehydration, hypovolemia, and

TABLE 9–7 Treatment of acute adrenal crisis.

Glucocorticoid replacement
(1) Administer hydrocortisone sodium phosphate or sodium succinate, 100 mg intravenously every 6 h for 24 h
(2) When the patient is stable, reduce the dosage to 50 mg every 6 h
(3) Taper to maintenance therapy by day 4 or 5 and add mineralocorticoid therapy as required
(4) Maintain or increase the dose to 200-400 mg/d if complications persist or occur

General and supportive measures
(1) Correct volume depletion, dehydration, and hypoglycemia with intravenous saline and glucose
(2) Evaluate and correct infection and other precipitating factors

electrolyte abnormalities; general supportive measures; and treatment of coexisting or precipitating disorders.

A. Cortisol (Hydrocortisone)   Parenteral cortisol in soluble form (hydrocortisone hemisuccinate or phosphate) is the glucocorticoid preparation most commonly used. When administered in supraphysiologic doses, hydrocortisone has sufficient sodium-retaining potency so that additional mineralocorticoid therapy is not required in patients with primary adrenocortical insufficiency.

Cortisol in intravenous doses of 100 mg is given every 6 hours for the first 24 hours. The response to therapy is usually rapid, with improvement occurring within 12 hours or less. If improvement occurs and the patient is stable, 50 mg every 6 hours is given on the second day, and in most patients the dosage may then be gradually reduced to approximately 10 mg two to three times daily by the fourth or fifth day (see section "Maintenance Therapy," later).

1. In severely ill patients, especially in those with additional major complications (eg, sepsis), higher cortisol doses (100 mg intravenously every 6-8 hours) are maintained until the patient is stable.
2. In primary Addison disease, mineralocorticoid replacement, in the form of fludrocortisone (see later), is usually added when hydrocortisone replacement is reduced to near physiological levels.
3. In secondary adrenocortical insufficiency with acute crisis, the primary requirement is glucocorticoid replacement and is satisfactorily supplied by the administration of cortisol, as outlined above. If the possibility of excessive fluid and sodium retention in such patients is of concern, equivalent parenteral doses of synthetic steroids such as prednisolone or dexamethasone may be substituted.

B. Intravenous fluids   Intravenous glucose and saline are administered to correct volume depletion, hypotension, and hypoglycemia. Volume deficits may be severe in Addison disease, and hypotension and shock may not respond to vasopressors unless glucocorticoids are administered. Hyperkalemia and acidosis are usually corrected with cortisol and volume replacement; however, an occasional patient may require specific therapy for these abnormalities (see also Chapter 24).

Maintenance Therapy (Table 9–8)

Patients with Addison disease require life-long glucocorticoid and mineralocorticoid therapy. Cortisol (hydrocortisone) is the glucocorticoid preparation of choice. The basal production rate of cortisol is approximately 8 to 12 mg/m^2/d. The maintenance dose of hydrocortisone is usually 15 to 25 mg daily in adults. The oral dose is usually divided into 10 to 15 mg in the morning on arising and 5 to 10 mg later in the day. Cortisol in twice-daily doses gives satisfactory responses in most patients; however, some patients may require only a single morning dose, and others may require three doses daily (eg, 10-5-5) to maintain well-being and normal energy levels. Insomnia is a side-effect of glucocorticoid

TABLE 9– 8 Regimen for maintenance therapy of primary adrenocortical insufficiency.

(1) Hydrocortisone, 10-15 mg in AM, 5-10 mg in the afternoon (4-5 PM)
(2) Fludrocortisone, 0.05-0.1 mg orally in AM
(3) Clinical follow-up: maintenance of normal weight, blood pressure, and electrolytes with regression of clinical features
(4) Patient education plus identification card, medical alert bracelet or necklace (*dog tag*). Useful patient education materials are available from the National Institutes of Health. http://www.cc.nih.gov/ccc/patient_education/pepubs/mngadrins.pdf
(5) Increase hydrocortisone dosage during stress. Double the oral dose for mild illness. Provide patient with injectable form of glucocorticoid for emergency use

administration and can usually be prevented by administering the last dose in the early afternoon.

Fludrocortisone (9α-fluorocortisol) is used for mineralocorticoid therapy; the usual doses are 0.05 to 0.2 mg/d orally in the morning. Because of the long half-life of this agent, divided doses are not required. About 10% of addisonian patients can be managed with cortisol and adequate dietary sodium intake alone and do not require fludrocortisone.

Secondary adrenocortical insufficiency is treated with the cortisol dosages described above for the primary form. Fludrocortisone is rarely required. The recovery of normal function of the HPA axis following suppression by exogenous glucocorticoids may take weeks to years, and its duration is not readily predictable. Consequently, prolonged replacement therapy may be required. Recent studies in women have pointed to the potential benefits of DHEA in doses of 50 mg/d in terms of improvement in well-being, although this remains controversial.

Response to Therapy

General clinical signs, such as good appetite and sense of well-being, are the guides to the adequacy of replacement. Obviously, signs of Cushing syndrome indicate overtreatment. It is generally expected that the daily dose of hydrocortisone should be doubled during periods of minor stress, and the dose needs to be increased to as much as 200 to 300 mg/d during periods of major stress, such as a surgical procedure. Patients receiving excessive doses of glucocorticoids are also at risk for increased bone loss and clinically significant osteoporosis. Therefore, the replacement dose of glucocorticoid should be maintained at the lowest amount needed to provide the patient with a proper sense of well-being. Two major factors have prompted a reassessment of the issue of appropriateness and possible excess glucocorticoid replacement for patients with adrenal insufficiency. First, there is a greater appreciation of the potential risks of overtreatment or undertreatment. Recent evidence suggests that subclinical Cushing syndrome associated with adrenal incidentalomas contributes to poor control of blood sugar and blood pressure in diabetic patients, decreased bone density, and increased serum lipid levels. The levels of cortisol secretion by many incidentalomas are similar to those observed in patients with adrenal insufficiency receiving mild cortisol overreplacement. In addition, studies in patients receiving glucocorticoid replacement therapy demonstrate an inverse relationship between dose and bone mineral density and a positive correlation between dose and markers of bone resorption. Second, there is recognition that there is considerable variation among individuals in terms of the plasma levels of cortisol achieved with orally administered hydrocortisone or cortisol.

The measurement of urine free cortisol does not provide a reliable index for appropriate glucocorticoid replacement. Similarly, ACTH measurements are not a good indication of the adequacy of glucocorticoid replacement; marked elevations of plasma ACTH in patients with chronic adrenal insufficiency are often not suppressed into the normal range despite adequate hydrocortisone replacement. In fact, plasma ACTH values that fall to low normal or low levels suggest overreplacement with glucocorticoids. Plasma cortisol day curves—multiple samples for plasma cortisol concentration—have been proposed but not yet widely adopted. Therefore, it is prudent to use clinical assessment of the patient's response to therapy, rather than biochemical criteria, to gauge the adequacy of steroid replacement.

Adequate treatment results in the disappearance of weakness, malaise, and fatigue. Anorexia and other gastrointestinal symptoms resolve, and weight returns to normal. The hyperpigmentation invariably improves but may not entirely disappear. Inadequate cortisol administration leads to persistence of these symptoms of adrenal insufficiency, and excessive pigmentation remains.

Adequate mineralocorticoid replacement may be determined by assessment of blood pressure and electrolyte composition. With adequate treatment, the blood pressure is normal without orthostatic change, and serum sodium and potassium remain within the normal range. Some endocrinologists monitor plasma renin activity (PRA) as an objective measure of fludrocortisone replacement. Upright PRA levels are usually less than 5 ng/mL/h in adequately replaced patients. Hypertension and hypokalemia result if the fludrocortisone dose is excessive. Conversely, undertreatment may lead to fatigue and malaise, orthostatic symptoms, and subnormal supine or upright blood pressure, with hyperkalemia and hyponatremia.

Prevention of Adrenal Crisis

The development of acute adrenal insufficiency in previously diagnosed and treated patients is almost entirely preventable in compliant individuals. The essential elements are patient education and increased glucocorticoid dosages during illness.

The patient should be informed about the necessity for lifelong therapy, the possible consequences of acute illness, and the necessity for increased therapy and medical assistance during acute illness. An identification card or bracelet should be carried or worn at all times.

The cortisol dose should be increased by the patient to 60 to 80 mg/d with the development of minor illnesses; the usual maintenance dosage may be resumed in 24 to 48 hours if improvement occurs. Increased mineralocorticoid therapy is not required.

If symptoms persist or become worse, the patient should continue increased cortisol doses and call the physician.

TABLE 9–9   Steroid coverage for surgery.

(1) Correct electrolytes, blood pressure, and hydration if necessary
(2) Give hydrocortisone sodium phosphate or sodium succinate, 100 mg intramuscularly, on call to operating room
(3) Give 50 mg intramuscularly or intravenously in the recovery room and then every 6 h for the first 24 h
(4) If progress is satisfactory, reduce dosage to 25 mg every 6 h for 24 h and then taper to maintenance dosage over 3-5 d. Resume previous fludrocortisone dose when the patient is taking oral medications
(5) Maintain or increase hydrocortisone dosage to 200-400 mg/d if fever, hypotension, or other complications occur

Reproduced, with permission, from Miller WL, Tyrrell JB. In: Felig P, Baxter JD, Frohman LA, eds. *Endocrinology and Metabolism.* 3rd ed. McGraw-Hill; 1995.

Vomiting may result in inability to ingest or absorb oral cortisol, and diarrhea in addisonian patients may precipitate a crisis because of rapid fluid and electrolyte losses. Patients must understand that if these symptoms occur, they should seek immediate medical assistance so that parenteral glucocorticoid therapy can be given.

Steroid Coverage for Surgery (Table 9–9)

The normal physiologic response to surgical stress involves an increase in cortisol secretion. The increased glucocorticoid activity may serve primarily to modulate the immunologic response to stress. Thus, patients with primary or secondary adrenocortical insufficiency scheduled for elective surgery require increased glucocorticoid coverage. This problem is most frequently encountered in patients with pituitary-adrenal suppression due to exogenous glucocorticoid therapy. The principles of management are outlined in Table 9–9.

PROGNOSIS OF ADRENOCORTICAL INSUFFICIENCY

Before glucocorticoid and mineralocorticoid therapy became available, primary adrenocortical insufficiency was invariably fatal, with death usually occurring within 2 years after onset. Survival now depends on the underlying cause of the adrenal insufficiency. In patients with autoimmune Addison disease, survival approaches that of the normal population, and most patients lead normal lives. In general, death from adrenal insufficiency now occurs only in patients with rapid onset of disease who may die before the diagnosis is established and appropriate therapy started.

Secondary adrenal insufficiency has an excellent prognosis with glucocorticoid therapy. Adrenal insufficiency due to bilateral adrenal hemorrhage may be fatal, with some cases being recognized only at autopsy.

CUSHING SYNDROME

Chronic glucocorticoid excess, whatever its cause, leads to the constellation of symptoms and physical features known as **Cushing syndrome**. It is most commonly iatrogenic, resulting

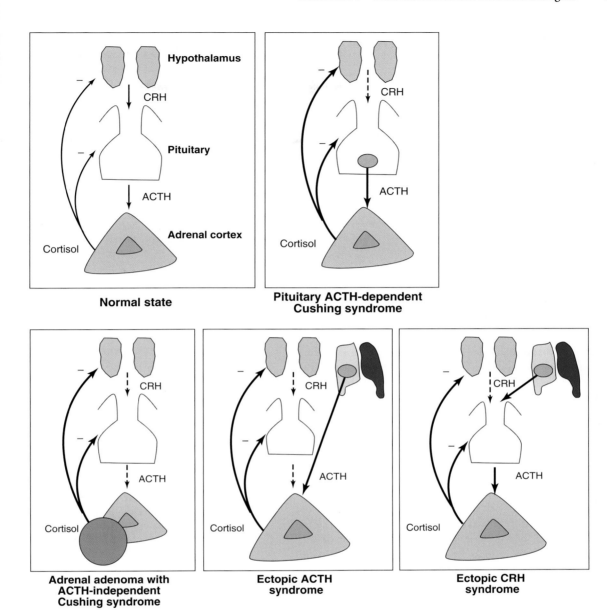

FIGURE 9–12 Hypothalamic-pituitary axis in Cushing syndrome of different causes. These panels illustrate hormone secretion in the normal state (upper left), and four types of cortisol excess: Pituitary ACTH-dependent (with an ACTH-secreting pituitary tumor) (upper right), adrenal tumor (lower left), ectopic ACTH syndrome due to an ACTH-secreting lung cancer (lower middle), and ectopic CRH syndrome due to a CRH-secreting lung tumor. In contrast to normal secretion and hormone levels, decreased hormonal secretion is indicated by a dotted line and increased secretion by a dark solid line.

from chronic glucocorticoid therapy. Spontaneous Cushing syndrome is caused by abnormalities of the pituitary or adrenal gland or may occur as a consequence of ACTH or CRH secretion by nonpituitary tumors (**ectopic ACTH syndrome; ectopic CRH syndrome**) (Figure 9–12). **Cushing disease** is defined as the specific type of Cushing syndrome due to excessive pituitary ACTH secretion from a pituitary tumor. This section will review the various types of spontaneous Cushing syndrome and discuss their diagnosis and therapy (see also Chapter 4).

Classification and Incidence

Cushing syndrome is conveniently classified as either ACTH dependent or ACTH independent (Table 9–10). The ACTH-dependent types of Cushing syndrome—ectopic ACTH syndrome and Cushing disease—are characterized by chronic ACTH hypersecretion, which results in hyperplasia of the adrenal zonae fasciculata and reticularis and, therefore, increased secretion of cortisol, androgens, and DOC.

TABLE 9–10 Cushing syndrome: differential diagnosis.

ACTH-dependent
Pituitary adenoma (Cushing disease)
Nonpituitary neoplasm (ectopic ACTH)

ACTH-independent
Iatrogenic (glucocorticoid, megestrol acetate)
Adrenal neoplasm (adenoma, carcinoma)
Nodular adrenal hyperplasia
  Primary pigmented nodular adrenal disease (PPNAD)
  Massive macronodular adrenonodular hyperplasia
  Food dependent (GIP mediated)
  Factitious

ACTH-independent Cushing syndrome may be caused by a primary adrenal neoplasm (adenoma or carcinoma) or nodular adrenal hyperplasia. In these cases, the cortisol excess suppresses pituitary ACTH secretion.

A. Cushing disease   This is the most frequent type of Cushing syndrome and is responsible for about 80% of reported cases. Cushing disease is much more common in women than in men (female-male ratio of about 5:1) and the age at diagnosis is usually 20 to 40 years but may range from childhood to 70 years.

B. Ectopic ACTH hypersecretion   This disorder accounts for approximately 10% of patients with ACTH-dependent Cushing syndrome. The production of ACTH from a tumor of nonpituitary origin may result in severe hypercortisolism, but many of these patients lack the classic features of glucocorticoid excess. This presumably reflects the acuteness of the clinical course in the ectopic ACTH syndrome. The clinical presentation of ectopic ACTH secretion is most frequently seen in patients with tumors of a thoracic origin. Bronchial carcinoid and small cell lung carcinoma are responsible for about 50% of cases of this syndrome. The prognosis in patients with the ectopic ACTH syndrome is generally poor and largely a function of the primary tumor. Individuals with ectopic ACTH syndrome from small cell lung carcinoma have a mean survival of less than 12 months. The ectopic ACTH syndrome may also present in a fashion identical to classic Cushing disease and pose a challenging diagnostic dilemma. A wide variety of tumors has been reported to produce ectopic ACTH and may be radiologically inapparent at the time of the presentation. The ectopic ACTH syndrome is more common in men, and the peak age incidence is 40 to 60 years.

C. Primary adrenal tumors   Primary adrenal tumors cause approximately 10% of cases of Cushing syndrome. Most of these patients have benign adrenocortical adenomas. Adrenocortical carcinomas are uncommon, with an incidence of approximately 2 per million per year. Both adrenocortical adenomas and carcinomas are more common in women. Autonomous cortisol secretion without the classic features of Cushing syndrome occurs in about 5% of patients with adrenal incidentalomas (see later).

D. Childhood cushing syndrome   Cushing disease is more common in the adolescent population than in younger children. Most pediatric cases occur in patients over 10 years of age with an equal distribution between the sexes. Cushing disease remains the most common cause accounting for more than 80% of cases. Primary adrenal disease accounts for an additional 10% to 15% of all pediatric cases.

Pathology

A. Anterior pituitary gland

1. **Pituitary adenomas**—Pituitary adenomas are present in over 90% of patients with Cushing disease. These tumors are typically smaller than those secreting GH or PRL; 80% to 90% are less than 10 mm in diameter. A small group of patients have larger tumors (>10 mm); these macroadenomas are frequently invasive, leading to extension outside the sella turcica. Malignant pituitary tumors occur rarely.

   Microadenomas are located within the anterior pituitary; they are not encapsulated but surrounded by a rim of compressed normal anterior pituitary cells. With routine histologic stains, these tumors are composed of compact sheets of well-granulated basophilic cells in a sinusoidal arrangement. ACTH, β-lipotropin (LPH), and β-endorphin have been demonstrated in these tumor cells by immunocytochemical methods. Larger tumors may appear chromophobic on routine histologic study; however, they also contain ACTH and its related peptides. These ACTH-secreting adenomas typically show Crooke changes (a zone of perinuclear hyalinization that is the result of chronic exposure of corticotroph cells to hypercortisolism). Electron microscopy demonstrates secretory granules that vary in size from 200 to 700 nm. The number of granules varies in individual cells; they may be dispersed throughout the cytoplasm or concentrated along the cell membrane. A typical feature of these adenomas is the presence of bundles of perinuclear microfilaments (average 7 nm in diameter) surrounding the nucleus; these are responsible for Crooke hyaline changes visible on light microscopy.

2. **Hyperplasia**—Diffuse hyperplasia of corticotroph cells has been reported rarely in patients with Cushing disease.

3. **Other conditions**—In patients with adrenal tumors or ectopic ACTH syndrome, the pituitary corticotrophs show prominent Crooke hyaline changes and perinuclear microfilaments. The ACTH content of corticotroph cells is reduced consistent with their suppression by excessive cortisol secretion present in these conditions.

B. Adrenocortical hyperplasia
Bilateral hyperplasia of the adrenal cortex occurs with chronic ACTH hypersecretion. Two types have been described: simple and bilateral nodular hyperplasia.

1. **Simple adrenocortical hyperplasia**—This condition is usually due to Cushing disease. Combined adrenal weight (normal, 8-10 g) is modestly increased, ranging from 12 to 24 g. On histologic study, there is equal hyperplasia of the compact cells of the zona reticularis and the clear cells of the zona fasciculata; consequently, the width of the cortex is increased. Electron microscopy reveals normal ultrastructural features. When ACTH levels are very high as in the ectopic ACTH syndrome, the adrenals are frequently larger, with combined weights up to or more than 50 g. The characteristic microscopic

feature is marked hyperplasia of the zona reticularis; columns of compact reticularis cells expand throughout the zona fasciculata and into the zona glomerulosa. The zona fasciculata clear cells are markedly reduced.

2. **Bilateral nodular hyperplasia**—Bilateral nodular hyperplasia with Cushing syndrome has been identified as a morphologic consequence of several unique pathophysiologic disorders. Longstanding ACTH hypersecretion—either pituitary or nonpituitary—may result in nodular enlargement of the adrenal gland. These focal nodules are often mistaken for adrenal neoplasms and have led to unnecessary as well as unsuccessful unilateral adrenal surgery. In occasional cases these nodules may, over a period of time, even become autonomous or semiautonomous. Removal of the ACTH-secreting neoplasm results in regression of the adrenal nodules as well as resolution of hypercortisolism unless the nodules have already developed significant autonomy.

Several types of ACTH-independent nodular adrenal hyperplasia have been described. ACTH-independent macronodular adrenal hyperplasia (and occasionally a unilateral adrenocortical tumor) may be under the control of abnormal or ectopic hormone receptors. Aberrant regulation of cortisol production and adrenal growth has been shown in some of these patients to be mediated by the abnormal adrenal expression of receptors for a variety of hormones. The best characterized appears to be the expression of glucose-dependent insulinotropic polypeptide (GIP), whose adrenal expression has resulted in the modulation of cortisol production after physiologic postprandial fluctuation of endogenous levels of GIP, causing a state of *food-dependent Cushing syndrome.* Other abnormal hormone receptors that have been described in association with endogenous hypercortisolism with this phenomenon include vasopressin, beta-adrenergic agonists, human chorionic gonadotropin-LH, serotonin, angiotensin II, and leptin (see also Chapter 21). The identification of an abnormal adrenal receptor raises the possibility of new pharmacologic approaches to control of hypercortisolism by suppressing the endogenous ligands or by blocking the abnormal receptor with specific antagonists.

Another unusual adrenal-dependent cause of Cushing syndrome associated with bilateral adrenal nodular hyperplasia has been referred to as primary pigmented nodular adrenocortical disease. This is a familial disorder with an autosomal dominant inheritance pattern usually presenting in adolescence or young adulthood. The disorder is associated with unusual conditions such as myxomas (cardiac, cutaneous, and mammary), spotty skin pigmentation, endocrine overactivity, sexual precocity, acromegaly, and schwannomas—the Carney complex. Activating mutations in protein kinase A have recently been shown to be present in many of these patients. Interestingly, the adrenal glands in this syndrome are often small or normal in size and have multiple black and brown nodules with intranodular cortical atrophy.

Finally, in McCune-Albright syndrome, activating mutations of $G_s\alpha$ leads to constitutive steroidogenesis in adrenal nodules carrying the mutation.

C. Adrenal tumors Adrenal tumors causing Cushing syndrome are independent of ACTH secretion and are either adenomas or carcinomas.

1. **Glucocorticoid-secreting adrenal adenomas**—These adenomas are encapsulated, weigh 10 to 70 g, and range in size from 1 to 6 cm. Microscopically, clear cells of the zona fasciculata type predominate, although cells typical of the zona reticularis are also seen.

2. **Adrenal carcinomas**—Adrenal carcinomas are usually greater than 4 cm when diagnosed and often weigh more than 100 g, occasionally exceeding 1 kg. They may be palpable as abdominal masses. Grossly, they are encapsulated and highly vascular; necrosis, hemorrhage, and cystic degeneration are common, and areas of calcification may be present. The histologic appearance of these carcinomas varies considerably; they may appear to be benign or may exhibit considerable pleomorphism. Vascular or capsular invasion is predictive of malignant behavior, as is local extension. These carcinomas invade local structures (kidney, liver, and retroperitoneum) and metastasize hematogenously to liver and lung.

3. **Uninvolved adrenal cortex**—The cortex contiguous to the tumor and that of the contralateral gland are atrophic in the presence of functioning adrenal adenomas and carcinomas. The cortex is markedly thinned, whereas the capsule is thickened. Histologically, the zona reticularis is virtually absent; the remaining cortex is composed of clear fasciculata cells. The architecture of the zona glomerulosa is normal.

Etiology and Pathogenesis

A. Cushing disease The causes and natural history of Cushing disease are reviewed in Chapter 4. Current evidence is consistent with the view that spontaneously arising corticotroph-cell pituitary adenomas are the primary cause and that the consequent ACTH hypersecretion and hypercortisolism lead to the characteristic endocrine abnormalities and hypothalamic dysfunction. This is supported by evidence showing that selective removal of these adenomas by pituitary microsurgery reverses the abnormalities and is followed by return of the HPA axis to normal. In addition, molecular studies have shown that nearly all corticotroph adenomas are monoclonal.

Although these primary pituitary adenomas are responsible for the great majority of cases, a few patients have been described in whom pituitary disease has been limited to corticotroph-cell hyperplasia; these may be secondary to excessive CRH secretion by rare, benign hypothalamic gangliocytoma.

B. Ectopic ACTH syndrome and ectopic CRH syndrome Ectopic ACTH syndrome arises when nonpituitary tumors synthesize and hypersecrete biologically active ACTH. The related peptides β-LPH and β-endorphin are also synthesized and secreted, as are inactive ACTH fragments. Production of CRH has also been demonstrated in ectopic tumors secreting ACTH, but whether CRH plays a role in pathogenesis is unclear. A few cases in which nonpituitary tumors produced only CRH have been reported.

Ectopic ACTH syndrome occurs predominantly in only a few tumor types (Figure 9–13); carcinoid tumors of lung and small cell carcinoma of the lung cause half of cases. Other tumors causing the syndrome originate from neuroendocrine tumors, thymus, gut, ovary, pancreatic islet cell tumors, or medullary thyroid

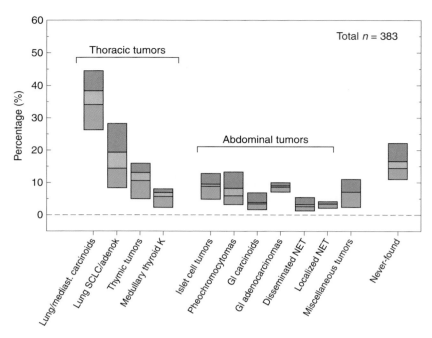

FIGURE 9-13 Prevalence of the most common tumors causing ectopic ACTH secretion. (K, carcinoma; NET, neuroendocrine tumor; SCLC, small cell lung carcinoma). (From: Isidori AM, Lenzi A. Ectopic ACTH syndrome. *Arq Bras Endocrinol Metab.* 2007;51:1217.)

carcinoma. Multiple other tumor types have also been reported to cause the ectopic ACTH syndrome, but are very rare (see Chapter 21).

C. Adrenal tumors   Glucocorticoid-producing adrenal adenomas and carcinomas arise spontaneously. They are not under hypothalamic-pituitary control and autonomously secrete adrenocortical steroids. Rarely, adrenal carcinomas develop in the setting of chronic ACTH hypersecretion in patients with either Cushing disease and nodular adrenal hyperplasia or congenital adrenal hyperplasia.

Pathophysiology (Figures 9–12, 9–13)

A. Cushing disease   In Cushing disease, ACTH hypersecretion is random and episodic and causes cortisol hypersecretion in the absence of the normal circadian rhythm. Feedback inhibition of ACTH (secreted from the pituitary adenoma) by physiologic levels of glucocorticoids is suppressed; thus, ACTH hypersecretion persists despite elevated cortisol secretion and results in chronic glucocorticoid excess. The episodic secretion of ACTH and cortisol results in variable plasma levels that may at times be within the normal range. However, elevation of urine free cortisol or demonstration of elevated late-night serum or salivary cortisol levels because of the absence of diurnal variability confirms cortisol hypersecretion (see sections on laboratory evaluation and diagnosis of Cushing syndrome). The overall increase in glucocorticoid secretion causes the clinical manifestations of Cushing syndrome. ACTH and β-LPH secretion are not usually elevated sufficiently to cause hyperpigmentation.

1. **Abnormalities of ACTH secretion**—Despite ACTH hypersecretion, stress responsiveness is absent; stimuli such as hypoglycemia or surgery fail to further elevate ACTH and cortisol secretion. This is probably due to suppression of hypothalamic function and CRH secretion by hypercortisolism, resulting in loss of hypothalamic control of ACTH secretion (see Chapter 4).

2. **Effect of cortisol excess**—Cortisol excess not only inhibits normal pituitary and hypothalamic function, affecting ACTH, TSH, GH, and gonadotropin release, but also results in all the systemic effects of glucocorticoid excess described in previous sections and in the section on clinical features later.

3. **Androgen excess**—Secretion of adrenal androgens is also increased in Cushing disease, and the degree of androgen excess parallels that of ACTH and cortisol. Thus, plasma levels of DHEA, DHEA sulfate, and androstenedione may be moderately elevated in Cushing disease; the peripheral conversion of these hormones to testosterone and dihydrotestosterone leads to androgen excess. In women, this causes hirsutism, acne, and amenorrhea. In men with Cushing disease, cortisol suppression of LH secretion decreases testosterone secretion by the testis, resulting in decreased libido and impotence. The increased adrenal androgen secretion is insufficient to compensate for the decreased gonadal testosterone production.

B. Ectopic ACTH syndrome   Hypersecretion of ACTH and cortisol is usually greater in patients with ectopic ACTH syndrome than in those with Cushing disease. ACTH and cortisol hypersecretion is randomly episodic, and the levels are often greatly elevated. Usually, ACTH secretion by ectopic tumors is not subject to negative feedback control; that is, secretion of ACTH and cortisol is nonsuppressible with pharmacologic doses of glucocorticoids (see section on diagnosis later).

Plasma levels, secretion rates, and urinary excretion of cortisol, the adrenal androgens, and DOC are often markedly elevated; despite this, the typical features of Cushing syndrome maybe absent, presumably because of rapid onset of hypercortisolism, anorexia, and other manifestations of the associated malignant disease. Features of mineralocorticoid excess (hypertension and hypokalemia) are frequently present and have been attributed to increased secretion of DOC and the mineralocorticoid effects of cortisol. With ectopic CRH secretion, pituitary corticotroph hyperplasia and ACTH hypersecretion are observed along with resistance to negative feedback by cortisol.

C. Adrenal tumors

1. **Autonomous secretion**—Primary adrenal tumors, both adenomas and carcinomas, autonomously hypersecrete cortisol. Circulating plasma ACTH levels are suppressed, resulting in cortical atrophy of the uninvolved adrenal. Secretion is randomly episodic, and these tumors are typically unresponsive to manipulation of the hypothalamic-pituitary axis with pharmacologic agents such as dexamethasone and metyrapone.

2. **Adrenal adenomas**—Adrenal adenomas causing Cushing syndrome typically present solely with clinical manifestations of glucocorticoid excess, because they usually secrete only cortisol. Thus, the presence of androgen or mineralocorticoid excess should suggest that the tumor is an adrenocortical carcinoma.

3. **Adrenal carcinomas**—Adrenal carcinomas frequently hypersecrete multiple adrenocortical steroids and their precursors. Cortisol and androgens are the steroids most frequently secreted in excess; 11-deoxycortisol is often elevated, and there may be increased secretion of DOC, aldosterone, or estrogens. Plasma cortisol and urine free cortisol are often markedly increased; androgen excess is usually even greater than that of cortisol. Thus, high levels of plasma DHEA, DHEA sulfate, and of testosterone typically accompany the cortisol excess. Clinical manifestations of hypercortisolism are usually severe and rapidly progressive in these patients. In women, features of androgen excess are prominent; virilism may occasionally occur. Hypertension and hypokalemia are frequent and most commonly result from the mineralocorticoid effects of cortisol; less frequently, DOC and aldosterone hypersecretion also contribute.

Clinical Features (Table 9–11)

A. Symptoms and signs

1. **Obesity**—Obesity is the most common manifestation, and weight gain is usually the initial symptom. It is classically central, affecting mainly the face, neck, trunk, and abdomen, with relative sparing of the extremities. Generalized obesity with central accentuation is equally common, particularly in children.

    Accumulation of fat in the face leads to the typical *moon facies*, which is present in 75% of cases and is accompanied by facial plethora in most patients. Fat accumulation around the neck is prominent in the supraclavicular and dorsocervical fat pads; the latter is responsible for the *buffalo hump*.

    Obesity is absent in a handful of patients who do not gain weight; however, they usually have central redistribution of fat and a typical facial appearance.

2. **Skin changes**—Skin changes are frequent, and their presence should arouse a suspicion of cortisol excess. Atrophy of the

TABLE 9–11 Clinical features of Cushing syndrome (% prevalence).

General
Obesity 90%
Hypertension 85%
Skin
Plethora 70%
Hirsutism 75%
Striae 50%
Acne 35%
Bruising 35%
Musculoskeletal
Osteopenia 80%
Weakness 65%
Neuropsychiatric 85%
Emotional lability
Euphoria
Depression
Psychosis
Gonadal dysfunction
Menstrual disorders 70%
Impotence, decreased libido 85%
Metabolic
Glucose intolerance 75%
Diabetes 20%
Hyperlipidemia 70%
Polyuria 30%
Kidney stones 15%

epidermis and its underlying connective tissue leads to thinning (a transparent appearance of the skin) and facial plethora. Easy bruisability following minimal trauma is present in about 40%. Striae occur in 50% but are very unusual in patients over 40 years of age. These are typically red to purple, depressed below the skin surface secondary to loss of underlying connective tissue, and wider (not infrequently 0.5-2 cm) than the pinkish-white striae that may occur with pregnancy or rapid weight gain. These striae are most commonly abdominal but may also occur over the breasts, hips, buttocks, thighs, and axillae.

Acne presenting as pustular or papular lesions may result from glucocorticoid excess or hyperandrogenism.

Minor wounds and abrasions may heal slowly, and surgical incisions sometimes undergo dehiscence.

Mucocutaneous fungal infections are frequent, including tinea versicolor, involvement of the nails (onychomycosis), and oral candidiasis.

Hyperpigmentation of the skin is rare in Cushing disease or adrenal tumors but is common in ectopic ACTH syndrome.

3. **Hirsutism**—Hirsutism is present in about 80% of female patients owing to hypersecretion of adrenal androgens. Facial hirsutism is most common, but increased hair growth may also occur over the abdomen, breasts, chest, and upper thighs. Acne and seborrhea usually accompany hirsutism. Virilism is unusual except in cases of adrenal carcinoma, in which it occurs in about 20% of patients.

4. **Hypertension**—Hypertension is a classic feature of spontaneous Cushing syndrome; it is present in about 75% of cases, and the diastolic blood pressure is greater than 100 mm Hg

in over 50%. Hypertension and its complications contribute greatly to the morbidity and mortality rates in spontaneous Cushing syndrome.

5. **Gonadal dysfunction**—This is very common as a result of elevated androgens (in females) and cortisol (in males and to a lesser extent in females). Amenorrhea occurs in 75% of premenopausal women and is usually accompanied by infertility. Decreased libido is frequent in males, and some have decreased body hair and soft testes.

6. **Central nervous system and psychologic disturbances**—Psychologic disturbances occur in the majority of patients. Mild symptoms consist of emotional lability and increased irritability. Anxiety, depression, poor concentration, and poor memory may also be present. Euphoria is frequent, and occasionally patients manifest overtly manic behavior. Sleep disorders are present in most patients, with either insomnia or early morning awakening.

    Severe psychologic disorders occur in a few patients and include severe depression, psychosis with delusions or hallucinations, and paranoia. Some patients have committed suicide. Loss of brain volume that is at least partially reversible following correction of hypercortisolism has been observed.

7. **Muscle weakness**—This occurs in about 60% of cases; it is more often proximal and is usually most prominent in the lower extremities. Hypercortisolism is associated with both low fat-free muscle mass and low total body protein.

8. **Osteoporosis**—Owing to the profound effects of glucocorticoids on the skeleton, patients with Cushing syndrome frequently have evidence of significant osteopenia and osteoporosis. Patients may present with multiple fragility fractures—typically of the feet, ribs, or vertebrae. Back pain may be the initial complaint. Compression fractures of the spine are demonstrated radiographically in 15% to 20% of patients. In fact, unexplained osteopenia in any young or middle-aged adult should always prompt an evaluation for Cushing syndrome, even in the absence of any other signs or symptoms of cortisol excess. Although avascular necrosis of bone has been associated with exogenous glucocorticoid administration, the problem is rarely observed in patients with endogenous hypercortisolism, suggesting a role for the underlying disorders in patients for whom glucocorticoids are prescribed.

9. **Renal calculi**—Calculi secondary to glucocorticoid-induced hypercalciuria occur in approximately 15% of patients, and renal colic may occasionally be a presenting complaint.

10. **Thirst and polyuria**—Polyuria is rarely due to overt hyperglycemia but is usually cause by glucocorticoid inhibition of vasopressin (antidiuretic hormone) secretion and the direct enhancement of renal free water clearance by cortisol.

11. **Growth deceleration**—In children, nearly all (>95%) show decreasing linear growth. Weight gain accompanying decreasing linear growth in a child should prompt an evaluation for Cushing syndrome.

B. Laboratory findings   Routine laboratory examinations are described here. Specific tests to establish the diagnosis of Cushing syndrome are discussed in the section on diagnosis.

High normal hemoglobin, hematocrit, and red cell counts are usual; polycythemia is rare. The total white count is usually normal; however, both the percentage of lymphocytes and the total lymphocyte count may be subnormal. Eosinophils are also depressed, and a total eosinophil count less than $100/\mu L$ is present in most patients. Serum electrolytes, with rare exceptions, are normal in Cushing disease; however, hypokalemic alkalosis occurs when there is marked steroid hypersecretion with the ectopic ACTH syndrome or adrenocortical carcinoma.

Although fasting hyperglycemia occurs in only 10% to 15% of patients, glucose intolerance is a relatively common finding and occurs in 60% of patients. Most patients have secondary hyperinsulinemia and abnormal glucose tolerance tests.

Serum calcium is normal; serum phosphorus is low normal or slightly depressed. Hypercalciuria is present in 40% of cases.

C. Imaging studies   Routine radiographs may reveal cardiomegaly due to hypertensive or atherosclerotic heart disease or mediastinal widening due to central fat accumulation. Vertebral compression fractures, rib fractures, and renal calculi may be present.

D. Electrocardiographic findings   Hypertensive, ischemic, and electrolyte-induced changes may be present on the electrocardiogram.

Features Suggesting a Specific Cause

A. Cushing disease   Cushing disease typifies the classic clinical picture: female predominance, onset generally between ages 20 and 40, and a slow progression over several years. Hyperpigmentation and hypokalemic alkalosis are rare; androgenic manifestations are limited to acne and hirsutism. Secretion of cortisol and adrenal androgens is only moderately increased.

B. Ectopic ACTH syndrome (carcinoma)   In contrast, this syndrome occurs predominantly in males, with the highest incidence between ages 40 and 60. The clinical manifestations of hypercortisolism are frequently limited to weakness, hypertension, and glucose intolerance; the primary tumor is usually apparent. Hyperpigmentation, hypokalemia, and alkalosis are common, as are weight loss and anemia. The hypercortisolism is of rapid onset, and steroid hypersecretion is frequently severe, with equally elevated levels of glucocorticoids, androgens, and DOC.

C. Ectopic ACTH syndrome (benign tumor)   A minority of patients with ectopic ACTH syndrome due to more benign tumors, especially bronchial carcinoids, present a more slowly progressive course, with typical features of Cushing syndrome. These patients may be clinically identical to those with pituitary-dependent Cushing disease, and the responsible tumor may not be apparent. Hyperpigmentation, hypokalemic alkalosis, and anemia are variably present. Further confusion may arise, since a number of these patients with occult ectopic tumors may have ACTH and steroid dynamics typical of Cushing disease (see below).

D. Adrenal adenomas   The clinical picture in patients with adrenal adenomas is usually that of glucocorticoid excess alone, and androgenic effects such as hirsutism are absent. Onset is gradual, and hypercortisolism is mild to moderate. Plasma androgens are usually in the low normal or subnormal range.

E. Adrenal carcinomas

In general, adrenal carcinomas have a rapid onset of the clinical features of excessive glucocorticoid, androgen, and mineralocorticoid secretion and are rapidly progressive. Marked elevations of both cortisol and androgens are usual; hypokalemia is common, as are abdominal pain, palpable masses, and hepatic and pulmonary metastases.

Diagnosis

The clinical suspicion of Cushing syndrome must be confirmed with biochemical studies. Initially, a general assessment of the patient regarding the presence of other illnesses, drugs, alcohol, or psychiatric problems must be done since these factors may confound the evaluation. In the majority of cases, the biochemical differential diagnosis of Cushing syndrome can be easily performed in the ambulatory setting (Figure 9–14).

A. Dexamethasone suppression test

The overnight 1-mg dexamethasone suppression test is a valuable screening test in patients with suspected hypercortisolism. This study employs the administration of 1 mg of dexamethasone at bedtime (11:00 PM), with determination of a plasma cortisol early the following morning. Normal subjects should suppress plasma cortisol to less than 1.8 µg/dL (50 nmol/L) following an overnight 1-mg test. Although a level of less than 5 µg/dL has been used in the past, several false-negative studies have been discovered using this test criterion. False-negative results may occur in some patients with mild hypercortisolism and exquisite negative feedback sensitivity to glucocorticoids and in those with intermittent hypercortisolism. This test should only be employed as a screening tool for the consideration of Cushing syndrome, and biochemical confirmation must rely on additional biochemical testing. False-positive results with the overnight 1-mg dexamethasone suppression test may be caused by patients receiving drugs that accelerate dexamethasone metabolism (phenytoin, phenobarbital, rifampin). False-positive results also occur in patients with renal failure, depression, alcoholism, or in patients undergoing a stressful event or serious illness.

B. Urine free cortisol

Another study in the confirmation of Cushing syndrome is the determination of urine free cortisol measured by HPLC or LC/MS/MS in a 24-hour urine collection.

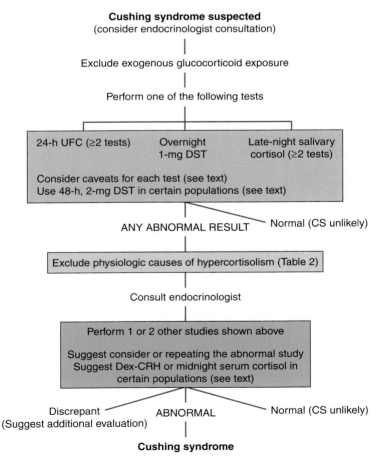

FIGURE 9–14 The diagnosis of Cushing syndrome. (Reproduced, with permission, from Nieman LK, et al. The diagnosis of Cushing syndrome: an Endocrine Society Clinical Practice Guideline. *J Clin Endocrinol Metab.* 2008;93:1526. Copyright 2008; The Endocrine Society.)

These methods are highly accurate and specific. Commonly used drugs and medications do not interfere; however, carbamazepine and fenofibrate can cause falsely elevated results with HPLC since they elute with cortisol. Urinary free cortisol is usually less than 50 µg/24 h (<135 nmol/24 h) when measured by HPLC or LC/MS/MS. Urine free cortisol determinations usually provide clear discrimination between patients with hypercortisolism and obese non-Cushing patients, although exceptions occur. Less than 5% of obese subjects have mild elevations of urine free cortisol. The major liability of urine free cortisol is its poor sensitivity for detecting patients with mild hypercortisolism (sensitivity <75%). Consequently, this modality should not be used alone to exclude Cushing syndrome.

C. Late-night serum and salivary cortisol   The absence of diurnal rhythm has been considered a hallmark of the diagnosis of Cushing syndrome. Normally, cortisol is secreted episodically with a diurnal rhythm paralleling the secretion of ACTH. Levels are usually highest early in the morning and decrease gradually throughout the day, reaching the nadir in the late evening between 11:00 PM and midnight. Several studies have demonstrated that an elevated midnight plasma cortisol level (>5.2-7.0 µg/dL [140-190 nmol/L]) is highly accurate in differentiating patients with Cushing syndrome from normal subjects and from patients with pseudo-Cushing conditions such as depression or alcoholism.

Because obtaining such plasma cortisol measurements is impractical on an ambulatory basis, the measurement of salivary cortisol provides a simple and more convenient means of probing nighttime cortisol secretion. Saliva can easily be sampled at home by the patient using a variety of techniques. Reference ranges for late-night salivary cortisol concentrations are dependent on the assay employed; however, using a radioimmunoassay, normal subjects should have values less than 0.15 µg/dL (4 nmol/L).

Problems in Diagnosis

A major diagnostic problem is distinguishing patients with mild Cushing syndrome from those with mild physiologic hypercortisolism due to conditions that are classified as **pseudo-Cushing syndrome**. These include the depressed phase of affective disorder, alcoholism, withdrawal from alcohol intoxication, or eating disorders such as anorexia and bulimia nervosa. These conditions may have biochemical features of Cushing syndrome, including elevations of urine free cortisol, disruptions in the normal diurnal pattern of cortisol secretion, and lack of suppression of cortisol after the overnight 1-mg dexamethasone suppression test. Although the history and physical examination may provide specific clues to the appropriate diagnosis, definitive biochemical confirmation may be difficult and may require repeated testing. Another study to distinguish mild Cushing syndrome from pseudo-Cushing conditions is the use of dexamethasone suppression followed by CRH stimulation. This test takes advantage of differential response of patients with Cushing syndrome and pseudo-Cushing syndrome to both dexamethasone and CRH by combining these tests to provide greater accuracy in the diagnosis. This study

involves the administration of dexamethasone, 0.5 mg every 6 hours for eight doses, followed immediately by a CRH stimulation test, starting 2 hours after the completion of the low-dose dexamethasone suppression. A plasma cortisol concentration greater than 1.4 µg/dL (38.6 nmol/L) measured 15 minutes after administration of CRH correctly identifies the majority of patients with Cushing syndrome. After administration of high-dose dexamethasone, patients with pseudo-Cushing syndrome do not have a rise in cortisol or ACTH in response to CRH. However, it is now appreciated that some patients with pseudo-Cushing syndrome (eg, anorexia nervosa) may have abnormal dexamethasone CRH suppression tests.

Differential Diagnosis

The differential diagnosis of Cushing syndrome is usually difficult and should always be performed with consultation by an endocrinologist. The introduction of several technologic advances, including a specific and sensitive IRMA or ICMA for ACTH, CRH stimulation test, inferior petrosal sinus sampling (IPSS), CT and magnetic resonance imaging (MRI) of the pituitary and adrenal glands have all provided means for an accurate differential diagnosis.

A. Plasma ACTH   Initially, the differential diagnosis for Cushing syndrome must distinguish between ACTH-dependent Cushing syndrome (pituitary or nonpituitary ACTH-secreting neoplasm) and ACTH-independent hypercortisolism. The best way to distinguish these forms of Cushing syndrome is measurement of plasma ACTH by IRMA or ICMA. The development of this sensitive and specific test has made it possible to reliably identify patients with ACTH-independent Cushing syndrome. The ACTH level is less than 5 pg/mL (1.1 pmol/L) and exhibits a blunted response to CRH (peak response <10 pg/mL [2.2 pmol/L]) in patients with cortisol-producing adrenal neoplasms, autonomous bilateral adrenal cortical hyperplasia, and factitious Cushing syndrome (Figure 9–15). Patients with ACTH-secreting neoplasms usually have plasma ACTH levels greater than 10 pg/mL (2.2 pmol/L) and frequently greater than 52 pg/mL (11.5 pmol/L). The major challenge in the differential diagnosis of ACTH-dependent Cushing syndrome is identifying the source of the ACTH-secreting tumor. The vast majority of these patients (90%) have a pituitary tumor, whereas the others harbor a nonpituitary neoplasm. Diagnostic studies needed to differentiate these two entities must yield nearly perfect sensitivity, specificity, and accuracy. Although plasma ACTH levels are usually higher in patients with ectopic ACTH than those with pituitary ACTH-dependent Cushing syndrome, there is considerable overlap between these two entities. Many of the ectopic ACTH-secreting tumors are radiologically occult at the time of presentation and may not become clinically apparent for many years after the initial diagnosis. However, an enhanced ACTH response for CRH administration is more frequently found in pituitary Cushing syndrome compared with ectopic ACTH syndrome.

B. Pituitary MRI   When ACTH-dependent Cushing syndrome is present, MRI of the pituitary gland with gadolinium enhancement

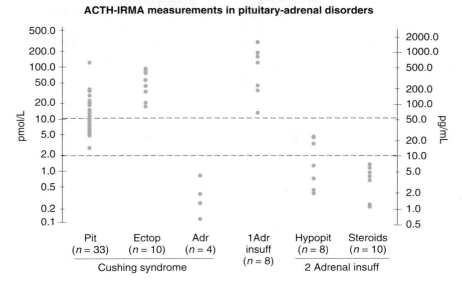

ACTH-IRMA measurements in pituitary-adrenal disorders

FIGURE 9–15 Plasma ACTH-IRMA (pmol/L or pg/mL) of patients with pituitary-adrenal disorders. Dashed horizontal lines indicate normal range. (Reproduced, with permission, from Findling JW. Clinical application of a new immunoradiometric assay for ACTH. *Endocrinologist*. 1992;2:360.)

should be performed and will identify an adenoma in at least 50% to 60% of the patients. If the patient has classic clinical laboratory findings of ACTH-dependent hypercortisolemia and an unequivocal pituitary lesion on MRI, the likelihood of Cushing disease is 98% to 99%. However, it must be emphasized that approximately 10% of the population in the age group from 20 to 50 years will have incidental tumors of the pituitary demonstrable by MRI. Therefore, some patients with ectopic ACTH syndrome will have radiographic evidence of a pituitary lesion.

C. High-Dose dexamethasone suppression   Traditionally, the high-dose dexamethasone suppression test has been utilized in the differential diagnosis of Cushing syndrome. However, the diagnostic accuracy of this procedure is only 70% to 80%, which is actually less than the pretest probability of Cushing disease—on average about 90%. As a result, this study is no longer recommended.

D. Inferior petrosal sinus sampling   The most definitive means of accurately distinguishing pituitary from nonpituitary ACTH-dependent Cushing syndrome is the use of bilateral simultaneous IPSS with CRH stimulation, and this procedure is the next step in the evaluation of patients with ACTH-dependent Cushing syndrome when MRI does not reveal a definite adenoma. This study takes advantage of the means by which pituitary hormones reach the systemic circulation. Blood leaves the anterior lobe of the pituitary and drains into the cavernous sinuses, which then empty into the inferior petrosal sinuses and subsequently into the jugular bulb and vein. Simultaneous inferior petrosal sinus and peripheral ACTH measurement before and after CRH stimulation can reliably confirm the presence or absence of an ACTH-secreting pituitary tumor. An inferior petrosal sinus to peripheral (IPS-P) ratio greater than 2.0 prior to CRH and greater

than 3.0 after CRH is consistent with a pituitary ACTH-secreting tumor, and an IPS-P ratio less than 1.8 supports the diagnosis of ectopic ACTH. Anatomical variants can cause false-negative studies; however, simultaneous measurement of PRL can be used to construct a PRL-normalized ACTH ratio which can eliminate false negatives caused by anatomical variants.

Bilateral IPSS with CRH stimulation does require a skilled interventional radiologist. However, in experienced hands, the procedure has yielded a diagnostic accuracy approaching 100% in identifying the source of ACTH-dependent Cushing syndrome.

E. Occult ectopic ACTH   If the IPSS study is consistent with a nonpituitary ACTH-secreting tumor, a search for an occult ectopic ACTH-secreting tumor is needed. Because the majority of these lesions are in the thorax, high-resolution CT of the chest may be useful; MRI of the chest may have even better sensitivity in finding these lesions, which are usually small bronchial carcinoid tumors. Unfortunately, utilization of a radiolabeled somatostatin analog scan (octreotide acetate scintigraphy) has met with only mixed results in localizing these tumors.

F. Adrenal localizing procedures   CT (Figure 9–16) and MRI are used to define adrenal lesions. Their primary use is to localize adrenal tumors in patients with ACTH-independent Cushing syndrome. Most adenomas exceed 2 cm in diameter; carcinomas are usually much larger.

TREATMENT

A. Cushing disease   The aim of treatment of Cushing syndrome is to remove or destroy the basic lesion and thus correct hypersecretion of adrenal hormones without inducing pituitary or

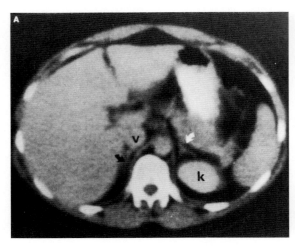 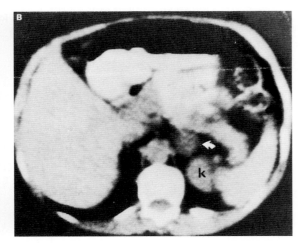

FIGURE 9–16 Adrenal CT scans in Cushing syndrome. **A**. Patient with ACTH-dependent Cushing syndrome. The adrenal glands are not detectably abnormal by this procedure. The curvilinear right adrenal (black arrow) is shown posterior to the inferior vena cava (V) between the right lobe of the liver and the right crus of the diaphragm. The left adrenal (white arrow) has an inverted Y appearance anteromedial to the left kidney (K). **B**. A 3-cm left adrenal adenoma (white arrow) is shown anteromedial to the left kidney (K). (Reproduced, with permission, from Korobkin M, et al. Computed tomography in the diagnosis of adrenal disease. *AJR Am J Roentgenol*. 1979;132:231.)

adrenal damage, which requires permanent replacement therapy for hormone deficiencies.

Treatment of Cushing disease is currently directed at the pituitary to control ACTH hypersecretion; available methods include microsurgery, various forms of radiation therapy, and pharmacologic inhibition of ACTH secretion. Treatment of hypercortisolism per se by surgical or medical adrenalectomy is less commonly used. These methods are discussed in Chapter 4.

B. Ectopic ACTH syndrome   Cure of ectopic ACTH syndrome is usually possible only in cases involving the more benign tumors such as bronchial or thymic carcinoids or pheochromocytomas. Treatment is made difficult by the presence of metastatic tumors and accompanying severe hypercortisolism. Therapy directed to the primary tumor is usually unsuccessful, and other means must be used to correct the steroid-excess state.

Severe hypokalemia may require potassium replacement in large doses and spironolactone to block mineralocorticoid effects.

Drugs that block steroid synthesis (ketoconazole and metyrapone) are useful, but they may produce hypoadrenalism, and steroid secretion must be monitored and replacement steroids given if necessary. The dosage of ketoconazole is 400 to 800 mg/d in divided doses and is usually well tolerated. Because of its slow onset of action, narrow therapeutic window, and possible serious side-effects, mitotane is less useful. If used, several weeks of therapy may be required before control of cortisol secretion is achieved.

Bilateral adrenalectomy may be necessary if hypercortisolism cannot be controlled in other ways.

C. Adrenal tumors

1. **Adrenal adenomas**— Patients with adrenal adenomas are successfully treated by unilateral adrenalectomy, and the outlook

is excellent. Laparoscopic adrenal surgery has become widely used in patients with benign or small adrenal tumors and has significantly reduced the duration of the hospital stay. Because the hypothalamic-pituitary axis and the contralateral adrenal are suppressed by prolonged cortisol secretion, these patients have postoperative adrenal insufficiency and require glucocorticoid therapy both during and following surgery until the remaining adrenal recovers.

2. **Adrenal carcinomas**—Therapy in cases of adrenocortical carcinoma is less satisfactory, because the tumor has frequently already metastasized (usually to the retroperitoneum, liver, and lungs) by the time the diagnosis is made.

   a. **Operative treatment**—Surgical cure is rare, but excision serves to reduce the tumor mass and the degree of steroid hypersecretion. Persisting nonsuppressible steroid secretion in the immediate postoperative period indicates residual or metastatic tumor.

   b. **Medical treatment**—Mitotane is the drug of choice. The dosage is 6 to 12 g/d orally in three or four divided doses. The dose must often be reduced because of side-effects in 80% of patients (diarrhea, nausea and vomiting, depression, somnolence). About 70% of patients achieve a reduction of steroid secretion, but only 35% achieve a reduction in tumor size.

Ketoconazole and metyrapone (singly or in combination) are useful in controlling steroid hypersecretion in patients who do not respond to mitotane. Radiotherapy and conventional chemotherapy have not been useful in this disease.

D. Nodular adrenal hyperplasia   When pituitary ACTH dependency can be demonstrated, macronodular hyperplasia may be treated like other cases of Cushing disease. When ACTH dependency is not present, as in micronodular hyperplasia and in some cases of macronodular hyperplasia, bilateral adrenalectomy is appropriate.

PROGNOSIS

A. Cushing syndrome Untreated Cushing syndrome is frequently fatal, and death may be due to the underlying tumor itself, as in the ectopic ACTH syndrome and adrenal carcinoma. However, in most cases, death is the consequence of sustained hypercortisolism and its complications, including hypertension, cardiovascular disease, stroke, thromboembolism, and susceptibility to infection.

B. Cushing disease In contrast to patients with untreated Cushing syndrome, individuals with Cushing disease who achieve normalization of cortisol levels as result of therapy have a standard mortality ratio (SMR) similar to age-matched populations. However, patients with persistent hypercortisolism despite treatment continue to have an increased SMR (3.8- to 5.0-fold), when compared to the general population.

With current refinements in pituitary microsurgery and irradiation, the great majority of patients with Cushing disease can be treated successfully, and the operative mortality and morbidity rates that attended bilateral adrenalectomy are no longer a feature of the natural history of this disease. Reduction in health-related quality of life, especially related to psychological functioning, may persist. Patients with Cushing disease, who have large pituitary tumors at the time of diagnosis, have a much less satisfactory prognosis and may die as a consequence of tumor invasion or persistent hypercortisolism.

C. Adrenal tumors The prognosis in adrenal adenomas is excellent. In adrenal carcinoma, the prognosis is almost universally poor, and the median survival from the date of onset of symptoms is about 4 years.

D. Ectopic ACTH syndrome Prognosis is also poor in patients with ectopic ACTH syndrome due to the nature of the malignancy producing the hormone, and in these patients with severe hypercortisolism, survival is frequently only days to weeks. Some patients respond to tumor resection or chemotherapy. The prognosis is better in patients with benign tumors producing the ectopic ACTH syndrome.

HIRSUTISM AND VIRILISM

Excessive adrenal or ovarian secretion of androgens or excessive conversion of weak androgens to testosterone and dihydrotestosterone in peripheral tissues leads to hirsutism and virilism (see Chapter 13). As previously discussed, the adrenal secretory products DHEA, DHEA sulfate, and androstenedione are weak androgens; however, the peripheral conversion to testosterone and dihydrotestosterone can result in a state of androgen excess.

Excessive androgen production is seen in both adrenal and ovarian disorders. Adrenal causes include Cushing syndrome, adrenal carcinoma, and congenital adrenal hyperplasia (see previous sections and Chapter 14). Mild adult-onset cases of congenital adrenal enzyme deficiencies have been described; these appear to be relatively uncommon. Biochemical diagnosis of late-onset 21-hydroxylase deficiency is best achieved by measurement of the 17-hydroxyprogesterone response to ACTH. Ovarian causes are discussed in Chapter 13.

In children, androgen excess is usually due to premature adrenarche, congenital adrenal hyperplasia, or adrenal carcinoma. In women, hirsutism accompanied by amenorrhea, infertility, ovarian enlargement, and elevated plasma LH levels is typical of the polycystic ovary syndrome, whereas in Cushing syndrome hirsutism is accompanied by features of cortisol excess. Late-onset 21-hydroxylase deficiency is accompanied by elevated levels of plasma 17-hydroxyprogesterone, especially following ACTH administration. Virilism and severe androgen excess in adults are usually due to androgen-secreting adrenal or ovarian tumors; virilism is unusual in the polycystic ovary syndrome and rare in Cushing disease. In the absence of these syndromes, hirsutism in women is usually idiopathic or due to milder forms of polycystic ovary syndrome. Exogenous androgen administration (eg, DHEA) should also be considered.

The diagnosis and therapy of hirsutism are discussed in Chapter 13.

INCIDENTAL ADRENAL MASS

The incidental adrenal mass has become a common diagnostic problem, because approximately 2% to 4% of patients undergoing CT studies of the abdomen are found to have focal enlargement of the adrenal gland. Adrenal masses in an adult may represent functional or nonfunctional cortical adenomas or carcinoma, pheochromocytomas, cysts, myelolipomas, or metastasis from other tumors. Congenital adrenal hyperplasia may also present as a focal enlargement of the adrenal gland, and adrenal hemorrhage also causes enlargement, although usually bilateral.

The appropriate diagnostic approach to patients with an incidentally discovered adrenal mass is unresolved. The roentgenographic appearance taken in context with the clinical setting may provide some insight. The size of the lesion is important. Primary adrenocortical carcinoma is rare in adrenal masses smaller than 4 cm. The presence of unilateral or bilateral adrenal masses (>3 cm) in a patient with a known malignancy (particularly lung, gastrointestinal, renal, or breast) probably represents metastatic disease. Adrenal lesions smaller than 3 cm in patients with a known malignancy actually represent metastases in only 20% to 30% of cases.

Other CT findings may be informative. The presence of fat within the adrenal mass may suggest a myelolipoma, which is usually a benign lesion. Adrenocortical adenomas are usually round masses with smooth margins, and adrenal cysts can also be identified with either CT or ultrasound examination. Lesions with low density (<10 Hounsfield units) on unenhanced CT scans are usually benign. Adrenal hemorrhage usually has irregular borders with some lack of homogeneity. Primary adrenocortical carcinoma usually presents as a lesion greater than 5 cm with irregular borders. MRI of the adrenal gland is usually not necessary but may be helpful in selected patients. Typically, malignancies and pheochromocytomas tend to have bright signal intensity with T2-weighted images, in contrast to benign lesions of the adrenal gland; however, exceptions to this rule have been seen, limiting the clinical utility of this technique.

Malignancy

Primary adrenocortical carcinoma usually presents with a large lesion, and most authorities recommend removing all adrenal masses greater than 4 cm. One series of 45 adrenal masses greater than 5 cm showed 30 benign lesions (16 pheochromocytomas, 6 adenomas, 4 adrenal cysts, 2 myelolipomas, 1 hematoma, 1 ganglioneuroma) and 15 malignancies (7 adrenocortical carcinomas, 5 adrenal metastases, and 3 adrenal lymphomas. Lesions less than 4 to 5 cm in diameter are of concern only in patients with a known malignancy or in those in whom there is a high index of suspicion based on other clinical information. In patients with primary malignancies of the lung, gastrointestinal tract, kidney, or breast, an ultrasound or CT-guided needle biopsy may be helpful in establishing the presence or absence of metastatic disease once pheochromocytoma has been excluded. Metastatic disease can be identified with an accuracy of 75% to 85% in such patients; however, there are both false-negative and false-positive findings. Percutaneous adrenal biopsy really has no demonstrated efficacy in patients with adrenal masses and no history of a malignancy. Percutaneous adrenal biopsy should be reserved for patients in whom the presence or absence of adrenal metastases may alter the therapy or prognosis of the patient.

Endocrine Evaluation

The appropriate biochemical evaluation of an incidental adrenal mass is also controversial. An expert panel from the National Institutes of Health found that the available evidence suggests that an overnight (1-mg) dexamethasone suppression test and determination of fractionated urinary or plasma metanephrines should be performed, and that in patients with hypertension, serum potassium and a plasma aldosterone concentration-PRA ratio should be determined to evaluate for primary aldosteronism. However, good clinical judgment is essential, and repeat CT imaging in 6 to 12 months was also recommended to exclude neoplastic disease. Hormonal abnormalities may develop over time, and follow-up testing has been recommended by some depending on the clinical context.

Cortisol-Producing Adenoma

The most common functioning lesion in patients with an incidentally discovered adrenal mass appears to be an adenoma with autonomous secretion of cortisol. Approximately 6% to 9% of patients with adrenal incidentalomas ranging from 2 to 5 cm in diameter have autonomous cortisol hypersecretion. These benign adrenal adenomas secrete small amounts of cortisol that are often not sufficient to elevate urine cortisol excretion but are able to cause some suppression of the hypothalamic-pituitary axis. These patients can be easily identified by their failure to suppress cortisol to less than 1.8 μg/dL (50 nmol/L) following an overnight 1-mg dexamethasone suppression test. In addition, the basal levels of ACTH in

these patients are subnormal or frankly suppressed. DHEA sulfate levels are also usually decreased in patients with cortisol-secreting adenomas, likely reflecting ACTH suppression. The cortisol secretion by the tumor probably results in blunting of diurnal variation and eventually in lack of suppression by dexamethasone. The low plasma ACTH level manifests in a blunted response to CRH administration. Removal of these silent adrenocortical adenomas may be followed by clinically significant secondary adrenal insufficiency. Therefore, an overnight dexamethasone suppression test or measurement of plasma ACTH should be performed before surgical removal of any unknown adrenal neoplasm. These patients have been described as having *preclinical* or *subclinical* Cushing syndrome. The natural history of this autonomous cortisol secretion is unknown. Many of these patients described with this problem have hypertension, obesity, or diabetes, and improvements in these clinical problems have been reported following resection of these cortisol-producing adenomas. Consequently, adrenalectomy is recommended in young patients with preclinical Cushing syndrome and in patients with clinical problems that might potentially be aggravated by glucocorticoid excess.

Pheochromocytoma

Pheochromocytoma is a potentially life-threatening tumor that may present as an incidental adrenal mass. Surprisingly, pheochromocytoma may account for as many as 2% to 3% of incidental adrenal lesions. Many of these patients have hypertension and symptoms associated with catecholamine excess such as headache, diaphoresis, palpitations, or nervousness (see Chapter 11).

Aldosterone-Producing Adenoma

Although aldosterone-producing adenomas are more common than either pheochromocytomas or cortisol-producing adenomas, they actually represent a very unusual cause of an incidentally discovered adrenal mass. This appears to be due to the fact that aldosterone-producing adenomas are usually small and frequently missed with CT imaging of the adrenal gland. Because most of these patients have hypertension, this diagnosis needs to be considered only in patients with hypertension. The presence of hypokalemia should arouse suspicion of this diagnosis, but hypokalemia is not invariably present. It is usually present in patients with aldosterone-producing adenomas greater than 3 cm. Hyperaldosteronism can be excluded by the measurement of aldosterone and PRA. If the aldosterone (ng/dL)-PRA (ng/mL/h) ratio is less than 30 and plasma aldosterone is less than 20 ng/dL, an aldosterone-producing adenoma is excluded.

GLUCOCORTICOID THERAPY FOR NONENDOCRINE DISORDERS

Principles

Glucocorticoids have been used for their anti-inflammatory and immunosuppressive activity in treatment of a wide variety of disorders. These include rheumatologic disorders (eg, rheumatoid arthritis and systemic lupus erythematosus), pulmonary diseases (eg, asthma), renal disease (eg, glomerulonephritis), and many others. Because of their side-effects, glucocorticoids should be used in the minimum effective dose and for the shortest possible duration of therapy.

Synthetic Glucocorticoids

Steroid compounds have been synthesized, taking advantage of chemical alterations to the steroid nucleus that enhances glucocorticoid activity relative to mineralocorticoid activity. For example, prednisone has a double bond between positions 1 and 2 of cortisol and an 11-keto group instead of a hydroxyl group. It has three to five times more glucocorticoid activity than cortisol and relatively little mineralocorticoid activity. It must be converted to prednisolone by reduction of the 11-keto group to a hydroxyl group in order to be biologically active, a process that may be reduced in the presence of liver disease. Dexamethasone has the same additional double bond, a fluoro atom in the 9α position and a 16α-methyl group. This results in 10 to 20 times the glucocorticoid activity of cortisol and negligible mineralocorticoid activity. Many other compounds have been synthesized. Although most synthetic glucocorticoids exhibit little binding to CBG, their plasma half-lives are longer than that of cortisol.

Modes of Administration

Glucocorticoids may be administered parenterally, orally, topically, and by inhalation. Absorption rates from intramuscular and intra-articular sites depend on the particular glucocorticoid and its formulation. Transdermal absorption also depends on the severity of the inflammatory disorder, the area of the body to which the drug is applied, the presence of vehicles that enhance absorption (eg, urea), and the use of an occlusive dressing. Inhaled glucocorticoids vary in their bioavailability; the technique of administration (eg, use of spacers) also affects the amount of drug delivered to the lungs.

Side-Effects

In general, the severity of the side-effects is a function of dose and duration of therapy, but there is marked individual variation.

A. Hypothalamic-pituitary-adrenal axis suppression
Glucocorticoids suppress CRH and ACTH secretion (negative feedback). Suppression of the HPA axis may occur with doses of prednisone greater than 5 mg/d. It is difficult, however, to predict the development or degree of suppression in any given individual. In general, patients who develop clinical features of Cushing syndrome or who have received glucocorticoids equivalent to 10 to 20 mg of prednisone per day for 3 weeks or more should be assumed to have clinically significant HPA axis suppression. Patients treated with alternate-day steroid regimens exhibit less suppression than those who receive steroids daily.

B. Cushing syndrome
Glucocorticoid administration results in the development of cushingoid features. Of special concern is steroid-induced osteoporosis, particularly in patients for whom a long course of steroid therapy is anticipated. The severity of systemic effects of inhaled glucocorticoids varies among different preparations. However, they are associated with both local effects (dysphonia and oral candidiasis) and systemic effects, especially glaucoma, cataracts, osteoporosis, and growth retardation in children. Protease inhibitors are now well recognized to decrease the metabolism of exogenous glucocorticoids. When the two are used in combination, the resultant increase in circulating glucocorticoid can lead to exogenous Cushing syndrome.

C. Steroid withdrawal
Because of their adverse effects, glucocorticoids must be tapered downward as the clinical situation permits. Tapering regimens are essentially empirical. Factors that may limit the ability to taper the dose down to physiologic replacement levels include recrudescence of disease and steroid withdrawal syndrome. The latter appears in a variety of patterns. Patients may develop fatigue, arthralgias, and desquamation of the skin. Psychologic dependence has also been described. Even after the dose has been reduced to physiologic levels, HPA axis suppression (ie, secondary adrenal insufficiency) persists for an average of 9 to 10 months but may continue for as long as 1 to 2 years.

REFERENCES

General

Arit W, Stewart PM. Adrenal corticosteroid biosynthesis, metabolism, and action. *Endocrinol Metab Clin North Am.* 2005;34:293. [PMID: 15850843]

Becker KL, Bilezikian JP, Bremner WJ, et al, eds. *Principles and Practice of Endocrinology and Metabolism.* 3rd ed. Philadelphia, PA: Lippincott Williams & Wilkins; 2001.

Bottner A, Bornstein SR. Lessons learned from gene targeting and transgenesis for adrenal physiology and disease. *Rev Endocr Metab Disord.* 2001;2:275. [PMID: 11705133]

DeGroot LJ, Jameson JL, eds. *Endocrinology.* 5th ed. vol. 3. Philadelphia, PA: Saunders; 2005.

Hammer GD, Parker KL, Schimmer BP. Minireview: transcriptional regulation of adrenocortical development. *Endocrinology.* 2005;146:1018. [PMID: 15604207]

Lindsay JR, Nieman LK. The hypothalamic-pituitary-adrenal axis in pregnancy: challenges in disease detection and treatment. *Endocr Rev.* 2005;6:775. [PMID: 15827110]

Miller WL, Tyrrell JB. The adrenal cortex. In: Felig P, Baxter JD, Frohman LA, eds. *Endocrinology and Metabolism.* 4th ed. New York: McGraw-Hill; 2002.

Payne AH, Hales DB. Overview of steroidogenic enzymes in the pathway from cholesterol to active steroid hormones. *Endocr Rev.* 2004;25:947. [PMID: 15131259]

Seckl JR. 11β-hydroxysteroid dehydrogenases: changing glucocorticoid action. *Curr Opin Pharm.* 2004;4:597. [PMID: 15525550]

Simard J, Ricketts ML, Gingras S, Soucy P, Feltus FA, Melner MH. Molecular biology of the 3β-hydroxysteroid dehydrogenase/Δ^5-Δ^4 isomerase gene family. *Endocr Rev.* 2005;26:525. [PMID: 15632317]

Van den Berghe G. Neuroendocrine pathobiology of chronic critical illness. *Crit Care Clin.* 2002;18:509. [PMID: 12140911]

Williams RH, et al, eds. Williams Textbook of Endocrinology. 11th ed. Philadelphia, PA: Saunders; 2007.

Biologic Effects and Glucocorticoid Therapy

Chrousos GP. The glucocorticoid receptor gene, longevity, and the complex disorders of Western societies. *Am J Med.* 2004;117:204. [PMID: 15300973]

Czock D, Keller F, Rasche FM, Häussler U. Pharmacokinetics and pharmacodynamics of systemically administered glucocorticoids. *Clin Pharmacokinet.* 2005;44:61. [PMID: 15634032]

Jones A, Fay JK, Burr ML, et al. Inhaled corticosteroid effects on bone metabolism in asthma and mild chronic obstructive pulmonary disease. *Cochrane Database Syst Rev.* 2002:CD003537. [PMID: 11869676]

Limbourg FP, Liao JK. Nontranscriptional actions of the glucocorticoid receptor. *J Mol Med.* 2003;81:168. [PMID: 12682725]

Reichardt HM, Tronchea F, Bergera S, Kellendonka C, Schütza G. New insights into glucocorticoid and mineralocorticoid signaling: lessons from gene targeting. *Adv Pharmacol.* 2000;47:1. [PMID 10582083]

Rosen J, Miner JN. The search for safer glucocorticoid receptor ligands. *Endocr Rev.* 2005;26:452. [PMID: 15814846]

Sizonenko PC. Effects of inhaled or nasal glucocorticosteroids on adrenal function and growth. *J Pediatr Endocrinol Metab.* 2002;15:5. [PMID: 11822580]

Tuckermann JP, Kleiman A, McPherson KG, Reichardt HM. Molecular mechanisms of glucocorticoids in the control of inflammation and lymphocyte apoptosis. *Crit Rev Clin Lab Sci.* 2005;42:71. [PMID: 15697171]

Vgontzas AN, Chrousos GP. Sleep, the hypothalamic-pituitary-adrenal axis, and cytokines: multiple interactions and disturbances in sleep disorders. *Endocrinol Metab Clin North Am.* 2002;31:15. [PMID: 12055986]

Wang M. Review: the role of glucocorticoid action in the pathophysiology of the metabolic syndrome. *Nutrit Metabol.* 2005;2:3. [PMID: 15689240]

Adrenal Insufficiency

Annane D, Bellissant E, Bollaert PE, et al. Corticosteroids for severe sepsis and septic shock: a systematic review and meta-analysis. *BMJ.* 2004;329:480. [PMID: 15289273]

Annane D, Sébille V, Charpentier C, et al. Effect of treatment with low doses of hydrocortisone and fludrocortisone on mortality in patients with septic shock. *JAMA.* 2002;288:862. [PMID: 12186604]

Arit W, Allolio B. Adrenal insufficiency. *Lancet.* 2003;361:1881. [PMID: 12788587]

Barker JM, Ide A, Hostetler C, et. al. Endocrine and immunogenetic testing in individuals with type 1 diabetes and 21-hydroxylase autoantibodies: Addison's disease in a high-risk population. *J Clin Endocrinol Metab.* 2005;90:128. [PMID: 15483092]

Bornstein SR. Predisposing factors for adrenal insufficiency. *N Engl J Med.* 2009;360:2328. [PMID: 19474430]

Buttgereit F, Burmester GR, Lipworth BJ. Optimised glucocorticoid therapy: the sharpening of an old spear. *Lancet.* 2005;365:801. [PMID: 15733723]

Cameron DR, Braunstein GD. The use of dehydroepiandrosterone therapy in clinical practice. *Treat Endocrinol.* 2005;4:95. [PMID: 15783247]

Charmandari E, Kino T, Chrousos GP. Familial/sporadic glucocorticoid resistance: clinical phenotype and molecular mechanisms. *Ann N Y Acad Sci.* 2004;1024:168. [PMID: 15265781]

Coursin DB, Wood KE. Corticosteroid supplementation for adrenal insufficiency. *JAMA.* 2002;287:236. [PMID: 11779267]

Dorin RI, Qualls CR, Crapo LM. Diagnosis of adrenal insufficiency. *Ann Intern Med.* 2003;139:194. [PMID 12899587]

Eisenbarth GS, Gottlieb PA. Autoimmune polyendocrine syndromes. *N Engl J Med.* 2005;350:2068. [PMID 15141045]

Glowniak JV, Loriaux DL. A double-blind study of perioperative steroid requirements in secondary adrenal insufficiency. *Surgery.* 1997;121:123. [PMID: 9037222]

Hamrahian AH, Oseni TS, Arafah BM. Measurements of serum free cortisol in critically ill patients. *N Engl J Med.* 2004;350:1629. [PMID: 15084695]

Inder WJ, Hunt PJ. Glucocorticoid replacement in pituitary surgery: guidelines for perioperative assessment and management. *J Clin Endocrinol Metab.* 2002;87:2745. [PMID: 12050244]

Libè R, Barbetta L, Dall'Asta C, et al. Effects of dehydroepiandrosterone (DHEA) supplementation on hormonal, metabolic and behavioral status in patients with hypoadrenalism. *J Endocrinol Invest.* 2004;27:736. [PMID: 15636426]

Richter B, Neises G, Clar C. Glucocorticoid withdrawal schemes in chronic medical disorders. A systematic review. *Endocrinol Metab Clin North Am.* 2002;31:751. [PMID: 12227130]

Sprung CL, Annane D, Keh D, et al. Hydrocortisone therapy for patients with septic shock. *N Engl J Med.* 2008;358:111. [PMID: 18184957]

Suliman AM, Smith TP, Labib M, Fiad TM, McKenna TJ. The low-dose ACTH test does not provide a useful assessment of the hypothalamic-pituitary-adrenal axis in secondary adrenal insufficiency. *Clin Endocrinol (Oxf).* 2002;56:533. [PMID: 11966747]

Widmer IE, Puder JJ, König C, et al. Cortisol response in relation to the severity of stress and illness—the "CORESSI"-Study. *J Clin Endocrinol Metab.* 2005;90:4579. [PMID: 15886236]

Cushing Syndrome

Elamin MD, Murad MH, Mullan R, et al. Accuracy of diagnostic tests for Cushing's syndrome: a systematic review and metaanalyses. *J Clin Endocrinol Metab.* 2008;94:741. [PMID: 19088166]

Findling JW, Raff H. Cushing's syndrome. *Endocrinol Metab Clin North Am.* 2005;34:257. [PMID: 15850849]

Findling JW, Raff H. Screening and diagnosis of Cushing's syndrome. *Endocrinol Metab Clin North Am.* 2005;34:385. [PMID:15850849]

Findling JW, Raff H, Aron DC. The low-dose dexamethasone suppression test: a reevaluation in patients with Cushing's syndrome. *J Clin Endocrinol Metab.* 2004;89:1222. [PMID: 15001614]

Hammer GD, Tyrrell JB, Lamborn KR, et al. Transsphenoidal microsurgery for Cushing's disease: initial outcome and long-term results. *J Clin Endocrinol Metab.* 2004;89:6348. [PMID: 15579802]

Iacobone M, Mantero F, Basso SM, Lumachi F, Favia G. Results and long-term follow-up after unilateral adrenalectomy for ACTH-independent hypercortisolism in a series of fifty patients. *J Endocrinol Invest.* 2005;28:327. [PMID: 15966505]

Isidori AM, Lenzi A. Ectopic ACTH syndrome. *Arq Bras Endocrinol Metab.* 2007;51:1217. [PMID: 18209859]

Lacroix A, Baldacchino V, Bourdeau I, Hamet P, Tremblay J. Cushing's syndrome variants secondary to aberrant hormone receptors. *Trends Endocrinol Metab.* 2004;15:375. [PMID: 15380809]

Newell-Price J, Morris DG, Drake WM, et al. Optimal response criteria for the human CRH test in the differential diagnosis of ACTH-dependent Cushing's syndrome. *J Clin Endocrinol Metab.* 2002;87:1640. [PMID: 11932295]

Nieman LK, Biller BM, Findling JW, et al. The diagnosis of Cushing's syndrome: an Endocrine Society Clinical Practice Guideline. *J Clin Endocrinol Metab.* 2008;93:1526. [PMID: 18334580]

Quddisi S, Browne P, Hirsch IB. Cushing's syndrome due to surreptitious glucocorticoid administration. *JAMA.* 1998;158:294. [PMID: 9472211]

Savage MO, Lienhardt A, Lebrethon MC, et al. Cushing's disease in childhood: presentation, investigation, treatment and long-term outcome. *Horm Res.* 2001;55(suppl 1):24. [PMID: 11408758]

Stratakis CA, Kirschner LS, Carney JA. Clinical and molecular features of the Carney complex: diagnostic criteria and recommendations for patient evaluation. *J Clin Endocrinol Metab.* 2001;86:4041. [PMID: 11549623]

van Aken MO, Pereira AM, Biermasz NR, et al. Quality of life in patients after long-term biochemical cure of Cushing's disease. *J Clin Endocrinol Metab.* 2005;90:3279. [PMID: 15741267]

Yaneva M, Mosnier-Pudar H, Dugué MA, et al. Midnight salivary cortisol for the initial diagnosis of Cushing's syndrome of various causes. *J Clin Endocrinol Metab.* 2004;89:3345. [PMID: 15240613]

Hirsutism and Virilization

Azziz R. The evaluation and management of hirsutism. *Obstet Gynecol.* 2003;101:995. [PMID: 12738163]

Cabrera MS, Vogiatzi MG, New MI. Long term outcome in adult males with classic congenital adrenal hyperplasia. *J Clin Endocrinol Metab.* 2001;86:3070. [PMID: 11443169]

Kelestimur F. Hirsutism of adrenal origin in adolescents: consequences in adults. *J Pediatr Endocrinol Metab.* 2001;14:1309. [PMID: 11964028]

Miller WL. Androgen biosynthesis from cholesterol to DHEA. *Mol Cell Endocrinol.* 2002;198:7. [PMID: 12573809]

New MI. Inborn errors of adrenal steroidogenesis. *Mol Cell Endocrinol.* 2003;211:75. [PMID: 14656479]

Speiser PW, White PC. Congenital adrenal hyperplasia. *N Engl J Med.* 2003;349:776. [PMID: 12930931]

Wilson JD, Leihy MW, Shaw G, Renfree MB. Androgen physiology: unsolved problems at the millennium. *Mol Cell Endocrinol.* 2002;198:1. [PMID: 12573808]

Incidentally Discovered Adrenal Masses and Adrenal Cancer

Aron DC, Howlett TA. Incidentalomas. *Endocrinol Metab Clin North Am.* 2000;29: 205. [PMID: 10732272]

Caoili EM, Korobkin M, Francis IR, et al. Adrenal masses: characterization with combined unenhanced and delayed enhanced CT. *Radiology.* 2002;222:629. [PMID: 11867777]

Grumbach MM, Biller BMK, Braunstein GD, et al. Management of the clinically inapparent adrenal mass ("incidentaloma"). *Ann Intern Med.* 2003;138:424. [PMID: 12614096]

Icard P, Goudet P, Charpenay C, et al. Adrenocortical carcinomas: surgical trends and results of a 253-patient series from the French Association of Endocrine Surgeons study group. *World J Surg.* 2001;25:891. [PMID: 11572030]

Ogilvie JB, Duh QY. New approaches to the minimally invasive treatment of adrenal lesions. *Cancer J.* 2005;11:64. [PMID: 15831226]

Sahdev A, Reznek RH. Imaging evaluation of the non-functioning indeterminate adrenal mass. *Trend Endocrinol Metab.* 2004;15:271. [PMID: 15358280]

Young WF. The incidentally discovered adrenal mass. *N Engl J Med.* 2007;356:601. [PMID: 17287480]

Endocrine Hypertension

William F. Young, Jr, MD, MSc

11β-HSD2	11β-Hydroxysteroid dehydrogenase type 2	**DOC**	Deoxycorticosterone
		FH	Familial hyperaldosteronism
ACE	Angiotensin-converting enzyme	**GH**	Growth hormone
ACTH	Corticotropin	**GRA**	Glucocorticoid-remediable aldosteronism
AME	Apparent mineralocorticoid excess		
ANP	Atrial natriuretic peptide	**HU**	Hounsfield units
APA	Aldosterone-producing adenoma	**IHA**	Idiopathic hyperaldosteronism
ARB	Angiotensin receptor blocker	**IVC**	Inferior vena cava
AVS	Adrenal venous sampling	**PAC**	Plasma aldosterone concentration
CAH	Congenital adrenal hyperplasia	**PAH**	Primary adrenal hyperplasia
CT	Computed tomography	**PRA**	Plasma renin activity

Hypertension affects one in four adults in the developed world. Although hypertension is *essential* or *idiopathic* in most cases, a cause can be detected in approximately 15% of the hypertensive population. The secondary causes of hypertension can be divided into renal (eg, renal vascular or parenchymal disease) and endocrine causes. There are at least 14 endocrine disorders in which hypertension may be the initial clinical presentation (Table 10–1). The diagnosis of endocrine hypertension presents the clinician an opportunity to provide a surgical cure or to achieve a marked response with targeted pharmacologic therapy. Pheochromocytoma and Cushing syndrome are reviewed in detail in Chapters 11 and 9, respectively. The renin-angiotensin-aldosterone system, the diagnostic and therapeutic approaches to mineralocorticoid hypertension (eg, primary aldosteronism), and less common forms of endocrine hypertension are reviewed in this chapter.

RENIN-ANGIOTENSIN-ALDOSTERONE SYSTEM

The components of the renin-angiotensin-aldosterone system are shown in Figure 10–1. Aldosterone is secreted from the zona glomerulosa under the primary control of angiotensin II, potassium, and corticotropin (ACTH). The secretion of aldosterone is restricted to the zona glomerulosa because of zonal-specific expression of aldosterone synthase (CYP11B2). Atrial natriuretic peptide (ANP), dopamine, and heparin inhibit aldosterone secretion.

Renin and Angiotensin

Renin is an enzyme produced in the juxtaglomerular apparatus of the kidney, stored in granules, and released in response to specific secretagogues. The first 43 amino acids of the 340 amino acid renin protein are a prosegment cleaved to produce the active enzyme. The release of renin into the circulation is the rate-limiting step in the activation of the renin-angiotensin-aldosterone system. Renal renin release is controlled by juxtaglomerular cells acting as pressure transducers that sense stretch of the afferent arteriolar wall and thus renal perfusion pressure; the macula densa, a specialized group of convoluted distal tubular cells that function as chemoreceptors for monitoring the sodium and chloride loads present in the distal tubule; the sympathetic nervous system, which modifies the release of renin, particularly in response to upright posture; and humoral factors, including potassium, angiotensin II, and ANPs. Thus, renin release is maximized in conditions of low renal perfusion pressure or low tubular sodium

TABLE 10–1   Endocrine causes of hypertension.

Adrenal Dependent
Pheochromocytoma
Primary aldosteronism
Hyperdeoxycorticosteronism
   Congenital adrenal hyperplasia
      11β-Hydroxylase deficiency
      17α-Hydroxylase deficiency
   Deoxycorticosterone-producing tumor
   Primary cortisol resistance
Cushing syndrome
Apparent Mineralocorticoid Excess (AME)/11β-Hydroxysteroid
Dehydrogenase Deficiency
Genetic
   Type 1 AME
Acquired
   Licorice or carbenoxolone ingestion (type 1 AME)
   Cushing syndrome (type 2 AME)
Thyroid Dependent
Hypothyroidism
Hyperthyroidism
Pituitary Dependent
Acromegaly
Cushing disease

which constitute a signal peptide that is cleaved prior to secretion. The action of renin on angiotensinogen produces angiotensin I. Angiotensin I is composed of the first 10 amino acid sequence following the signal peptide and does not have biologic activity. Angiotensin II, the main form of biologically active angiotensin, is formed by cleavage of the two carboxyl-terminal amino acids of angiotensin I by angiotensin-converting enzyme (ACE) (Figure 10–2). ACE is localized to cell membranes in the lung and intracellular granules in certain tissues that produce angiotensin II. Amino peptidase A removes the amino-terminal aspartic acid to produce the heptapeptide, angiotensin III. Angiotensin II and angiotensin III have equivalent efficacy in promoting aldosterone secretion and modifying renal blood flow. The half-life in the circulation of angiotensin II is short (<60 seconds). Elements of the renin-angiotensin-aldosterone system are present in the adrenal glands, the kidneys, the heart, and the brain. For example, the adrenal glomerulosa cells contain the proteins needed to produce and secrete angiotensin II. Other tissues contain one or more components of the renin-angiotensin system and require other cells or circulating components, or both, to generate angiotensin II.

Angiotensin II functions through the angiotensin receptor to maintain normal extracellular volume and blood pressure by (a) increasing aldosterone secretion from the zona glomerulosa by increasing transcription of CYP11B2; (b) constriction of vascular smooth muscle, thereby increasing blood pressure and reducing renal blood flow; (c) enhancing the release of norepinephrine and epinephrine from the adrenal medulla; (d) enhancement of the activity of the sympathetic nervous system by increasing central sympathetic outflow, thereby increasing norepinephrine discharge from sympathetic nerve terminals; and (e) promotion of the release of vasopressin.

content (eg, renal artery stenosis, hemorrhage, dehydration). Renin release is suppressed by elevated perfusion pressure at the kidney (eg, hypertension) and high sodium diets. Renin release is increased directly by hypokalemia and decreased by hyperkalemia.

Angiotensinogen, an α_2-globulin synthesized in the liver, is the substrate for renin and is broken down into the angiotensin peptides. Angiotensinogen consists of 485 amino acids, 33 of

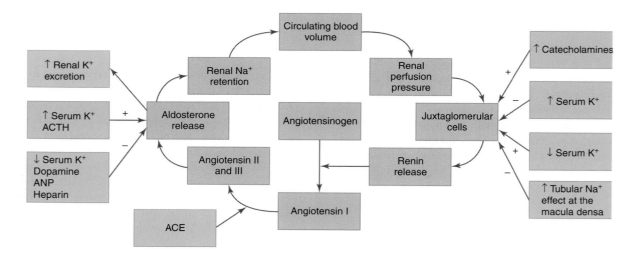

FIGURE 10–1 Renin-angiotensin-aldosterone and potassium-aldosterone feedback loops. Zona glomerulosa aldosterone production and secretion are determined by input from each loop (ACE, angiotensin-converting enzyme; ACTH, cortocotropin; ANP, atrial natriuretic peptide; BP, blood pressure; K⁺, potassium; Na⁺, sodium).

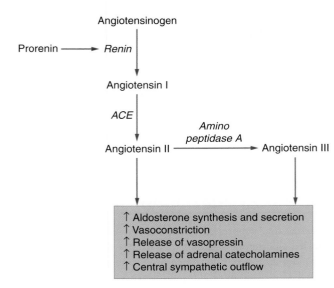

FIGURE 10–2 Steps in the production of angiotensin peptides by the renin-angiotensin system (ACE, angiotensin-converting enzyme).

Aldosterone

Aldosterone is produced in the zona glomerulosa of the adrenal cortex. Approximately 50% to 70% of aldosterone circulates bound to either albumin or corticosteroid-binding globulin; 30% to 50% of total plasma aldosterone is free. Aldosterone is rapidly inactivated to tetrahydroaldosterone in the liver and has a half-life of 15 to 20 minutes. Aldosterone regulates extracellular volume and potassium homeostasis by binding to renal cortical collecting duct principal epithelial cell mineralocorticoid receptors (Figure 10–3). The mineralocorticoid receptor—a member of the nuclear receptor family and also found in the heart, colon, and hippocampus—is localized to the cytoplasm prior to activation, undergoes a conformation change on binding to aldosterone, and translocates into the nucleus where it functions as a transcription factor. The aldosterone-regulated serum- and glucocorticoid-inducible kinase appears to be a key intermediary (see Figure 10–3). Aldosterone increases expression of this kinase which phosphorylates and inactivates neural-precursor-cell-expressed, developmentally down regulated (Nedd) 4-2, a ubiquitin ligase which is responsible for degrading the epithelial sodium channel. This, in turn, leads to an increased number of open

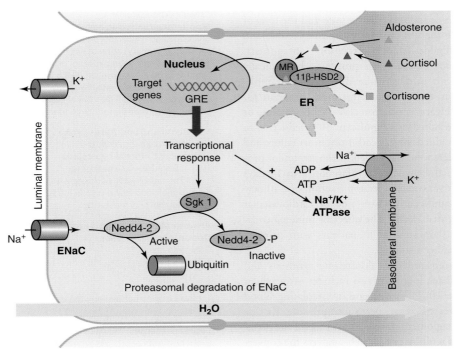

FIGURE 10–3 Aldosterone regulates extracellular volume and potassium homeostasis by binding to the renal cortical collecting duct principal epithelial cell mineralocorticoid receptor (MR). The activated MR translocates into the nucleus where it binds to the glucocorticoid response element (GRE) and functions as a transcription factor. Aldosterone increases expression of serum- and glucocorticoid-inducible kinase (Sgk1), which phosphorylates and inactivates neural-precursor-cell-expressed, developmentally downregulated gene (Nedd) 4-2, a ubiquitin ligase which is responsible for degrading the epithelial sodium channel (ENaC). Another mediator of mineralocorticoid receptor transcriptional response is the activation is the sodium-potassium ATPase (Na$^+$/K$^+$ ATPase) at the basolateral membrane, which drives the uptake of potassium and export of sodium. Although glucocorticoids and mineralocorticoids bind equally to the mineralocorticoid receptor, specificity of action is due to the glucocorticoid-degrading enzyme, 11β-hydroxysteroid dehydrogenase type 2 (11β-HSD2), which prevents glucocorticoids from interacting with the receptor. (Adapted from Odermatt A, Atanasov AG. Mineralocorticoid receptors: Emerging complexity and functional diversity. *Steroids* 2009; 74:163-171.)

sodium channels in the luminal membrane of the principal cells in the cortical collecting tubule, resulting in increased sodium ion reabsorption. The sodium loss increases luminal electronegativity, which augments tubular secretion of potassium by the renal tubular cells and hydrogen ion by the renal interstitial cells. Another mediator of the mineralocorticoid receptor transcriptional response is the activation is the sodium-potassium ATPase at the basolateral membrane, which drives the uptake of potassium and export of sodium (see Figure 10–3). Although glucocorticoids and mineralocorticoids bind equally to the mineralocorticoid receptor, specificity of action is due to the glucocorticoid-degrading enzyme, 11β-hydroxysteroid dehydrogenase, which is strongly expressed in the kidney and prevents glucocorticoids from interacting with the receptor.

Aldosterone has nonclassic effects that, although probably genomic and therefore mediated by activation of the cytosolic mineralocorticoid receptor, do not include modification of sodium-potassium balance. Aldosterone-mediated actions include the expression of several collagen genes; activation of genes controlling tissue growth factors, such as transforming growth factor β and plasminogen activator inhibitor type 1; or increased expression of genes mediating inflammation. The resultant actions lead to microangiopathy, necrosis (acutely), and fibrosis in various tissues such as the heart, the vasculature, and the kidney. Increased levels of aldosterone are not necessary to cause this damage; an imbalance between the volume or sodium balance state and the level of aldosterone appear to be the critical factors. Spironolactone and eplerenone are mineralocorticoid receptor antagonists. Mineralocorticoid receptor blockade has proven to be clinically important in patients with cardiovascular disease. For example, when spironolactone was added to the treatment program for patients with New York Heart Association class IV heart failure or class III heart failure, it resulted in a significant 30% reduction in overall mortality due to reductions in death from heart failure and sudden death. When eplerenone was added to the treatment program for patients who had a myocardial infarction 3 to 14 days previously and had a left ventricular ejection fraction of ≤40 percent, it resulted in a significantly lower rate of cardiovascular mortality and sudden cardiac death. The effect of mineralocorticoid receptor antagonists on survival in patients with primary aldosteronism has not yet been studied.

The action of angiotensin II on aldosterone synthesis and secretion involves a feedback loop that also includes extracellular fluid volume (see Figure 10–1). A decrease in circulating blood volume results in decreased renal perfusion pressure that is detected by the renal juxtaglomerular cells. Activation of the juxtaglomerular cells increases renin release, which catalyzes the conversion of angiotensinogen to angiotensin I. Angiotensin-converting enzyme (ACE) in the pulmonary and renal endothelium catalyzes the conversion of angiotensin I to angiotensin II and III, which act on the adrenal zona glomerulosa angiotensin receptor to stimulate aldosterone release. Aldosterone acts at the renal mineralocorticoid receptors to stimulate sodium and water retention to preserve the circulating blood volume. Renin release can also be triggered by catecholamines, hypokalemia, and a decrease in sodium chloride absorption in the macula densa cells. Aldosterone secretion can be directly stimulated by ACTH and hyperkalemia. Thus,

sodium restriction activates and sodium overload suppresses the renin-angiotensin-aldosterone axis. Mineralocorticoid escape refers to the counterregulatory mechanisms that occur after 3 to 5 days of excessive mineralocorticoid administration. Several mechanisms contribute to this escape, including renal hemodynamic factors and increased release of ANP.

Excess aldosterone secretion causes hypertension through two main mechanisms: (1) mineralocorticoid-induced expansion of plasma and extracellular fluid volume; and (2) increase in total peripheral vascular resistance.

PRIMARY ALDOSTERONISM

Hypertension, suppressed plasma renin activity (PRA), and increased aldosterone excretion characterize the syndrome of primary aldosteronism. Aldosterone-producing adenoma (APA) and bilateral idiopathic hyperaldosteronism (IHA) are the two most common subtypes of primary aldosteronism (Table 10–2).

TABLE 10–2 Adrenocortical causes of hypertension.

Low Renin and High Aldosterone
PRIMARY ALDOSTERONISM
Aldosterone-producing adenoma (APA) ≈35% of cases
Bilateral idiopathic hyperplasia (IHA) ≈60% of cases
Unilateral (primary) adrenal hyperplasia ≈2% of cases
Aldosterone-producing adrenocortical carcinoma <1% of cases
Familial hyperaldosteronism (FH)
Glucocorticoid-remediable aldosteronism (FH type I) <1% of cases
FH type II (APA or IHA) <2% of cases
Ectopic aldosterone-producing adenoma or carcinoma <0.1% of cases
Low Renin and Low Aldosterone
HYPERDEOXYCORTICOSTERONISM
Congenital adrenal hyperplasia
11β-Hydroxylase deficiency
17α-Hydroxylase deficiency
Deoxycorticosterone-producing tumor
Primary cortisol resistance
APPARENT MINERALOCORTICOID EXCESS (AME)/11β-HYDROXYSTEROID DEHYDROGENASE DEFICIENCY
Genetic
Type 1 AME
Type 2 AME
Acquired
Licorice or carbenoxolone ingestion (type 1 AME)
Cushing syndrome (type 2 AME)
CUSHING SYNDROME
Exogenous glucocorticoid administration–most common cause
Endogenous
ACTH-dependent ≈85% of cases
Pituitary
Ectopic
ACTH-independent ≈15% of cases
Unilateral adrenal disease
Bilateral adrenal disease
Massive macronodular hyperplasia (rare)
Primary pigmented nodular adrenal disease (rare)

ACTH, corticotropin; AME, apparent mineralocorticoid excess; APA, aldosterone-producing adenoma; FH, familial hyperaldosteronism; IHA, idiopathic hyperaldosteronism.

A much less common form, unilateral hyperplasia, is caused by micronodular or macronodular hyperplasia of the zona glomerulosa of predominantly one adrenal gland. Unilateral hyperplasia is referred to as primary adrenal hyperplasia (PAH). Familial hyperaldosteronism (FH) is also rare and two types have been described: FH type I and FH type II. FH type I, or glucocorticoid-remediable aldosteronism (GRA), is autosomal dominant in inheritance and associated with variable degrees of hyperaldosteronism, high levels of hybrid steroids (eg, 18-hydroxycortisol and 18-oxocortisol), and suppression with exogenous glucocorticoids. FH type II refers to the familial occurrence of APA or IHA or both.

Prevalence

In the past, clinicians would not consider the diagnosis of primary aldosteronism unless the patient presented with spontaneous hypokalemia, and then the diagnostic evaluation would require discontinuing antihypertensive medications for at least 2 weeks. The *spontaneous hypokalemia/no antihypertensive drug* diagnostic approach resulted in predicted prevalence rates of less than 0.5% of hypertensive patients. However, it is now recognized that most patients with primary aldosteronism are not hypokalemic and that case-detection testing can be completed with a simple blood test (plasma aldosterone concentration [PAC]-to-plasma renin activity [PRA] ratio) while the patient is taking most antihypertensive drugs. Using the PAC-PRA ratio as a case-detection test, followed by aldosterone suppression confirmatory testing, has resulted in much higher prevalence estimates (5%-10% of all patients with hypertension) for primary aldosteronism.

Clinical Presentation

The diagnosis of primary aldosteronism is usually made in patients who are in the third to sixth decade of life. Few symptoms are specific to the syndrome. Patients with marked hypokalemia may have muscle weakness and cramping, headaches, palpitations, polydipsia, polyuria, nocturia, or a combination of these. Periodic paralysis is a very rare presentation in Caucasians, but it is not an infrequent presentation in patients of Asian descent. The polyuria and nocturia are a result of a hypokalemia-induced renal concentrating defect and the presentation is frequently mistaken for prostatism in men. There are no specific physical findings. Edema is not a common finding because of mineralocorticoid escape. The degree of hypertension is usually moderate to severe and may be resistant to usual pharmacologic treatments. Although not common, primary aldosteronism may present with hypertensive urgencies. Patients with APA tend to have higher blood pressures than those with IHA. Hypokalemia is frequently absent; thus, all patients with hypertension are candidates for this disorder. In other patients, the hypokalemia only becomes evident with addition of a potassium-wasting diuretic (eg, hydrochlorothiazide, furosemide). Aldosterone excess also leads to a mild metabolic alkalosis because of increased urinary hydrogen excretion mediated both by hypokalemia and by the direct stimulatory effect of aldosterone on distal renal tubule acidification. Because of a reset osmostat, the serum sodium concentration tends to be high-normal or slightly above the upper limit of normal—this clinical finding is very useful when initially assessing the potential for primary aldosteronism.

Several studies have shown that patients with primary aldosteronism may be at higher risk than other patients with hypertension for target organ damage of the heart and kidney. When matched for age, blood pressure, and duration of hypertension, patients with primary aldosteronism have greater left ventricular mass by echocardiographic measurements than patients with other types of hypertension (eg, pheochromocytoma, Cushing syndrome, or essential hypertension). In patients with APA, the left ventricular wall thickness and mass decreases markedly 1 year after adrenalectomy. Patients presenting with either APA or IHA have a significantly higher rate of cardiovascular events (eg, stroke, atrial fibrillation, and myocardial infarction) than matched patients with essential hypertension who have similar degrees of hypertension duration and control.

Diagnosis

The diagnostic approach to primary aldosteronism can be considered in three parts: case-detection tests, confirmatory tests, and subtype evaluation tests.

A. Case-detection tests Spontaneous hypokalemia is uncommon in patients with uncomplicated hypertension and, when present, strongly suggests associated mineralocorticoid excess. However, most patients with primary aldosteronism have baseline serum levels of potassium in the normal range. Therefore, hypokalemia is not and should not be the only criterion used to determine whom to test for primary aldosteronism. Patients with hypertension and hypokalemia (regardless of presumed cause), treatment-resistant hypertension (three antihypertensive drugs and poor control), severe hypertension (≥160 mm Hg systolic or ≥100 mm Hg diastolic), hypertension and an incidental adrenal mass, and onset of hypertension at a young age should undergo case-detection testing for primary aldosteronism (Figure 10–4). In addition, primary aldosteronism should be tested for when considering a secondary hypertension evaluation (eg, when testing for renovascular disease or pheochromocytoma).

In patients with suspected primary aldosteronism, case detection can be accomplished by measuring a morning (preferably between 8 AM and 10 AM) ambulatory paired random PAC and PRA (see Figure 10–4). This test may be performed while the patient is taking most antihypertensive medications and without posture stimulation. Hypokalemia reduces the secretion of aldosterone, and it is optimal in patients with hypokalemia to restore the serum level of potassium to normal before performing diagnostic studies. Mineralocorticoid receptor antagonists (eg, spironolactone and eplerenone) are the only medications that absolutely interfere with interpretation of the ratio and should be discontinued at least 6 weeks before testing. ACE-inhibitors and angiotensin receptor blockers (ARB) have the potential to falsely elevate PRA. Therefore, in a patient treated with an ACE inhibitor or ARB, the finding of a detectable PRA level or a low PAC-PRA ratio does not exclude the diagnosis of primary aldosteronism. However, a very

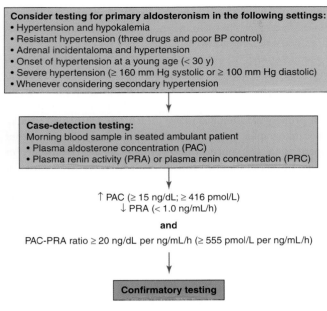

Consider testing for primary aldosteronism in the following settings:
• Hypertension and hypokalemia
• Resistant hypertension (three drugs and poor BP control)
• Adrenal incidentaloma and hypertension
• Onset of hypertension at a young age (< 30 y)
• Severe hypertension (≥ 160 mm Hg systolic or ≥ 100 mm Hg diastolic)
• Whenever considering secondary hypertension

Case-detection testing:
Morning blood sample in seated ambulant patient
• Plasma aldosterone concentration (PAC)
• Plasma renin activity (PRA) or plasma renin concentration (PRC)

↑ PAC (≥ 15 ng/dL; ≥ 416 pmol/L)
↓ PRA (< 1.0 ng/mL/h)
and
PAC-PRA ratio ≥ 20 ng/dL per ng/mL/h (≥ 555 pmol/L per ng/mL/h)

Confirmatory testing

FIGURE 10–4 When to consider testing for primary aldosteronism and use of the plasma aldosterone concentration to plasma renin activity ratio as a case-finding tool (BP, blood pressure, PAC, plasma aldosterone concentration, PRA, plasma renin activity, PRC, plasma renin concentration).

useful clinical point is that when a PRA level is undetectably low in a patient taking an ACE inhibitor or ARB, primary aldosteronism is likely. A second important clinical point is that PRA is suppressed (<1.0 ng/mL/h) in almost all patients with primary aldosteronism, regardless of concurrent medications.

The PAC-PRA ratio is based on the concept of paired hormone measurements. For example, in a hypertensive hypokalemic patient: (a) secondary hyperaldosteronism should be considered when both PRA and PAC are increased and the PAC-PRA ratio is less than 10 (eg, renovascular disease); (b) an alternate source of mineralocorticoid receptor agonism should be considered when both PRA and PAC are suppressed (eg, hypercortisolism); and (c) primary aldosteronism should be suspected when PRA is suppressed (<1.0 ng/mL/h) and PAC is increased (Figure 10–5). Although there is some uncertainty about test characteristics and lack of standardization, the PAC-PRA ratio is widely accepted as the case-detection test of choice for primary aldosteronism. It is important to understand that the lower limit of detection varies among different PRA assays and can have a dramatic effect on the PAC-PRA ratio. As an example, if the lower limit of detection for PRA is 0.6 ng/mL/h and the PAC is 18 ng/dL, then the PAC-PRA ratio would be 30; however, if the lower limit of detection for PRA is 0.1 ng/mL/h and the PAC is 18 ng/dL, then the PAC-PRA ratio would be 180. Thus, the cutoff for a high PAC-PRA ratio is laboratory dependent and, more specifically, PRA assay dependent. At Mayo Clinic, a PAC (in ng/dL)-PRA (in ng/mL/h) ratio of 20 or more and PAC of at least 15 ng/dL are found in more than 90% of patients with surgically confirmed APA. In patients without primary aldosteronism, most of the variation occurs within the normal range. The sensitivity and specificity of the PAC-PRA ratio in the diagnosis of primary aldosteronism are approximately 80% and 75%, respectively. A high PAC-PRA ratio with a PAC of at least 15 ng/dL is a positive case-detection test result, a finding that warrants further testing. Other initial case-detection strategies include measurement of isolated plasma renin activity or 24-hour urinary aldosterone excretion.

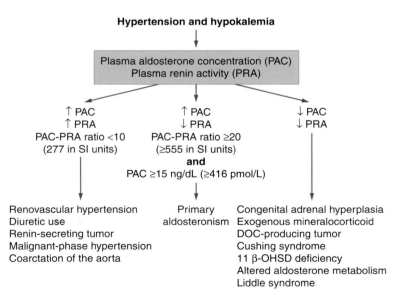

Hypertension and hypokalemia

Plasma aldosterone concentration (PAC)
Plasma renin activity (PRA)

↑ PAC
↑ PRA
PAC-PRA ratio <10
(277 in SI units)

↑ PAC
↓ PRA
PAC-PRA ratio ≥20
(≥555 in SI units)
and
PAC ≥15 ng/dL (≥416 pmol/L)

↓ PAC
↓ PRA

Renovascular hypertension
Diuretic use
Renin-secreting tumor
Malignant-phase hypertension
Coarctation of the aorta

Primary aldosteronism

Congenital adrenal hyperplasia
Exogenous mineralocorticoid
DOC-producing tumor
Cushing syndrome
11 β-OHSD deficiency
Altered aldosterone metabolism
Liddle syndrome

FIGURE 10–5 Use of the plasma aldosterone concentration-to-plasma renin activity ratio to differentiate among different causes of hypertension and hypokalemia (DOC, deoxycorticosterone; OHSD, hydroxysteroid dehydrogenase; PAC, plasma aldosterone concentration; PRA, plasma renin activity; SI units, International System of Units). (Adapted from Young WF Jr, Hogan MJ. Renin-independent hypermineralocorticoidism. *Trends Endocrinol Metab.* 1994;5:97-106.)

B. Confirmatory tests   An increased PAC-PRA ratio is not diagnostic by itself, and primary aldosteronism must be confirmed by demonstrating lack of normal suppressiblity of aldosterone secretion. The list of drugs and hormones capable of affecting the renin-angiotensin-aldosterone axis is extensive and frequently a medication-contaminated evaluation is unavoidable. Calcium channel blockers and α_1-adrenergic receptor blockers do not affect the diagnostic accuracy in most cases. It is impossible to interpret data obtained from patients receiving treatment with mineralocorticoid receptor antagonists (eg, spironolactone, eplerenone) when PRA is not suppressed. Therefore, treatment with a mineralocorticoid receptor antagonist should not be initiated until the evaluation has been completed and the final decisions about treatment have been made. If primary aldosteronism is suspected in a patient receiving treatment with spironolactone or eplerenone, the treatment should be discontinued for at least 6 weeks before further diagnostic testing. Aldosterone suppression testing can be performed with orally administered sodium chloride and measurement of urinary aldosterone or with intravenous sodium chloride loading and measurement of PAC:

a. **Oral sodium loading test**—After hypertension and hypokalemia are controlled, patients should receive a high-sodium diet (supplemented with sodium chloride tablets if needed) for 3 days, with a goal sodium intake of 5000 mg of sodium (equivalent to 12.8 g sodium chloride or 218 mEq of sodium). The risk of increasing dietary sodium in patients with severe hypertension must be assessed in each case. Because the high-sodium diet can increase kaliuresis and hypokalemia, vigorous replacement of potassium chloride may be needed, and the serum level of potassium should be monitored daily. On the third day of the high-sodium diet, a 24-hour urine specimen is collected for measurement of aldosterone, sodium, and creatinine. To document adequate sodium repletion, the 24-hour urinary sodium excretion should exceed 200 mEq. Urinary aldosterone excretion more than 12 mcg/24 h is consistent with autonomous aldosterone secretion. The sensitivity and specificity of the oral sodium loading test are 96% and 93%, respectively.

b. **Intravenous saline infusion test**—The intravenous saline infusion test has also been used for the confirmation of primary aldosteronism. Normal subjects show suppression of PAC after volume expansion with isotonic saline; subjects with primary aldosteronism do not show this suppression. The risks associated with rapid intravenous volume expansion should be assessed in each case. The test is done after an overnight fast. Two liters of 0.9% sodium chloride solution are infused intravenously with an infusion pump over 4 hours into the recumbent patient. Blood pressure and heart rate are monitored during the infusion. At the completion of the infusion, blood is drawn for measurement of PAC. PAC levels in normal subjects decrease to less than 5 ng/dL; most patients with primary aldosteronism do not suppress to less than 10 ng/dL; postsaline infusion PAC values between 5 and 10 ng/dL are indeterminate and can be seen in patients with IHA.

C. Subtype studies   Following case-detection and confirmatory testing, the third management step guides the therapeutic approach by distinguishing APA and PAH from IHA and GRA. Unilateral adrenalectomy in patients with APA or PAH results in normalization of hypokalemia in all; hypertension is improved in all and is cured in approximately 30% to 60% of them. In IHA and GRA, unilateral or bilateral adrenalectomy seldom corrects the hypertension. IHA and GRA should be treated medically. APA is found in approximately 35% of cases and bilateral IHA in approximately 60% of cases (see Table 10–2). APAs are usually hypodense nodules (<2 cm in diameter) on CT and are golden yellow in color on cut section. IHA adrenal glands may be normal on CT or show nodular changes. Aldosterone-producing adrenal carcinomas are almost always greater than 4 cm in diameter and have a suspicious imaging phenotype on CT. Patients with aldosterone-producing adrenocortical carcinomas usually have severe aldosterone excess with serum potassium concentrations frequently less than 2.0 mEq/L.

a. **Adrenal CT**—Primary aldosteronism subtype evaluation may require one or more tests, the first of which is imaging the adrenal glands with CT (Figure 10–6). This imaging test is usually ordered as CT of the abdomen limited to the adrenal glands with 2-mm contiguous cuts. Although contrast enhancement is not necessary, contrast administration result in improved discrimination between normal adrenal cortex and the small lipid-rich cortical adenoma. When a solitary unilateral hypodense (Hounsfield units [HU] <10) macroadenoma (>1 cm) and normal contralateral adrenal morphology are found on CT in a young patient (adrenal incidentalomas are uncommon in patients <40 years) with primary aldosteronism, unilateral adrenalectomy is a reasonable therapeutic option (Figure 10–7). However, in many cases, CT may show normal-appearing adrenals, minimal unilateral adrenal limb thickening, unilateral microadenomas (<1 cm), bilateral macroadenomas, or a large (eg, >2 cm) unilateral macroadenoma that would be atypical for primary aldosteronism. In these cases, when the patient wants to pursue the surgical treatment option for primary aldosteronism, additional testing is required to determine the source of excess aldosterone secretion (Figure 10–8). Small APAs may be labeled incorrectly as IHA on the basis of CT findings of bilateral nodularity or normal-appearing adrenals. Also, apparent adrenal microadenomas may actually represent areas of hyperplasia, and unilateral adrenalectomy would be inappropriate. In addition, nonfunctioning unilateral adrenal macroadenomas are not uncommon, especially in individuals more than 40 years of age. Unilateral PAH may be visible on CT or the PAH adrenal may appear normal on CT. In general, patients with APAs have more severe hypertension, more frequent hypokalemia, higher plasma (>25 ng/dL) and urinary (>30 mcg/24 h) levels of aldosterone than those with IHA.

Adrenal CT is not accurate in distinguishing between APA and IHA. In one study of 203 patients with primary aldosteronism who were evaluated with both CT and adrenal venous sampling (AVS), CT was accurate in only 53% of patients; based on CT findings, 42 patients (22%) would have been incorrectly excluded as candidates for adrenalectomy and 48 (25%) might have had unnecessary or inappropriate surgery. Therefore, AVS is essential to direct appropriate therapy in patients older than 40 years of age with primary aldosteronism who have a high probability of

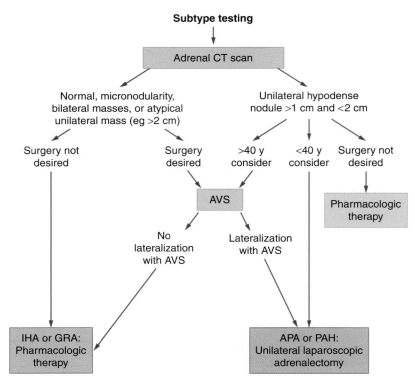

FIGURE 10–6 Subtype evaluation of primary aldosteronism. For patients who want to pursue a surgical treatment for their hypertension, adrenal venous sampling is frequently a key diagnostic step. See text for details (APA, aldosterone-producing adenoma; AVS, adrenal venous sampling; CT, computed tomography; IHA, idiopathic hyperaldosteronism; PAH, primary adrenal hyperplasia). (Adapted from Young WF Jr, Hogan MJ. Renin-independent hypermineralocorticoidism. *Trends Endocrinol Metab*. 1994;5:97-106).

APA and who seek a potential surgical cure. However, it is important to recognize that the surgical option is not mandatory in patients with APA—pharmacologic therapy with a mineralocorticoid receptor antagonist is the medication equivalent of adrenalectomy (see later).

b. Adrenal venous sampling—AVS is the criterion standard test to distinguish between unilateral and bilateral disease in patients with primary aldosteronism who want to pursue surgical management for their hypertension. AVS is an intricate procedure because the right adrenal vein is small and may be difficult to locate and cannulate—the success rate depends on the proficiency of the angiographer. The five keys to a successful AVS program are (1) appropriate patient selection; (2) careful patient preparation; (3) focused technical expertise; (4) defined protocol; and (5) accurate data interpretation. A center-specific, written protocol is mandatory. The protocol should be developed by an interested group of endocrinologists, hypertension specialists, internists, radiologists, and laboratory personnel. Safeguards should be in place to prevent mislabeling of the blood tubes in the radiology suite and to prevent sample mix-up in the laboratory. At Mayo Clinic, we use continuous cosyntropin infusion during AVS (50 μg/h started 30 minutes before sampling and continued throughout the procedure) for the following reasons: (a) to minimize stress-induced fluctuations in aldosterone secretion during nonsimultaneous AVS; (b) to maximize the gradient in cortisol from adrenal vein to inferior vena cava (IVC) and thus confirm successful

sampling of the adrenal veins; and (c) to maximize the secretion of aldosterone from an APA. The adrenal veins are catheterized through the percutaneous femoral vein approach, and the position of the catheter tip is verified by gentle injection of a small amount of nonionic contrast medium and radiographic documentation (see Figure 10–8). Blood is obtained from both adrenal veins and the IVC below the renal veins and assayed for aldosterone and cortisol concentrations. To be sure there is no cross-contamination, the IVC sample should be obtained from the external iliac vein. The venous sample from the left side typically is obtained from the common phrenic vein immediately adjacent to the entrance of the adrenal vein. The cortisol concentrations from the adrenal veins and IVC are used to confirm successful catheterization; the adrenal vein-IVC cortisol ratio is typically more than 10:1.

Dividing the right and left adrenal vein PACs by their respective cortisol concentrations corrects for the dilutional effect of the inferior phenic vein flow into the left adrenal vein; these are termed **cortisol-corrected ratios** (see Figure 10–8). In patients with APA, the mean cortisol-corrected aldosterone ratio (APA-side PAC/cortisol:normal adrenal PAC/cortisol) is 18:1. A cutoff of the cortisol-corrected aldosterone ratio from high side to low side more than 4:1 is used to indicate unilateral aldosterone excess (see Figure 10–8). In patients with IHA, the mean cortisol-corrected aldosterone ratio is 1.8:1 (high side:low side); a ratio less than 3:1 is suggestive of bilateral aldosterone

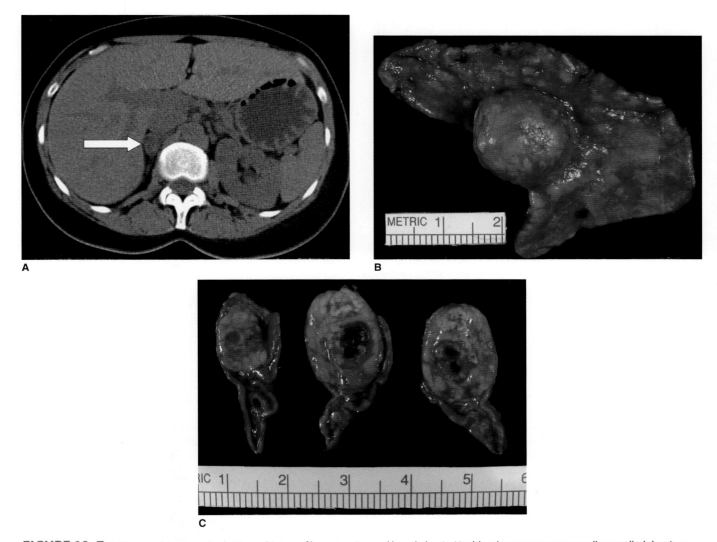

FIGURE 10–7 A 30-year-old woman had a 7-year history of hypertension and hypokalemia. Her blood pressure was not well controlled despite a four-drug program that included a calcium channel blocker, ACE-inhibitor, thiazide diuretic, and a β-adrenergic blocker. To correct her hypokalemia, she took 420 mEq of potassium per day. The case-detection test for primary aldosteronism was positive, with a plasma aldosterone concentration (PAC) of 34 ng/dL and low plasma renin activity (PRA) at less than 0.6 ng/mL/h (PAC-PRA ratio >56). The confirmatory test for primary aldosteronism was also positive, with 24-hour urinary excretion of aldosterone of 77 μg on a high-sodium diet (urinary sodium, 205 mEq/24 h). **A.** Adrenal CT axial image showing a 15-mm low-density mass (arrow) within the right adrenal gland. She underwent laparoscopic right adrenalectomy. **B.** Right adrenal gland (6.2 g, 6.1 cm × 3.7 cm × 1.4 cm) with a 1.8-cm cortical adenoma arising from the surface. **C.** Cut sections of the yellow adrenal cortical adenoma forming a 1.8 cm × 1.7 cm × 1.3 cm nodule. The postoperative plasma aldosterone concentration was less than 1.0 ng/dL. Hypokalemia was resolved. Four years after surgery, her blood pressure was normal without the aid of antihypertensive medications.

hypersecretion. Therefore, most patients with a unilateral source of aldosterone will have cortisol-corrected aldosterone lateralization ratios greater than 4.0; ratios greater than 3.0 but less than 4.0 represent a zone of overlap. Ratios no more than 3.0 are consistent with bilateral aldosterone secretion. The test characteristics of AVS for detecting unilateral aldosterone hypersecretion (APA or PAH) have sensitivity of 95% and specificity of 100%. However, since all patients who undergo AVS are not sent to surgery, the true diagnostic sensitivity of AVS is unknown. At centers with experience with AVS, the complication rate is 2.5% or less. Complications can include symptomatic groin hematoma, adrenal hemorrhage, and dissection of an adrenal vein.

Some centers and clinical practice guidelines recommend that AVS should be performed in all patients who have the diagnosis of primary aldosteronism. However, a more practical approach is to consider the use of AVS based on patient preferences, patient age, clinical comorbidities, and clinical probability of finding an APA (see Figure 10–6).

c. **Glucocorticoid-remediable aldosteronism—familial hyperaldosteronism type I**—This syndrome is inherited in an autosomal dominant fashion and is extremely rare (responsible for fewer than 1% of cases of primary aldosteronism) (see Table 10–2). GRA is characterized by hypertension of early onset that is usually severe and refractory to conventional antihypertensive therapies, aldosterone excess,

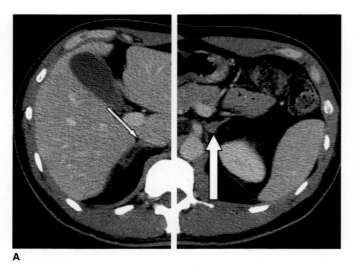
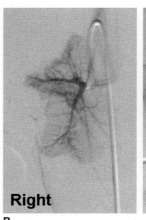
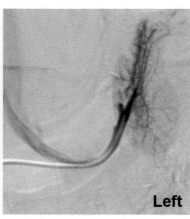

A   **B**

Bilateral adrenal venous sampling

Vein	Aldosterone (A), ng/dL	Cortisol (C), μg/dL	A/C ratio	Aldosterone ratio*
R adrenal vein	8450	1669	5.1	8.5
L adrenal vein	923	1599	0.6	
Inferior vena cava	13	22	0.6	

*R adrenal vein A/C ratio divided by L adrenal vein A/C ratio.

C

FIGURE 10–8 A 48-year-old man had a 7-year history of hypertension that was not optimally controlled on four antihypertensive drugs (β-adrenergic blocker, peripheral α₁-antagonist, angiotensin receptor blocker, and a thiazide diuretic). He was not hypokalemic. Resistant hypertension prompted case-detection testing for primary aldosteronism with a plasma aldosterone concentration (PAC) of 15 ng/dL and low plasma renin activity (PRA) at less than 0.6 ng/mL/h (PAC-PRA ratio >25). The confirmatory test for primary aldosteronism was also positive, with 24-hour urinary excretion of aldosterone of 16 μg on a high-sodium diet (urinary sodium, 356 mEq/24 h). **A.** Adrenal CT split section axial images show a 12-mm thickening (large arrow) in the inferior aspect of the left adrenal gland and a tiny nodule (small arrow) in the right adrenal gland. The patient wanted to pursue a surgical approach to the resolution of or improvement in hypertension. **B.** Adrenal venous sampling images showing the catheter in the right and left adrenal veins. The delicate venous architecture is demonstrated. **C.** Adrenal venous sampling lateralized aldosterone secretion to the right adrenal gland, and a 3-mm yellow cortical adenoma was found at laparoscopic right adrenalectomy. The postoperative plasma aldosterone concentration was less than 1.0 ng/dL. One year after surgery, his blood pressure was in the normal range with the aid of one antihypertensive medication. (Reproduced with permission from: Young WF. Endocrine Hypertension: Then and Now. Endocr Pract. 2010;16:888-902.)

suppressed PRA, and excess production of 18-hydroxycortisol and 18-oxycortisol. GRA is caused by a chimeric gene duplication that results from unequal crossing over between the promoter sequence of *CYP11B1* gene (encoding 11β-hydroxylase) and the coding sequence of *CYP11B2* (encoding aldosterone synthase). This chimeric gene contains the 3′ ACTH-responsive portion of the promoter from the *11β-hydroxylase* gene fused to the 5′ coding sequence of the aldosterone synthase gene. The result is ectopic expression of aldosterone synthase activity in the cortisol-producing zona fasciculata. Thus, mineralocorticoid production is regulated by ACTH instead of the normal secretagogue, angiotensin II. Aldosterone secretion can be suppressed by glucocorticoid therapy. In the absence of glucocorticoid therapy, this mutation results in overproduction of aldosterone and the hybrid steroids 18-hydroxycortisol and 18-oxycortisol, which can be measured in the urine to make the diagnosis.

Genetic testing is a sensitive and specific means of diagnosing GRA and obviates the need to measure the urinary

levels of 18-oxocortisol and 18-hydroxycortisol or to perform dexamethasone suppression testing. Genetic testing for GRA should be considered for primary aldosteronism patients with a family history of primary aldosteronism or onset of primary aldosteronism at a young age (eg, <20 years), or in primary aldosteronism patients who have a family history of strokes at a young age. Cerebrovascular complications (eg, hemorrhagic stroke) associated with intracranial aneurysms affect approximately 20% of all patients with GRA—a frequency of cerebral aneurysm similar to that found in adult polycystic kidney disease.

d. Familial hyperaldosteronism type II—FH type II is autosomal dominant and may be monogenic. The hyperaldosteronism in FH type II does not suppress with dexamethasone, and GRA mutation testing is negative. FH type II is more common than FH type I, but it still represents less than 2% of all patients with primary aldosteronism. The molecular basis for FH type II is unclear, although a recent linkage analysis study showed an association with chromosomal region 7p22.

Treatment

The treatment goal is to prevent the morbidity and mortality associated with hypertension, hypokalemia, and cardiovascular damage. The cause of the primary aldosteronism helps to determine the appropriate treatment. Normalization of blood pressure should not be the only goal in managing a patient who has primary aldosteronism. In addition to the kidney and colon, mineralocorticoid receptors occur in the heart, brain, and blood vessels. Excessive secretion of aldosterone is associated with increased risk of cardiovascular disease and morbidity. Therefore, normalization of circulating aldosterone or mineralocorticoid receptor blockade should be part of the management plan for all patients with primary aldosteronism. However, clinicians must understand that most patients with long-standing primary aldosteronism have some degree of renal insufficiency that is masked by the glomerular hyperfiltration associated with aldosterone excess. The true degree of renal insufficiency may only become evident after effective pharmacologic or surgical therapy.

A.   Surgical treatment of aldosterone-producing adenoma and unilateral hyperplasia   Unilateral laparoscopic adrenalectomy is an excellent treatment option for patients with APA or PAH (unilateral hyperplasia). Although blood pressure control improves in nearly 100% of patients postoperatively, average long-term cure rates of hypertension after unilateral adrenalectomy for APA range from 30% to 60%. Persistent hypertension following adrenalectomy is correlated directly with having more than one first-degree relative with hypertension, use of more than two antihypertensive agents preoperatively, older age, increased serum creatinine level, and duration of hypertension.

Laparoscopic adrenalectomy is the preferred surgical approach and is associated with shorter hospital stays and less long-term morbidity than the open approach. Because APAs are small and may be multiple, the entire adrenal gland should be removed. To decrease the surgical risk, hypokalemia should be corrected with potassium supplements and/or a mineralocorticoid receptor antagonist preoperatively. The mineralocorticoid receptor antagonist and potassium supplements should be discontinued postoperatively. PAC should be measured 1 to 2 days after the operation to confirm a biochemical cure. Serum potassium levels should be monitored weekly for 4 weeks after surgery and a generous sodium diet should be followed to avoid the hyperkalemia of hypoaldosteronism that may occur because of the chronic suppression of the renin-angiotensin-aldosterone axis. In approximately 5% of APA patients clinically significant hyperkalemia may develop after surgery and short-term fludrocortisone supplementation may be required. Typically, the component of hypertension that was associated with aldosterone excess resolves in 1 to 3 months postoperatively.

B.   Pharmacologic treatment   IHA and GRA should be treated medically. In addition, APA patients may be treated medically if the medical treatment includes mineralocorticoid receptor blockade. A sodium-restricted diet (<100 mEq of sodium per day), maintenance of ideal body weight, tobacco avoidance, and regular aerobic exercise contribute significantly to the success of pharmacologic treatment. No placebo-controlled randomized trials have evaluated the relative efficacy of drugs in the treatment of primary aldosteronism. Spironolactone, available as 25-, 50-, and 100-mg tablets, has been the drug of choice to treat primary aldosteronism for more than four decades. The initial dosage is 12.5 to 25 mg/d and is increased to 400 mg/d if necessary to achieve a high-normal serum potassium concentration without the aid of oral potassium chloride supplementation. Hypokalemia responds promptly, but hypertension may take as long as 4 to 8 weeks to correct. After several months of therapy, this dosage often can be decreased to as little as 25 to 50 mg/d; dosage titration is based on a goal serum potassium level in the high-normal range. Serum potassium and creatinine should be monitored frequently during the first 4 to 6 weeks of therapy (especially in patients with renal insufficiency or diabetes mellitus). Spironolactone increases the half-life of digoxin, and for patients taking this drug, the dosage may need to be adjusted when treatment with spironolactone is started. Concomitant therapy with salicylates should be avoided because they interfere with the tubular secretion of an active metabolite and decrease the effectiveness of spironolactone. Spironolactone is not selective for the mineralocorticoid receptor. For example, antagonism at the testosterone receptor may result in painful gynecomastia, erectile dysfunction, and decreased libido in men; agonist activity at the progesterone receptor results in menstrual irregularity in women.

Eplerenone is a steroid-based antimineralocorticoid that acts as a competitive and selective mineralocorticoid receptor antagonist. It has a marked reduction in progestational and antiandrogenic actions compared with spironolactone. Treatment trials comparing the efficacy of eplerenone versus spironolactone for the treatment of primary aldosteronism have not been published. Eplerenone is available as 25- and 50-mg tablets. For primary aldosteronism, it is reasonable to start with a dose of 25 mg twice daily (twice daily because of the shorter half-life of eplerenone compared to spironolactone) and titrated upward for a target high-normal serum potassium concentration without the aid of potassium supplements. Potency studies with eplerenone show 50% less milligram per milligram potency when compared with spironolactone. As with spironolactone, it is important to follow blood pressure, serum potassium, and serum creatinine levels closely.

Patients with IHA frequently require a second antihypertensive agent to achieve adequate blood pressure control. Hypervolemia is a major reason for resistance to drug therapy, and low doses of a thiazide (eg, 12.5-50 mg of hydrochlorothiazide daily) or a related sulfonamide diuretic are effective in combination with the mineralocorticoid receptor antagonist. Because these agents often lead to further hypokalemia, serum potassium levels should be monitored.

Before initiating treatment, GRA should be confirmed with genetic testing. In the GRA patient, chronic treatment with physiologic doses of a glucocorticoid normalizes blood pressure and corrects hypokalemia. The clinician should avoid iatrogenic Cushing syndrome with excessive doses of glucocorticoids, especially with the use of dexamethasone in children. The smallest effective dose of shorter acting agents such as prednisone or hydrocortisone should be prescribed in relation to body surface area (eg, hydrocortisone, 10-12 mg/m^2/d). Target blood pressure in children should be guided by age-specific blood pressure percentiles. Children should be monitored by pediatricians with expertise in glucocorticoid therapy, with careful attention paid to preventing retardation of linear growth by overtreatment. Treatment with mineralocorticoid receptor antagonists in these patients may be just as effective and avoids the potential disruption of the hypothalamic-pituitary-adrenal axis and risk of iatrogenic side effects. In addition, glucocorticoid therapy or mineralocorticoid receptor blockade may even have a role in normotensive GRA patients.

OTHER FORMS OF MINERALOCORTICOID EXCESS OR EFFECT

The medical disorders associated with excess mineralocorticoid effect from 11-deoxycorticosterone (DOC) and cortisol are listed in Table 10–2. These diagnoses should be considered when PAC and PRA are low in patients with hypertension and hypokalemia.

Hyperdeoxycorticosteronism

A. Congenital adrenal hyperplasia   Congenital adrenal hyperplasia (CAH) is caused by enzymatic defects in adrenal steroidogenesis that result in deficient secretion of cortisol (see Chapter 14). The lack of inhibitory feedback by cortisol on the hypothalamus and pituitary produces an ACTH-driven buildup of cortisol precursors proximal to the enzymatic deficiency. A deficiency of 11β-hydroxylase (CYP11B) or 17α-hydroxylase (CYP17) causes hypertension and hypokalemia because of hypersecretion of the mineralocorticoid DOC. The mineralocorticoid effect of increased circulating levels of DOC also decreases PRA and aldosterone secretion. These defects are autosomal recessive in inheritance and typically are diagnosed in childhood. However, partial enzymatic defects have been shown to cause hypertension in adults.

  a. 11β-Hydroxylase deficiency—Approximately 5% of all cases of CAH are due to 11β-hydroxylase deficiency; the prevalence in Caucasians is 1 in 100,000. More than 40 mutations have been described in *CYP11B1*, the gene encoding 11β-hydroxylase. There is an increased prevalence among Sephardic Jews from Morocco, suggestive of a founder effect. The impaired conversion of DOC to corticosterone results in high levels of DOC, 11-deoxycortisol, and adrenal androgens (see Chapter 14). Females present in infancy or childhood with hypertension, hypokalemia, acne, hirsutism, and virilization. Males present with pseudoprecocious puberty. Approximately two-thirds of patients have mild to moderate hypertension. Markedly increased levels of DOC, 11-deoxycortisol, and adrenal androgens confirm the diagnosis. Glucocorticoid replacement normalizes the steroid abnormalities and hypertension.

  b. 17α-Hydroxylase deficiency—17α-Hydroxylase deficiency is a rare cause of CAH. 17α-Hydroxylase is essential for the synthesis of cortisol and gonadal hormones, and deficiency results in decreased production of cortisol and sex hormones. Genetic 46,XY males present with either pseudohermaphroditism or as phenotypic females, and 46,XX females present with primary amenorrhea. Therefore, a person with this form of CAH may not come to medical attention until puberty. Patients present with eunuchoid proportions and appearance. The biochemical findings include low concentrations of plasma adrenal androgens, plasma 17α-hydroxyprogesterone and cortisol. The plasma concentrations of DOC, corticosterone, and 18-hydroxycorticosterone (all produced in the zona fasciculata) are increased. Aldosterone (produced in zona glomerulosa) and PRA are suppressed. Although rare, there is an increased prevalence among Dutch Mennonites. As with 11β-hydroxylase deficiency, glucocorticoid replacement normalizes the steroid abnormalities and hypertension.

B. Deoxycorticosterone-producing tumor   DOC-producing adrenal tumors are usually large and malignant. Some of them secrete androgens and estrogens in addition to DOC, which may cause virilization in women and feminization in men. A high level of plasma DOC or urinary tetrahydrodeoxycorticosterone and a large adrenal tumor seen on CT confirm the diagnosis. Aldosterone secretion in these patients is typically suppressed. Optimal treatment is complete surgical resection.

C. Primary cortisol resistance   Increased cortisol secretion and plasma cortisol concentrations without evidence of Cushing syndrome are found in patients with primary cortisol resistance (or glucocorticoid resistance), a rare familial syndrome. Cortisol resistance leads to elevations in ACTH secretion which, in turn, increases adrenal steroid production. The syndrome is characterized by hypokalemic alkalosis, hypertension, increased plasma concentrations of DOC, as well as cortisol, and increased adrenal androgen secretion. The hypertension and hypokalemia are likely due to the combined effects of excess DOC and increased cortisol access to the mineralocorticoid receptor (high rates of cortisol production that overwhelm 11β-hydroxysteroid dehydrogenase type 2 [11β-HSD2] activity). Primary cortisol resistance is caused by defects in glucocorticoid receptors and assembly of the steroid–receptor complex. The treatment for the mineralocorticoid-dependent hypertension is blockade of the mineralocorticoid receptor with a mineralocorticoid receptor antagonist or suppression of ACTH secretion with dexamethasone.

Apparent Mineralocorticoid Excess Syndrome

Type 1 apparent mineralocorticoid excess (AME) is the result of impaired activity of the microsomal enzyme 11β-HSD2, which normally inactivates cortisol in the kidney by converting it to cortisone (Figure 10–9). Cortisol can be a potent mineralocorticoid, and as a result of the enzyme deficiency, high levels of cortisol accumulate in the kidney. Thus, 11β-HSD2 normally excludes physiologic glucocorticoids from the nonselective mineralocorticoid receptor by converting them to the inactive 11-keto compound, cortisone. The characteristic abnormal urinary cortisol-cortisone

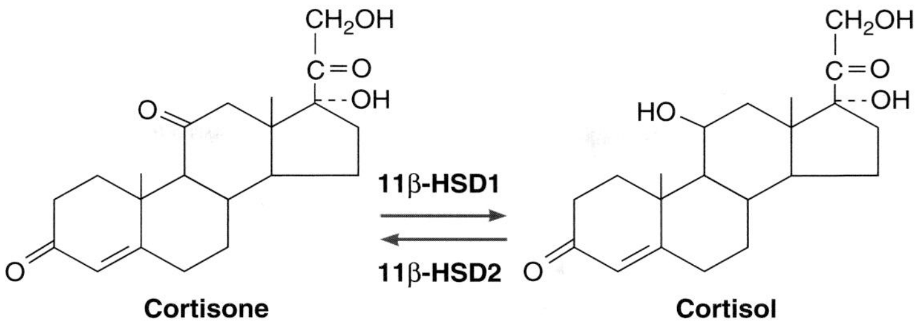

FIGURE 10–9   Interconversion of hormonally active cortisol to inactive cortisone is catalyzed by two isozymes of 11β-hydroxysteroid dehydrogenase (11β-HSD). 11β-HSD1 converts cortisone to cortisol and 11β-HSD2 inactivates cortisol to cortisone.

metabolite profile seen in apparent mineralocorticoid excess reflects decreased 11β-HSD2 activity (ratio of cortisol to cortisone increased 10-fold from normal).

Decreased 11β-HSD2 activity may be hereditary or secondary to pharmacologic inhibition of enzyme activity by glycyrrhizic acid, the active principle of licorice root (*Glycyrrhiza glabra*) and some chewing tobaccos. The congenital form is a rare autosomal recessive disorder, and children present with low birth weight, failure to thrive, hypertension, polyuria and polydipsia, and poor growth. The clinical phenotype of patients with AME includes hypertension, hypokalemia, metabolic alkalosis, low PRA, low PAC, and normal plasma cortisol levels. The diagnosis is confirmed by demonstrating an abnormal ratio of cortisol to cortisone in a 24-hour urine collection. Treatment includes blockade of the mineralocorticoid receptor with a mineralocorticoid receptor antagonist or suppression of endogenous cortisol secretion with dexamethasone.

Carbenoxolone (18β-glycyrrhetinic acid sodium hemisuccinate) is a glycyrrhizic acid metabolite that is used in some countries to treat gastroesophageal reflux disorder. Carbenoxolone acts by protecting the gastrointestinal mucosal barrier from acid-pepsin attack and increasing mucosal mucin production. However, carbenoxolone is also an inhibitor of 11β-HSD2 and side effects include sodium retention, hypokalemic alkalosis, suppressed plasma renin, and hypertension.

Type 2 AME caused by ectopic ACTH secretion, seen in patients with Cushing syndrome, is related to the high rates of cortisol production that overwhelm 11β-HSD2 activity. DOC levels may also be increased in severe ACTH-dependent Cushing syndrome and contribute to the hypertension and hypokalemia in this disorder.

Liddle Syndrome—Abnormal Renal Tubular Ionic Transport

In 1963, Liddle described an autosomal dominant renal disorder that appeared to be primary aldosteronism with hypertension, hypokalemia, and inappropriate kaliuresis. However, PAC and PRA were very low in patients with Liddle syndrome; thus, another name for this disorder is "pseudoaldosteronism." Liddle syndrome is caused by mutations in the β or γ subunits of the amiloride-sensitive epithelial sodium channel—resulting in enhanced activity of the epithelial sodium channel with increased

sodium reabsorption, potassium wasting, hypertension, and hypokalemia. Clinical genetic testing is available (www.genetests.org). As would be predicted, amiloride and triamterene are very effective agents to treat the hypertension and hypokalemia. However, spironolactone is ineffective in these patients. Liddle syndrome can easily be distinguished from AME based on a good clinical response to amiloride or triamterene, lack of efficacy of spironolactone and dexamethasone, and normal 24-hour urine cortisone-cortisol ratio.

Hypertension Exacerbated by Pregnancy

Hypertension exacerbated by pregnancy is a rare autosomal dominant disorder found in women with early-onset hypertension with suppressed levels of aldosterone and renin. During pregnancy, both the hypertension and hypokalemia are severely exacerbated. These patients have an activating mutation in the gene encoding the mineralocorticoid receptor which allows progesterone and other mineralocorticoid antagonists to become agonists.

OTHER ENDOCRINE DISORDERS ASSOCIATED WITH HYPERTENSION

Cushing Syndrome

Hypertension occurs in 75% to 80% of patients with Cushing syndrome (see Chapter 9). Most patients with endogenous Cushing syndrome have ACTH-dependent disease due to a corticotroph pituitary adenoma (see Table 10–2). Ectopic ACTH secretion is the second most common cause of endogenous Cushing syndrome. The ACTH-independent causes (eg, adrenal cortisol-secreting adenoma or carcinoma) of Cushing syndrome are less common. ACTH-independent macronodular hyperplasia is associated with massive hyperplasia of both adrenal glands—usually a result of activation of one or several G protein–coupled receptors aberrantly expressed in the adrenal cortex. ACTH-independent primary pigmented nodular adrenal disease (PPNAD) is a bilateral form of micronodular adrenal hyperplasia that leads to Cushing syndrome. Germline mutations in *PRKAR1A* cause PPNAD in the setting of Carney complex (see Chapter 9). The mechanisms of hypertension in the setting of Cushing syndrome include increased production of DOC, enhanced pressor sensitivity to endogenous vasoconstrictors (eg, epinephrine and angiotensin II), increased cardiac output, activation of the renin-angiotensin system by increasing the hepatic production of angiotensinogen, and overload of the cortisol inactivation system with stimulation of the mineralocorticoid receptor. The source of excess glucocorticoids may be exogenous (iatrogenic) or endogenous. Mineralocorticoid production is usually normal in endogenous Cushing syndrome; aldosterone and renin levels are usually normal and DOC levels are normal or mildly increased. In patients with adrenal carcinoma, DOC and aldosterone may be elevated.

The case-detection studies for endogenous cortisol excess include: (a) measurement of free cortisol in a 24-hour urine collection; (b) midnight salivary cortisol measurement; and (c) 1-mg overnight dexamethasone suppression test. Further studies to confirm Cushing syndrome and to determine the cause of the cortisol excess state are outlined in Chapter 9.

The hypertension associated with Cushing syndrome should be treated until a surgical cure is obtained. Mineralocorticoid receptor antagonists, at dosages used to treat primary aldosteronism, are effective in reversing the hypokalemia. Second-step agents (eg, thiazide diuretics) may be added for optimal control of blood pressure. The hypertension associated with the hypercortisolism usually resolves over several weeks after a surgical cure, and antihypertensive agents can be tapered and withdrawn.

Thyroid Dysfunction

A. Hyperthyroidism   When excessive amounts of circulating thyroid hormones interact with thyroid hormone receptors on peripheral tissues, both metabolic activity and sensitivity to circulating catecholamines increase. Thyrotoxic patients usually have tachycardia, high cardiac output, increased stroke volume, decreased peripheral vascular resistance, and increased systolic blood pressure. The initial management of patients with hypertension who have hyperthyroidism includes a β-adrenergic blocker to treat hypertension, tachycardia, and tremor. The definitive treatment of hyperthyroidism is cause specific (see Chapter 7).

B. Hypothyroidism   The frequency of hypertension, usually diastolic, is increased three fold in hypothyroid patients and may account for as much as 1% of cases of diastolic hypertension in the population. The mechanisms for the elevation in blood pressure include increased systemic vascular resistance and extracellular volume expansion. Treatment of thyroid hormone deficiency decreases blood pressure in most patients with hypertension and normalizes blood pressure in one-third of them. Synthetic levothyroxine is the treatment of choice for hypothyroidism (see Chapter 7).

Acromegaly

Chronic growth hormone (GH) excess from a GH-producing pituitary tumor results in the clinical syndrome of acromegaly. The effects of chronic excess of GH include acral and soft tissue overgrowth, progressive dental malocclusion, degenerative arthritis related to chondral and synovial tissue overgrowth within joints, low-pitched sonorous voice, excessive sweating and oily skin, perineural hypertrophy leading to nerve entrapment (eg,

carpal tunnel syndrome), cardiac dysfunction, and hypertension (see Chapter 4). Hypertension occurs in 20% to 40% of the patients and is associated with sodium retention and extracellular volume expansion. Pituitary surgery is the treatment of choice; if necessary, it is supplemented with medical therapy or irradiation or both. The hypertension of acromegaly is treated most effectively by eliminating GH excess. If a surgical cure is not possible, the hypertension usually responds well to diuretic therapy.

REFERENCES

Primary Aldosteronism

Funder JW, Carey RM, Fardella C, et al. Case detection, diagnosis, and treatment of patients with primary aldosteronism: an endocrine society clinical practice guideline. *J Clin Endocrinol Metab*. 2008;93:3266. [PMID: 18552288]

Kempers MEJ, Lenders JWM, van Outheusden L, et al. Systematic review: diagnostic procedures to differentiate unilateral from bilateral adrenal abnormality in primary aldosteronism. *Ann Intern Med*. 2009;151:329. [PMID: 19721021]

Reincke M, Rump LC, Quinkler M, et al. Risk factors associated with a low glomerular filtration rate in primary aldosteronism. *J Clin Endocrinol Metab*. 2009;94:869. [PMID: 19116235]

Sechi LA, Novello M, Lapenna R, et al. Long-term renal outcomes in patients with primary aldosteronism. *JAMA*. 2006;295:2638. Erratum in: *JAMA*. 2006;296:1842. [PMID: 16772627]

Stowasser M. Update in primary aldosteronism. *J Clin Endocrinol Metab*. 2009;94:3623. [PMID: 19737921]

Young WF, Jr. Primary aldosteronism—one picture is not worth a thousand words. *Ann Intern Med*. 2009;151:357. Comment on: *Ann Intern Med*. 2009;151:329-337. [PMID: 19721025]

Young WF. Primary aldosteronism: renaissance of a syndrome. *Clin Endocrinol (Oxf)*. 2007;66:607. [PMID: 17492946]

Young WF, Stanson AW. What are the keys to successful adrenal venous sampling (AVS) in patients with primary aldosteronism? *Clin Endocrinol (Oxf)*. 2009;70:14. [PMID: 19128364]

Other Forms of Mineralocorticoid Excess or Effect

Charmandari E, Kino T, Souvatzoglou E, Vottero A, Bhattacharyya N, Chrousos GP. Natural glucocorticoid receptor mutants causing generalized glucocorticoid resistance: molecular genotype, genetic transmission, and clinical phenotype. *J Clin Endocrinol Metab*. 2004;89:1939. [PMID: 15070967]

Geller DS, Farhi A, Pinkerton N, et al. Activating mineralocorticoid receptor mutation in hypertension exacerbated by pregnancy. *Science*. 2000;289:119. [PMID: 10884226]

Hammer F, Stewart PM. Cortisol metabolism in hypertension. *Best Pract Res Clin Endocrinol Metab*. 2006;20:337. [PMID: 16980198]

Merke DP, Bornstein SR. Congenital adrenal hyperplasia. *Lancet*. 2005;365:2125. [PMID: 15964450]

Morineau G, Sulmont V, Salomon R, et al. Apparent mineralocorticoid excess: report of six new cases and extensive personal experience. *J Am Soc Nephrol*. 2006;17:3176. [PMID: 17035606]

New MI, Geller DS, Fallo F, Wilson RC. Monogenic low renin hypertension. *Trends Endocrinol Metab*. 2005;16:92. [PMID: 15808805]

Stewart PM, Corrie JE, Shackleton CH, et al. Syndrome of apparent mineralocorticoid excess. A defect in the cortisol-cortisone shuttle. *J Clin Invest*. 1988;82:340. [PMID: 303514]

Snyder PM. Minireview: regulation of epithelial Na$^+$ channel trafficking. *Endocrinology*. 2005;146:5079. [PMID: 16150899]

Warnock DG. Liddle's syndrome: genetics and mechanisms of Na$^+$ channel defects. *Contrib Nephrol*. 2001;136:1-10. [PMID: 11688373]

Other Endocrine Disorders Associated with Hypertension

Danzi S, Klein I. Thyroid hormone and blood pressure regulation. *Curr Hypertens Rep*. 2003;5:513. [PMID: 14594573]

Magiakou MA, Smyrnaki P, Chrousos GP. Hypertension in Cushing's syndrome. *Best Pract Res Clin Endocrinol Metab.* 2006;20:467. [PMID: 16980206]

Sacerdote A, Weiss K, Tran T, Rokeya Noor B, McFarlane SI. Hypertension in patients with Cushing's disease: pathophysiology, diagnosis, and management. *Curr Hypertens Rep.* 2005;7:212. [PMID: 15913497]

Streeten DH, Anderson GH Jr, Howland T, Chiang R, Smulyan H. Effects of thyroid function on blood pressure. Recognition of hypothyroid hypertension. *Hypertension.* 1988;11:78. [PMID: 3338842]

Terzolo M, Matrella C, Boccuzzi A, et al. Twenty-four hour profile of blood pressure in patients with acromegaly. Correlation with demographic, clinical and hormonal features. *J Endocrinol Invest.* 1999;22:48. [PMID: 10090137]

Adrenal Medulla and Paraganglia

Paul A. Fitzgerald, MD

ACE	Angiotensin-converting enzyme
ACTH	Adrenocorticotropic hormone
AM	Adrenomedullin
APMO	Adnexal cystadenomas of probable mesonephric origin
ARDS	Acute respiratory distress syndrome
ATP	Adenosine triphosphate
cAMP	Cyclic adenosine monophosphate
CgA	Chromogramin A
CGRP	Calcitonin gene–related peptide
COMT	Catecholamine-O-methyltransferase
DBH	Dopamine-β-hydroxylase
FDG	Fluorodeoxyglucose
DHMA	Dihydroxymandelic acid
DHPG	Dihydroxyphenylglycol
ECD	Electrochemical detection
HIF	Hypoxia-inducible factor
HPLC	High-pressure liquid chromatography
IP₃	Inositol triphosphate
MAO	Monoamine oxidase
MEN	Multiple endocrine neoplasia

MHBA	3-methoxy-4-hydroxybenzylamine
MIBG	Metaiodobenzylguanidine
NF-1	Neurofibromatosis type 1
NSE	Neuron-specific enolase
PBSC	Peripheral blood stem cell
PNMT	Phenylethanolamine-N-methyltransferase
PTHrP	Parathyroid hormone–related peptide
RECIST	Response evaluation criteria in solid tumors
SDH	Succinate dehydrogenase
SDHB	Succinate dehydrogenase subunit B
SDHC	Succinate dehydrogenase subunit C
SDHD	Succinate dehydrogenase subunit D
SPECT	Single photon emission computed tomography
SRI	Somatostatin receptor imaging
VEGF	Vascular endothelial growth factor
VHL	Von Hippel-Lindau
VIP	Vasoactive intestinal polypeptide
VMA	Vanillylmandelic acid (3-methoxy-4-hydroxymandelic acid)

The adrenal medulla and paraganglia are part of the autonomic/sympathetic nervous system. The endocrine and nervous systems are alike in that they exert their actions by releasing hormones/neurotransmitters that bind to cell surface receptors in the target tissue, thereby inducing an effect.

Autonomic nerves are not under conscious control. They innervate the heart, adrenal medulla, vascular smooth muscle, and smooth muscle in visceral organs, thereby controlling cardiac rate and output, adrenal medullary secretion of catecholamines, blood pressure, the genitourinary tract, and intestinal motility. Autonomic nerves originate within the central nervous system and have two major divisions according to their anatomic locations:

(1) **Parasympathetic** preganglionic nerves exit the central nervous system via the cranial nerves and sacral spinal nerves. They terminate in nonchromaffin paraganglia that are most numerous in the neck and associated with the glossopharyngeal and vagus nerves. These ganglia serve as chemoreceptors that are involved in the control of respiration. An important paraganglion at the carotid bifurcation is known as the **carotid body**. They are also found along the jugular vein and in the jugulo-tympanic region. Head-neck paragangliomas are tumors that arise from these parasympathetic paraganglia.

(2) **Sympathetic** preganglionic nerves exit the central nervous system via the thoracic and lumbar spinal nerves. The

sympathetic nervous system coordinates the body's automatic *fight-flight* response by stimulating the adrenal medulla to secrete catecholamines and by directly stimulating cardiac output and blood flow to muscles while diverting blood flow away from visceral organs.

Sympathetic preganglionic nerves terminate mainly in paravertebral and prevertebral nerve ganglia where they secrete acetylcholine as their neurotransmitter; they are, therefore, known as *cholinergic* nerves. These nerve ganglia are collectively known as **paraganglia** and contain neuroendocrine cells that are similar to adrenal medullary cells on light microscopy by chromaffin and immunohistochemical staining. Paraganglia are also found in the mediastinum, particularly adjacent to the cardiac atria, and in the abdomen along the sympathetic nerve chains in paravertebral and prevertebral positions. Paraganglia are plentiful along the aorta, particularly around the celiac axis, adrenal glands, renal medullae, and aortic bifurcation (organ of Zuckerkandl). Paraganglia are also abundant in the pelvis, particularly adjacent to the bladder. Preganglionic nerves also terminate in the adrenal medulla, which is basically a sympathetic ganglion that is surrounded by adrenal cortex.

Sympathetic postganglionic nerve fibers originate from the paraganglia and run to the tissues being innervated. They secrete norepinephrine as their neurotransmitter at synaptic junctions. Adrenal medullary cells are basically modified postganglionic nerves that lack axons and secrete their neurotransmitter (mainly epinephrine) directly into the blood; thus, the bloodstream acts like a giant synapse, carrying epinephrine to receptors throughout the body. Synonyms for epinephrine and norepinephrine are *adrenalin* and *noradrenaline*, respectively (see later).

Although the adrenal medulla is not essential for survival, its secretion of epinephrine and other compounds helps maintain the body's homeostasis during stress. Investigations of the adrenal medulla and the sympathetic nervous system have led to the discovery of different catecholamine receptors and the production of a wide variety of sympathetic agonists and antagonists with diverse clinical applications.

Pheochromocytomas are tumors that arise from the adrenal medulla, whereas non–head-neck **paragangliomas** arise from extra-adrenal sympathetic ganglia. Pheochromocytomas can secrete excessive amounts of both epinephrine and norepinephrine, whereas paragangliomas secrete only norepinephrine. The excessive secretion of catecholamines can result in a dangerous exaggeration of the stress response.

ANATOMY

Embryology (Figure 11–1)

The sympathetic nervous system arises in the fetus from the primitive cells of the neural crest (sympathogonia). At about the fifth week of gestation, these cells migrate from the spinal ganglia in the thoracic region to form the sympathetic chain posterior to the dorsal aorta. They then begin to migrate anteriorly to form the remaining ganglia.

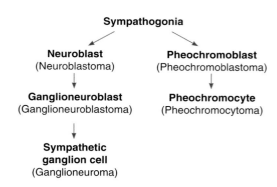

FIGURE 11–1 The embryonic development of adrenergic cells and tumors that develop from them (in parentheses). Sympathogonia are primitive cells derived from the neural crest. Neuroblasts are also called sympathoblasts; ganglion cells are the same as sympathocytes; and pheochromocytes are mature chromaffin cells.

At 6 weeks of gestation, groups of these primitive cells migrate along the central vein and enter the fetal adrenal cortex to form the adrenal medulla, which is detectable by the eighth week. The adrenal medulla at this time is composed of sympathogonia and pheochromoblasts, which then mature into pheochromocytes. The cells appear in rosette-like structures, with the more primitive cells occupying a central position. Storage granules can be found in these cells at 12 weeks. The adrenal medullas are very small and amorphous at birth but develop into recognizable adult form by the sixth month of postnatal life.

Pheochromoblasts and pheochromocytes also collect on both sides of the aorta to form the paraganglia. These cells collect principally at the origin of the mesenteric arteries and at the aortic bifurcation where they fuse anteriorly to form the organ of Zuckerkandl, which is quite prominent during the first year of life. Pheochromocytes (chromaffin cells) also are found scattered throughout the abdominal sympathetic plexi as well as in other parts of the sympathetic nervous system.

Gross Structure

The anatomic relationships between the adrenal medulla and the adrenal cortex differ in different species. In mammals, the medulla is surrounded by the adrenal cortex, and in humans, the adrenal medulla occupies a central position in the widest part of the gland, with only small portions extending into the narrower parts. The mass of adrenal medullary tissue in both adult adrenal glands averages about 1000 mg (about 15% of the total weight of both adrenal glands), although the proportions vary from individual to individual. There is no clear demarcation between cortex and medulla. A cuff of adrenal cortical cells usually surrounds the central vein within the adrenal medulla, and there may be islands of cortical cells elsewhere in the medulla.

Microscopic Structure

The **chromaffin cells** or **pheochromocytes** of the adrenal medulla are large ovoid columnar cells arranged in nests, alveoli, or cords around a rich network of capillaries and venous sinusoids that drain blood from the adrenal cortex. Pheochromocytes have large nuclei and a well-developed Golgi apparatus. Their cytoplasm contains large numbers of vesicles (granules) that measure 100 to 300 nm in diameter and appear similar to the neurosecretory granules seen in peripheral sympathetic nerves. Catecholamines (epinephrine and/or norepinephrine) comprise about 20% of the mass of neurosecretory vesicles. Vesicles containing norepinephrine appear darker than those containing epinephrine. The vesicles also contain proteins, lipids, and adenosine triphosphate (ATP), as well as chromogranins, neuropeptide Y, enkephalins, and proopiomelanocortin (along with related peptides such as adrenocorticotropic hormone [ACTH] and β-endorphin).

Nerve Supply

The cells of the adrenal medulla are innervated by preganglionic fibers of the sympathetic nervous system, which release acetylcholine and enkephalins at the synapses. Most of these fibers arise from a plexus in the capsule of the posterior surface of the gland and enter the adrenal glands in bundles of 30 to 50 fibers without synapsing. They follow the course of the blood vessels into the medulla without branching into the adrenal cortex. Some reach the wall of the central vein, where they synapse with small autonomic ganglia. However, most fibers end in relationship to the pheochromocytes.

Blood Supply

The adrenal gland is perfused by the superior, middle, and inferior adrenal branches of the inferior phrenic artery, directly from the aorta and from the renal arteries. On reaching the adrenal gland, these arteries branch to form a plexus under the capsule supplying the adrenal cortex. A few of these vessels, however, penetrate the cortex, passing directly to the medulla. The medulla is also nourished by branches of the arteries supplying the central vein and cuff of cortical tissue around the central vein. Capillary loops passing from the subcapsular plexus of the cortex also supply blood as they drain into the central vein. Most of the blood supply to adrenal medullary cells is via a portal vascular system that arises from the capillaries in the cortex. There is also a capillary network of lymphatics that drain into a plexus around the central vein.

Norepinephrine is converted to epinephrine by the enzyme phenylethanolamine-*N*-methyltransferase (PNMT). In mammals, the expression of PNMT is induced by cortisol. Chromaffin cells that produce epinephrine are exposed to higher concentrations of cortisol from capillaries draining adrenocortical cells, whereas chromaffin cells containing norepinephrine are supplied by arteries that course directly to the adrenal medulla (see sections on biosynthesis and decretion, later).

The central vein of the right adrenal is short and drains directly into the vena cava with about 5% having multiple veins. About 5% of right adrenal veins drain into the hepatic vein. For the left adrenal gland, the vein is somewhat longer and drains into the left renal vein.

HORMONES OF THE ADRENAL MEDULLA AND PARAGANGLIA

CATECHOLAMINES

Biosynthesis (Figure 11–2)

Catecholamines are molecules that have a catechol nucleus consisting of benzene with two hydroxyl side groups plus a side-chain amine. Catecholamines include dopamine, norepinephrine, and epinephrine (see Figure 11–2).

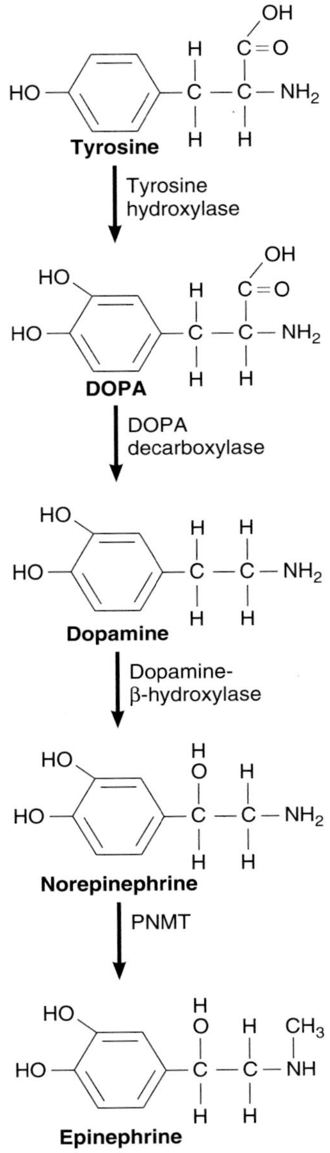

FIGURE 11–2 Biosynthesis of catecholamines (DOPA: L-dihydroxyphenylalanine; PNMT: phenylethanolamine-*N*-methyltransferase). Epinephrine is not produced in paraganglia.

Epinephrine is the main hormone secreted by the normal adrenal medulla. The proportions of epinephrine and norepinephrine found in the adrenal medulla vary with the species; in humans, the adrenal medulla contains 15% to 20% norepinephrine.

Norepinephrine is found primarily in the central nervous system and in peripheral sympathetic paraganglia and nerves. Dopamine is found in the adrenal medulla and in sympathetic neurons as a precursor to norepinephrine. It is present in high concentrations in the brain, in specialized neurons in the sympathetic ganglia, and in the carotid body, where it serves as a neurotransmitter. Dopamine is also present in the proximal renal tubule where it promotes sodium excretion and in the gastrointestinal tract where it serves a paracrine function.

Chromogranin A (CgA) is a peptide that is stored and released with catecholamines during exocytosis; catestatin is a fragment of the CgA prohormone that inhibits further catecholamine release by acting as an antagonist at the neuronal cholinergic receptor. CgA levels tend to be somewhat higher in patients with hypertension than in matched normotensive individuals. CgA has become a valuable tumor marker, particularly for patients with paragangliomas that are otherwise nonsecretory.

A. Conversion of tyrosine to DOPA

The catecholamines are synthesized from tyrosine, which may be derived from ingested food or synthesized from phenylalanine in the liver. Tyrosine circulates at a concentration of 1 to 1.5 mg/dL of blood. It enters neurons and chromaffin cells by an active transport mechanism and is converted to L-dihydroxyphenylalanine (L-DOPA). The reaction is catalyzed by *tyrosine hydroxylase*, which is transported via axonal flow to the nerve terminal. Tyrosine hydroxylase is the rate-limiting step in catecholamine synthesis. It is transcriptionally activated by acetylcholine through the nicotinic cholinergic receptor, which in turn activates protein kinase A via cAMP. Tyrosine hydroxylase activity may be inhibited by a variety of compounds; alpha methyltyrosine (metyrosine) is an inhibitor that is sometimes used in the therapy of metastatic or unresectable pheochromocytomas.

B. Conversion of DOPA to dopamine

DOPA is converted to dopamine by the enzyme aromatic L-amino acid decarboxylase (DOPA decarboxylase). This enzyme is found in all tissues, with the highest concentrations in liver, kidney, brain, and vas deferens. The various enzymes have different substrate specificities depending on the tissue source. Competitive inhibitors of DOPA decarboxylase, such as methyldopa, are converted to substances (an example is α-methylnorepinephrine) that are then stored in granules in the nerve cell and released in place of norepinephrine. These products (false transmitters) were thought to mediate the antihypertensive action of drugs at peripheral sympathetic synapses but are now believed to stimulate the alpha receptors of the inhibitory corticobulbar system, reducing sympathetic discharge peripherally.

C. Conversion of dopamine to norepinephrine

Dopamine enters granulated storage vesicles where it is hydroxylated to norepinephrine by the enzyme dopamine-β-hydroxylase (DBH), which is found within the vesicle membrane. Norepinephrine is then actively transported into the vesicle by vesicular monoamine transferase (VMAT), which is located in the lipid bilayer of the vesicle wall. Norepinephrine constantly diffuses out of the vesicle, so it is best to consider it being concentrated in the vesicle, rather than being stored there. The granulated storage vesicle migrates to the cell surface and secretes its contents via exocytosis; both norepinephrine and DBH are released during exocytosis. After secretion, most norepinephrine is avidly recycled back into the nerve. Normally, about 93% of circulating norepinephrine originates from diffusion out of nonadrenal sympathetic nerve cells and synapses, while only 7% originates from the adrenal medulla.

D. Conversion of norepinephrine to epinephrine

Norepinephrine constantly diffuses out from storage granules into the cytoplasm. In most cells of the adrenal medulla, cytoplasmic norepinephrine is converted to epinephrine, catalyzed by PNMT. Epinephrine can then return to the vesicle, diffuse from the cell, or undergo catabolism. High concentrations of cortisol enhance the expression of the gene encoding PNMT. Cortisol is present in high concentrations in most areas of the adrenal medulla due to venous blood flow from the adjacent adrenal cortex. This accounts for the fact that in the normal human adrenal medulla, about 80% of the catecholamine content is epinephrine and only 20% is norepinephrine. In mouse models, the administration of exogenous corticosteroids appears to increase adrenal medullary PNMT expression, despite suppression of ACTH and endogenous adrenal cortisol production.

Paragangliomas rarely secrete epinephrine, because they do not have high local concentrations of cortisol to induce PNMT expression. Pheochromocytomas secrete epinephrine and norepinephrine in various ratios. Interestingly, after adrenalectomy, recurrent pheochromocytoma can secrete epinephrine without any surrounding adrenal cortex, indicating that the induction of PNMT may continue in subsequent cell lineages without high local levels of cortisol. After both adrenal glands are resected, serum epinephrine levels abruptly fall to nearly zero, whereas norepinephrine concentrations do not decline significantly, since most circulating norepinephrine originates from leakage out of sympathetic nerves and synapses.

The enzyme PNMT is found in many tissues outside the adrenal medulla. PNMT that is identical to adrenal PNMT has been found in the lung, kidney, pancreas, and cancer cells. Therefore, nonadrenal tissue is capable of synthesizing epinephrine if norepinephrine is available as a substrate. However, nonadrenal production of epinephrine usually contributes minimally to circulating levels. PNMT is found in human lung, and glucocorticoids increase its expression, thereby increasing lung epinephrine. This may possibly contribute to the bronchial dilation that is induced by glucocorticoids (inhaled or systemic). PNMT activity is also found in red blood cells, where its activity is increased in hyperthyroidism and decreased in hypothyroidism. Renal PNMT activity is such that up to one-half of the epinephrine found in normal urine may be the product of renal conversion from norepinephrine.

In the adrenal medulla, catecholamine stores can be depleted during prolonged hypoglycemia. Biosynthesis of catecholamines increases during nerve stimulation by activation of tyrosine hydroxylase. Prolonged stimulation leads to the induction of increased amounts of this rate-limiting enzyme.

Storage of Catecholamines

Catecholamines are not truly stored in intracellular vesicles. Rather, they exist in a dynamic equilibrium between the vesicle and the surrounding cytoplasm. Catecholamines continuously leak out of the vesicles into the cytoplasm but reenter and become concentrated in the vesicles by the action of two vesicular monoamine transporters: VMAT-1 and VMAT-2. Both are expressed in the adrenal medulla, but only VMAT-2 is expressed in sympathetic nerves.

In the adrenal medulla, the percentage of stored epinephrine (vs total catecholamines) varies widely among different species. In the human adrenal medulla, epinephrine comprises about 80% of stored catecholamines. Epinephrine and norepinephrine are stored in different cells. Morphologic differences in epinephrine and norepinephrine storage vesicles are visible on light microscopy after proper staining. Cells that store predominantly epinephrine tend to be adjacent to intramedullary sinusoidal vessels that bathe the cells in blood from the adrenal cortex; such blood contains cortisol that induces the enzyme PNMT that catalyzes the conversion of norepinephrine to epinephrine in the cytoplasm such that these vesicles contain predominantly epinephrine. Adrenal medullary cells that contain predominantly norepinephrine tend to be farther away from such vessels.

Norepinephrine is also found in the synaptic vesicles of postganglionic autonomic nerves in organs that have rich sympathetic innervations: the heart, salivary glands, vascular smooth muscle, liver, spleen, kidneys, and muscles. A single sympathetic nerve cell may have up to 25,000 synaptic bulges along the length of its axon; each synapse synthesizes norepinephrine and stores it in adrenergic synaptic vesicles adjacent to target cells.

Catecholamine biosynthesis is coupled to secretion, so that the stores of norepinephrine at the nerve endings remain relatively unchanged even in the presence of marked nerve activity. The adrenal medulla contains catecholamines at a concentration of about 0.5 mg/g; the spleen, vas deferens, brain, spinal cord, and heart contain 1 to 5 μg/g; and the liver, gut, and skeletal muscle contain 0.1 to 0.5 μg/g. Catecholamines are stored in electron-dense granules approximately 1 μm in diameter that contain catecholamines and ATP in a 4:1 molar ratio, as well as several neuropeptides, calcium, magnesium, and water-soluble proteins called **chromogranins** (see earlier). The interior surface of the membrane contains DBH and ATPase. The Mg^{2+}-dependent ATPase facilitates the uptake and inhibits the release of catecholamines by the granules. Adrenal medullary granules appear to contain and release a number of active peptides including adrenomedullin, ACTH, vasoactive intestinal peptide (VIP), chromogranins, and enkephalins. The peptides derived from chromogranins are physiologically active and may modulate catecholamine release.

Secretion of Catecholamines (Figure 11–3 and Table 11–1)

Preganglionic nerve fibers terminate in adrenal medullary cells, where they release acetylcholine at synapses and stimulate adrenal medullary receptors. Activation of the receptors depolarizes the cell membranes and causes an influx of calcium ions. The increased intracellular concentration of calcium triggers exocytosis of the neurosecretory vesicles with consequent release of their contents: catecholamines, chromogranins, and soluble DBH. Vesicular membrane-bound DBH is not released during exocytosis.

Adrenal medulla. In the adrenal medulla, exocytosis of the neurosecretory vesicles releases epinephrine and norepinephrine into the circulation. In normals, over 90% of circulating epinephrine is derived from the adrenal medulla, whereas adrenal medullary secretion accounts for only about 7% of circulating norepinephrine. Catecholamines also diffuse out of the neurosecretory vesicles into the cytoplasm. Catecholamines in the cytoplasm may reenter a vesicle via VMAT or may be metabolized by COMT into catecholamine metabolites: metanephrine and normetanephrine, which gradually diffuse out of the cell and enter the circulation.

Adrenal medullary catecholamine secretion increases with exercise, angina pectoris, myocardial infarction, hemorrhage, ether anesthesia, surgery, hypoglycemia, anoxia and asphyxia, and many other stressful stimuli. The rate of secretion of epinephrine increases more than that of norepinephrine in the presence of hypoglycemia and most other stimuli. However, during hypoxia, the adrenal medullary cells preferentially release norepinephrine. Such release is mainly not by exocytosis but rather by leakage of norepinephrine from neurosecretory vesicles into the cytoplasm and out of the cell into the circulation. The preferential release of norepinephrine may be because the adrenal medullary cells that concentrate norepinephrine are located farther from blood vessels and may be more susceptible to hypoxic injury. (See Storage of Catecholamines, earlier.)

Sympathetic neurons. In sympathetic neurons, exocytosis of the neurosecretory vesicle releases norepinephrine into the synapse. Norepinephrine that has been secreted into a synapse by exocytosis is either reabsorbed via norepinephrine transporters (NETs) or leaks out of the synapse into the circulation. Such synaptic leakage accounts for the majority of circulating norepinephrine in normal individuals.

Metabolism and Excretion of Catecholamines (Figure 11–4)

A. Catecholamine metabolism in cells of origin

Adrenal medulla. In the adrenal medulla, catecholamines are metabolized to metanephrines primarily by membrane-bound catecholamine-*O*-methyltransferase (COMT): epinephrine to metanephrine and norepinephrine to normetanephrine. The metanephrine metabolites subsequently leak into the circulation.

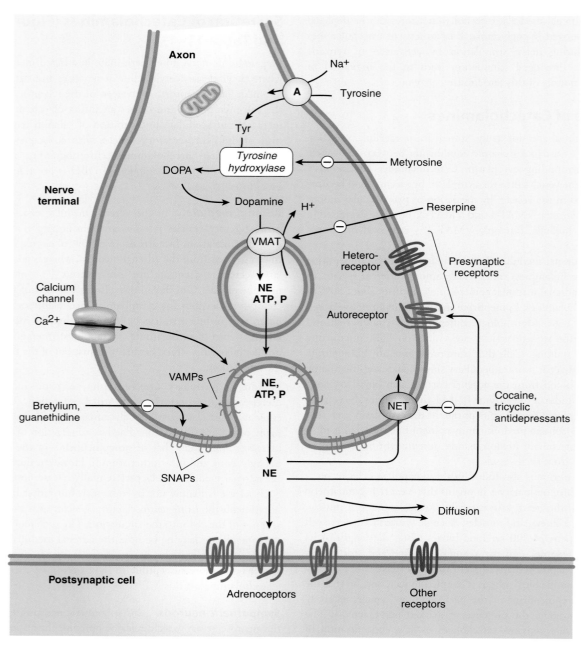

FIGURE 11–3 Schematic diagram of a noradrenergic junction of the peripheral sympathetic nervous system (not to scale). The neural axons form synaptic junctions with cells in target organs. The neurotransmitter is norepinephrine, which originates through de novo synthesis from tyrosine or from norepinephrine that has been secreted and reabsorbed by a norepinephrine transporter (NET). Tyrosine is transported into the noradrenergic endings or varicosities by a sodium-dependent carrier (A). In the cytoplasm, tyrosine hydroxylase converts tyrosine to DOPA that is converted by DOPA decarboxylase to dopamine. Dopamine, as well as norepinephrine (NE) is transported into the vesicles by vesicular monoamine transferase (VMAT). Dopamine is converted to NE in the vesicle by dopamine-β-hydroxylase. Exocytosis of the neurosecretory vesicle with release of transmitter occurs when an action potential opens voltage-sensitive calcium channels and increases intracellular calcium. Fusion of vesicles with the surface membrane results in expulsion of norepinephrine, cotransmitters, and dopamine-β-hydroxylase. After release, norepinephrine diffuses out of the cleft or is transported into the cytoplasm of the nerve itself (uptake 1) or transported into the postjunctional target cell (uptake 2). Regulatory receptors are present on the presynaptic terminal (SNAPs, synaptosome-associated proteins; VAMPs, vesicle-associated membrane protein). **Not shown:** In adrenal medullary and pheochromocytoma cells, norepinephrine constantly diffuses from the vesicle into the cytoplasm where it may be converted to epinephrine by phenylethanolamine-N-methyltransferase (PNMT). Alternatively, cytoplasmic membrane-bound catecholamine-O-methyltransferase (COMT) can metabolize epinephrine and norepinephrine directly into metanephrine and normetanephrine, respectively, which are then released. (Reproduced, with permission, from Katzung BJ, ed. *Basic & Clinical Pharmacology.* 11th ed. McGraw-Hill; 2009.)

TABLE 11–1   Range of plasma catecholamine levels observed in healthy subjects and patients.

	Norepinephrine	Epinephrine
Healthy Subjects		
Basal	150-400 pg/mL (0.9-2.4 nmol/L)	25-100 pg/mL (0.1-0.6 nmol/L)
Ambulatory	200-800 pg/mL (1.2-4.8 nmol/L)	30-100 pg/mL (0.1-1 nmol/L)
Exercise	800-4000 pg/mL (4.8-24 nmol/L)	100-1000 pg/mL (0.5-5 nmol/L)
Symptomatic hypoglycemia	200-1000 pg/mL (1.2-6 nmol/L)	1000-5000 pg/mL (5-25 nmol/L)
Patients		
Hypertension	200-500 pg/mL (1.2-3 nmol/L)	20-100 pg/mL (0.1-0.6 nmol/L)
Surgery	500-2000 pg/mL (3-12 nmol/L)	199-500 pg/mL (0.5-3 nmol/L)
Myocardial infarction	1000-2000 pg/mL (6-12 nmol/L)	800-5000 pg/mL (4-25 nmol/L)

Over 90% of circulating metanephrine and about 40% of circulating normetanephrine is produced by the adrenal medulla.

Sympathetic nerves.   Catecholamines that are released at the synapse bind to their receptors with relatively low affinity and dissociate rapidly (see Figure 11–4). About 10% of norepinephrine escapes from synapses into the systemic circulation (see later). About 90% of synaptic norepinephrine is reabsorbed by the nerves from which they were released or by the target cells. Cytoplasmic norepinephrine is metabolized to 3,4-dihydroxyphenylglycol (DHPG) at the outer mitochondrial membrane by the enzyme monoamine oxidase (MAO) that regulates the norepinephrine content of neurons. DHBG leaks from the neuron and is absorbed by the liver and other tissues that convert it to VMA (see later) that is excreted in the urine. In normals, most urinary VMA is derived from DHPG that leaks from sympathetic nerves.

Sympathetic nerves in abdominal organs, particularly the intestines and pancreas, account for nearly half the body's production of norepinephrine. Intestinal cells contain sulfatases that conjugate norepinephrine to norepinephrine-SO$_4$ that enters the portal vein and bypasses the liver to be excreted in the urine. Intestinal cells also conjugate normetanephrine to normetanephrine-SO$_4$.

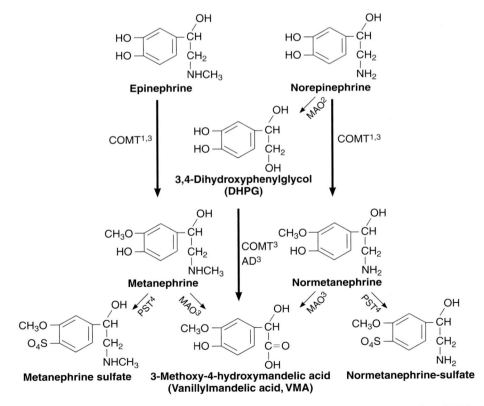

FIGURE 11–4 Metabolism of catecholamines by catechol-O-methyltransferase (COMT), monoamine oxidase (MAO), aldehyde dehydrogenase (AD), and phenol-sulfotransferase (PST). (1) Adrenal medulla or pheochromocytoma; (2) sympathetic nerves; (3) liver and kidneys; (4) GI, platelets, lungs.

Pheochromocytomas. In pheochromocytomas, catecholamines that leak out of the neurosecretory vesicles are methylated by membrane-bound COMT: epinephrine to metanephrine and norepinephrine to normetanephrine. These metanephrine metabolites continuously leak directly into the circulation, in contrast to catecholamines that are secreted intermittently. The pheochromocytoma's continuous excretion of metanephrines accounts for the superior sensitivity of plasma or urine-fractionated free metanephrine testing in the diagnosis of pheochromocytoma. In patients with pheochromocytoma, over 90% of circulating total metanephrines are derived from the tumor itself, rather than from peripheral metabolism.

B. Circulating catecholamine uptake and metabolism

Following release into the circulation, catecholamines bind to albumin and other proteins with low affinity and high capacity. Catecholamines are quickly removed from the bloodstream and have a circulating half-life of less than 2 minutes. Although some free catecholamines are excreted directly into the urine, most are actively transported from the circulation into other cells where they are metabolized. Organic cation transporters (OCTs) are largely responsible for removing catecholamines from the circulation; they are expressed in many tissues, particularly the liver. Following active transport into a cell, catecholamines and their immediate metabolites undergo further metabolism. The main extra-adrenal/neuronal catecholamine metabolic pathway is initially via the enzyme MAO that converts both epinephrine and norepinephrine to DHPG. DHPG is further metabolized by soluble COMT to 3-methoxy-4-hydroxyphenylglycol (MHPG) that is converted by aldehyde dehydrogenase (AD) to vanillylmandelic acid (VMA) that is excreted in the urine.

Catecholamines, metanephrines, and MHPG also undergo conjugation of their phenolic hydroxyl group with sulfate or glucuronide; this reaction occurs mainly in gastrointestinal cells. To a lesser extent, catecholamines are also converted to metanephrines via a soluble form of COMT, an enzyme found in most tissues, especially blood cells, liver, kidney, and vascular smooth muscle. The soluble form of COMT is less active than the membrane-bound form of COMT found in the adrenal medulla and pheochromocytomas.

Catecholamines, their metabolites, and conjugates are excreted in the urine. Normally, the proportions of urine catecholamines and metabolites are approximately 50% metanephrines, 35% VMA, 10% conjugated catecholamines and other metabolites, and less than 5% free catecholamines.

CATECHOLAMINE (ADRENERGIC) RECEPTORS (TABLES 11–2 AND 11–3; FIGURES 11–5 AND 11–6)

The adrenergic receptors are G protein–coupled receptors activated by norepinephrine and epinephrine. They mediate the sympathetic *fight or flight* response. The finding that most cells in the body have adrenergic receptors has led to an appreciation of

TABLE 11–2 Catecholamine receptor types and subtypes.

Receptor	Relative Agonist Potency	Effects
Alpha₁ Type	Norepinephrine > epinephrine	$\uparrow$IP₃, DAG common to all
Alpha₁ₐ		
Alpha₁ᵦ		
Alpha₁ᴅ		
Alpha₂ Type	Norepinephrine > epinephrine; clonidine	$\downarrow$cAMP; $\uparrow$K⁺ channels; $\downarrow$Ca²⁺ channels
Alpha₂ₐ		
Alpha₂ᵦ	Norepinephrine > epinephrine	$\downarrow$cAMP; $\downarrow$Ca²⁺ channels
Alpha₂ᴄ		$\downarrow$cAMP
Beta Type		
Beta₁	Epinephrine = norepinephrine	$\uparrow$cAMP
Beta₂	Epinephrine >>> norepinephrine	$\uparrow$cAMP
Beta₃	Norepinephrine > epinephrine	$\uparrow$cAMP

Adapted, with permission, from Katzung B, ed. *Basic and Clinical Pharmacology.* 9th ed. McGraw-Hill; 2004.

the important regulatory role of the peripheral sympathetic nervous system and circulating catecholamines.

Adrenergic receptors were originally classified into two groups: α and β. This classification has been expanded as subtypes of the α and β receptors have been discovered and includes α_{1A}, α_{1B}, α_{1C}, α_{2A}, α_{2B}, α_{2C} as well as β_1 and β_2, and β_3. Each receptor subtype is encoded by a different gene. Adrenergic receptors are variably distributed in the central nervous system and peripheral tissues.

Norepinephrine and epinephrine are roughly equipotent in activating α and β_1 receptors. Epinephrine is much more potent in activating β_2 receptors and norepinephrine is more potent in activating β_3 receptors (Table 11–2). The physiologic effects mediated by them are summarized in Table 11–3.

Adrenergic receptors are transmembrane proteins with an extracellular amino terminus and an intracellular carboxyl terminus. Each of their seven hydrophobic regions spans the cell membrane. Although these regions of the adrenergic receptor subtypes exhibit significant amino acid homology, differences in the fifth and sixth segments determine the specificity of agonist binding. Differences in the fifth and seventh segments determine which of the guanylyl nucleotide binding proteins (G proteins) is coupled to the receptor. G proteins consist of α, β, and γ subunits. When a hormone binds to the receptor, the β and γ subunits dissociate from the α subunits, allowing GDP to be replaced by GTP on the α subunits and causing the β and γ subunits to dissociate from it. The GTP-bound α subunits activate the postreceptor pathways (see Figure 11–5).

A. Alpha-adrenergic receptors

Alpha₁ receptors are G_q-coupled receptors with three homologous subtypes: α_{1A}, α_{1B}, and α_{1C}. When an agonist binds to the α_1 receptor, the alpha subunit

TABLE 11-3 Catecholamine receptors: location and actions.

Catecholamine Receptor	Tissue Location	Action Following Receptor Activation
Alpha$_1$	Vascular smooth muscle	Increases vasoconstriction (increases blood pressure)
	Liver	Increases glycogenolysis and gluconeogenesis
	Eye	Increases ciliary muscle contraction (pupil dilation)
	Skin	Increases pilomotor smooth muscle contraction (erects hairs)
	Prostate	Increases contraction and ejaculation
	Uterus	Increases gravid uterus contraction
	Intestines	Increases sphincter tone and relaxes smooth muscle
	Spleen capsule	Contracts spleen volume, expelling blood
Alpha$_2$	Preganglionic nerves	Decreases release of neurotransmitter
	Vascular smooth muscle	Increases vasoconstriction (increases blood pressure)
	Pancreatic islet cells	Decreases release of insulin and glucagon
	Blood platelets	Increases platelet aggregation
	Adipose cells	Decreases lipolysis
	Brain	Decreases norepinephrine release
Beta$_1$	Myocardium	Increases force and rate of contraction
	Kidney (juxtaglomerular apparatus)	Increases secretion of renin
	Adipose cells	Increases lipolysis
	Most tissues	Increases calorigenesis
	Nerves	Increases conduction velocity
Beta$_2$	Vascular smooth muscle	Decreases vasoconstriction (increases blood flow)
	Bronchiolar smooth muscle	Decreases contraction (bronchial dilation)
	Liver	Increases glycogenolysis and gluconeogenesis
	Intestinal smooth muscle	Decreases intestinal motility; increases sphincter tone
	Pancreatic islet cells	Increases release of insulin and glucagon
	Adipose tissue	Increases lipolysis
	Muscles	Increases muscle contraction speed and glycogenolysis
	Liver and kidney	Increases peripheral conversion of T_4 to T_3
	Uterus smooth muscle	Decreases nongravid uterine contraction (uterine relaxation)
Beta$_3$	Adipose cells	Increases lipolysis
	Intestinal smooth muscle	Increases intestinal motility
Dopamine$_1$	Vascular smooth muscle	Decreases vasoconstriction (vasodilation);
	Renal tubule	Enhances natriuresis
Dopamine$_2$	Sympathetic nerves	Inhibits synaptic release of norepinephrine
	Pituitary lactotrophes	Inhibits prolactin release
	Gastrointestinal tract	Paracrine functions

of the guanylyl nucleotide-binding protein, G_q, is released and activates phospholipase C. This enzyme catalyzes the conversion of phosphatidylinositol phosphate to 1,4,5-inositol triphosphate (IP_3) and diacylglycerol. IP_3 releases calcium ion from intracellular stores to stimulate physiologic responses. Diacylglycerol activates protein kinase C, which in turn phosphorylates a series of other proteins that initiate or sustain effects stimulated by the release of IP_3 and calcium ion (see Figure 11–5). Prazosin and phenoxybenzamine are selective antagonists of the α_1 receptor.

Alpha$_1$ receptors are postsynaptic (target organ) receptors that mediate diverse effects, particularly arteriolar vasoconstriction. Hepatic α_1 receptors stimulate glycogenolysis and gluconeogenesis. In the eye, α_1 receptors stimulate contraction of the radial muscle of the iris that dilates the pupil. In the skin, α_1 receptors mediate apocrine sweating and pilomotor contraction. In the genitourinary tract, α_1 receptors mediate ejaculation, gravid uterine contraction, and contraction of the bladder sphincter and trigone. In the intestines, α_1 receptors reduce smooth muscle contraction and increase sphincter tone, thereby promoting

constipation. Alpha$_1$ receptors are also found in the splenic capsule and mediate the contraction of the capsule (particularly during hypoxia), which contracts the splenic volume up to 20% and can expel up to 125 mL of packed red blood cells into the circulation within 3 seconds of apnea.

Sympathetic nerves secrete norepinephrine into synaptic junctions where the concentration of norepinephrine is high, thereby stimulating synaptic effector organ α_1 receptors. Epinephrine has a similar effect upon α_1 receptors but is secreted only by the adrenal medulla such that circulating concentrations are usually much lower than concentrations of synaptic norepinephrine. At low plasma concentrations, epinephrine predominantly stimulates β_2-adrenergic receptors (causing vasodilation, see later), whereas at higher plasma concentrations, epinephrine stimulates α_1 receptors sufficiently to override vasodilation and cause vasoconstriction.

Alpha$_2$ receptors are G_i coupled receptors with three highly homologous subtypes: α_{2A}, α_{2B}, and α_{2C}. Agonist binding to the α_2 receptor releases G_i alpha, which inhibits the enzyme adenylyl cyclase and reduces the formation of cAMP (Figure 11–6).

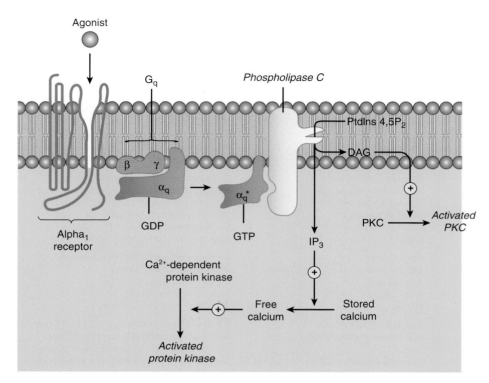

FIGURE 11–5 Activation of α_1-adrenergic responses. Stimulation of α_1 receptors by catecholamines leads to the activation of a G_q-coupling protein. The activated α_q subunit of this G protein activates phospholipase C, which catalyzes the conversion of PtdIns 4,5-P_2 (phosphatidylinositol 4,5-bisphosphate) to IP_3 (inositol 1,4,5-trisphosphate) and DAG (diacylglycerol). IP_3 stimulates the release of sequestered stores of calcium, leading to an increased concentration of cytoplasmic Ca^{2+} that may then activate Ca^{2+}-dependent protein kinases that phosphory-late their substrates. DAG activates protein kinase C (PKC) (GDP, guanosine diphosphate; GTP, guanosine triphosphate). See Table 11–3 and text for physiologic effects of α_1 receptor activation. (Reproduced, with permission, from Katzung BG, ed. *Basic & Clinical Pharmacology*. 11th ed. McGraw-Hill; 2009.)

Presynaptic (nerve) α_2 receptors are located near the synapses of sympathetic nerves. Synaptic norepinephrine binds to this receptor, resulting in feedback inhibition of its own release. Alpha$_2$ receptors are also found in vascular smooth muscle where they mediate vasoconstriction. Alpha$_2$ receptors in platelets stimulate platelet aggregation and clotting. In the brain, α_2 receptors are found in the locus ceruleus, cerebral cortex, and limbic system. Although their location is postsynaptic, stimulation of the α_2 receptors results in reduced release of norepinephrine. Clonidine is a central α_2 agonist. Yohimbine is a selective antagonist for the α_2 receptor. Phentolamine is an antagonist for both α_1 and α_2 receptors.

In the pancreatic beta cells, activation of α_2 receptors inhibits insulin secretion. This causes glucose intolerance in patients with pheochromocytoma. The gene *Adra2a* encodes the adrenergic α_{2A} receptor. A polymorphism in *Adra2a* increases the number of α_{2A} receptors on beta cells, which reduces insulin secretion and increases the risk of type 2 diabetes mellitus.

B. Beta-adrenergic receptors Beta-adrenergic receptors are postsynaptic (target organ) cell surface glycoproteins. Agonist binding to β-adrenergic receptors activates adenylyl cyclase via the G_s alpha subunit to increase the production of cAMP, which in turn converts protein kinase A to its active form. Kinase A then phosphorylates a variety of proteins, including enzymes, ion channels, and receptors (see Figure 11–6).

Beta$_1$-adrenergic receptors are located primarily in the heart, kidneys, and adipose tissue. In the heart, β_1 receptors are located in the SA and AV nodes, atrium, ventricle, and conduction system; activation of these receptors mediates an increase in heart rate and cardiac contraction with an overall increase in cardiac output. Stimulation of β_1 receptors in the ventricles also increases the firing of idioventricular pacemakers such that excessive stimulation predisposes to ventricular ectopy. Triiodothyronine (T_3) increases the total number of cardiac β_1 receptors; this may contribute to the forceful cardiac contraction and tachyarrhythmias that are characteristic of hyperthyroidism. Beta$_1$ receptors in the renal juxtaglomerular apparatus stimulate the release of renin that, in turn, activates the renin-angiotensin system. In fat cells, activation of β_1 receptors increases lipolysis. In nerve cells, activation of β_1 receptors increases nerve conduction velocity. In the brain, β_1 receptors are found particularly in the nucleus accumbens and the ventral putamen (striatum).

Beta$_2$-adrenergic receptors are particularly activated by epinephrine. They are located mainly in the smooth muscles of arterioles, veins, and bronchi where they mediate relaxation. In the

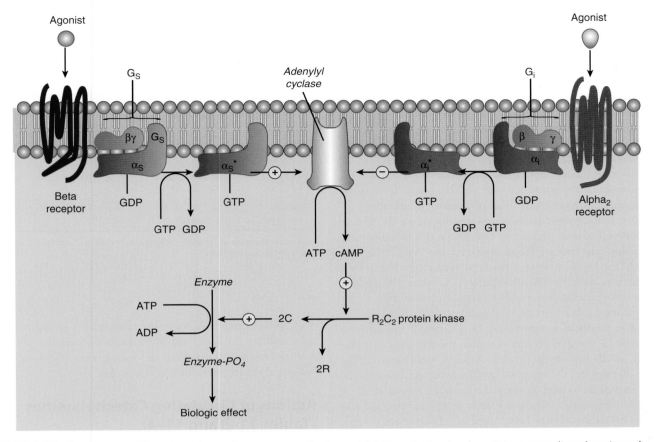

FIGURE 11–6 Activation of β- and α_2-adrenergic responses: activation vs inhibition of adenyl cyclase. Beta receptor ligands activate the stimulatory G protein, G_s, which leads to the dissociation of its $G\alpha_s$ subunit, charged with GTP. The activated $G\alpha_s$ subunit directly activates adenyl cyclase, resulting in increased cAMP that binds to the regulatory subunit (R) of the cAMP-dependent protein kinase, leading to the liberation of active catalytic subunits (C) that phosphorylate specific enzyme substrates and modify their activity. These catalytic units also phosphorylate the cAMP response element–binding protein (CREB), which modifies gene expression. Alpha$_2$ adrenoreceptor ligands inhibit adenyl cyclase by causing dissociation of the inhibitory G protein (G_i) into its subunits; that is, the α_i subunit charged with GTP and a βγ unit. The mechanism by which these subunits inhibit adenyl cyclase is uncertain. See Table 11–3 and text for physiologic effects of β and α_2 receptor activation. (Reproduced, with permission, from Katzung BG, ed. *Basic and Clinical Pharmacology.* 11th ed. McGraw-Hill; 2009.)

heart, β_2 receptors are located in the same locations as β_1 receptors (see earlier) and likewise mediate increases in cardiac rate and contraction. β_2 Receptors are also located in smaller coronary arteries where they mediate dilation of the coronaries, thereby increasing blood flow to cardiac muscle. Vascular β_2 receptors mediate vasodilation of arterioles, particularly in skeletal muscle and the hepatic artery. Stimulation of venous β_2 receptors mediates venous dilation. Stimulation of β_2 receptors also causes relaxation of other smooth muscles, resulting in bronchial dilation and relaxation of the nonpregnant uterus. During exercise or hypoglycemia, epinephrine is secreted and activates hepatic β_2 receptors. This stimulates glycogenolysis and gluconeogenesis for the increased glucose production that is needed for increased cardiac and skeletal muscle activity. Beta$_2$ receptors in skeletal muscle promote increased contraction speed, glycogenolysis, and tremor. The net effect of β_2 agonists (eg, epinephrine) upon liver and skeletal muscle is to increase serum glucose. Beta$_2$-adrenergic receptors are also expressed in various areas of the brain,

particularly the right hippocampus, which normally has a higher density of β_2 receptors than the left hippocampus.

Beta$_2$ receptor polymorphisms have been associated with obesity in women and differences in sensitivity to albuterol in asthmatics. Other β_2 receptor polymorphisms appear to account for individual differences in the vascular response to stress and increased risk for development of hypertension-induced left ventricular hypertrophy.

Beta$_3$-adrenergic receptors are expressed mainly in adipose tissue but also in the gallbladder, colon, central nervous system, and heart. Activation of this receptor increases energy expenditure, lipolysis, and intestinal motility. β_3 receptor activation promotes lipolysis in adipose tissue and increased thermogenesis in skeletal muscle. Although β_3-adrenergic receptors are found in the brains of infants, by adulthood their concentration decreases by 100-fold. Pima Indians, who are homozygous for inactivating mutations in the β_3 gene, have an earlier onset of type 2 diabetes.

C. Dopamine receptors   Five different dopamine receptors have been identified (D_1 to D_5), each encoded by a different gene. Dopamine receptors are found throughout the brain (including the anterior pituitary), arteries, proximal renal tubules, and gastrointestinal tract. D_1 and D_2 receptors are the predominant subtypes.

D_1-like family of receptors (D_1 and D_5) couples to G_s that activates adenyl cyclase, thereby increasing intracellular cyclic AMP (cAMP). D_1 receptors mediate vasodilation in the coronary, renal, cerebrovascular, and mesenteric arteries. D_1 receptors in the proximal renal tubule enhance natriuresis. The D_1 receptor is the most abundant dopamine receptor in the brain. Intravenous therapeutic dopamine at low doses predominantly stimulates D_1 receptors, causing vasodilation. (However, high-dose therapeutic dopamine sufficiently occupies α and β receptors to cause vasoconstriction and increase blood pressure.) The A48G polymorphism of the D_1 receptor gene has been associated with essential hypertension, with the 48G allele being found more frequently in hypertensive patients, presumably through a negative effect on the proximal renal tubule's excretion of sodium.

D_2-like family of receptors (D_2, D_3, D_4) couple to a different G protein, G_i that inhibits adenyl cyclase, thereby reducing intracellular cAMP, opening potassium channels, and decreasing the influx of calcium. D_2 receptors are predominately presynaptic receptors that are located on sympathetic nerves. Activation of D_2 receptors inhibits the synaptic release of norepinephrine and also inhibits the transmission of nerve impulses at sympathetic ganglia. Pituitary lactotroph cells also express D_2 receptors, whose activation inhibits the secretion of prolactin. Activation of other D_2 receptors in the brain causes vomiting. D_2 receptors are also found throughout the stomach, small intestines, and proximal colon, where the dopaminergic system is believed to work in a paracrine fashion.

Regulation of Sympathoadrenal Activity

The rate of catecholamine secretion largely determines sympathoadrenal activity. However, adrenergic receptors and postreceptor events are sites of fine regulation.

As noted earlier, norepinephrine and epinephrine released during nerve stimulation bind to presynaptic alpha$_2$ receptors and reduce the amount of norepinephrine released. CgA is secreted from neurosecretory vesicles, along with catecholamines. Catestatin, a fragment of CgA, blocks postreceptor cells' cholinergic receptors, thereby inhibiting sympathoadrenal activity.

The binding of a catecholamine agonist to its receptor reduces the number of receptors on the effector cell surface by a process called down regulation. Catecholamine receptor antagonists do not cause down regulation of receptor expression. The mechanisms involved in some of these changes are known. For example, phosphorylation of the β-adrenergic receptor by β-adrenergic receptor kinase results in sequestration of the receptors into membrane vesicles, where they are internalized and degraded. The phosphorylated receptor also has a greater affinity for β-arrestin, another regulatory protein, which prevents its interaction with $G_s\alpha$.

TABLE 11–4 Plasma levels of catecholamines required to produce hemodynamic and glucose effects.

	Norepinephrine	Epinephrine
Systolic blood pressure	↑ at 2500 pg/mL (15 nmol/L)	↑ at 500 pg/mL (3 nmol/L)
Diastolic blood pressure	↑ at 2500 pg/mL (15 nmol/L)	↓ at 500 pg/mL (3 nmol/L)
Pulse	↓ at 2500 pg/mL (15 nmol/dL)	↑ at 250 pg/mL (1.5 nmol/L)
Plasma glucose	↑ at 2500 pg/mL (15 nmol/L)	↑ at 250-500 pg/mL (1.5-3 nmol/L)

Data from Silverberg AB, et al. *Am J Physiol.* 1978;234:E252; and from Clutter WE, et al. *J Clin Invest.* 1980;66:94.

Thyroid hormone increases the number of β receptors in the myocardium. Estrogen, which increases the number of alpha receptors in the myometrium, also increases the affinity of some vascular alpha receptors for norepinephrine.

Actions of Circulating Catecholamines (Tables 11–3 and 11–4)

Norepinephrine activates α_1-adrenergic receptors, increasing the influx of calcium into the target cell. Vascular α_1-adrenergic receptors are found in the heart, papillary dilator muscles, and smooth muscle. Activation of α_1-adrenergic receptors causes hypertension, increased cardiac contraction, and dilation of the pupils. Alpha$_1$-adrenergic activation stimulates sweating from nonthermoregulatory apocrine stress sweat glands, which are located on the palms, axillae, and forehead. Norepinephrine also activates β_1-adrenergic receptors that increase cardiac contraction and rate; stimulation of the heart rate is opposed by simultaneous vagal stimulation. Norepinephrine has less affinity for β_2-adrenergic receptors. However, with higher circulating norepinephrine levels, hypermetabolism and hyperglycemia are noted. Norepinephrine also activates β_3-adrenergic receptors on fat cells, causing lipolysis and an increase in serum levels of free fatty acids.

Epinephrine also stimulates α_1- and β_1-adrenergic receptors, with the same effects noted above for norepinephrine. However, epinephrine also activates β_2 receptors, causing vasodilation in skeletal muscles. Epinephrine thus has a variable effect on blood pressure ranging from hypertension to hypotension (rare). Hypoglycemia is a strong stimulus for the adrenal medulla to secrete epinephrine, which increases hepatic glycogenolysis. Epinephrine stimulates lipolysis, resulting in increased serum levels of free fatty acids. Epinephrine also increases the basal metabolic rate. Epinephrine does not cross the blood–brain barrier well. However, high serum levels of epinephrine do stimulate the hypothalamus, resulting in unpleasant sensations ranging from nervousness to an overwhelming sense of impending doom.

Dopamine is an important central neurotransmitter and a precursor to norepinephrine and epinephrine. However, most circulating dopamine is actually derived from the gastrointestinal tract from local synthesis and dietary sources. Dopamine that is synthesized by the intestines does not function as a neurotransmitter but rather as a paracrine hormone, affecting intestinal motility, blood flow, and sodium transport. Dopamine is also synthesized in the proximal renal tubule where it is a natriuretic hormone. Dopamine synthesis is increased by a high-salt diet. The renal dopamine-paracrine system accounts for the relatively large amounts of dopamine that are normally found in the urine. Circulating dopamine is not normally a significant catecholamine. High serum concentrations of dopamine stimulate vascular D_1 receptors, causing vasodilation and increased renal blood flow. Extremely high serum levels of dopamine are required to sufficiently activate vascular α_1 receptors to cause vasoconstriction.

Physiologic Effects of Catecholamines

A. Cardiovascular effects   The release or injection of catecholamines generally increases heart rate and cardiac output and causes peripheral vasoconstriction, leading to an increase in blood pressure. The infusion of catecholamines also leads to a rapid reduction in plasma volume. These events are modulated by reflex mechanisms, so that, as the blood pressure increases, reflex vagal parasympathetic stimulation may slow the heart rate and tend to reduce cardiac output. Although norepinephrine usually has these effects, the effect of epinephrine may vary depending on the smooth muscle tone of the vascular system at the time. For example, in an individual with increased vascular tone, the net effect of small amounts of epinephrine may be to reduce the mean blood pressure through vasodilation, despite an increase in heart rate and cardiac output. In an individual with a reduction in vascular tone, epinephrine increases blood pressure. In addition cardiovascular function is integrated by the central nervous system, so that, under appropriate circumstances, one vascular bed may be dilated while others remain unchanged. The central organization of the sympathetic nervous system is such that its basal regulatory effects are quite discrete—in contrast to periods of stress, when stimulation may be rather generalized and accompanied by release of catecholamines into the circulation.

B. Effects on extravascular smooth muscle   Catecholamines have effects on smooth muscle in tissues other than blood vessels. These effects include contraction (α_1) and relaxation (β_2) of uterine myometrium, relaxation of intestinal and bladder smooth muscle (β_2), contraction of the smooth muscle in the bladder (α_1) and intestinal sphincters, relaxation of tracheal smooth muscle (β_2), and pupillary dilation (α_1).

C. Metabolic effects   Catecholamines increase oxygen consumption and heat production. This effect is mediated by β_1 receptors. Catecholamines also regulate glucose and fat mobilization from storage depots. Glycogenolysis in heart muscle and liver leads to an increase in available carbohydrate for utilization. Stimulation of adipose tissue leads to lipolysis and the release of

TABLE 11–5   Disorders causing epinephrine or norepinephrine deficiency.

Diabetes mellitus autonomic neuropathy (glucose toxicity or autoimmunity): serum norepinephrine low
Recurrent hypoglycemia-associated autonomic failure: serum norepinephrine low
Wolfram syndrome: diabetes insipidus, diabetes mellitus, optic atrophy, deafness (DIDMOAD): serum norepinephrine low
Neurological diseases associated with autonomic neuropathy: serum norepinephrine low
Pure autonomic failure: serum norepinephrine <u>and</u> epinephrine low
Primary adrenocortical insufficiency: serum epinephrine low
Congenital adrenal hyperplasia: serum epinephrine low
Allgrove syndrome: achalasia, ACTH resistance, alacrima (AAA syndrome): serum epinephrine low

free fatty acids and glycerol into the circulation. In humans, these effects are mediated by the β receptor. Both α_1 and β_2 receptors stimulate hepatic glycogenolysis and gluconeogenesis, which causes the release of glucose into the circulation. Both receptors are activated by epinephrine, which is particularly effective in raising hepatic glucose production. Plasma levels of catecholamines required to produce some cardiovascular and metabolic effects in humans are shown in Table 11–5.

Catecholamines have effects on water, sodium, potassium, calcium, and phosphate excretion in the kidney. Stimulation of the β_1 receptor increases the secretion of renin from the renal juxtaglomerular apparatus, thereby activating the renin-angiotensin system. This leads to stimulation of aldosterone secretion.

DISORDERS OF THE ADRENAL MEDULLA AND PARAGANGLIA

EPINEPHRINE AND NOREPINEPHRINE DEFICIENCY

Epinephrine is the major catecholamine secreted by the normal adrenal medulla, and its secretion is unique to the adrenal medulla. Epinephrine is usually deficient in cortisol deficiency of any cause, because high local concentrations of cortisol in the adrenal medulla are necessary for transcription of the enzyme PNMT, which catalyzes the conversion of norepinephrine to epinephrine in the catecholamine biosynthetic pathway. Primary autoimmune adrenal cortical insufficiency produces epinephrine deficiency. Hypothalamic/pituitary ACTH deficiency also causes cortisol deficiency and consequently epinephrine deficiency.

Autonomic Insufficiency (Table 11–5 and Figure 11–6)

Autonomic insufficiency is also know as dysautonomia. It refers to a general reduction in autonomic activity. Since the adrenal medulla is part of the autonomic nervous system, there is usually an associated deficiency in circulating epinephrine. Autonomic

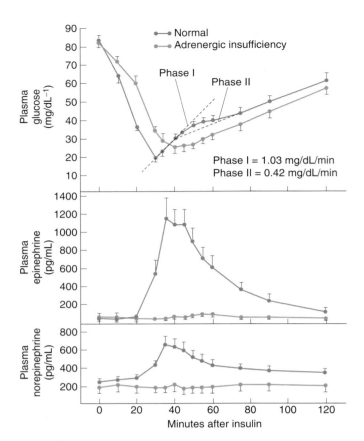

FIGURE 11–7 Plasma glucose, epinephrine, and norepinephrine levels after insulin administration in 14 normal subjects (•—•) and 7 patients with idiopathic orthostatic hypotension (•—•) with low or absent epinephrine responses. Results are expressed as mean ± SEM. (Reproduced, with permission, from Polinsky RJ, et al. The adrenal medullary response to hypoglycemia in patients with orthostatic hypotension. *J Clin Endocrinol Metab.* 1980;51:1404.)

insufficiency most commonly occurs in patients with long-standing type 1 diabetes mellitus. Diabetic autonomic neuropathy may be due to glucose neurotoxicity, but may also be due to autoimmunity. In one study of middle-aged patients with type 1 diabetes mellitus, 52% had complement-fixing antibodies against the sympathetic ganglia and 35% had antibodies against the adrenal medulla. They have minor defects in recovery from insulin-induced hypoglycemia (Figure 11–7), but in patients with diabetes mellitus in whom the glucagon response is also deficient, the additional loss of adrenal medullary response leaves them more susceptible to bouts of severe hypoglycemia. This is the result of a decrease in the warning symptoms as well as an impaired response to the hypoglycemia (see Chapters 17 and 18). Patients with generalized autonomic insufficiency usually have orthostatic hypotension. Familial dysautonomia can manifest as orthostatic tachycardia; norepinephrine transporter deficiency has been determined to be one cause of this condition. The causes of disorders associated with autonomic insufficiency are listed in Table 11–5.

When a normal individual stands, a series of physiologic adjustments occur that maintain blood pressure and ensure adequate circulation to the brain. The initial lowering of the blood pressure stimulates the baroreceptors, which then activate central reflex mechanisms that cause arterial and venous constriction, increase cardiac output, and activate the release of renin and vasopressin. Interruption of afferent, central, or efferent components of this autonomic reflex results in autonomic insufficiency.

Patients with generalized autonomic insufficiency usually have orthostatic hypotension; the reduction in blood pressure on standing that causes visual disturbances, lightheadedness, and even syncope. Symptoms tend to be worse upon awakening, after meals, in hot weather, and at high altitude. Many patients have supine hypertension, even when not taking hypertensive medication. Affected patients often have a fixed heart rate, sinus tachycardia, diminished sweating, reduced metabolic rate, heat intolerance, nocturia, and erectile dysfunction. Angina pectoris can sometimes occur in the absence of coronary atherosclerosis. Patients frequently have a neurogenic bladder with associated symptoms of frequency, nocturia, hesitancy, reduced urine stream, and recurrent urinary tract infections. Patients may also have gastroparesis and disordered gastrointestinal motility. Sleep apnea is common and death can occur during sleep from reduced respiratory drive.

The diagnosis of autonomic insufficiency can usually be made clinically in patients with typical symptoms and orthostatic blood pressure changes on examination. Additionally, plasma and urine norepinephrine levels are usually very low, sometimes only 10% of average normal in severely affected individuals. Plasma epinephrine levels are often low as well.

The treatment of symptomatic orthostatic hypotension is dependent on maintenance of an adequate blood volume. Physical measures should be employed, such as raising the foot of the bed at night, crossing the legs when sitting, and wearing full-leg fitted support stockings. Adequate hydration is important. Volume expansion with fludrocortisone is the most effective drug treatment. However, fludrocortisone can cause hypokalemia, supine hypertension, and edema. Midodrine is an α_1-receptor agonist that must be administered every 8 hours, due to its short half-life of 3 to 4 hours. Midodrine's use is limited by common side effects that include severe supine hypertension, bradycardia, and erythema multiforme. Therefore, midodrine should only be used for patients with very symptomatic orthostatic hypotension who have failed other therapies. Octreotide has been used, either alone or in combination with midodrine, for patients with severe autonomic failure where other treatment measures have failed.

PHEOCHROMOCYTOMA AND PARAGANGLIOMA

Both pheochromocytoma and non–head-neck paraganglioma are tumors of the sympathetic nervous system. Although they are similar tumors, they warrant distinction from each other to emphasize their differences in the following: (1) locations, (2) manifestations, (3) secretion profiles, (4) genetic syndromes, (5) difficulty of surgical resection, and (6) propensity to metastasize.

Pheochromocytomas are tumors that arise from the adrenal medulla, whereas non–head-neck paragangliomas arise from the ganglia of the sympathetic nervous system. Pheochromocytomas are more common (85%), and may be bilateral (17%). Patients with adrenal pheochromocytomas are less likely to develop detectable metastases (11%) compared to paragangliomas (30%).

Incidence

The yearly incidence of diagnosed pheochromocytoma/paraganglioma tumors is about 2 to 8 per million; nearly half of these present as an unexplained death. The National Cancer Registry in Sweden has reported that pheochromocytomas/paragangliomas are discovered in about 2 patients per million people yearly. However, autopsy series suggest a higher incidence. The reported incidence in autopsy series has varied from about 250 cases per million to 1300 cases per million in a Mayo Clinic autopsy series. Retrospectively, 61% of pheochromocytoma/paraganglioma tumors at autopsy occurred in patients who were known to have had hypertension; about 91% had the nonspecific symptoms associated with secretory pheochromocytoma/paraganglioma tumors. In one autopsy study, a large number of patients with these tumors had nonclassic symptoms such as abdominal pain, vomiting, dyspnea, heart failure, hypotension, or sudden death (Table 11–6). Considering these autopsy data, it is clear that the majority of pheochromocytoma/paraganglioma tumors are not diagnosed during life. Tumors occur in both sexes and at any age but are most commonly diagnosed in the fourth and fifth decades.

Pheochromocytomas are chromaffin tumors that arise from the adrenal medulla. They account for 90% of all pheochromocytoma/paraganglioma tumors in adults and 70% in children. Adrenal pheochromocytomas are usually unilateral (90%). Unilateral pheochromocytomas occur more frequently in the right (65%) versus the left adrenal (35%). Right-sided pheochromocytomas have been described as producing paroxysmal hypertension more often than sustained hypertension, whereas the opposite was true for tumors arising from the left adrenal. Adrenal pheochromocytomas are bilateral in about 10% of adults and 35% of children. Bilateral pheochromocytomas are particularly common (24% overall) in patients with familial pheochromocytoma syndromes caused by certain germline mutations (see later).

Basically, the adrenal medulla is a sympathetic ganglia whose neurons secrete neurotransmitters (epinephrine and norepinephrine) into capillaries instead of synapses. The adrenal medulla is surrounded by the adrenal cortex, with which it shares a portal system that bathes it in high concentrations of cortisol. Cortisol stimulates expression of the gene encoding PNMT, the enzyme that catalyzes the conversion of norepinephrine to epinephrine. Adrenal pheochromocytomas nearly always secrete catecholamines with variable amounts of epinephrine as well as norepinephrine and their metanephrine metabolites. Metastases from adrenal pheochromocytomas usually secrete only norepinephrine and its metabolite normetanephrine; they may rarely secrete epinephrine.

Pheochromocytomas are typically encapsulated by a true capsule or a pseudocapsule, the latter being the adrenal capsule. Pheochromocytomas are firm in texture. Hemorrhages that occur within a pheochromocytoma can give the tumor a mottled or dark red appearance. A few *black* pheochromocytomas have been described, with the dark pigmentation believed to be due to an accumulation of neuromelanin, a catecholamine metabolite. Larger tumors frequently contain large areas of hemorrhagic necrosis that have undergone cystic degeneration; viable tumor may be found in the cyst wall. Calcifications are often present. Pheochromocytomas can invade adjacent organs, and tumors may extend into the adrenal vein and the vena cava, resulting in pulmonary tumor emboli. Pheochromocytomas vary tremendously in size, ranging from microscopic to 3600 g. The average pheochromocytoma weighs about 100 g and is 4.5 cm in diameter.

Non–head-neck paragangliomas arise from sympathetic ganglia (Figure 11–8). They account for about 10% of all pheochromocytoma/paraganglioma tumors in adults and about 30% in

TABLE 11–6 Causes of death in patients with unsuspected pheochromocytomas.

Myocardial infarction
Cerebrovascular accident
Arrhythmias
Irreversible shock
Renal failure
Dissecting aortic aneurysm
Acute respiratory distress syndrome

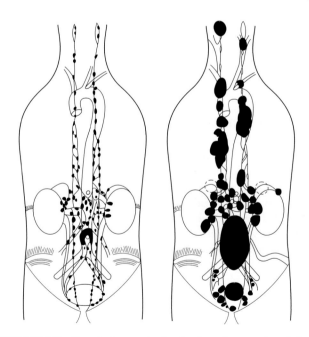

FIGURE 11–8 Left: Anatomic distribution of extra-adrenal chromaffin tissue in the newborn. **Right:** Locations of extra-adrenal pheochromocytomas reported before 1965. (Reproduced, with permission, from Coupland R. *The Natural History of the Chromaffin Cell.* Longmans Green; 1965).

children. About 75% are intra-abdominal where they are often mistaken for adrenal pheochromocytomas. Paragangliomas are sometimes nonsecretory and may be confused with other neuroendocrine tumors. They arise most commonly in the perinephric, periaortic, and bladder regions but often found in the chest (25%), arising in the anterior or posterior mediastinum or the heart. Pelvic paragangliomas may involve the bladder wall, obstruct the ureters, and metastasize to regional lymph nodes. About 36% to 60% of paragangliomas are functional, secreting norepinephrine and normetanephrine. Functional status is not known to affect survival. Nonfunctional paragangliomas can often concentrate metaiodobenzylguanidine (MIBG) or secrete CgA. Paragangliomas of the bladder can cause symptoms associated with micturition. Large perinephric tumors can cause renal artery stenosis and elevations in plasma renin activity. Vaginal tumors may cause dysfunctional vaginal bleeding. Paragangliomas can rarely arise in central nervous system locations, including the sella turcica, petrous ridge, and pineal region. Cauda equina paragangliomas can cause increased intracranial pressure.

Paragangliomas commonly metastasize (30%-50%) and present with pain or a mass. They tend to metastasize to the liver, lungs, lymph nodes, and bone. PGLs can be locally invasive and may destroy adjacent vertebrae and cause spinal cord and nerve root compression. PGL metastases usually secrete norepinephrine and normetanephrine. They do not secrete epinephrine and therefore do not typically cause significant weight loss, hyperglycemia, anxiety, or tremor.

Nonchromaffin parasympathetic paragangliomas are typically found in the head and neck. Unlike chromaffin sympathetic paragangliomas, only about 5% of these tumors secrete catecholamines. **Carotid body tumors** are paragangliomas that arise near the carotid bifurcation. They usually present as a painless neck mass, but can injure the vagus or hypoglossal nerves. **Glomus tympanicum** paragangliomas arise in the middle ear and cause tinnitus and hearing loss. The tumor may be seen as a reddish mass behind an intact tympanic membrane (*red drum*) that blanches when pressure is applied with a pneumatic ear speculum (Brown sign). **Glomus jugulare paragangliomas** arise in the jugular foramen. They often cause tinnitus and hearing loss as well as compression of cranial nerves, resulting is dysphagia. Vagal paragangliomas are rare, usually presenting as a painless neck mass often associated with hoarseness or dysphagia. Head-neck paragangliomas can also arise in the larynx, nasal cavity, nasal sinuses, and thyroid gland. Head-neck PGLs themselves are of more interest to otolaryngologists than endocrinologists. But they may be seen along with sympathetic paragangliomas in familial paraganglioma syndromes, particularly those with germline succinate dehydrogenase subunit D (SDHD) mutations (see later).

Nonchromaffin paragangliomas behave differently from sympathetic paragangliomas and pheochromocytomas, although they are embryologically related to chromaffin sympathetic paragangliomas and may arise concurrently with sympathetic paragangliomas in familial paraganglioma syndromes. These tumors are less likely to be malignant, although their indolence can be deceiving; recurrence and metastases may not appear for many years. Metastases to local nodes, lungs, and bone can occur. Long-term

surveillance for recurrence or metastases is recommended for all patients. These tumors can produce CgA, and preoperative determination of CgA is recommended to determine if it will be a good serum marker for tumor recurrence. Patients with cervical paragangliomas often have an underlying germline mutation in the gene encoding succinate dehydrogenase (SDH); *SDHD*, *SDHC*, and *SDHB* gene sequencing is recommended for all these patients (see later). Individuals harboring a germline mutation must be screened for the existence of other paragangliomas and pheochromocytomas (see "Genetic Conditions Associated with Pheochromocytomas and Paragangliomas," later).

Neuroblastomas, ganglioneuroblastomas, and **ganglioneuromas** are sympathetic nervous system tumors that are related to pheochromocytomas and likewise arise from embryonal sympathogonia (see Figure 11–1). Neuroblastoma is the most common malignant disease of infancy and the third most common pediatric cancer, accounting for 15% of childhood cancer deaths. Neuroblastomas are embryonal cancers of the postganglionic sympathetic nervous system and develop from sympathetic tissue in the adrenal gland, neck, posterior mediastinum, retroperitoneum, or pelvis. These tumors differ in their degree of maturation and malignancy. Neuroblastoma tumors derive from immature neuroblasts, are generally aggressive, tend to occur in very young children, and display clinical heterogeneity. The prognosis for neuroblastoma depends on age at diagnosis, with infants under age 1 year having a high likelihood of cure with surgical excision. Similarly, children with a localized neuroblastoma may be cured surgically. Some tumors can regress spontaneously or differentiate into benign ganglioneuromas. However, older children with widespread hematogenous metastases have a very poor prognosis, as do those whose neuroblastoma harbors an amplification of the *Myc* proto-oncogene. Some neuroblastomas are more indolent, depending on the nature of their oncogene mutations.

Ganglioneuroblastomas are composed of a mixture of neuroblasts and more mature gangliocytes; these develop in older children and tend to run a more benign course. Ganglioneuromas are the most benign of these tumors and are composed of gangliocytes and mature stromal cells.

Despite catecholamine secretion, children with neuroblastomas tend to be more symptomatic from their primary tumor or metastases than from catecholamine secretion. Tumors tend to concentrate radiolabeled MIBG, making it a useful imaging and therapeutic agent. Treatment of malignant tumors consists of surgery, chemotherapy, external beam radiation to skeletal metastases, and high-dose ^{131}I-MIBG therapy for patients with MIBG-avid tumors.

Screening for Pheochromocytomas and Paragangliomas

Hypertension, defined as either a systolic or diastolic blood pressure over 140/90 mm Hg, is an extremely common condition, affecting about 20% of all American adults and over 50% of adults over 60 years of age. The incidence of pheochromocytoma is estimated to be less than 0.1% of the entire hypertensive population, but it is higher in certain subgroups whose hypertension is

TABLE 11–7 Patients to be screened for pheochromocytoma and paraganglioma.

Young hypertensives
Hypertensive patients with:
  Symptoms listed in Table 11–13
  Weight loss
  Seizures
  Orthostatic hypotension
  Unexplained shock
  Family history of pheochromocytoma or medullary carcinoma of thyroid
  Neurofibromatosis and other neurocutaneous syndromes
  Mucosal neuromas
  Hyperglycemia
  Cardiomyopathy
Marked lability of blood pressure
Family history of pheochromocytoma
Shock or severe pressor responses with:
  Induction of anesthesia
  Parturition
  Surgery
  Invasive procedures
Radiologic evidence of adrenal mass
Radiologic evidence of mass in area of paraganglia

labile or severe. Screening for pheochromocytomas should be considered for such patients with severe hypertension and also for hypertensive patients with suspicious symptoms (eg, headaches, palpitations, sweating episodes, or unexplained bouts of abdominal or chest pains; Table 11–7).

Genetic Conditions Associated with Pheochromocytomas and Paragangliomas (Tables 11–8 through 11–11)

Most pheochromocytomas occur sporadically, although a substantial proportion of these tumors are found to have developed a somatic mutation similar to those germline mutations that give rise to familial syndromes. Based on family history, it was formerly thought that only about 10% of patients with these tumors developed it as part of a genetic syndrome. With genetic testing, it is now clear that about 26% of patients with pheochromocytomas or paragangliomas carry a germline mutation associated with a familial syndrome. About 19% of patients with an apparently sporadic single pheochromocytoma and no known family history of pheochromocytoma harbor a germline mutation. For example, about 9% of patients with apparently sporadic, unilateral pheochromocytoma have been found to have von Hippel-Lindau (VHL) mutations. Genetic testing is advisable for all patients with a pheochromocytoma or paraganglioma. Genetic testing is strongly recommended for patients with extra-adrenal paragangliomas or multifocal tumors; onset of symptoms before age 45 years; prior history of head-neck paraganglioma; family history of paraganglioma, pheochromocytoma, or other tumors associated with MEN 2 or VHL. Genetic screening is also performed for patients with other manifestations of genetic syndromes noted later. Genetic screening can be done for MEN 2 *RET* proto-oncogene mutations, *VHL* mutations, and *SDH* (*SDHB*, *SDHD*, and *SDHC*) gene mutations. *Neurofibromatosis* is usually diagnosed clinically without genetic testing, since the NF-1 gene is very large.

A. Multiple endocrine neoplasia type 2: *RET* proto-oncogene (10q11.2)
The first description of a pheochromocytoma was in a patient with MEN 2. In 1882, Felix Fränkel described pheochromocytomas in an 18-year-old woman with bilateral adrenal tumors; genetic testing of four living relatives has revealed a germline RET mutation.

The prevalence of MEN 2 has been estimated at 1 in 30,000. MEN 2 is an autosomal dominant disorder that causes a predisposition to medullary thyroid carcinoma, pheochromocytoma, and other abnormalities described later. MEN 2 is caused by an activating mutation in the *RET* proto-oncogene on chromosome 10q11.2. *RET* consists of 21 exons that encode a transmembrane receptor tyrosine kinase that is expressed in neural crest tissues. The constitutive activation of *RET* causes hyperplasia in affected tissues, including the adrenal medulla. Additional mutation(s) are believed to be required for a pheochromocytoma to develop. The somatic loss of a tumor suppressor gene on chromosome 1p appears to be necessary for pheochromocytoma formation. Additionally, reduced expression of *NF-1* has been reported in a minority of pheochromocytomas arising in patients with MEN 2 mutations.

TABLE 11–8 Surveillance protocol for individuals carrying a *RET* protooncogene mutation.

Twice yearly: physical examination with blood pressure and neck examination; plasma free metanephrine; serum calcium and albumin (serum PTH if *RET* codon 634 mutation); serum calcitonin (patients with intact thyroid or with medullary thyroid carcinoma)
Prophylactic thyroidectomy: by age 5 years for MEN 2A and by 6 months for codon 918 mutations (MEN 2B)
Yearly thyroid ultrasound for patients with an intact thyroid
For rising or elevated serum calcitonin levels after thyroidectomy: close surveillance for medullary thyroid carcinoma is required. [18]FDG-PET-CT fusion scans are particularly helpful
For suspicious symptoms and before major surgical procedures and pregnancy: biochemical screening for pheochromocytoma with plasma free metanephrine
For abnormal biochemical screening for pheochyromocytoma: MRI or CT scan of the abdomen (nonionic contrast) with thin-section adrenal cuts; ^{123}I-MIBG SPECT or ^{18}F-FDA PET scan to confirm the identity of small masses

MEN 2 kindreds can be grouped into two distinct subtypes: MEN 2A (90%) and MEN 2B (10%). Patients with MEN 2A have various single amino acid missense mutations affecting the extracellular *RET* domain that cause *RET* homodimerization and constitutive activation of its tyrosine kinase. Patients with MEN 2B have a particular missense mutation (codon 918, exon 16) affecting the intracellular domain at the *RET* tyrosine kinase's catalytic site, causing constitutive activation. In either subtype, pheochromocytomas usually develop in the adrenals (96%); extra-adrenal paragangliomas are rare (4%). About 42% of patients with pheochromocytoma in MEN 2 have hypertension, usually paroxysmal. Overall, only about 53% exhibit symptoms of pheochromocytoma. Each specific type of mutation in the *RET* codon determines each kindred's idiosyncrasies, such as the age at onset and the aggressiveness of medullary thyroid carcinoma.

A limited number of *RET* gene exons have been found to harbor mutations that are capable of causing constitutive activation of the tyrosine kinase. *RET* exons 10, 11, 13, 14, 15, and 16 are usually involved. Therefore, routine genetic screening searches for mutations only in these exons. If no mutation is found in these exons, the remaining 15 exons can be sequenced in a research laboratory. When an affected kindred's *RET* mutation is already known, an individual in the kindred is screened for that specific mutation.

Pheochromocytomas arise in the adrenals, and extra-adrenal paragangliomas are rare in MEN 2. In patients with MEN 2, only about 4% of pheochromocytomas are found to be metastatic, possibly because of earlier detection. When pheochromocytomas develop in patients with MEN 2, they are bilateral in about two-thirds of cases; however, with close surveillance of affected kindreds, pheochromocytomas are discovered earlier and are more likely to be unilateral. After a unilateral adrenalectomy for pheochromocytoma in a patient with MEN 2, a contralateral pheochromocytoma develops in about 50% of patients an average of 12 years after the first adrenalectomy. In patients with MEN 2, adrenal pheochromocytomas produce norepinephrine and epinephrine (with its metabolite metanephrine). When screening for small pheochromocytomas, plasma catecholamine concentrations may be normal but plasma metanephrine concentrations are usually elevated, making plasma free metanephrines the screening test of choice for these patients. However, some pheochromocytomas are detected only by a 24-hour urine determination for fractionated metanephrines, catecholamines, and creatinine.

1. **MEN 2A (Sipple syndrome)**—Patients with this genetic condition develop medullary thyroid carcinoma (95%-100%), hyperparathyroidism due to multiglandular hyperplasia (35%), and pheochromocytoma (50%; range 6%-100% depending on the kindred) or adrenal medullary hyperplasia. Patients with MEN 2A also have an increased incidence of cutaneous lichen amyloidosis and Hirschsprung disease. Pheochromocytomas tend to present in middle age, often without hypertension. The incidence of hyperparathyroidism has also varied, averaging 35%.

   Individuals belonging to an MEN 2A kindred should have genetic testing for *RET* proto-oncogene mutations by 5 years of age to determine if they carry the genetic mutation that will require prophylactic thyroidectomy and close surveillance for pheochromocytoma and hyperparathyroidism.

   More than 85% of the mutations in MEN 2A families affect codon 634 in exon 11 of the *RET* proto-oncogene. Individuals with mutations in RET codon 630 also have a high incidence of pheochromocytoma. Pheochromocytomas also occur in most other kindreds with MEN 2A. Screening for pheochromocytoma should commence with the routine blood pressure measurements that are performed during examinations in childhood for medullary thyroid carcinoma and follow-up of hypothyroidism following thyroidectomy. At about age 15 years, affected individuals should commence yearly screening for pheochromocytoma with plasma free metanephrine determinations.

   Certain *RET* mutations (codons 609, 768, val804met, and 891) rarely produce pheochromocytomas. Less intense screening for pheochromocytomas is required in patients with these mutations.

2. **MEN 2B**—Over 90% of patients with MEN 2B have a single amino acid substitution of methionine to threonine on codon 918 in exon 16 that affects the intracellular domain of tyrosine kinase. About 50% of such mutations are familial while the rest arise de novo and are sporadic. Patients with this genetic condition are prone to develop mucosal neuromas, pheochromocytoma, adrenal medullary hyperplasia, and aggressive medullary thyroid carcinoma. About 50% of affected patients develop all three manifestations of the syndrome. Mucosal neuromas tend to develop first and occur in most patients. They appear as small bumps on the tongue, lips and buccal mucosa, eyelids, cornea, and conjunctivae. The lips and eyelids may become diffusely thickened. Intestinal ganglioneuromatosis occurs and alters intestinal motility, causing diarrhea or constipation and occasionally megacolon. Affected individuals have a marfanoid habitus with associated spinal scoliosis or kyphosis, pectus excavatum, a high-arched foot and talipes equinovarus (club foot) deformities. In patients with MEN 2B, medullary thyroid carcinoma tends to be aggressive and occurs at an earlier age than in patients with MEN 2A. Members of kindred with MEN 2B should immediately have genetic testing for their family's *RET* proto-oncogene mutation. If an individual is found to carry the family's *RET* mutation, early prophylactic thyroidectomy is advisable. In kindreds with MEN 2B, infants are screened for the mutation at birth. For affected infants, prophylactic thyroidectomy is performed by 6 months of age.

All individuals carrying a *RET* proto-oncogene mutation must have close medical surveillance (see Table 11–8). See Chapter 22: Multiple Endocrine Neoplasia.

B. Von Hippel-Lindau disease: *VHL* gene (3p25-26)

VHL disease is inherited as an autosomal dominant trait that predisposes its carriers to develop tumors in multiple tissues. Although certain VHL kindreds are predisposed to develop pheochromocytomas, it is not the dominant tumor of this syndrome. Pheochromocytomas develop only in patients with type 2 VHL (see later), and these are different from sporadic pheochromocytomas in that they are less likely to be malignant, more likely to be bilateral, and more likely to present at an earlier age. Although most VHL-associated pheochromocytomas arise in the adrenal, extra-adrenal paragangliomas sometimes arise; these usually occur along the sympathetic chain, but head-neck parasympathetic paragangliomas have been described. The mean age of presentation for a pheochromocytoma in type 2 VHL is 28 years; the youngest reported patient was 5 years old.

The different types and subtypes of VHL are as follows:

1. **Type 1 VHL**—Affected members of families with type 1 VHL do not develop pheochromocytomas. They tend to have loss-of-function *VHL* gene mutations, particularly gene deletions, frameshifts, or truncations.
2. **Type 2 VHL**—Affected members of families with type 2 VHL mutations are prone to develop pheochromocytomas. These patients carry VHL missense mutations. Type 2 VHL may be divided into subtypes as follows:
   a. **Type 2A VHL**—Pheochromocytomas, hemangioblastomas, *low* risk of renal cell carcinoma.
   b. **Type 2B VHL**—Pheochromocytomas, hemangioblastomas, *high* risk of renal cell carcinoma.
   c. **Type 2C VHL**—Pheochromocytomas, *no* hemangioblastomas, *no* renal cell carcinomas.

The prevalence of VHL is about 1 in 30,000 persons. VHL disease carriers are predisposed to multicentric hemangioblastomas in the retina (retinal angiomas), cerebellum, and spinal cord. Renal cysts and renal clear-cell carcinoma commonly develop.

Multiple cysts and nonfunctional neuroendocrine tumors may develop in the pancreas. Endolymphatic sac tumors may occur, resulting in hearing loss, vertigo, or ataxia. Adnexal cystadenomas of probable mesonephric origin (APMO) are found in many women with VHL. APMOs may develop in the ovary, broad ligament, vagina, uterine cervix, and vulva. Equivalent epididymal cystadenomas occur in men with VHL.

Genetic testing for VHL disease should be done in children born to a parent with known VHL disease. If VHL disease is suspected, but the family's VHL mutation is not known, the patient must be screened for point mutations by direct *VHL* gene sequencing of the entire coding region and splice junctions.

The clinical diagnosis of VHL disease is made when a patient with a known *VHL* gene mutation develops one tumor typical of VHL. In patients without a known family history of VHL, a presumptive diagnosis of VHL is made when they develop two or more hemangioblastomas or a hemangioblastoma in association with a pheochromocytoma or clear-cell renal carcinoma. Similarly, VHL disease should be suspected in patients with multiple VHL-associated tumors or one VHL-associated tumor that presents at a young age (<50 years for pheochromocytoma or hemangioblastoma; <30 years for clear-cell renal carcinoma). Such patients should have *VHL* gene sequencing.

The *VHL* gene is a tumor suppressor gene whose locus is 3p25/26. It encodes two different proteins (pVHL) of 213 and 160 amino acids. Both gene products have a role in the degradation of the hypoxia-inducible factors (HIF-1α and HIF-2α) as follows: The pVHL proteins have an α domain that binds with the protein elongin. The β domain of pVHL is open to bind HIF that has been hydroxylated, a reaction that requires oxygen. This complex then binds ubiquitin that targets HIF for intracellular destruction by proteases. In this manner, well-oxygenated cells destroy HIF. Conversely, cells that are either oxygen-deprived or that lack functional pVHL cause an intracellular accumulation of HIF. HIF is a transcription factor that induces the production of vascular endothelial growth factor (VEGF), erythropoietin, erythropoietin receptor, glucose transporter-1, and platelet-derived growth factor-B; these proteins allow an adaptation to hypoxia, but, in excess, are believed to enhance tumorigenesis.

For a tumor to develop in a patient harboring a VHL germline mutation, an additional somatic mutation must develop in the patient's remaining wild-type VHL allele. This second-hit mutation must occur in a cell in susceptible somatic tissue (eg, vascular tissue) in order for the cell to grow into a VHL-associated tumor.

In patients with VHL disease, vascular tumors, particularly hemangioblastomas, renal cysts, and renal cell carcinomas, develop when there is a somatic second-hit on the wild-type allele in one cell; this can be caused by various spontaneous mutations (loss of heterozygosity) or promoter hypermethylation of the wild-type VHL allele. In these vascular tumors, a second-hit is usually necessary to cause sufficient accumulation of HIF to promote tumorigenesis. In contrast, pheochromocytomas that develop in patients with type 2 VHL typically have a normal wild-type VHL allele. However, most VHL-associated pheochromocytomas also demonstrate a somatic loss of chromosome 3 (94%) or chromosome 11 (86%).

A germline mutation in the VHL tumor suppressor gene has been identified in most families with VHL disease. About 60% of affected families have loss-of-function mutations (30% with truncated pVHL and 30% with large *VHL* gene deletions), resulting in type 1 VHL. About 40% have missense mutations, resulting in an amino acid substitution in pVHL, causing type 2 VHL.

In a French series of 36 patients with pheochromocytomas and VHL disease, pheochromocytomas were the presenting tumor in 53%. Pheochromocytomas tended to develop at an early age and were bilateral in 42%; concurrent paragangliomas were present in 11%. Three of the 36 patients had a malignant pheochromocytoma. In 18% of these patients with VHL disease, pheochromocytoma was the only known manifestation. Approximately 9% of patients with apparently sporadic, unilateral pheochromocytoma have been found to harbor a germline VHL mutation. In certain regions of Europe, the percentage is up to 20%, due to a founder effect for the Tyr98His *black forest* mutation that is more common in kindreds with German ancestry.

Pheochromocytomas in VHL disease produce exclusively norepinephrine. Therefore, the metabolite of norepinephrine (normetanephrine) is also produced in these tumors. Plasma normetanephrine levels are usually elevated when patients with VHL disease develop a pheochromocytoma. Therefore, it is advisable for patients with a type 2 *VHL* gene missense mutation to be screened regularly with plasma normetanephrine levels.

In patients with VHL, a major risk to life is the development of a renal cell carcinoma. When an abdominal computed tomography (CT) scan detects a solid renal lesion, it must be removed. Even simple cystic renal lesions are considered premalignant, and their removal is advisable if renal function can be preserved. If renal cysts are observed, they must be followed every 6 months with dynamic thin-section CT scanning to search for characteristics of malignancy: growth, wall irregularity, or septation. Individuals carrying

TABLE 11–9 Surveillance protocol for individuals carrying a type 2 VHL mutation.

Yearly: retinal examination; plasma free normetanephrine levels yearly from age 10 to 15 years
Twice yearly: physical examination with blood pressure beginning at age 5 years; plasma free normetanephrine levels beginning at age 15 years
Every 2 years: MRI scanning (with intravenous contrast) of the entire brain and spinal cord (VHL types 2A and 2B VHL); MRI scanning of the abdomen
For suspicious symptoms and before major surgical procedures and pregnancy: biochemical screening for pheochromocytoma with plasma free metanephrine
For abnormal biochemical screening: MRI or CT scan of the abdomen (nonionic contrast) with thin-section adrenal cuts; ^{123}I-MIBG SPECT or ^{18}F-FDA PET scan to confirm the identity of small masses

a VHL mutation must have close medical surveillance. A surveillance protocol is recommended in Table 11–9.

C. Von Recklinghausen (type 1) neurofibromatosis: NF-1 gene (17q11.2)

Pheochromocytomas are ultimately diagnosed in 0.1–5.7% of patients with von Recklinghausen neurofibromatosis type 1 (*NF-1*). Most of these pheochromocytomas are not diagnosed during life, since the autopsy incidence of pheochromocytoma in NF-1 patients is 3.3% to 13%. Pheochromocytomas that develop in patients with NF-1 are similar to sporadic pheochromocytomas: 84% have solitary adrenal tumors, 10% have bilateral adrenal tumors, 6% have extra-adrenal paragangliomas, and 12% have metastases or local invasion.

Pheochromocytomas are present in 20% to 50% of NF-1 patients with hypertension, and all NF-1 patients with hypertension must be screened for pheochromocytoma. It is prudent to screen all patients with NF-1 for pheochromocytoma yearly, with interval testing if hypertension or symptoms develop that are suggestive of pheochromocytoma (headache, perspiration, palpitations). Similarly, all patients with NF-1 should be screened for pheochromocytoma before major surgical procedures and pregnancy.

In patients with NF-1, pheochromocytomas can present anytime during life, from infancy to old age, with a mean age of 42 years at diagnosis. These pheochromocytomas can grow to large size. Although patients with pheochromocytomas may develop hypertension, many patients are surprisingly asymptomatic despite increased catecholamine secretion. Patients with NF-1 are prone to develop vascular anomalies such as coarctation of the aorta and renal artery dysplasia, which can produce hypertension and mimic a pheochromocytoma.

Von Recklinghausen disease is caused by a mutation in the NF-1 tumor suppressor gene mapped to chromosome 17q11.2. The *NF-1* gene encodes a 2818 amino acid protein called neurofibromin, which inhibits *Ras* oncogene activity; loss of neurofibromin leads to *Ras* activation and tumor formation. It is a common

autosomal dominant genetic disorder (although 50% of cases seem sporadic), with an approximate incidence of 300 to 400 cases per million population. Although genetic testing for NF-1 is available, the diagnosis is usually made clinically during childhood or adolescence.

Patients with NF-1 can present in childhood with optic gliomas that impair vision or in adolescence with plexiform neurofibromas. Patients develop visible subcutaneous neurofibromas and schwannomas of cranial and vertebral nerve roots. Skeletal abnormalities are common. Hypothalamic hamartomas may occur and cause precocious puberty. Iris hamartomas may occur and are known as Lisch nodules. NF-1 patients have an increased risk of developing other tumors, especially malignant peripheral nerve sheath tumors and leukemia (particularly juvenile chronic myelogenous leukemia). Patients may also have freckles in their axillae and skin folds. Multiple cutaneous pigmented café au lait spots develop and grow in size and number with age; most patients ultimately develop more than six spots (smooth bordered) measuring more than 1.5 cm in diameter.

Individuals carrying an NF-1 mutation must have close medical surveillance. A surveillance protocol is recommended in Table 11–10.

D. Familial paraganglioma/pheochromocytoma syndromes: succinate dehydrogenase gene mutations

Certain kindreds have a proclivity to develop multicentric head-neck paragangliomas, sympathetic paragangliomas, and adrenal pheochromocytomas. These autosomal dominant syndromes were originally called familial paraganglioma syndromes, although some patients develop adrenal pheochromocytomas. The paraganglioma syndromes are caused by mutations in three of the four genes encoding mitochondrial complex II: SDH subunit B (*SDHB, PGL 4*), SDH subunit C (*SDHC, PGL 3*), and SDH subunit D (*SDHD, PGL 1*). (Note that *PGL 2* is not caused by an *SDH* mutation.) SDHB encodes a catalytic subunit, while *SDHC* and *SDHD* encode membrane-anchoring subunits involved in electron transport. *SDHC* and *SDHD* (paternal) have an autosomal dominant proclivity to develop paragangliomas; those with *SDHB* and *SDHD* mutations can also develop adrenal pheochromocytomas. Individuals with *SDHD* mutations develop paragangliomas only if the mutated gene is inherited from the father (see later). Overall, about 12% of patients with paragangliomas and

TABLE 11–10 Surveillance protocol for individuals carrying a NF-1 gene mutation.

Twice yearly: physical and neurologic examination and blood pressure, and a careful examination of the skin for development or growth of neurofibromas
Yearly: CBC with WBC differential; plasma-fractionated free metanephrines; complete eye examination with visual fields
Before major surgical procedures and pregnancy: plasma-fractionated free metanephrines to screen for pheochromocytoma
For abnormal biochemical screening: MRI or CT scan of the abdomen (nonionic contrast); ^{123}I-MIBG SPECT or ^{18}F-FDA PET scan

pheochromocytomas have been found to have germline *SDH* gene mutations.

Head-neck paragangliomas occur with an incidence of 10 to 33 cases per million persons. In one series of 34 patients with head-neck paragangliomas, 41% were found to have *SDH* germline mutations. Of those patients with germline mutations, 79% had *SDHD* mutations, and 21% had *SDHB* mutations.

These syndromes are caused by mutations in nuclear genes that encode three of the four subunits that comprise mitochondrial complex II (*SDH*) that oxidizes succinate to fumarate (Krebs cycle). The four subunits of the tetrameric *SDH* consist of a 70-kDa flavoprotein (*SDHA*), a 30-kDa iron-sulfur protein (*SDHB*), a 15-kDa subunit of cytochrome b (*SDHC*), and a 12-kDa subunit of cytochrome b (*SDHD*). SDHC and SDHD components of cytochrome b are integral mitochondrial membrane subunits anchoring the catalytic subunits *SDHA* and *SDHB* that are involved with the electron transport chain, transferring an electron to coenzyme Q (ubiquinone). *SDH* is essential for aerobic energy production and the tricarboxylic acid cycle. Genetic defects cause mitochondrial dysfunction making the cells functionally hypoxic. This leads to increased secretion of VEGF that is necessary for tumor growth. (SDHA germline mutations do not cause paragangliomas but rather cause Leigh syndrome, a fatal early-onset mitochondrial neurodegenerative disease.)

All patients with paragangliomas and pheochromocytomas ideally should be tested for germline mutations in *SDH*; such testing is highly recommended for patients with neck paragangliomas (>15% have germline mutations), other paragangliomas (particularly multifocal paragangliomas or pheochromocytomas), a family history of paraganglioma or pheochromocytoma, and paragangliomas arising in patients with Dutch ancestry.

Carney-Stratakis syndrome: Some patients with loss-of-function mutations in SDHB, SDHC, or SDHD can develop the dyad of paragangliomas and gastric stromal sarcomas, which is known as **Carney-Stratakis syndrome**. Tumors present relatively early, with an average age of 24 years at diagnosis. Women and men are affected equally. The paragangliomas that develop in this syndrome are usually functional and develop in the abdomen, rather than head-neck region. In this syndrome, the condition is familial and affected kindreds do not develop pulmonary chondromas, factors that distinguish it from Carney triad.

1. ***SDHB* gene mutations**—The *SDHB* gene has been mapped to chromosome 1p36. This has also been described as familial paraganglioma syndrome type 4 or *PGL 4*. Affected individuals are prone to develop paragangliomas all along the sympathetic chains, from the neck to the pelvis, and can develop pheochromocytomas as well; they are less prone to glomus tumors of the neck than individuals with *SDHD* mutations. Paragangliomas that arise in patients with *SDHB* germline mutations are much more likely to be metastatic (35%) at the time of diagnosis than tumors seen in patients with *SDHD* germline mutations. In one kindred with a large *SDHB* exon 1 deletion, the phenotypic penetrance of paraganglioma was 35% by age 40. There have been no clear genotype-phenotype correlations with different *SDHB* mutations. However, certain kindreds have a distinctly higher penetrance. Also, some point *SDHB* mutations

may be relatively benign genetic polymorphisms rather than pathological mutations. Due to the rarity of these tumors, the precise penetrance for each *SDHB* mutation has not been fully determined. Other malignancies may possibly be more common in patients with *SDHB* mutations. In one series of 53 patients, renal cell carcinoma was detected in two patients. Pediatric neuroblastoma has been described in a child with an *SDHB* exon deletion.

2. ***SDHC* gene mutations**—The *SDHC* gene has been mapped to chromosome 1q2. Affected individuals are prone to develop parasympathetic head-neck paragangliomas, but not pheochromocytomas. This is the least common *SDH* mutation. About 4% of patients with head-neck paragangliomas harbor an *SDHC* germline mutation.

3. ***SDHD* gene mutations**—The *SDHD* gene has been mapped to chromosome 11q23. Only patients with paternally inherited *SDHD* gene mutations are predisposed to develop paragangliomas and pheochromocytomas. Affected individuals are particularly prone to develop parasympathetic head-neck paragangliomas that do not typically secrete catecholamines. About 15% of patients with head-neck paragangliomas harbor this germline mutation.

In kindreds with *SDHD* gene mutations, only paternal transmission of the mutated gene causes the susceptibility to paragangliomas and pheochromocytomas; this phenomenon is known as **maternal genomic imprinting**, meaning that the maternally inherited mutant gene does not cause the syndrome in the mother's offspring. A male who inherits an *SDHD* mutation from his mother does not express the phenotype (ie, no paragangliomas) but can pass on the gene to his children, who can express the phenotype (paragangliomas). A female who inherits an *SDHD* mutation from her father develops paragangliomas, but her children who inherit the *SDHD* mutation are not affected.

Head-neck paragangliomas: Individuals with *SDHD* germline mutations are particularly prone to develop head-neck paragangliomas that arise from parasympathetic ganglia that are embryologically related to sympathetic paraganglia. These tumors do not usually secrete catecholamines and are known as **nonchromaffin** paragangliomas. **Carotid body tumors** are also known as **chemodectomas** and arise near the carotid bifurcation. They usually present as a painless neck mass but can injure the vagus or hypoglossal nerves. **Glomus tympanicum paragangliomas** arise in the middle ear and cause tinnitus and hearing loss. The tumor may be seen as a reddish mass behind an intact tympanic membrane. **Glomus jugulare paragangliomas** arise in the jugular foramen that often causes tinnitus and hearing loss as well as compression of cranial nerves, resulting is dysphagia. **Vagal paragangliomas** are rare, usually presenting as a painless mass in the neck that may cause hoarseness or dysphagia. Head-neck paragangliomas can also arise in the larynx, nasal cavity, nasal sinuses, and thyroid gland. Multicentric tumors have been reported in about 74% of paraganglioma patients with *SDHD* mutations. About 50% of patients with seemingly isolated pheochromocytomas and a germline *SDHD* mutation harbor a hidden paraganglioma. Sympathetic paragangliomas and adrenal pheochromocytomas (8%) also occur in affected individuals.

A founder *SDHD* mutation has been noted in families of Italian descent: *Q109X*. Three *SDHD* founder mutations have

TABLE 11–11   Surveillance protocol for individuals carrying a SDHB, SDHC, or paternally-inherited SDHD mutation.

Twice yearly: physical examination and blood pressure; plasma-fractionated free metanephrines and serum chromogranin A
Yearly: scanning with ultrasound of the neck and abdomen on odd years and MRI or CT (nonionic contrast) of the neck, chest, abdomen, and pelvis on even years
For suspicious symptoms and before major surgical procedures and pregnancy: complete biochemical screening for pheochromocytoma with fractionated plasma metanephrines and serum chromogranin A
For abnormal biochemical screening: CT scan (nonionic contrast) of the chest, abdomen, and pelvis or ^{18}F-FDG-PET with CT fusion scan; to confirm ambiguous results: ^{123}I-MIBG SPECT or ^{18}F-FDA PET scan

been discovered in families of Dutch ancestry: *Leu95Pro*, *Asp92Tyr*, and *Asp92Tyr*. An investigation of 243 family members with a paternally inherited *Asp92Tyr* mutation in SDHD reported the following. The risk of developing a paraganglioma or pheochromocytoma was 54% by age 40 years, 68% by 60 years, and 87% by 70 years. Most patients had head-neck paragangliomas, while some had sympathetic paragangliomas and 8% had pheochromocytomas. Multiple tumors were found in 65%.

Malignancy appears to be uncommon in patients with SDHD-associated paragangliomas. However, cervical paragangliomas can be indolent, and metastases to neck nodes, lungs, and bones may not be clinically evident for many years. Therefore, lifelong surveillance is necessary (Table 12–11).

E. Other genetic syndromes associated with pheochromocytoma or paraganglioma

1. **Carney triad**—Multicentric paragangliomas occur in patients with Carney triad. While this is not a familial syndrome, it is believed to be genetic in origin. The underlying genetic defect is not known. Affected individuals can develop indolent gastric leiomyosarcomas, pulmonary chondromas, and paragangliomas (or adrenal pheochromocytomas). Only one-fifth of reported cases have had all three tumors, while most patients have had two of the three tumors, usually gastric sarcomas and pulmonary chondromas. Other tumors can develop in this syndrome, including adrenocortical adenomas (12%) and esophageal leiomyomas. Women account for 86% of the cases. Tumors tend to develop early in life, with an average age of 21 years at diagnosis.

2. **Beckwith-Wiedemann syndrome**—Pheochromocytomas have been reported in patients with Beckwith-Wiedemann syndrome and may be bilateral. Affected individuals also have other abnormalities, particularly neonatal hypoglycemia, omphalocele, umbilical hernia, macroglossia, and gigantism, and they are prone to develop malignancies.

3. *Prolyl hydroxylase domain 2 (PHD2)* **gene mutations**—PDH proteins regulate HIF. Germline mutations in *PHD2* cause congenital erythrocytosis. An additional mutation of the wild-type *PHD2* allele in paraganglia can give rise to a sympathetic

paraganglioma. This gene mutation is different from *VHL* gene mutations, although both gene mutations cause an increase in HIF as a probable mechanism for paraganglioma tumor production.

4. *KIF1B* **gene mutations**—*KIF1B* is a gene that is believed to be a proapoptotic factor for sympathetic cell precursors. The gene is located on 1p36, where gene deletions have been noted in neural crest tumors. Mutations in *KIF1B* have been associated with pheochromocytomas, paragangliomas, and neuroblastomas, as well as other tumors that are not of neural crest origin. These tumors are transcriptionally related to *NF-1* and *RET* tumors.

5. **Familial paraganglioma syndrome type 2**—One known kindred has a familial paraganglioma syndrome that has been labeled *PGL2*, but which is not due to an SDH mutation. This kindred harbors a mutation in the succinate dehydrogenase assembly factor 2 (*SDHAF2*) gene at 11q13.1.

Physiology of Pheochromocytoma and Paraganglioma

Pheochromocytomas are tumors that arise from the adrenal medulla, whereas paragangliomas arise from sympathetic nerve ganglia. Although some pheochromocytomas do not secrete catecholamines, most synthesize catecholamines at increased rates that may be up to 27 times the synthetic rate of the normal adrenal medulla (Figure 11–9). The persistent hypersecretion of catecholamines by most pheochromocytomas is probably due to lack of feedback inhibition at the level of tyrosine hydroxylase. Catecholamines are produced in quantities that greatly exceed the vesicular storage capacity and accumulate in the cytoplasm. Catecholamines that are in the cytoplasm are subject to intracellular metabolism to metanephrines; excess catecholamines and their metabolites diffuse out of the pheochromocytoma cell into the circulation.

In contrast to the normal adrenal medulla, most adrenal pheochromocytomas produce more norepinephrine than epinephrine, while many produce both hormones. Some pheochromocytomas produce epinephrine almost exclusively. Most paragangliomas produce mostly norepinephrine with some dopamine and no epinephrine. Paragangliomas that produce large amounts of dopamine tend to be metastatic. Some paragangliomas secrete no catecholamines or metanephrines.

Serum levels of catecholamines correlate only modestly with tumor size. On average, large tumors secrete more catecholamines than smaller tumors. However, large tumors are much more variable in their secretion of tumor markers. This may be due to the fact that larger tumors tend to develop hemorrhagic necrosis and cysts that are not functional. Additionally, about 20% of large, malignant paragangliomas are less differentiated and are nonsecretory.

Severe hypertensive episodes occur in most patients with pheochromocytomas. Exocytosis of catecholamines from the pheochromocytoma can play a role in such paroxysms, but most pheochromocytomas have minor sympathetic innervation. Instead, hypertensive crises are often caused by spontaneous hemorrhages within the tumor or by pressure on the tumor causing the release of blood from venous sinusoids that are rich in catecholamines.

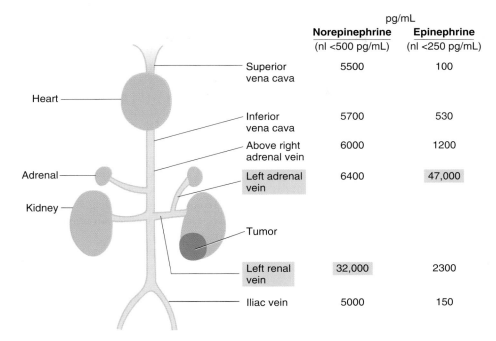

	pg/mL	
	Norepinephrine (nl <500 pg/mL)	**Epinephrine** (nl <250 pg/mL)
Superior vena cava	5500	100
Inferior vena cava	5700	530
Above right adrenal vein	6000	1200
Left adrenal vein	6400	47,000
Left renal vein	32,000	2300
Iliac vein	5000	150

FIGURE 11-9 Plasma norepinephrine and epinephrine levels in venous samples of blood from a patient with a secretory left perinephric paraganglioma. Note that the level of epinephrine is very high in the left adrenal vein sample, distinguishing it from the drainage of the paraganglioma that secretes norepinephrine into the left renal vein. Note the relatively normal peripheral levels of epinephrine (seen in the iliac vein or the superior vena cava). Such venous sampling is rarely required for diagnosis and localization of pheochromocytoma or paraganglioma.

Thus, catecholamines can be released by physical stimuli such as bending or twisting or by micturition in patients with bladder paragangliomas. Of course, surgical manipulation of such tumors releases catecholamines and can cause life-threatening hypertensive crises.

Chronically high circulating levels of catecholamines may cause normal sympathetic axons to become saturated with catecholamines due to active catecholamine neuronal uptake. This may account for the paroxysms of hypertension that are triggered by pain, emotional upset, intubation, anesthesia, or surgical skin incisions. Adrenergic catecholamine saturation may also explain the elevations in plasma and urine catecholamines that can occur for 10 days or longer after a successful surgical resection of a pheochromocytoma.

Secretion of Other Peptides by Pheochromocytomas and Paragangliomas (Table 11–12)

Although pheochromocytomas secrete mainly catecholamines and their metabolites, they also secrete many other peptide hormones, many of which contribute to a patient's clinical symptoms. Secretion of parathyroid hormone–related peptide (PTHrP) can cause hypercalcemia. Ectopic ACTH production can cause Cushing syndrome. Erythropoietin secretion can cause erythrocytosis. Leukocytosis is frequently seen in patients with pheochromocytoma, probably caused by cytokine release from the tumor.

TABLE 11-12 Other proteins and peptides that may be secreted by pheochromocytomas, in addition to catecholamines and metanephrines.[a]

Adrenocorticotropic hormone
Adrenomedullin
Atrial natriuretic factor
Beta-endorphin
Calbindin
Calcitonin
Cholecystokinin
Chromogranin A
Cytokines
Enkephalins
Erythropoietin
Galanin
Gonadotropin-releasing hormone
Growth hormone
Interleukin-6
Motilin
Neuron-specific enolase
Neuropeptide Y
Neurotensin
Parathyroid hormone–related peptide
Peptide histidine-isoleucine
Renin
Serotonin
Somatostatin
Substance P
Vasoactive intestinal polypeptide

[a]Pheochromocytomas variably secrete different peptides. Not all peptides have been documented to produce clinical manifestations. See text.

Interleukin-6 secretion can cause fevers and acute respiratory distress syndrome (ARDS).

Chromogranin A: Chromogranins are acidic single-chain glycoproteins that are found in neurosecretory granules. They have been categorized into three classes: chromogranins A (CgA), CgB (secretogranin I), and CgC (secretogranin II). In humans, the gene for CgA is on chromosome 14 and encodes a molecule with 431 to 445 amino acids. CgA molecules aggregate with low pH or high calcium concentrations and promote the formation of secretory vesicles and the concentration of hormones within these vesicles.

CgA also acts as a prohormone. It is cleaved by endopeptidases into smaller peptides. CgA is the prohormone for the amino terminal fragments vasostatin I (CgA 1-76) and vasostatin II (CgA 1-115), which appear to inhibit vasoconstriction. CgA is also the prohormone for catestatin (CgA 352-372), which blocks acetylcholine receptors and thus inhibits adrenosympathetic activity.

Most pheochromocytomas secrete CgA, and serum CgA levels may be assayed as a tumor marker for pheochromocytoma. However, CgA is not unique to the adrenal medulla. It is produced in neuroendocrine cells outside the adrenal medulla that secrete peptide hormones. CgA is found in the pituitary gland, parathyroid gland, central nervous system, and pancreatic islet cells.

Neuropeptide Y (NPY): Many pheochromocytomas secrete significant amounts of NPY. The molecule is a 36 amino acid peptide (see primary sequence later) that is found in neurosecretory granules and is secreted along with catecholamines. It is a very potent nonadrenergic vasoconstrictor that contributes to hypertension in some patients with pheochromocytoma.

Tyr-Pro-Ser-Lys-Pro-Asp-Asn-Pro-Gly-Glu-Asp-AlaPro-Ala-Glu-Asp-Met-Ala-Arg-Tyr-Tyr-Ser-Ala-LeuArg-His-Tyr-Ile-Asn-Leu-Ile-Thr-Arg-Gln-Arg-Tyr-NH$_2$

NPY acts on G protein–coupled receptors, which belong to the pancreatic polypeptide family of cell-surface receptors called peptide YY (PYY). Six subtypes of these receptors have been identified (Y$_1$R-Y$_6$R). NPY has particular affinity for the Y$_1$-R, Y$_2$-R, Y$_3$-R, and Y$_5$-R receptors. Some PYY receptors are found in vascular smooth muscle and mediate NPY-induced vasoconstriction. Other PYY receptors are found on the pheochromocytes themselves and mediate NPY's autocrine effects: NPY appears to inhibit catecholamine synthesis via Y$_3$R, a receptor which blocks L-type Ca^{2+} channels. It inhibits catecholamine release via Y$_2$R, a receptor which blocks N-type Ca^{2+} channels.

NPY also has paracrine effects, stimulating endothelial cell proliferation and angiogenesis that may foster tumor growth. Patients with essential hypertension have normal levels of NPY. However, in a series of eight patients with pheochromocytomas, NPY levels were elevated 2- to 465-fold above the normal reference range. In another series, 59% of adrenal pheochromocytomas were found to secrete NPY during surgical resection; high serum levels of NPY were observed to correlate with vascular resistance, independent of norepinephrine. NPY appears to contribute to hypertension and left ventricular hypertrophy in most patients with pheochromocytoma. In contrast, few paragangliomas secrete NPY.

Adrenomedullin (AM): It was originally isolated from a pheochromocytoma, thus its misleading name. Although AM is produced by the adrenal medulla, it is also produced in the adrenal cortex (zona glomerulosa). It is produced by so many other tissues that the adrenal gland is actually a minor source for circulating AM.

AM is a 52 amino acid peptide cleavage product of a prohormone, preproadrenomedullin, encoded on chromosome 11. AM has some homology with *calcitonin* gene–related peptide (CGRP), and exerts its effects as a ligand for CGRP1 receptors and specific AM receptors. Ligand binding to the G protein–coupled receptors causes adenylate cyclase activation and an elevation of cellular cAMP levels.

AM is a pluripotent hormone. In the adrenal, AM appears to suppress aldosterone secretion. It is also secreted by the heart, lung, kidney, and brain as well as vascular endothelium, where it causes vasodilation. AM is also a natriuretic peptide and is secreted by the heart in congestive heart failure. AM is expressed in pheochromocytomas and a variety of other tumors, where it appears to stimulate tumor growth, reduce apoptosis, and suppress the immune response to the tumor.

Neuron-specific enolase (NSE): It is a neuroendocrine glycolytic enzyme. Serum levels of NSE have been reported to be normal in patients with benign pheochromocytoma but are elevated in about half of patients with malignant pheochromocytomas. Therefore, an elevated serum level of NSE increases the likelihood that a given pheochromocytoma is malignant.

Manifestations of Pheochromocytoma and Paraganglioma (Table 11–13)

More than one-third of pheochromocytomas cause death prior to diagnosis. Death usually results from a fatal cardiac arrhythmia, myocardial infarction, or stroke. Adult patients with a pheochromocytoma usually have paroxysmal symptoms, which may last minutes or hours; symptoms usually begin abruptly and subside slowly. The particular constellation of symptoms varies considerably among patients. One cause for the differences in symptoms is the variable production of epinephrine and norepinephrine by these tumors. Pheochromocytomas that produce epinephrine tend to cause paroxysmal β-adrenergic manifestations, particularly anxiety, tremor, diaphoresis, tachycardia, palpitations, and hyperglycemia. Epinephrine and cytokine secretion can cause pulmonary edema and ARDS. Paragangliomas do not secrete epinephrine but most secrete norepinephrine that causes hypertension. Paragangliomas are more likely to metastasize.

Manifestations and their approximate incidence include hypertension (90%), headaches (80%), diaphoresis (70%), and palpitations or tachycardia (60%). Other common symptoms include episodic anxiety (60%), tremor (40%), abdominal or chest pain (35%), pallor (30%), and nausea or vomiting (30%). Hyperglycemia occurs in about 30% but is usually asymptomatic; diabetic ketoacidosis has been reported but is very rare. Patients may also experience fever (28%), fatigue (25%), flushing (18%), and dyspnea (15%).

TABLE 11–13   Clinical manifestations of pheochromocytomas and paraganglioma.

Blood pressure	Hypertension: severe or mild, paroxysmal or sustained; orthostasis; hypotension/shock; normotension
Vasospasm	Cyanosis, Raynaud syndrome, gangrene; severe radial artery vasospasm with thready pulse; falsely low blood pressure by radial artery transducer
Multisystem crisis	Severe hypertension/hypotension, fever, encephalopathy, renal failure, ARDS, death
Cardiovascular	Palpitations, dysrhythmias, chest pain, acute coronary syndrome, cardiomyopathy, heart failure, cardiac paragangliomas
Gastrointestinal	Abdominal pain, nausea, vomiting, weight loss, intestinal ischemia; pancreatitis, cholecystitis, jaundice; rupture of abdominal aneurysm; constipation, toxic megacolon
Metabolic	Hyperglycemia/diabetes; lactic acidosis; fevers
Neurologic	Headache, paresthesias, numbness, dizziness, CVA, TIA, hemiplegia, hemianopsia, seizures, hemorrhagic stroke; skull metastases may impinge on brain structures, optic nerve, or other cranial nerves; spinal metastases may impinge on cord or nerve roots
Pulmonary	Dyspnea; hypoxia from ARDS
Psychiatric	Anxiety (attacks or constant); depression; chronic fatigue; psychosis
Renal	Renal insufficiency, nephrotic syndrome, malignant nephrosclerosis; large tumors often involve the kidneys and renal vessels
Skin	Apocrine sweating during paroxysms, drenching sweats as attack subsides; eczema; mottled cyanosis during paroxysm
Ectopic hormone production	ACTH (Cushing syndrome); VIP (Verner-Morrison syndrome); PTHrP (hypercalcemia)
Children	More commonly have sustained hypertension, diaphoresis, visual changes, polyuria/polydipsia, seizures, edematous or cyanotic hands; more commonly harbor germline mutations, multiple tumors, and paragangliomas
Women	More symptomatic than men: more frequent headache, weight loss, numbness, dizziness, tremor, anxiety, and fatigue
Pregnancy	Hypertension mimicking eclampsia; hypertensive multisystem crisis during vaginal delivery; postpartum shock or fever; high mortality
General laboratory	Leukocytosis, erythrocytosis, eosinophilia

Change in bowel habits occurs frequently with either constipation (13%) or diarrhea (6%). Visual changes occur in 12% with either transient blurring or field loss during attacks; metastases to the orbit or skull base may directly impinge on the optic nerve. See Table 11–13.

Triggers for paroxysms: Episodic paroxysms may not recur for months or may recur many times daily. Each patient tends to have a different pattern of symptoms, with the frequency or severity of episodes usually increasing over time. Attacks can occur spontaneously or may occur with bladder catheterization, anesthesia, and surgery. Acute attacks may also be triggered by eating foods containing tyramine (the precursor to catecholamines): aged cheeses, meats, fish, beer, wine, chocolate, or bananas. Hypertensive crises can also be triggered by certain drugs: ionic radiocontrast media, MAO inhibitors, tricyclic antidepressants, sympathomimetics, decongestants, glucagon, chemotherapy, prednisone, ACTH, opiates, methyldopa, metoclopramide, nicotine, and cocaine. Phenothiazines have been reported to cause shock and pulmonary edema in patients with pheochromocytoma.

Paroxysms can be induced by seemingly benign activities such as bending, rolling over in bed, exertion, abdominal palpation, or micturition (with bladder paragangliomas). There is an amazing interindividual variability in the manifestations of pheochromocytomas.

Most patients have dramatic symptoms, but other patients with incidentally discovered secretory pheochromocytomas are completely asymptomatic. Patients who develop pheochromocytomas as part of MEN 2 or VHL disease are especially prone to be normotensive and asymptomatic.

Blood pressure: Hypertensive crisis is the quintessential manifestation of pheochromocytoma. Blood pressure that exceeds 200/120 mm Hg is an immediate threat to life, being associated with encephalopathy or stroke, cardiac ischemia or infarction, pulmonary edema, aortic dissection, rhabdomyolysis, lactic acidosis, and renal insufficiency.

Definition of hypertension: In adults, hypertension is considered to be present when blood pressure exceeds 140 mm Hg systolic or 90 mm Hg diastolic. In children, blood pressure increases with age, such that maximal normal ranges are age dependent; hypertension is considered to be present when blood pressure measurements exceed the following: younger than 6 months, 110/60 mm Hg; 3 years, 112/80 mm Hg; 5 years, 115/84 mm Hg; 10 years, 130/90 mm Hg; and 15 years, 138/90 mm Hg.

Presentation of hypertension: Hypertension is present in 90% of patients in whom a pheochromocytoma is diagnosed. Hypertension occurs primarily from the secretion of norepinephrine. Epinephrine secretion variably increases blood pressure. Also, pheochromocytomas often secrete neuropeptide Y that is a potent vasoconstrictor. Some tumors may grow so large that they impinge upon the renal artery, causing increased renin production and secondary renovascular hypertension. Blood pressure patterns vary among patients with pheochromocytomas. Adults most commonly have sustained but variable hypertension, with severe hypertension during symptomatic episodes. Paroxysms of severe hypertension occur in about 50% of adults and in about 8% of children with pheochromocytoma. Other patients may be completely normotensive, may be normotensive between paroxysms, or may have stable sustained hypertension.

Hypertension can be mild or severe and resistant to treatment. Severe hypertension may be noted during induction of anesthesia for unrelated surgeries. Although hypertension usually accompanies paroxysmal symptoms and may be elicited by the above activities, this is not always the case.

Orthostasis: Patients with sustained hypertension frequently exhibit orthostatic changes in blood pressure, often with orthostatic tachycardia. Patients may complain of orthostatic faintness. Blood pressure may drop, even to hypotensive levels, after the patient arises from a supine position and stands for 3 minutes; such orthostasis, especially when accompanied by a rise in heart rate, is suggestive of pheochromocytoma. Epinephrine secretion from a pheochromocytoma may cause episodic hypotension and even syncope.

Hypotension and shock: Although hypertension is usually the key symptom in pheochromocytoma patients, hypotension and shock can occur. Some pheochromocytomas produce purely epinephrine that can produce mild hypertension from alpha stimulation but can also produce hypotension from predominantly beta-stimulated vasodilation. After a especially intense and prolonged attack of hypertension, shock may ultimately occur. This may be due to loss of vascular tone, low plasma volume, arrhythmias, or cardiac damage. Spontaneous necrosis within a pheochromocytoma can lead to severe hypotension when norepinephrine levels suddenly drop. Similarly, surgical resection of a pheochromocytoma often precipitates sudden and severe intraoperative hypotension, particularly in the presence of alpha blockade and other antihypertensives. Cardiogenic shock can occur as a result of cardiac ischemia or infarction as well as catecholamine cardiomyopathy. (See "Cardiac Manifestations," later.)

Peripheral vasospasm and gangrene: Vasoconstriction is responsible for the pallor and mottled cyanosis that can occur with paroxysms of hypertension. Raynaud phenomenon can occur. Peripheral pulses may become thready or even nonpalpable during paroxysms. Catheters inserted into the radial artery and connected to continuous blood pressure monitoring transducers can give misleadingly low-pressure readings during paroxysms of vasospasm, a condition known as **pseudoshock.** Prolonged severe peripheral vasospasm has rarely caused gangrene of the skin, fingers, or toes. Reflex vasodilation usually follows an attack and can cause facial flushing.

Multisystem crisis: Massive release of catecholamines can occur spontaneously during tumor necrosis or can be triggered by any of the factors noted earlier. This can cause multisystem crisis that can be the presenting manifestation of pheochromocytoma, with hypertension or hypotension, high fever, encephalopathy,

renal failure, ARDS, and death. Multisystem crisis resembles septic shock, so the diagnosis of pheochromocytoma may be missed entirely.

Cardiac manifestations: The heart is affected in most patients with pheochromocytoma, either directly from excessive catecholamines or indirectly from hypertension. Palpitation is one of the most frequent complaints.

Dysrhythmias: Tachycardia or dysrhythmias occur in about 60% of patients with pheochromocytoma. Patients may note palpitations, described variably as episodes of excessive heart pounding at rest or a fluttering sensation, during which they may become lightheaded. Supraventricular tachycardia is common, particularly in patients with epinephrine-secreting pheochromocytomas. The heart rate will often increase when standing. There can be an initial tachycardia during a paroxysm, followed by a reflex bradycardia. Atrial fibrillation may occur. Other dysrhythmias described with pheochromocytoma include nodal tachycardia, torsades de pointes, sick sinus syndrome, and Wolff-Parkinson-White (WPW) syndrome. Atrioventricular dissociation can occur and right bundle branch block has been reported. Ventricular tachycardia or ventricular fibrillation can occur suddenly and is a common cause of death.

Acute coronary syndrome (ACS): During a paroxysm, severe coronary vasospasm can cause myocardial ischemia or infarction, even in the absence of coronary atherosclerosis. This typically occurs simultaneously with increased myocardial oxygen demand caused by catecholamine-induced increases in heart rate and contractility. Patients may experience crushing chest pain or pressure with referred pain, usually to the jaw or the left shoulder or arm. Acute heart failure may occur along with severe hypotension or shock.

It can be difficult to distinguish ACS due to coronary stenosis/thrombosis from ACS due to a pheochromocytoma. Changes in the electrocardiogram and serum levels of troponin and creatine kinase-MB (CK-MB) are the same for both conditions. Patients with coronary disease can have tachycardia, cardiomyopathy, hypertension, dysrhythmias, diaphoresis, anxiety, and increased plasma catecholamine levels. However, patients with pheochromocytoma usually do not have critical coronary artery stenosis on coronary angiogram and usually have severe hypertension, headache, and other paroxysmal symptoms.

Cardiomyopathy: Left ventricular hypertrophy and hypertensive cardiomyopathy can occur in patients with chronic hypertension from pheochromocytoma. High levels of catecholamines can also directly cause myocarditis and a dilated cardiomyopathy. This is known as **catecholamine cardiomyopathy.** Takotsubo cardiomyopathy is the term used to describe asymmetric cardiac contractility with apical and midventricular akinesis or dyskinesis with hyperkinesis at the base. Other patterns of cardiac hypokinesis can occur. Most patients with catecholamine cardiomyopathy develop pulmonary edema and die. However, full recovery from cardiomyopathy may occur after treatment and surgical resection of a pheochromocytoma. In some patients, myocardial scarring and fibrosis lead to irreversible cardiomyopathy and heart failure. Fatal Takotsubo cardiomyopathy has been reported after dobutamine stress echocardiography.

There can be multiple causes of cardiomyopathy in patients with pheochromocytoma: hypertensive, ischemic, and catecholamine. The underlying pathophysiology of catecholamine cardiomyopathy appears to involve high levels of intracellular calcium in cardiac myocytes. Postmortem histopathology typically reveals intracardiac hemorrhages, edema, and concentrations of lymphocytes and leukocytes in cardiac muscle with areas of myocardial fibrosis.

Cardiac paragangliomas: These are rare tumors that arise at the base of the heart near the trunks of the aortic and pulmonary arteries and may be asymptomatic or cause hypertension and palpitations. They typically involve the left atrium or interatrial groove and often protrude into the atrium, resembling an atrial myxoma. Cardiac paragangliomas often have an invasive intramural component, making tumor resection difficult.

Diaphoresis and fever: During a paroxysm, sweating usually occurs initially from apocrine glands, affecting the palms, axillae, head, and shoulders. Reflex thermoregulatory eccrine sweating occurs later in an attack, dissipating the heat that was acquired during the prolonged vasoconstriction that occurred during the paroxysm. This can cause drenching sweats, usually as a paroxysm subsides. Patients with pheochromocytoma commonly develop fevers that may be mild or severe, even as high as 41°C. Up to 70% of patients have unexplained low-grade elevations in temperature of 0.5°C or more. Such fevers have been attributed to the secretion of interleukin-6 and respond to NSAID therapy.

Gastrointestinal manifestations: Many patients with pheochromocytoma exhibit gastrointestinal symptoms such as abdominal pain, nausea, and vomiting. Most patients lose some weight, even if appetite is preserved. More severe weight loss (>10% of basal weight) occurs in about 15% of patients overall and in 41% of those with sustained and prolonged hypertension. Abdominal pain may be due to splanchnic vasoconstriction (*intestinal angina*) and prolonged vasospasm can cause ischemic enterocolitis. Vasospasm can rarely cause ischemic gangrene of the bowel. Pain may also be caused by the growth of a large intra-abdominal tumor. Intestinal motility disorders are also common. Catecholamines relax gastrointestinal smooth muscle while increasing contraction of the pyloric and ileocecal sphincters. Constipation is common, and abdominal distention and even toxic megacolon can occur. Other abdominal emergencies can be seen with pheochromocytoma, including the rupture of an aortic aneurysm, acute cholecystitis, and acute pancreatitis.

Neurologic manifestations: Headache is a common manifestation during an acute paroxysms. Patients frequently complain of paresthesia, numbness, or dizziness. Affected patients have an increase risk of experiencing a cerebrovascular accident (CVA) or transient ischemic attack (TIA). Hemiplegia can occur, sometimes with homonymous hemianopsia, and may be transient or permanent. Although most CVAs are ischemic in origin, hemorrhagic stroke can also occur during hypertensive paroxysms. Rupture of the internal carotid artery into the cavernous sinus can occur, causing a third nerve palsy. Some patients develop confusion or even psychosis during paroxysms. Paresthesias can occur.

Pulmonary manifestations: Patients may complain of dyspnea during a paroxysm. Patients with catecholamine cardiomyopathy may also present with dyspnea. Some patients develop ARDS, which can develop acutely or over several days. This is a life-threatening condition but may be self-limited during an attack. Isolated adrenal pheochromocytomas can produce ARDS. Patients with large hepatic metastases may be more prone to develop this complication. It may be mistaken for pneumonia, pulmonary edema, pulmonary emboli, or congestive heart failure. It is hypothesized that ARDS is caused by interleukin-6 produced by the tumor. Congestive heart failure may also cause pulmonary edema and can be distinguished from ARDS by echocardiogram.

Renal manifestations: Some degree of renal insufficiency is common in patients with pheochromocytoma. Hypertensive nephrosclerosis occurs in patients with a long history of severe hypertension. Nephrotic syndrome may occur with significant proteinuria, possibly due to secretion of interleukin-6 by the tumor. Malignant nephrosclerosis can occur with severe hypertension damaging renal arterioles, resulting in rapidly progressive renal failure. Large pheochromocytomas and perirenal paragangliomas can impinge upon the renal artery, causing increased renin production and a Goldblatt kidney, resulting in renovascular hypertension that is additive to norepinephrine-induced hypertension. The tumor may directly invade the renal vein and extend into the inferior vena cava, causing pulmonary emboli and an increased risk of lower extremity deep vein thrombosis. Severe hypertensive paroxysms can cause muscle ischemic damage and rhabdomyolysis with release of myoglobin that causes myoglobinuric renal failure. Acute tubular necrosis can occur after a severe hypotensive episode.

Ectopic hormone production: Pheochromocytomas can rarely produce ACTH that stimulates the adrenal cortex to produce excessive cortisol, resulting in Cushing syndrome. Tumors can also produce VIP that can cause watery diarrhea, hypokalemia, and achlorhydria, the WHDA (Verner-Morrison) syndrome. Some tumors produce PTHrP that causes hypercalcemia. Although pheochromocytomas can secrete renin directly, elevated plasma renin levels are usually derived from the juxtaglomerular apparatus, whose β_1 receptors are stimulated by both epinephrine and norepinephrine.

Manifestations in children: The symptoms of pheochromocytomas in children are different from those in adults. Over 80% of children exhibit hypertension that is usually sustained and less frequently (10%) paroxysmal. Children are more prone to diaphoresis and visual changes. Children are more likely to have paroxysms of nausea, vomiting, and headache, which often occur after exertion. They are also prone to weight loss, polydipsia, polyuria, and convulsions. Affected children may also exhibit reddish-blue mottled skin along with edematous and cyanotic-appearing hands, a symptom rarely seen in adults. Children are more likely to have multiple tumors and extra-adrenal paragangliomas. In one series, 39% of affected children had bilateral adrenal pheochromocytomas, an adrenal pheochromocytoma plus a paraganglioma, or multiple paragangliomas; a single paraganglioma occurred in an additional 14% of children. Affected children often have genetic conditions associated with pheochromocytomas and paragangliomas. Thus, they may harbor the other tumors associated with these conditions. All affected children should have genetic testing for mutations in VHL, RET, SDHB, and SDHD (see earlier).

Manifestations in women: There are sex differences in pheochromocytoma symptomatology, with women tending to be more symptomatic than men. Women report significantly more headache (80% vs 52%), weight change (88% vs 43%), numbness (57% vs 24%), dizziness (83% vs 39%), tremor (64% vs 33%), anxiety (85% vs 50%), and changes in energy level (89% vs 64%).

Manifestations in pregnancy: A pheochromocytoma during pregnancy can cause sustained hypertension or paroxysmal hypertension that is typically mistaken for eclampsia. Hypertensive paroxysms tend to occur more frequently as the uterus enlarges, triggered by direct pressure upon the tumor by shifts in position or movement of the fetus. Hypertensive crisis typically occurs at the time of vaginal delivery and is commonly associated with cardiac arrhythmia, ARDS, and death. Postpartum women may develop shock or fever that can mimic uterine rupture, amniotic fluid embolus, or infection (puerperal sepsis). A tumor that is unrecognized carries a grave prognosis, with a reported 40% maternal mortality and a 56% fetal mortality. If the diagnosis of pheochromocytoma is made before delivery, the maternal mortality rate drops to about 10%. (See "Pregnancy and Pheochromocytoma," later in the chapter.)

Manifestations of malignancy: Metastases occur in about 10% of pheochromocytomas and 30% of non–head-neck sympathetic paragangliomas. Since histopathology cannot distinguish whether a given pheochromocytoma is malignant, the term malignant is dependent upon whether metastases are detectable at presentation (50%) or months to years later (50%). Metastases are usually (80%) functional and can cause recurrent hypertension and symptoms many months or years after an operation that had been thought to be curative. (See "Metastatic Pheochromocytoma and Paraganglioma" discussed later.)

Normotension despite high plasma levels of norepinephrine   Interestingly, about 14% of patients with pheochromocytomas and paragangliomas have no hypertension despite having chronically elevated serum norepinephrine levels. This phenomenon has been variably called desensitization, tolerance, or tachyphylaxis.

Patients can be genetically prone to adrenergic desensitization. Adrenergic desensitization is caused by adrenergic receptors undergoing sequestration, downregulation, or phosphorylation. Adrenergic desensitization appears to be one cause of the cardiovascular collapse that can occur abruptly following the removal of a pheochromocytoma in some patients.

Desensitization does not account for all patients who are normotensive in the face of elevated serum levels of norepinephrine, because some such patients can still have hypertensive responses to norepinephrine. Secretion of epinephrine can have a hypotensive effect and may account, at least in part, for this phenomenon. Some patients are homozygous for certain polymorphisms of β_2-adrenergic receptors that allow continued β_2-adrenergic-mediated vasodilation, thus counteracting the pressor effects of circulating epinephrine and norepinephrine caused by stimulation of vascular α_1-adrenergic receptors.

Cosecretion of DOPA may reduce blood pressure through a central nervous system action. Similarly, cosecretion of dopamine may directly dilate mesenteric and renal vessels and thus modulate the effects of norepinephrine.

Biochemical Testing for Pheochromocytoma

No single test is absolutely sensitive and specific for pheochromocytoma. Plasma-fractionated free metanephrines or urinary 24-hour metanephrines have a sensitivity of about 97%. Sensitivities of other tests are somewhat lower: urinary norepinephrine 93%, plasma norepinephrine 92%, urinary VMA 90%, plasma epinephrine 67%, urinary epinephrine 64%, and plasma dopamine 63%. However, some malignant tumors secrete only dopamine and no catecholamines and no metanephrines at all. Also, the determination of plasma catecholamines-metanephrine ratios can be of value in discriminating false-positive from true-positive results (see later). Therefore, assays for plasma catecholamines, dopamine, and serum chromogranin A are often warranted.

Pheochromocytomas are deadly tumors and missing the diagnosis can be disastrous, so screening tests must be very sensitive. The secretion of catecholamines can be paroxysmal, with low secretion rates between paroxysms. In contrast, the secretion of metanephrine or normetanephrine metabolites is relatively high and constant. Tumors secrete metanephrines in their unconjugated (free) form. Thus, plasma-fractionated free metanephrines is the single most sensitive screening tests for these tumors. Urinary 24-hour fractionated metanephrines has a similar sensitivity but is less convenient. Some rare tumors (usually malignant) have a defect in the conversion of dopamine to norepinephrine by DBH, such that serum dopamine levels are very high while catecholamines are normal or mildly elevated and metanephrines are totally normal. Additionally, some paragangliomas secrete no catecholamines or metanephrines but do secrete chromogranin A.

The establishment of normal reference ranges is problematic for catecholamines and metanephrines, since levels vary with sex, age, and medical conditions:

1. **Sex**—Women have lower plasma epinephrine and metanephrine levels than men; their urinary excretion of catecholamines and metanephrines is also lower.
2. **Age**—Children, especially boys, have somewhat higher levels of plasma epinephrine and metanephrine than do adults. Conversely, children's average 24-hour urine epinephrine and norepinephrine excretion rates are lower than those of adults and increase through childhood as weight increases. Therefore, children's 24-hour urine tests are best assessed by using ratios of catecholamines to creatinine and metanephrines to creatinine. In adults, plasma norepinephrine and normetanephrine levels increase with advancing age.
3. **Medical conditions**—On average, hospitalized patients and those with essential hypertension have higher levels of catecholamines and metanephrines (plasma and urine) than do

matched nonhospitalized and normotensive individuals. Therefore, many laboratories have separate reference ranges for hypertensives and nonhypertensives.

Patients with illness, trauma, or sleep apnea have increased excretion of both catecholamines and metanephrines. Patients with renal failure on dialysis have elevated levels of plasma catecholamines (58%), plasma free metanephrines (25%), and plasma total (deconjugated) metanephrines (100%). Patients with partial renal insufficiency also have misleadingly elevated levels of plasma catecholamines (32%), plasma free metanephrines (26%), and plasma total metanephrines (50%). Thus, in patients with renal failure, the best screening test is plasma free metanephrines, but the test still lacks specificity when elevated. Serum chromogranin A levels are also elevated in renal insufficiency.

Misleading elevations of at least one metanephrine or catecholamine determination occur in 10% to 20% of tested individuals without pheochromocytoma. These elevations are typically less than 50% above the maximum normal and often normalize on retesting. Patients with pheochromocytomas usually have elevations of metanephrines or catecholamines that are more than three times normal. In one large series, a false-positive elevation in at least one test occurred in 22% and marked elevations in at least one test occurred in 3.5% of patients with no pheochromocytoma. False-positive test results were judged to have occurred from physiologic variation (33%), laboratory errors (29%), or drug interference (21%).

Plasma normetanephrines reflect disease activity in patients with secretory paragangliomas or metastases. Normal ranges for plasma metanephrines in children are different from those of adults and have been reported by Weise et al, 2002. Plasma normetanephrine levels typically increase with age; about 16% of older patients being evaluated for pheochromocytoma have levels above the published normal range for young adults (false positives); only 3% of young adults have false-positive plasma normetanephrine concentrations. Plasma concentrations of norepinephrine do not correlate with blood pressure. Stimulation tests are not recommended (see later).

A. Metanephrines and catecholamines

Plasma-fractionated free metanephrines.   The most sensitive test for pheochromocytoma is an assay for plasma-fractionated (metanephrine and normetanephrine) free metanephrines. This assay is particularly useful when screening for a small pheochromocytoma in patients with established MEN 2 (metanephrine) or VHL disease (normetanephrine). For younger children, plasma testing is preferred to urine testing due to the relative ease of collection.

Normal references ranges for plasma-fractionated metanephrines vary by sex (children), age, and laboratory. For boys ages 5 to 17 years, the upper limit of normal (ULN) for plasma free metanephrine is ≤0.52 nmol/L and the ULN for plasma free normetanephrine is ≤0.53 nmol/L. For girls ages 5 to 17 years, the ULN for plasma free metanephrine is ≤0.37 nmol/L and the ULN for plasma free normetanephrine is ≤0.42 pmol/L. For adults, the

reported ULN for plasma free metanephrine has ranged from 0.30 to 0.47 nmol/L and the reported ULN for plasma free normetanephrine has ranged from 0.60 to 1.1 nmol/L. In conventional units, the adult ULN reported by Quest Diagnostics Laboratory is ≤57 pg/mL for plasma free metanephrine and ≤148 pg/mL for plasma free normetanephrine.

In the United States, most reference laboratories assays for metanephrines use high-pressure liquid chromatography (HPLC) with tandem mass spectrometry (MS/MS). This test is 97% sensitive and about 87% specific for pheochromocytoma in a referred patient population. MS/MS reduces drug interference that can be a problem with assays that employ HPLC with electrochemical detection (ECD). Metanephrine assays are more sensitive and specific for pheochromocytoma than plasma or urinary catecholamine determinations.

The 3% of affected patients with normal plasma-fractionated free metanephrines usually have very small tumors, nonsecreting tumors, or dopamine-secreting tumors such that they are not hypertensive. Since the test's specificity is much lower than its sensitivity, most patients with levels above the reference range do not harbor a tumor. This is particularly true when plasma levels are less than three times higher than the upper limit of the reference range. Conversely, it is extremely likely that a patient harbors a pheochromocytoma when the plasma metanephrine is above 236 pg/mL (1200 nmol/mL) or the plasma normetanephrine is above 400 pg/mL (2200 nmol/mL).

Normally, about 90% of circulating metanephrine and about 50% of circulating normetanephrine originate directly from the adrenal medulla. The term **total metanephrines** refers to both normetanephrine and metanephrine. There are two circulating forms of normetanephrine and metanephrines: free and sulfate-conjugated metanephrines. The free metanephrines produced in the adrenal medulla and paraganglia are sulfate conjugated by intestinal tissue; the sulfated form represents 97% of circulating metanephrines. Only 3% of total circulating metanephrine is free. Plasma metanephrine levels are sometimes measured after a deconjugation step, such that both free and conjugated metanephrines are measured; this assay is termed **deconjugated metanephrines** and reflects mostly the sulfate-conjugated species. The plasma free metanephrines assay is superior to the total (deconjugated) metanephrine assay.

In the United States, when plasma metanephrines are requested, most reference laboratories test for free (nondeconjugated) metanephrines. Most reference laboratories assay metanephrines using MS/MS, which avoids interference by drugs and foods. Blood specimens for plasma-fractionated free metanephrines can be collected at any time, but are best drawn after an overnight fast while the patient is seated and relaxed.

The sensitivity of the plasma free metanephrines is due to the tumor's continuous secretion of metanephrines. Catecholamines in secretory vesicles exist in a dynamic equilibrium with the surrounding cytoplasm, with catecholamine uptake into the vesicles being balanced by their leakage into the cytoplasm. In the cytoplasm, the enzyme COMT converts epinephrine to metanephrine and converts norepinephrine to normetanephrine. The catecholamine metabolites then leak out of the cell continuously to become free metanephrines. While catecholamines are secreted in bursts associated with exocytosis of neurosecretory vesicles, free metanephrines are produced continuously. This eliminates the need to catch a paroxysmal hypertensive event. Plasma free metanephrine levels are within the reference range in 75% of patients on dialysis and 74% of patients with renal insufficiency. In contrast, plasma deconjugated metanephrines are within the reference range in 0% of patients on dialysis and in 50% of patients with renal insufficiency.

Factors causing misleading plasma free metanephrine levels.
Smoking can elevate plasma free metanephrine assays. The patient must not smoke for at least 4 hours before collection. Epinephrine-like drugs should be discontinued for at least 7 days before the test. Other drugs that can interfere with the plasma free metanephrine assay include local anesthetics, cocaine, lidocaine, halothane anesthesia, MAO inhibitors, and acetaminophen. Drug withdrawal and severe stress can also increase plasma free metanephrine levels. Misleading elevations in plasma free metanephrines occur in children (especially boys), renal failure, and stressful illness. Physical exercise raises plasma free metanephrine and normetanephrine by over 80%. Assumption of a supine resting position reduces plasma metanephrine by an average of 34% and reduces normetanephrine by 19%, compared to standing at rest. Coffee increases plasma normetanephrine by 20% and food increases plasma normetanephrine by 8%; but they have no effect upon metanephrine levels. Blood samples should ideally be drawn from an indwelling heparin-locked intravenous line while the patient is fasting and resting supine. Blood should be centrifuged immediately and stored at 4°C to improve stability.

In patients with adrenal pheochromocytoma, over 90% of circulating metanephrine originates from the tumor, while variable percentages of circulating normetanephrine originate from the tumor. Patients with elevated plasma metanephrine are likely to have an adrenal pheochromocytoma, since paragangliomas do not secrete epinephrine or metanephrine. Metastases from epinephrine-secreting pheochromocytomas may sometime continue to secrete epinephrine and metanephrine.

24-Hour urine-fractionated metanephrines.
This assay, which measures the sum of both conjugated and free urinary metanephrines, rivals plasma free metanephrines in sensitivity. In the United States, most reference laboratories employ tandem mass spectrometry (MS/MS), which eliminates interference by drugs and foods. Urinary metanephrines are rather stable compounds, so it is not necessary to collect the specimen with acid preservative. Conversely, acid preservative (used for collection of urinary catecholamines) does not adversely affect metanephrines. The disadvantages of 24-hour urine collections include: (1) the inconvenience to the patient; (2) the likelihood that there will be an error in the patient's collection or in the laboratory's handling of the specimen; (3) the inaccuracy for patients with renal failure. (See Appendix for normal reference ranges for 24-hour metanephrines.)

Like plasma-fractionated metanephrines, urinary metanephrines are much more sensitive than they are specific. Most patients with elevated levels of fractionated metanephrines do not harbor a pheochromocytoma if their levels are less than three times the upper limit of the reference range. Conversely, patients are very likely to have a pheochromocytoma if the 24-hour urine metanephrine excretion is above 600 µg/d (3.0 µmol/d) or normetanephrine excretion is above 1500 µg/d (8.2 µmol/d).

As with plasma metanephrines, patients with elevated urinary metanephrine are likely to harbor an adrenal pheochromocytoma, since paragangliomas do not secrete epinephrine or metanephrine.

Plasma-fractionated catecholamines.
Misleading elevations in plasma catecholamines commonly occur from the stress of having the phlebotomy. Normal plasma levels of catecholamines are listed in the Appendix.

Although plasma metanephrines are more sensitive than plasma catecholamines for detecting a pheochromocytoma, plasma catecholamines are of value in helping distinguish true-positive from false-positive results. In normal individuals, about 100% of circulating epinephrine originates from the adrenal medulla, while over 90% of circulating norepinephrine originates from peripheral sympathetic synapses. In both normals and those with pheochromocytomas, plasma norepinephrine levels fluctuate with the degree of peripheral sympathetic activation and both epinephrine and norepinephrine levels can increase during pheochromocytoma paroxysms. In patients with pheochromocytomas, the tumor's production of metanephrine metabolites is rather constant and relatively unrelated to peripheral sympathetic activity or a tumor's paroxysmal catecholamine secretion. Patients with false-positive test results due to sympathetic activation tend to have the following pattern: a higher percentage increase of plasma norepinephrine above the upper limit of the reference range compared to plasma normetanephrine; a higher percentage increase of plasma epinephrine above the upper limit of the reference range compared to plasma metanephrine.

Plasma catecholamines are of limited value in patients on dialysis and in those with renal insufficiency. About 58% of dialysis patients have plasma catecholamines above the normal reference range; about 32% of renal insufficiency patients have catecholamines above the normal reference range.

Most assays for plasma catecholamines currently employ HPLC with ECD; assays using tandem mass spectrometry (MS/MS) have not become generally available.

Urine-fractionated catecholamines and dopamine.
Adult normal maximal urinary concentrations for catecholamines and their metabolites are listed in the Appendix. A single 24-hour urine specimen is collected for fractionated catecholamines, fractionated metanephrines, dopamine, and creatinine. The container is acidified with 10 to 25 mL of 6 N HCl for preservation of the catecholamines; the acid does not interfere with metanephrine and creatinine assays. The acid preservative may be omitted for children for safety reasons, in which case the specimen should be kept cold and processed immediately. The laboratory requisition form should request that assays for fractionated catecholamines, fractionated metanephrines, and creatinine be performed on the same specimen.

A single-void urine specimen may be collected on first morning void or following a paroxysm. No acid preservative is used on single-void specimens, because it dilutes the specimen and is not required. For single-void collections, patients are instructed to void and discard the urine immediately at the onset of a paroxysm and then collect the next voided urine. The laboratory requisition should request spot urine for total metanephrine (by HPLC and ECD) and creatinine concentrations. It is prudent to contact the laboratory technician and explain that the specimen is meant to be a single-void urine and not a 24-hour specimen or else the specimen may be rejected. Patients with pheochromocytomas generally excrete over 2.2 μg total metanephrine/mg creatinine.

Urinary dopamine determination is not a sensitive test for pheochromocytomas. However, in patients with established pheochromocytomas, a normal urine dopamine is fairly predictive of benignity, whereas elevated urine dopamine excretion is seen in both benign and malignant pheochromocytomas.

B. Serum chromogranin A   Some tumors (mostly paragangliomas) fail to secrete catecholamines or metanephrines. Serum chromogranin A (CgA) is a useful test to diagnose and monitor such nonsecretory tumors. CgA may be determined by immunoradiometric assays. The serum CgA assay has become useful for the diagnosis of pheochromocytoma. However, CgA undergoes extensive tumor-specific cleavages so that only certain serum assays are useful for clinical diagnosis.

Serum CgA levels have a circadian rhythm in normal individuals, with lowest levels found at 8 AM and higher levels in the afternoon and at 11 PM. CgA levels are not elevated in essential hypertension. CgA is also secreted from extra-adrenal sympathetic nerves. Serum CgA levels are elevated in the great majority of patients with pheochromocytomas. The serum levels of CgA correlate with tumor mass, making CgA a useful tumor marker. However, smaller tumors may not be diagnosed. Serum CgA levels tend to be particularly elevated in patients with metastatic pheochromocytoma.

Serum CgA can be elevated even in patients with biochemically silent tumors. In patients with normal renal function, serum CgA has a sensitivity of 83% to 90% and a specificity of 96% for diagnosis of these tumors. However, the usefulness of serum CgA levels is negated by any degree of renal failure because of its excretion by the kidneys; even mild azotemia causes serum levels to be elevated. However, in patients with normal renal function, a high serum level of CgA along with high urine or plasma catecholamines or metanephrines is virtually diagnostic of pheochromocytoma.

Since CgA is also cosecreted with gastrin, serum CgA levels are also elevated in conditions with elevated serum gastrin: atrophic gastritis, pernicious anemia, postvagotomy, gastrinoma, gastric carcinoma, carcinoid tumor, and small cell lung carcinoma. CgA levels are elevated in about 60% of patients taking proton pump inhibitors (PPIs), but not H_2 blockers. Serum CgA levels rise variably after meals, so blood for CgA should be drawn after an overnight fast or repeated fasting if a nonfasting level is elevated. False-positive testing has also occurred in patients with inflammatory bowel disease, liver disease, hepatocellular carcinoma, prostate cancer, pituitary tumors, rheumatoid arthritis, and stress. False-positives have been reported to be due to heterophile antibody interference with the assay. Serum CgA levels can also be elevated without any discernable cause.

C. Suppression and stimulation testing   Glucagon stimulation testing is no longer used since it can cause dangerous hypertension.

Clonidine suppression test: This test may help distinguish patients with pheochromocytoma from normals with elevated normetanphrine levels. Clonidine is a central a 2-adrenergic blocker that suppresses the release of norepinephrine at sympathetic nerve synapses, thereby reducing circulating levels of norepinephrine and its metabolite, normetanephrine. In contrast, in patients with pheochromocytoma, most circulating normetanephrine is derived from continuous leakage from the tumor, such that clonidine is less able to suppress it. This test is most accurate when free normetanephrine is assayed, rather than norepinephrine.

To perform the clonidine suppression test, the patient must be fasting overnight and avoid smoking or interfering medications such as phenoxybenzamine, b-blockers, tricyclics and diuretics for at least 48 hours. An indwelling venous catheter is inserted, and the patient should remain recumbent. Thirty minutes later, blood is drawn for baseline plasma free normetanephrine. Clonidine is then given orally in a dose of 0.3 mg/kg; 3 hours afterward, blood is again drawn for plasma free normetanephrine.

In 1 study of 49 normals without pheochromocytoma, clonidine suppressed plasma normetanephrine levels more than 40% or to below 112 pg/mL in 100%. However, clonidine failed to suppress normetanephrine in 46 of 48 patients with pheochromocytoma. Despite the potential helpfulness of the clonidine suppression test, it cannot be completely relied upon. Unnecessary surgeries have been performed on the basis of misleading clonidine suppression testing.

D. Other laboratory tests

1. **Urine VMA**—Urinary VMA determinations have an overall diagnostic sensitivity for pheochromocytoma of only about 63% and do not improve the sensitivity or specificity of other tests for the diagnosis of pheochromocytoma. However, some centers have traditionally used a combination of 24-hour urinary VMA, metanephrine, and creatinine determinations with good results. VMA is stable for 5 days at room temperature; 6 N HCl is used to preserve urine specimens that are stored for longer than 5 days before analysis. Before urine collections for VMA testing, patients must avoid salicylates, caffeine, phenothiazines, and antihypertensive drugs for 72 hours. Coffee, tea, chocolate, bananas, and vanilla must also be avoided. Normal ranges for VMA vary by age (see Appendix).

2. **Plasma renin activity**—Levels of plasma renin activity are not typically suppressed in patients with pheochromocytomas because catecholamines stimulate renin release, and some tumors may secrete renin ectopically.

3. **Other tests**—Patients with pheochromocytoma are frequently found to have an increased white blood count with a high absolute neutrophil count. Counts as high as 23,600/μL

TABLE 11–14 Factors that can cause misleading catecholamine or metanephrine results.[a]

Drugs	Foods	Conditions
Acetaminophen[b]	Bananas[c]	Amyotrophic lateral sclerosis[c]
Aldomet[b]	Caffeine[c]	Brain lesions[c]
Amphetamines[c]	Coffee[b]	Carcinoid[c]
Bronchodilators[c]	Peppers[b]	Eclampsia[c]
Buspirone[b]		Emotion (severe)[c]
Captopril[b]		Exercise (vigorous)[c]
Cimetidine[b]		Guillain-Barré syndrome[c]
Cocaine[c]		Hypoglycemia[c]
Codeine[b]		Lead poisoning[c]
Contrast media		Myocardial infarction (acute)[c]
(meglumine		Pain (severe)[c]
acetrizoate,		Porphyria (acute)[c]
meglumine		Psychosis (acute)[c]
diatrizoate)[e]		Quadriplegia
Decongestants[c]		Renal failure[d]
Ephedrine[c]		Sleep apnea[c]
Fenfluramine[d]		
Isoproterenol[c]		
Labetalol[b,c]		
Levodopa[b]		
Mandelamine[b]		
Metoclopramide[b]		
Monoamine oxidase		
inhibitors[f]		
Nitroglycerin[c]		
Phenoxybenzamine[c]		
Smoking[f]		
Tricyclic		
antidepressants[c]		
Viloxazine[b]		

[a]Note that assays for metanephrine employing tandem mass spectroscopy (MS/MS) are not prone to interference from drugs or foods, except those that increase catecholamine excretion. Reproduced, with permission, from McPhee SJ, Papadakis MA, ed. *Current Medical Diagnosis & Treatment 2010*. McGraw Hill; 2010.

[b]May cause confounding peaks on HPLC chromatograms.

[c]Increases catecholamine excretion.

[d]Decreases catecholamine excretion.

[e]May decrease urine metanephrine excretion.

[f]Increases plasma and urinary normetanephrine and metanephrine.

have been reported. Marked eosinophilia may sometimes occur. Hyperglycemia is noted in about 35% of patients with pheochromocytoma, but frank diabetes mellitus is uncommon. The erythrocyte sedimentation rate is elevated in some patients. Hypercalcemia is common and may be caused by bone metastases or tumoral secretion of PTHrP. Hypocalcemia occurs rarely. Erythrocytosis sometimes occurs, usually due to volume contraction and rarely due to ectopic secretion of erythropoietin.

Factors That May Cause Misleading Biochemical Testing for Pheochromocytoma

Several different methods may be employed for assay of urine and plasma catecholamines and metanephrines. Each assay uses different methods and internal standards. Most assays for catecholamines now employ HPLC with ECD. Such assays can be affected by interference from a diverse range of drugs and foods. These substances cause unusual shapes in the peaks on the chromatogram. Not all of these assays are the same, and the potential for interference depends on the particular method employed. Therefore, it is best to check with the reference laboratory that runs the test or provides the test kit.

A. Drugs (see Table 11–14) Certain radiopaque contrast media, including those that contain meglumine acetrizoate or meglumine diatrizoate (eg, Renografin, Hypaque-M, Renovist, Cardiografin, Urografin, and Conray), can falsely lower urinary metanephrine determinations in some assays for up to 12 hours following administration. However, diatrizoate sodium is an intravenous contrast agent that does not cause such interference and should be requested if a CT scan must be performed prior to testing for metanephrines. Many other drugs cause interference in the older fluorometric assays for VMA and metanephrines. Tandem mass spectrometry for metanephrines virtually eliminates direct drug interference in the assay.

B. Foods Even while using HPLC-ECD assay techniques, certain foods can cause misleading results in assays for catecholamines and metanephrines (see Table 11–16). Coffee (even if decaffeinated) contains substances that can be converted into a catechol metabolite (dihydrocaffeic acid) that may cause confusing peaks on HPLC. Caffeine inhibits the action of adenosine; one action of adenosine is to inhibit the release of catecholamines. Heavy caffeine consumption causes a persistent elevation in norepinephrine production and raises blood pressure an average of 4 mm Hg systolic. Bananas contain considerable amounts of tyrosine, which can be converted to dopamine by the central nervous system; dopamine is then converted to epinephrine and norepinephrine. Dietary peppers contain 3-methoxy-4-hydroxybenzylamine (MHBA), a compound that can interfere with the internal standard used in some assays for metanephrines.

C. Diseases Any severe stress can elicit increased production of catecholamines and metanephrines. Urinary excretion of catecholamines and metanephrines is reduced in renal failure.

Differential Diagnosis of Pheochromocytoma (Table 11–15)

Pheochromocytomas have such protean manifestations that many conditions enter into the differential diagnosis. Essential hypertension is extremely common, and it is not practical to screen for pheochromocytoma in all patients with elevated blood pressure. However, pheochromocytoma should enter the differential diagnosis for any hypertensive patient having blood pressures above 180 mm Hg systolic and for any hypertensive patient who has one of the following symptoms: headaches, palpitations, sweating episodes, or unexplained bouts of abdominal or chest pains.

Anxiety (panic) attacks begin abruptly and can be associated with tachycardia, tachypnea, and chest discomfort, symptoms that

TABLE 11–15 Differential diagnosis of pheochromocytoma.

Acute intermittent porphyria
Autonomic epilepsy
Cardiac arrhythmias
Clonidine withdrawal
Coronary vasospasm
Encephalitis
Erythromelalgia
Essential hypertension
Hypertensive crisis associated with:
  Cerebrovascular accidents
  Surgery
  Acute pulmonary edema
  Severe pain
  Hypertensive crisis of MAO inhibitors
Hypoglycemia
Hypogonadal hot flushes
Lead poisoning
Mastocytosis
Migraine and cluster headache
Renovascular hypertension
Sleep apnea
Sympathomimetic drug ingestion
Thyrotoxicosis
Toxemia (eclampsia) of pregnancy

are commonly seen with pheochromocytomas. However, patients with panic attacks are more likely to have a precipitating social situation, tend to be exhausted for more than 2 hours following an attack, live in dread of the next attack, and often change their activities to avoid situations that might trigger anxiety.

Renal artery stenosis and renal parenchymal disease can cause increased secretion of renin resulting in severe hypertension. However, a detectable serum renin level does not exclude pheochromocytoma, because catecholamines can stimulate renin secretion and pheochromocytomas can secrete renin ectopically. Furthermore, large pheochromocytomas and paragangliomas arising near the renal hilum can occlude the renal artery, causing concomitant renovascular hypertension.

Hypogonadism can cause vasomotor instability in both women and men; attacks of flushing, sweating, and palpitations can mimic symptoms seen with pheochromocytoma. Factitious symptoms may be caused by surreptitious self-administration of various drugs such as epinephrine. Hyperthyroidism can cause heat intolerance, sweating, palpitations, and systolic hypertension with a widened pulse pressure. Carcinoid syndrome causes flushing during attacks but usually without pallor, hypertension, palpitations, or diaphoresis.

Obstructive sleep apnea can cause systemic hypertension; recurrent nocturnal hypoxia results in repeated episodes of stressful arousal that cause bursts of secretion of catecholamines, particularly epinephrine. Sleep apnea has been reported to cause misleading increases in the urinary excretion of catecholamines.

Patients with erythromelalgia can have episodic hypertension, but it is associated with flushing of the face and legs during the attack; patients with pheochromocytoma typically have facial pal-

lor during attacks. With erythromelalgia, patients have painful erythema and swelling in the legs that is relieved by application of ice; such symptoms are not characteristic of pheochromocytoma.

Patients who have intermittent bizarre symptoms may have their blood pressure and pulse checked during a symptomatic episode with a home blood pressure meter or an ambulatory blood pressure monitor. Those who are normotensive during an attack are not likely to harbor a pheochromocytoma.

Pheochromocytomas often present with abdominal pain and vomiting. Such symptoms are similar to those of an intra-abdominal emergency, particularly in the presence of leukocytosis and fever, which can also be seen with pheochromocytomas. Abdominal pain usually prompts a CT scan of the abdomen, which generally shows the pheochromocytoma or paraganglioma. Even after detection on CT scan, pheochromocytomas and juxtarenal paragangliomas may be mistaken for renal carcinoma. Large left-sided pheochromocytomas are often mistaken for carcinoma of the tail of the pancreas.

Neuroblastoma is the most common extra-cranial solid malignancy of childhood. It is also the most common malignancy in infants under 18 months old. Neuroblastomas are derived from the embryonic neural crest of the peripheral sympathetic nervous system. They most often arise in the adrenal gland, but can also develop in sympathetic nerve ganglia near the cervical or thoracic vertebrae or in the pelvis. They metastasize to bones, lymph nodes, liver, and skin. Symptoms depend upon the age of the patient, site of origin, degree of metastatic involvement, and the systemic response to the tumor. Infants usually present with localized disease (Stage 1 or 2) or with a special disseminated pattern of disease (Stage 4S—infants with metastatic disease to liver and/or skin) associated with a favorable outcome. In contrast, most children over 1 year of age present with advanced disease (Stage 3 or 4). Unfavorable biologic features include amplification of myelomatosis viral-related oncogene, neuroblastoma (MYCN), deletion or loss of heterozygosity of chromosome 1p or 11q and gains at 17q. Favorable biologic features include hyperdiploidy and overexpression of the gene encoding the nerve growth factor receptor, tyrosine kinase A (TrkA). About 85% of affected children secrete excessive catecholamines—but rarely in sufficient amounts to cause symptomatic hypertension or the paroxysms typical of pheochromocytomas. Most neuroblastomas concentrate ^{123}I-MIBG but they can be distinguished from pheochromocytomas and paragangliomas by clinical and histologic criteria.

Localization Studies for Pheochromocytoma

There are several available imaging modalities for pheochromocytoma and paraganglioma, each having unique sensitivity and specificity. There is no single imaging study that is 100% sensitive and specific. Generally, when a pheochromocytoma or paraganglioma is suspected, the initial diagnosis is best made biochemically. The initial localization scan is with CT or MRI of the abdomen and pelvis, which will detect about 95% of these tumors. However, since paragangliomas can arise in the chest, further scanning of the chest may be required. Diagnostic confirmation that

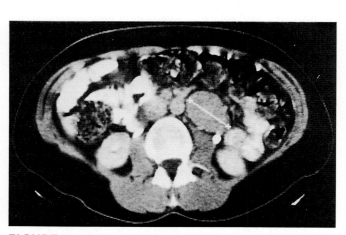

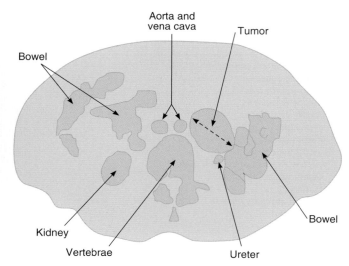

FIGURE 11–10 Left infrarenal paraganglioma shown by CT scanning. The diagram on the right identifies many of the visible structures.

the tumor is a pheochromocytoma or paraganglioma may be done with either ^{123}I-MIBG or ^{18}F-FDA positron emission tomography (PET) scanning; unfortunately, these scans are only 78% sensitive for these tumors. Scanning with ^{18}F-FDG or ^{18}F-FDA PET is more sensitive for detecting metastases than is ^{123}I-MIBG.

A. Computed tomography (Figure 11–10)

After a pheochromocytoma has been diagnosed by clinical and biochemical criteria, hypertension must first be controlled (see later), because intravenous ionic contrast can precipitate a hypertensive crisis. The pheochromocytoma must then be localized. It is useful to perform an initial nonenhanced (without intravenous contrast) CT of the adrenals because the density of an adrenal tumor can be better approximated without intravenous contrast. An adrenal mass with a density of less than 10 Hounsfield units (HU) is unlikely to be a pheochromocytoma. CT scanning of the entire abdomen (from the diaphragm through the pelvis) is obtained with intravenous contrast-enhanced and delayed contrast-enhanced imaging. Thin-section (2-5 mm) cuts should be obtained through the adrenals with an adrenal protocol that specifically looks for a vascular tumor blush and determines rate of contrast washout. Pheochromocytomas tend to have a tumor blush and slower contrast washout than adrenocortical adenomas. Hypertensive crises have been provoked in pheochromocytoma patients receiving ionic intravenous contrast agents; this has prompted the tradition of initiating an alpha-blocking agent before the CT scan. However, nonionic intravenous contrast poses much less of threat. No increases in blood pressure or plasma catecholamines were noted in a series of 10 pheochromocytoma patients who received iohexol intravenous nonionic contrast. Glucagon should not be used during a CT because it may provoke a hypertensive crisis.

If no mass is discovered, ^{123}I-MIBG imaging may be obtained or the CT scan may be extended into the chest in search of a paraganglioma—or both procedures may be employed. The great majority of pheochromocytomas are over 2 cm in diameter, well within the resolution capacity of the CT scan.

The overall sensitivity of CT scanning for an adrenal pheochromocytoma is about 90%—and over 95% for pheochromocytomas that are over 0.5 cm in diameter. However, CT scanning is less sensitive for the detection of small adrenal pheochromocytomas or adrenal medullary hyperplasia; this becomes an important issue in patients with MEN 2 or VHL disease. CT is also less sensitive for detecting extra-adrenal paragangliomas and early recurrent tumors in the adrenal surgical bed. CT will not detect small metastases or some metastases that strictly involve the bone marrow without osteoclastic activity. Metal surgical clips pose problem for CT scanning, causing distortion artifact and reducing the resolution of the scan.

B. Magnetic resonance imaging

MRI is useful in the diagnosis of adrenal pheochromocytomas, paragangliomas, and metastatic disease. It may be used with or without gadolinium contrast. Intravenous gadolinium contrast does not cause hypertensive crisis. MRI scanning with intravenous gadolinium contrast is also useful for patients with a known allergy to intravenous iodinated CT contrast agents. MRI is the scanning technique of choice in children and during pregnancy, because it involves no radiation exposure. Since MRI scanning delivers no radiation, it is preferred for serially scanning patients known to harbor a gene mutation predisposing them to PHEO/PGL.

MRI can help determine whether an adrenal mass is a pheochromocytoma when biochemical studies are inconclusive. On MRI T1-weighted images, pheochromocytomas have a dull signal (due to lack of fat cells), similar to kidney and muscle, distinguishing it from adrenal cortical adenomas, which contain fat and therefore have an intensely bright signal on T1-weighted images. The hypervascularity of pheochromocytomas makes them appear bright on MRI T2-weighted images, without signal loss on opposed phase imaging. However, other adrenal malignancies, adrenal adenomas, and hemorrhages can also appear bright on MRI T2-weighted images. Therefore, MRI scanning cannot definitively identify an adrenal mass as a pheochromocytoma. MRI of the abdomen has a sensitivity of about 95% for adrenal pheochromocytomas over 0.5 cm in diameter. Like CT scanning, MRI is less sensitive for the detection of extra-adrenal paragangliomas, metastatic disease, and recurrent small tumors in the adrenal surgical bed. MRI is helpful in visualizing paragangliomas that are intracardiac, juxtacardiac, or juxtavascular; MRI is particularly important for patients with paragangliomas adjacent to the vena cava or renal vein to detect vascular invasion. MRI is superior to CT in visualizing paragangliomas of the bladder wall. MRI can visualize some metastases to bone suspected on ^{123}I-MIBG imaging or PET scanning. Another advantage of MRI scanning is that retained internal metallic surgical clips do not cause the distorting reflection artifacts that occur with CT scanning.

The disadvantages of MRI scanning include expense and its inability to crisply image lungs (due to movement artifact). Also, morbidly obese patients may not be able to fit into a standard helical MRI scanner; open MRI scanners can be used but are generally less sensitive. Claustrophobic patients require a sedative before the scan or an open MRI. Patients with internal pacemakers or defibrillators may not have MRI scans; nor may patients with implanted neural stimulators, cochlear implants, Swan-Ganz catheters, insulin pumps, cerebral aneurysm clips, ocular metallic foreign bodies, or retained metal shrapnel or bullets. Patients with retained surgical clips, artificial heart valves and joints may have MRI imaging; the spine may be imaged in patients with spinal hardware, but the imaging can be distorted.

C. Metaiodobenzylguanidine scanning (Figure 11–11 and Table 11–16)

MIBG is a guanidine derivative that resembles norepinephrine and is actively transported into adrenal medullary cells via the norepinephrine transporter system, selectively accumulating in neurosecretory granules. Unlike norepinephrine, MIBG has low affinity for catecholamine receptors and is not metabolized.

Scintigraphy using ^{123}I-MIBG or ^{131}I-MIBG is useful for determining whether an adrenal mass is a pheochromocytoma, for

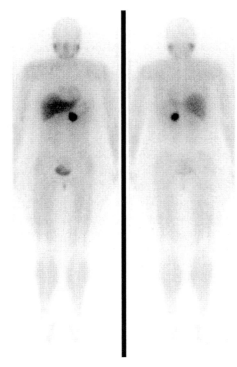

FIGURE 11–11 ^{123}I-metaiodobenzylguanidine (^{123}I-MIBG) scan of a woman with a large left pheochromocytoma. Normal ^{123}I-MIBG uptake is seen in the liver, salivary glands, and heart. ^{123}I-MIBG is renally excreted and is visible in the bladder.

imaging occult paragangliomas, and for confirming whether a certain extra-adrenal mass is a paraganglioma or neuroblastoma. MIBG scanning is also useful for screening patients for metastases. MIBG uptake can often be seen in apparently nonfunctioning pheochromocytomas.

The isotope that is preferable for precise imaging is ^{123}I-MIBG, because ^{123}I emits γ radiation at lower energy (159 keV) than does [131]I (364 keV). The lower-energy γ emissions allows crisper images with ^{123}I-MIBG scanning as well as single photon emission computed tomography (SPECT). ^{123}I-MIBG SPECT scanning is more sensitive than ^{123}I-MIBG planar imaging for detecting small metastases and has the advantage of being able to do the scanning on the day following injection of the isotope. SPECT scanning with ^{123}I-MIBG can be combined with CT to produce a three-dimensional fusion scan; the resultant combined images can help distinguish whether a given mass has ^{123}I-MIBG uptake.

^{123}I-MIBG is administered intravenously in doses of 3 mCi (children) to 10 mCi (adults), whereas ^{131}I-MIBG is administered intravenously in doses of 0.5 to 1 mCi. [123]I emits lower energy γ radiation and less heavy particle radiation over a shorter period than ^{131}I, so ^{123}I-MIBG scanning results in a somewhat lower absorbed radiation dose than ^{131}I-MIBG scanning. However, most centers still use ^{131}I-MIBG due to its longer half-life, lower expense, and better commercial availability.

TABLE 11–16 Drugs that inhibit MIBG uptake by pheochromocytomas (time that inhibition persists after stopping drug).

Inhibitors of type I catecholamine uptake: cocaine, tricyclic drugs, labetalol (2-6 wk), renlafaxine, mirtazapine, reboxetine, bupropion

Stimulants of catecholamine discharge: reserpine (2 wk)

Displacement of catecholamines from intracellular stores and competition with uptake of MIBG: all amphetamines; nasal decongestants, oral or nasal (2 wk)

Others: phenothiazines, haloperidol, thiothixene (2 wk)

^{123}I-MIBG scanning has an overall sensitivity of 82% and a specificity of 82% for pheochromocytomas and paragangliomas combined. The sensitivity of ^{123}I-MIBG scanning is 88% for primary adrenal pheochromocytomas and 67% for paragangliomas, with an overall sensitivity of 78% for primary PHEO/PGL tumors. The sensitivity of ^{123}I-MIBG scanning for metastases is lower at only 57%. Scanning with ^{123}I-MIBG is more sensitive for pheochromocytomas that are benign, unilateral, adrenal, capsule-invasive, and sporadic. Scanning with ^{123}I-MIBG is less sensitive for bilateral, malignant, extra-adrenal, noninvasive, and MEN 2-related or VHL-related pheochromocytomas.

To block the thyroid's uptake of free radioiodine, saturated solution of potassium iodide, five drops orally three times daily, is given before the injection and daily for 4 days after ^{123}I-MIBG and for 7 days after ^{131}I-MIBG. Scanning is performed 24 to 48 hours after ^{123}I-MIBG infusion and 48 to 72 hours after ^{131}I-MIBG infusion.

False-negative MIBG scans are seen in about 15% of cases of either benign or malignant pheochromocytoma. False-negative scans can occur in patients who have taken certain drugs (eg, tricyclic antidepressants or cyclobenzaprine) within 6 weeks. Other drugs that can cause false-negative scans when taken within 2 weeks include amphetamines, phenylpropanolamine, haloperidol, phenothiazines, thiothixene, reserpine, nasal decongestants, cocaine, and diet pills. Labetalol reduces MIBG uptake, but the scan can still be done, albeit with suboptimal sensitivity (Table 11–16). When plasma norepinephrine levels are over 500 pg/mL (3 nmol/L), cardiac visualization is reduced on ^{18}F-dopamine PET scanning. This phenomenon is believed due to competitive inhibition of uptake-1 by high levels of circulating norepinephrine. Therefore, it is likely that very high endogenous norepinephrine levels may reduce the sensitivity of ^{123}I-MIBG scanning as well as PET scanning that employs ^{18}F-DA or ^{19}F-DOPA because these compounds are transported into pheochromocytomas, paragangliomas, and their metastases by the same uptake mechanism.

False-positive MIBG scans occur infrequently. Following ^{123}I-MIBG, some uptake in a normal adrenal medulla is seen in 32% to 75% of patients at 24 hours. Following ^{131}I-MIBG, uptake in a normal adrenal medulla is seen in 16% of normals at 48 hours. Adrenal uptake is often asymmetric and can be misinterpreted as showing a tumor. MIBG has renal excretion, so the renal pelvis and bladder are usually visualized on scanning and must be distinguished from tumor. If a patient is being evaluated for a bladder mass (ie, to exclude a paraganglioma), a bladder catheter may be inserted and the bladder flushed with saline to distinguish tumor from renal excretion of isotope. Urine contamination with ^{123}I-MIBG can also cause a false-positive scan. False-positive results have been reported with adrenal carcinomas and infections such as actinomycosis. The salivary glands are typically visualized since they are richly innervated. The heart, liver, and spleen normally take up some ^{123}I-MIBG. Some isotope is excreted in the stool, and intracolonic collections can be mistaken for tumor. When there is doubt about whether an area of uptake is a tumor, scanning can be repeated the next day, preceded by a laxative if required.

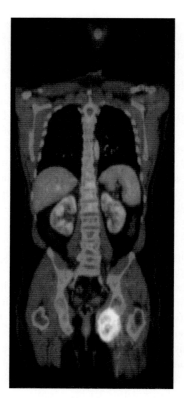

FIGURE 11–12 ^{18}F-deoxyglucose ([18]FDG) PET/CT fusion scan. Patient had a retroperitoneal paraganglioma that was resected. [18]FDG-PET/CT fusion scan shows a large metastasis involving the left acetabulum and inferior pubic ramus. The metastasis had negligible ^{123}I-MIBG uptake. A metastasis causing an L4 compression had been treated previously with radiation therapy.

D. Positron emission tomography (Figure 11–12)   PET scanning can be performed shortly after the intravenous infusion of short-lived isotopes that are tagged to a compound that is preferentially absorbed by tumor tissue. These isotopes emit positrons (anti-matter) during their decay, causing positron-electron collisions that emit γ photons traveling in precisely opposite directions (180 degrees out of phase). In the PET scanner, sensitive gamma detectors surround the patient; simultaneous activation of two gamma detectors indicates that the source is located directly between them. Multiple such detections of this nature allow three-dimensional imaging of tumors and can accurately determine their location. Advanced scanners can perform PET and CT scanning simultaneously to produce particularly sensitive and accurate three-dimensional anatomic imaging.

PET scanning has certain advantages over MIBG scanning. PET scanning can be done almost immediately. This gives it some advantage over MIBG scanning, which must be delayed for 24 to 48 hours after the injection to allow dissipation of background radiation. PET scanning does not require pretreatment with iodine to protect the thyroid, as is necessary with MIBG scanning. However, PET scanning is very expensive. The isotope ^{18}F has a half-life of just 2 hours and must be produced in a cyclotron, so ^{18}F-FDG or ^{18}F-FDA PET scanning is practical only at medical centers that have a cyclotron nearby.

1. **PET scanning with ^{18}F-FDG**—Deoxyglucose (DG) is absorbed by tissues with active metabolism, including tumors. For PET scanning, DG is tagged with ^{18}F to produce fluorodeoxyglucose, or ^{18}F-FDG. This scan is widely available as a fusion scan with CT, ^{18}F-FDG PET/CT. This scan's sensitivity is 88% for nonmetastatic pheochromocytoma/paraganglioma and 76% for metastatic pheochromocytoma/paraganglioma. The sensitivity of ^{18}F-FDG-PET/CT is lower for indolent tumors and for patients who are diabetic or who are not fasting before the scan. ^{18}F-FDG-PET localizes in other tissues with a high metabolic rate, including areas of inflammation, brown fat, shivering muscles, but such areas of PET uptake can be distinguished from tumors by the lack of a CT correlate. However, ^{18}F-FDG-PET/CT detects other tumors besides pheochromocytoma/paraganglioma and is, therefore, less specific for pheochromocytoma/paraganglioma than is ^{18}F-FDA-PET or ^{123}I-MIBG scanning.

2. **PET scanning with ^{18}F-FDA**—PET scanning may also be performed using radioisotope-tagged dopamine: 6-[^{18}F] fluorodopamine (^{18}F-FDA-PET). This scan is more specific for paraganglioma and metastatic pheochromocytoma than is ^{18}F-FDG-PET/CT, because dopamine is a substrate for the norepinephrine transporter in tumor tissue. The sensitivity of ^{18}F-FDA-PET is 78% for nonmetastatic pheochromocytoma/paraganglioma and 76% for metastatic pheochromocytoma/paraganglioma. It is widely available and is generally more sensitive than ^{123}I-MIBG scanning, particularly in patients who harbor VHL or MEN 2 germline mutations.

3. **PET scanning with ^{18}F-DOPA**—PET scanning may be performed using radioisotope-tagged DOPA: 6-[^{18}F]fluoro-L-dihydroxyphenylalanine (^{18}F-DOPA). The sensitivity of ^{18}F-DOPA-PET is about 81% for nonmetastatic PHEO/PGL and 45% for metastatic pheochromocytoma/paraganglioma. For SDHB-associated metastatic paraganglioma, its sensitivity is only 20%. This scan is not widely available and is not recommended because of its lack of sensitivity for metastatic pheochromocytoma or paraganglioma.

E. Somatostatin receptor imaging with ^{111}In-octreotide Somatostatin receptors are cell surface, transmembrane, and G protein–coupled receptors, and there are five subtypes. About 70% of pheochromocytomas express somatostatin receptors, particularly types 2 and 4. Octreotide is a stable 8 amino acid analog of somatostatin with a high affinity for type 2 receptors. For imaging, octreotide is coupled with ^{111}In-diaminetriaminepentacetate (DTPA). ^{111}In has a half-life of 2.8 days and γ emissions of 173 keV and 247 keV. Scanning with ^{111}In-labeled octreotide, known as somatostatin receptor imaging (SRI), has a sensitivity of only 25% for adrenal pheochromocytomas and juxtarenal paragangliomas. This low sensitivity is due to high uptake of ^{111}In-octreotide by the kidneys as well as renal excretion. However, SRI detects 87% of pheochromocytoma metastases and is also a sensitive technique for detecting paragangliomas of the head and neck (chemodectomas). SRI also detects some metastases not visible on MIBG scanning, and vice versa. SRI has been reported to detect a cardiac paraganglioma that was not visible on MIBG scanning. When paragangliomas or metastases are suspected, SRI may be useful, particularly when MIBG scanning is negative.

^{111}In-octreotide has physiologic uptake in the kidneys, thyroid, pituitary, salivary glands, gallbladder, bowels, spleen, liver, and mammary glands. Infection and recent surgery sites can also have misleading uptake of ^{111}In-octreotide.

F. Ultrasound imaging On transabdominal ultrasound, an adrenal pheochromocytoma typically appears as a well-defined mass. Large pheochromocytomas tend to develop internal hemorrhagic necrotic cysts, making the tumor appear heterogenous. Transabdominal ultrasound is most sensitive in slender individuals, in whom 85% of adrenal pheochromocytomas can be visualized. However, ultrasound lacks specificity, such that a pheochromocytoma is not distinguishable from an adrenal adenoma or a mass in the superior pole of a kidney. Likewise, a left adrenal pheochromocytoma may be mistaken for a pancreatic tail tumor, and a right adrenal pheochromocytoma may be mistaken for a hepatic mass. Ultrasound may be used for initial imaging for pheochromocytomas in pregnant women, infants, and young children, although MRI is superior. Ultrasound is also useful for imaging and surveillance of neck paragangliomas. Ultrasound examinations have also been performed endoscopically, from the stomach and duodenum, with a longitudinal sector array, yielding sensitive detection of small adrenal pheochromocytomas, lymphangitic metastases, and local recurrences. For pelvic and bladder paragangliomas, pelvic transvaginal ultrasound is very helpful for tumor localization and surveillance.

G. Venous sampling for catecholamines (see Figure 11–9) Selective venous sampling for catecholamines is dangerous, since the required venography can provoke a pheochromocytoma crisis. Venous sampling can help distinguish whether a mass is a secretory pheochromocytoma or paraganglioma. However, venous sampling it is rarely required and seldom indicated.

INCIDENTALLY DISCOVERED ADRENAL MASSES

Clinically inapparent adrenal nodules are commonly discovered incidentally on abdominal CT or MRI scans that are performed for unrelated reasons. (See "Computed Tomography," earlier.) Such nodules are known as **adrenal incidentalomas.** The incidence of adrenal nodules is about 3% in middle-aged, rising to 10% in the elderly. Most such nodules are small, benign adrenal adenomas, with densities below 10 HU on noncontrast CT. However, pheochromocytomas can produce nonspecific symptoms of abdominal pain, nausea, and weight loss, for which CT scans may be performed. Pheochromocytomas account for about 4% of incidentally discovered adrenal masses. In the United States nearly half of the pheochromocytomas diagnosed during life are detected incidentally on an abdominal or chest CT scan performed for other reasons. Therefore, all patients with adrenal nodules, even normotensives, should be screened for pheochromocytoma with plasma-fractionated free metanephrines. A problem arises with metanephrines that are marginally elevated. Such patients with metanephrines that are one to two times higher than the reference range's ULN have about a 30% chance of harboring a pheochromocytoma. Those with metanephrines more than twice the ULN have a very high risk of having a pheochromocytoma. For apparently nonfunctioning adrenal nodules, it is generally reasonable to observe those that are under 3 cm in maximum diameter. Nonfunctioning nodules that are 3 to 5 cm in maximum diameter require especially close surveillance. Adrenal nodules that are over 5 cm in diameter are generally resected, except for obvious myelolipomas. When pheochromocytoma has been ruled out, patients with an adrenal nodule should be screened for hyperaldosteronism and Cushing syndrome.

Adrenal Percutaneous Fine-Needle Aspiration Biopsy

Most pheochromocytomas can be readily diagnosed on the basis of their clinical, biochemical, and radiologic presentation. Fine-needle aspiration biopsy (FNAB) is not usually required for the diagnosis of a pheochromocytoma. However, some pheochromocytomas are discovered incidentally on abdominal CT or ultrasound and may be clinically or biochemically silent. Although there may be a temptation to biopsy such masses, patients with a suspicious adrenal or retroperitoneal mass require testing for pheochromocytoma before any biopsy. There is a 70% risk of complications after percutaneous FNAB of pheochromocytomas and paragangliomas. Such complications include: increased difficulty in the tumor's resection (41%), severe hypertension (15%), hematoma (30%), severe pain (25%), and incorrect or inadequate biopsy (25%). FNAB cytology can be misinterpreted as a different primary malignancy or a metastasis from another malignancy; this potential for confusion is due to the fact that pheochromocytomas are rare tumors and have pleomorphic and hyperchromic nuclei. Large left-sided pheochromocytomas have been misdiagnosed as carcinoma of the tail of the pancreas based on CT scanning and biopsy. Percutaneous biopsy can also disrupt the pheochromocytoma capsule and cause seeding of the tumor within the peritoneum.

Medical Management of Pheochromocytoma and Paraganglioma

Patients need to be treated with oral antihypertensives and stabilized hemodynamically prior to surgery. Patients receiving increasing doses of antihypertensive medications should have daily measurements of blood pressure and pulse rate in the lying, sitting, and standing positions. Additionally, patients are taught to determine their own blood pressure and pulse rate during any paroxysmal symptoms. Most clinicians gradually increase antihypertensive medications over 2 or more weeks. However, prolonged preoperative preparation has not proven more effective for preventing intraoperative hypertension than are shorter preparation periods. Some hypertensive patients have been admitted emergently for hypertension control and hydration, stabilized, and operated on successfully with intravenous infusion of a vasodilator drug (eg, nicardipine, nitroprusside, nitroglycerin; see discussed later). Ideally, the blood pressure should be reduced to an average of 130/85 mm Hg or less prior to surgery, while avoiding symptomatic orthostasis.

A. Alpha-adrenergic blockers   Alpha-adrenergic blockers have historically been used for most patients with pheochromocytoma in preparation for surgical resection. Patients who are normotensive are also usually treated (carefully) preoperatively. Phenoxybenzamine (10-mg capsules) is an oral nonselective alpha blocker that is the most commonly used alpha-blocking agent. It has a long half-life of about 24 hours. Patients with mild hypertension may be given phenoxybenzamine at a starting dosage of 10 mg once daily, while those with more severe hypertension may receive a starting dosage of 10 mg twice daily. The dose of phenoxybenzamine may be increased by 10 mg every 2 days until the blood pressure falls to an average of 130/85 mm Hg sitting or until symptomatic orthostatic hypotension occurs. Patients who have been normotensive between paroxysms are particularly prone to develop hypotension with phenoxybenzamine. Phenoxybenzamine does not block the synthesis of catecholamines; in fact, the synthesis of catecholamines and metanephrines tends to increase during alpha blockade. Therapy with phenoxybenzamine increases the heart rate but decreases the frequency of ventricular arrhythmias. Patients are encouraged to hydrate themselves well. Patients must be monitored daily for symptomatic orthostatic hypotension. Certain adverse effects are common, including dry mouth, headache, diplopia, inhibition of ejaculation, and nasal congestion. Nasal decongestants should not be used if urinary catecholamine determinations or ^{123}I-MIBG scanning is planned, but antihistamines are acceptable. Phenoxybenzamine is not well tolerated as chronic therapy for hypertension in patients with unresectable or metastatic pheochromocytoma, and such patients are better treated with calcium channel blockers (see later), sometimes together with low-dose phenoxybenzamine.

Phenoxybenzamine crosses the placenta and accumulates to levels that are 60% higher in the fetus than in the maternal circulation; this can cause hypotension and respiratory depression in the newborn for several days following birth. Most patients require 30 to 60 mg/d, but the dosage is sometimes escalated to as high as 140 mg/d. Excessive alpha blockade with phenoxybenzamine is undesirable because it worsens postoperative hypotension. Furthermore, excessive alpha blockade may deny a critical surgical indicator (ie, a drop in blood pressure after complete resection of the tumor and aggravation of hypertension during palpation of the abdomen in case of multiple tumors or metastases).

Doxazosin is another alpha blocker with a half-life of about 22 hours. It is effective in the medical management of pheochromocytomas when given orally in doses of 2 to 16 mg daily. In one series, there was no difference in hemodynamic instability during surgery in patients pretreated with doxazosin versus phenoxybenzamine. Alternatively, prazosin is a short-acting selective alpha blocker with a half-life of about 3 hours. It appears to cause less reflex tachycardia and less postoperative hypotension. With chronic use, it has been reported to cause less ejaculatory disturbance in men, compared to phenoxybenzamine. The starting dose of prazosin is 0.5 mg/d, increasing up to 10 mg twice or three times daily, if necessary.

B. Calcium channel blockers

Calcium channel blockers are excellent antihypertensive agents for patients with pheochromocytomas. Patients tend to tolerate calcium channel blockers better than alpha blockers. Patients who are normotensive between paroxysms are less likely to become hypotensive with calcium channel blockers compared to alpha blockers. Patients with angina from coronary vasospasm are also best treated with calcium channel blockers. Perioperative fluid requirements have been lower among patients who were pretreated with calcium channel blockers instead of alpha blockers. In a French series, 70 patients with pheochromocytoma were successfully prepared for surgery using oral calcium channel blockers (usually nicardipine). Nicardipine may be given in doses of 20 to 40 mg orally every 8 hours; nicardipine is also available as a sustained-release preparation that may be given in doses of 30 to 60 mg orally every 12 hours.

Nifedipine is a calcium channel blocker that is administered as a slow-release preparation in doses of 30 to 60 mg orally once or twice daily. For hypertensive paroxysms, nifedipine 10 mg (chewed pierced capsule) is usually a fast and effective treatment. Chewed nifedipine is generally safe for use by patients with pheochromocytoma, who may self-administer the drug at home during paroxysms but only with close blood pressure monitoring. In one small study, nifedipine therapy appeared to improve the uptake of MIBG into pheochromocytomas in four of eight patients at scanning doses. It is possible that nifedipine might reduce the growth of pheochromocytomas and metastases, because in vitro nifedipine added to cultured pheochromocytoma cells reduces their mitotic index and proliferation. The effect of nifedipine on pheochromocytoma tumor growth in vivo has not been studied. Amlodipine may also be used for patients with pheochromocytoma in doses of 10 to 20 mg daily.

Other calcium channel blockers are reported to be less effective for patients with pheochromocytoma. Verapamil has been used in a sustained-release preparation, but has been reported to be associated with postoperative pulmonary edema after pheochromocytoma resection. Diltiazem has been reported to provide inadequate intraoperative blood pressure control.

Intravenous calcium channel blockers are useful for hypertensive crisis, particularly during surgery. Nicardipine and clevidipine are both available as intravenous preparations. (See "Surgical Management of Pheochromocytoma and Paraganglioma" later.)

C. Angiotensin-converting enzyme inhibitors

ACE inhibitors have successfully treated hypertension in patients with pheochromocytomas but not as the sole agent. Angiotensin receptor blockers have also been successfully added to multidrug antihypertensive therapy. Catecholamines stimulate renin production. In turn, renin stimulates the production of angiotensin I, which is converted by ACE to angiotensin II; this can be blocked by ACE inhibitors. Furthermore, pheochromocytomas have been demonstrated to have angiotensin II–binding sites. ACE inhibitors are contraindicated in pregnancy, because their use in the second and third trimesters has been associated with fetal malformations, including skull hypoplasia, renal failure, limb and craniofacial deformation, lung hypoplasia, intrauterine growth retardation, patent ductus arteriosus, and death.

D. Beta-adrenergic blockers

These agents are generally not prescribed for patients with pheochromocytomas until treatment has been started with antihypertensive medications such as α-adrenergic blockers or calcium channel blockers. Beta-adrenergic blockade should then be used for treatment of β-adrenergic symptoms such as flushing, pounding heart, or tachycardia. It is important to institute alpha blockade first, because blocking vasodilating β_2 receptors without also blocking vasoconstricting α_1 receptors can lead to hypertensive crisis if serum norepinephrine levels are high.

Nonselective beta blockers block both β_1- and β_2-adrenergic receptors. The inhibition of vasodilating arterial β_2 receptors causes unopposed vasoconstrictive α-adrenergic stimulation that aggravates hypertension. Therefore, nonselective beta blockers should ordinarily not be administered to patients with pheochromocytoma or paraganglioma. Nonselective beta blockers include: nadolol, pindolol, propranolol, and timolol. Labetalol and carvedilol are different nonselective β blockers that additionally block α_1 receptors. Labetalol has been used to treat patients with pheochromocytoma; however, it can initially aggravate hypertension, produce false elevations of catecholamines in some assays, and reduce MIBG uptake.

Selective beta blockers specifically block β_1-adrenergic receptors at low doses. This leads to a rather selective reduction in heart rate without unopposed alpha receptor dependent hypertension. However, at higher doses, these beta blockers also block β_2-adrenergic receptors and can cause a paradoxical worsening of hypertension. Selective beta blockers include: atenolol, betaxolol, bisoprolol, nebivolol, esmolol, and metoprolol. Atenolol has a half-life of only 6 hours, so it does not produce satisfactory 24-hour blockade. Nebivolol has vasodilating activity through enhancement of nitric oxide release. Esmolol is the preferred intravenous preparation. Extended-release metoprolol (metoprolol ER) is the preferred oral preparation.

E. Metyrosine (α-methylparatyrosine)

Metyrosine inhibits the enzyme tyrosine hydroxylase, which catalyzes the first reaction in catecholamine biosynthesis. Because of its potential side effects, it is usually used only to treat hypertension in patients with metastatic pheochromocytoma. Metyrosine is administered orally as 250-mg capsules, beginning with one every 6 hours; the dose is titrated upward every 3 to 4 days according to blood pressure response and side effects. Most patients can tolerate 2 g/d, but higher doses usually cause side effects. The maximum dosage is 4 g/d. Catecholamine excretion is usually reduced by 35% to 80%.

Preoperative treatment with metyrosine tends to reduce intraoperative hypertension and arrhythmias; however, postoperative hypotension is likely to be more severe for several days. Side effects of metyrosine include sedation, psychiatric disturbance, extrapyramidal symptoms, and potentiation of sedatives and phenothiazines. Crystalluria and urolithiasis can occur, so adequate hydration is mandatory. Metyrosine does not inhibit MIBG uptake by the tumor, allowing concurrent ^{123}I-MIBG scanning or treatment with high-dose ^{131}I-MIBG.

F. Octreotide   Octreotide has not been formally studied or approved for use in patients with pheochromocytoma. However, octreotide (100 μg subcutaneously three times daily), has been reported to reduce hypertensive episodes and catecholamine excretion in a man with pheochromocytoma whose hypertensive paroxysms were uncontrolled using other means. Octreotide therapy has been observed to reduce bone pain in a woman with a malignant paraganglioma whose skeletal metastases were avid for ^{111}In-labeled octreotide. Octreotide therapy is usually begun at a dose of 50 to 100 μg injected subcutaneously every 8 hours. Side effects are common and may include nausea, vomiting, abdominal pain, and dizziness. If the drug is tolerated, the dose can be titrated upward to a maximum of 1500 μg daily. Octreotide LAR can be given as subcutaneous injections in doses of 10 to 30 mg every 4 weeks.

G. Activities to avoid   Vigorous exercise, particularly involving bending or heavy lifting, can aggravate hypertension in some individuals with pheochromocytoma, so mild exertion or rest is best during preparation for surgery. Emotional stress can provoke hypertensive attacks, so arguments and stressful situations are best avoided.

H. Foods to avoid   Tyramine is a precursor to catecholamines and intravenous tyramine causes hypertension in most patients with pheochromocytoma. While dietary tyramine has not been studied in patients with pheochromocytoma, it is known that dietary tyramine can provoke hypertensive crisis in patients taking MAO inhibitor antidepressants. Therefore, although strict dietary precautions are not required, it is reasonable for patients with a known pheochromocytoma to avoid consuming large amounts of foods with high tyramine content during preparation for surgery such as red wine, tap beers, aged dairy products, aged meats, fermented or pickled fish, liver, protein extracts, overripe fruit, soybeans, tofu, fava bean pods, bean pastes, brewer's yeast pills, marmite, and vegemite.

Surgical Management of Pheochromocytoma and Paraganglioma

A. Perioperative preparation   Prior to surgery, patients should be reasonably normotensive on medication, with an average blood pressure of 130/85 mm Hg or less, without symptomatic orthostasis (see earlier). They should also be well hydrated.

It is ideal for patients to be admitted for administration of intravenous fluids at least 1 day prior to surgery. Patients may predonate blood for autologous transfusion. The transfusion of two units of blood within 12 hours before surgery reduces the risk of postoperative hypotension. Blood pressure must be monitored continuously during surgery. This requires placement of an arterial line, preferably in a large artery that is not prone to spasm (eg, femoral artery). A central venous pressure line helps determine the volume of fluid replacement. For certain high-risk patients with congestive heart failure or coronary artery disease, a pulmonary artery (Swan-Ganz) line may be inserted preoperatively to further optimize fluid replacement. Constant electrocardiographic monitoring is mandatory. Severe hypertension can occur—even in fully blocked patients—during bladder catheterization, intubation, or surgical incision. During laparoscopic surgery, catecholamine release is typically stimulated by pneumoperitoneum and by tumor manipulation. However, laparoscopic procedures cause less fluctuation of catecholamine levels and blood pressure than do open surgeries. All antihypertensive medications (see later) that might be required should be available and should be in the operating room well in advance.

Arterial embolization of the tumor can be performed immediately prior to surgery. This may be beneficial to the surgeon, particularly for the open resection of very large paragangliomas that tend to be extremely vascular and difficult to resect, due to blood loss and venous oozing. Embolization of neck paragangliomas is an established intervention. Secretory paragangliomas can also be embolized preoperatively. An experienced interventional radiologist must perform such embolizations with full monitoring and an anesthesia team in attendance.

The major problem during surgery for pheochromocytoma is hemodynamic instability. Serious blood pressure variations are more common in patients whose blood pressure has not been adequately pretreated. Intraoperative hemodynamic instability is also more common in patients with higher plasma norepinephrine levels and larger tumor size.

B. Antihypertensive and antiarrhythmic drugs

1. **Calcium channel blockers**—These are effective therapies for intraoperative hypertension. They can cause reflex tachycardia that can be controlled with intravenous beta blockers (eg, esmolol). Nicardipine is administered as an intravenous infusion, starting at a dose of 5 mg/h and increasing by 2.5 mg/h every 5 to 15 minutes up to 15 mg/h. Nicardipine was successfully used as the sole intraoperative vasodilating agent in one French series of 70 patients and in another series of 19 patients. Its half-life is 9 hours. Clevidipine has a shorter half-life of 1 to 15 minutes. It is available for intravenous infusion at a dose of 1 to 2 mg/h, doubling the dose after 90 seconds, then increasing in smaller increments at longer intervals (5-10 minutes) up to 4 to 6 mg/h or a maximum of 16 mg/h.

2. **Phentolamine**—It is a parenteral α-adrenergic blocker that has a short half-life of 19 minutes. It can be given intravenously in bolus doses, starting with 5 mg (children, 1-3 mg) and repeating in doses of 5 to 15 mg as needed for blood pressure control. Phentolamine may also be given by intravenous infusion at a rate of 0.5 to 1 mg/min. Side effects include

hypotension, tachycardia, cardiac arrhythmias, nasal stuffiness, nausea, and vomiting.

3. **Nitroprusside**—It is given by intravenous infusion and is an effective drug for managing hypertensive episodes; advantages include widespread familiarity with its use and its short half-life of 2 minutes. Nitroprusside is initiated at 0.25 to 0.3 μg/kg/min and titrated for the desired effect. The maximum infusion rate is 10 μg/kg/min for 10 minutes. High infusion rates should not be given for prolonged periods; long-duration (over 6 hours) nitroprusside infusion rates above 2 μg/kg/min cause cyanide accumulation and toxicity. Cyanide toxicity causes metabolic acidosis and an increase in venous oxygen saturation (>90%) in severe cases. If cyanide toxicity is suspected, the nitroprusside infusion must be stopped or slowed. In the United States, there are two different cyanide antidote kits available. (1) The conventional kit contains amyl nitrite, sodium nitrite, and thiosulfate. Administer an amyl nitrite crushed ampule at the end of the endotracheal tube or under the patient's nose and give 10 mL 3% sodium nitrite intravenously. Also administer 25% sodium thiosulfate solution (50 mL) intravenously. (2) Additionally, hydroxocobalamin (Cyanokit) is available for intravenous administration at a dose of 5 g (children, 70 mg/kg). Coadministration of sodium thiosulfate (1 g/100 mg nitroprusside) prevents cyanide accumulation. Nitroprusside must be administered cautiously, since it can cause precipitous and profound hypotension, resulting in irreversible ischemic injuries.

4. **Nitroglycerin**—It is given by intravenous infusion and is effective therapy for perioperative hypertension. Nitroglycerin infusions are initiated at 5 μg/min and increased by 5 μg/min every 3 to 5 minutes until target blood pressure is achieved or a dose of 20 μg/min is reached; if the response has been insufficient, the dose can be increased by 10 to 20 μg/min every 5 minutes to a maximum of 100 μg/min. Because nitroglycerin adheres to polyvinyl chloride tubing, non-PVC infusion sets must be used. Nitroglycerin infusions can cause headache and hypotension. Methemoglobinemia has occurred during prolonged high-dose infusions and is manifested by cyanosis in the presence of a normal arterial pO$_2$. The therapy for methemoglobinemia consists of immediately stopping the nitroglycerin and giving methylene blue, 1 to 2 mg/kg intravenously.

5. **Magnesium sulfate**—It is given intravenously in a bolus of 4 g over 15 minutes and has been reported to be effective in managing hypertension during resection of a pheochromocytoma during pregnancy.

6. **Lidocaine**—It may be used to treat cardiac ventricular arrhythmias. In adults, lidocaine is administered with a loading dose of 150 to 200 mg over about 15 minutes, or as a series of smaller boluses. This is followed by a maintenance infusion of 2 to 4 mg/min in order to achieve a therapeutic plasma level of 2 to 6 μg/mL.

7. **Beta blockers**—Atrial tachyarrhythmias may be treated with intravenous atenolol in 1-mg boluses or by constant intravenous infusion of esmolol, a short-acting beta blocker. Esmolol is given as an initial dose of 500 μg/kg intravenously over 1 minute, then continued at 50 μg/kg/min. If required, the infusion rate may be increased by 50 μg/kg/min every 4 minutes.

8. **Drugs to avoid**—*Atropine* should not be used as preoperative medication for patients with pheochromocytomas because it can precipitate arrhythmias and severe hypertension. Metoclopramide and glucagon can also precipitate a hypertensive crisis. *MAO* inhibitor antidepressants can provoke hypertensive crisis by blocking the metabolism of catecholamines. Other medications that can elicit hypertensive crisis include decongestants (eg, pseudoephedrine), epinephrine, amphetamines and amphetamine derivatives, and cocaine.

Labetalol is not recommended for preoperative or intraoperative management of pheochromocytomas because it aggravates postresection hypotension as a consequence of its long half-life. It can also paradoxically initially aggravate hypertension, because its beta-blocking effect may occur initially, allowing a brief period of unopposed α-receptor stimulation. Labetalol also inhibits MIBG uptake and causes misleading elevations in catecholamine determinations in certain assays. *Diazoxide* is ineffective against hypertension caused by pheochromocytoma.

C. Anesthesia   Anesthetic agents such as intravenous propofol, enflurane, isoflurane, sufentanil, alfentanil, and nitrous oxide appear to be safe and effective. Atropine should not be used. Muscle relaxants with the least hypertensive effect should be employed (eg, vecuronium). Intraoperative hypertension can be managed by increasing the depth of anesthesia and by intravenous vasodilators for blood pressures over 160/90 mm Hg. Serum catecholamine levels drop sharply after adrenal vein ligation and profound hypotension can occur suddenly after resection of a pheochromocytoma. Therefore, it is prudent to stop the vasodilator infusion just prior to adrenal vein ligation.

D. Operative management   Perioperative mortality is about 2.4% overall, but morbidity rates of up to 24% have been reported. Surgical complications do occur and include splenectomy, which is more common with open abdominal exploration than with laparoscopic surgery. Reported surgical complication rates have been higher in patients with severe hypertension and in patients having reoperations. Surgical morbidity and mortality risks can be minimized by adequate preoperative preparation, accurate tumor localization, and meticulous intraoperative care.

1. **Laparoscopy**—Most pheochromocytomas can be resected laparoscopically, which has become the procedure of choice for removing most adrenal neoplasms that are under 6 cm in diameter. Adrenal laparoscopic surgery is usually performed through 4 subcostal ports of 10 to 12 mm. Laparoscopic surgery is widely used now that preoperative localization of the tumor is possible. However, tumors that are invasive or over 6 cm in diameter are more difficult to resect laparoscopically and may require open surgery. For larger pheochromocytomas, a lateral laparoscopic approach can be used, because it affords greater opportunity to explore the abdomen and inspect the liver for metastases. For patients with small adrenal pheochromocytomas and for those who have had prior abdominal surgery, a posterior laparoscopic approach may be preferred.

The laparoscope allows unsurpassed magnified views of the pheochromocytoma and its vasculature. Pheochromocytomas are bagged to reduce the risk of fragmentation and spread of tumor cells within the peritoneum or at the port site. Larger tumors can be removed through laparoscopic incisions that can be widened for the surgeon's hand (laparoscopic-assisted adrenalectomy). With laparoscopic surgery, hypotensive episodes are less frequent and less severe. Laparoscopic adrenalectomy has other advantages also compared with open adrenalectomy: less postoperative pain, faster return to oral foods, and shorter hospital stays (median 3 days vs 7 days for the open approach). This approach is the least invasive for the patient, who can usually begin eating and ambulating the next day. The laparoscopic approach may be used during pregnancy. The technique has also been used successfully for certain extra-adrenal paragangliomas. Surgical mortality is under 3% at referral centers.

2. **Needlescopic adrenalectomy**—This procedure uses three subcostal ports of 3 mm, with a larger umbilical port for tumor removal. In one series of 15 patients, this technique reduced surgical times and recovery time compared with the standard laparoscopic approach. However, more extensive experience with this technique is required.

3. **Adrenal cortex-sparing surgery**—All patients undergoing bilateral total adrenalectomies require life-long glucocorticoid and mineralocorticoid hormone replacement. To avoid adrenal insufficiency, patients with benign familial or bilateral pheochromocytomas have had successful selective laparoscopic resection of small pheochromocytomas, sparing the adrenal cortex. Such adrenal-sparing surgery has unfortunately resulted in a pheochromocytoma recurrence rate of about 24%.

4. **Open laparotomy**—Open laparotomy is indicated for patients with particularly large pheochromocytomas or paragangliomas, or for those with intra-abdominal metastases that require debulking. Large vascular paragangliomas can be considered for preoperative arterial embolization, but its efficacy is uncertain. An open anterior midline or subcostal approach usually yields adequate exposure. For patients with paragangliomas of the urinary bladder, a partial cystectomy can sometimes be curative. Other patients with larger bladder paragangliomas require a total cystectomy and construction of a diverting ureteroenterostomy if the tumor has not been fully resected. For patients with a curative total cystectomy, construction of a new ileal neobladder is possible.

E. Therapy for shock occurring after pheochromocytoma resection   Severe shock and cardiovascular collapse can occur immediately following ligation of the adrenal vein during resection of a pheochromocytoma, particularly in patients having norepinephrine-secreting tumors. Such hypotension may be due to desensitization of α_1-adrenergic receptors, persistence of antihypertensives, and low plasma volume. Preoperative preparation with calcium channel blockers or alpha blockade plus intravenous hydration or blood transfusions reduces the risk of shock. Intravenous antihypertensives are held just prior to ligation of the adrenal vein. Treatment of shock consists of large volumes of intravenous saline or colloid. Intravenous norepinephrine is sometimes required in very high doses.

F. Intravenous dextrose   Immediately following removal of a pheochromocytoma, intravenous 5% dextrose should be infused at a constant rate of about 100 mL/h to prevent the postoperative hypoglycemia that is otherwise frequently encountered.

Pregnancy and Pheochromocytoma

Pheochromocytomas occur in about 1 in every 50,000 pregnancies and are unrecognized antepartum in about 50% of cases. Such unsuspected pheochromocytomas result in a maternal mortality of 40% and a fetal mortality of 56%. However, if the diagnosis is made antepartum, the mortality is much lower. Hypertension is often misdiagnosed as eclampsia. Hypertensive crisis usually occurs during labor and can be associated with cardiac arrhythmias or pulmonary edema. Although maternal catecholamines do not cross the placenta, maternal hypertensive crisis is very dangerous for the fetus, causing uteroplacental insufficiency and fetal death.

Pregnant hypertensive patients are often treated with methyldopa that can cause false-positive testing for catecholamines by older fluorometric methodologies, but not by HPLC. Methyldopa does not cause interference with plasma or urine metanephrine measurements performed with tandem mass spectrometry. The localization of a pheochromocytoma in pregnancy is best done with MRI.

As soon as a pheochromocytoma is diagnosed, alpha blockade is commenced. Phenoxybenzamine is usually used. However, phenoxybenzamine crosses the placenta and accumulates in the fetus. After 26 days of maternal phenoxybenzamine therapy, cord blood levels in the newborn are 60% higher than the mother's serum levels. Therefore, some perinatal depression and hypotension may occur in newborns of mothers receiving phenoxybenzamine. For maternal treatment near term, a short-acting selective alpha blocker (eg, prazosin) would have an obvious theoretical advantage over long-acting alpha blockers; chronic use increases the risk of fetal demise. The starting dose of prazosin is 0.5 mg/d orally, increasing up to 10 mg orally twice daily if necessary.

There has been little experience with the use of calcium channel blockers to treat hypertension in pregnant women with pheochromocytoma. However, calcium channel blockers can be safely used during pregnancy and are not teratogenic in the first trimester. Therefore, nifedipine or nicardipine may be used to supplement or replace alpha blockade as needed.

If possible, beta blockade should not be used at all during pregnancy. Propranolol crosses the placenta and can cause intrauterine growth restriction. Newborns of mothers taking propranolol at delivery exhibit bradycardia, respiratory depression, and hypoglycemia. Therefore, during cesarean delivery, serious atrial tachyarrhythmias should be controlled by a short infusion of esmolol, a beta blocker with a very short half-life.

During the first 6 months of pregnancy, it is often possible to treat a woman with alpha blockade, followed by laparoscopic resection of the tumor. Although the fetus usually survives, spontaneous abortion is common despite a successful resection of the tumor. If a pheochromocytoma is not discovered until the last trimester, treatment consists of alpha blockade followed by elective cesarean delivery as early as feasible. Intravenous magnesium sulfate is a useful antihypertensive during surgery. Intravenous calcium channel blockers may be used to treat patients with hypertensive crisis caused by pheochromocytoma in pregnancy. The tumor is resected after the cesarean delivery. In the presence of an active pheochromocytoma, vaginal delivery should never be allowed, since life-threatening hypertensive crisis will predictably occur.

Pathology of Pheochromocytoma and Paraganglioma

On histopathology, pheochromocytomas are extremely vascular tumors with neurosecretory granules. Central necrosis is often present. The cells may be arranged in nests (zellballen pattern), anastomosing cords (trabecular pattern), or a combination of both. Cells vary in size with pleomorphic and eccentric nuclei that are often large and bizarre in appearance. The cells exhibit immunofluorescence staining for CgA and synaptophysin.

No single characteristic of pheochromocytoma or paraganglioma can determine whether a given tumor is malignant. Therefore, the definition of malignancy is based upon whether metastases are present. Metastases must be distinguished from additional paragangliomas by their location (liver, lung, bone) where sympathetic paraganglia are rare. Metastases must also be distinguished from intraperitoneal seeding, a phenomenon known as pheochromocytomatosis. Metastases can vary in virulence from relatively indolent to extremely aggressive (see discussion on malignant pheochromocytoma later).

Overall, about 26% of these tumors arise in patients with identifiable germline mutations. Individuals with no known family history of these tumors have about a 17% risk of harboring a known germline mutation. About 18% of cases develop in children. The earlier a tumor presents, the more likely that individual harbors a germline mutation. (See discussion on genetics of pheochromocytoma and paraganglioma, earlier.)

Adrenal pheochromocytomas and paragangliomas appear very similar on microscopy. Paragangliomas are often large and arise near the adrenal, making the distinction particularly difficult based upon preoperative localization scans. But it is important to distinguish these two tumors because paragangliomas are more likely to metastasize. One way to distinguish these tumors preoperatively is to evaluate their secretions. Tumors that secrete epinephrine (or its metabolite, metanephrine) are predictably adrenal pheochromocytoma. However, tumors that secrete strictly norepinephrine (or its metabolite normetanephrine) may be either pheochromocytoma or paraganglioma. Intraoperatively, the surgeon may be able to identify the adrenal gland as separate from the tumor. On pathology, it is often possible to visualize the adrenal cortex lying in close proximity to the pheochromocytoma or even arising out of the adrenal medulla. An intact adrenal gland may be included in the surgical specimen, indicating that the tumor was a juxta-adrenal paraganglioma. On microscopy, paragangliomas may have visible nerve ganglia.

Composite pheochromocytomas are rare tumors that exhibit histopathologic features of both pheochromocytoma and neuroblastoma. Such tumors have generally not recurred and have not exhibited *N-myc* amplification, which distinguishes them from typical neuroblastomas. Therefore, composite pheochtomoctyomas are considered to be a histological variant of pheochromocytomas.

Metastatic Pheochromocytoma and Paraganglioma (Table 11–17)

No pheochromocytoma or paraganglioma should be labeled *benign*. Histopathology cannot reliably determine whether a given tumor has metastasized. Such metastases can be microscopic and indolent, eluding detection with the most sensitive scanning and biochemical screening. Therefore, it is best to think of these tumors as either having detectable metastases (metastatic pheochromocytoma) or having *no detectable* metastases.

It is conceivable that *all* pheochromocytomas and paragangliomas metastasize single cells but that such cells will only grow if certain genes are downregulated and other genes upregulated. This concept is supported by genome-wide expression profiling of pheochromocytomas. These profiles have identified candidate genes that are differentially expressed in tumors with detectable metastases versus those with no detectable metastases. Gene expression arrays of pheochromocytomas with detectable metastases have demonstrated that five genes are differentially upregulated in these tumors.

Research in malignant pheochromocytoma has been hampered by the absence of a viable human cell line. However, a highly malignant mouse pheochromocytoma model has been developed in which a gene expression array has demonstrated the upregulation of 8 genes and the downregulation of 38 genes.

The risk for detectable metastases is higher under the following circumstances: extra-adrenal location (paraganglioma) or extensive local invasion. One surgical observation is that tumors that are stickier and more difficult to dissect from adjacent tissue are more likely to recur or metastasize. Tumors are also more likely to metastasize if they contain high levels of Ki-67, a protein expressed in proliferating cells that can be detected by the monoclonal antibody MIB-1 and quantified as a high MIB-1 score. Metastatic pheochromocytomas also have increased activity of telomerase. Tumors with high c-*myc* gene expression are more likely to be malignant. In one series, 50% of patients with malignant pheochromocytoma were found to have high serum levels of NSE, but in none of 13 patients in another series with benign pheochromocytomas.

Metastases are evident at the time of diagnosis in about 10% of patients with an adrenal pheochromocytoma. Another 5% to 10% are found to have metastatic disease or local recurrence within 20 years. In genetic syndromes, pheochromocytomas have been found to be metastatic or locally invasive at the time of diagnosis as follows: MEN 2A, 4%; VHL, 8%; and NF-1, 12%. Extra-adrenal paragangliomas commonly metastasize. In a Mayo Clinic series of paragangliomas, 15% had local invasion and 21% had detectable distant metastases at the time of initial surgery, with an overall 36% risk of local or distant metastasis.

Malignancy is determined only by the presence of metastases. CT or MRI scanning may not detect small metastases within their field and will certainly not visualize metastases outside their field. Therefore, following the resection of an apparently benign PHEO or PGL, long-term surveillance is required because metastases may not become clinically apparent for years or decades. Such surveillance includes regular lifetime clinical assessment and biochemical testing as indicated. Plasma-fractionated metanephrines is the most sensitive test to detect early recurrence or metastases. However, screening for metastases from nonsecretory paragangliomas should include serum CgA determinations. Plasma metanephrines and serum CgA usually fall into the normal range by 2 weeks following successful resection of a single benign pheochromocytoma. However, normal postoperative tests are not reliable indicators of benignancy, because small or nonsecretory metastases may still be present.

The differential diagnosis for apparent metastases includes second paragangliomas, multicentric paragangliomas, second pheochromocytomas, false-positive scanning, and intraperitoneal seeding of tumor (pheochromocytomatosis).

Sites of metastasis (see Table 11–17): Metastases from pheochromocytomas or paragangliomas typically involve bones (82%), liver (30%), lungs (36%), lymph nodes, the contralateral adrenal, and sometimes muscle. The bones most frequently involved include vertebrae, pelvis and ischium, clavicles, cranium, and proximal femurs and humeri. Tibia, radius, and ulna are occasionally involved. Patients with metastases and an SDHB mutation have a higher prevalence of metastases involving long bones compared to those without the mutation. PHEO/PGL metastases have a proclivity for the skull where they may form a dumbbell-type lesion, sometimes being palpable as a soft cyst-like bump; they also may grow inside the skull to impinge upon the brain. Prevertebral paragangliomas may destroy adjacent vertebrae, and spinal cord compression may occur. Most bone metastases affect the cortical bone; they may be indolent, but are often osteolytic and cause progressive bone destruction. Other bone metastases primarily involve trabecular bone and marrow; such metastases are usually visible on MRI but may be invisible on CT. Metastases to lymph nodes outside the abdomen are most frequent in the supraclavicular and inguinal regions. Metastases to muscle are usually indolent. These tumors have not been reported to metastasize to brain, although metastases to the cranium and skull base may impinge upon the brain, pituitary, and cranial nerves.

TABLE 11–17 Distribution of metastases in 50 cases of metastatic pheochromocytoma.

Region of Metastasis	Percentage
Bones	82%
Abdomen (nodes, peritoneum, local recurrence)	56%
Lung parenchyma	36%
Liver	30%
Pelvis (soft tissue)	20%
Mediastinum and lung hila	18%
Lymph nodes (extra-abdominal) especially supraclavicular and inguinal	14%
Chest wall	12%
Muscle	6%
Brain	0%

Gonias S, et al. Phase II study of high-dose [^{131}I]metaiodobenzylguanidine therapy for patients with metastatic pheochromocytoma and paraganglioma. *J Clin Oncol.* 2009;27:6162.

Note: One case of abdominal recurrence was peritoneal seeding (pheochromocytomatosis).

Metastases usually secrete norepinephrine and normetanephrine. Some metastases secrete predominantly dopamine. Metastases rarely secrete epinephrine or metanephrine, with the exception of some metastases from epinephrine-secreting adrenal pheochromocytomas. About 20% of primary paragangliomas and their metastases do not secrete catecholamines or metanephrines, but most continue to secrete CgA, which becomes a valuable tumor marker.

Assessing the growth rate of PHEO/PGL metastases: Treatment can be tailored to the tumor's rate of growth. Knowledge of the growth rate of a patient's metastases may be obtained through close biochemical surveillance and serial volumetric imaging with CT or MRI. Patients who are asymptomatic with a few indolent osseous metastases may elect to receive bisphosphonate therapy and delay life-threatening chemotherapy or radioisotope therapy, as long as they remain under close surveillance. Even patients with a symptomatic osteolytic metastasis may elect to receive targeted therapy rather than systemic treatment if their overall tumor burden is low.

Surveillance: A series of 110 Swedish patients with PHEO/PGL, treated surgically, found an unexpectedly high relative risk for developing non-PHEO/PGL malignancies (RR ≅2.0). Therefore, additional tumors should not be presumed to be metastases unless they have uptake on MIBG scanning or [18]FDA-PET scanning. Suspicious lesions without such uptake should be considered for biopsy. Patients with hereditary forms of PHEO or PGL can present with bilateral disease or develop second primaries, distinct from metastatic disease.

Biochemical surveillance: Such screening is best done with plasma-fractionated metanephrines and catecholamines (with dopamine), along with serum CgA. While this is sensitive for secretory metastases, false-positive testing occurs commonly. Adrenal PHEOs usually secrete both norepinephrine and epinephrine; metastases from adrenal PHEOs may sometimes continue to produce epinephrine, but more commonly produce norepinephrine and its metabolite normetanephrine. Extra-adrenal PGLs ordinarily produce only norepinephrine and normetanephrine and sometimes only CgA; their metastases do likewise.

Scan surveillance: CT or MRI scanning is the most sensitive for recurrence; however, they will not detect metastases that are outside their field and obtaining full-body CT or MRI scanning is logistically difficult. Radionuclide scanning is advantageous in that the entire body may be included in the scan. However, no radionuclide scan is 100% sensitive. PHEO/PGL metastases have variable avidity for MIBG. Even when the primary tumor is avid for MIBG, some or all of the metastases may not be visible on MIBG scanning. Some metastases are deficient in norepinephrine transporter (NET) expression and are invisible on ^{123}I-MIBG scanning, such that the scan's sensitivity for metastasis is only 57%. In a given individual, some metastases may be avid for MIBG, while others show virtually no uptake. When patients have a recurrence or progression of metastases after ^{131}I-MIBG therapy, metastases with less MIBG-avid are usually the ones that emerge or progress in size. When such imaging is negative, metastases may be detected with MRI or CT scanning. Metabolically active metastases are usually visible with ^{18}F-FDG-PET scanning, which has the additional advantage of being a whole-body scan with a sensitivity of about 76% for metastases. ^{18}F-FDA-PET has a sensitivity of about 78% for metastases. Octreoscan will often detect metastases that are not visible with other scans.

A. Surgery   It is usually best to resect the primary tumor as well as large metastases. This is especially true of secretory tumors that are causing hypertension and other symptoms that can be a threat to life. Even lung metastases may be resected. However, the decision about whether to resect metastases is a difficult one and must be based upon very thorough staging of the patient's tumor. Of course, when resecting secretory metastases, preoperative preparation is mandatory and hypertension must be adequately controlled.

B. Chemotherapy   Due to the rarity of pheochromocytoma and paraganglioma, there have been no large-scale series comparing available chemotherapies. However, there have been small series of patients and case reports from which to derive recommendations.

In vitro studies have found that cultured pheochromocytoma cells are protected from cytotoxic insult by amitriptyline and fluoxetine, possibly through upregulation of superoxide dismutase. Therefore, patients being treated for metastatic pheochromocytoma or paraganglioma should probably not take tricyclic antidepressants or selective serotonin reuptake inhibitors, although there have been no in vivo studies of their effect on survival.

Cyclophosphamide, vincristine, dacarbazine (CVD): In one series, 8 of 14 patients responded to this regimen, with a median remission of 21 months. CVD was delivered over 2 days and the cycles repeated every 3 to 4 weeks, indefinitely. After controlling symptoms of catecholamine excess, cycles of CVD were administered as follows: cyclophosphamide 750 mg/m^2, vincristine 1.4 mg/m^2, and dacarbazine 600 mg/m^2 on day 1, followed by dacarbazine 600 mg/m^2 on day 2. Metastases progressed in 9 of the 14 patients, and there were 6 deaths with short-term follow-up. About one-third of patients appear to have a sustained remission or stable disease, as long as CVD is continued. When chemotherapy is stopped, the tumors usually recur. Many patients cannot tolerate such a long-term regimen, due to fatigue, cytopenias, neuropathy, and other adverse reactions. However, some patients tolerate it reasonably well and may experience a complete biochemical remission. Once in remission, CVD cycles are continued at gradually increasing intervals. If complete biochemical remission is achieved, chemotherapy may be stopped, while the patient is kept under close surveillance for progressive disease.

Sunitinib: Partial remissions in metastatic pheochromocytoma have been reported with sunitinib, a tyrosine kinase inhibitor. Sunitinib is administered orally, usually in a dose of 50 mg daily in cycles of 4 weeks on, then 2 weeks off. The dosage may be adjusted in 12.5-mg increments according to response and toxicity. Sunitinib is metabolized in the liver by CYP3A4, so dose adjustments should be made for patients taking the wide variety of drugs that are inhibitors or inducers of CYP3A4. Sunitinib can cause serious adverse reactions, including heart failure, cardiac arrhythmias, marrow suppression, pancreatitis, hypo- or hyperthyroidism, nephrotic syndrome, and rhabdomyolysis with acute renal failure. Patients treated with sunitinib also commonly experience nausea, vomiting, diarrhea, hypertension, skin discoloration, mucositis, asthenia, dyspnea, myalgias, and arthralgias. The use of sunitinib has been limited by its expense.

C. Bisphosphonates   No controlled clinical trials have assessed the efficacy of bisphosphonates against osteolytic bone metastases from paragangliomas and pheochromocytomas. However, bisphosphonates have demonstrated effectiveness in other osteolytic solid tumors to reduce skeletal-related adverse events. Zoledronic acid is usually administered every 1 to 2 months as an intravenous infusion to patients with osteolytic bone metastases. Patients unable to tolerate zoledronic acid may tolerate intravenous pamidronate.

D. Radiation therapy   When administered to patients with symptomatic spinal or cranial metastases, radiation therapy can reduce pain and produce neurologic improvement. Although conventional radiation therapy is usually administered, Gamma Knife can be given to smaller symptomatic bone metastases. Conventional radiation therapy to large primary tumors or intra-abdominal metastases is not advisable, because it is usually ineffective and causes morbidity such as radiation enteritis and a proclivity to later surgical complications such as wound dehiscence, infections, and fistulas. However, small recurrent tumors can be treated with CyberKnife stereotactic radiosurgery. Radiation therapy to tumors reduces their uptake of ^{131}I-MIBG. Surgical debulking of large abdominal or thoracic tumors (or other therapies) is usually preferable to radiation therapy.

E. Arterial embolization and radiofrequency ablation   Before arterial embolization or radiofrequency ablation, patients with secretory pheochromocytomas or paragangliomas must be fully prepared such that their blood pressure is near normal as described earlier. Pretreatment includes alpha blockade and/or other measures such as beta blockade, calcium channel blockers, or metyrosine. Patients are monitored with arterial blood pressure transducers and given a central line before endotracheal general anesthesia. Anesthesia standby is necessary in case severe hypertension occurs, and it becomes necessary to administer intravenous antihypertensive drugs.

Arterial embolization has been used on rare occasions to reduce blood flow to paragangliomas and pheochromocytomas, either in preparation for surgery or for inoperable cases. These tumors are usually very vascular and preoperative embolization may reduce intraoperative hemorrhage. Also, embolizing the tumor's blood supply may slow its growth. However, there have been no controlled clinical trials as to its effectiveness. A major potential risk of embolization is that of pheochromocytoma crisis. However, embolization has been used successfully on secretory tumors where the patient has been fully prepared with alpha blockade and/or other measures. Localization arteriograms should use nonionic contrast.

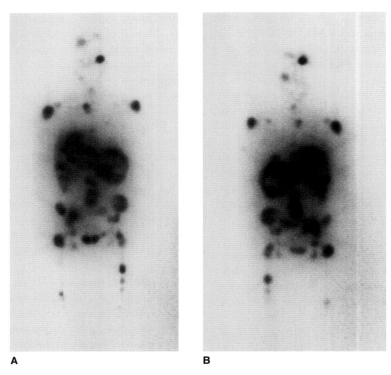

A   **B**

FIGURE 11–13 Posttherapy scan 1 week after administration of 500 mCi ^{131}I-MIBG. Patient is a 22-year-old woman with a large unresect-able pheochromocytoma in the left adrenal that has central hemorrhagic necrosis. There are widespread metastases to liver and bones. A metastasis to the left orbit has caused optic nerve compression and a visual field defect. A large metastasis to the left pelvis has caused pain and required prior external beam radiation therapy. **A.** Anterior image; **B.** Posterior image.

Radiofrequency (RF) thermal ablation has been success-fully for patients with metastatic PHEO/PGL, particularly for liver and bone metastases. Most reported RF ablations of bone metastases have targeted rib or ischial/pelvic lesions. Before RF ablations, the RF electrode(s) is guided into the tumor with ultra-sound and CT guidance. Single electrodes may be used for small lesions, while metastases over 2.5 cm diameter usually require triple parallel cluster needle electrodes.

F. ^{131}I-MIBG therapy (Figure 11–13)

^{131}I-MIBG is a treat-ment option for patients with metastatic or unresectable pheo-chromocytoma or paraganglioma whose tumors are avid for the isotope. ^{131}I-MIBG therapy was developed at the University of Michigan and first administered to patients with metastatic pheo-chromocytomas in 1983. Subsequently, many other patients have been treated with ^{131}I-MIBG. Treatment protocols have employed repeated doses of 100 to 200 mCi (3.7-7.4 GBq) or larger single doses of 500 to 1000 mCi (18.5-37 GBq). Uptake occurs in many nonfunctioning pheochromocytomas and metastases, and such treatment can be effective for these tumors as long as scanning demonstrates that they are avid for MIBG. Following therapy with ^{131}I-MIBG, once background radiation has dissipated, a posttreatment whole-body scan is obtained.

High-dose ^{131}I-MIBG therapy (≥500 mCi) is available at sev-eral medical centers in the United States and Europe. Precautions must be taken before giving ^{131}I-MIBG that exceeds 500 mCi or 12 mCi/kg body weight, since high doses of radioactive isotope

can cause serious bone marrow suppression. Before ^{131}I-MIBG therapy, patients are premedicated with potassium iodide to reduce the risk of thyroid damage that could be caused by any free ^{131}I generated through metabolism of ^{131}I-MIBG. Patients are pretreated with nonphenothiazine antiemetics; they remain hospi-talized in lead-shielded rooms until the emitted gamma radiation declines to acceptable levels, which usually requires about 5 to 7 days.

Complete or partial remissions, defined by strict RECIST (Response Evaluation Criteria in Solid Tumors), occur in about 22% of patients treated with ^{131}I-MIBG, while an additional 35% have minor responses and 8% have stable disease. However, 35% of patients experience progressive disease within a year after ther-apy. High-dose ^{131}I-MIBG appears to improve 5-year survival. It predictably causes some degree of bone marrow suppression that commences about 2.5 weeks after therapy. Other adverse reactions include nausea, occasional sialadenitis, and transient hair, hypogo-nadism, infertility, and an increased lifetime risk of second malig-nancies, particularly myelodysplasia and leukemia. ARDS and bronchiolitis obliterans organizing pneumonia (BOOP) are rare complications of treatment with ^{131}I-MIBG that have rarely occurred in patients treated with doses over 800 mCi. Repeated treatments may be required.

About 30% to 40% of patients with metastatic PHEO or PGL have insufficient uptake of MIBG for treatment to be effective. Also, there can be variable MIBG uptake into metastases in a given patient. So, theoretically, therapy with ^{131}I-MIBG could be made more effective if the tumor's uptake of MIBG could be increased. Pretreatment with nifedipine increased MIBG retention in four of eight patients in one report. Some patients with good uptake of MIBG on diagnostic scanning have disappointingly poor uptake of large therapeutic doses of ^{131}I-MIBG, possibly caused by competitive inhibition by large amounts of nonradioactive [127]I-MIBG that are present in most formulations of ^{131}I-MIBG.

Prognosis

The mortality rate for patients undergoing pheochromocytoma resection has dropped to under 3% due to improved medical preparation and surgical technique. Laparoscopic resections have reduced perioperative morbidity and shortened the length of hospitalization. However, even after complete resection of the pheochromocytoma, hypertension persists or recurs in 25% of patients. Recurrent hypertension is an indication for reevaluation for pheochromocytoma.

Following surgical resection of a benign pheochromocytoma, patients have a 5-year survival rate of 96%. Risk factors for death from pheochromocytoma include tumor size over 5 cm, metastatic disease, and local tumor invasion. However, the long-term mortality rate is much higher than expected. In a Swedish long-term outcome study of 121 patients with pheochromocytoma, there was no perioperative mortality, but 50% of patients remained hypertensive postoperatively. Of the 121 patients, 42 died during an observation period averaging 15 years, versus an expected 24 deaths in an age-matched control population. Thus, their relative risk of mortality was increased 78% (1.78). Of the 42 patients who died, 20 deaths were due to cardiovascular disease, 6 from associated neuroectodermal tumors, 5 from other malignancies, 7 from unrelated causes, and 4 from malignant pheochromocytoma.

Patients with pheochromocytoma or paraganglioma metastases have an average 5-year survival of about 50% from the time that metastases are detected. However, for patients in whom close surveillance and scanning find presymptomatic metastases, the average 5-year survival is probably longer, simply because the metastases are diagnosed at an earlier stage. Also, metastases are variably aggressive, between patients and within a given patient. Some metastases are quite indolent and may present clinically one or two decades after resection of the primary tumor. However, other metastases are exceptionally aggressive. Asymptomatic patients with only a few bone metastases tend to have the best prognosis, while those with a heavy burden of liver and lung metastases tend to have the most malignant disease.

Pheochromocytoma: Postoperative Long-Term Surveillance

All patients with pheochromocytomas require long-term postoperative surveillance. They require lifetime surveillance and aggressive treatment of all cardiovascular risk factors, due to their increased long-term risk of death from cardiovascular causes.

Additionally, patients should be tested for familial genetic syndromes and appropriately screened for associated malignancies (see "Genetic Conditions Associated with Pheochromocytomas and Paragangliomas," Tables 11–8 through 11–11). Persistent symptoms or hypertension can signify recurrence at the surgical site, seeding of the peritoneum, a contralateral pheochromocytoma, a paraganglioma, or possibly metastatic disease. About 10% of pheochromocytomas have metastasized at the time of diagnosis or soon postoperatively. However, occult metastatic disease is detected up to 20 years later in another 5%. Other patients develop multiple recurrent intra-abdominal tumors (pheochromocytomatosis) probably caused by tumor seeding that may occur spontaneously from the original tumor or during surgery.

Patients with secretory tumors are usually followed with plasma-fractionated free metanephrine determinations. Plasma-fractionated catecholamines and dopamine may also be obtained if they were predominantly secreted by the primary tumor. The first determination of postoperative plasma-fractionated free metanephrines is obtained at least 2 weeks after surgery, because catecholamine excretion often remains high for up to 10 days after successful surgery. Testing is obtained quarterly during the first year following surgery, then annually or semiannually for at least 5 years. Serum CgA is a useful tumor marker for patients with pheochromocytomas whose primary tumor secreted CgA and whose renal function is normal; elevated and rising levels of CgA usually indicate tumor recurrence or metastases. (See Chromogranin A, earlier.) Rarely, nonfunctioning tumors may later develop functioning metastases. Lifetime medical follow-up is required. Patients should continue to have annual physical examinations for life. Long-term biochemical follow-up is tailored to the individual patient.

For hypertensive patients, weekly home blood pressure monitoring is recommended for the first year postoperatively and monthly afterward. A rising blood pressure or recurrence of symptoms should trigger a full work-up for recurrent or metastatic pheochromocytoma.

A postoperative ^{123}I-MIBG scan or PET scan is recommended for all patients—but especially for those in whom there is any doubt about complete resection of the pheochromocytoma and for any patients with paraganglioma or multiple tumors. The postoperative scan is usually obtained several months after surgery. PET scanning is particularly useful for patients with metastatic PHEO/PGL or nonsecreting paragangliomas.

REFERENCES

Adrenal Medulla and Adrenergic Physiology

Biaggioni I, Robertson D. Adrenoceptor agonists and sympathomimetic drugs. In: Katzung BG, ed. *Basic and Clinical Pharmacology*. 11th ed. New York: McGraw Hill; 2009.

Bylund DB. Alpha- and beta-adrenergic receptors: Ahlquist's landmark hypothesis of a single mediator with two receptors. *Am J Physiol Endocrinol Metab.* 2007;29:E1479. [PMID: 17957033]

Goldstein DS, Eisenhofer G, Kopin IJ. Clinical catecholamine neurochemistry: a legacy of Julius Axelrod. *Cell Mol Neurobiol.* 2006;26:695. [PMID: 16871444]

Katzung BG. Introduction to autonomic pharmacology. In: Katzung BG, ed. *Basic and Clinical Pharmacology*. 11th ed. New York: McGraw Hill; 2009.

Rosengren AH, Jokubka R, Tojjar D, et al. Overexpression of alpha2A-adrenergic receptors contributes to type 2 diabetes. *Science.* 2010;327:217. [PMID: 19965390]

Autonomic Insufficiency

Bornstein SR, Breidert M, Ehrhart-Bornstein M, Kloos B, Scherbaum WA. Plasma catecholamines in patients with Addison's disease. *J Clin Endocrinol (Oxf).* 1995;42:215. [PMID: 7704967]

Granberg V, Ejskjaer N, Peakman M, Sundkvist G. Autoantibodies to autonomic nerves associated with cardiac and peripheral autonomic neuropathy. *Diabetes Care.* 2005;28:1959. [PMID: 16043739]

Gupta V, Lipsitz LA. Orthostatic hypotension in the elderly: diagnosis and treatment. *Am J Med.* 2007;120:841. [PMID: 17904451]

Pheochromocytoma and Paranglioma Reviews

Cohade C, Broussaud S, Louiset E, Bennet A, Huyghe E, Caron P. Ectopic Cushing's syndrome due to a pheochromocytoma: a new case in the post-partum and review of literature. *Gynecol Endocrinol.* 2009;10:1. [PMID: 19591016]

Guerrero MA, Schreinemakers JM, Vriens MR, et al Clinical spectrum of pheochromocytoma. *J Am Coll Surg.* 2009;209:727. [PMID: 19959041]

Lai EW, Perera SM, Havekes B, et al. Gender-related differences in the clinical presentation of malignant and benign pheochromocytoma. *Endocrine.* 2008;34:96. [PMID: 18982461]

Manger WM. The protean manifestations of pheochromocytoma. *Horm Metab Res.* 2009;41:658. [PMID: 19242899]

Pacak K, Lenders JWM, Eisenhofer G, eds. *Pheochromocytoma: Diagnosis, Localization, and Treatment.* Oxford: Blackwell Publishing; 2007.

Sutton MG, Sheps SG, Lie JT. Prevalence of clinically unsuspected pheochromocytoma. review of a 50-year autopsy series. *Mayo Clin Proc.* 1981;56:354. [PMID: 6453259]

Pheochromocytoma Pathophysiology

Kantorovich V, Pacak K. A new concept of unopposed beta-adrenergic overstimulation in a patient with pheochromocytoma. *Ann Intern Med.* 2005;142:1026. [PMID: 15968023]

Knauf F, Desir GV, Perazella MA. A case of extreme hemodynamic lability and hypocalcemia. *Am J Med Sci.* 2009;338:241. [PMID: 19590425]

Olson SW, Deal LE, Piesman M. Epinephrine-secreting pheochromocytoma presenting with cardiogenic shock and profound hypocalcemia. *Ann Intern Med.* 2004;140:849. [PMID: 15148085]

Schifferdecker B, Kodali D, Hausner E, Aragam J. Adrenergic shock—an overlooked clinical entity? *Cardiol Rev.* 2005;13:69. [PMID: 15705255]

Genetic Aspects of Pheochromocytoma and Paraganglioma

Boedeker CC, Erlic Z, Richard S, et al. Head and neck paragangliomas in von Hippel-Lindau and multiple endocrine neoplasia, type 2. *J Clin Endocrinol Metab.* 2009;94:1938. [PMID: 19336503]

Ladroue C, Carcenac R, Leporrier M, et al. PHD2 mutation and congenital erythrocytosis with paraganglioma. *N Engl J Med.* 2008;359:25. [PMID: 19092153]

McNeill A, Rattenberry E, Barber R, Killick P, MacDonald F, Maher ER. Genotype-phenotype correlations in VHL exon deletions. *Am J Med Genet A.* 2009;149A:2147. [PMID: 19764026]

Neumann HP, Vortmeyer A, Schmidt D, et al. Evidence of MEN-2 in the original description of classic pheochromocytoma. *N Engl J Med.* 2007;357:1311. [PMID: 17898100]

Neumann HP, Eng C. The approach to the patient with paraganglioma. *J Clin Endocrinol Metab.* 2009;94:2677. [PMID: 19657044]

Pasini B, McWhinney SR, Bei T, et al. Clinical and molecular genetics of patients with the Carney-Stratakis syndrome and germline mutations of the genes coding for the succinate dehydrogenase subunits SDHB, SDHC, and SDHD. *Eur J Hum Genet.* 2008;16:79. [PMID: 17667967]

Ricketts CJ, Forman JR, Rattenberry E, et al. Tumour risks and genotype-phenotype-proteotype analysis in 358 patients with germline mutations in SDHB and SDHD. *Hum Mutat.* 2010;31:41. [PMID: 19802898]

Rybicki EZ, Rybicki L, Peczkowska M, et al. Clinical predictors and algorithm for the genetic diagnosis of pheochromocytoma patients. *Clin Cancer Res.* 2009;15:6378. [PMID: 19825962]

Solis DC, Burnichon N, Timmers HJ, et al. Penetrance and clinical consequences of a gross SDHB deletion in a large family. *Clin Genet.* 2009;75:354. [PMID: 19389109]

Timmers HJ, Kozupa A, Eisenhofer G, et al. Clinical presentations, biochemical phenotypes, and genotype-phenotype correlations in patients with succinate dehydrogenase subunit B-associated pheochromocytomas and paragangliomas. *J Clin Endocrinol Metab.* 2007;92:779. [PMID:17200167]

Yeh IT, Lenci RE, Qin Y, et al. A germline mutation of the KIF1B beta gene on 1p36 in a family with neural and nonneural tumors. *Hum Genet.* 2008;124:279. [PMID:18726616]

Diagnostic Tests and Differential Diagnosis for Pheochromocytoma

De Jong WH, Eisenhofer G, Post WJ, et al. Dietary influences on plasma and urinary metanephrines: implications for the diagnosis of catecholamine-producing tumors. *J Clin Endocrinol Metab.* 2009;94:2841. [PMID: 19567530]

Deutschbein T, Unger N, Jaeger A, Broecker-Preuss M, Mann K, Petersenn S. Influence of various confounding variables and storage conditions on metanephrine and normetanephrine levels in plasma. *Clin Endocrinol (Oxf).* 2009;Dec 18. [PMID: 20039892]

Eisenhofer G, Goldstein DS, Walther MM, et al. Biochemical diagnosis of pheochromocytoma: how to distinguish true- from false-positive test results. *J Clin Endocrinol Metab.* 2003;88:2656. [PMID: 12788870]

Kim BW, Lee BI, Kim HK, et al. Influence of long-term gastric acid suppression therapy on the expression of serum gastrin, chromogranin A, and ghrelin. *Korean J Gastroenterol.* 2009;53:126. [PMID: 19237833]

Sethi PS, Hiser W, Gaffar H, et al. Fatal pheochromocytoma crisis precipitated by dobutamine stress echocardiography. *Eur J Echocardiogr.* 2008;9:819. [PMID: 18579490]

Vanderveen KA, Thompson SM, Callstrom MR, et al. Biopsy of pheochromocytoma and paraganglioma: potential for disaster. *Surgery.* 2009;146:1158. [PMID: 19958944]

Weise M, Merke DP, Pacak K, Walther MM, Eisenhofer G. et al. Utility of plasma free metanephrines for detecting childhood pheochromocytoma. *J Clin Endocrinol Metab.* 2002;87:1955. [PMID: 11994324]

Yu R, Weu N. False positive test results for pheochromocytoma from 2000 to 2008. *Exp Clin Endocrinol Diabetes.* 2009;Dec 8. [PMID: 19998239]

Localizing Scans for Pheochromocytoma and Paraganglioma

Baid SK, Lai EW, Wesley RA, et al. Brief communication: radiographic contrast infusion and catecholamine response in patients with pheochromocytoma. *Ann Intern Med.* 2009;150:27. [PMID: 19124817]

Havekes B, Lai EW, Corssmit EP, Romijn JA, Timmers HJ, Pacak K. Detection and treatment of pheochromocytomas and paragangliomas: current standing of MIBG scintigraphy and future role of PET imaging. *Q J Nucl Med Mol Imaging.* 2008;52:419. [PMID: 19088695]

Imani F, Agopian VG, Auerbach MS, et al. 18F-FDOPA PET and PET/CT accurately localize pheochromocytoma. *J Nucl Med.* 2009;50:513. [PMID: 19289420]

Kaji P, Carrasquillo JA, Linehan WM, et al. The role of 6-[18F]fluorodopamine positron emission tomography in the localization of adrenal pheochromocytoma associated with von Hippel-Lindau syndrome. *Eur J Endocrinol.* 2007;156:483. [PMID: 17389464]

Koopmans KP, Jager PL, Kema IP, Kerstens MN, Albers F, Dullaart RP. ^{111}In-octreotide is superior to ^{123}I-metaiodobenzylguanidine for scintigraphic detection of head and neck paragangliomas. *J Nucl Med.* 2008;48:1232. [PMID: 18632829]

Timmers HY, Chen CC, Carrasquillo JA, et al. Comparison of ^{18}F-fluro-L-DOPA, ^{18}F-fluoro-deoxyglucose, and ^{18}F-fluorodopamine PET and ^{123}I-MIBG scintigraphy in the localization of pheochromocytoma and paraganglioma. *J Clin Endocrinol Metab.* 2009;94:4757. [PMID: 19864450]

Wiseman GA, Pacak K, O'Dorisio MS, et al. Usefulness of ^{123}I-MIBG scintigraphy in the evaluation of patients with known or suspected primary or metastatic pheochromocytoma or paraganglioma: results from a prospective multicenter trial. *J Nucl Med.* 2009;50:1448. [PMID: 19690028]

Incidental Adrenal Tumors

Gross MD. Contemporary imaging of incidentally discovered adrenal masses. *Nat Rev Urol.* 2009;6:363. [PMID: 19506582]

Johnson PT, Horton KM, Fishman EK. Adrenal mass imaging with multidetector CT: pathologic conditions, pearls, and pitfalls. *Radiographics.* 2009;29:1333. [PMID: 19755599]

Kopetschke R, Slisko M, Kilisli A, et al. Frequent incidental discovery of phaeochromocytoma: data from a German cohort of 201 phaeochromocytoma. *Eur J Endocrinol.* 2009;16:355. [PMID:19497985]

Mazzaglia PJ, Monchik JM. Limited value of adrenal biopsy in the evaluation of adrenal neoplasm: a decade of experience. *Arch Surg.* 2009;144:465. [PMID: 19451490]

Vanderveen KA, Thompson SM, Callstrom MR, et al. Biopsy of pheochromocytoma and paragangliomas: potential for disaster. *Surgery.* 2009;146:1158. [PMID: 19958944]

Wagnerova H, Dudasova D, Lazurova I. Hormonal and metabolic evaluation of adrenal incidentalomas. *Neoplasma.* 2009;56:521. [PMID: 19728761]

Medical Therapy for Pheochromocytoma

Che Q, Schreiber MJ Jr, Rafey MA. Beta-blockers for hypertension: are they going out of style? *Curr Drug Ther.* 2009;76:533. [PMID: 19726558]

Pacak K. Approach to the patient. Preoperative management of the pheochromocytoma patient. *J Clin Endocrinol Metab.* 2007;92:4069. [PMID: 17989126]

Westaby S, Shahir A, Sadler G, Flynn F, Ormerod O; Medscape. Mechanical bridge to recovery in pheochromocytoma myocarditis. *Nat Rev Cardiol.* 2009;6:482. [PMID: 19554007]

Pheochromocytoma in Pregnancy

Desai AS, Chutkow WA, Edelman E, Economy KE, Dec GW Jr. Clinical problem-solving. A crisis in late pregnancy. *N Engl J Med.* 2009;361:2271. [PMID: 19955528]

Oliva R, Angelos P, Kaplan E, Bakris G. Pheochromocytoma in pregnancy: a case series. *Hypertension.* 2010; 55:600. [PMID: 20083723]

Ross JJ, Desai AS, Chutkow WA, Economy KE, Dec GW Jr. Interactive medical case. A crisis in late pregnancy. *N Engl J Med.* 2009;361:e45. [PMID: 19916244]

Sarathi V, Lila AR, Bandgar TR, Menon PS, Shah NS. Pheochromocytoma and pregnancy: a rare but dangerous combination. *Endocr Pract.* 2010;16:300. [PMID: 20061281]

Surgery for Pheochromocytoma and Paraganglioma

Berber E, Tellioglu G, Harvey A, Mitchell J, Milas M, Siperstein A. Comparison of laparoscopic transabdominal lateral versus posterior retroperitoneal adrenalectomy. *Surgery.* 2009;146:621. [PMID: 19789020]

Bruynzeel H, Feelders RA, Groenland TH, et al. Risk factors for hemodynamic instability during surgery for pheochromocytoma. *J Clin Endocrinol Metab.* 2010;95:678. [PMID: 19965926]

Kazaryan AM, Marangos IP, Rosseland AR, et al. Laparoscopic adrenalectomy: Norwegian single-center experience of 242 procedures. *J Laparoendosc Adv Surg Tech A.* 2009;19:181. [PMID: 19216698]

Liao CH, Lai MK, Li HY, Chen SC, Chueh SC. Laparoscopic adrenalectomy using needlescopic instruments for adrenal tumors less than 5 cm in 112 cases. *Eur Urol.* 2008;54:640. [PMID: 18164803]

Meyer-Rochow GY, Soon PS, Delbridge LW, et al. Outcomes of minimally invasive surgery for phaeochromocytoma. *ANZ J Surg.* 2009;79:367. [PMID: 19566519]

Zhou J, Chen HT, Xiang J, Qu XH, Zhou YQ, Zang WF. Surgical treatment of cardiac pheochromocytoma: a case report. *Ann Thorac Surg.* 2009;88:278. [PMID: 19559246]

Radiation, Embolization and Radiofrequency Ablation of Paragangliomas, Pheochromocytomas, and Metastases

Baguet JP, Hammer L, Tremel F, Mangin L, Mallion JM. Metastatic phaeochromocytoma: risks of diagnostic needle puncture and treatment by arterial embolization. *J Hum Hypertens.* 2001;15:209. [PMID: 11317207]

Beland MD, Mayo-Smith WW. Ablation of adrenal neoplasms. *Abdom Imaging.* 2009;34:588. [PMID: 18830736]

Guss ZD, Batra S, Li G, et al. Radiosurgery for glomus jugulare: history and recent progress. *Neurosurg Focus.* 2009;27:E5. [PMID: 19951058]

Huy PT, Kania R, Duet M, Dessard-Diana B, Mazeron JJ, Benhamed R. Evolving concepts in the management of jugular paraganglioma: a comparison of radiotherapy and surgery in 88 cases. *Skull Base.* 2009;19:83. [PMID: 19568345]

Tasar M, Yetiser S. Glomus tumors: therapeutic role of selective embolization. *J Craniofac Surg.* 2004;15:497. [PMID: 15111818]

Venkatesan AM, Locklin J, Lai EW, et al. Radiofrequency ablation of metastatic pheochromocytoma. *J Vasc Interv Radiol.* 2009;20:1483. [PMID: 19875067]

Metastatic Pheochromocytoma and Paraganglioma

Adjallé R, Plouin PF, Pacak K, Lehnert H. Treatment of malignant pheochromocytoma. *Horm Metab Res.* 2009;41:687. [PMID: 19672813]

Coleman RE, Stubbs JB, Barrett JA, de la Guardia M, Lafrance N, Babich JW. Radiation dosimetry, pharmacokinetics, and safety of ultratrace iobenguane I-131 in patients with malignant pheochromocytoma/paraganglioma or metastatic carcinoid. *Cancer Biother Radiopharm.* 2009;24:469. [PMID: 19694582]

Goldsby R, Fitzgerald P. Meta[^{131}I]iodobenzylguanidine therapy for patients with metastatic and unresectable pheochromocytoma and paraganglioma. *Nuc Med Biol.* 2008;35:S1:49.

Gonias S, Goldsby R, Matthay KK, et al. Phase II study of high-dose [^{131}I] metaiodobenzylguanidine therapy for patients with metastatic pheochromocytoma and paraganglioma. *J Clin Oncol.* 2009;27:6162. [PMID: 19636009]

He J, Makey D, Fojo T, et al. Successful chemotherapy of hepatic metastases in a case of succinate dehydrogenase subunit B-related paraganglioma. *Endocrine.* 2009;36:189. [PMID: 19618298]

Huang H, Abraham J, Hung E, et al. Treatment of malignant pheochromocytoma/paraganglioma with cyclophosphamide, vincristine, and dacarbazine: recommendation from a 22-year follow-up of 18 patients. *Cancer.* 2008;113:2020. [PMID: 18780317]

Jimenez C, Cabanillas ME, Santarpia L, et al. Use of the tyrosine kinase inhibitor sunitinib in a patient with von Hippel-Lindau disease: targeting angiogenic factors in pheochromocytoma and other Hippel-Lindau disease-related tumors. *J Clin Endocrinol Metab.* 2009;94:386. [PMID: 19017755]

Joshua AM. Rationale and evidence for sunitinib in the treatment of malignant paraganglioma/pheochromocytoma. *J Clin Endocrinol Metab.* 2009;94:5. [PMID: 19001511]

Lai EW, Joshi BH, Martiniova L, et al. Overexpression of interleukin-13 receptor-$\alpha 2$ in neuroendocrine malignant pheochromacytoma: a novel target for receptor directed anti-cancer therapy. *J Clin Endocrinol Metab.* 2009;94:2952. [PMID: 19491224]

Martiniova L, Lai EW, Elkahloun AG, et al. Characterization of an animal model of aggressive pheochromocytoma linked to a specific gene signature. *Clin Exp Metastasis.* 2009;26:239. [PMID:19169894]

Park KS, Lee JL, Ahn H, et al. Sunitinib, a novel therapy for anthracycline- and cisplatin-refractory malignant pheochromocytoma. *Jpn J Clin Oncol.* 2009;39:327. [PMID: 19264767]

Wu D, Tischler AS, Lloyd RV, et al. Observer variation in the application of the Pheochromocytoma of the Adrenal Gland Scaled Score. *Am J Surg Pathol.* 2009;33:599. [PMID: 19145205]

Zelinka T, Timmers HJ, Kozupa A, et al. Role of positron emission tomography and bone scintigraphy in the evaluation of bone involvement in metastatic pheochromocytoma and paraganglioma: specific implications for succinate dehydrogenase enzyme subunit B gene mutations. *Endocr Relat Cancer.* 2008;15:311. [PMID: 18310297]

Testes

Glenn D. Braunstein, MD

ACTH	Adrenocorticotropic hormone	**IVF**	In vitro fertilization
cAMP	Cyclic adenosine monophosphate	**LH**	Luteinizing hormone
DHEA	Dehydroepiandrosterone	**mRNA**	Messenger ribonucleic acid
DHT	Dihydrotestosterone	**PDE5**	Type 5 phosphodiesterase
FSH	Follicle-stimulating hormone	**PRL**	Prolactin
GnRH	Gonadotropin-releasing hormone	**SHBG**	Sex hormone–binding globulin
hCG	Human chorionic gonadotropin	**TGFβ**	Transforming growth factor β
ICSI	Intracytoplasmic sperm injection		

The testes contain two major components that are structurally separate and serve different functions. The **Leydig cells**, or **interstitial cells**, comprise the major endocrine component. The primary secretory product of these cells, testosterone, is responsible either directly or indirectly for embryonic differentiation along male lines of the external and internal genitalia, male secondary sexual development at puberty, and maintenance of libido and potency in the adult male. The **seminiferous tubules** comprise the bulk of the testes and are responsible for the production of approximately 30 million spermatozoa per day during male reproductive life (puberty to death).

Both of these testicular components are interrelated, and both require an intact hypothalamic-pituitary axis for initiation and maintenance of their function. In addition, several accessory genital structures are required for the functional maturation and transport of spermatozoa. Thus, disorders of the testes, hypothalamus, pituitary, or accessory structures may result in abnormalities of androgen or gamete production, infertility, or a combination of these problems.

ANATOMY AND STRUCTURE-FUNCTION RELATIONSHIPS (FIGURE 12–1)

TESTES

The adult testis is a prolate spheroid with a mean volume of 18.6 ± 4.8 mL. The average length is 4.6 cm (range, 3.6-5.5 cm), and the average width is 2.6 cm (range, 2.1-3.2 cm). The testes are located within the scrotum, which not only serves as a protective envelope but also helps to maintain the testicular temperature approximately 2°C (35.6°F) below abdominal temperature. Three layers of membranes—visceral tunica vaginalis, tunica albuginea, and tunica vasculosa—comprise the testicular capsule. Extensions of the tunica albuginea into the testicle as fibrous septa result in the formation of approximately 250 to 300 pyramidal lobules, each of which contains coiled seminiferous tubules. Within each testis there are over 400 meters of seminiferous tubules, and these structures account for about half of the testicular mass. The approximately 200 million androgen-producing Leydig cells, as well as the blood and lymphatic vessels, nerves, and fibroblasts, are interspersed between the seminiferous tubules.

The blood supply to the testes is derived chiefly from the testicular arteries, which are branches of the internal spermatic arteries. After traversing a complicated capillary network, blood enters multiple testicular veins that form an anastomotic network, the pampiniform plexus. The pampiniform plexuses coalesce to form the internal spermatic veins. The right spermatic vein drains directly into the vena cava; the left enters the renal vein.

The seminiferous tubules in the adult average 165 μm in diameter and are composed of Sertoli cells and germinal cells. The Sertoli cells line the basement membrane and form tight junctions with other Sertoli cells. These tight junctions prevent the passage of proteins from the interstitial space into the lumens of the seminiferous tubules, thus establishing a *blood–testis barrier*. Through extension of cytoplasmic processes, the Sertoli cells surround developing germ cells and provide an environment essential for germ cell differentiation. In addition, these cells have been shown to be responsible for the movement of germ cells from the

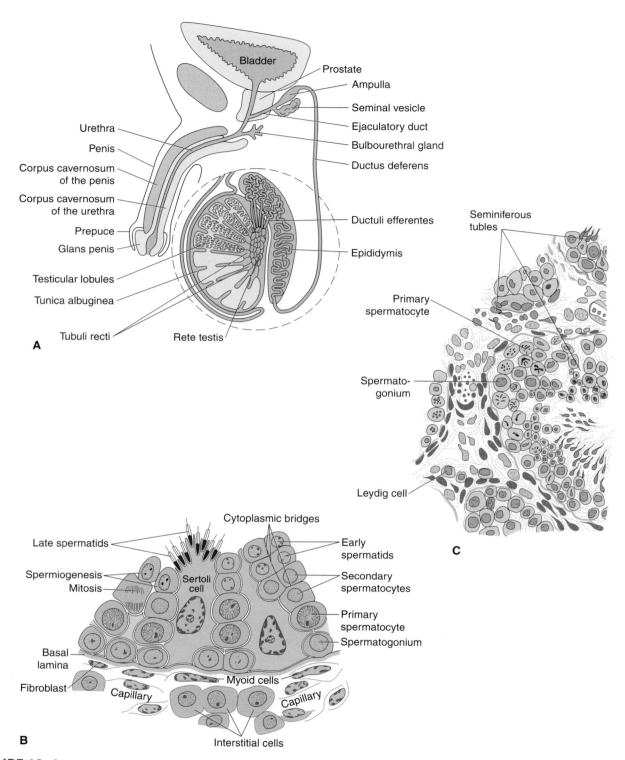

FIGURE 12–1 Male genital system. **A.** The testis and the epididymis are in different scales from the other parts of the reproductive system. Observe the communication between the testicular lobules. **B.** Structural organization of the human seminiferous tubule and interstitial tissue. This figure does not show the lymphatic vessels frequently found in the connective tissue. (**A** and **B** reproduced, with permission, from Junqueira LC, Carneiro J, Kelley RO. *Basic Histology*. 9th ed. McGraw-Hill; 1999.)
C. Section of human testis. (**C** reproduced, with permission, from Ganong WF. *Review of Medical Physiology*. 20th ed. McGraw-Hill; 2001.)

base of the tubule toward the lumen and for the release of mature sperm into the lumen. These cells also actively phagocytose damaged germ cells and residual bodies, which are portions of the germ cell cytoplasm not used in the formation of spermatozoa. Finally, in response to follicle-stimulating hormone (FSH) or testosterone, the Sertoli cells secrete androgen-binding protein, a molecule with high affinity for androgens. This substance, which enters the tubular lumen, provides a high concentration of testosterone to the developing germinal cells during the process of spermatogenesis.

More than a dozen different types of germ cells have been described in males. Broadly, they can be classified as spermatogonia, primary spermatocytes, secondary spermatocytes, spermatids, and spermatozoa. Spermatogenesis occurs in an orderly fashion, with the spermatocytes being derived from the spermatogonia via mitotic division. Through meiotic (or reduction) division, the spermatids are formed; they contain a haploid number of chromosomes (23). The interval from the beginning of spermatogenesis to release of mature spermatozoa into the tubular lumen is approximately 64 days. Although there is little variation in the duration of the spermatogenic cycle, a cross-section of a seminiferous tubule demonstrates several stages of germ cell development.

ACCESSORY STRUCTURES

The seminiferous tubules empty into a highly convoluted anastomotic network of ducts called the **rete testis**. Spermatozoa are then transported through efferent ductules and into a single duct, the epididymis, by testicular fluid pressure, ciliary motion, and contraction of the efferent ductules. During the approximately 12 to 14 days required for transit through the epididymis, spermatozoa undergo morphologic and functional changes essential to confer on the gametes the capacity for fertilizing an ovum. The epididymis also serves as a reservoir for sperm. Spermatozoa stored in the epididymis enter the vas deferens, a muscular duct 35 to 50 cm long that propels its contents by peristaltic motion into the ejaculatory duct.

In addition to the spermatozoa and the secretory products of the testes, retia testis, and epididymides, the ejaculatory ducts receive fluid from the seminal vesicles. These paired structures, 4.5 to 5.5 cm long, are composed of alveolar glands, connective tissue, and muscle. They are the source of seminal plasma fructose, which provides nourishment to the spermatozoa. In addition, the seminal vesicles secrete seminogelin I, phosphorylcholine, ergothioneine, flavins, prostaglandins, and antioxidants, including superoxide dismutase, catalase, and ascorbic acid. About 60% of the total volume of seminal fluid is derived from the seminal vesicles.

The ejaculatory ducts terminate in the prostatic urethra. There additional fluid (~20% of total volume) is added by the prostate, a tubuloalveolar gland with a fibromuscular stroma that weighs about 20 g and measures 4 cm × 2 cm × 3 cm. The constituents of the prostate fluid include spermine, citric acid, cholesterol, phospholipids, fibrinolysin, fibrinogenase, zinc, acid phosphatase, and prostate-specific antigen, a 34-kDa kallikrein-like serine protease. Fluid is also added to the seminal plasma by the bulbourethral (Cowper) glands and urethral (Littre) glands during its transit through the penile urethra.

PHYSIOLOGY OF THE MALE REPRODUCTIVE SYSTEM

GONADAL STEROIDS (FIGURE 12–2)

The three steroids of primary importance in male reproductive function are testosterone, dihydrotestosterone, and estradiol. From a quantitative standpoint, the most important androgen is testosterone. Over 95% of the testosterone is secreted by the testicular Leydig cells. In addition to testosterone, the testes secrete small amounts of the potent androgen dihydrotestosterone and the weak androgens dehydroepiandrosterone (DHEA) and androstenedione. The Leydig cells also secrete small quantities of estradiol, estrone, pregnenolone, progesterone, 17α-hydroxypregnenolone, and 17α-hydroxyprogesterone. The steps in testicular androgen biosynthesis are illustrated in Figure 12–2.

Dihydrotestosterone and estradiol are derived not only by direct secretion from the testes but also by conversion in peripheral tissues of androgen and estrogen precursors secreted by both the testes and the adrenals. Thus, about 80% of the circulating concentration of these two steroids is derived from such peripheral conversion. Table 12–1 summarizes the approximate contributions of the testes, adrenals, and peripheral tissues to the circulating levels of several sex steroid hormones in men.

In the blood, androgens and estrogens exist in either a free (unbound) state or as bound to serum proteins. Although about 38% of testosterone is weakly bound to albumin, the major binding protein is *sex hormone–binding globulin* (SHBG), a high affinity, low capacity binding protein, which binds 60% of the testosterone. This glycosylated dimeric protein is homologous to, yet distinct from, the androgen-binding protein secreted by the Sertoli cells. SHBG is synthesized in the liver, with the gene located on the short arm of chromosome 17. The serum concentrations of this protein are increased by estrogen, tamoxifen, phenytoin, or thyroid hormone administration and by hyperthyroidism and cirrhosis and are decreased by exogenous androgens, glucocorticoids, or growth hormone and by hypothyroidism, acromegaly, obesity, and hyperinsulinemic states. About 2% of the circulating testosterone is not bound to serum proteins and is able to enter cells and exert its metabolic effects. In addition, some of the albumin-bound testosterone may dissociate from the protein and enter target tissues; thus, the amount of bioavailable testosterone may be greater than just the amount of non–protein-bound testosterone.

As noted later, testosterone may be converted to dihydrotestosterone within specific androgen target tissues. Most circulating testosterone is converted primarily by the liver into various metabolites such as androsterone and etiocholanolone, which, after conjugation with glucuronic or sulfuric acid, are excreted in the urine as 17-ketosteroids. However, it should be noted that only 20% to 30% of the urinary 17-ketosteroids are derived from testosterone metabolism. The majority of the 17-ketosteroids are

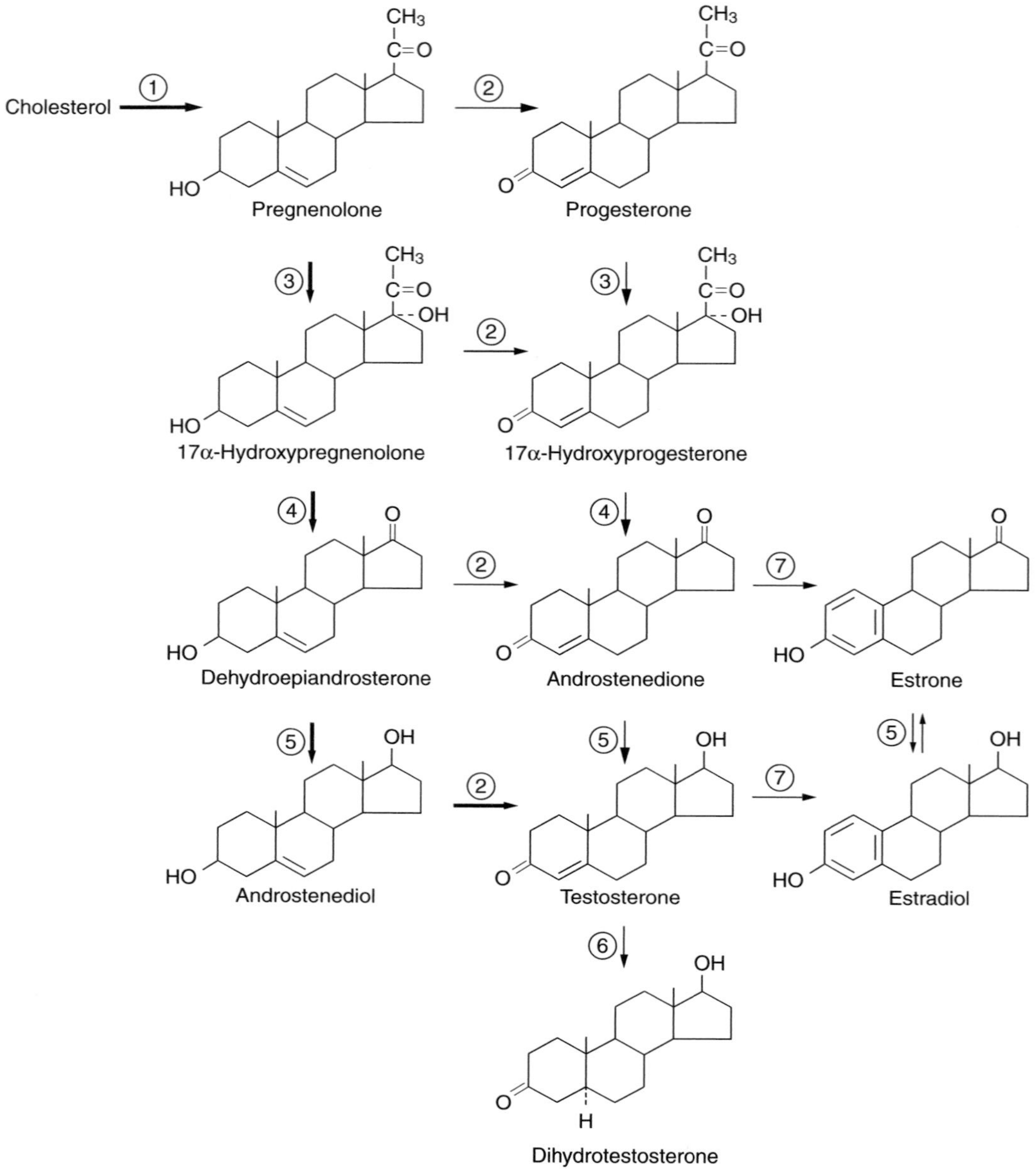

FIGURE 12–2 Pathways for testicular androgen and estrogen biosynthesis. Heavy arrows indicate major pathways. Circled numbers represent enzymes as follows: ①, CYP11A1 (20,22-desmolase; P450scc); ②, 3β-hydroxysteroid dehydrogenase and Δ^5,Δ^4-isomerase II (3βHSDII); ③, CYP17 (17α-hydroxylase; P450c17); ④, CYP17 (17,20-lyase; P450c17); ⑤, 17α-HSD3 (17α-hydroxysteroid dehydrogenase 3; 17-ketoreductase); ⑥, 5α-reductase; ⑦, CYP19 (aromatase). StAR, steroidogenic acute regulatory protein. (See also Figures 9–4, 13–4, and 14–13.)

formed from the metabolism of adrenal steroids. Therefore, 17-ketosteroid determinations do not reliably reflect testicular steroid secretion.

Testosterone leaves the circulation and rapidly traverses the cell membrane (Figure 12–3). In most androgen target cells, testosterone is enzymatically converted to the more potent androgen dihydrotestosterone by the microsomal isoenzyme 5α-reductase-2, which has a pH optimum of 5.5. Another isoenzyme, 5α-reductase-1, has a pH optimum near 8.0 and may involve androgen action in the skin, but it is not active in the urogenital tract. Dihydrotestosterone as well as testosterone then binds to the

same specific intracellular receptor protein (R_c in Figure 12–3) that is distinct from both androgen-binding protein and SHBG. The genes that encode for this protein are located on the X chromosome. The androgen receptor is a member of the steroid-thyroid hormone nuclear superfamily. It is synthesized in the cytoplasm and is associated with several heat shock proteins and immunophilins. When testosterone or dihydrotestosterone binds to the receptor, it dissociates from the multiprotein complex, and conformational changes take place that allow it to form a homodimer with another hormone-androgen receptor molecule and to be translocated into the nucleus through binding to

TABLE 12–1 Relative contributions (approximate percentages) of the testes, adrenals, and peripheral tissues to circulating levels of sex steroids in men.

Hormone	Testicular Secretion	Adrenal Secretion	Peripheral Conversion of Precursors
Testosterone	95	<1	<5
Dihydrotestosterone	<20	<1	80
Estradiol	<20	<1	80
Estrone	<2	<1	98
DHEA sulfate	<10	90	—

importins (R_n in Figure 12–3). In the nucleus, the androgen–androgen receptor complex binds to androgen response elements in DNA through the DNA-binding domain of the receptor and interacts with protein coactivators, which allows the polymorphic transactivating domain of the receptor to initiate transcriptional activity. This results in the synthesis of messenger RNA (mRNA), which is eventually transported to the cytoplasm, where it directs new protein synthesis and other changes that together constitute androgen action. In addition to this classical genomic pathway of androgen action, which brings about action in hours to days, androgens may exhibit a rapid effect through nonclassical signaling pathways involving cell surface actions that alter cellular calcium influx.

A variety of biologic effects of androgens have been defined in males. As discussed in Chapter 14, they are essential for appropriate differentiation of the internal and external male genital system during fetal development. During puberty, androgen-mediated growth of the scrotum, epididymis, vas deferens, seminal vesicles, prostate, and penis occurs. The functional integrity of these organs requires androgens. Androgens stimulate skeletal muscle growth and growth of the larynx, which results in deepening of the voice, and of the epiphysial cartilaginous plates, which results in the pubertal growth spurt. Both ambisexual (pubic and axillary) hair growth and sexual (beard, mustache, chest, abdomen, and back) hair growth are stimulated, as is sebaceous gland activity. Other effects include stimulation of erythropoiesis and social behavioral changes.

CONTROL OF TESTICULAR FUNCTION

Hypothalamic-Pituitary-Leydig Cell Axis (Figure 12–4)

The hypothalamus synthesizes a decapeptide, gonadotropin-releasing hormone (GnRH), and secretes it in pulses every 30 to 120 minutes into the hypothalamohypophysial portal blood. After

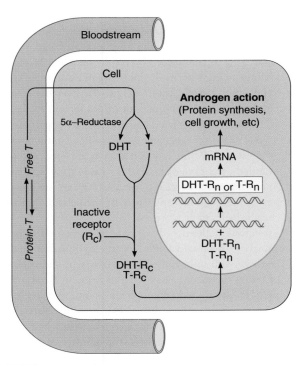

FIGURE 12–3 Mechanisms of androgen action (DHT, dihydrotestosterone; mRNA, messenger RNA; Rc, inactive receptor; R_n, activated nuclear receptor; T, testosterone).

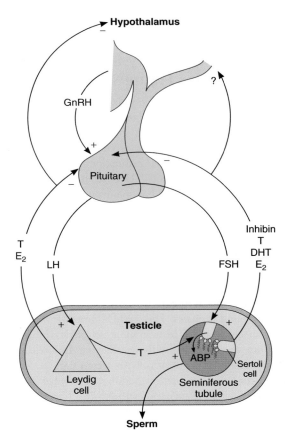

FIGURE 12–4 Hypothalamic-pituitary-testicular axis (ABP, androgen-binding protein; DHT, dihydrotestosterone; E_2, estradiol; FSH, follicle-stimulating hormone; GnRH, gonadotropin-releasing hormone; LH, luteinizing hormone; T, testosterone; +, positive influence; –, negative influence).

reaching the anterior pituitary, GnRH binds to the gonadotrophs and stimulates the release of both luteinizing hormone (LH) and, to a lesser extent, FSH into the general circulation. LH is taken up by the Leydig cells, where it binds to specific membrane receptors. The LH receptor is a G protein–coupled receptor containing seven transmembrane domains with a serine- and threonine-rich cytoplasmic region containing a phosphorylation site and a 350- to 400 amino acid extracellular hormone-binding domain. The binding of LH to the receptor leads to activation of adenylyl cyclase and generation of cAMP and other messengers. It also stimulates the synthesis of a steroidogenic acute regulatory protein. This enhances the transfer of cholesterol into the inner mitochondrial membrane, leading to the synthesis and secretion of androgens. In turn, the elevation of androgens inhibits the secretion of LH from the anterior pituitary through a direct action on the pituitary and an inhibitory effect at the hypothalamic level. Both the hypothalamus and the pituitary have androgen and estrogen receptors. Experimentally, pure androgens such as dihydrotestosterone (DHT) reduce LH pulse frequency, whereas estradiol reduces LH pulse amplitude. However, the major inhibitory effect of androgen on the hypothalamus appears to be mediated principally by estradiol, which may be derived locally through the aromatization of testosterone. Leydig cells also secrete small quantities of cytokines and other peptides, which may be important for paracrine regulation of testicular function.

Hypothalamic-Pituitary-Seminiferous Tubular Axis (See Figure 12–4)

After stimulation by GnRH, the gonadotrophs secrete FSH into the systemic circulation. This glycoprotein hormone binds to specific receptors in the Sertoli cells and stimulates the production of androgen-binding protein. FSH is necessary for the initiation of spermatogenesis. However, full maturation of the spermatozoa appears to require not only an FSH effect but also testosterone. Indeed, the major action of FSH on spermatogenesis may be via the stimulation of androgen-binding protein production, which allows a high intratubular concentration of testosterone to be maintained.

In addition to androgen-binding protein, the Sertoli cell secretes several other substances, including insulin-like growth factor-I, transferrin, Müllerian duct inhibitory factor, and inhibin. At least three genes have been found to direct inhibin synthesis. Although two forms of inhibin have been identified, only inhibin B has been found in males. This 32-kDa protein, which is composed of an alpha and a beta subunit, selectively inhibits FSH release from the pituitary without affecting LH release. FSH directly stimulates the Sertoli cells to secrete inhibin B. Serum inhibin B concentrations reflect Sertoli cell number and sperm production. They correlate with testicular size. There is a reciprocal relationship between serum inhibin B and FSH levels, and inhibin B is therefore probably a physiologic regulator of pituitary FSH secretion, possibly together with the gonadal steroids. Inhibin levels decline with advancing age.

Two additional inhibin-related proteins that have been identified in porcine follicular fluid may also be present in the testes. These factors, designated follicle regulatory protein and activin,

are composed of inhibin beta subunit dimers and can selectively stimulate pituitary FSH secretion in vitro. They are structurally similar to transforming growth factor β (TGFβ), which can also stimulate pituitary FSH release. The physiologic role, if any, that follicle regulatory protein, activin, and TGFβ have in the regulation of FSH secretion is unknown.

EVALUATION OF MALE GONADAL FUNCTION

CLINICAL EVALUATION

Clinical Presentation

The clinical presentation of patients with deficient testosterone production or action depends on the age at onset of hypogonadism. Androgen deficiency during the second to third months of fetal development results in varying degrees of ambiguity of the genitalia and male pseudohermaphroditism. If the deficiency develops during the third trimester, defects in testicular descent leading to cryptorchidism as well as micropenis may occur. These topics are covered in Chapters 14 and 15.

Prepubertal androgen deficiency leads to poor secondary sexual development and eunuchoid skeletal proportions. The penis fails to enlarge, the testes remain small, and the scrotum does not develop the marked rugae characteristic of puberty. The voice remains high-pitched and the muscle mass does not develop fully, resulting in less than normal strength and endurance. The lack of appropriate stimulation of sexual hair growth results in sparse axillary and pubic hair (which receive some stimulation from adrenal androgens) and absent or very sparse facial, chest, upper abdominal, and back hair. Although the androgen-mediated pubertal growth spurt fails to take place, the epiphysial plates of the long bones continue to grow under the influence of insulin-like growth factor-I and other growth factors. Thus, the long bones of the upper and lower extremities grow out of proportion to the axial skeleton. Healthy white men have an average upper segment (crown to pubis) to lower segment (pubis to floor) ratio of greater than 1, whereas prepubertal hypogonadism results in a ratio of less than 1. Similarly, the ratio of total arm span to total height averages 0.96 in white men. Because of the relatively greater growth in the upper extremities, the arm span of eunuchoid individuals exceeds height by 5 cm or more.

If testosterone deficiency develops after puberty, the patient may complain of decreased libido, erectile dysfunction, and low energy. Patients with mild androgen deficiency or androgen deficiency of recent onset may not note a decrease in facial or body hair growth; it appears that although adult androgen levels must be achieved to *stimulate* male sexual hair growth, relatively low levels of androgens are required to *maintain* sexual hair growth. With long-standing hypogonadism, the growth of facial hair will diminish, and the frequency of shaving may also decrease (Figure 12–5). In addition, fine wrinkles may appear in the corners of the mouth and eyes and, together with the sparse beard growth, result in the classic hypogonadal facies.

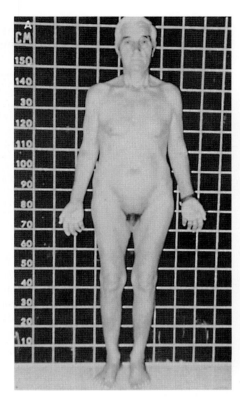
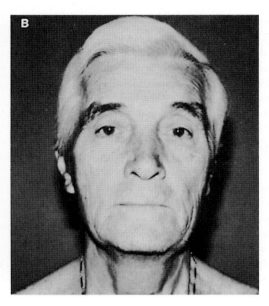

FIGURE 12–5 **A.** Hypogonadal habitus. Note absence of body and facial hair as well as feminine body distribution. **B.** Hypogonadal facies. Note absence of facial hair and fine wrinkles around the corners of the eyes and lips.

Genital Examination

Adequate assessment of the genitalia is essential in the evaluation of male hypogonadism. The examination should be performed in a warm room in order to relax the dartos muscle of the scrotum. The penis should be examined for the presence of hypospadias, epispadias, and chordee (abnormal angulation of the penis due to a fibrotic plaque), which may interfere with fertility. The fully stretched dorsal penile length should be measured in the flaccid state from the pubopenile skin junction to the tip of the glans. The normal range in adults is 12 to 16 cm (10th and 90th percentiles, respectively).

Assessment of testicular volume is also vital to the evaluation of hypogonadism. Careful measurement of the longitudinal and transverse axes of the testes may be made and testicular volume (V) calculated from the formula for a prolate spheroid: $V = 0.52 \times$ length $\times$ width^2. The mean volume for an adult testis is 18.6 ± 4.8 mL. Alternatively, volume may be estimated with the Prader orchidometer, which consists of a series of plastic ellipsoids ranging in volume from 1 to 25 mL. Each testis is compared with the appropriate ellipsoid. Adults normally have volumes greater than 15 mL by this method.

Because about half of testicular volume is composed of seminiferous tubules, decrease in volume indicates lack of tubular development or regression of tubular size. The consistency of the testicle should be noted. Small, firm testes are characteristic of hyalinization or fibrosis, as may occur in Klinefelter syndrome.

Small, rubbery testes are normally found in prepubertal males; in an adult, they are indicative of deficient gonadotropin stimulation. Testes of soft consistency are characteristically found in individuals with postpubertal testicular atrophy.

The epididymis and vas deferens should also be examined. One of the most important parts of the examination is evaluation for the presence of varicocele resulting from incompetence of the internal spermatic vein. As will be discussed later, this is an important and potentially correctable cause of male infertility. The patient should be examined in the upright position while performing the Valsalva maneuver. The examiner should carefully palpate the spermatic cords above the testes. A varicocele can be felt as an impulse along the posterior portion of the cord. About 85% of varicoceles are located on the left side, and 15% are bilateral.

LABORATORY TESTS OF TESTICULAR FUNCTION

Semen Analysis

With some exceptions, a normal semen analysis excludes gonadal dysfunction. However, a single abnormal semen analysis is not a sufficient basis for a diagnosis of disturbance of testicular function, because marked variations in several of the parameters may be seen in normal individuals: at least three semen samples should be examined over a 2- to 3-month interval in order to evaluate this facet of male gonadal function. As noted earlier, approximately 3 months are required for completion of the spermatogenic cycle and movement of the mature spermatozoa through the ductal system. Therefore, when an abnormal semen sample is produced, one must question the patient about prior fever, trauma, drug exposure, and other factors that may temporarily damage spermatogenesis.

The semen should be collected by masturbation after 2 to 7 days of sexual abstinence and examined within 1 hour after collection. Normal semen has a volume of more than 2 to 4 mL, with 20×10^6 or more sperms per milliliter. Over half of the spermatozoa should exhibit progressive motility, and 30% or more should have normal morphology.

Steroid Measurements

Each of the gonadal steroids may be measured by specific assays. Although single determinations may distinguish between normal individuals and patients with severe hypogonadism, mild defects in androgen production may be missed. In normal individuals, there are frequent, rapid pulsatile changes in serum testosterone concentration as well as a slight early morning elevation. Therefore, at least three separate blood samples should be collected at 20- to 40-minute intervals during the morning for testosterone measurement. The testosterone may be measured in each of the serum samples, or equal aliquots of each of the three serum samples may be combined, mixed, and subjected to testosterone analysis. The latter procedure provides a savings in cost as well as a mean serum testosterone concentration that takes into account the pulsatile release of testosterone.

Androgen and estrogen immunoassays measure total serum steroid concentrations. This is the sum of the free, biologically active hormone and the protein-bound moiety. There is a great deal of variability with different testosterone immunoassays, especially in the lower ranges. The most reliable methods are specific immunoassays following extraction of serum or gas chromatography (GC)- or liquid chromatography (LC)-tandem mass spectroscopy. Although in most circumstances it is not necessary to determine the actual quantity of free steroid hormones, in some situations alterations in the binding protein concentration may occur. Lowered concentrations of SHBG are seen in patients with hypothyroidism, obesity, and acromegaly. In these circumstances, the free testosterone concentration should be measured, because it may be normal when the total serum testosterone level is decreased. The normal male serum concentrations of gonadal steroids collected in the basal state are given in Table 12–2.

Gonadotropin and Prolactin Measurements

LH and, to a lesser extent, FSH are released in pulsatile fashion throughout the day. In addition, there is a diurnal variation with higher levels in the morning than in the evening. Therefore, as with testosterone, at least three blood samples should be obtained at 20- to 40-minute intervals during the morning. FSH and LH may be measured in each of the samples or in a single pooled

TABLE 12–2 Normal ranges for gonadal steroids, pituitary gonadotropins, and prolactin in men.

Hormone	Ranges
Testosterone, total	260-1000 ng/dL (9.0-34.7 nmol/L)
Testosterone, free	50-210 pg/mL (173-729 pmol/L)
Dihydrotestosterone	27-75 ng/dL (0.9-2.6 nmol/L)
Androstenedione	50-250 ng/dL (1.7-8.5 nmol/L)
Estradiol	10-50 pg/mL (3.67-18.35 pmol/L)
Estrone	15-65 pg/mL (55.5-240 pmol/L)
FSH	1.6-8 mIU/mL (1.6 8 IU/L)
LH	1.5-9.3 mIU/mL (1. 5-9.3 IU/L)
PRL	2-18 ng/mL (87-780 nmol/L)

specimen. Although many laboratories give a numerical value for the lower limits of normal for gonadotropins, some normal males have undetectable concentrations of FSH and LH by presently available immunoassay techniques. Furthermore, the concentrations of gonadotropins measured in one laboratory may not be directly comparable to those measured in another because of differences in the reference preparations used. The primary use of basal FSH and LH concentrations is to distinguish between hypergonadotropic hypogonadism, in which either or both of the gonadotropins are elevated, and hypogonadotropic hypogonadism, in which the gonadotropins are low or inappropriately normal in the presence of decreased androgen production.

Elevations of serum prolactin (PRL) inhibit the normal release of pituitary gonadotropins (shown by a reduced LH pulse frequency), probably through an effect on the hypothalamus. Thus, serum PRL measurements should be performed in any patient with hypogonadotropic hypogonadism. Serum PRL concentrations are generally stable throughout the day; therefore, measurement of this hormone in a single sample is usually sufficient. However, the patient should abstain from eating for 3 hours before the blood sample is obtained, because a protein meal may acutely stimulate the release of PRL from the pituitary. The normal ranges for serum PRL and gonadotropins are shown in Table 12–2.

Chorionic Gonadotropin Stimulation Test

Human chorionic gonadotropin (hCG) is a glycoprotein hormone with biologic actions similar to those of LH. Following an injection of chorionic gonadotropin, this hormone binds to the LH receptors on the Leydig cells and stimulates the synthesis and secretion of testicular steroids. Therefore, the Leydig cells may be directly assessed by the intramuscular injection of 4000 IU of chorionic gonadotropin daily for 4 days. A normal response is a doubling of the testosterone level following the last injection. Alternatively, a single intramuscular dose of chorionic gonadotropin (5000 IU/1.7 m^2 in adults or 100 IU/kg in children) may be given, with blood samples taken for testosterone measurements 72 and 96 hours later. Patients with primary gonadal disease have a diminished response following administration of chorionic gonadotropin, whereas patients with Leydig cell failure secondary to pituitary or hypothalamic disease have a qualitatively normal response.

Testicular Biopsy

Testicular biopsy in hypogonadal men is primarily indicated in patients with normal-sized testes and azoospermia in order to distinguish between spermatogenic failure and ductal obstruction. Although germinal aplasia, hypoplasia, maturation arrest, and other abnormalities of spermatogenesis may be diagnosed by examination of testicular tissue in oligospermic males, knowledge of the type of defect does not alter therapy. Therefore, testicular biopsy is not usually indicated for evaluation of mild to moderate oligospermia. If a testicular biopsy is carried out, testicular sperm extraction for possible intracytoplasmic sperm injection (ICSI) into ova may be performed at the same time.

Evaluation for Male Hypogonadism

Figure 12–6 outlines an approach to the diagnosis of male gonadal disorders. Semen analysis and determination of the basal concentrations of testosterone, FSH, and LH allow the clinician to distinguish patients with primary gonadal failure who have poor semen characteristics, low or normal testosterone, and elevated FSH or LH from those with secondary gonadal failure and abnormal semen analysis, decreased testosterone, and low or inappropriately normal gonadotropins.

In patients with elevations of gonadotropins resulting from primary testicular disease, chromosomal analysis helps to differentiate between genetic abnormalities and acquired testicular defects. Because no therapy exists that restores spermatogenesis in an individual with severe testicular damage, androgen replacement is the treatment of choice. Patients with isolated seminiferous tubule failure may have normal or elevated FSH concentrations in association with normal LH and testosterone levels and usually severe oligospermia. Patients with azoospermia require evaluation for the possible presence of ductal obstruction, because this defect may be surgically correctable. Fructose is added to seminal plasma by the seminal vesicles, and an absence of fructose indicates that the seminal vesicles are absent or bilaterally obstructed. The combination of a poor semen analysis with low testosterone, FSH, and LH is indicative of a hypothalamic or pituitary defect. Such patients need further evaluation of anterior and posterior pituitary gland function with appropriate pituitary function tests, as well as neuroradiologic and neuro-ophthalmologic studies (Chapter 4).

PHARMACOLOGY OF DRUGS USED TO TREAT MALE GONADAL DISORDERS

ANDROGENS

A variety of drugs are available for the treatment of androgen deficiency. Preparations for sublingual or oral administration such as methyltestosterone, oxymetholone, and fluoxymesterone have the advantage of ease of administration but the disadvantage of erratic absorption, potential for cholestatic jaundice, and decreased effectiveness when compared to the intramuscular preparations.

Testosterone propionate is a short-acting androgen. Its main use is in initiating therapy in older men, whose prostate glands may be exquisitely sensitive to testosterone. A dose of 50 mg two or three times per week is adequate. Obstructive symptoms due to benign prostatic hypertrophy following therapy with this androgen usually resolve rapidly because of its short duration of action.

Androgen deficiency may be treated with testosterone enanthate or cyclopentylpropionate (cypionate) given intramuscularly. Unlike the oral androgen preparations, both of these agents are capable of completely virilizing the patients. Therapy may be initiated with 50 mg intramuscularly every 4 weeks and gradually increased to a maintenance dose of 75 to 100 mg every week or 150 to 200 mg every 2 weeks. Testosterone undecanoate, a long-acting form of testosterone given intramuscularly every 3 months, is available in many countries, but is not yet approved by the FDA for use in the United States. Testosterone pellets may be implanted subcutaneously for a longer duration of effect. However, this therapy has not enjoyed much popularity. Transdermal delivery via membranes impregnated with testosterone (Androderm) is another method of replacement therapy. The patches can be placed on the skin of the back, shoulder, or abdomen and provide normal androgen concentrations. A testosterone gel (AndroGel 1%; Testim 1%) that is applied daily to the abdomen, shoulders, or upper arms also results in physiologic concentrations of testosterone. A buccal preparation (Striant) applied twice daily under the upper lip also is available, but is not widely used due to gum irritation.

Androgens, both oral and intramuscular, have been used (illegally) by some athletes to increase muscle mass and strength. Although this may achieve the anticipated result in some individuals, adverse effects include oligospermia and testicular atrophy—in addition to some of the complications noted below.

Androgen therapy is currently contraindicated in patients with prostatic carcinoma. About 1% to 2% of patients receiving oral methyltestosterone or fluoxymesterone develop intrahepatic cholestatic jaundice that resolves when the drug is discontinued. Rarely, these methylated or halogenated androgens have been associated with benign and malignant hepatocellular tumors.

Androgen therapy also may cause premature fusion of the epiphyses in an adolescent, and this may result in some loss of potential height. Therefore, androgen therapy is usually withheld until a hypogonadal male reaches 13 years of age. Sodium and water retention may induce hypertension or congestive heart failure in susceptible individuals. Because androgens stimulate erythropoietin production, erythrocytosis may occur during therapy. This is not usually clinically significant. Inhibition of spermatogenesis is mediated through suppression of gonadotropins by the androgens. Gynecomastia may develop during initiation of androgen therapy but usually resolves with continued administration of the drug. Sleep apnea may be precipitated. Priapism, acne, and aggressive behavior are dose-related adverse effects and generally disappear after reduction of dosage. Androgens decrease the production of thyroxine-binding globulin and corticosteroid-binding globulin by the liver. Therefore, total serum thyroxine and cortisol concentrations may be decreased, although the free hormone concentrations remain normal. High-density lipoprotein concentrations may also be reduced with oral androgens.

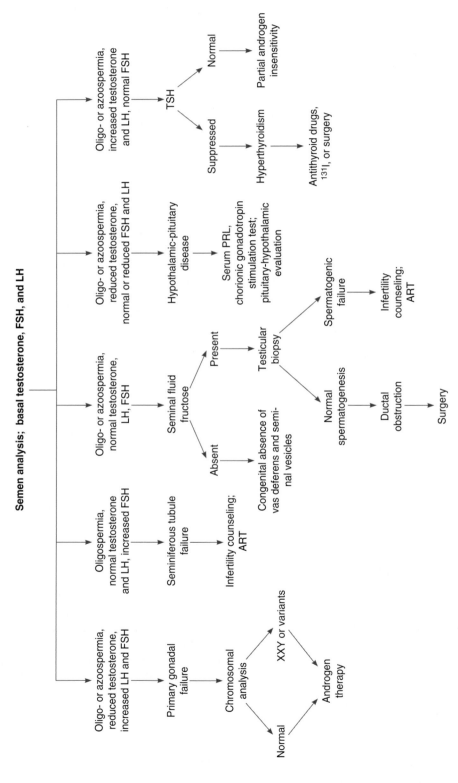

FIGURE 12–6 Scheme for evaluation of clinical hypogonadism (ART, assisted reproductive technologies such as in vitro fertilization and sperm injection into ova).

GONADOTROPINS

In patients with hypogonadism due to inadequate gonadotropin secretion, spermatogenesis and virilization may be induced by exogenous gonadotropin injections. Because the gonadotropins are proteins with short half-lives, they must be administered parenterally two or three times a week.

The expense and inconvenience of this type of therapy preclude its routine use for the treatment of androgen deficiency. The two major indications for exogenous gonadotropins are treatment of cryptorchidism (see later) and induction of spermatogenesis in hypogonadal males who wish to father children.

To induce spermatogenesis, 2000 IU of chorionic gonadotropin may be given intramuscularly three times a week for 9 to 12 months. In some individuals with partial gonadotropin deficiencies, this may induce adequate spermatogenesis. In patients with more severe deficiencies, menotropins, available in vials containing 75 IU each of FSH and LH, or highly purified urinary FSH (urofollitropin) or FSH produced by recombinant DNA technology (follitropin beta), each containing 75 IU of FSH, is added to chorionic gonadotropin therapy after 9 to 12 months and is administered in a dosage of one vial intramuscularly three times a week.

Adverse reactions with such therapy are minimal. Acne, gynecomastia, or prostatic enlargement may be noted as a result of excessive Leydig cell stimulation. Reduction of the chorionic gonadotropin dosage or a decrease in the frequency of chorionic gonadotropin injections generally results in resolution of the problem.

GONADOTROPIN-RELEASING HORMONE

GnRH (gonadorelin acetate), administered in pulses every 60 to 120 minutes by portable infusion pumps, effectively stimulates the endogenous release of LH and FSH in hypogonadotropic hypogonadal patients. This therapy does not currently appear to offer any major advantage over the use of exogenous gonadotropins for induction of spermatogenesis or the use of testosterone enanthate or cypionate for virilization, and is no longer available in the United States. A long-acting analog of GnRH, leuprolide acetate, is available for the treatment of advanced prostatic carcinoma. Daily subcutaneous administration of 1 mg or monthly intramuscular injections of 7.5 mg of a depot preparation—22.5 mg for 3 months or 30 mg for 4 months—results in desensitization of the pituitary GnRH receptors, which reduces LH and FSH levels and so ultimately testosterone concentrations. Similar results are produced with a subcutaneous injection of the depot form of the GnRH analog goserelin or monthly intramuscular injections of triptorelin. With these therapies, initial remission rates for prostatic carcinoma are similar to those found with orchiectomy or treatment with diethylstilbestrol (about 70%). A long-acting GnRH antagonist, abarelix, also is an effective means of inducing medical castration by reducing LH, FSH, and testosterone secretion. Although GnRH agonists may produce an initial rise in LH, FSH, and testosterone levels, no such rise is seen with GnRH antagonists, making them better agents to use in the presence of metastasis in sensitive areas such as the spinal cord.

TABLE 12–3 Classification of male hypogonadism.

Hypothalamic-Pituitary Disorders
Panhypopituitarism
Isolated LH deficiency (fertile eunuch)
Isolated FSH deficiency
LH and FSH deficiency
  a. With normal sense of smell
  b. With hyposmia or anosmia (Kallmann syndrome)
  c. With complex neurologic syndromes
    Prader-Willi syndrome
    Laurence-Moon, Bardet-Biedl syndromes
    Möbius syndrome
    Lowe syndrome
    Cerebellar ataxia
Biologically inactive LH
Hyperprolactinemia

Gonadal Abnormalities
Klinefelter syndrome
Other chromosomal defects (XX male, XY/XXY, XX/XXY, XXXY, XXXXY, XXYY, XYY)
Bilateral anorchia (vanishing testes syndrome)
Leydig cell aplasia
Cryptorchidism
Noonan syndrome
Myotonic dystrophy
Adult seminiferous tubule failure
Adult Leydig cell failure
Defects in androgen biosynthesis

Defects in Androgen Action
Complete androgen insensitivity (testicular feminization)
Incomplete androgen insensitivity

Nafarelin acetate is a GnRH agonist that is administered intranasally for the treatment of endometriosis and central precocious puberty. Central precocious puberty also may be treated with leuprolide acetate and another analog, histrelin acetate. Long-acting GnRH agonists also are used to suppress endogenous gonadal steroid production as part of the endocrine treatment of transsexual persons. Long-acting GnRH agonists combined with testosterone have been studied as a possible male contraceptive, but they do not uniformly induce azoospermia.

CLINICAL MALE GONADAL DISORDERS

Hypogonadism may be subdivided into three general categories (Table 12–3). A thorough discussion of the hypothalamic-pituitary disorders that cause hypogonadism is presented in Chapters 4 and 15. The defects in androgen biosynthesis and androgen action are described in Chapter 14. The following section emphasizes the primary gonadal abnormalities.

KLINEFELTER SYNDROME (XXY SEMINIFEROUS TUBULE DYSGENESIS)

Klinefelter syndrome is the most common genetic cause of male hypogonadism, occurring in one of 600 male births. An extra X chromosome is present in about 0.2% of male conceptions and

0.1% to 0.2% of live-born males. Sex chromosome surveys of mentally retarded males have revealed an extra X chromosome in 0.45% to 2.5% of such individuals. Patients with an XXY genotype have classic Klinefelter syndrome; those with an XXXY, XXXXY, or XXYY genotype or with XXY/chromosomal mosaicism are considered to have variant forms of the syndrome.

Etiology and Pathophysiology

The XXY genotype is usually due to meiotic nondisjunction during parental gametogenesis, which results in an egg with two X chromosomes or a sperm with an X and a Y chromosome. After fertilization, nondisjunction during mitotic division results in mosaicism.

At birth there are generally no physical stigmas of Klinefelter syndrome, and during childhood there are no specific signs or symptoms. The chromosomal defect is expressed chiefly during puberty. As the gonadotropins increase, the seminiferous tubules do not enlarge but rather undergo fibrosis and hyalinization, which results in small, firm testes. Obliteration of the seminiferous tubules results in azoospermia.

In addition to dysgenesis of the seminiferous tubules, the Leydig cells are also abnormal. They are present in clumps and appear to be hyperplastic on initial examination of a testicular biopsy. However, the Leydig cell mass is not increased, and the apparent hyperplasia is actually due to the marked reduction in tubular volume. Despite the normal mass of tissue, the Leydig cells are functionally abnormal. The testosterone production rate is reduced, and there is a compensatory elevation in serum LH. Stimulation of the Leydig cells with exogenous chorionic gonadotropin results in a subnormal rise in testosterone. The clinical manifestations of androgen deficiency vary considerably from patient to patient and may be related to the degree of diminished testosterone production and alterations in the androgen receptor. Exon 1 of the androgen receptor gene contains a polymorphism with a variable number of CAG repeats. As the number of repeats increases, there is a progressive decrease in androgen action and more phenotypic abnormalities. Thus, some individuals have virtually no secondary sexual developmental changes, whereas others are indistinguishable from healthy individuals.

The elevated LH concentrations also stimulate the Leydig cells to secrete increased quantities of estradiol and estradiol precursors. The relatively high estradiol: testosterone ratio is responsible for the variable degrees of feminization and gynecomastia seen in these patients. The elevated estradiol also stimulates the liver to produce SHBG. This may result in total serum testosterone concentrations that are within the low-normal range for adult males. However, the free testosterone level may be lower than normal.

The pathogenesis of the eunuchoid proportions, personality, and intellectual deficits and associated medical disorders is presently unclear.

Testicular Pathology

Most of the seminiferous tubules are fibrotic and hyalinized, although occasional Sertoli cells and spermatogonia may be

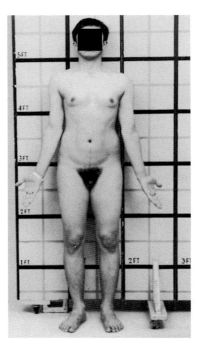

FIGURE 12-7 Klinefelter syndrome in a 20-year-old man. Note relatively increased lower/upper body segment ratio, gynecomastia, small penis, and sparse body hair with a female pubic hair pattern.

present in some sections. Absence of elastic fibers in the tunica propria is indicative of the dysgenetic nature of the tubules. The Leydig cells are arranged in clumps and appear hyperplastic, although the total mass is normal.

Clinical Features (Figure 12–7)

A. Symptoms and signs   There are usually no symptoms before puberty other than poor school performance in some affected individuals. Puberty may be delayed but not usually by more than 1 to 2 years. During puberty, the penis and scrotum undergo varying degrees of development, with some individuals appearing normal. Most patients (80%) have diminished facial and torso hair growth. The major complaint is often persistent gynecomastia, which is clinically present in over half of patients. The testes are uniformly small (<2 cm in longest axis and <4 mL in volume) and firm as a result of fibrosis and hyalinization. Other complaints include infertility or insufficient libido and potency. The patient may have difficulty putting into words his embarrassment in situations where he must disrobe in the presence of other men, and the subnormal development of the external genitalia along with gynecomastia may lead to feelings of inadequacy that may be partly responsible for the maladjusted social behavior some patients exhibit. Bone mineral density may be dramatically reduced in patients with long-standing androgen deficiency.

Patients with Klinefelter syndrome have abnormal skeletal proportions that are not truly eunuchoid. Growth of the lower extremities is relatively greater than that of the trunk and upper extremities; therefore, pubis-to-floor height (which represents appendicular bone growth) is greater than crown-to-pubis height (which predominantly represents axial bone growth), and span is less than total height. Thus, the abnormal skeletal proportions are not the result of androgen deficiency per se (which results in span greater than height).

Intellectual impairment is noted in many patients with Klinefelter syndrome, but the true proportion of affected individuals with subnormal intelligence is not known. Deficits in language and higher intellectual functions, such as concept formation and problem solving, have been noted. Poor social skills also are common (see earlier). Patients generally show lack of ambition and difficulties in maintaining permanent employment.

Several clinical and genotypic variants of Klinefelter syndrome have been described. In addition to small testes with seminiferous tubular hyalinization, azoospermia, deficient secondary sexual development, and elevated gonadotropins, patients with three or more X chromosomes uniformly have severe mental retardation. The presence of more than one Y chromosome tends to be associated with aggressive antisocial behavior and macronodular acne. Skeletal deformities such as radioulnar synostosis, flexion deformities of the elbows, and clinodactyly are more commonly seen in Klinefelter variants. Patients with sex chromosome mosaicism (XX/XXY) may have only a few of the Klinefelter stigmas. These patients may have normal testicular size and may be fertile if their testes contain the XY genotype.

Medical disorders found to be associated with Klinefelter syndrome with more than chance frequency include chronic pulmonary disease (emphysema, chronic bronchitis), varicose veins, extragonadal germ cell tumors, cerebrovascular disease, glucose intolerance, primary hypothyroidism, and taurodontism—with early tooth decay. Some studies suggest that there is a 20-fold increased risk of breast cancer, while others do not.

B. Laboratory findings   Serum testosterone is low or normal, and FSH and LH concentrations are elevated. Azoospermia is present. The buccal smear is chromatin-positive (20% of cells having a Barr body), and chromosomal analysis reveals a 47,XXY karyotype.

Differential Diagnosis

Klinefelter syndrome should be distinguished from other causes of hypogonadism. Small, firm testes should suggest Klinefelter syndrome. Hypothalamic-pituitary hypogonadism may be associated with small, rubbery testes if puberty has not occurred or atrophic testes if normal puberty has occurred. The consistency of the testes in Klinefelter syndrome is also different from that noted in acquired forms of adult seminiferous tubular damage. The elevated gonadotropins place the site of the lesion at the testicular level, and chromosomal analysis confirms the diagnosis. Chromosomal analysis is also required to differentiate classic Klinefelter syndrome from the variant forms.

Treatment

A. Medical treatment   Androgen deficiency should be treated with testosterone replacement. Patients with personality

defects should be virilized gradually to decrease the risk of aggressive behavior. Testosterone enanthate or cypionate, 100 mg intramuscularly, may be given every 2 to 4 weeks initially and increased to 200 mg every 2 weeks if well tolerated. Patients with low-normal androgen levels may not require androgen replacement therapy. For those desiring fertility, sperm may be extracted directly from the testes in about half of the patients and used for ICSI with a live birth rate of up to 20%.

B. Surgical treatment   If gynecomastia presents a cosmetic problem, mastectomy may be performed.

Course and Prognosis

Patients generally feel better after androgen replacement therapy has begun. However, the personality defects do not improve, and these patients often require long-term psychiatric counseling. Life expectancy is not affected.

BILATERAL ANORCHIA (VANISHING TESTES SYNDROME)

Approximately 3% of phenotypic boys undergoing surgery to correct unilateral or bilateral cryptorchidism are found to have absence of one testis, and in about 1% of cryptorchid males both testes are absent. Thus, bilateral anorchia is found in approximately one out of every 20,000 males.

Etiology and Pathophysiology

Functional testicular tissue must be present during the first 14 to 16 weeks of embryonic development in order for Wolffian duct growth and Müllerian duct regression to occur and for the external genitalia to differentiate along male lines. Absence of testicular function before this time results in varying degrees of male pseudohermaphroditism with ambiguous genitalia. Prenatal testicular injury occurring after 16 weeks of gestation as a result of trauma, vascular insufficiency, infection, or other mechanisms may result in loss of testicular tissue in an otherwise normal phenotypic male; hence the term **vanishing testes syndrome**.

Testicular Pathology

In most instances, no recognizable testicular tissue has been identified despite extensive dissections. Wolffian duct structures are generally normal, and the vas deferens and testicular vessels may terminate blindly or in a mass of connective tissue in the inguinal canal or scrotum.

Clinical Features

A. Symptoms and signs   At birth, patients appear to be normal phenotypic males with bilateral cryptorchidism. Growth and development are normal until secondary sexual development fails to occur at puberty. The penis remains small; pubic and axillary hair does not fully develop despite the presence of adrenal androgens; and the scrotum remains empty. If the patient does not receive androgens, eunuchoid proportions develop. Gynecomastia does not occur.

An occasional patient undergoes partial spontaneous virilization at puberty. Although anatomically no testicular tissue has been identified in such patients, catheterization studies have demonstrated higher testosterone concentrations in venous blood obtained from the spermatic veins than in the peripheral venous circulation. This suggests that functional Leydig cells are present in some patients, although they are not associated with testicular germinal epithelium or stroma.

B. Laboratory findings Serum testosterone concentrations are generally quite low, and both LH and FSH are markedly elevated. Serum testosterone concentrations do not rise following a chorionic gonadotropin stimulation test. Serum Müllerian duct inhibitory factor levels are low. Chromosomal analysis discloses a 46,XY karyotype.

C. Imaging studies Testicular artery arteriograms, spermatic venograms, and gadolinium-infusion magnetic resonance venography show vessels that taper and end in the inguinal canal or scrotum without an associated gonad.

D. Special examinations Thorough inguinal and abdominal laparoscopic examination or retroperitoneal examination at laparotomy may locate the testes. If testicular vessels and the vas deferens are identified and found to terminate blindly together, it may be assumed that the testis is absent.

Differential Diagnosis

Bilateral cryptorchidism must be differentiated from congenital bilateral anorchia. A normal serum testosterone concentration that rises following stimulation with chorionic gonadotropin is indicative of functional Leydig cells and probable bilateral cryptorchidism. Elevated serum LH and FSH and a low testosterone that fails to rise after administration of exogenous chorionic gonadotropin indicate bilateral absence of functional testicular tissue.

Treatment

Androgen replacement therapy is discussed in the section on pharmacology (see "Androgens," earlier in the chapter).

Implantation of testicular prostheses for cosmetic purposes may be beneficial after the scrotum has enlarged in response to androgen therapy.

LEYDIG CELL APLASIA

Defective development of testicular Leydig cells is a rare cause of male pseudohermaphroditism with ambiguous genitalia.

Etiology and Pathophysiology

Testes are present in the inguinal canal and contain prepubertal-appearing tubules with Sertoli cells and spermatogonia without germinal cell maturation. The interstitial tissue has a loose myxoid appearance with an absence of Leydig cells. The syndrome is caused by inactivating mutations in the LH receptor that alters receptor signal transduction. The presence of a vas deferens and epididymis in these patients indicates that the local concentration of testosterone was high enough during embryogenesis to result in differentiation of the Wolffian duct structures. However, the ambiguity of the genitalia indicates that the androgen concentration in these patients was insufficient to bring about full virilization of the external genitalia. The absence of Müllerian duct structures is compatible with normal fetal secretion of Müllerian duct inhibitory factor from the Sertoli cells.

Clinical Features

A. Symptoms and signs These patients may present in infancy with variable degrees of genital ambiguity, including a bifid scrotum, clitoral phallus, urogenital sinus, and blind vaginal pouch. Alternatively, they may appear as normal phenotypic females and escape detection until adolescence, when they present with primary amenorrhea, with or without normal breast development. The gonads are generally located in the inguinal canal. Axillary and pubic hair, although present, may be sparse. Mild defects may result in Leydig cell hypoplasia, a disorder whose clinical manifestations include micropenis, hypospadias, and variable suppression of fertility.

B. Laboratory findings Serum gonadotropins are elevated, and testosterone levels are below normal limits for a male and within the low-normal range for females. There is no increase in testosterone following chorionic gonadotropin administration.

Differential Diagnosis

Leydig cell aplasia should be differentiated from the vanishing testes syndrome, testosterone biosynthetic defects, disorders of androgen action, and 5α-reductase deficiency. The differential diagnostic features of these disorders are discussed in Chapter 14.

Treatment

Patients with Leydig cell aplasia respond well to the exogenous administration of testosterone, and it would be anticipated that they would be fully virilized and even develop some degree of spermatogenesis with exogenous testosterone administration. However, because the few patients who have been reported have been discovered either late in childhood or as adolescents and have been raised as females, it would be inappropriate to attempt a gender reversal at such a late period. Removal of the cryptorchid testes and feminization with exogenous estrogens would appear to be the most prudent course of therapy.

CRYPTORCHIDISM

Cryptorchidism is unilateral or bilateral absence of the testes from the scrotum because of failure of normal testicular descent from the genital ridge through the external inguinal ring. Between 2% and 4% of full-term and 20% to 25% of premature male infants have cryptorchidism. In most cases of cryptorchidism noted at birth, spontaneous testicular descent occurs during the first year of life, reducing the incidence to 0.2% to 0.8% by 1 year of age. Approximately 0.75% of adult males are cryptorchid. Unilateral cryptorchidism is 5 to 10 times more common than bilateral cryptorchidism.

Almost 50% of cryptorchid testes are located at the external inguinal ring or in a high scrotal position; 19% lie within the inguinal canal between the internal and external inguinal rings (canalicular); 9% are intra-abdominal; and 23% are ectopic (ie, located away from the normal pathway of descent from the abdominal cavity to the scrotum). Most ectopic testes are found in a superficial inguinal pouch above the external inguinal ring.

Etiology and Pathophysiology

Testicular descent usually occurs between the 12th week of fetal development and birth. Both mechanical and hormonal factors appear to be important for this process. Cryptorchidism is common in patients with congenital defects in androgen synthesis or action and in patients with congenital gonadotropin deficiency, and experimental studies have demonstrated that DHT is required for normal testicular descent. These observations suggest that prenatal androgen deficiency may be of etiologic importance in the development of cryptorchidism. Environmental endocrine disruptors with estrogen or antiandrogen activity, such as phthalates or bisphenol A, have been proposed as a cause of the increased incidence of cryptorchidism seen in recent years.

It is not known whether pathologic changes in the testes are due to the effects of cryptorchidism or to intrinsic abnormalities in the gonad. Experimental studies in animals have shown that an increase in the temperature of the testes by 1.5°C to 2°C (34.7°F -35.6°F) (the temperature differential between the abdomen and scrotum) results in depression of spermatogenesis. Serial testicular biopsies in cryptorchid patients have demonstrated partial reversal of the histologic abnormalities following surgical correction, suggesting that the extra-scrotal environment is partly responsible for the observed pathologic abnormalities.

An intrinsic abnormality in the testes in patients with unilateral cryptorchidism is suggested by the observation that such patients are at increased risk for development of germ cell neoplasms in the scrotal testis. Similarly, the observation that adults with unilateral cryptorchidism surgically corrected before puberty had low sperm counts, high basal serum LH and FSH concentrations, and an exaggerated FSH response to GnRH suggests either that both testes are intrinsically abnormal or that the cryptorchid gonad somehow suppresses the function of the scrotal testis.

Pathology

Histologic studies on cryptorchid testes have demonstrated a decrease in the size of the seminiferous tubules and number of spermatogonia and an increase in peritubular tissue. The Leydig cells usually appear normal. It is unclear at what age these changes first appear. Abnormalities have been detected as early as 6 months. It is well established that the longer a testis remains cryptorchid, the more likely it is to show pathologic changes. More severe changes are generally found in intra-abdominal testes than in canalicular testes.

Clinical Features

A. Symptoms and signs There are usually no symptoms unless a complication such as testicular torsion, trauma, or malignant degeneration occurs. School-age children may have gender identity problems. Adults may complain of infertility, especially if they have a history of bilateral cryptorchidism.

Absence of one or both testes is the cardinal clinical finding. This may be associated with a small scrotum (bilateral cryptorchidism) or hemiscrotum (unilateral cryptorchidism). Signs of androgen deficiency are not present.

B. Laboratory findings Basal or stimulated serum FSH, LH, and testosterone concentrations are not helpful in evaluating prepubertal unilaterally cryptorchid males. However, serum FSH and LH concentrations and the testosterone response to exogenous chorionic gonadotropin are useful in differentiating cryptorchid patients from those with congenital anorchia. The latter have high basal gonadotropins, low serum testosterone, and absent or diminished testosterone rise following chorionic gonadotropin stimulation. Alternatively, measurement of the serum concentration of Müllerian duct inhibitory factor can be used; children with no testicular tissue have very low levels in comparison to those with bilateral cryptorchidism.

Postpubertal adults may have oligospermia, elevated basal serum FSH and LH concentrations, and an exaggerated FSH increase following GnRH stimulation. Such abnormalities are more prevalent in patients with a history of bilateral cryptorchidism than with unilateral cryptorchidism.

C. Imaging studies Gadolinium-infusion magnetic resonance venography is a sensitive method for localizing the nonpalpable cryptorchid testes. Intravenous urography discloses an associated abnormality of the upper urinary tract in 10% of cases—horseshoe kidney, renal hypoplasia, ureteral duplication, hydroureter, and hydronephrosis.

Differential Diagnosis

Retractile testis (pseudocryptorchidism) is due to a hyperactive cremasteric reflex, which draws the testicle into the inguinal canal. Cold temperature, fear, and genital manipulation commonly activate the reflex, which is most prominent between the ages of 5 and 6 years. The child should be examined with warm hands in a warm room. The testis can usually be milked into the scrotum with gentle pressure over the lower abdomen in the direction of the inguinal canal.

Bilateral anorchia is associated with elevated gonadotropins, decreased testosterone, and an absent or subnormal response to stimulation with chorionic gonadotropin.

The virilizing forms of congenital adrenal hyperplasia may result in prenatal fusion of the labial-scrotal folds and clitoral hypertrophy (Chapter 14). Severely affected females have the appearance of phenotypic males with bilateral cryptorchidism. Because of the potentially disastrous consequences (acute adrenal insufficiency) if this diagnosis is missed, a chromosomal analysis should be performed on bilaterally cryptorchid phenotypic male infants.

Complications and Sequelae

A. Hernia   Approximately 90% of cryptorchid males have associated ipsilateral inguinal hernia resulting from failure of the processus vaginalis to close. This is rarely symptomatic.

B. Torsion   Because of the abnormal connection between the cryptorchid testis and its supporting tissues, torsion may occur. This should be suspected in any patient with abdominal or pelvic pain and an ipsilateral empty scrotum.

C. Trauma   Testes that lie above the pubic tubercle are particularly susceptible to traumatic injury.

D. Neoplasms   A cryptorchid testis is four to six times more likely to undergo malignant degeneration than a normal testis. The incidence of such tumors is greater in patients with intra-abdominal testes than in patients with canalicular testes. Seminomas are the neoplasms most commonly associated with maldescended testes. In addition, there is an increased risk for development of testicular intraepithelial neoplasia (carcinoma in situ). Orchiopexy before or during puberty decreases the risk of malignancy. Because of the increased risk of neoplasia, many urologists recommend orchiectomy for a unilaterally undescended testicle in a patient first seen after puberty. Patients who present with bilateral cryptorchidism after puberty should have bilateral orchiopexy and testicular biopsies to preserve testicular endocrine function and to make palpation for detection of neoplasia easier.

E. Infertility   Over 75% of untreated bilaterally cryptorchid males are infertile. About 30% to 50% of bilaterally cryptorchid patients who undergo prepubertal orchiopexy have been found to be fertile. About half of patients with untreated unilateral cryptorchidism are infertile, whereas infertility is found in less than one-fourth of such patients whose cryptorchidism is surgically repaired before puberty.

Prevention

Although cryptorchidism cannot be prevented, the complications can be avoided. It is clear that the adverse changes that take place in the testes are related in part to the location of the maldescended testis and the duration of the cryptorchidism. Most testes that are undescended at birth enter the scrotum during the first year of life. However, it is rare for a cryptorchid testis to descend spontaneously after the age of 6 months. Because adverse histologic changes have been noted around the age of 2 years, hormonal or surgical correction should be undertaken at or before that time, ideally between 6 and 12 months.

Treatment

A. Medical

1. **Intramuscular chorionic gonadotropin therapy**—Because growth of the vas deferens and testicular descent are at least partially dependent on androgens, stimulation of endogenous testosterone secretion by chorionic gonadotropin may correct the cryptorchidism. Cryptorchidism is corrected in less than 25% of patients treated with a course of chorionic gonadotropin, and recent studies suggest that patients with conditions that respond to hormonal therapy may actually have retractile testes rather than true cryptorchidism. Nevertheless, this therapy may be tried prior to orchiopexy, because it is innocuous and may avoid the need for surgery. For bilateral cryptorchidism, give a short course of chorionic gonadotropin consisting of 3300 U intramuscularly every other day over a 5-day period (three injections). For unilateral cryptorchidism, give 500 U intramuscularly three times a week for 6½ weeks (20 injections).

2. **Intranasal GnRH therapy**—GnRH given three times a day for 28 days by nasal spray has been shown to be as effective as chorionic gonadotropin injections in correcting cryptorchidism in some patients. This therapy is not approved for treatment of cryptorchidism in the United States.

B. Surgical treatment   Several procedures have been devised to place the maldescended testis into the scrotum (orchiopexy). The operation may be performed in one or two stages. Inguinal hernia should be repaired if present. As noted earlier, the surgery is best performed between 6 and 12 months of age.

NOONAN SYNDROME (MALE TURNER SYNDROME)

Phenotypic and genotypic males with many of the physical stigmas of classic Turner syndrome have been described under a variety of names, including Noonan syndrome and male Turner syndrome. It has an incidence of 1:1000 to 1:2500 live births and may occur sporadically or may be familial—inherited in an autosomal dominant fashion with variable penetrance. Approximately half of the patients have a gain-of-function mutation in the protein-tyrosine phosphatase, nonreceptor type II (*PTPN11*) gene on chromosome 12, which encodes for Src homology region two-domain phosphatase (SHP-2), a signaling protein that modulates cellular proliferation, differentiation, and migration. A number of pathologic features have been noted, including reduced seminiferous tubular size with or without sclerosis, diminished or absent germ cells, and Leydig cell hyperplasia.

Clinical Features

A. Symptoms and signs   The most common clinical features are short stature, webbed neck, hypertelorism, cubitus valgus, and bleeding diathesis. Other somatic defects are variably observed in these patients. Congenital cardiac anomalies are common and involve primarily the right side of the heart—in contrast to patients with XO gonadal dysgenesis.

Cryptorchidism is frequently present. Although some affected individuals are fertile, with normal testes, most have small testes and mild to moderate hypogonadism.

B. Laboratory findings   Serum testosterone concentrations are usually low or low-normal, and serum gonadotropins are high. The karyotype is 46,XY.

Differential Diagnosis

The clinical features of Noonan syndrome are sufficiently distinct so that confusion with other causes of hypogonadism is usually not a problem. However, a rare individual with XY/XO mosaicism may have similar somatic anomalies requiring chromosomal analysis for differentiation. Some of the phenotypic features are shared with the Costello and cardiofaciocutaneous syndromes.

Treatment

If the patient is hypogonadal, androgen replacement therapy is indicated.

MYOTONIC DYSTROPHY

Myotonic dystrophies types 1 (DM1) and 2 (DM2) are autosomal dominant disorders of muscle with multisystem clinical features including primary hypogonadism. The underlying lesion in DM1 is an expansion of the CTG repeat in the 3′ untranslated region of a gene that encodes a serine-threonine protein kinase located on chromosome 19. The cause of DM2 is expansion of a CCTG repeat in intron 1 of the *zinc finger protein-9* gene on chromosome 3.

Testicular histology varies from moderate derangement of spermatogenesis with germinal cell arrest to regional hyalinization and fibrosis of the seminiferous tubules. The Leydig cells are usually preserved and may appear in clumps.

The testes are normal in affected prepubertal individuals, and puberty generally proceeds normally. Testosterone secretion is normal, and secondary sexual characteristics develop appropriately. After puberty, seminiferous tubular atrophy results in a decrease in testicular size and change of consistency from firm to soft or mushy. Infertility is a consequence of disrupted spermatogenesis. If testicular hyalinization and fibrosis are extensive, Leydig cell function may also be impaired.

Clinical Features

A. Symptoms and signs   The disease usually becomes apparent in adulthood. Progressive weakness and atrophy of the facial, neck, hand, and lower extremity muscles is commonly observed. Severe atrophy of the temporalis muscles, ptosis due to weakness of the levator muscles of the eye with compensatory wrinkling of the forehead muscles, and frontal baldness comprise the myopathic facies characteristic of the disorder. Myotonia is present in several muscle groups and is characterized by inability to relax the muscle normally after a strong contraction.

Testicular atrophy is not noted until adulthood, and most patients develop and maintain normal facial and body hair growth and libido. Gynecomastia is usually not present.

Associated features include mental retardation (type 1 disease only), cataracts, diabetes mellitus, cardiac arrhythmias, and primary hypothyroidism.

B. Laboratory findings   Serum testosterone is normal to slightly decreased. FSH is uniformly elevated in patients with atrophic testes. LH is also frequently elevated, even in patients with normal serum testosterone levels. Leydig cell reserve is generally diminished, with subnormal increases in serum testosterone following stimulation with chorionic gonadotropin. An excessive rise in FSH and, to a lesser extent, LH is found following GnRH stimulation.

Treatment

There is no therapy that will prevent progressive muscular atrophy in this disorder. Testosterone replacement therapy is not indicated unless serum testosterone levels are subnormal.

ADULT SEMINIFEROUS TUBULE FAILURE

Adult seminiferous tubule failure encompasses a spectrum of pathologic alterations of the seminiferous tubules that results in hypospermatogenesis, germinal cell arrest, germinal cell aplasia, and tubular hyalinization. Almost half of infertile males exhibit some degree of isolated seminiferous tubule failure.

Etiology, Pathology, and Pathophysiology

Etiologic factors in seminiferous tubule failure include mumps or gonococcal orchitis, leprosy, cryptorchidism, irradiation, uremia, alcoholism, paraplegia, lead poisoning, and therapy with antineoplastic agents such as cyclophosphamide, chlorambucil, vincristine, methotrexate, and procarbazine. Vascular insufficiency resulting from spermatic artery damage during herniorrhaphy, testicular torsion, or sickle cell anemia may also selectively damage the tubules. Similar pathologic changes may be found in oligospermic patients with varicoceles. Deletions of portions of the Y chromosome may also present as adult seminiferous tubule failure. In many patients, no etiologic factors can be identified, and the condition is referred to as **idiopathic**.

The rapidly dividing germinal epithelium is more susceptible to injury than are the Sertoli or Leydig cells. Thus, pressure necrosis (eg, mumps or gonococcal orchitis), increased testicular temperature (eg, cryptorchidism and perhaps varicocele and paraplegia), and the direct cytotoxic effects of irradiation, alcohol, lead, and chemotherapeutic agents primarily injure the germ cells. Although the Sertoli and Leydig cells appear to be morphologically normal, severe testicular injury may result in functional alterations in these cells.

Several different lesions may be found in testicular biopsy specimens. The pathologic process may involve the entire testes or may appear in patches. The least severe lesion is hypospermatogenesis, in which all stages of spermatogenesis are present but there is a decrease in the number of germinal epithelial cells. Some degree of peritubular fibrosis may be present. Cessation of development at the primary spermatocyte or spermatogonial stage of the spermatogenic cycle is classified as germinal cell arrest. More severely affected testes may demonstrate a complete absence of germ cells with maintenance of morphologically normal Sertoli cells (Sertoli cell–only syndrome). The most severe lesion is fibrosis or hyalinization of the tubules. This latter pattern may be indistinguishable from that seen in Klinefelter syndrome.

Irrespective of the etiologic factors involved in damage to the germinal epithelium, the alterations in spermatogenesis result in oligospermia. If the damage is severe, as in the Sertoli cell–only syndrome or tubular hyalinization, azoospermia may be present. Because testicular volume consists chiefly of tubules, some degree of testicular atrophy is often present in these patients. Some patients have elevations in basal serum FSH concentrations and demonstrate a hyperresponsive FSH rise following GnRH, suggesting that the Sertoli cells are functionally abnormal despite their normal histologic appearance.

Clinical Features

A. Symptoms and signs   Infertility is usually the only complaint. Mild to moderate testicular atrophy may be present. Careful examination should be made for the presence of varicocele by palpating the spermatic cord during Valsalva maneuver with the patient in the upright position. The patients are fully virilized, and gynecomastia is not present.

B. Laboratory findings   Semen analysis shows oligospermia or azoospermia, and serum testosterone and LH concentrations are normal. Basal serum FSH levels may be normal or high, and an excessive FSH rise following GnRH may be present. Serum inhibin B levels generally are low, but they add little information beyond that of the serum FSH measurement.

Differential Diagnosis

Patients with hypothalamic or pituitary disorders may have oligospermia or azoospermia and testicular atrophy. The serum FSH and LH concentrations are often in the low-normal range, and the testosterone level is usually (not always) diminished. The presence of neurologic and ophthalmologic abnormalities, diabetes insipidus, anterior pituitary trophic hormone deficiencies, or an elevated serum PRL concentration distinguishes these patients from those with primary seminiferous tubule failure. Other causes of primary testicular failure are associated either with clinical signs and symptoms of androgen deficiency or with enough somatic abnormalities to allow differentiation from isolated seminiferous tubule failure.

Prevention

In many instances, damage to the seminiferous tubules cannot be prevented. Early correction of cryptorchidism, adequate shielding of the testes during diagnostic radiologic procedures or radiotherapy, and limitation of the total dose of chemotherapeutic agents may prevent or ameliorate the adverse effects.

Treatment

A. Medical   Attempts to treat oligospermia and infertility medically have included low-dose testosterone, exogenous gonadotropins, thyroid hormone therapy, vitamins, bromocriptine, aromatase inhibitors, tamoxifen, and clomiphene citrate. None of these agents have been found to be uniformly beneficial, and several may actually lead to a decrease in the sperm count.

B. Surgical   Some of the pathologic changes in the testes have been reversed by early orchiopexy in cryptorchid individuals. If a varicocele is found in an oligospermic, infertile male, it should be ligated.

Course and Prognosis

Patients who have received up to 300 cGy of testicular irradiation may show partial or full recovery of spermatogenesis months to years following exposure. The prognosis for recovery is better for individuals who receive the irradiation over a short interval than for those who are exposed over several weeks. Radiation therapy for prostate cancer may cause an acute reduction in spermatogenesis and testosterone followed in most patients by partial or full recovery.

Recovery of spermatogenesis may also occur months to years following administration of chemotherapeutic agents. The most important factor determining prognosis is the total dose of chemotherapy administered.

Improvement in the quality of the semen is found in 60% to 80% of patients following successful repair of varicocele. Restoration of fertility has been reported in about half of such patients.

The prognosis for spontaneous improvement of idiopathic oligospermia due to infection or infarction is poor.

ADULT LEYDIG CELL FAILURE (ANDROPAUSE)

In contrast to the menopause in women, men do not experience an abrupt decline or cessation of gonadal function. However, a gradual diminution of testicular function does occur in many men as part of the aging process (see Chapter 23). It is not known how many men develop symptoms directly attributable to this phenomenon.

Etiology, Pathology, and Pathophysiology

After age 50, there is a gradual decrease in the total serum testosterone concentration, although the actual values remain within the normal range. The levels of free testosterone decrease to a greater extent because of an increase in SHBG. The testosterone production rate declines and Leydig cell responsiveness to hCG also decreases. A gradual compensatory increase in serum LH levels has also been noted. Aging also is associated with alterations in the hypothalamic-pituitary portion of the axis.

Histologic studies of the aging testes have shown patchy degenerative changes in the seminiferous tubules with a reduction in number and volume of Leydig cells. The pathologic changes are first noted in the regions most remote from the arterial blood supply. Thus, microvascular insufficiency may be the etiologic basis for the histologic tubular changes and the decrease in Leydig cell function noted with aging. In addition, virtually all of the conditions that cause adult seminiferous tubule failure may lead to Leydig cell dysfunction if testicular injury is severe enough.

Clinical Features

A. Symptoms and signs A great many symptoms have been attributed to the male climacteric (andropause), including decreased libido and potency, emotional instability, fatigue, decreased strength, decreased concentrating ability, vasomotor instability (palpitations, hot flushes, diaphoresis), and a variety of diffuse aches and pains. There are usually no associated signs unless the testicular injury is severe. In such patients, a decrease in testicular volume and consistency may be present as well as gynecomastia.

B. Laboratory findings Serum testosterone may be low or low-normal. Serum LH concentration is usually high-normal or slightly high, but a number of men have a normal LH and borderline low total and free testosterone. Oligospermia is usually present. Bone mineral density may be decreased.

C. Special examinations Because many men with complaints compatible with Leydig cell failure have borderline low testosterone concentrations and LH concentrations within the normal adult range, a therapeutic testosterone/placebo trial may be attempted. The test is best performed double-blind over an 8-week period. During the first or last 4 weeks, the patient receives testosterone enanthate, 100 mg intramuscularly per week; during the other 4-week period, placebo injections are administered. The patient is interviewed by the physician 2 weeks after the last course of injections. After the interview, the code is broken; if the patient notes amelioration of symptoms during the period of androgen administration but not during the placebo period, the diagnosis or adult Leydig cell failure is substantiated. If the patient experiences no subjective improvement following testosterone, or if improvement is noted following both placebo and testosterone injections, Leydig cell failure is effectively ruled out.

Differential Diagnosis

Erectile dysfunction from vascular, neurologic, or psychologic causes must be distinguished from Leydig cell failure. A therapeutic trial of androgen therapy does not help erectile dysfunction that is not due to androgen deficiency.

Treatment

Androgen replacement therapy is the treatment of choice for both symptomatic and asymptomatic Leydig cell failure. This results in increases in lean body mass, bone mineral density, hemoglobin, libido, strength, and sense of well-being and decreases in total and high-density lipoprotein cholesterol and markers of bone resorption.

MALE INFERTILITY

About 15% of married couples are unable to produce off spring. Male factors are responsible in about 30% of cases, female factors in about 45%, and couple factors in 25%.

Etiology and Pathophysiology

In order for conception to occur, spermatogenesis must be normal, the sperm must complete its maturation during transport through patent ducts, adequate amounts of seminal plasma must be added to provide volume and nutritional elements, and the male must be able to deposit the semen near the female's cervix. Any defect in this pathway can result in infertility due to a male factor problem. The spermatozoa must also be able to penetrate the cervical mucus and reach the uterine tubes, where conception takes place. These latter events may fail to occur if there are female reproductive tract disorders or abnormalities of sperm motility or fertilizing capacity.

Table 12–4 lists the identified causes of male infertility. Disturbances in the function of the hypothalamus, pituitary, adrenals, or thyroid are found in approximately 4% of males evaluated for infertility. Sex chromosome abnormalities, cryptorchidism, adult seminiferous tubule failure, and other forms of primary testicular failure are found in 15% of infertile males. Congenital or acquired ductal problems are found in approximately 6% of such patients, and poor coital technique, sexual dysfunction, ejaculatory disturbances, and anatomic abnormalities such as hypospadias are causative factors in 4% to 5% of patients evaluated for infertility. Idiopathic infertility, in which no cause can be identified with certainty, accounts for approximately 35% of patients. Some of these patients may have mild forms of androgen receptor defects, microdeletions of the Y chromosome, or mutations in the cystic fibrosis gene. Autoimmune disturbances that lead to sperm agglutination and immobilization causes infertility in only a small fraction of patients. Varicoceles are found in 25% to 40% of patients classified as having idiopathic infertility, and experimental studies have shown an adverse effect of varicoceles on spermatogenesis. However, it is unclear why some individuals appear to be more susceptible to testicular problems from

TABLE 12–4 Causes of male infertility.

Endocrine
    Hypothalamic-pituitary disorders
    Testicular disorders
    Defects of androgen action
    Hyperthyroidism
    Hypothyroidism
    Adrenal insufficiency
    Congenital adrenal hyperplasia
Systemic illness
Defects in spermatogenesis
    Immotile cilia syndrome
    Drug induced
    Adult seminiferous tubule failure
    Microdeletions within Y chromosomes
Ductal obstruction
    Congential
    Acquired
Seminal vesicle disease
Prostatic disease
Varicocele
Retrograde ejaculation
Antibodies to sperm or seminal plasma
Anatomic defects of the penis
Poor coital technique
Sexual dysfunction
Idiopathic

varicoceles, as the presence of a varicocele is not uniformly associated with infertility and they are found in 8% to 20% of healthy males in the general population.

Clinical Features

A. Symptoms and signs The clinical features of the hypothalamic-pituitary, thyroid, adrenal, testicular, and sexual dysfunctional disorders have been discussed in preceding sections of this chapter. Evaluation for the presence of varicocele has also been described.

Patients with immotile cilia syndrome have associated mucociliary transport defects in the lower airways that result in chronic pulmonary obstructive disease. Some patients with this disorder also have Kartagener syndrome, with sinusitis, bronchiectasis, and situs inversus. Infections of the epididymis or vas deferens may be asymptomatic or associated with scrotal pain that may radiate to the flank, fever, epididymal swelling and tenderness, and urethral discharge. The presence of thickened, enlarged epididymis and vas is indicative of chronic epididymitis. Chronic prostatitis is usually asymptomatic, although a perineal aching sensation or low back pain may be described. A boggy or indurated prostate may be found on rectal palpation. A careful examination for the presence of penile anatomic abnormalities such as chordee, hypospadias, or epispadias should be made, because these defects may prevent the deposit of sperm in the vagina.

B. Laboratory findings A carefully collected and performed semen analysis is mandatory. A normal report indicates normal

endocrine function and spermatogenesis and an intact transport system. Sperm function can be further evaluated through sperm penetration assays, the inducibility of the acrosome reaction, and motility evaluation on a postcoital test. Immunologic infertility can be examined with a mixed antiglobulin reaction test for antisperm antibodies.

If semen analysis shows abnormalities, at least two more specimens should be obtained at monthly intervals. Persistent oligospermia or azoospermia should be evaluated by studies outlined in Figure 12–6. Patients with severe oligospermia or azoospermia should undergo chromosome analysis and testing for Yq microdeletions. If congenital absence of the vas deferens is present, testing for cystic fibrosis transmembrane conductance regulator gene mutations should be performed.

The female partner should be thoroughly examined to verify patency of the uterus and uterine tubes, normal ovulation, and normal cervical mucus. This examination must be performed even in the presence of a male factor abnormality, because infertility is due to a combination of male and female factors in about 20% of cases.

C. Imaging studies In patients with azoospermia or severe oligospermia, transscrotal ultrasound allows an assessment of the seminal vesicles and ejaculatory ducts. Patency of the ducts can be examined with scrotal vasography or seminovesiculography.

Treatment

A. Endocrine disorders Correction of hyperthyroidism, hypothyroidism, adrenal insufficiency, and congenital adrenal hyperplasia generally restores fertility. Patients with hypogonadotropic hypogonadism may have spermatogenesis initiated with gonadotropin therapy. Chorionic gonadotropin (2000 units intramuscularly three times per week) with urofollitropin or follitropin beta (75 units intramuscularly three times per week) added after 12 to 18 months if sperm cells do not appear in the ejaculate, restores spermatogenesis in most hypogonadotropic men. The sperm count following such therapy usually does not exceed 10 million/mL but may still allow impregnation. Patients with isolated deficiency of LH may respond to chorionic gonadotropin alone. There is no effective therapy for adult seminiferous tubule failure not associated with varicocele or cryptorchidism. However, if the oligospermia is mild (10-20 million/mL), cup insemination of the female partner with concentrates of semen may be tried. In vitro fertilization (IVF) and other assisted reproductive techniques, including direct injection of a spermatozoon into an egg (intracytoplasmic sperm injection; ICSI), are increasingly being utilized as a method for achieving pregnancy in couples in which the male is oligospermic.

B. Defects of spermatogenesis There is no treatment for immotile cilia syndrome or for chromosomal abnormalities associated with defective spermatogenesis. Drugs that interfere with spermatogenesis should be discontinued. These include the antimetabolites, phenytoin, marijuana, alcohol, monoamine oxidase inhibitors, sulfasalazine, and nitrofurantoin. Discontinuing use of these agents may be accompanied by restoration of normal sperm production. In some patients with maturation arrest, severe hypospermatogenesis or incomplete Sertoli cell only, retrieval of sperm through testicular aspiration or testicular biopsy followed by IVF or ICSI have resulted in pregnancies.

C. Ductal obstruction Localized obstruction of the vas deferens may be treated by vasovasostomy. Sperm are detected in the ejaculate of 60% to 80% of patients following this procedure. However, the subsequent fertility rate is only 40% to 50%; the presence of antisperm antibodies that agglutinate or immobilize sperms probably accounts for the high failure rate.

Epididymovasostomy may be performed for epididymal obstruction. Sperm in the postoperative ejaculate have been found in approximately half of patients treated with this procedure, but subsequent fertility has been demonstrated in only 20% of cases.

D. Genital tract infections Acute prostatitis may be treated with daily sitz baths, prostatic massage, and antibiotics. A combination of trimethoprim (400 mg) and sulfamethoxazole (2000 mg), twice a day for 10 days followed by the same dosage once a day for another 20 days, has been used with some success. Chronic prostatitis requires a longer period of treatment or a switch to a fluoroquinolone, such as ciprofloxacin 500 mg orally twice daily for 4 weeks. Acute epididymitis may respond to injections of local anesthetic into the spermatic cord just above the testicle. Appropriate antibiotic therapy should also be given. The prognosis for fertility following severe bilateral chronic epididymitis or extensive scarring from acute epididymitis is poor.

E. Varicocele The presence of varicocele in an infertile male with oligospermia is considered an indication for surgical ligation of the incompetent spermatic veins or radiographic embolization of the veins. Improvement in the semen is noted in 60% to 80% of treated patients, and about half are subsequently fertile.

F. Retrograde ejaculation Ejaculation of semen into the urinary bladder may occur following disruption of the internal bladder sphincter or with neuropathic disorders such as diabetic autonomic neuropathy. Normal ejaculation has been restored in a few patients with the latter problem following administration of phenylpropanolamine, 15 mg orally twice daily in timed-release capsules. Sperm can also be recovered from the bladder following masturbation for the purpose of direct insemination of the female partner.

G. Antibodies to sperm or seminal plasma Antibodies in the female genital tract that agglutinate or immobilize sperm may be difficult to treat. Older methods such as condom therapy or administration of glucocorticoids have not been uniformly successful. Currently, intrauterine insemination with washed spermatozoa, IVF, and gamete intrafallopian transfer are considered the most effective treatments.

H. Anatomic defects of the penis Patients with hypospadias, epispadias, or severe chordee may collect semen by masturbation for use in insemination.

I. Poor coital technique Couples should be counseled not to use vaginal lubricants or postcoital douches. In order to maximize the sperm count in cases of borderline oligospermia, intercourse should not be more frequent than every other day. Exposure of the cervix to the seminal plasma is increased by having the woman lie supine with her knees bent up for 20 minutes after intercourse.

Course and Prognosis

The prognosis for fertility depends on the underlying cause. It is good for patients with nontesticular endocrine abnormalities, varicoceles, retrograde ejaculation, and anatomic defects of the penis. If fertility cannot be restored, the couple should be counseled regarding intrauterine insemination with concentrated sperm, artificial insemination, IVF, ICSI, or adoption.

ERECTILE DYSFUNCTION

Erectile dysfunction is the inability to achieve or maintain an erection of sufficient duration and firmness to complete satisfactory sexual activity in more than 25% of attempts. It may occur with or without associated disturbances of libido or ejaculation. Approximately 5% of men have complete erectile dysfunction by age 40 and 15% by age 70. Some degree of erectile dysfunction is present in about 50% of men between ages 40 and 70.

Etiology and Pathophysiology

Penile erection occurs when blood flow to the penile erectile tissue (corpora cavernosa and spongiosum) increases as a result of dilation of the urethral artery, the artery of the bulb of the penis, the deep artery of the penis, and the dorsal artery of the penis following psychogenic or sensory stimuli transmitted to the limbic system and then to the thoracolumbar and sacral autonomic nervous system. The relaxation of the cavernosal arterial and cavernosal trabecular sinusoidal smooth muscle occurs following stimulation of the sacral parasympathetic (S2-4) nerves, which results in the release of acetylcholine, vasoactive intestinal peptide, and an endothelial cell-derived nitric oxide, which activates guanylyl cyclase. As the sinusoids become engorged, the subtunical venous plexus is compressed against the tunica albuginea, preventing egress of blood from the penis. Contraction of the bulbocavernosus muscle through stimulation of the somatic portion of the S2 to S4 pudendal nerves further increases the intracavernosal pressure. These processes result in the distention, engorgement, and rigidity of the penis that constitute erection.

Broadly speaking, erectile dysfunction may be divided into psychogenic and organic causes. Major epidemiologic factors that have been associated with erectile dysfunction include diabetes, hypertension, depression, smoking, aging, low high-density lipoprotein cholesterol, metabolic syndrome, cardiovascular disease, lower urinary tract symptoms of benign prostatic hyperplasia, and a low serum DHEA sulfate level. Table 12–5 lists various pathologic conditions and drugs that may be associated with erectile dysfunction.

TABLE 12–5 Organic causes of erectile dysfunction.

Neurologic
Anterior temporal lobe lesions
Spinal cord lesions
Autonomic neuropathy

Vascular
Leriche syndrome
Pelvic vascular insufficiency
Sickle cell disease
Venous leaks
Aging

Endocrine
Diabetes mellitus
Hypogonadism
Hyperprolactinemia
Adrenal insufficiency
Feminizing tumors
Hypothyroidism
Hyperthyroidism

Urogenital
Trauma
Castration
Priapism
Peyronie disease

Systemic Illness
Cardiac insufficiency
Cirrhosis
Uremia
Respiratory insufficiency
Lead poisoning

Postoperative
Aortoilliac or aortofemoral reconstruction
Lumbar sympathectomy
Perineal prostatectomy
Retroperitoneal dissection

Drugs
Endocrinologic
Antiandrogens
Estrogens
5α-Reductase inhibitors
GnRH agonists
Antihypertensives
Diuretics
Antidepressants
   Selective serotonin-reuptake inhibitors
   Lithium
   Monamine oxidase inhibitors
   Tricyclic antidepressants
Other
   Tobacco
   Alcohol
   Opioids
   H$_2$-receptor antagonists
   Gemfibrozil
   Amphetamines
   Cocaine
   Interferon-α
   Anticonvulsants
   Disopyramide

Most organic causes of erectile dysfunction result from disturbances in the neurologic pathways essential for the initiation and maintenance of erection or in the blood supply to the penis. Many of the endocrine disorders, systemic illnesses, and drugs associated with erectile dysfunction affect libido, the autonomic pathways essential for erection, or the blood flow to the penis. Venous incompetence because of anatomic defects in the corpora cavernosa or subtunical venous plexus is being recognized with increasing frequency. Local urogenital disorders such as Peyronie disease (idiopathic fibrosis of the covering sheath of the corpus cavernosum) may mechanically interfere with erection. In some patients, the cause of erectile dysfunction is multifactorial. For example, some degree of erectile dysfunction is reported by over 50% of men with diabetes mellitus. The basis of the erectile dysfunction is usually autonomic neuropathy. However, vascular insufficiency, antihypertensive medication, uremia, and depression may also cause or contribute to the problem in diabetics.

Clinical Features

A. Symptoms and signs   Patients may complain of constant or episodic inability to initiate or maintain an erection, decreased penile turgidity, decreased libido, or a combination of these difficulties. The degree of erectile dysfunction can be assessed by questionnaires such as the International Index of Erectile Function or the Sexual Health Inventory for men. Besides the specific sexual dysfunction symptoms, symptoms and signs of a more pervasive emotional or psychiatric problem may be elicited. If an underlying neurologic, vascular, or systemic disorder is the cause of erectile dysfunction, additional symptoms and signs referable to the anatomic or metabolic disturbances may be present. A history of claudication of the buttocks or lower extremities should direct attention toward arterial insufficiency. Lower urinary tract disorders may be screened for through the use of the International Prostate Symptom Score questionnaire. A thorough history of medication, herb, illicit drug and alcohol use should be obtained.

The differentiation between psychogenic and organic erectile dysfunction can usually be made on the basis of the history. Even though the patient may be selectively unable to obtain or maintain a satisfactory erection to complete sexual intercourse, a history of repeated normal erections at other times is indicative of psychogenic erectile dysfunction. Thus, a history of erections that occur nocturnally, during masturbation, or during foreplay or with other sexual partners eliminates significant neurologic, vascular, or endocrine causes of erectile dysfunction. Patients with psychogenic erectile dysfunction often note a sudden onset of sexual dysfunction concurrently with a significant event in their lives such as loss of a friend or relative, an extramarital affair, or the loss of a job.

Patients with organic erectile dysfunction generally note a more gradual and global loss of potency. Initially, such individuals may be able to achieve erections with strong sexual stimuli, but ultimately they may be unable to achieve a fully turgid erection under any circumstances. In contrast to patients with psychogenic erectile dysfunction, patients with organic erectile dysfunction generally maintain a normal libido. However, patients with systemic illness may have a concurrent diminution of libido and potency. Hypogonadism should be suspected in a patient who has never had an erection (primary erectile dysfunction).

During the physical examination, the patient's secondary sexual characteristics should be assessed and examination performed for gynecomastia, discordant or diminished femoral pulses, reduced testicular volume or consistency, penile plaques, and evidence of peripheral or autonomic neuropathy. The bulbocavernosus reflex tests the integrity of the S2 to S4 nerves. It is performed by inserting a finger into the patient's rectum while squeezing his glans penis. Contraction of the anal musculature represents a normal response.

B. Laboratory findings and special examinations

Serum testosterone measurements may uncover a mild and otherwise asymptomatic androgen deficiency. If the testosterone level is low, serum PRL should be measured because hyperprolactinemia—whether drug-induced or due to a pituitary or hypothalamic lesion—may inhibit androgen production. Diabetes mellitus is a relatively common cause of erectile dysfunction and erectile dysfunction may be the presenting symptom of diabetes; therefore, fasting and 2-hour postprandial blood glucose measurements should be ordered.

In a patient with a normal physical examination and screening blood tests, many clinicians elect to begin with a therapeutic trial of a type 5 phosphodiesterase (PDE5) inhibitor that potentiates the effects of nitric oxide by inhibiting the breakdown of cyclic guanosine monophosphate. The initial oral dose is usually 50 mg of sildenafil (Viagra), 10 mg of tadalafil (Cialis), or 10 mg vardenafil (Levitra). This should be tried only if the patient is not taking nitrates, has not had a myocardial infarction in the last 6 months, and does not have unstable angina, hypotension, severe congestive heart failure, or retinitis pigmentosa.

The integrity of the neurologic pathways and the ability of the blood vessels to deliver a sufficient amount of blood to the penis for erection to occur may be objectively examined by placement of a strain gauge behind the glans penis and at the base of the penis at the time the patient retires for sleep. The occurrence of nocturnal penile tumescence can thus be recorded. Healthy men and those with psychogenic erectile dysfunction have three to five erections a night associated with rapid eye movement sleep. Absence or reduced frequency of nocturnal tumescence indicates an organic lesion. Penile rigidity as well as tumescence can be evaluated with an ambulatory monitor called RigiScan. The vascular integrity of the penis may be examined by Doppler ultrasonography with spectral analysis following intracorporeal injection of a vasoactive drug. This method allows detection of venous leaks with a sensitivity of 55% to 100% and specificity of 69% to 88%. Arterial problems are also detected with a sensitivity of 82% to 100% and specificity of 64% to 96%. The choice of other laboratory tests such as cavernosometry, cavernosography, or arteriography depends on associated organic symptoms or signs.

Treatment

Discontinuation of an offending drug usually results in a return of potency. Similarly, effective therapy of an underlying systemic or endocrine disorder may cure the erectile dysfunction. For psychogenic erectile dysfunction, simple reassurance and explanation, formal psychotherapy, and various forms of behavioral therapy have a reported 40% to 70% success rate. Sildenafil, 25 to 100 mg taken orally about 1 hour before anticipated intercourse is approximately 70% to 80% effective in patients with a wide variety of causes of erectile dysfunction, including psychogenic ones. This agent is absolutely contraindicated in men receiving oral or transdermal nitrates for vascular disease. Side effects include headache (16%) and visual disturbances (3%). Other PDE5 inhibitors that are available include vardenafil (2.5-20 mg) and tadalafil (2.5-20 mg).

Vasoactive drugs including prostaglandin E_1, papaverine hydrochloride, and phentolamine mesylate, either alone or in combination, may induce an erection following intracavernous injection. Of these, the only Food and Drug Administration-approved agent is prostaglandin E_1 (alprostadil), which needs to be individualized within the dosage range of 2.5 to 60 μg per injection. In clinical studies, up to 90% of men with erectile dysfunction developed erections with intracavernosal injections. Side effects include penile pain (33% of patients), hematoma (3%), penile fibrosis (3%), and priapism (0.4%). Intraurethral insertion of a 1.4-mm pellet containing alprostadil leads to satisfactory erections in two-thirds of patients, with effects beginning within 10 minutes and lasting 30-60 minutes. The major side effects are penile pain (36%), urethral pain (13%), and dizziness (4%).

Devices have been developed that use suction to induce penile engorgement and constrictive bands to maintain the ensuing erection. Erections are achieved in 90% of patients with an approximately 70% couple satisfaction rate. Alternatively, a surgically implanted semirigid or inflatable penile prosthesis provides satisfactory results in 85% to 90% of cases, but the device must be replaced every 5 to 10 years.

Repair of venous leaks and microsurgical revascularization of arterial lesions have had variable success rates. Patients with permanent erectile dysfunction due to organic lesions that cannot be corrected should be counseled in noncoital sensate focus techniques.

GYNECOMASTIA

Gynecomastia is common during the neonatal period and is present in about 70% of pubertal males (Chapter 15). Clinically apparent gynecomastia has been noted at autopsy in almost 1% of adult males, and 40% of autopsied males have histologic evidence of gynecomastia.

Etiology and Pathophysiology

The causes of gynecomastia are listed in Table 12–6. Several mechanisms have been proposed to account for this disorder. All involve a relative imbalance between estrogen and androgen concentrations or action at the mammary gland level. Decrease in free testosterone may be due to primary gonadal disease or an increase

TABLE 12–6 Causes of gynecomastia.

Physiologic
Neonatal
Pubertal
Involutional

Drug Induced
Hormones
  Androgens and anabolic steroids
  Chorionic gonadotropin
  Estrogens and estrogen agonists
  Growth hormone
  Environmental estrogens
Antiandrogens or inhibitors of androgen synthesis
  Cyproterone
  Flutamide
  Biclutamide
Antibiotics
  Isoniazid
  Ketoconazole
  Metronidazole
Antiulcer medications
  Cimetidine
  Omeprazole
  Ranitidine
Cancer chemotherapeutic agents (especially alkylating agents)
Cardiovascular drugs
  Amiodarone
  Captopril
  Enalapril
  Nifedipine
  Spironolactone
  Verapamil
Psychoactive agents
  Diazepam
  Haloperidol
  Phenothiazines
  Tricyclic antidepressants
Drugs of abuse
  Alcohol
  Amphetamines
  Heroin
  Marijuana
Other
  Highly active antiretroviral therapy (HAART)
  Phenytoin
  Penicillamine

Endocrine
Primary hypogonadism with Leydig cell damage
Hyperprolactinemia
Hyperthyroidism
Androgen receptor disorders
Excessive aromatase activity

Systemic Diseases
Hepatic cirrhosis
Uremia
Recovery from malnourishment

Neoplasms
Testicular germ cell or Leydig cell tumors
Feminizing adrenocortical adenoma or carcinoma
HCG-secreting nontrophoblastic neoplasms

Idiopathic

in SHBG as is found in hyperthyroidism and some forms of liver disease (eg, alcoholic cirrhosis). Decreased androgen action in patients with the androgen insensitivity syndromes results in unopposed estrogen action on the breast glandular tissue. Acute or chronic excessive stimulation of the Leydig cells by pituitary gonadotropins alters the steroidogenic pathways and favors excessive estrogen and estrogen precursor secretion relative to testosterone production. This mechanism may be responsible for the gynecomastia found with hypergonadotropic states such as Klinefelter syndrome and adult Leydig cell failure. The rise of gonadotropins during puberty may lead to an estrogen-androgen imbalance by similar mechanisms. Patients who are malnourished or have systemic illness may develop gynecomastia during refeeding or treatment of the underlying disorder. Malnourishment and chronic illness are accompanied by a reduction in gonadotropin secretion, and during recovery the gonadotropins rise and may stimulate excessive Leydig cell production of estrogens relative to testosterone.

Excessive stimulation of Leydig cells may also occur in patients with hCG-producing trophoblastic or nontrophoblastic tumors. In addition, some of these tumors are able to convert estrogen precursors into estradiol. Feminizing adrenocortical and Leydig cell neoplasms may directly secrete excessive quantities of estrogens. The mechanisms by which PRL-secreting pituitary tumors and hyperprolactinemia produce gynecomastia are unclear. Elevated serum PRL levels may lower testosterone production and diminish the peripheral actions of testosterone, which may result in an excessive estrogen effect on the breast that is not counteracted by androgens.

Drugs may reduce androgen production (eg, spironolactone, ketoconazole), peripherally antagonize androgen action (spironolactone, cimetidine), or interact with breast estrogen receptors (spironolactone and phytoestrogens in marijuana).

Finally, it has been proposed that patients with idiopathic and familial gynecomastia have breast glandular tissue that is inordinately sensitive to normal circulating levels of estrogen or excessively converts estrogen precursors to estrogens.

Pathology

Three histologic patterns of gynecomastia have been recognized. The florid pattern consists of an increase in the number of budding ducts, proliferation of the ductal epithelium, periductal edema, and a cellular fibroblastic stroma. The fibrous type has dilated ducts, minimal duct epithelial proliferation, no periductal edema, and a virtually acellular fibrous stroma. An intermediate pattern contains features of both types.

Although it has been proposed that different causes of gynecomastia are associated with either the florid or the fibrous pattern, it appears that the duration of gynecomastia is the most important factor in determining the pathologic picture. Approximately 75% of patients with gynecomastia of 4 months' duration or less exhibit the florid pattern, whereas 90% of patients with gynecomastia lasting a year or more have the fibrous type. Between 4 months and 1 year, 60% of patients have the intermediate pattern.

Clinical Features

A. Symptoms and signs The principal complaint is unilateral or bilateral concentric enlargement of breast glandular tissue. Nipple or breast pain is present in one-fourth of patients and objective tenderness in about 40%. A complaint of nipple discharge can be elicited in 4% of cases. Histologic examination has demonstrated that gynecomastia is almost always bilateral, although grossly it may be detected only on one side. The patient often complains of discomfort in one breast despite obvious bilateral gynecomastia. Breast or nipple discomfort generally lasts less than 1 year. Chronic gynecomastia is usually asymptomatic, with the major complaint being the cosmetic one. Symptoms and signs of underlying disorders may be present. Gynecomastia may be the earliest manifestation of an hCG-secreting testicular tumor; therefore, it is mandatory that careful examination of the testes be performed in any patient with gynecomastia. Enlargement, asymmetry, and induration of a testis may be noted in such patients.

B. Laboratory findings Once pubertal and drug-induced gynecomastia have been excluded, a biochemical screen for liver and renal abnormalities should be performed. If those are normal and the gynecomastia is of recent onset, then serum hCG, LH, testosterone, and estradiol levels should be measured. The interpretation of the results is outlined in Figure 12–8. For chronic, asymptomatic gynecomastia detected on physical examination, measurement of a morning serum testosterone level is a reasonable screen for hypogonadism.

Differential Diagnosis

Gynecomastia should be differentiated from lipomas, neurofibromas, carcinoma of the breast, and obesity. Breast lipomas, neurofibromas, and carcinoma are usually unilateral, painless, and eccentric, whereas gynecomastia characteristically begins in the subareolar areas and enlarges concentrically. The differentiation between gynecomastia and enlarged breasts due to obesity may be difficult. The patient should be supine. Examination is performed by spreading the thumb and index fingers and gently palpating the breasts during slow apposition of the fingers toward the nipple. In this manner, a concentric ridge of tissue can be felt in patients with gynecomastia but not in obese patients without glandular tissue enlargement. The examination may be facilitated by applying soap and water to the breasts.

Complications and Sequelae

There are no complications other than possible psychologic damage from the cosmetic defect. With the possible exclusion of patients with Klinefelter syndrome, individuals with gynecomastia do not have an increased risk of development of breast carcinoma.

Treatment

A. Medical treatment The underlying disease should be corrected if possible, and offending drugs should be discontinued. Antiestrogens or selective estrogen receptor modulators, such as tamoxifen or raloxifene, have been found useful in relieving pain and reversing gynecomastia in some patients. Whether these

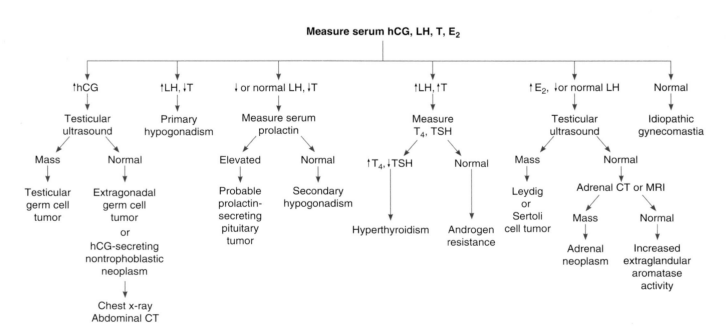

FIGURE 12–8 Diagnostic evaluation for endocrine causes of gynecomastia (E_2, estradiol; hCG, human chorionic gonadotropin; LH, luteinizing hormone; T, testosterone; T_4, thyroxine; TSH, thyrotropic hormone). (Reproduced, with permission, from Braunstein GD. Gynecomastia. *N Engl J Med.* 1993;328:490).

therapies will be useful in most patients with gynecomastia remains to be seen. Aromatase inhibitors have also been tried but are not as beneficial as tamoxifen. Tamoxifen is also useful in preventing development of gynecomastia in many patients who are starting therapy for prostate cancer with antiandrogens.

B. Surgical treatment   Reduction mammoplasty should be considered for cosmetic reasons in any patient with long-standing gynecomastia that is in the fibrotic stage.

C. Radiologic treatment   Patients with prostatic carcinoma may receive low-dose radiation therapy (900 cGy or less) to the breasts before initiation of antiandrogen monotherapy for prostate cancer. This may prevent or diminish the gynecomastia that usually results from such therapy, although tamoxifen is more effective. Radiotherapy should not be given to other patients with gynecomastia.

Course and Prognosis

Pubertal gynecomastia usually regresses spontaneously over 1 to 2 years. Patients who develop drug-induced gynecomastia generally have complete or near-complete regression of the breast changes if the drug is discontinued during the early florid stage. Once gynecomastia from any cause has reached the fibrotic stage, little or no spontaneous regression occurs, and medical therapy is ineffective.

TESTICULAR TUMORS

Testicular neoplasms account for 1% to 2% of all male-specific malignant neoplasms and 4% to 10% of all genitourinary neoplasms. They are the most frequent type of cancer in men between 20 and 34 years of age. The incidence is 5.4 per 100,000 men in the United States and 4.6 to 7.3 per 100,000 men in Europe. The incidence is lower in nonwhite than in white populations. Ninety-five percent of testicular tumors are of germ cell origin; 5% are composed of stromal or Leydig cell neoplasms.

Etiology and Pathophysiology

The cause of germ cell testicular tumors is not known. Predisposing factors include testicular maldescent and dysgenesis. About 4% to 12% of testicular tumors are found in association with cryptorchidism, and such a testicle has a 20- to 30-fold greater risk of developing a neoplasm than does a normally descended one. Almost 20% of testicular tumors associated with cryptorchidism arise in the contralateral scrotal testis, suggesting that testicular dysgenesis may be of etiologic importance in the development of germ cell neoplasms. Although trauma is frequently cited as an etiologic factor in testicular tumors, no causal relationship has been established. What is more likely is that testicular trauma serves to call the patient's attention to the presence of a testicular mass. Familial predisposition is found in 1% to 2% of patients. An increased incidence has been noted in patients with Down and Klinefelter syndromes and prenatal exposure to exogenous estrogens. Increased risk also has been associated with smoking and possibly HIV infection. Extra copies of a portion of chromosome 12 (isochromosome 12p) have been found in testicular germ cell tumors.

Bilateral gynecomastia is uncommon in patients who present with germ cell tumors. It is generally associated with production of hCG by the trophoblastic elements in the tumor. The hCG stimulates the Leydig cells to produce excessive estrogens relative to androgen production, resulting in estrogen-androgen imbalance and gynecomastia. In addition, the trophoblastic tissue in some of the germ cell tumors may convert estrogen precursors to estrogens, as can Leydig and Sertoli cell tumors.

Pathology

A. Germ cell tumors   Seminomas account for 33% to 50% of all germ cell tumors. They are composed of round cells with abundant cytoplasm, prominent nuclei, and large nucleoli. The cells are arranged in cords and nests and have a thin delicate network of stromal connective tissue. Embryonal cell neoplasms comprise 20% to 33% of germ cell tumors. These tumors have multiple histologic patterns composed of cuboidal pleomorphic cells. One distinct pattern of cellular arrangement is the endodermal sinus tumor (yolk sac tumor), the most frequent germ cell neoplasm found in infants. Immunohistochemical techniques have localized alpha-fetoprotein to the embryonal cells. About 10% of germ cell tumors are teratomas, which are composed of well-differentiated cells derived from all three germ layers. When one or more of the teratoid elements are malignant or are mixed with embryonal carcinoma cells, the term teratocarcinoma is applied. These tumors account for one-tenth to one-third of germ cell neoplasms. Choriocarcinoma is the rarest form of germ cell tumor (2%) and is composed of masses of large, polymorphic, multinucleated syncytiotrophoblastic cells. Although pure choriocarcinoma is rare, many testicular tumors contain an occasional trophoblastic giant cell. Immunohistochemical techniques have shown that these cells are the source of hCG in such tumors.

B. Leydig and Sertoli cell tumors   Leydig cell (interstitial cell) tumors are rare. Most are benign and are composed of sheets of oval to polygonal cells arranged in lobules separated from one another by thin strands of connective tissue. Malignant Leydig cell tumor disseminates by both lymphatic and venous channels, with initial metastatic deposits being found in the regional lymph nodes, followed by metastases to liver, lung, and bone. Sertoli cell tumors also are rare, are generally benign, and are composed of large tubules, a thick basement membrane with enlarged cuboidal Sertoli cells. There may be extensive calcification within the tumors and the tumors may be multifocal and bilateral.

Clinical Features

A. Symptoms and signs

1. **Germ cell tumors**—Testicular tumors usually present as painless enlargement of a testicle with an associated feeling of fullness or heaviness in the scrotum. Thus, about 80% of

patients note a testicular swelling or mass, whereas only 25% complain of testicular pain or tenderness. About 6% to 25% of patients give a history of testicular trauma that brought the testicular mass to their attention. Gynecomastia may be present initially in 2% to 4% of patients and develops subsequently in another 10%. About 5% to 10% of patients present with symptoms of distant metastatic disease, including backache, skeletal pains, gastrointestinal symptoms and abdominal pains, inguinal adenopathy, cough, hemoptysis, and neurological dysfunction.

A testicular mass or generalized enlargement of the testis is often present on examination. In 5% to 10% of patients, a coexisting hydrocele may be present. In the presence of metastatic disease, supraclavicular and retroperitoneal lymph node enlargement may be present.

2. **Leydig and Sertoli cell tumors**—In children, Leydig cell tumors of the testes may produce sexual precocity, with rapid skeletal growth and development of secondary sexual characteristics. Adults with such tumors usually present with a testicular mass and occasionally gynecomastia. Decreased libido may also be present in such patients. Sertoli cell tumors are associated with gynecomastia and feminization due to excessive aromatase activity. In addition, these tumors are associated with the autosomal dominant Peutz-Jeghers syndrome (gastrointestinal polyposis and oval, irregularly pigmented lip macules) and the Carney complex (cardiac myxomas, spotty cutaneous pigmentation, primary pigmented nodular adrenocortical disease with hypercortisolism).

B. Laboratory findings

1. **Germ cell tumors**—The tumor markers hCG, alpha-fetoprotein, and lactate dehydrogenase (LDH) should be measured in every male presenting with a testicular mass. hCG is found in the sera of 5% to 10% of males with seminoma, over half of patients with teratocarcinoma or embryonal cell carcinoma, and all patients with choriocarcinoma. hCG should be measured as the beta subunit or other hCG-specific immunoassay method. Elevated serum immunoreactive alpha-fetoprotein concentrations are found in almost 70% of patients with nonseminomatous forms of germ cell neoplasms. Both markers are elevated in over 50% of patients with nonseminomatous germ cell tumors, and at least one of the markers is elevated in 85% of such patients. These markers can also be used to monitor the results of therapy. LDH measurements have an independent prognostic significance and reflect tumor growth rate and cellular proliferation. It is increased in about 80% of patients with advanced seminomas and 60% of advanced nonseminomatous tumors. The results of the three marker measurements are included in the formal staging classification from the American Joint Committee on Cancer.

2. **Leydig and Sertoli cell tumors**—Serum DHEA sulfate, urinary 17-ketosteroid, and both urinary and serum estrogen levels may be increased, while serum testosterone concentrations tend to be low or within the normal adult range in patients with Leydig cell tumors. Individuals with Sertoli cell tumors have elevated estradiol levels.

C. Imaging studies

Testicular ultrasonography may be required to visualize small tumors. Staging of testicular tumors requires chest and abdominal CT scans and other radiologic procedures depending on the type of tumor and the symptoms.

Differential Diagnosis

Testicular tumors are sometimes misdiagnosed as epididymitis or epididymo-orchitis. An inflammatory reaction of the epididymis often involves the vas deferens. Therefore, both the vas and the epididymis are thickened and tender on examination during the acute disease. Pyuria and fever also help to differentiate between epididymitis and testicular tumor. Because hydrocele may coexist with testicular tumor, the testes should be carefully examined following aspiration of the hydrocele.

Other conditions that can cause confusion with testicular tumors include inguinal hernia, hematocele, hematoma, torsion, spermatocele, varicocele, and (rarely) sarcoidosis, tuberculosis, and syphilitic gumma. Ultrasonic examination of the scrotum may help distinguish between testicular tumors and extratesticular disease such as acute or chronic epididymitis, spermatocele, or hydrocele.

Benign Leydig cell tumors of the testes must be differentiated from adrenal rest tumors in patients with congenital adrenal hyperplasia. Because the testes and the adrenals are derived from the same embryologic source, ectopic adrenal tissue may be found to migrate with the testes. This tissue can enlarge under the influence of ACTH in patients with congenital adrenal hyperplasia or Cushing disease. Adrenal rest tumors tend to be bilateral, whereas patients with Leydig cell tumors generally have unilateral disease. Both may be associated with elevated urine 17-ketosteroids and elevated serum DHEA sulfate concentrations. Elevated serum and urinary estrogen concentrations are found with both disorders. However, patients with congenital adrenal hyperplasia or Cushing disease have a decrease in 17-ketosteroids, DHEA sulfate, and estrogen concentrations, as well as a decrease in tumor size, following administration of dexamethasone, while those with Leydig cell tumors do not.

Treatment

A. Germ cell tumors   Seminomas are quite radiosensitive, and disease localized to the testes is usually treated with radical inguinal orchiectomy and 2000 to 4000 cGy of conventional radiotherapy delivered to the ipsilateral inguinal-iliac and bilateral para-aortic lymph nodes to the level of the diaphragm. For disease that has spread to the lymph nodes below the diaphragm, additional whole abdominal radiotherapy and prophylactic mediastinal and supraclavicular lymph node irradiation are usually given. Widely disseminated disease is generally treated with a combination of radiotherapy and chemotherapy, especially with bleomycin, etoposide, and cisplatin.

Nonseminomatous tumors are treated with orchiectomy, retroperitoneal lymph node dissection, and, if necessary, radiotherapy or chemotherapy (or both). Although many chemotherapeutic agents have been used, combinations of etoposide, bleomycin, and cisplatin currently appear to produce the best overall results. Patients with nonseminomatous tumors treated by these means should be monitored with serial measurements of serum hCG and alpha-fetoprotein.

B. Leydig and Sertoli cell tumors   Leydig and Sertoli cell tumors of the testes are treated by unilateral radical inguinal orchiectomy. Objective remissions of malignant Leydig cell tumors have been noted following treatment with mitotane.

Course and Prognosis

A. Germ cell tumors   In patients with seminoma confined to the testicle, the 5-year survival rates after orchiectomy and radiotherapy are 98% to 100%. Disease in the lymph nodes below the diaphragm also has an excellent prognosis, with 5-year survival rates of 80% to 85%. Disease above the diaphragm and disseminated disease have overall 5-year survival rates of about 70%.

In patients with nonseminomatous germ cell tumors, aggressive surgery and combination chemotherapy have raised the 5-year survival rates from less than 20% to 60% to 90%.

B. Leydig and Sertoli cell tumors   Removal of a benign Leydig or Sertoli cell tumor is accompanied by regression of iso- or heterosexual precocious puberty in children or feminization in adults. The prognosis for malignant Leydig cell tumor is poor, with most patients surviving less than 2 years from the time of diagnosis.

REFERENCES

Physiology

Agarwal A, Bragais FM, Sabanegh E. Assessing sperm function. *Urol Clin N Amer.* 2008;35:157. [PMID: 18423237]

Amory JK, Bremner WJ. Regulation of testicular function in men: implications for male hormonal contraceptive development. *J Steroid Biochem Mol Biol.* 2003;85:357. [PMID: 12943722]

Josso N, Picard JY, Rey R, Clemente N. Testicular anti-Mullerian hormone: history, genetics, regulation and clinical application. *Pediat Endocrinol Rev.* 2006;3:347. [PMID: 16816803]

Rajender S, Singh L, Thangaraj K. Phenotypic heterogeneity of mutations in androgen receptor gene. *Asian J Androl.* 2007;9:147. [PMID: 17334586]

Rosner W, Auchus RJ, Azziz R, Sluss PM, Raff H. Position statement: utility, limitations, and pitfalls in measuring testosterone: an Endocrine Society Position Statement. *J Clin Endocrinol Metab.* 2007;92:405. [PMID: 17090633]

Sofikitis N, Giotitsas N, Tsounapi P, Baltogiannis D, Giannakis D, Pardalidis N. Hormonal regulation of spermatogenesis and spermiogenesis. *J Steroid Biochem Molecular Biol.* 2008;109:323. [PMID: 18400489]

Androgen Therapy

Seftel A. Testosterone replacement therapy for male hypogonadism: part III. Pharmacologic and clinical profiles, monitoring, safety issues, and potential future agents. *Int J Impotence Res.* 2007;19:2. [PMID: 16193074]

Hypogonadism

Bhasin S, Cunningham GR, Hayes FJ, et al. Testosterone therapy in adult men with androgen deficiency syndromes: an Endocrine Society Clinical Practice Guideline. *J Clin Endocrinol Metab.* 2006;91:1995. [PMID: 16720669]

Foresta C, Cunningham GR, Hayes FJ, Role of hormones, genes, and environment in human cryptorchidism. *Endocrine Rev.* 2008;29:560. [PMID: 18436703]

Lanfranco F, Kamischke A, Zitzmann M, Nieschlag E. Klinefelter's syndrome. *Lancet.* 2004;364:273. [PMID: 15262106]

Practice Committee of the American Society for Reproductive Medicine in collaboration with the Society for Male Reproduction and Urology. Androgen deficiency in the aging male. *Fertil Steril.* 2008;90(suppl 3):S83. [PMID: 19002654]

Ranum LPW, Day JW. Myotonic dystrophy: RNA pathogenesis comes into focus. *Am J Hum Genet.* 2004;74:793. [PMID: 15065017]

Ritzen EM, Bergh A, Bjerknes R, et al. Nordic consensus on treatment of undescended testes. *Acta Paediatrica.* 2007;96:638. [PMID: 17326260]

Seftel A. Male hypogonadism. Part II: etiology, pathophysiology, and diagnosis. *Int J Impotence Res.* 2006;18:223. [PMID: 16094414]

Van der Burgt I. Noonan syndrome. *Orphanet J Rare Dis.* 2007;2:4. [PMID: 17222357]

Wang C, Nieschlag E, Swerdloff R, et al. ISA, ISSAM, EAU, EAA and ASA recommendations: investigation, treatment and monitoring of late-onset hypogonadism in males. *Int J Impotence Res.* 2009;21:1. [PMID: 18923415]

Infertility

Bhasin S. Approach to the infertile man. *J Clin Endocrinol Metab.* 2007;92:1995. [PMID: 17554051]

French DB, Desai NR, Agarwal A. Varicocele repair: does it still have a role in infertility treatment? *Curr Opin Obstet Gynecol.* 2008;20:269. [PMID: 18460942]

Kim HH, Schlegel PN. Endocrine manipulation in male infertility. *Urol Clin N Am.* 2008;35:303. [PMID: 18423250]

Oates RD. The genetic basis of male reproductive failure. *Urol Clin N Am.* 2008;35:257. [PMID: 18423246]

Pauli SA, Berga SL, Shang W, Session DR. Current status of the approach to assisted reproduction. *Pediatr Clin N Am.* 2009;56:467. [PMID: 19501687]

Practice Committee of the American Society for Reproductive Medicine. Report on varicocele and infertility. *Fertil Steril.* 2008;90 (suppl 3):S247. [PMID: 19007639]

Practice Committee of the American Society for Reproductive Medicine. Sperm retrieval for obstructive azoospermia. *Fertil Steril.* 2008;90 (suppl 3):S213. [PMID: 19007634]

Practice Committee of the American Society for Reproductive Medicine in collaboration with the Society for Male Reproduction and Urology. The management of infertility due to obstructive azoospermia. *Fertil Steril.* 2008;90 (suppl 3):S121. [PMID: 19007607]

Practice Committee of the American Society for Reproductive Medicine in collaboration with the Society for Male Reproduction and Urology. Evaluation of the azoospermic male. *Fertil Steril.* 2008;90 (suppl 3):S74. [PMID: 19007652]

Tournaye H. Evidence-based management of male subfertility. *Curr Opin Obstet Gynecol.* 2006;18:253. [PMID: 167355823]

Erectile Dysfunction

McVary KT. Clinical practice. Erectile dysfunction. *N Engl J Med.* 2007;357:2472. [PMID: 18077811]

Montague DK, Jarow JP, Broderick GA, et al. The management of erectile dysfunction: an AUA update. *J Urol.* 2005;174:230. [PMID: 15947645]

Gynecomastia

Braunstein GD. Clinical practice. Gynecomastia. *N Engl J Med.* 2007;357:1229. [PMID: 17881754]

Niewoehner CB, Schorer AE. Gynaecomastia and breast cancer in men. *BMJ.* 2008;336:709. [PMID: 18369226]

Testicular Cancer

American Cancer Society: Detailed Guide: Testicular Cancer. http://www.cancer.org/docroot/CRI/CRI_2_3x.asp?dt=41.

Carmignani L, Salvioni R, Gadda F, et al. Long-term followup and clinical characteristics of testicular Leydig cell tumor: experience with 24 cases. *J Urol.* 2006;176:2040. [PMID: 17070249]

Gori S, Porrozzi S, Roila F, Gatta G, De Giorgi U, Marangolo M. Germ cell tumours of the testis. *Crit Rev Oncol/Hematol.* 2005;53:141. [PMID: 15661565]

Female Reproductive Endocrinology and Infertility

Mitchell P. Rosen, MD and Marcelle I. Cedars, MD

ACTH	Adrenocorticotropic hormone		**IGF-BP**	Insulin-like growth factor binding protein
AFC	Antral follicle count		**IUI**	Intrauterine insemination
AIRE	Autoimmune regulator gene		**LDL**	Low-density lipoprotein
AIS	Androgen insensitivity syndrome		**LH**	Luteinizing hormone
AMH	Anti-Müllerian hormone		**MBH**	Medial basal hypothalamus
APS	Autoimmune polyglandular syndrome		**MCR**	Metabolic clearance rate
ArKO	Aromatase knockout		**MMP**	Matrix metalloproteinase
ART	Assisted reproductive therapy		**MPA**	Medroxyprogesterone acetate
BBT	Basal body temperature		**MT**	Menopausal transition
BMD	Bone mineral density		**OMI**	Oocyte maturation inhibitor
BMP	Bone morphogenic protein		**PCOS**	Polycystic ovarian syndrome
cAMP	Cyclic adenosine monophosphate		**POF**	Premature ovarian failure
CEE	Conjugated equine estrogen		**PR**	Production rate
CRH	Corticotropin-releasing hormone		**PRL**	Prolactin
DHEAS	Dehydroepiandrosterone sulfate		**SERM**	Selective estrogen receptor modulator
DHT	Dihydrotestosterone		**SF-1**	Steroidogenic factor-1
DXA	Dual-energy x-ray absorptiometry		**SHBG**	Sex hormone–binding globulin
ERA	Estrogen Replacement and Atherosclerosis Trial		**SNRI**	Serotonin-norepinephrine reuptake inhibitor
FGFR1	Fibroblast growth factor receptor 1		**SR**	Secretion rate
FMR1	*Fragile X* gene		***SRY***	Sex-determining region of the Y gene
FSH	Follicle-stimulating hormone		**SSRI**	Selective serotonin reuptake inhibitor
FXTAS	Fragile-*X* tremor ataxia syndrome		**StAR**	Steroidogenic acute regulatory protein
GH	Growth hormone		**STRAW**	Stages of Reproductive Aging Workshop
GnRH	Gonadotropin-releasing hormone		**SWAN**	Study of Women's Health Across the Nation
hCG	Human chorionic gonadotropin			
HDL	High-density lipoprotein		**Tg**	Thyroglobulin
HERS	Heart and Estrogen-Progestin Replacement Study		**TGF**	Transforming growth factor
			TPO	Thyroid peroxidase
HPO	Hypothalamic pituitary ovarian		**TRH**	Thyrotropin-releasing hormone
HRT	Hormone replacement therapy		**TSH**	Thyroid-stimulating hormone
HSD	Hydroxysteroid dehydrogenase		**VEGF**	Vascular endothelial growth factor
HT	Hormone therapy		**WHI**	Women's Health Initiative

EMBRYOLOGY AND ANATOMY

No gene has yet been identified that generates an ovary from an undifferentiated gonad. It is only in the absence of the sex-determining region of the Y gene *(SRY)* that the gonad develops into an ovary. (For more details, see the discussion of sexual differentiation in Chapter 14.) Primordial germ cells, which give rise to oocytes or spermatogonia, are first identifiable in the yolk sac endoderm (hindgut) at 3 to 4 weeks' gestation. Once specified, they migrate and proliferate en route through the dorsal mesentery into the gonadal ridge, which is located lateral to the dorsal mesentery of the gut and medial to the mesonephros (Figure 13–1). Studies in mice have suggested that the process of proliferation and navigation to the gonad depends on several genes, including *Steel* (kit ligand and receptor), β_1 *integrin, pog* (proliferation of germ cells), and many cytokines. Failure of primordial germ cells to develop or migrate into the gonadal ridge results in failure of ovarian development. In contrast, it is suggested that male gonadal development may continue to develop into functional testis despite the absence of germ cells.

The germ cells that reach the gonadal ridge (6 weeks' gestation) continue to proliferate and are referred to as oogonia (premeiotic germ cells). At 10 to 12 weeks' gestation, some oogonia leave the mitotic pool and begin meiosis, where they arrest in prophase I (dictyotene stage). These arrested germ cells are now called primary oocytes. By 16 weeks, primordial follicles are first identified, making a clear distinction for gonadal differentiation into an ovary. At approximately 20 weeks' gestation, a peak of 6 to 7 million germ cells (two-thirds of them primary oocytes and one-third oogonia) are present in the ovaries. During the second half of gestation, the rate of mitosis rapidly decreases and the rate of oogonial and follicular atresia increases. Those oogonia that are not transformed into primary oocytes will undergo atresia before birth. This leads to a reduction in the number of germ cells, resulting in a total of 1 to 2 million germ cells at birth. No germ cell mitosis occurs after birth, whereas follicular atresia continues, with the result that the average girl entering puberty has only 300,000 to 400,000 germ cells.

The ovary is organized into an outer cortex and an inner medulla. The germ cells are located within the cortex. Along the outer surface of the cortex is the germinal epithelium. This cell layer is composed of cuboidal cells resting on a basement membrane and forms a continuous layer with the peritoneum. Even though it is called the germinal epithelium, there are no germ cells within this layer. During embryonic development, the epithelial cells proliferate and enter the underlying tissue of the ovary to form cortical cords. When the primordial germ cells arrive at the genital ridge, they are incorporated into these cortical cords. At the same time the germ cells migrate from the yolk sac, the stromal cells of the ovary (granulosa and interstitial cells) migrate from the mesonephric tubules into the gonad. **Primordial follicles** form within the cortical cords. They are composed of a primary oocyte and one layer of granulosa cells with its basement membrane. Oocytes not surrounded by granulosa cells are lost, probably by apoptosis. This finite follicle population represents the pool of germ cells that will ultimately be available to enter the follicular cycle.

During fetal development, the gonad is held in place by the suspensory ligament at the upper pole and the gubernaculum at the lower pole. The final location of the gonad is dependent on hormone production. In the presence of testosterone, the gubernaculum grows while the suspensory ligament regresses. As the gubernaculum continues to grow, the gonad (testis) descends into the scrotum. In contrast, when testosterone is absent, the suspensory ligament remains and the gubernaculum regresses. This process maintains the gonad (ovary) in the pelvis.

The remainder of the female internal reproductive organs are formed from the paramesonephric (Müllerian) ducts. In the absence of anti-Müllerian hormone (AMH), the paramesonephric system develops into the uterine (fallopian) tubes, uterus, cervix, and upper third of the vagina. Unlike Wolffian duct differentiation, the development of the female reproductive tract is not

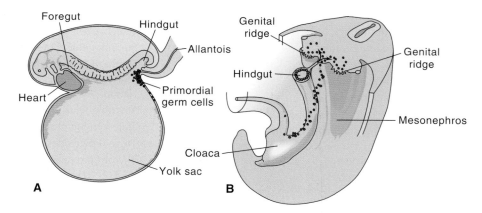

FIGURE 13–1 **A.** Schematic drawing of a 3-week-old embryo showing the primordial germ cells in the wall of the yolk sac, close to the attachment of the allantois. **B.** Drawing to show the migrational path of the primordial germ cells along the wall of the hindgut and the dorsal mesentery into the genital ridge. (Reproduced, with permission, from Langman J, Sadler TW. *Langman's Medical Embryology.* 8th ed. Lippincott Williams & Wilkins; 2000.)

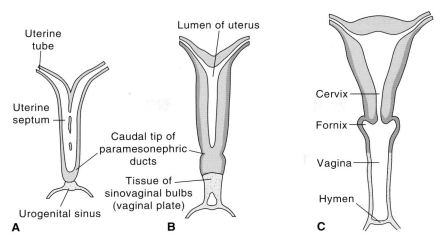

FIGURE 13–2 Schematic drawing showing the formation of the uterus and vagina. **A.** At 9 weeks. Note the disappearance of the uterine septum. **B.** At the end of the third month. Note the tissue of the sinovaginal bulbs. **C.** Newborn. The upper portion of the vagina and the fornices are formed by vacuolization of the paramesonephric tissue and the lower portion by vacuolization of the sinovaginal bulbs. (Reproduced, with permission, from Langman J, Sadler TW. *Langman's Medical Embryology*. 8th ed. Lippincott Williams & Wilkins; 2000.)

dependent on hormone production. (For more details, see "Human Sex Differentiation" in Chapter 14.) Briefly, the Müllerian buds are formed lateral to the Wolffian ducts and the gonadal ridge after 37 days' gestation (Figure 13–2). These buds elongate, extend caudally, and cross medially to the Wolffian ducts by 8 weeks' gestation. By 10 weeks, the adjacent paired Müllerian ducts meet in the midline as they join the Müllerian tubercle (urogenital sinus). Over the next couple of weeks, the Wolffian ducts degenerate, and the paired Müllerian ducts fuse and begin to canalize. The intervening septum resorbs between the 12th and 16th weeks of gestation, resulting in a single uterine cavity. The most cranial parts of the Müllerian ducts remain unfused and form the uterine tubes, which remain patent with the coelom (future peritoneal cavity). The caudal segments stimulate solid cords to extend from the Müllerian tubercle to the sinovaginal bulbs from the posterior aspect of the urogenital sinus. In turn, the sinovaginal bulbs extend cranially and fuse with the vaginal cords, forming the vaginal plate. The vagina is subsequently formed by canalization of the vaginal plate. It is ultimately the cervix and the upper one-third of the vagina that are derived from the Müllerian structures, and the remaining lower two-thirds are formed from the urogenital sinus.

The uterus is composed of endometrium (innermost lining), myometrium, and serosa. The adult uterus is a pear-shaped hollow organ. The cervical portion extends approximately 2 cm into the vagina, and the remaining corpus extends approximately 6 cm into the abdomen. The normal adult uterus weighs 40 to 80 g.

The uterus is located in the pelvis and rests on the pelvic floor. Seventy percent to 80% of the time, the uterine position is anteflexed (cervical-uterine corpus angle) and anteverted (cervical-vaginal angle). Therefore, when a woman is standing, the corpus of the uterus is horizontal and resting on top of the bladder. The uterus has several paired ligaments that develop from thickenings

of the peritoneum and serve to maintain this anatomic position. The cardinal ligament (Mackenrodt) is the main supporting ligament. It attaches to the lateral margins of the cervix at the upper vagina and extends to the lateral pelvic wall. The remaining ligaments—uterosacral, round, and broad—have a lesser role in supporting the uterus.

The uterine artery originates from the anterior division of the internal iliac artery (hypogastric), enters the cardinal ligament, and supplies the uterus. The uterine artery divides into a descending branch and an ascending branch known as the vaginal and arcuate arteries, respectively. The arcuate arteries anastomose with each other and form a vascular network around the uterus. The radial arteries branch off from the arcuate network and penetrate the uterus to supply the myometrium. Smaller basal branches and spiral arteries supply the endometrium.

The ovary is suspended in the pelvis and has three associated ligaments. The average adult ovary is 2.5 to 5 cm × 2.5 cm × 1 cm in size and weighs 3 to 8 g. The position of the ovary is variable, but in a nulliparous woman it is often located in a peritoneal depression on the pelvic sidewalls between the ureter and external iliac vein. The suspensory (infundibulopelvic) ligament attaches to the cranial pole of the ovary and extends to the pelvic brim. This ligament suspends the ovary in the pelvis and contains the ovarian vessels, lymphatics, and nerves. The utero-ovarian ligament attaches to the inferior pole of the ovary and extends to the uterus. The mesovarium connects the anterior portion of the ovary to the posterior leaf of the broad ligament. The blood supply of the ovary originates from the abdominal aorta, passes through the suspensory ligament, and enters the mesovarium to form an anastomotic network with branches from the uterine artery. The ovarian artery enters the ovarian hilum and branches into spiral arteries that enter the medulla and extend to the ovarian cortex. Other branches from the anastomotic network, located in the mesovarium, supply the uterine tubes.

OVARIAN STEROIDOGENESIS

The ovaries are not only the store for germ cells—they also produce and secrete hormones that are vital for reproduction and the development of secondary sexual characteristics. The next section will briefly discuss the biosynthesis of ovarian hormones.

In the ovary, the major source of hormone production is the maturing follicle. The components of the follicle are the theca cells, the granulosa cells, and the primary oocyte. The theca cells produce androgens, and the granulosa cells produce estrogens. The other stromal cells that contribute to androgen production can be divided into two populations of cells: the secondary interstitial cells (derived from theca) and the hilum cells. These cells are the major ones involved in ovarian hormone production during menopause (see below).

The ovarian hormones are derived from cholesterol. Steroidogenic cells acquire the cholesterol substrate from one of three sources. The most common source is plasma lipoprotein-carrying cholesterol, primarily in the form of low-density lipoprotein (LDL). Other minor sources include de novo synthesis from acetate and liberation from stored lipid droplets (cholesterol esters). Stimulation of ovarian cells by trophic hormones such as follicle-stimulating hormone (FSH) and luteinizing hormone (LH) facilitate uptake of cholesterol by increasing the number of LDL receptors on the cell surface. The LDL particle is subsequently internalized and degraded in the lysosome. The free cholesterol that is liberated from the lysosome is delivered to the mitochondria by an unknown mechanism, possibly via microfilaments and microtubules. The cholesterol is then translocated into the mitochondria by the steroidogenic acute regulatory protein (StAR). Thus, StAR is the rate-limiting step regulating substrate availability for steroidogenesis.

Although acute alterations in steroid production result from changes in delivery of cholesterol to the mitochondria, the long-term control of steroid synthesis results from regulation of gene expression. Most of the genes involved in steroidogenesis contain at least one steroidogenic factor-1 (SF-1) response element in the promoter region. These elements are critical for the regulation of steroidogenic genes as well as the development of adrenal gland, ovary, and testis. The importance of SF-1 for steroidogenesis is highlighted in knockout mice deficient in this transcription factor which lack adrenal glands and gonads. Although SF-1 is essential, the specific expression of each gene involves many other transcription factors that work independently or in concert with SF-1.

The rate-determining step that commits cholesterol to steroid synthesis is the cholesterol side chain cleavage enzyme reaction (P450scc) (Figure 13–3). This reaction converts cholesterol to pregnenolone, the precursor of steroid hormones, and takes place in the mitochondria. Pregnenolone is transported out of the mitochondrion, and the remaining steps in sex steroid production take place primarily within the smooth endoplasmic reticulum (SER).

Once pregnenolone is formed, the particular hormones that are synthesized are dependent on the endocrine organ and cell type. For example, the main sources of sex steroids in the female

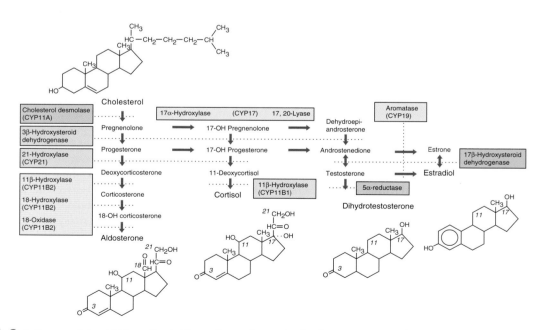

FIGURE 13–3 Pathways of steroid biosynthesis. The pathways for synthesis of progesterone and mineralocorticoids (aldosterone), glucocorticoids (cortisol), androgens (testosterone and dihydrotestosterone), and estrogens (estradiol) are arranged left to right. The enzymatic activities catalyzing each bioconversion are written in the boxes. For those activities mediated by specific cytochrome P450, the systematic name of the enzyme (*CYP* followed by a number) is listed in parentheses. CYPB2 and CYP17 have multiple activities. The planar structures of cholesterol, aldosterone, cortisol, dihydrotestosterone, and estradiol are placed near the corresponding labels. (Reproduced, with permission, from White PC, Speiser PW. Congenital adrenal hyperplasia due to 21-hydroxylase deficiency. *Endocr Rev.* 2000;21:245.)

come from the adrenal gland, ovary, and the periphery. The specific type of hormone synthesized is dependent on the specific gene expression within each cell type.

In the adrenal gland, there are three zones: zona glomerulosa, zona fasciculata, and zona reticularis. The cells in the different zones start with the same hormone precursor but differ in their secretory products. The glomerulosa produces mainly aldosterone, whereas cortisol and androgen are produced by the zona fasciculata and zona reticularis, respectively. The major androgen produced by the adrenal gland is dehydroepiandrosterone sulfate (DHEAS). Differences in enzymatic activity among cells in the various zones are what regulate hormone production. The zona reticularis and zona fasciculata lack 11β-hydroxylase, which is necessary for aldosterone synthesis (see Figure 13–3; see Chapters 9 and 10). The zona glomerulosa lacks 17-hydroxylase and 17,20-lyase (CYP17), which are necessary for sex steroid synthesis.

Ovarian cells similarly secrete different hormones due to differential enzyme activity. The theca interstitial and secondary interstitial cells lack aromatase and hence are the androgen producers in the ovarian cortex. The granulosa cells, on the other hand, lack CYP17 and, therefore, secrete estrogens—mainly estradiol—from thecal cell-derived androgens in the proliferative phase and progesterone in the luteal phase (see later).

Adipose and skin make significant contributions to plasma concentrations of some sex steroids. Adipose tissue is able to sequester most steroids due to their lipid solubility. Fat also expresses genes capable of sex steroid metabolism (ie, aromatase). Skin significantly contributes to the plasma concentration of testosterone by utilizing circulating DHEAS and androstenedione as precursors.

The major circulating androgens include DHEAS, androstenedione, and testosterone. During the reproductive years, the ovaries are directly responsible for one-third of the testosterone production. The remaining two-thirds come from the periphery (17β-hydroxysteroid dehydrogenase [HSD] types 3 and 5) and is derived from ovarian and adrenal gland precursors—notably androstenedione, which is produced in equal proportions by the adrenal gland and the ovary. The adrenal gland may directly secrete testosterone, but its major contribution is derived from its production of precursors. Therefore, the ovaries are responsible for nearly two-thirds of the circulating testosterone. This differs from males, in whom only 5% of the circulating testosterone is derived from peripheral conversion of androstenedione. It is also estimated that more than 60% of the most potent androgen, dihydrotestosterone (DHT) in women, is produced in the skin (5α-reductase type 1 and 2) and originates from androstenedione. DHEAS is the major androgen produced by the adrenal gland. The adrenal gland is responsible for more than 95% of the circulating DHEAS levels. Although it is the most abundant androgen circulating in the body, it contributes minimally to serum testosterone levels. The relative strengths of androgens are listed in Table 13–1.

The circulating estrogens include estrone, estrone sulfate, estradiol, and estriol (pregnancy). More than 95% of estradiol in the circulation is produced from the ovary. In contrast to estradiol, approximately one-half of the circulating estrone is secreted from the ovary, while the remaining is derived from peripheral conversion. The most significant precursor, androstenedione, is aromatized

TABLE 13–1 Relative androgenic activity of androgens.

Steroid	Activity
Dihydrotestosterone	300
Testosterone	100
Androstenedione	10
DHEA, DHEAS	5

Reproduced, with permission, from Yen SSC, Jaffe RB, Barbieri RL, eds. *Reproductive Endocrinology*. Saunders; 1999.

in the adipose tissue, hair follicles, and the liver to estrone. Estrone is also derived from estradiol through 17β-HSD type 2 activity or from estrone sulfate (steroid sulfatase). Almost all estriol is produced during pregnancy and is secreted from the placenta (see Chapter 16).

Ultimately, the serum concentration of sex steroids is dictated by the secretion rate (SR), production rate (PR), and metabolic clearance rate (MCR), as shown in Table 13–2. The SR of sex steroids from each organ determines the PR of the hormone. If the SR for a specific hormone in the ovary equals the PR, then there is no extragonadal formation. However, if there is extra-gonadal formation, then the PR exceeds the SR.

MCR is the volume of blood per unit of time cleared of the hormone. The metabolic clearance rate of sex steroids is inversely related to the affinity for sex hormone–binding globulin (SHBG) and/or albumin. Prior to excretion, steroids are conjugated to make them water soluble. The bulk of testosterone is bound to SHBG (~65%) and to a lesser extent albumin (~35%); only 1% (*free* hormone) is active and available for metabolism. The remaining androgens have negligible binding affinity for SHBG. Free testosterone may be converted to more potent androgens such as DHT or may be metabolized through androstenedione. Metabolites of androstenedione and DHT are conjugated with a sulfate or glucuronide and are excreted in the urine. The majority of estradiol is also bound, although it has less binding affinity than testosterone for SHBG (38%) and more for albumin (60%); approximately 2% is unbound. Estradiol may be directly conjugated (16α-hydroxylated or 2-hydroxylated) or is metabolized to estrone prior to conjugation. The remaining estrogens are weakly bound to proteins. Progesterone is metabolized into many intermediates prior to conjugation. Pregnanediol glucuronide is the major metabolite observed in the urine.

A variety of clinical conditions result from or cause deviations in normal secretion rates, leading to disturbances in the menstrual cycle. This chapter discusses the normal physiology and touches on several of these hormonal disturbances.

PHYSIOLOGY OF FOLLICULOGENESIS AND THE MENSTRUAL CYCLE

The menstrual cycle is regulated by complex interactions between the hypothalamic-pituitary-ovarian (HPO) axis and the uterus. Briefly, the hypothalamus secretes gonadotropin-releasing hormone

TABLE 13-2 Production rate (PR), secretion rate (SR), and metabolic clearance rate (MCR) of plasma steroids in women.

Compound	MCR of Compound in Peripheral Plasma (L/d)	Phase of Menstrual Cycle	Concentration in Plasma		PR of Circulating Compound (mg/d)	SR by Both Ovaries (mg/d)
			(nmol/L)	(µg/dL)		
Estradiol	1350	Early follicular	0.2	0.006	0.081	0.07
		Late follicular	1.2–2.6	0.033-0.070	0.445-0.945	0.4-0.8
		Midluteal	0.7	0.020	0.270	0.25
Estrone	2210	Early follicular	0.18	0.005	0.110	0.08
		Late follicular	0.5-1.1	0.015-0.030	0.331-0.662	0.25-0.50
		Midluteal	0.4	0.011	0.243	0.16
Progesterone	2200	Follicular	3.0	0.095	2.1	1.5
		Luteal	36	1.13	25.0	24.0
20α-Hydroxyprogesterone	2300	Follicular	1.5	0.05	1.1 5.8	0.8
		Luteal	7.5	0.25		3.3
17-Hydroxyprogesterone	2000	Early follicular	0.9	0.03	0.6	0-0.3
		Late follicular	6 6	0.20	4.0	3-4
		Midluteal		0.20	4.0	3-4
Androstenedione	2010		5.6	0.159	3.2	0.8-1.6
Testosterone	690		1.3	0.038	0.26	
Dehydroepiandrosterone	1640		17	0.490	8.0	0.3-3

From Tagatz GE, Gurpride E. Hormone secretion by the normal human ovary. In: Greep RP, Astwood EP, eds. *Handbook of Physiology*. Section 7, Vol. II, Part 1 American Physiological Society. Williams and Wilkins; 1973:603.

(GnRH), which stimulates the pituitary to release FSH and LH. These gonadotropins then trigger the ovary to release an oocyte that is capable of fertilization. Concurrently, the ovary secretes hormones, which act on the endometrial lining of the uterus to prepare for implantation. In addition, the ovarian hormones feed back to the hypothalamus and pituitary, regulating the secretion of gonadotropins during the phases of the menstrual cycle. This complex interaction will be discussed in greater detail below. The hormonal changes associated with menstruation are summarized in Figure 13–4.

The Hypothalamic-Pituitary Axis

GnRH is the central initiator of reproduction. GnRH is a 10 amino acid peptide with a short half-life of 2 to 4 minutes. It is processed in specialized secreting neurons that originate in the olfactory placode during development and migrate to the arcuate nucleus of the medial basal hypothalamus (MBH). These neurons project from the median eminence and secrete GnRH, with inherent rhythmic behavior (pulse generator), into the portal vessels to reach the gonadotropes within the anterior pituitary. GnRH binds to its receptor, a member of the G protein–coupled seven-transmembrane-spanning receptor superfamily. 1,4,5–inositol triphosphate and diacylglycerol act as second messengers for GnRH. The pulsatile frequency of GnRH secretion regulates gonadotropin synthesis and the secretion of pituitary gonadotropes (see Chapter 4).

During the late luteal-follicular phase, the slower pulsatile release of GnRH—every 90 to 120 minutes—favors FSH secretion. In

response to FSH, the maturing follicle in the ovary secretes estradiol. This hormone is involved in a negative feedback loop that inhibits the release of FSH by indirectly decreasing the production of GnRH via gamma-aminobutyric acid neurons, in addition to possibly having a direct effect on the pituitary gland. Estradiol is also involved in a positive feedback loop that increases the frequency of GnRH pulses to every 60 minutes during the follicular phase and acts directly on the pituitary to stimulate LH secretion. LH stimulates the ovary to further increase estradiol production (see two-cell theory, later). There is no further change in GnRH pulsatility at this point in the cycle; however, estradiol and other regulatory factors (see later) increase pituitary sensitivity to GnRH. This increased sensitivity results in a rapid elevation of LH production—the LH surge—which stimulates ovulation. After ovulation, the ruptured follicle (corpus luteum) secretes progesterone. This hormone is involved in a negative-feedback loop, indirectly through increased endogenous opioid activity and possibly directly through a reduction in GnRH pulsatility to every 3 to 5 hours. This favors FSH synthesis during the luteal-follicular transition. As progesterone levels fall again, GnRH pulsatility increases, favoring FSH release.

Role of the Pituitary

Gonadotropes are located in the adenohypophysis and make up approximately 10% of the cells in the pituitary. These cells synthesize and secrete FSH and LH. These hormones, thyroid-stimulating hormone (TSH) and human chorionic gonadotropin (hCG), all belong to a family of glycoprotein hormones. Gonadotropins

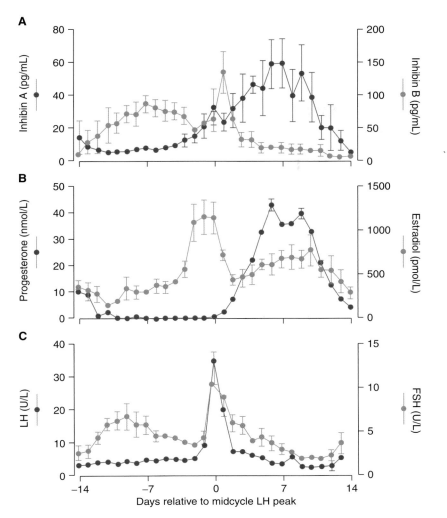

FIGURE 13–4 The endocrinology of the luteal-follicular transition in women. Data are mean ± SE of daily serum concentrations of FSH, LH, estradiol, progesterone, and immunoreactive inhibin in women with normal cycles. Note the secondary rise in plasma FSH in the late luteal phase (~2 days before menses). (Reproduced with permission from Erickson GF. Ovarian anatomy and physiology. In: Lobo R, ed. *Menopause: Biology and Pathobiology.* Academic Press; 2000.)

are functional as heterodimers and are composed of an alpha and a beta subunit. The alpha subunit amino acid sequence is identical for all of the glycoprotein hormones while the beta subunits contain different amino acid sequence and confer unique specificity on the glycoproteins.

The synthesis of FSH and LH mostly occur in the same cell, yet their secretion patterns differ. The secretion of FSH is tightly linked to the expression of the FSH beta subunit. This suggests that there is minimal storage of FSH within the gonadotropes, and the majority of secretion follows more of a constitutive pathway. This is in contrast to LH secretion, in which it is first stored in organelles and then released with the appropriate trigger (regulated pathway). The different oligosaccharides on the beta subunits likely facilitate the intracellular sorting that results in different mechanisms of secretion.

The differential gene expression that leads to the production and release of gonadotropins by cells in the pituitary is influenced by GnRH and ovarian hormones through feedback loops. Slower

GnRH pulse frequency enhances FSH beta subunit expression and increases LH amplitude. In turn, increased GnRH pulse frequency stimulates LH beta subunit expression while promoting FSH release. As a result, LH amplitude decreases while the mean concentration rises. Thus, ovarian steroid modification of hypothalamic GnRH pulsatility controls pituitary gonadotrophin production.

An intrapituitary network involves several factors that play a role in regulating gonadotropin synthesis and secretion. The gonadotropes produce and secrete peptides that are in the transforming growth factor (TGF) family. Activin is a local regulatory protein that is involved in control of gonadotrope function. Slow pulses of GnRH enhance activin synthesis, which subsequently enhances FSH transcription. Follistatin, another TGF-related protein that binds to activin, is stimulated by rapid pulses of GnRH. This decreases the bioavailability of activin and consequently reduces FSH synthesis. In addition to these local modifiers, ovarian transforming growth factors such as inhibin also modulate the expression of gonadotropins (see later).

Role of the Ovary

The ovary is intimately involved in regulating the menstrual cycle via steroid feedback to alter gonadotropin secretion. In addition, the ovary contains an intraovarian network involving factors that are synthesized locally and have a paracrine and autocrine role in the modulation of gonadotropin activity. The intraovarian regulators include the insulin-like growth factor (IGF) family, TGF superfamily, and epidermal growth factor (EGF) family. Furthermore, it is these factors that assist in the coordination of follicular development, steroidogenesis, and ovulation.

The menstrual cycle of the ovary includes a follicular phase and a luteal phase. The follicular phase is characterized by growth of the dominant follicle and ovulation. It typically lasts 10 to 14 days. It is, however, this phase that is variable in duration and most often accounts for the variability in menstrual cycle length in ovulatory women. The luteal phase starts after ovulation and is the period when the ovary secretes hormones that are essential to accommodate conceptus implantation. This phase is relatively constant and averages 14 days (range, 12-15 days) in duration. The next section will describe the two phases in some detail.

Primordial follicles are the fundamental reproductive units that comprise the pool of resting oocytes. Morphologically, they are composed of a primary oocyte that is surrounded by a single layer of squamous granulosa cells and a basement membrane. They have no blood supply. These primordial follicles develop between the sixth and ninth months of gestation and harbor the complete supply of ovarian follicles.

The initiation of follicular growth begins with the transition of the dormant primordial follicle into the growth phase. The exact mechanisms controlling the initial recruitment of the primordial follicle are under investigation. It is suggested that the resting follicular pool is probably under tonic inhibitory control. The initial recruitment process induces growth in some primordial follicles; other neighboring follicles remain quiescent for many months or years. It is thought that the recruitment of these follicles is a continuous process that begins once the germ pool is created and ends with follicular exhaustion. This complex process is gonadotropin independent. Several studies have suggested that an intraovarian signaling network, involving members of the TGF superfamily, is responsible for primordial follicle recruitment. It is also known that recruitment and growth of the follicle absolutely requires cell-to-cell contact with neighboring granulosa cells and the oocyte. These cells transfer various factors, nutrients, and waste to and from the oocyte through gap junctions derived from connexins.

One theory proposes that the oocyte actively influences its own fate by secreting various factors. These include two particular growth factors related to TGF-β, which are produced by the oocyte early in follicular development, growth differentiation factor (GDF)-9 and bone morphogenic protein (BMP)-15. Knockout mouse studies suggest that the oocyte induces granulosa cell proliferation through these growth factors, and the granulosa cell responds with factors (eg, follistatin, c-kit) to decrease the inhibitory influences (eg, activin A, Müllerian-inhibiting substance) and promote stimulators of oocyte growth (Figure 13–5).

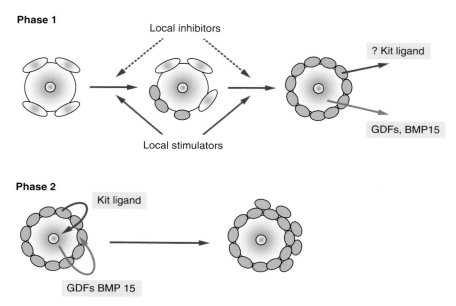

FIGURE 13–5 A theoretical model of follicular recruitment into the growth phase. Initiation of follicular growth may be regulated by many local inhibitory and stimulatory factors (ie, inhibin A, follistatin, kit ligand) and begins with transformation of the granulosa cells from squamous to cuboidal shape. Oocytes subsequently commence growth and regulate proliferation and differentiation of granulosa cells with members of the transforming growth factor β superfamily (ie, GDF-9, BMP15). Phase 1: transition of granulosa cells from flattened to cuboidal. Phase 2: oocyte growth and proliferation and differentiation of granulosa cells. (Redrawn with permission of Braw-Tal R. The initiation of follicle growth: the oocyte of the somatic cells? *Mol Cell Endocrinol.* 2002;187:11.)

Several other local factors have been described to date, and many more will be identified in the future. The ongoing search for these growth factors and hormones will ultimately elucidate the physiology of primordial follicle recruitment. There is a finite number of germ cells, and each successive recruitment further depletes the germ pool. Any abnormality that alters the number of germ cells or accelerates recruitment could perhaps lead to early ovarian follicular depletion and, therefore, early reproductive failure (see section on infertility, later).

Primary follicle development is the first stage of follicular growth (Figure 13–6). Primary follicles differ from primordial follicles in several ways. The oocyte begins to grow. As growth progresses, the zona pellucida is formed. This is a thick layer of glycoprotein that is most likely synthesized by the oocyte. It completely surrounds the oocyte and forms a barrier between the oocyte and the granulosa cell layer. It serves a number of biologic functions that are critical for protection of the oocyte and conception. Finally, the granulosa cells undergo a morphologic change from squamous to cuboidal. This stage of development may last 150 days.

The progression to a **secondary follicle** includes attainment of maximal oocyte growth (120 μm in diameter), proliferation of granulosa cells, and acquisition of theca cells. The exact mechanism involved in acquiring theca cells is not completely understood, but they are thought to be derived from the surrounding ovarian mesenchyme (stromal fibroblasts) as the developing follicle migrates to the medulla. It is the development of this layer that gives rise to the theca interna and theca externa. With theca cell development, these follicles gain an independent blood supply, although the granulosa cell layer remains avascular. In addition, the granulosa cells in the secondary follicle develop FSH, estrogen, and androgen receptors. This phase of follicular development may take as long as 120 days, probably because of the long doubling time (>250 hours) of granulosa cells.

Further follicular development leads to the tertiary follicle or early antral phase. This phase is characterized by the formation of an antrum or cavity in the follicle. The antral fluid contains steroids, proteins, electrolytes, proteoglycans, and an ultrafiltrate that forms from diffusion through the basal lamina. Other changes in this phase include further theca cell differentiation. Subpopulations

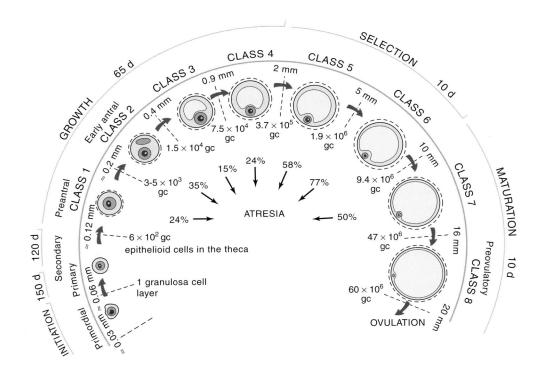

FIGURE 13–6 The chronology of folliculogenesis in the human ovary. Folliculogenesis is divided into two major periods, preantral (gonadotropin independent) and antral (FSH dependent). In the preantral period, a recruited primordial follicle develops into the primary/secondary (class 1) and early tertiary (class 2) stages, at which time cavitation or antrum formation begins. The antral period includes the small graafian (0.9-5 mm, classes 4 and 5), medium graafian (6-10 mm, class 6), large graafian (10-15 mm, class 7), and preovulatory (16-20 mm, class 8) follicles. Time required for completion of preantral and antral periods is approximately 300 and 40 days, respectively. Number of granulosa cells (gc), follicle diameter (mm), and atresia (%) are indicated. (Reproduced, with permission, from Gougeon A. Regulation of ovarian follicular development in primates: facts and hypotheses. *Endocr Rev.* 1996;17:121.)

of thecal interstitial cells develop within the theca interna, acquire LH receptors, and are capable of steroidogenesis. The granulosa cells begin to differentiate into distinct cell layers. Starting from the basal lamina, the cells can be stratified into the membrana, periantral, cumulus oophorus, and corona radiata layers. This developmental process is influenced by FSH and unidentified signals originating from the oocyte. It is suggested that oocyte-derived GDF-9, is an important factor in this process, where the relative concentration of GDF-9 dictates the specific subtype of granulosa cell. In addition, the granulosa cell—most likely in response to FSH—starts producing activin, a member of the TGF family. Activin is composed of two types of beta subunits, βA and βB, which are held together by disulfide bonds. It is the combination of these subunits that generates the various activins (activin A [βA,βA], AB [βA,βB], or BB [βB,βB]). It is unlikely that activin has an endocrine role, because serum activin levels do not change throughout the menstrual cycle and the free activin level in the serum is negligible. Activin's primary activity is within the ovary, where it plays an autocrine role by enhancing FSH receptor gene expression in the granulosa cells and accelerating folliculogenesis.

Follicular growth during the early antral phase occurs at a slow and constant pace. The follicle achieves a diameter of 400 μm. FSH-stimulated mitosis of granulosa cells is the major contributor to follicular growth at this stage. Until this point, follicular growth and survival are largely independent of gonadotropins. In fact, prepubertal females and women taking oral contraceptives may have follicles arrested at various phases up until this point. It is at this phase in follicular development that FSH is critical for growth and survival. If FSH does not rescue these follicles, they undergo atresia.

The morphologic follicular unit, consisting of theca cells and granulosa cells, is also a functional hormonal unit capable of substantial estrogen production (two-cell theory; Figure 13–7). The thecal interstitial cells and granulosa cells are under the direct influence of LH and FSH, respectively. The gonadotropins increase cyclic adenosine monophosphate (cAMP) production and the activity of the transcription factor SF-1 in the respective cell types.

In the theca cell, LH increases the number of LH receptors on the cell surface and the expression and activity of StAR, P450scc, 3β-HSD-II, and P450c17 to increase androgen production. FSH increases the expression of aromatase and 17β-HSD within the granulosa cell.

The pathway of androgen synthesis is shown in Figure 13–3. Androgens may be formed in one of two ways: (1) Δ5 pathway, which entails dehydroepiandrosterone (DHEA) as the precursor to androgens, and (2) Δ4 pathway, which synthesizes androgen through 17-OH progesterone. However, in the human, the contribution of the Δ4 pathway for androgen production appears minimal. This is due to 17,20-lyase activity having a much higher affinity for 17-OH pregnenolone than 17-OH progesterone. Therefore, the main precursor to sex steroids in the human is DHEA.

The androgens—mainly androstenedione—then diffuse through the basal lamina of the follicle and are the main precursors that granulosa cells utilize for estrogen production through

the activity of the aromatase enzyme. However, the pathway of estradiol biosynthesis is dictated by the type of 17β-HSD that is expressed. In humans, seven 17β-HSDs have been identified, each having different affinities for particular steroids. In the granulosa cell, it is type 1 17β-HSD that is expressed preferentially reducing estrone to yield estradiol. Type 3 17β-HSD preferentially reduces androstenedione to testosterone and is expressed in the Leydig cells and not in the ovary. However, type 5 17β-HSD is expressed in the theca cells and is likely the catalyst for the final step in testosterone synthesis from androstenedione in the ovary. In summary, the major pathway of estradiol biosynthesis within the granulosa cell entails androstenedione aromatization to estrone by aromatase, followed with a reduction to estradiol by type 1 17β-HSD.

The importance of estradiol on folliculogenesis with respect to its negative and positive feedback effects on gonadotropin secretion is well established. However, the role of estradiol in local oocyte maturation and follicular growth remains controversial. There is evidence that estrogen is synergistic with FSH during the follicular phase by increasing FSH and LH receptors, stimulating proliferation of granulosa cells and gap junctions as well as aromatase activity. The aromatase knockout (ArKO) mouse suggests a local role for estrogen. The ArKO mouse initially has large antral follicles, but after the first year, there are no remaining antral follicles or secondary follicles and atresia is evident among the remaining primary follicles. However, the ArKO oocytes are capable of in vitro maturation and blastocyst formation. There is evidence that both estrogen receptors are expressed in the granulosa and theca cells. Studies with the estrogen receptor α knockout mice show these mice are infertile and lack graafian follicles. However, the estrogen receptor β knockouts are fertile but produce smaller litters. In humans, there are cases where follicular development has occurred in the absence of estradiol secretion. This was observed in a woman with CYP17α deficiency where promotion of follicular growth was noted with gonadotropins. Embryo development followed in vitro fertilization, but unfortunately no pregnancy resulted.

Intraovarian factors play a major modulatory role in both folliculogenesis and steroidogenesis. The oocyte-derived factor GDF-9 is expressed throughout folliculogenesis. It is thought not only to promote granulosa cell differentiation but also to have a stimulatory effect on theca cells and an inhibitory effect on luteal cell formation. The IGFs enhance the response to FSH. In vitro studies have shown that both IGF-1 and IGF-2 increase granulosa cell proliferation and estradiol secretion. However, it is suggested that IGF-2 rather than IGF-1 plays a dominant role in follicular maturation. This may be explained by the absence of IGF-1 expression in the granulosa cells of dominant follicles. Furthermore, women with Laron syndrome (IGF-1 deficiency) can be induced to ovulate by ovarian stimulation with gonadotropins. This scenario suggests that IGF-1 is not critical for folliculogenesis.

The granulosa cells produce other hormones (members of the TGF-β family), that regulate folliculogenesis (see activin earlier). The granulosa cells synthesize the alpha subunit, which combines with beta subunits to create a heterodimer known as inhibin A (αβA) or inhibin B (αβB). The role of inhibins in folliculogenesis

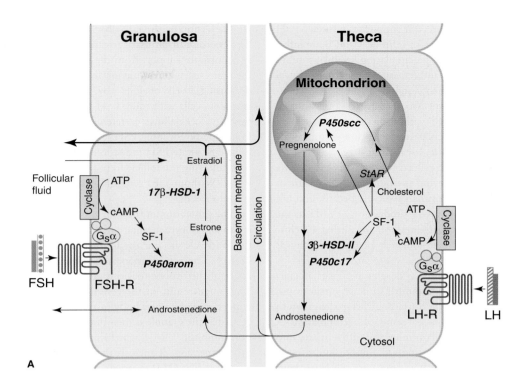

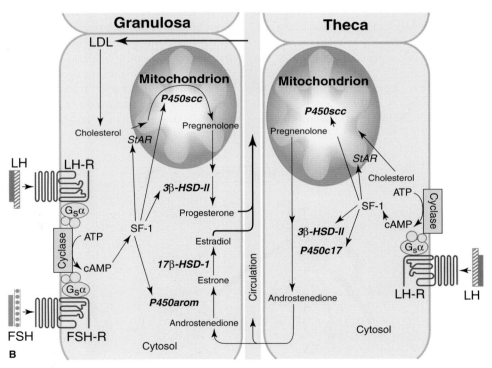

FIGURE 13-7 Two-cell hypothesis. **A.** The preovulatory follicle produces estradiol through a paracrine interaction between theca and granulosa cells. The theca cells provide the substrate, androstenedione, to the granulosa cell for estradiol production. The granulosa cells express the enzymes necessary for transformation of androstenedione to estradiol (P450 aromatase, 17β hydroxysteroid dehydrogenase-1). **B.** In the corpus luteum, granulosa-lutein cells gain vascularity, LH receptors, and the enzymes necessary for progesterone synthesis. The theca-lutein cells remain the source of androstenedione for estradiol production in granulosa-lutein cells. Gonadotropins, steroidogenic factor-1 (SF-1), and steroidogenic acute regulatory protein (StAR) play crucial roles in steroidogenesis with the ovary (ATP, adenosine triphosphate; cAMP, cyclic adenosine monophosphate; FSH-R, follicle-stimulating hormone receptor; LH-R, luteinizing hormone receptor; P450 arom, P450 aromatase; 17β- HSD-I, 17-β hydroxysteroid dehydrogenase-I). (Redrawn with permission from Larsen et al, eds. The physiology and pathology of the female reproductive axis. In: *Williams Textbook of Endocrinology*. Saunders; 2003; 604.)

and steroidogenesis is largely indirect; it suppresses pituitary FSH secretion. The serum concentrations of inhibin A and B are influenced by the menstrual rhythm. The circulating levels of inhibin A rise late in the follicular phase and remain elevated in the luteal phase whereas the concentration of inhibin B mirrors the menstrual pattern of serum FSH levels (see Figure 13–4). Although inhibin B expression is increased within the granulosa cell on stimulation with FSH, the follicular concentration of inhibin B does not change with follicular size. It has been suggested that the serum concentration of inhibin B reflects the volume of granulosa cells within the ovary, thereby serving as an indicator of the size of the growing cohort of follicles (ovarian reserve). Because inhibin B is the primary inhibitor of pituitary production of FSH in the follicular phase in the absence of estradiol, measuring baseline FSH circulating levels early in the follicular phase (cycle day 3) serves as indirect marker of ovarian reserve (see infertility).

The antral growth phase of follicular development is characterized by rapid follicle growth (1-2 mm/d) and is gonadotropin dependent. In response to FSH, the antral follicle rapidly grows to a diameter of 20 mm, primarily as a result of accumulation of antral fluid. The theca interna continues to differentiate into interstitial cells that produce increasing amounts of androstenedione for aromatization to estrone. The granulosa cell layers have continued to differentiate from each other. The membrana layer, through the action of FSH, acquires LH receptors. This differs from the cumulus layer, which lacks LH receptors. The final progression to a mature graafian follicle is a selection process that in most cases generates one dominant follicle destined for ovulation.

The selection process actually begins in the midluteal phase of the previous cycle. The rise in estrogen level that is generated by the preovulatory follicle augments FSH activity within the follicle while exerting negative feedback on the pituitary release of FSH. The decrease in pituitary release of FSH results in withdrawal of gonadotropin support from the smaller antral follicles, promoting their atresia. The dominant follicle continues to grow, despite decreasing levels of FSH, by accumulating a greater mass of granulosa cells with more FSH receptors. Increased vascularity of the theca cells allows preferential FSH delivery to the dominant follicle despite waning FSH levels. Increased estrogen levels in the follicle facilitate FSH induction of LH receptors on the granulosa cells, allowing the follicle to respond to the ovulatory surge of LH levels. Without estrogen, LH receptors do not develop on the granulosa cells.

The generation of the LH surge is absolutely required for ovulation and oocyte maturation. The amplified production of LH in the midcycle is due to an increase in pituitary sensitivity to GnRH. The sensitization is mediated by the positive feedback effect of the exponential rise in estrogen and possibly inhibin A. This surge results in the resumption of meiosis I in the oocyte with release of a polar body just prior to ovulation. Evidence suggests that the granulosa membrana cells secrete an oocyte maturation inhibitor (OMI), which interacts with the cumulus to block the progression of meiosis during most of folliculogenesis. It is theorized that OMI exerts its inhibitory influence by stimulating the cumulus to increase cAMP production, which diffuses into the oocyte and halts meiotic maturation. The LH surge overcomes the arrest of meiosis by inhibiting OMI secretion; thereby decreasing cAMP levels and increasing intracellular calcium, allowing the resumption of meiosis (Figure 13–8).

Just prior to the ovulation, progesterone production increases, and this may be responsible, at least in part, for the midcycle peak in FSH and the coordination of the LH surge. The FSH peak stimulates the production of an adequate number of LH receptors

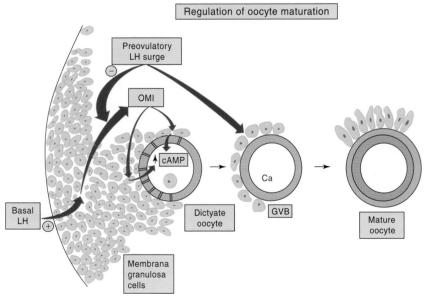

FIGURE 13–8 Current concepts of control of meiotic maturation. (Reproduced, with permission, from Felig P, Frohman LA, eds. *Endocrinology and Metabolism.* 4th ed. McGraw-Hill; 2001.)

on the granulosa cells for luteinization. FSH, LH, and progesterone induce expression of proteolytic enzymes that degrade the collagen in the follicular wall, thereby making it prone to rupture. Prostaglandin (PG) production increases and may be responsible for contraction of smooth muscle cells in the ovary, aiding the extrusion of the oocyte.

The LH surge lasts approximately 48 to 50 hours. Thirty-six hours after onset of the LH surge, ovulation occurs. The feedback signal to terminate the LH surge is not known. Perhaps the rise in progesterone production results in a negative feedback loop and inhibits pituitary LH secretion by decreasing the pulsatility of GnRH. In addition, just prior to ovulation LH downregulates its own receptors, which decreases the activity of the functional hormonal unit. As a result, estradiol production decreases.

Following ovulation and in response to LH, the granulosa cells (membrana) and thecal interstitial cells that remain in the ovulated follicle differentiate into granulosa lutein and theca lutein cells, respectively, to form the corpus luteum. In addition, LH induces the granulosa lutein cells to produce vascular endothelial growth factor (VEGF), which plays an important role in developing the corpus luteum vascularization. This neovascularization penetrates the basement membrane and provides the granulosa lutein cells with LDL for progesterone biosynthesis. After ovulation, the luteal cells upregulate their LH receptors by an unknown mechanism. This is critical in that it allows basal levels of LH to maintain the corpus luteum. Rescue of the corpus luteum with hCG from the developing conceptus works through the LH receptor, which is vital for embryonic life.

Hormone production by the corpus luteum requires the cooperation of theca lutein and granulosa lutein cells, much like the preovulatory follicle (see Figure 13–7). In response to LH and hCG, the theca lutein cells increase the expression of all the enzymes responsible for androstenedione production (see earlier). Aromatase activity is increased in the granulosa lutein cells by LH to aromatize the androgens to estrogen. A notable difference in the granulosa lutein cells, as opposed to the preovulatory granulosa cells, is that LH also induces the expression of P450scc and 3β-HSD, which enables the cell to synthesize progesterone. The secretion of progesterone and estradiol is episodic and correlates with the LH pulses. FSH has minimal influence on progesterone production but continues to stimulate estrogen production during the luteal phase. The progesterone levels rise and reach a peak on approximately day 8 of the luteal phase. The luteal phase lasts approximately 14 days.

The corpus luteum starts to undergo luteolysis (programmed cell death) approximately 9 days after ovulation. The mechanism of luteal regression is not completely known. Once luteolysis begins, there is a rapid decline in progesterone levels. A number of studies suggest that estrogen has a role in luteolysis. It has been shown that direct injection of estrogen into the ovary containing a corpus luteum induces luteolysis and a fall in progesterone levels. Experimental data suggest that there is increased aromatase activity in the corpus luteum just prior to luteolysis. The rise in aromatase activity is secondary to gonadotropin (FSH and LH) stimulation, although later in the luteal phase, FSH probably plays a more important role. Consequently, estrogen production

increases, and this decreases 3β-HSD activity. This may result in a decline in progesterone levels and lead to luteolysis. Furthermore, local modifiers such as oxytocin, which is secreted by luteal cells, have been shown to modulate progesterone synthesis. Other evidence supports the role of PGs in luteolysis. Experimental data suggest that $PGF_{2\alpha}$, which is secreted from the uterus or ovary during the luteal phase, stimulates the synthesis of cytokines such as tumor necrosis factor; this causes apoptosis and, therefore, may be linked to corpus luteum degeneration.

The process of luteolysis is known to involve proteolytic enzymes. Evidence suggests that matrix metalloproteinase (MMP) activity is increased during luteolysis. hCG is a known modulator of MMP activity. This may play an important role in early pregnancy, when hCG rescues the corpus luteum and prevents luteal regression. However, in the absence of pregnancy, the corpus luteum regresses, resulting in a decrease in progesterone, estradiol, and inhibin A levels. The decrease in these hormones allows for increased GnRH pulsatility and FSH secretion. The rise in FSH will rescue another cohort of follicles and initiate the next menstrual cycle.

Role of the Uterus

The sole function of the uterus is to accommodate and support a fetus. Furthermore, it is the endometrium, the lining of the uterine cavity, that differentiates during the menstrual cycle so that it can support and nourish the conceptus. Histologically, the endometrium is made up of an epithelium composed of glands and a stroma that contains stromal fibroblasts and extracellular matrix. The endometrium is divided into two layers based on morphology: the basalis layer and the functionalis layer. The basalis layer lies adjacent to the myometrium and contains glands and supporting vasculature. It provides the components necessary to develop the functionalis layer. The functionalis is the dynamic layer that is regenerated every cycle. More specifically, it is this layer that can accommodate implantation of the blastocyst.

During the menstrual cycle, the endometrium responds to hormones secreted from the ovaries. Somewhat like the other endocrine organs, it contains a network of local factors that modulate hormonal activity. The endometrial phases are coordinated with ovulatory phases. During the follicular phase, the endometrium goes through the proliferative phase. It begins with the onset of menses and ends at ovulation. During the luteal phase, the endometrium undergoes the secretory phase. It starts at ovulation and ends just before menses. If implantation does not occur, a degenerative phase follows the secretory phase within the endometrium. It is this phase that results in menstruation. The next section will discuss the phases of the endometrium in more detail.

During the follicular phase, the ovary secretes estrogen, which stimulates the glands in the basalis to initiate formation of the functionalis layer. Estrogen promotes growth by enhancing gene expression of cytokines and a variety of growth factors, including EGF, TGFα, and IGF. These factors provide a microenvironment within the endometrium to modulate the effects of hormones. At the beginning of the menstrual cycle, the endometrium is thin— usually less than 2 mm in total thickness. The endometrial glands are straight and narrow and extend from the basalis toward the surface of the endometrial cavity. As the epithelium and the underlying stroma develop, they acquire estrogen and progesterone receptors. The spiral blood vessels from the basalis layer extend through the stroma to maintain blood supply to the epithelium. Ultimately, the lining (functionalis) surrounds the entire uterine cavity and achieves a thickness of 3 to 5 mm in height (total thickness 6 to 10 mm). This phase is known as the proliferative phase.

After ovulation, the ovary secretes progesterone, which inhibits further endometrial proliferation. This mechanism may be mediated by antagonizing estrogen effects. Progesterone downregulates estrogen receptors in the epithelium and mediates estradiol metabolism within the endometrium by stimulating 17β-HSD activity and converting estradiol into the weaker estrogen, estrone. During the luteal phase, the glandular epithelium accumulates glycogen and begins to secrete glycopeptides and proteins—along with a transudate from plasma—into the endometrial cavity. It is this fluid that provides nourishment to the free-floating blastocyst. Progesterone also stimulates differentiation of the endometrium and causes characteristic histologic changes. The glands become progressively more tortuous, and the spiral vessels coil and acquire a corkscrew appearance. The underlying stroma becomes very edematous as a result of increased capillary permeability, and the cells begin to appear large and polyhedral, with each cell developing an independent basement membrane. This process is termed predecidualization. These cells are very active and respond to hormonal signals. They produce PGs along with other factors that play an important role in menstruation, implantation, and pregnancy. This phase is known as the secretory phase.

If there is no implantation of an embryo, the endometrium enters the degenerative phase. Estrogen and progesterone withdrawal promotes prostaglandin production—$PGF_{2\alpha}$ and PGE_2. These PGs stimulate progressive vasoconstriction and relaxation of the spiral vessels. These vasomotor reactions lead to endometrial ischemia and reperfusion injury. Eventually, there is hemorrhage within the endometrium with subsequent hematoma formation. The progesterone withdrawal triggers MMP activity, which facilitates degradation of the extracellular matrix. As ischemia and degradation progress, the functionalis becomes necrotic and sloughs away as menstruum consisting of endometrial tissue and blood. The amount of blood lost in normal menses ranges from 25 mL to 60 mL. Although $PGF_{2\alpha}$ is a potent stimulus for myometrial contractility and limits postpartum bleeding, it has minimal impact on cessation of menstrual bleeding. The major mechanisms responsible for limiting blood loss involve the formation of thrombin-platelet plugs and estrogen-induced healing of the basalis layer by reepithelialization of the endometrium, which begins in the early follicular phase of the next menstrual cycle.

If conception takes place, implantation can occur in the endometrium during the midsecretory (midluteal) phase, at which time it is of sufficient thickness and full of sustenance. The syncytiotrophoblast subsequently secretes hCG, which rescues the corpus luteum and maintains progesterone secretion, essential for complete endometrial decidual development.

In summary, the ovary has two phases during the menstrual cycle: the follicular phase and the luteal phase. The endometrium has three phases and is synchronized by the ovary. The complex feedback loops between the ovary and the hypothalamic-pituitary axis regulate the menstrual cycle. During the follicular phase, the ovary secretes estradiol, which stimulates the endometrium to undergo the proliferative phase. After ovulation (luteal phase), the ovary secretes estrogen and progesterone, which maintains the endometrial lining and promotes the secretory phase. In a nonpregnant cycle, luteolysis occurs, resulting in cessation of hormone production. This hormone withdrawal results in the degenerative phase and the onset of menses.

MENSTRUAL DISTURBANCES

AMENORRHEA

The mean age of menarche is 12.8 years. Normally, this event marks the completion of puberty. The onset of regular cyclicity in the menstrual cycle is determined by the duration of the maturation process of the HPO axis, which is quite variable. As a result, anovulation can occur in 50% to 80% of girls 2 years after menarche, and in more than 20% of girls, it can persist until 5 years after menarche. This period of time can be frustrating for many girls and their parents. The evaluation should include a clinical examination and reassurance. If positive findings are noted, limited, pertinent diagnostic tests (see later) are indicated.

Amenorrhea can be defined as either the absence of menarche by age 16 or no menses for more than three cycles in an individual who has previously had cyclic menses. The definition, although arbitrary, nonetheless gives a general guideline to the clinician for further evaluation. Although amenorrhea does not cause harm, in the absence of pregnancy, it may be a sign of genetic, endocrine, and/or anatomic abnormalities. If the outflow tract is intact, amenorrhea is most likely the result of disruption in the HPO axis. These aberrations can affect any level of control in the menstrual cycle and, thus, result in menstrual abnormalities.

Amenorrhea was formerly classified as primary or secondary depending on whether the individual had experienced menses in the past. This classification may lead to misdiagnosis of the cause of amenorrhea. Although primary amenorrhea is more often associated with genetic and anatomic abnormalities, each individual should be assessed by means of the history and clinical findings, including the presence or absence of secondary sexual characteristics (Table 13–3). The causes of amenorrhea are grouped according to the level of involvement in the regulatory systems that govern normal menstrual activity (ie, hypothalamic, pituitary, ovarian, and uterine). An algorithm for the workup of amenorrhea or oligomenorrhea in the presence of secondary sexual characteristics is illustrated in Figure 13–9.

TABLE 13-3 Assessment of patients with amenorrhea.

I. Absent breast development; uterus present 　A. Gonadal failure 　　1. Gonadal agenesis 　　2. Gonadal dysgenesis 　　　a. 45,X (Turner syndrome) 　　　b. 46,X abnormal X (eg, short- or long-arm deletion) 　　　c. Mosaicism (eg, X/XX, X/XX/XXX) 　　　d. 46,XX or 46,XY (Swyer syndrome) gonadal dysgenesis 　B. Defects in estrogen biosynthesis (46, XX) 　　1. 17,20-Lyase deficiency 　　2. CYP17α deficiency 　C. Hypothalamic failure secondary to inadequate GnRH release 　　1. Insufficient GnRH secretion 　　　a. FHA 　　　b. Anorexia nervosa and bulimia 　　　c. CNS neoplasm (craniopharyngioma, gliomas) 　　　d. Excessive exercise 　　　e. Constitutional delay 　　2. Inadequate GnRH synthesis (Kallmann syndrome) 　　3. Developmental anatomic abnormalities in central nervous system 　D. Pituitary failure 　　1. Isolated gonadotropin insufficiency 　　2. GnRH resistance 　　3. Pituitary tumors (hyperprolactinemia) 　　4. Pituitary insufficiency 　　　a. Infections (mumps, encephalitis) 　　　b. Newborn kernicterus 　　5. Prepubertal hypothyroidism **II. Breast development; uterus absent** 　A. Androgen resistance (androgen insensitivity syndrome) 　B. Congenital absence of uterus (utero-vaginal agenesis) **III. Absent breast development; uterus absent** 　A. Defects in testosterone biosynthesis (46,XY) 　　1. 17,20-Lyase deficiency 　　2. CYP17α deficiency 　　3. 17β-Hydroxysteroid dehydrogenase deficiency 　B. Testicular regression syndrome (46,XY)	**IV. Breast development; uterus present** 　A. Pregnancy 　B. Hypothalamic etiology 　　1. FHA 　　2. Anorexia nervosa and bulimia 　　3. Psychogenic (depression) 　　4. CNS neoplasm 　　5. Chronic disease 　C. Pituitary etiology 　　1. Pituitary tumors (hyperprolactinemia) 　　2. Pituitary insufficiency 　　　a. Hypotensive event (Sheehan syndrome) 　　　b. Infections 　　　c. Autoimmune destruction 　　　d. Iatrogenic (surgery, radiation) 　D. Ovarian etiology 　　1. POF 　　　a. Mosaicism (46,XX/XO,XX/XY) 　　　b. Autoimmune destruction 　　　c. Iatrogenic (radiation, chemotherapy) 　　　d. Fragile X syndrome 　　　e. Infections 　　2. Resistant ovarian syndrome (Savage syndrome) 　E. Chronic estrogenized anovulation 　　1. Hyperandrogenic 　　　a. PCOS 　　　b. Nonclassical congenital adrenal hyperplasia 　　　c. Cushing syndrome 　　　d. Androgen secreting tumors 　　2. Other 　　　a. Adrenal insufficiency 　　　b. Thyroid disorders 　F. Outflow tract 　　1. Congenital abnormalities 　　　a. Transvaginal septum 　　　b. Imperforate hymen 　　2. Asherman syndrome

HYPOTHALAMIC AMENORRHEA

Isolated GnRH Deficiency

The hypothalamus is the source of GnRH, which directs the synthesis and secretion of pituitary gonadotropins. Dysfunction at this level leads to hypogonadotropic hypogonadism or eugonadotropic hypogonadism. Disorders of GnRH production can result in a wide range of clinical manifestations. The individual's appearance is dependent on the age at onset and the degree of dysfunction.

Isolated GnRH deficiency results in hypogonadotropic hypogonadism. Female patients present with amenorrhea, and females and males present with absent or incomplete pubertal development secondary to absent or diminished sex steroids (estradiol in females, testosterone in males). They have normal stature with a eunuchoidal body habitus. Because the adrenal glands are unaffected by the absence of GnRH, body hair distribution is not affected.

A. Genetic origin Several genetic lesions associated with GnRH deficiency have been described. The best characterized form of GnRH deficiency is Kallmann syndrome, which involves the *Kal-1* gene as well as a number of other genes. The *Kal-1* gene normally codes for anosmin, an adhesion molecule that appears to be involved in the migration of GnRH and olfactory neurons from the olfactory placode to the hypothalamus. The *Kal-1* gene is located on the short arm of the X chromosome. Most cases of Kallmann syndrome are sporadic, although the disorder has also been observed to have a familial pattern, and most often it is transmitted by X-linked recessive inheritance. Autosomal recessive and dominant patterns have been reported but are much less common. When mutations exist in the *Kal-1* gene, there may be associated defects, including anosmia and, less frequently, midline facial defects, renal anomalies, and neurologic deficiency. The disorder affects both sexes, but because of the X-linked inheritance pattern it is more common in boys. Unlike males, the specific genetic mutations in the *Kal-1* gene in females with hypogonadotropic hypogonadism have not been identified, suggesting there

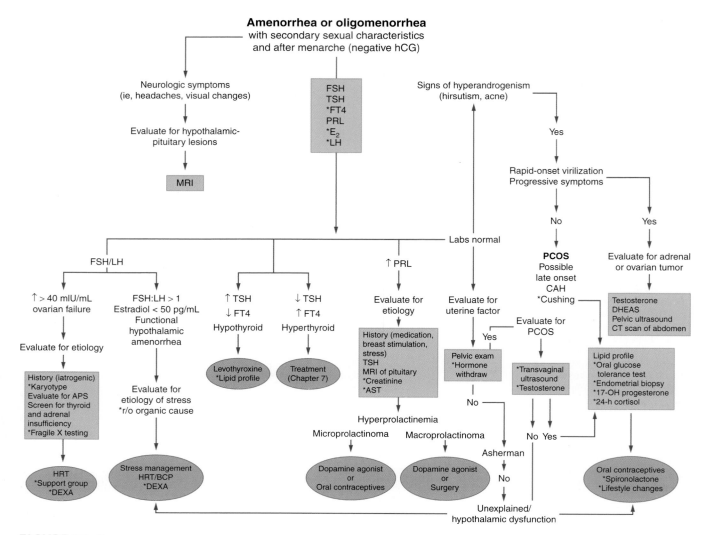

FIGURE 13–9 An algorithm for women who have developed secondary sexual characteristics, have experienced menarche, and are presenting with amenorrhea or oligomenorrhea. A negative human chorionic gonadotropin test documents the nonpregnant state. All women should be screened for known causes of oligomenorrhea, whether or not hyperandrogenism is present. Hyperandrogenism suggests either polycystic ovarian syndrome (PCOS) or late-onset congenital adrenal hyperplasia (CAH). If rapid in onset, progressive virilization requires an evaluation for an androgen-secreting tumor. Management of late-onset CAH and PCOS is similar. Clinical history and physical findings suggesting hypoestrogenism, stress, or thyroid dysfunction are indications for measurement of estradiol (E₂), luteinizing hormone (LH), and free thyroid hormone (FT4) levels in plasma (APS, autoimmune polyglandular syndrome). *As indicated (refer to text).

are other genetic mutations that cause this disorder. Recently, it was determined that heterozygous mutations in fibroblast growth factor receptor 1 (*FGFR1*) gene, known as the *Kal-2*, were identified in cases of Kallmann syndrome. *FGFR1* and *Kal-1* are coexpressed at the same sites during development and are thought to have a functional interaction. Mutations in the *Kiss-1* derived peptide receptor, GPR54, have also been identified in these patients. Several mechanisms of how GPR54 may regulate gonadotropin production via GnRH function or production have been proposed. Several studies have shown that females with presumed Kallmann syndrome demonstrate variable responses to exogenous GnRH administration, which suggests a GnRH receptor defect. In fact, mutations in the GnRH receptor have been identified in both sexes and are inherited in an autosomal recessive fashion.

Management of hypogonadotropic hypogonadism involves scheduled hormone replacement therapy (HRT) to stimulate the development of secondary sexual characteristics and increase bone mineral density. If pregnancy is desired, treatment involves the administration of pulsatile GnRH or gonadotropin treatment.

B. Endocrine causes

1. **Functional hypothalamic amenorrhea**—Functional hypothalamic amenorrhea is one of the most common types of amenorrhea and accounts for 15% to 35% of cases. It is an endocrine disorder, although the exact mechanism has not been definitively determined. It is characterized by a reduced GnRH drive (decrease in pulse frequency and amplitude), leading to low or low-normal serum levels of FSH and LH and

resulting in anovulation. The ratio of serum FSH to LH in these patients is often equivalent to that of a prepubertal female with a relative FSH dominance.

The adipocyte hormone, leptin, has been implicated in the development of this disorder. Leptin is an important nutritional satiety factor, but it is also necessary for maturation of the reproductive system. The potential link to the reproductive system is thought to be through leptin receptors, which have been identified in the hypothalamus and gonadotropes. This is supported by the observation that leptin can stimulate GnRH pulsatility and gonadotropin secretion. Several studies suggest that women with functional hypothalamic amenorrhea have lower serum leptin levels in comparison with eumenorrheic controls. This relative deficiency may lead to dysfunctional release of GnRH and subsequent development of functional hypothalamic amenorrhea.

Abnormal, and often subtle, activation of the hypothalamic-pituitary-adrenal axis is associated with functional hypothalamic amenorrhea. The inciting event may be excessive production of corticotropin-releasing hormone (CRH), which has been shown to decrease the pulse frequency of GnRH and increase cortisol levels in vivo. In contrast, another study suggests that although acute elevations of CRH can suppress GnRH release, this suppression cannot be maintained with CRH alone. The cause of functional hypothalamic amenorrhea often remains unclear, but the associated hypercortisolemia suggests that it is preceded by psychologic stress, strenuous exercise, or poor nutrition. There is support for the concept that these factors may act synergistically to further suppress GnRH drive. In fact, patients with functional hypothalamic amenorrhea resulting from psychologic stress are usually high achievers who have dysfunctional coping mechanisms when dealing with daily stress. The severity of hypothalamic suppression is reflected by the clinical manifestations. The significant interpatient variability in the degree of psychologic or metabolic stress required to induce a menstrual disturbance explains the heterogeneity of clinical presentations, ranging from luteal phase defects to anovulation with erratic bleeding to amenorrhea.

Functional hypothalamic amenorrhea is reversible. Interestingly, the factors that have predicted the rate of recovery are body mass index and basal cortisol levels. When patients recover, ovulation is preceded by return of cortisol levels to baseline. Some experts have shown that cognitive behavioral therapy, teaching the patient how to cope with stress—and nutritional consultation—reverse this condition. Complete reversal may be less likely if the functional insult occurs during the period of peripubertal maturation of the HPO axis.

The diagnosis of functional hypothalamic amenorrhea can be made if the FSH-LH ratio is greater than 1 in the presence of hypoestrogenemia. However, a minor disturbance of hypothalamic dysfunction may present with normal laboratory findings, a clinical history that coincides with stress, and a negative evaluation for other causes of anovulation. Interestingly, most of these patients, despite hypoestrogenism, do not have symptoms. The estrogen status should still be evaluated given the strong correlation between hypoestrogenemia and the development of osteoporosis. Estrogen status can be determined by means of the progesterone withdrawal test or by measurement of serum estradiol (<50 pg/mL). If there is no withdrawal or the estradiol is less than 50 pg/mL, HRT with combination contraceptive hormones (or traditional HRT) should be instituted. If withdrawal bleeding occurs, any cyclic progestin-containing therapy is adequate to combat unopposed estrogen and the development of endometrial hyperplasia.

2. **Amenorrhea in the female athlete**—Hypothalamic dysfunction has been observed in female athletes. Competitors in events such as gymnastics, ballet, marathon running, and diving can show menstrual irregularities ranging from luteal phase defects to amenorrhea. The **female athletic triad** as defined by the American College of Sports Medicine is characterized by disordered eating, amenorrhea, and osteoporosis. The associated nutritional deficiencies can lead to impaired growth and delayed sexual maturation. The neuroendocrine abnormalities are similar to those of women with functional hypothalamic amenorrhea.

These patients have very low body fat, often below the tenth percentile. There is evidence that a negative correlation between body fat and menstrual irregularities exists. In addition, there appears to be a critical body fat level that must be present in order to have a functioning reproductive system. Several studies have shown that these amenorrheic athletes have significantly lower serum leptin levels, which further supports leptin's role as a mediator between nutritional status and the reproductive system. The strenuous exercise these athletes engage in amplifies the effects of the associated nutritional deficiency. This synergism causes severe suppression of GnRH, leading to the low estradiol levels.

Amenorrhea alone is not harmful. However, low serum estradiol over a period of time may lead to osteoporosis and delayed puberty. An analysis of estrogen status may be obtained with measurement of serum estradiol levels or with the progestin withdrawal test (see earlier). If estrogen is low, bone mineral density (BMD) should be assessed by dual-energy x-ray absorptiometry (DXA) scan. All patients diagnosed with female athletic triad need combination contraceptive therapy or HRT.

3. **Amenorrhea associated with eating disorders**—**Anorexia nervosa** is a disorder characterized by relentless dieting in pursuit of a thin body habitus. Approximately 95% of cases occur in females, and the onset is chiefly in adolescence. The clinical features include extreme weight loss leading to a body weight less than 85% of normal for age and height, a distorted body image, and intense fear of gaining weight. These patients usually have a preoccupation with food and are hyperactive, with an obsessive-compulsive personality. The associated symptoms include hypothermia, mild bradycardia, dry skin, constipation, and symptoms of hypoestrogenemia. Furthermore, as part of the diagnostic criteria, they must experience at least 3 months of no menses.

The dysfunction in the neuroendocrine system is similar to but often more severe than that described in association with functional hypothalamic amenorrhea. The severe reduction in GnRH pulsatility leads to suppression of FSH and LH secretion, possibly to undetectable levels, and results in anovulation and low serum estradiol levels. Given the severe psychologic and metabolic stress experienced by these individuals, the hypothalamic-pituitary-adrenal axis is activated. The circadian rhythm of adrenal secretion is maintained, but both cortisol production and plasma cortisol levels are persistently elevated secondary to increased pituitary secretion of adrenocorticotropic hormone (ACTH). Serum leptin levels in these individuals are significantly lower than normal healthy controls and correlate with percentage of body fat and body weight. A rise in leptin levels in response to dietary treatment is associated with a subsequent rise in gonadotropin levels. This further suggests leptin's role as a potential link between energy stores and the reproductive system.

The self-induced starvation state associated with anorexia nervosa leads to additional endocrine abnormalities not observed in other causes of hypothalamic amenorrhea. For instance, thyroid hormone metabolism is altered. TSH and T_4 levels are in the low-normal range, but T_3 levels are usually below normal. This is attributable to decreased peripheral conversion of T_4 to T_3 and increased conversion of T_4 to the metabolically inactive thyroid hormone, reverse T_3—a change that often resembles other states of starvation. This may be a protective mechanism in that the relative hypothyroid state attempts to reduce basal metabolic function in response to a highly catabolic state.

Bulimia occurs in about half of patients with anorexia and is defined as binge eating followed by self-induced purging. Not all bulimics have low body weight—in fact, normal-weight bulimic individuals are much more common. These patients also have a variety of neuroendocrine aberrations—often to a lesser degree than those with anorexia—which also lead to menstrual disturbances. Leptin levels are lower than in matched controls but not as low as in individuals with anorexia nervosa. They also have neurotransmitter abnormalities—notably low serotonin levels—which might help explain the often coexisting psychologic difficulties.

Anorexia nervosa is a life-threatening illness with a significant mortality rate due to its metabolic consequences. Anorexic patients should be considered for inpatient therapy and management with a multidisciplinary approach that includes nutritional counseling and psychotherapy. Force-feeding may be necessary in some patients. If weight gain cannot be achieved with oral intake, meals may need to be supplemented by enteral or parenteral feeding. Because anorexia nervosa is a hypoestrogenic state and there is a high potential for the development of osteoporosis, all patients should receive hormone therapy either in the form of HRT or combination contraceptive pills. It is important to note that many patients with anorexia will continue to have reduced bone size regardless of sex steroid administration presumably due to the concurrent malnutrition and metabolic compromise. Weight rehabilitation and recovery is associated with bone accretion; however, the loss of bone may not be completely reversible.

In summary, the hypothalamic amenorrhea endocrine syndromes are probably a continuum of disordered eating and nutritional deficiencies resulting in increasingly severe abnormalities in the reproductive system. Furthermore, the age at onset affects the potential complications of these disorders. If low estradiol levels are present before age 20, bone mineralization may be profoundly affected, because this period is critical for building peak bone mass. In addition, if these conditions occur prior to puberty, it may result in stunted growth and delayed development of secondary sexual characteristics.

C. Anatomic causes Numerous anatomic abnormalities within the central nervous system can result in menstrual disturbances. These include developmental defects, brain tumors, and infiltrative disorders. The most common anatomic lesion associated with

delayed puberty and amenorrhea is a craniopharyngioma. It is derived from Rathke pouch and extends into the hypothalamus, pituitary, and third ventricle. The symptoms include headaches, visual loss, and hypoestrogenism.

Infiltrative disorders that involve the hypothalamus are uncommon but can result from systemic diseases, including sarcoidosis, histiocytosis, hemochromatosis, and lymphoma. These diseases do not initially present with amenorrhea. However, in the presence of these diseases, the hypothalamus may be affected, so they should be part of the differential diagnosis of amenorrhea.

PITUITARY AMENORRHEA

There are a few genetic mutations affecting the pituitary that cause amenorrhea. Rare autosomal recessive mutations may cause deficiencies in FSH, LH, TSH, prolactin (PRL), and growth hormone (GH). The clinical manifestations may include delayed puberty, a hypoestrogenic state, and infertility.

A. Genetic causes A deficiency in FSH and LH may be a result of GnRH receptor gene mutations. Such mutations are primarily compound heterozygous mutations that affect GnRH receptor–dependent signal transduction. The phenotype of these individuals is similar to that of those with isolated GnRH deficiency. In fact, some investigators speculate that these receptor mutations may be the cause of isolated GnRH deficiency in women, given that no mutations have yet been identified in the ligand or *Kal-1* gene. The estimated prevalence of GnRH receptor mutations in women with hypothalamic amenorrhea is 2%. In a family with other affected females, the prevalence is 7%.

Other rare genetic defects have been associated with amenorrheic women. Mutations in the *FSHβ* gene have been reported. These have an autosomal recessive pattern of inheritance and lead to low serum FSH and estradiol levels and high plasma LH levels. The clinical features include minimal development of secondary sexual characteristics and amenorrhea with no history of menses. Combined hormone deficiencies have also been described. Mutations in Prop-1, a pituitary transcription factor for Pit-1, lead to deficiencies in gonadotropins, TSH, PRL, and GH. These patients present with stunted growth, hypothyroidism, and delayed puberty in addition to amenorrhea.

B. Endocrine causes **Hyperprolactinemia** is one of the most common causes of amenorrhea, accounting for 15% to 30% of cases. In the absence of pregnancy or postpartum lactation, persistently elevated PRL is almost always associated with a hypothalamic-pituitary disorder. Normal PRL secretion is regulated by several stimulatory and inhibitory factors (see Chapter 4). PRL secretion is primarily under tonic inhibition by dopamine, so that any interference with dopamine synthesis or transport from the hypothalamus may result in elevated PRL levels. In addition to menstrual disturbances, individuals with hyperprolactinemia may present with galactorrhea. In fact, hyperprolactinemia is a common cause of galactorrhea, and up to 80% of patients with amenorrhea and galactorrhea have elevated PRL levels. Other associated symptoms include headaches, visual field defects, infertility, and osteopenia.

The mechanism whereby hyperprolactinemia causes amenorrhea is not completely known. Studies have shown that PRL can affect the reproductive system in several ways. PRL receptors have been identified on GnRH neurons and may directly suppress GnRH secretion. Others have postulated that elevated PRL levels inhibit GnRH pulsatility indirectly by increasing other neuromodulators such as endogenous opioids. There is also evidence that GnRH receptors on the pituitary may be downregulated in the presence of hyperprolactinemia. Furthermore, PRL may affect the ovaries by altering ovarian progesterone secretion and estrogen synthesis. The best data now available suggest that hyperprolactinemia causes amenorrhea primarily by suppression of GnRH secretion.

Approximately half of patients with elevated PRL levels have radiologic evidence of a pituitary tumor. The most common type is a PRL-secreting tumor (prolactinoma), accounting for 40% to 50% of pituitary tumors. Prolactinomas are composed mainly of lactotrophs, and they secrete PRL. Occasionally these tumors secrete both GH and PRL.

The diagnosis of a pituitary adenoma is usually made by examination of the pituitary with magnetic resonance imaging (MRI). These tumors are categorized into two groups based on their dimensions—microadenomas are those less than 10 mm in diameter and macroadenomas are larger than 10 mm. These tumors are usually located in the lateral wings of the anterior pituitary. Microadenomas are typically wholly contained within the confines of the pituitary gland. Very rarely, a microadenoma infiltrates the surrounding tissue, including the dura, cavernous sinus, or adjacent skull base. A macroadenoma may expand farther and grow out of the sella to impinge on surrounding structures, such as the optic chiasm or may extend into the sphenoid sinus. As a result, macroadenomas are more frequently associated with severe headaches, visual field defects, and ophthalmoplegia. The incidence of a microadenoma progressing to a macroadenoma is relatively low, only 3% to 7%. During pregnancy the risk of a microprolactinoma enlarging is also low, but in the presence of a macroprolactinoma, the chance of tumor growth is up to 25%.

Some investigators have found a correlation between pituitary adenoma size and serum PRL levels. If the serum PRL is less than 100 ng/mL, a microprolactinoma is more likely, whereas if it is greater than 100 ng/mL, a macroprolactinoma is often present. Although this correlation has been reported, the evidence supporting it is not strong. In fact, low PRL levels may also be associated with nonfunctioning macroadenomas. This is thought to reflect impingement of the adenoma on the pituitary stalk leading to reduced dopamine secretion and loss of the tonic suppression of prolactin secretion. These nonfunctioning tumors may synthesize glycoproteins such as FSH, LH, or their free alpha subunits. Rarely, functioning tumors may arise from other pituitary cells, resulting in excessive hormone secretion. If a macroadenoma is present, measurement of IGF-I, alpha subunit,

TSH, and 24-hour urinary cortisol will begin to exclude other functioning adenomas.

Other tumors of nonpituitary origin may also result in delayed puberty and amenorrhea. The most common of these is a craniopharyngioma. Although craniopharyngiomas are commonly located in the suprasellar region, they can also involve the sella. These tumors have not been shown to produce hormones, but because they may compress the infundibulum, they can interfere with the tonic inhibition of PRL secretion and result in mildly elevated PRL levels.

Hyperprolactinemia in a patient with amenorrhea is defined as a PRL level greater than 20 ng/mL, although the limit of normal may vary between laboratories. Normal PRL release follows a sleep-circadian rhythm, but PRL may also be secreted in response to stress, physical exercise, breast stimulation, or a meal. Therefore, PRL should be measured in the midmorning hours and in the fasting state. Other causes of mildly elevated PRL include medications such as oral contraceptives, neuroleptics, tricyclic antidepressants, metoclopramide, methyldopa, and verapamil. Hyperprolactinemia has also been observed in several chronic diseases, including cirrhosis and renal disease. Furthermore, inflammatory diseases such as sarcoidosis and histiocytosis can infiltrate the hypothalamus or pituitary and result in hyperprolactinemia. Elevated PRL levels may be a physiologic response. During pregnancy, PRL levels may be two to four times baseline. With postpartum breast-feeding, the PRL level should be below 100 ng/mL after 7 days and below 50 ng/mL after 3 months. If a woman is not breast-feeding, PRL levels should return to baseline by 7 days postpartum.

Persistently elevated PRL levels may also be present in primary hypothyroidism. Approximately 40% of patients with primary hypothyroidism present with a minimal increase in prolactin (25-30 ng/mL), and 10% present with even higher serum levels. Individuals with primary hypothyroidism have an increase in thyrotropin-releasing hormone (TRH) from the hypothalamus, which stimulates TSH and PRL release and leads to hyperprolactinemia. Patients with long-standing primary hypothyroidism may eventually manifest profound pituitary enlargement due to hypertrophy of thyrotrophs. This mass effect with elevated PRL levels mimics a prolactinoma. Therefore, all patients with hyperprolactinemia should have their thyroid function investigated to exclude hypothyroidism as the cause.

Prolactinomas are the most common cause of persistent hyperprolactinemia. All patients with elevated PRL levels should have the test repeated for verification. In addition to blood tests, a careful clinical and pharmacologic history and physical examination should be performed to exclude other causes of hyperprolactinemia. If elevated PRL levels persist or if any measurement is found to be above 100 ng/mL, MRI of the hypothalamic-pituitary region should be performed. If a microadenoma is observed, the diagnosis of microprolactinoma can be made. If a macroadenoma is observed, other pituitary hormones should be measured to exclude other functioning adenomas or hypopituitarism. All patients diagnosed with macroadenoma should have a visual field examination.

The treatment of choice for prolactinoma is dopamine agonist therapy. These drugs (bromocriptine, cabergoline, pergolide, quinagolide) are very effective at lowering PRL levels, resolving symptoms, and causing tumor shrinkage. Treatment results in a rapid reduction in PRL levels in 60% to 100% of cases. Following reduction of PRL levels, 60% to 100% of women resume ovulatory menses within 6 weeks, and galactorrhea disappears within 1 to 3 months after starting treatment. Reduction in tumor size is usually evident after 2 to 3 months of drug therapy, but it may occur within days after initiation of treatment. The extrasellar portion of the tumor appears to be particularly sensitive to drug therapy, which explains the improvement in symptoms such as visual impairment or ophthalmoplegia with drug therapy. In patients diagnosed with a microadenoma that is manifested only as a menstrual disturbance, observation should only be considered if the patient does not desire conception. These individuals should be offered oral contraceptives to control the bleeding pattern and to protect bone from estrogen deficiency. However, the long-term sequelae of persistently elevated PRL levels are unknown. If dopamine agonist treatment is initiated for a microadenoma, therapy may be continued long term. If the tumor responds, the dose may be tapered and stopped after menopause. Many individuals with a macroadenoma take dopamine agonist therapy indefinitely. All patients diagnosed with a prolactinoma should have follow-up imaging, determination of serum PRL levels, and visual field examinations. Alternatively, patients with a micro- or macroprolactinoma may be offered discontinuation of therapy. Dopamine agonist therapy may be tapered and ultimately discontinued if follow-up PRL levels are normal, and follow-up MRI scans show no evidence of tumor (or tumor reduction of at least 50%, with the tumor at a distance of more than 5 mm from the optic chiasm and no evidence for tumor invasion of adjacent structures), and if follow-up after withdrawal is assured.

An alternative to medical management of pituitary tumors is transsphenoidal surgery, after which resolution of symptoms may be immediate. However, the success and recurrence rates vary and are dependent on the size of the tumor and the depth of invasion. The larger and more invasive the tumor is, the less chance there is for complete resection and the greater the chance of recurrence. In general, the success rate of surgery for a microadenoma in some centers may be 70% or higher; surgical cure rates for macroadenomas are generally less than 40%. Overall, the recurrence rate following surgery is approximately 50%. Surgery is a good alternative for resistant tumors or for patients intolerant of medical treatment. Because non-PRL-secreting pituitary tumors often do not respond well to medical therapy, operation is the treatment of choice for these tumors as well. The risks of surgery include infection, diabetes insipidus, and panhypopituitarism. Complete pituitary testing should be performed prior to surgery.

Women with hyperprolactinemia who desire to conceive should be administered dopamine agonist therapy. Elevated PRL levels can lead to anovulation and hormonal disturbances that can result in difficulty in achieving pregnancy. Once pregnant, patients with microadenomas may have their medication discontinued. If a macroadenoma is present, thought should be given to continuing dopamine agonist therapy throughout pregnancy. Women with prolactinomas may breast-feed since there is no evidence that it stimulates tumor growth. If breast-feeding, dopamine agonist therapy should be discontinued since these agents will interfere with lactation.

C. Anatomic causes

1. **Pituitary destruction**—Amenorrhea may be the result of not only pituitary neoplasms but also pituitary destruction. Infiltrative disorders that involve the hypothalamus can affect the pituitary. Other disorders that cause pituitary insufficiency may be situational. A rare autoimmune disease, lymphocytic hypophysitis, can cause pituitary destruction during the puerperium and ultimately results in panhypopituitarism. Pituitary necrosis may also occur secondary to a hypotensive event. Typically, 80% to 90% of the pituitary must be damaged before pituitary failure ensues, and the robust blood supply to the pituitary makes this an uncommon event. If pituitary ischemia and necrosis are related to postpartum hemorrhage, it is known as Sheehan syndrome; otherwise, it is called Simmond disease. Because this type of injury typically affects the entire pituitary, most often more than one or all the pituitary hormones may be deficient. Observation has suggested that hormone loss follows a pattern, starting with the gonadotropins, followed by GH and PRL; however, this is highly variable.

OVARIAN AMENORRHEA

The physiologic period in a woman's life when there is permanent cessation of menstruation and regression of ovarian function is known as menopause (see later). The cause of ovarian failure is thought to be depletion of ovarian follicles. The median age at menopause is 51.1 years. Premature menopause is defined as ovarian failure prior to age 40, which is reported to occur in 1% of the population. The etiology of premature ovarian failure (POF) may have a genetic basis. Several mutations that affect gonadal function have been identified and include defects in hormone receptors and steroid synthesis. Other potential causes include autoimmune ovarian destruction, iatrogenic ovarian injury, and idiopathic ovarian failure. The most severe form of POF presents with absent secondary sexual characteristics and is most often due to gonadal agenesis or dysgenesis (see Chapter 14). Less severe forms may result only in diminished reproductive capacity.

The other ovarian cause of amenorrhea is repetitive ovulation failure or anovulation. Other than menopause, it is the most common cause of amenorrhea. Chronic anovulation may be secondary to disorders of the hypothalamic-pituitary axis and has been previously discussed. Anovulation may also be due to systemic disorders. The causes of ovarian failure and anovulation due to peripheral disorders will be discussed later.

Ovarian failure is diagnosed based on the clinical picture of amenorrhea and the demonstration of elevated FSH (>40 IU/L). This may occur at any time from embryonic development onward. If it occurs prior to age 40, it is called POF. The presence or absence of secondary sexual characteristics defines whether ovarian activity was present in the past. The most common cause of hypergonadotropic amenorrhea, in the absence of secondary sexual characteristics, is abnormal gonadal development, which occurs in more than half of these individuals. When the gonad fails to develop, this is known as **gonadal agenesis.** The karyotype of these individuals is 46,XX, and the cause of failure is usually unknown. If streak gonads are present, this indicates at least partial gonadal development and is called **gonadal dysgenesis.** The karyotype of these individuals may be normal, but it is more likely that there are alterations in sex chromosomes (see Chapter 14).

Premature Ovarian Failure

A. Genetic origin of POF Two intact X chromosomes are necessary for the maintenance of oocytes during embryogenesis, and the loss of or any alteration in the sex chromosome leads to accelerated follicular loss. This implies that two intact alleles are required for the normal function of some genes on the X chromosome. Turner syndrome is a classic example of complete absence of one X chromosome. It manifests as short stature, sexual infantilism, amenorrhea, and ovarian dysgenesis. This is a well-recognized condition that occurs in 1:2000 to 1:5000 females at birth. Turner syndrome is associated with a number of other phenotypic abnormalities, including a webbed neck, broad chest, low hairline, and cardiovascular and renal defects. It is interesting that fewer than half of patients with Turner syndrome have a single cell line with the karyotype 45,X. The majority of patients actually present with a mosaic karyotype such as 45,X/46,XX. These patients have varying degrees of the Turner syndrome phenotype and may display some secondary sexual development or may have a history of menstrual function. Some pregnancies have been reported.

The term **mixed gonadal dysgenesis** is used to describe chromosomal aneuploidies with a Y-chromosome component. The most common type is a mosaic pattern that has been associated with Turner syndrome (45,X/46,XY). These patients may have some functional testicular tissue and present with varying degrees of genital ambiguity. If enough testicular tissue is present to produce AMH, these patients may also present with abnormalities of the internal genitalia. Individuals who have both ovarian tissue and testicular tissue along with Wolffian and Müllerian structures internally are termed **true hermaphrodites.** Interestingly, most true hermaphrodites have 46,XX karyotypes (see Chapter 14) but others may have a 46,XY or 46,XX/46,XY chimerism.

Patients with gonadal dysgenesis may be phenotypically normal, and the abnormality may be manifest only as delayed pubertal development and amenorrhea. They probably have normal Müllerian structures and streak gonads. These individuals can display an array of karyotypes, including 46,XY (Swyer syndrome). Patients with a male karyotype but a female phenotype presumably underwent testicular failure prior to internal or external genitalia differentiation. If a dysgenetic gonad contains a Y chromosome or a fragment of the Y chromosome, there is a 10% to 30% risk for future gonadal malignancy, and the risk is higher if a mutation in the *SRY* gene is present. These tumors may be hormonally active. The onset of spontaneous pubertal development in girls with mixed gonadal dysgenesis may be a clinical marker of tumor development. Gonadal extirpation is extirpation at the time of diagnosis.

POF is defined as ovarian failure before age 40 but after puberty. Because complete absence of an X chromosome results in

a dysgenetic gonad, candidate genes for POF are probably those that escape X inactivation. In mammals, X inactivation occurs in all cells in order to provide dosage compensation for *X-linked* genes between males and females (Lyon hypothesis). Further observation has illustrated that terminal deletions in Xp lead to the classic stigmata of Turner syndrome, whereas other deletions in Xp or Xq present with varying degrees of early reproductive failure. Most of the genes involved in folliculogenesis appear to be located on the long arm of the X chromosome. Several regions on the X chromosome, including POF 1 and POF 2, have been evaluated with knockout models in animals and have shown varying effects on ovarian development (Figure 13–10).

Limited observations have found that deletions occurring closer to the centromere of the X chromosome manifest a more severe phenotype that includes disruption of pubertal development. In contrast, deletions that occur in the distal regions tend to present with early reproductive aging and infertility. An example of a distal mutation on the long arm of the X chromosome is that in the *FMR1* gene (*fragile X* gene). An association has been described between the *FMR1* permutation state and POF. The prevalence of *FMR1* gene permutations accounts for approximately 2% to 3% of patients who present with sporadic POF and may be as high as 15% in familial cases. This permutation is also associated with the occurrence of a late-onset neurological disorder in male carriers designated as fragile-X tremor ataxia syndrome (FXTAS). Although a number of genes on the X chromosome have demonstrated involvement in ovarian physiology, the majority of patients with POF have no identifiable mutations on the X chromosome.

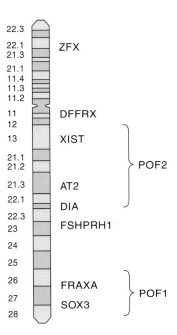

FIGURE 13–10 Candidate genes on the X chromosome for premature ovarian failure (POF). (Reproduced, with permission, from Davison RM, Davis CJ, Conway GS. The X chromosome and ovarian failure. *Clin Endocrinol.* 1999;51:673.)

Autosomal recessive genes that have been shown to contribute to POF are very rare. FSH receptor mutations have been identified in humans with POF. These individuals present with a phenotype that ranges from absent secondary sexual development to normal development and early reproductive failure. The prevalence of FSH receptor mutations varies but is most common in the Finnish population (1% carriers). This mutation has not been observed in North America. An inactivated LH receptor has been identified in patients with normal puberty and amenorrhea but is quite rare. Mutations in genes involved in steroidogenesis have also been associated with POF. These enzymes include CYP17α and aromatase. Patients with CYP17α mutations may have a 46,XX or 46,XY karyotype. They have a similar phenotype except that those with 46,XY have absent Müllerian structures because AMH is produced from their testes. Individuals with aromatase deficiency present with sexual ambiguity and clitoromegaly. Several other autosomal mutations have been discovered that may have a role in ovarian physiology. However, at this time, most cases of POF with normal pubertal development have not been associated with any specific mutation (see Chapter 14).

B. Autoimmune origin of POF

Autoimmune ovarian destruction is another potential cause of POF. This diagnosis is difficult to make unless it presents with one of the autoimmune polyglandular syndromes (see Chapter 2). The circumstantial evidence supporting the diagnosis is found in the high incidence of concomitant autoimmune disease—20% or more in patients with POF. The strongest association is with autoimmune thyroid disease. In addition, 10% to 20% of individuals with autoimmune adrenal disease experience POF. Conversely, 2% to 10% of patients with idiopathic POF develop adrenal insufficiency.

Autoimmune-associated POF is often diagnosed based on the presence of another autoimmune disease or detection of autoantibodies. Thyroid antibodies are most frequently screened. However, these antibodies are present in 15% to 20% of reproductive-aged women. Others have suggested measuring ovarian-specific autoantibodies. There is, however, significant inconsistency in the testing methodology, and this is not recommended. Although the diagnosis is imprecise, all patients suspected of having POF should be screened regularly for thyroid dysfunction. In addition, these patients should be evaluated for the autoimmune polyglandular syndrome (APS) and particularly tested for adrenal insufficiency, especially if there is no identifiable cause of POF. Testing for Addison disease can be performed using provocative ACTH testing or alternatively adrenal antibodies to identify patients at risk. There are commercially available tests for both antiadrenal antibodies and antibodies to 21-hydroxylase. The sensitivity of these tests for the diagnosis of adrenal insufficiency is 100%, the specificity 98%, and the PPV is 67%. If a patient has either of these antibodies they have a 25% to 50% risk of developing adrenal insufficiency within 5 to 10 years.

C. Iatrogenic causes of POF

Iatrogenic causes of POF include radiation therapy, chemotherapy, and ovarian insults resulting from torsion or surgery. The risk of POF following radiation and chemotherapy is proportionate to the patient's age. If the radiation dose is higher than 800 Gy, all women experience ovarian failure. Displacing the ovaries out of the radiation field (ovarian transposition) has shown to be very effective at preserving ovarian function in patients receiving pelvic radiation. Therefore, patients wishing to preserve their fertility should be offered this procedure. Chemotherapy alone, particularly with alkylating agents, may induce temporary or permanent ovarian failure. Studies have shown that the likelihood of experiencing amenorrhea during treatment is 50% to 100%, and on average 40% of patients experience irreversible menopause. In general, younger individuals with chemotherapy-induced ovarian injury are more likely to recover. In women older than age 40, the chance of recovery is less 10%. Modifications of chemotherapy drugs, duration of treatment, and dosing are modifiers of permanent ovarian injury.

D. Resistant ovary syndrome

A rare cause of hypergonadotropic amenorrhea associated with numerous unstimulated ovarian follicles is the resistant ovary syndrome. These patients classically have no history of ovulatory dysfunction and present with secondary sexual characteristics and symptoms suggestive of estrogen deficiency. This diagnosis was established in an era when ovarian biopsy was used to determine the cause of menstrual disturbances. However, the definition of resistant ovary syndrome is not universally accepted. In fact, in the original series, cases were included in which patients had demonstrated ovulatory function in the past but later developed a clinical picture suggestive of ovarian resistance. This pattern is more typical of ovarian aging and follicular depletion.

The cause is not known. Histologic features of ovarian biopsy demonstrate that there is no plasma cell or lymphocytic infiltration, indicating that it is not caused by autoimmune destruction. The presence of numerous follicles indicates that POF is not due to follicular depletion. Several studies have looked at gonadotropins, FSH receptors, and antibodies that serve as blockers to the gonadotropin receptors, and the literature to date is inconclusive about the cause.

Diagnosis can be established with certainty only with ovarian biopsy. However, current recommendations for management of amenorrhea do not include surgery to make a diagnosis. The diagnosis is, therefore, one of exclusion. In the absence of autoimmune disease and of any history of ovulation, karyotyping should be performed to exclude chromosomal abnormalities. In patients with normal karyotypes, the diagnosis of POF and resistant ovary syndrome is difficult to make without biopsy. Improvements in ultrasound technology may make it possible to differentiate these entities by the measurement of ovarian volumes and antral follicle counts.

E. Summary

In more than half of patients with POF, no specific cause can be identified. The age defining POF is somewhat arbitrary. By definition, menopause is preceded by reproductive failure. It is thought that the time interval between menopause and the end of fertility may be approximately 10 years, and we know that approximately 10% of women reach menopause by

46 years of age and 1% by 40 years. Therefore, women who experience menopause at 45 years of age probably encounter a decline in reproductive potential or even reproductive failure at 35 years of age. This has obvious implications for women who are delaying childbearing. Several studies have described a significant association between the menopausal ages of mothers and daughters, twins, and sisters. A number of studies have identified new genes that are involved in ovarian physiology. It is hoped that these investigations will help in the treatment of subfertility and result in a reduction in infertility. At a minimum, they may allow better prospective individual prediction of reproductive risk.

Women diagnosed with POF that is not readily explained must have an evaluation that consists of a karyotype, testing for fragile-X (FMR) permutation, and evaluation for APS. If a patient has an FMR permutation, one should offer screening to her father. If there is no identifiable cause of POF, screening for adrenal insufficiency is obligatory. All patients with POF should be considered for combination HRT. The increased risks associated with breast cancer are likely no greater than the age-adjusted risk of women with intact ovaries. Patients with absent secondary sexual characteristics should initially be given estrogen-only therapy in low doses and titrated every 3 to 6 months (see Chapters 14 and 15 and see below for management of menopause).

ANOVULATION

Chronic anovulation may be defined as repetitive ovulation failure, which differs from ovarian failure in that viable oocytes remain in the ovary. Anovulation is the most common cause of amenorrhea during the reproductive years. There are several causes; those associated with hypothalamic and pituitary disorders have previously been mentioned and will not be considered in this section. Other conditions that cause anovulation include the peripheral endocrinopathies. These disorders result in a hormonal imbalance—mainly elevated androgens or estrogens—and lead to inappropriate feedback mechanisms and ovulatory failure. The peripheral endocrine disorders will be discussed later in greater detail.

Hyperandrogenism and Anovulation

A. Polycystic ovarian syndrome
Hyperandrogenic anovulation accounts for more than 30% of cases of amenorrhea and up to 75% of all cases of anovulation. Most often it is due to polycystic ovarian syndrome (PCOS). The reported prevalence of PCOS depends on the criteria used to define it. Although there is considerable controversy over the definition, most investigators, until recently, have focused on the 1990 National Institutes of Health-National Institute for Child and Human Development (NIH-NICHD) diagnostic criteria (Table 13–4). This definition puts forth ovarian hyperandrogenism and anovulation as the cardinal features of PCOS. The criteria include ovulatory dysfunction with evidence of hyperandrogenism, either clinically or by laboratory testing, in the absence of identifiable causes of hyperandrogenism. Using these criteria, the prevalence of unexplained hyperandrogenic

TABLE 13–4 Revised diagnostic criteria for polycystic ovary syndrome.

1990 criteria (both 1 and 2)
1. Chronic anovulation
2. Clinical and/or biochemical signs of hyperandrogenism and exclusion of other etiologies
Revised 2003 criteria (2 of 3)
1. Oligo or anovulation
2. Clinical and/or biochemical signs of hyperandrogenism
3. Polycystic ovaries and exclusion of other etiologies (congenital adrenal hyperplasia, androgen-secreting tumors, Cushing syndrome)

From Rotterdam ESHRE/ASRM-Sponsored PCOS Consensus Workshop Group. Revised 2003 consensus on diagnostic criteria and long-term health risks related to polycystic ovary syndrome. *Fertil Steril.* 2004;81:19.

chronic anovulation approximates 4% to 6%, and it is considered the most common endocrine disorder in women of reproductive age. However, in 2003 the diagnostic criteria were revised by the Rotterdam consensus conference (see Table 13–4). The Rotterdam criteria consider a broader spectrum of ovarian dysfunction than previous definitions. Some experts criticize the new definition, because it encompasses many more women, notably those with hyperandrogenism and ovulatory cycles, in addition to women with anovulation without androgen excess. This is contrast to the 1990 NIH-NICHD definition, which required *both* androgen excess and irregular cycles. Most recently, the Androgen Excess Society task force proposed the criteria should be defined by the presence of hyperandrogenism and ovarian dysfunction (see Table 13–4). This definition expands upon the 1990 NIH-NICHD criteria and requires that all patients with PCOS are hyperandrogenic at some level. Although the revised criteria can include women with ovulatory cycles, the remaining discussion on PCOS focuses on women who have anovulatory cycles.

Approximately 50% of women diagnosed with PCOS are obese, and most have polycystic ovaries present on sonography (see later). Underlying these features are numerous biochemical abnormalities that have been associated with this syndrome, including elevated circulating total testosterone, free testosterone, DHEAS, and insulin as well as decreased SHBG and an elevated LH-FSH ratio. However, these abnormalities are not present in all PCOS patients. In fact, 40% of women who present with only hirsutism have elevated total testosterone levels, and 30% to 70% have elevated DHEAS levels. Similarly, the evaluation of increased LH pulsatility, in association with low-normal FSH levels (LH-FSH ratio), is not a reliable diagnostic test. Although elevated LH-FSH ratios are common findings in thin women, in obese patients with PCOS, the ratio is within the normal range about half of the time. The short half-life of LH (~20 minutes) is likely another major contributor to the inaccuracy of LH testing. Hyperinsulinemia has recently been hypothesized to play a major role in the pathogenesis of PCOS (see later). The prevalence of insulin resistance may approximate 50% to 60%, compared with 10% to 25% observed in the general population. However, insulin resistance is difficult to measure in the clinical setting. Part of the difficulty is that there is no universally agreed on definition of insulin resistance, and the laboratory tests are not standardized. Furthermore, baseline insulin levels vary depending on population and body weight. For example, up to 60% of ovulatory obese patients have demonstrated some form of insulin resistance. Nonetheless, there is good evidence that a subset of normal-weight women and obese women with PCOS have a greater degree of insulin resistance and compensatory hyperinsulinemia compared with weight-matched controls.

There is increasing evidence for a strong genetic component in the etiology of PCOS. Several candidate genes have been investigated, including genes involved in steroidogenesis and carbohydrate metabolism, but none has been conclusively linked with the disease. PCOS is heterogeneous clinically, raising the possibility of different genetic causes and a variable environmental contribution to the syndrome.

1. **Diagnosis of PCOS**—The diagnosis of PCOS is typically based on clinical features (irregular menstrual cycles, acne, hirsutism), although additional information may be obtained with biochemical testing and sonographic examination. Known causes of hyperandrogenism and anovulation should be excluded in all patients (ie, androgen-secreting tumors, thyroid and adrenal gland dysfunction, hyperprolactinemia).

In most situations, the manifestations of PCOS emerge in the peripubertal years, occasionally with premature pubarche, and likely irregular cycles that persist through much of reproductive life. The diagnosis may be challenging, however, because adolescent girls commonly display irregular cycles during the 5 years following menarche. Ultrasonography may help to solidify the diagnosis of PCOS in children given that the likelihood of restoration of normal ovarian morphology is small as long as irregular menses persist.

Polycystic ovaries tend to be enlarged and have been defined in multiple ways: (1) the presence of 10 or more cystic follicles that are between 2 and 8 mm in diameter and arranged along the subcapsular edge of the ovary in a string of pearls fashion; and (2) 12 or more follicles 2 to 9 mm in either ovary and/or an ovarian volume of 10 cm^3 or greater. The increased ovarian volume and displacement of follicles toward the periphery may be explained by the hyperplastic stroma. The stroma contains hilar cells and secondary interstitial cells (theca cells) that are capable of androgen synthesis.

Polycystic-appearing ovaries are very common in women with clinical features suggestive of hyperandrogenism, independent of menstrual disturbances. This finding suggests that ovarian hyperandrogenism can occur in ovulatory states and should be considered in the spectrum of PCOS, if polycystic ovaries are present. However, the finding of polycystic ovaries alone does not establish the diagnosis of PCOS. In fact, based on the Rotterdam definition, more than 30% of normal women have this ovarian morphologic feature. The prevalence is significantly impacted by age. Approximately 60% of women with regular cycles between the ages of 25 to 30 have morphologic characteristics consistent with polycystic ovaries compared to 7% of women between the ages of 41 to 45. Furthermore, the morphogenesis of polycystic ovaries is not unique to PCOS as it has been observed in other scenarios (ie, late-onset congenital adrenal hyperplasia, HIV, epilepsy).

2. **Hyperandrogenism**—The origin of sex steroids is from two sources: the gonads and the adrenal gland. The adrenal gland is responsible for most of the precursor hormones in the general circulation, which serve as reservoirs for the more potent androgens and estrogens. The ovary produces bioactive androgens and estrogens as well as precursor hormones. Figure 13–11 illustrates the relative contribution of each organ to the pool of circulating sex steroids. DHEAS is the most abundant steroid in the circulation, and serves as a precursor to the more potent androgens and estrogens. Over 98% of DHEAS is secreted from the adrenal gland. Approximately half of the circulating levels of androstenedione are equally derived from the adrenal gland and gonads and the remaining half from conversion of DHEAS (DHEA) in the periphery. DHEAS also serves as a substrate for the ovary to produce bioactive sex steroids. It is evident that the majority of bioactive androgen is derived from precursor steroids that undergo peripheral conversion. It is suggested over 60% of the testosterone is derived from circulating androstenedione, and the remaining is by direct secretion. The contribution of testosterone from the ovary and the adrenal gland is not completely known. The fact that the various methods to obtain secretion rates are difficult and that assays used to measure testosterone can be unreliable with resultant variability contributes to the uncertain interpretation.

A common clinical sign of hyperandrogenism is hirsutism. Hirsutism affects approximately 5% to 15% of the population. The prevalence depends on the population and the method used to establish the diagnosis. The most common scoring method used to diagnose hirsutism is based on the Ferriman and Gallwey system. It is based on evaluating 9 to 11 body areas and assigning a score of 0 to 4 based on the density of hair. This method is primarily used for research purposes. Clinically, it is often diagnosed by history and the presence of excess hair growth in centrally located regions, not commonly found in women. For example, those areas most affected are the face (sideburns, mustache, and beard), chest, linea alba, or the inner aspect of the thighs. The characteristics and distribution of body hair may be influenced by ethnic or racial factors. Alternatively, hyperandrogenism may present as acne or alopecia.

The diagnostic evaluation of hirsutism should include a thorough history and physical examination (Figure 13–12). The etiology can be divided between nonandrogenic and androgenic causes. Organic causes of hyperandrogenism must be excluded. Nonandrogenic causes include chronic skin irritation, anabolic medications, and rarely acromegaly. The most common androgenic cause is PCOS which affects at least 70% of hirsute women. Less common is late-onset congenital adrenal hyperplasia, which affects approximately 5% of patients. PCOS is a diagnosis of exclusion—measurements of serum androgen levels should play only a limited role in the evaluation. Most patients who have hyperandrogenemia present with obvious clinical manifestations, and the presence of normal androgen levels in a patient with hirsutism or acne does not exclude the diagnosis of PCOS. However, there are subsets of amenorrheic patients (ie, Asians) who are hyperandrogenemic without clinical manifestations, most likely as a result of their relative insensitivity to circulating androgens. It is in these patients that assessing androgen levels may be of value in determining the cause of amenorrhea. More commonly, androgens such as DHEAS and testosterone are measured to exclude other causes of hyperandrogenic anovulation such as nonclassic adrenal hyperplasia and androgen-secreting tumors (see later).

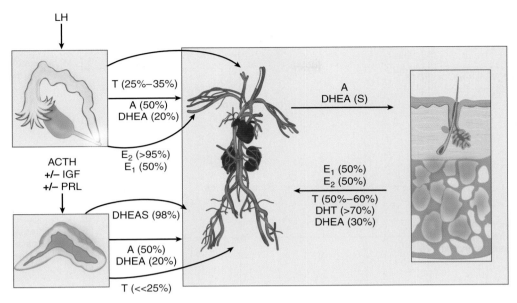

FIGURE 13–11 The origin of circulating sex steriods: the relative contribution of each organ to the pool of circulating sex steroids.

Another cause of hirsutism, made only after excluding other diagnoses, is characterized by regular menstrual cycles, normal androgen levels, and the absence of polycystic-appearing ovaries; it is termed idiopathic hirsutism. This common disorder occurs more frequently in certain ethnic populations, particularly those of Mediterranean descent. It is thought that the etiology of hirsutism in these patients is related to higher 5α-reductase activity (increased sensitivity) within the pilosebaceous unit.

3. **Mechanism of anovulation**—The mechanism of anovulation in PCOS remains unclear. It is evident that the population of antral follicles is increased and that follicular development is arrested. It is also known that the development of preantral follicles is not primarily under hormonal control. Evidence supports the components of the intraovarian network as regulators of antral follicle development. It is known that many of the accumulated follicles in PCOS remain steroidogenically competent and are capable of producing estrogen and progesterone. In fact, it is interesting that women with PCOS produce both androgens and estrogen (estrone) in excess.

One of the most frequently described characteristics of PCOS is the functional derangement of LH secretion. Numerous studies have shown that frequency, amplitude, and mean levels of LH are increased. The aberration in LH secretion may be a result of heightened pituitary responsiveness and increased hypothalamic GnRH activity. Under normal conditions, follicles respond to LH after they reach approximately 10 mm in diameter. However, polycystic ovarian follicles acquire responsiveness to LH at a much smaller diameter, which may lead to inappropriate terminal differentiation of granulosa cells and result in disorganized follicular development. It has been suggested that the theca cells increase their expression of steroidogenic enzymes following stimulation by LH, whereas the granulosa display resistance to FSH (see later). The elevated LH levels and relative hyperinsulinemia that exist in some PCOS patients may synergistically potentiate disordered folliculogenesis. Although hyperandrogenism is part of the diagnostic criteria for PCOS, its direct impact on folliculogenesis is not clear. It is conceivable that androgens contribute to the effects of LH and insulin on follicular maturation. It is also possible that the excess estrogens may result in a negative-feedback loop to inhibit FSH release and prevent further follicular development.

Most experts are of the opinion that excess androgen production is a fundamental abnormality in women with PCOS. Androgens within the ovary are produced mainly by the thecal interstitial cells that surround the follicle and to a lesser extent by the secondary interstitial cells located in the stroma (see earlier). The CYP17α complex is thought to be the key enzyme in biosynthesis of ovarian androgens. Under normal conditions, a large proportion of the androgens produced by the theca cells diffuses into the granulosa cell layer of the follicle where they are rapidly converted to estrogen as shown in Figures 13–7 and 13–11 (two-cell theory). The intrinsic control of androgen production in the ovary is modulated by intraovarian factors and hormones (see section on ovarian steroidogenesis at the beginning of this chapter). It is the dysregulation of hormone production that is most likely responsible for PCOS.

Several studies have shown that women with PCOS have an exaggerated ovarian androgen response to various stimuli. To illustrate, hyperstimulation of 17-hydroxyprogesterone levels was noted when women diagnosed with PCOS were given a GnRH agonist or hCG, suggesting increased CYP17α activity. This study is supported by in vitro studies in which measurement of steroids in cultured human theca cells from polycystic ovaries revealed concentrations of androstenedione, 17α-hydroxyprogesterone, and progesterone that were respectively 20-fold, 10-fold, and 5-fold higher than levels in control cells. Additional studies have found increased expression of the genes encoding CYP17α hydroxylase, P450scc, the LH receptor, and StAR. These findings reflect a global enhancement of

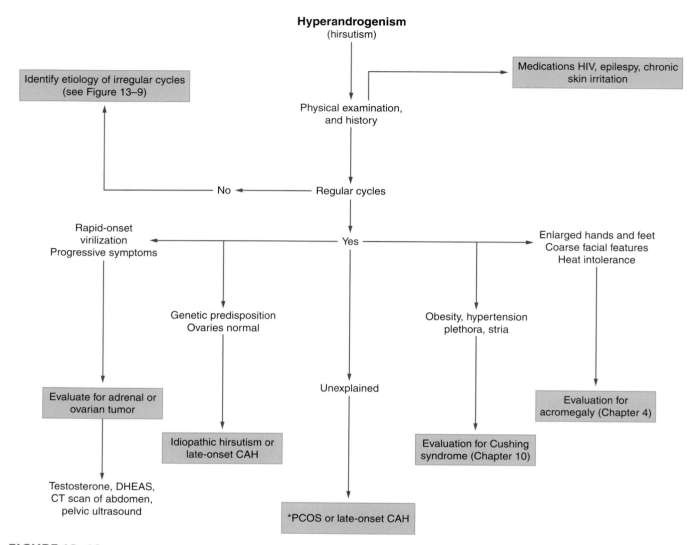

FIGURE 13–12 An algorithm for women with hirsutism. All women should be screened for known causes of hyperandrogenism. Hyperandrogenism suggests either PCOS or late-onset congenital adrenal hyperplasia (CAH). If hirsutism is rapid in onset or rapidly progressive in nature or the patient is frankly virilized, an evaluation for an androgen-secreting tumor is required. Management of hirsutism in late-onset CAH or PCOS is similar. *Late-onset CAH can present with regular cycles. Depending on the specific criteria (see Table 13–4), PCOS can present with regular cycles. Serum hormones are not required for the diagnosis of idiopathic hirsutism or PCOS.

steroidogenesis. This situation is compounded by the hypertrophy of theca cells that is present in women with PCOS.

Several studies have evaluated intraovarian modulators as participants in the pathogenesis of PCOS (Figure 13–13). IGF-binding proteins (IGFBPs), especially IGFBP-2 and IGFBP-4, are found to be increased in the follicular fluid of polycystic ovaries. They may act locally to decrease free IGF-2 and, thus, decrease the effects of FSH on the oocyte and granulosa cells. Alternatively, the granulosa cells may down-regulate their insulin receptors as a result of hyperinsulinemia. This would deprive the granulosa cells of their co-gonadotropin, IGF-2, and account for the relative FSH insensitivity. Inhibin is also a likely candidate, because a large proportion of women with PCOS have relative FSH suppression (Figure 13–13). However, studies have not shown consistent results, suggesting that if inhibin is involved, the effect is minimal. Follistatin, the

activin-binding protein, was in the past thought to play an important role in the development of PCOS. It was initially implicated because activin functions to inhibit androgen production and enhance FSH expression. However, current studies do not demonstrate a significant association between abnormalities in follistatin and PCOS.

The adrenal gland may be significantly involved in the pathogenesis of some cases of PCOS. The connection seems plausible because adrenal androgens can be converted to more potent androgens in the ovary. Furthermore, a significant portion of women with congenital adrenal hyperplasia have polycystic ovaries (see later). Several studies have shown that DHEAS is elevated in 25% to 60% of patients with PCOS. However, ACTH levels are normal in PCOS women. Interestingly, it has been reported that there is an increased response of androstenedione and 17α-hydroxyprogesterone to exogenous ACTH. These

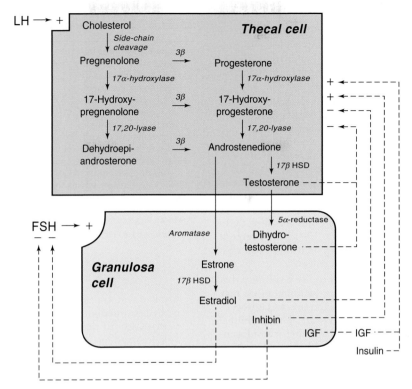

FIGURE 13–13 Regulation of sex steroid production in the theca and granulosa cells of the ovary. Several autocrine and paracrine factors such as insulin and insulin-like growth factors (IGFs) work synergistically with luteinizing hormone (LH) to stimulate androgen production through increased 17α-hydroxylase activity. (Redrawn with permission from Ehrmann DA, Barnes RB, Rosenfeld RL. Polycystic ovary syndrome as a form of functional ovarian hyperandrogenism due to dysregulation of androgen secretion. *Endocr Rev.* 1995;16:322.)

findings suggest an underlying abnormality in the CYP17α expressed in the adrenal gland as well as in the ovary. However, minimal data support CYP17α dysfunction in the adrenal gland. It has also been shown that ovarian steroids can stimulate adrenal androgen production; however, additional findings suggest that the ovary is not the primary cause of adrenal hyperresponsiveness. The critical role played by adrenal androgens during the pubertal transition has not been fully investigated as a potential contributor to the development of PCOS.

4. **Hyperinsulinemia and PCOS**—A relationship between insulin and hyperandrogenism has been postulated based on several observations. This association may be demonstrated in the peripubertal years with premature pubarche, which is more commonly associated with insulin resistance than with congenital adrenal hyperplasia or androgen excess. Various case reports have shown that **acanthosis nigricans**—hyperpigmentation of skin in the intertriginous areas—is associated with severe insulin resistance. A number of these patients also presented with hyperandrogenism and anovulation. The relationship was substantiated when it was observed that the degree of hyperinsulinemia was correlated with the degree of hyperandrogenism. Further studies revealed that hyperinsulinemia is frequently identified in women with PCOS.

It has been shown that the cause of hyperinsulinemia is insulin resistance and that the defect lies in the postreceptor signaling pathway. The frequency and degree of hyperinsulinemia in women with PCOS is amplified in the presence of obesity. Although many women with PCOS exhibit insulin resistance, some do not. However, insulin resistance is also observed in some thin PCOS patients.

Insulin may cause hyperandrogenism in several different ways, although the exact mechanism has not been well defined. It has been suggested that insulin has a stimulatory effect on CYP17α. There is evidence from in vitro models that insulin may act directly on the ovary (see Figure 13–13). It has been shown that the ovary possesses insulin receptors and IGF receptors. In addition, several studies have reported that insulin stimulates ovarian estrogen, androgen, and progesterone secretion and that its effects are greatly enhanced by the addition of gonadotropins. Administration of an insulin-sensitizing agent (eg, metformin or a thiazolidinedione) to obese women with PCOS leads to a substantial reduction in 17α-hydroxyprogesterone levels, reflecting decreased CYP17α activity. However, clinical studies, in which insulin infusions were administered to normal women, failed to demonstrate increased testosterone production, and there were no changes in androgen levels when normal women were given insulin-sensitizing agents. These observations suggest that insulin has more of a modifying rather than a predisposing effect on androgen production.

The relationship between insulin and adrenal androgen production is less clear. Some studies have shown that insulin increases secretion of 17α-hydroxyprogesterone and DHEAS in response to ACTH. Other studies have shown that DHEAS decreases after acute insulin infusions are administered to normal men and women. Furthermore, when insulin-sensitizing agents were administered to women with PCOS, a decrease in DHEAS was observed. Although there is less evidence to support the association of insulin and adrenal androgen production, if there is an insulin effect, it is as a modulator of adrenal secretory activity.

Insulin may indirectly affect androgen levels. Several studies have reported that insulin directly inhibits SHBG production. There is an inverse correlation between insulin levels and SHBG, so that decreasing insulin levels would decrease the circulating bioavailable androgen level (via increases in SHBG). It has also been shown that insulin decreases IGFBP-1. This would increase free IGF-1, which could modulate ovarian androgen production in a fashion similar to insulin (see Figure 13–13). Although these indirect mechanisms may play a role, the literature suggests that insulin acts directly to augment androgen production (see Figure 13–13). However, it appears that a dysregulation in steroidogenesis must also exist in order for insulin to cause hyperandrogenism.

Increasing attention is being directed to the possibility that PCOS begins before adolescence. In fact, the initial insult may begin in utero, where there is ample exposure to androgens derived from the fetal adrenal gland and ovary. This hormonal environment may reprogram the ovary and alter steroidogenesis in a manner that predisposes to PCOS. The phenotypic expression of PCOS would then be determined by environmental factors such as diet and exercise.

The various biochemical abnormalities associated with PCOS have led to studies investigating metabolic sequelae of this syndrome. Long-term health problems such as the development of cardiovascular disease and diabetes have been linked to PCOS. In fact, several studies have suggested that the metabolic syndrome is significantly more prevalent in women with PCOS. However, studies looking at whether women with PCOS actually experience increased cardiovascular events are limited. Several observational studies have demonstrated that women with PCOS have alterations in their lipid profiles, including increased triglycerides and LDL and decreased high-density lipoprotein (HDL) compared with weight-matched controls. Furthermore, the degree of dyslipidemia has been correlated with the magnitude of insulin resistance. The fact that insulin resistance occurs with greater frequency in women with PCOS suggests that they are at higher risk for the development of diabetes mellitus. It is known that up to 30% to 40% of women with PCOS have impaired glucose tolerance, although it is most often seen in patients who are obese. Limited retrospective studies have suggested that women with PCOS have an increased frequency of developing type 2 diabetes. In summary, as demonstrated by surrogate markers, the available data show that these patients have increased risk factors for cardiovascular events and diabetes. Long-term prospective studies will be required to determine if these patients are actually at risk for increased mortality and morbidity.

The fact that hyperinsulinemia underlies many of the potential adverse sequelae raises a question about whether insulin resistance should be assessed in all patients diagnosed with PCOS. There are several methods of measuring insulin resistance (Table 13–5). However, the potential impact of hyperinsulinemia is unknown. Furthermore, there is no universal laboratory criterion or standardization for establishing the diagnosis of insulin resistance, which raises doubts about whether any potential adverse sequelae can be prevented if

TABLE 13–5 Measurements of insulin resistance.

Frequently sampled intravenous glucose tolerance test (FSIGT)[a]
Euglycemic insulin clamp[a]
Insulin tolerance test (ITT)
Fasting insulin levels
Oral glucose tolerance test (OGTT) + insulin levels and calculating area under the curve
Glucose-insulin ratio
Derivatives of glucose-insulin ratio[b]
Insulin resistance index = glucose × insulin/25
Homeostasis model assessment of insulin resistance HOMA-IR = 22.5 × 18/glucose × or log (HOMA-IR)
Quantitative insulin sensitivity check index (QUICKD = 1/log (glucose) + log (insulin)

[a]American Diabetes Association (ADA) gold standard; not practical for clinical use.
[b]Calculations based on fasting glucose and insulin levels.

insulin resistance is identified. Further data are necessary, prior to widespread use of medications such as metformin or a thiazolidinedione to reduce insulin resistance in patients with PCOS to determine (1) if these patients are indeed at risk for cardiovascular events, (2) if hyperinsulinemia is an independent risk factor, and (3) whether long-term treatment with any insulin-sensitizing agent will decrease the potential sequelae.

5. **Additional risks associated with PCOS**—Another concern is that women who are anovulatory do not produce a significant amount of progesterone. This leads to a situation in which the uterine lining is stimulated by unopposed estrogens, which is a significant risk factor for development of endometrial cancer. In fact, an association has been found between endometrial cancer and PCOS. There is also evidence to suggest an association of PCOS with both breast cancer and ovarian cancer, but PCOS has not been conclusively shown to be an independent risk factor for either disease.

6. **Management of PCOS**—The management of PCOS should be dictated by the patients' risk factors for cardiovascular disease, diabetes, malignant sequelae, and symptomatology (see also "Infertility"). All patients should have a lipid profile measured. In addition, oral glucose tolerance tests should be performed—at least in obese women. In patients who have a long history of irregular cycles (>1 year), an endometrial biopsy should be considered.

Cardiovascular risk factors, weight loss, and progression to diabetes can be improved with diet and exercise. In the subset of patients with glucose intolerance, administration of insulin-sensitizing agents should be considered. Metformin, a biguanide, is the most widely studied. Several studies have shown modest transitory weight loss, and possibly a decreased incidence of diabetes in patients with PCOS due to its use. Metformin is not effective for treatment of hyperandrogenic symptomatology. The use of metformin is not recommended unless there is evidence of metabolic derangements that are not fixed with diet and exercise alone.

Irregular bleeding can be improved by the administration of oral contraceptives which induce scheduled withdrawal bleeding. However, another benefit of oral contraceptives has been the significant reduction in endometrial cancer in the general population. It is rational to expect that a similar benefit would accrue to women with PCOS, because the ovarian stimulation is minimized and the progestin would counteract the estrogenic environment.

Acne and hirsutism in women diagnosed with PCOS or of idiopathic origin can be treated with oral contraceptives. The mechanism is not completely known, but oral contraceptives decrease the amount of bioavailable androgens by increased SHBG production and by ovarian suppression. It has also been shown that progestins can inhibit 5α-reductase activity, which further decreases the production of dihydrotestosterone, the major androgen that stimulates hair growth. The maximal effect is evident after 6 months of treatment (the hair cycle length is estimated to be 4 months). If hirsutism is severe or if oral contraceptives alone are not effective, the addition of spironolactone may be beneficial. Spironolactone is an anti-mineralocorticoid agent that inhibits androgen biosynthesis in the adrenal gland and ovary, inhibits 5α-reductase, and is a competitive inhibitor of the androgen receptor. Side-effects are minimal and include diuresis in the first few days; dyspepsia; nausea; skin hypersensitivity; breast tenderness; and abnormal bleeding, which can be alleviated by increasing the dose to desired amount over 3 weeks. Spironolactone is used concomitantly with oral contraceptives. Because oral contraceptives and spironolactone act by different mechanisms, the combined effect is synergistic.

If oral contraceptives are not desired or have not improved the excess hair growth, there are several other methods that can be used in conjuction with oral contraceptives or administered alone. The only topical agent approved for hirustism by the FDA is Vaniqa (Eflornithine) cream, which is an inhibitor of L-ornithine decarboxylase. It has been shown to be effective for control of facial hair. Long-acting GnRH agonists and 5α-reductase inhibitors (finasteride) have been used for refractory cases with some success. Shaving, bleaching, chemical depilation, plucking, or waxing are temporary measures to control unwanted hair growth. However, several of these methods can cause skin irritation and result in progressive hair growth. Permanent techniques such as electrolysis or laser depilation have shown promising results.

B. Congenital adrenal hyperplasia Congenital adrenal hyperplasia is another disorder that may cause hyperandrogenism. It presents in a wide range of clinical forms, ranging from severe—which may be classified as *classic, salt-wasting,* or *simple virilizing*—to milder forms known as *acquired, adult-onset, nonclassic,* or *late-onset* congenital hyperplasia. The clinical manifestations reflect the severity of the enzymatic defect. Severe or classic forms are discussed in Chapter 14 and will not be considered here. This section will discuss the nonclassic forms, which affect 1% to 10% of the population, depending on the ethnicity of the patient. The clinical features are similar to those of patients diagnosed with PCOS and include menstrual irregularities, hyperandrogenism, and infertility, and up to 50% have polycystic ovaries.

The adrenal gland consists of a cortex and a medulla. The cortex is divided into three functional zones based on location and the principal hormone secreted (see Chapter 9). The zona glomerulosa is the outermost zone and lies adjacent to the adrenal capsule. It is primarily responsible for aldosterone production. The zona fasciculata lies immediately below the glomerulosa. It

principally secretes glucocorticoids, although it is capable of producing androgens. The zona reticularis is located beneath the zona fasciculata and overlies the adrenal medulla. It is this zone that principally secretes androgens. Both the zona fasciculata and the zona reticularis are regulated by ACTH. It is the secretory activity of these two zones that results in nonclassic adrenal hyperplasia.

Congenital adrenal hyperplasia is an autosomal recessive disorder that is caused by mutations of genes involved with adrenal steroidogenesis. The mutations mostly occur in the 21-hydroxylase gene *(P450c21B)* and rarely in the 3β-hydroxysteroid dehydrogenase gene or 11β-hydroxylase genes *(P450c11B* and *P450c11AS).* In classic forms, the enzymatic defects are severe, affect both alleles, and result in cortisol deficiency diagnosed at birth. Owing to the cortisol deficiency, there is ACTH excess and hyperstimulation of the adrenal gland. The adrenal precursors produced proximal to the enzymatic defect accumulate and promote the synthesis of DHEA and androstenedione through the androgen synthetic pathway. These are converted in the periphery to more potent androgens, resulting in symptoms of hyperandrogenism. Approximately 50% of patients diagnosed with nonclassic congenital adrenal hyperplasia are compound heterozygotes with one of the mutant alleles coding for a severe defect. Typically, patients who are carriers have a normal phenotype. Therefore, most patients with nonclassic adrenal hyperplasia do not demonstrate deficient cortisol production or excess ACTH. It is suggested that most of the androgen excess in nonclassic adrenal hyperplasia arises as a consequence of subtle alterations in enzyme kinetics. Furthermore, some studies report a generalized adrenocortical hyperactivity rather than deficient enzyme activity.

The diagnosis can be established by measuring early morning basal 17-hydroxyprogesterone levels. Levels greater than 800 ng/dL (24.24 pmol/L) are diagnostic of 21-hydroxylase deficiency. However, the elevation in 17-hydroxyprogesterone is often not impressive and does not differ from that observed in PCOS. If the basal 17-hydroxyprogesterone levels are greater than 200 ng/dL (6.06 pmol/L) and less than 800 ng/dL (24.2 pmol/L), a provocative test with ACTH (250 μg intravenously) should be performed. If 17-hydroxyprogesterone levels are greater than 1000 ng/dL (30.30 pmol/L) 1 hour after administration of ACTH, the diagnosis of 21-hydroxylase deficiency can be made. Elimination of a false elevation in 17-hydroxyprogesterone due to ovulation must be excluded by simultaneous measurement of progesterone. A 17-hydroxyprogesterone screening level greater than 200 ng/dL has 100% sensitivity, but only 7% positive predictive value for the diagnosis of nonclassic adrenal hyperplasia. The other rare enzymatic defects that result in nonclassic adrenal hyperplasia can be assessed with measurements of steroid products proximal to the blockade following provocative testing.

Treatment of nonclassic adrenal hyperplasia is similar to that of PCOS, raising a question about whether an etiologic diagnosis is necessary. It is certainly an expense, leading to no change in management except with regard to infertility treatment and management of subsequent pregnancies (see later). Establishing a specific diagnosis may be advisable to facilitate genetic counseling in the woman with adrenal hyperplasia who intends future childbearing and to prepare for in utero treatment should an affected fetus be identified by amniocentesis. Although some experts suggest dexamethasone treatment for symptoms of hyperandrogenism, studies show inconsistent results, and there is concern about the consequent adrenal suppression.

C. Cushing syndrome Chronic glucocorticoid excess, whatever its cause, leads to the constellation of symptoms and physical features known as Cushing syndrome. The most common cause is iatrogenic as a result of glucocorticoid treatment. However, an ACTH-secreting microadenoma (Cushing disease) accounts for more than 70% of cases of endogenous hypercortisolism. Less common causes include primary adrenal disease (tumors or hyperplasia) and ectopic (not hypothalamic-pituitary) ACTH-producing or CRH-producing tumors. Patients with Cushing syndrome have a range of clinical manifestations that vary with age at onset and etiology. This section will discuss the adult clinical presentation briefly. For a more detailed discussion, see Chapter 9.

Cushing syndrome (noniatrogenic) is rare and occurs in approximately 2.6 patients per million individuals in the population. It is responsible for less than 1% of those individuals who present with hirsutism. Although Cushing syndrome is uncommon, it presents in a manner similar to PCOS and congenital adrenal hyperplasia and needs to be considered in the differential diagnosis of hyperandrogenism and anovulation. Patients with ACTH excess typically have additional clinical features suggestive of glucocorticoid or mineralocorticoid hypersecretion. The most common features include obesity with increased centripetal fat, moon facies, muscle weakness, and striae. Other manifestations may include diabetes, hypertension, and osteoporosis. Women with primary tumors tend to have a rapid onset of symptoms and often manifest with severe hyperandrogenism (frank virilization) that includes male pattern baldness, deepening voice, clitoromegaly, and defeminization.

Hirsutism or acne is present in about 60% to 70% of women with Cushing syndrome. However, the exact mechanism of hyperandrogenic effects is not completely known. It is evident that excess ACTH causes hyperstimulation of the zona fasciculata and zona reticularis and results in hypersecretion of cortisol and androgens. It is also known that adrenal tumors may selectively overproduce androgens.

Menstrual irregularities occur in more than 80% of patients with Cushing syndrome. The exact cause of anovulation is unclear. It has already been observed that hyperandrogenemia may have a significant impact on ovulation. However, several studies have shown that glucocorticoids can also suppress the hypothalamic-pituitary axis. Thus, the elevated glucocorticoids may be an additional factor in the pathophysiology of anovulation associated with this syndrome (see Chapters 4 and 9 for the diagnosis and treatment of Cushing syndrome).

D. Androgen-secreting tumor If there is a rapid onset of androgenic symptoms, an androgen-secreting adrenal tumor should be suspected. Elevated testosterone (>200 ng/dL; 6.9 nmol/L) and DHEAS (>700 ng/mL; 19 μmol/L) levels should raise the suspicion of a tumor. However, more than 50% of adrenal androgen-secreting tumors have testosterone levels below

200 ng/dL (6.9 nmol/L). Furthermore, the majority of patients with high testosterone levels do not have tumors. Testosterone levels above 250 ng/dL are only 10% predictive for androgen-secreting tumor. Measurement of DHEAS levels in these patients yields similar inconsistencies. This suggests that laboratory tests have limited value in screening for androgen-secreting tumors, and a clinical history and physical examination are better predictors. The presence of systemic symptoms such as weight loss, anorexia, bloating, and back pain favor an androgen-secreting tumor. If suspicion is high, an abdominal computed tomography (CT) scan confirms the diagnosis. The treatment involves surgical resection, mitotane (adrenolytic), and steroid synthesis inhibitors.

Androgen-secreting tumors can also originate from the ovary. The incidence approximates 1:500 to 1:1000 hyperandrogenic patients. Testosterone levels >200 ng/dL (6.9 nmol/L) arouse suspicion, although in 20% of patients with ovarian androgen-producing tumors, testosterone levels are below this value. Again, the best screening procedures are the clinical history and physical examination. In the absence of Cushingoid features, adrenal and ovarian tumors present similarly. Ovarian tumors often have unilateral ovarian enlargement that can be palpated on pelvic examination. Ultrasonography often confirms the diagnosis. In selected cases, selective venous sampling may be performed if CT or sonography cannot identify the source of androgen production.

OBESITY

Obesity is the most prevalent chronic disease in the United States. Adverse health events are dramatically increased in obese subjects (see Chapter 20). These include cardiovascular disease, diabetes, joint disease, respiratory dysfunction, and colon, endometrial, and ovarian cancers. Obesity is often also associated with menstrual irregularities, and the relationship between the two is strengthened the earlier the onset of the obesity. Alterations in sex steroid metabolism are clearly evident in obese females, and the consequences are attenuated release of gonadotropins, which manifests as anovulation. Obese patients have increased production rates and MCRs of androgens; therefore, their serum levels of androgens are largely within the normal range. However, free testosterone levels tend to be in the high-normal range due to the decreased SHBG levels. A portion of androgen metabolism occurs in body fat. The excess adipose tissue aromatizes these androgens and increases the amount of circulating estrone causing a state of functional hyperestrogenism. In fact, studies have shown that the rate of peripheral conversion of androstenedione to estrone is correlated with body weight. Other studies have illustrated that the conversion of estrone to estradiol in adipose tissue is higher in visceral fat than subcutaneous fat. The increased visceral fat associated with obesity is also associated with hyperinsulinemia, which may have independent effects on ovarian function.

Management of Obesity

The management of obesity includes diet and exercise (see Chapter 20). In patients who have irregular uterine bleeding, an endometrial biopsy must be performed to rule out endometrial cancer. Oral contraceptives are effective at treating the irregular bleeding and reduce the incidence of endometrial cancer. Weight loss reestablishes normal menstrual cycles in the majority of these women.

Anovulation Unrelated to Excess Sex Steroid Production

A. Adrenal insufficiency   Adrenocortical insufficiency may be categorized as primary or secondary. Primary adrenal insufficiency (Addison disease) is caused by destruction of adrenal cortical tissue. Secondary adrenal insufficiency is due to defects in the hypothalamic-pituitary axis resulting in a deficiency in ACTH. Both types lead to cortisol deficiency, which is life threatening.

The main cause of primary adrenal failure is autoimmune destruction of the adrenal cortex. In fact, in the industrialized world, an autoimmune pathogenesis accounts for more than 60% of cases of primary adrenocortical deficiency. The symptoms are typically those of chronic insufficiency and include weakness, fatigue, menstrual disturbances, and gastrointestinal symptoms such as nausea, abdominal pain, and diarrhea. Additional signs may include weight loss, hypotension, and hyperpigmentation of the skin and mucous membranes. These symptoms may appear insidiously with a mean duration of approximately 3 years. Symptoms usually wax and wane until there is complete decompensation.

Autoimmune adrenal failure may occur as an isolated event, but estimates link more than 70% of cases to an autoimmune polyglandular syndrome (APS) of two subtypes (type 1 and 2). APS-1 usually presents in childhood with hypoparathyroidism, chronic mucocutaneous candidiasis, adrenal insufficiency, and other autoimmune disorders such as celiac disease and ovarian failure. It is caused by mutations in the autoimmune regulator gene *(AIRE)* and has an autosomal recessive inheritance. APS-2 (Schmidt syndrome) has its onset in adulthood (usually the third decade). Common manifestations include type 1 diabetes mellitus, myasthenia gravis, Hashimoto thyroiditis, ovarian failure, and adrenal insufficiency. Susceptibility to this disorder seems to be inherited as a dominant trait in linkage dysequilibrium with the HLA-B region of chromosome 6. Autoimmune adrenal insufficiency is associated with autoantibodies that are directed toward enzymes involved with steroidogenesis. Several studies suggest that the antigens in this disorder include 17α-hydroxylase, 21-hydroxylase, and P450scc. Detection of antibodies directed at these enzymes is helpful in making the diagnosis of autoimmune adrenal failure (see Chapters 2 and 9).

Worldwide, infection—especially tuberculosis—is the most common cause of primary adrenal failure. The adrenal cortex and medulla are involved and may be completely replaced by caseating granulomas. This phenomenon is always associated with other evidence of a tuberculosis infection. Fungal, viral, and bacterial pathogens are less common causes.

The most common cause of secondary adrenal insufficiency is adrenal suppression after exogenous glucocorticoid administration.

Adrenal insufficiency is also seen following treatment of Cushing disease and with a variety of hypothalamic-pituitary lesions that result in hypopituitarism. These patients more commonly present with symptoms suggestive of acute adrenal insufficiency. The clinical features include abdominal pain, hypotension, fever, severe volume depletion, and possibly profound shock.

Menstrual disturbances are a frequent presentation in patients with adrenal insufficiency. Autoimmune adrenal insufficiency is often accompanied by gonadal failure. In the two forms of APS, POF develops in APS-1 in 50% of patients and in APS-2 in 10% of patients. It has been shown that antibodies—particularly to CYP17α and P450scc—are associated with POF. Other causes of adrenal failure are associated with menstrual disorders more than 25% of the time. The cause of anovulation is not known with certainty, but chronic illness itself is probably responsible.

Diagnosis and treatment are discussed in Chapter 9. The screening process includes blood chemistries and basal cortisol levels. The diagnosis is confirmed with provocative tests using exogenous ACTH.

B. Thyroid disorders   The prevalence of overt thyroid dysfunction is 1% to 2% in women of reproductive age. Thyroid disorders can develop secondary to an insult in the hypothalamus, pituitary, or thyroid, the latter being most common. In order to understand the pathophysiology of these disorders, it is important to be familiar with the normal physiologic regulation (see Chapter 7). This section will briefly review the common causes of hyperthyroidism and hypothyroidism, their manifestations after the onset of puberty, and their impact on reproductive function.

1. Hyperthyroidism—Hyperthyroidism is the clinical syndrome associated with excessive thyroid hormone activity. The clinical presentation of hyperthyroidism (thyrotoxicosis) depends on the age at onset and the degree of thyrotoxicosis. The clinical manifestations can involve most organ systems, and the presentation ranges from asymptomatic to thyroid storm. Typical features include nervousness, malaise, palpitations, heat intolerance, weight loss, and inability to concentrate. Additional features may involve the eyes and include lid lag, proptosis, and ophthalmoplegia. The reproductive abnormalities include menstrual abnormalities, infertility, and spontaneous abortions.

The most common cause of hyperthyroidism is an autoimmune process that affects thyroid hormone production (Graves disease). Antibodies bind to the TSH receptor and stimulate the thyroid gland to secrete increased amounts of thyroid hormone. Less common causes include subacute thyroiditis, toxic multinodular goiter, and struma ovarii.

Excess thyroid hormone has an impact on sex steroids. Thyroid hormones stimulate hepatic production of SHBG. As a result, total serum estradiol, estrone, testosterone, and dihydrotestosterone are increased, yet free levels of these hormones remain within the normal range. The metabolic clearance pathways appear to be altered, which can be explained in part by the increased binding. The conversion rates of androstenedione to estrogen and testosterone are increased. The significance of the alterations in metabolism has not been determined.

Menstrual irregularities frequently occur in hyperthyroid states. The exact mechanism is unclear. Altered levels of TRH and TSH do not appear to have a significant impact on the HPO axis. The LH surge may be impaired, although studies have shown that hyperthyroid patients have normal FSH and LH responses to exogenous GnRH. It is possible that the weight loss and psychologic disturbances associated with this disease may contribute to the menstrual abnormalities. It is interesting to note that endometrial biopsies of many amenorrheic patients with hyperthyroidism have demonstrated a secretory endometrium, indicating that many of these women remain ovulatory. Menstrual abnormalities return to normal with treatment.

2. **Hypothyroidism**—A more common disorder than hyperthyroidism in women of reproductive age, hypothyroidism results from inadequate thyroid hormone production. Manifestations can involve almost any organ system, and the presentation can range from asymptomatic to myxedema coma. Common symptoms include lethargy, memory defects, cold intolerance, dry skin, hair loss or occasionally excess hair growth, deepening of the voice, nausea, and constipation. Physical findings include somnolence; bradycardia; mild hypertension; dry skin; periorbital puffiness; nonpitting edema of the hands, face, and ankles; and decreased tendon reflexes. Reproductive abnormalities include menstrual disorders, infertility, and spontaneous abortions.

The most common cause is autoimmune destruction of the thyroid (Hashimoto thyroiditis). It is mediated by humoral and cell-mediated processes. The antibodies are directed toward thyroglobulin (anti-Tg) and thyroid peroxidase (anti-TPO antibody). Histologic specimens show lymphocytic infiltration. Other causes include ablative therapy of the thyroid gland (postsurgery or radioactive iodine), end-stage Graves disease, and transient thyroiditis (viral, drug-induced, or postpartum).

Inadequate thyroid hormone levels influence the metabolism of sex steroids. The production of SHBG is decreased. As a result, serum estradiol and testosterone concentrations are decreased, but free hormone levels remain within the normal range. However, the metabolism of these steroids is altered and differs from that found in individuals with hyperthyroidism.

The mechanism underlying menstrual abnormalities in hypothyroidism is incompletely understood. Because primary hypothyroidism is associated with elevated serum PRL in up to one-third of patients, it is plausible that hyperprolactinemia is a contributing factor (see Chapter 4). However, menstrual abnormalities are also observed in the absence of elevated PRL. Alterations in FSH and LH levels have been investigated, and studies have shown inconclusive results, although several studies suggest that the midcycle surge is absent. Menstrual function returns to normal with thyroid hormone replacement.

Thyroid dysfunction often presents with nonspecific symptoms, which delays the diagnosis. If only menstrual abnormalities are present, it is prudent to screen for thyroid abnormalities. Most cases are detected by TSH assays. Confirmation is obtained with a repeat TSH level and serum thyroid hormone levels.

OUTFLOW TRACT DISORDERS

The true prevalence of Müllerian tract abnormalities is not known. It is reported in as many as 45% of women. The reproductive consequences depend on the type of abnormality identified. A septate uterus is the most common defect described. These patients often present with infertility or obstetric complications. Other abnormalities include unicornous, bicornous, and didelphic uteri. These abnormalities present most commonly with reproductive or obstetric complications. Müllerian agenesis, androgen insensitivity syndrome, and congenital outflow obstruction defects are abnormalities that present with primary amenorrhea with no history of menses. In the following section these two abnormalities are discussed in greater detail.

A. Müllerian agenesis   Müllerian agenesis (Mayer-Rokitansky-Küster-Hauser syndrome) is the second most common cause of primary amenorrhea. It is a congenital condition that occurs in one in 5000 female births. These individuals have normal ovarian development, normal endocrine function, and normal female sexual development. The physical findings are a shortened or absent vagina in addition to absence of the uterus, although small masses resembling a rudimentary uterus may be noted (see the section "Embryology and Anatomy" at the beginning of this chapter). About one-third of patients have renal abnormalities, and several have had bone abnormalities and eighth nerve deafness. These individuals have a 46,XX karyotype.

The exact cause has not been identified. It is known that regression of Müllerian structures in males is controlled by AMH, which is secreted by the Sertoli cells of the testis. One hypothesis assigns the underlying defect to an activating mutation of either the *AMH* gene or its receptor. The genes for both AMH and AMH receptor have been investigated, but no mutations have yet been identified in patients with this syndrome.

B. Androgen insensitivity syndrome   Androgen insensitivity syndrome (AIS) presents in somewhat the same way as Müllerian agenesis. The presentation differs in that individuals with complete AIS have minimal sexual hair. These patients have a male karyotype with a mutation of the androgen receptor on the X chromosome. They have normal testicular development and endocrine function. However, because the internal and external male sexual structures need testosterone for development, they are absent. This results in a female phenotype. Because the testis still secretes AMH, Müllerian regression does occur. Secondary sexual characteristics (female) develop as a result of peripheral conversion of testosterone to estradiol, effectively resulting in unopposed estrogen stimulation.

The diagnosis of either disorder is entertained when pelvic examination reveals a short or absent vagina and no uterus on rectal examination. Confirmation of absent uterus can be obtained with ultrasound, MRI, or laparoscopy. These two disorders can usually be differentiated based on physical examination; patients with AIS have no pubic hair. However, the differential diagnosis becomes more difficult when patients have incomplete AIS. A testosterone level and karyotype can easily differentiate the two syndromes. This disorder is further discussed in Chapter 14.

C. Congenital outflow obstruction   Transvaginal septum and imperforate hymen are typical obstructive abnormalities.

These patients usually present with cyclic lower abdominal pain and amenorrhea. The physical findings are a shortened or absent vagina. However, this syndrome differs from Müllerian agenesis in that the pelvic organs are present. Behind either defect is old blood that has not escaped with menses. The differential diagnosis is sometimes difficult, although bulging of the introitus suggests imperforate hymen, because the defect is thinner than a transvaginal septum.

The embryologic formations of the transvaginal septum and imperforate hymen are similar but not identical. Transvaginal septum is due to failure of complete canalization of the vaginal plate (see the section "Embryology and Anatomy" at the beginning of this chapter). The septum can vary in thickness and can be located at any level in the vagina. The hymen represents the junction of the sinovaginal bulbs and urogenital sinus. Typically, the hymen is perforated during fetal development. The hymen is thin and is always at the junction of the vestibule and vagina. It is important to distinguish these defects because the surgical correction procedures are different and require different levels of expertise.

D. Asherman syndrome   Intrauterine adhesions or synechiae (Asherman syndrome) are an acquired condition that may obliterate the endometrial cavity. These patients usually present with a range of menstrual disturbances, infertility, and recurrent spontaneous abortions. The most frequent symptom is amenorrhea.

Intrauterine adhesions result from damage to the endometrial basal layer. A common antecedent factor is a surgical procedure within the uterine cavity, and most often it is endometrial curettage that occurs shortly after pregnancy. The concurrent presence of infection or heavy bleeding increases the risk. Endometrial tuberculosis and septic abortion are rare causes.

The diagnosis is entertained after demonstrating no withdrawal bleeding after administration of estrogen and progesterone. Confirmation is made with a hysterosalpingogram, saline sonogram, or hysteroscopy. Treatment involves lysis of adhesions and hormonal therapy.

MENOPAUSE

The ovary is unique in that the age at which it ceases to function in women appears to have remained constant despite the increase in longevity experienced by women over the last century. Because the loss of ovarian function has a profound impact on the hormonal milieu in women and the subsequent risk of the development of disease resulting from the loss of estrogen production, improving our understanding of reproductive aging is critical for optimal female health.

Human follicles begin development in the fourth gestational month. Approximately 1000 to 2000 germ cells migrate to the gonadal ridge and multiply, reaching a total of 6 to 7 million around the fifth month of intrauterine life. At this point, multiplication stops and follicle loss begins, declining to approximately 1 million by birth. In the human male, the germ cells become quiescent and maintain their stem cell identity. In contrast, in the human female, between weeks 12 and 18, the germ cells enter meiosis and differentiate. Thus, in the female, all germ stem cells have differentiated prior to birth. In the adult woman, the germ cells may remain quiescent, may be recruited for further development and ovulation, or may be destroyed by apoptosis. Over time, the population of oocytes is depleted (without regeneration) through recruitment and apoptosis until less than a thousand oocytes remain and menopause ensues. Approximately 90% of women experience menopause at a mean age of 51.2 years (range, 46-55). The remainder experiences menopause prior to age 46 (often termed early menopause), with 1% of women experiencing menopause before age 40 years (POF, as discussed above).

Understanding ovarian aging has been difficult. The variability in definitions has made comparisons from study to study difficult. The participants in the Stages of Reproductive Aging Workshop (STRAW) developed criteria for staging female reproductive aging. They utilized menstrual cyclicity and early follicular FSH levels as the primary determinants for this staging system. Five stages precede the final menstrual period and two stages follow it. Stages –5 to –3 include the reproductive interval; stages –2 to –1 are termed the menopausal transition; and stages +1 and +2 are the postmenopause (Figure 13–14). The menopausal transition begins with increased variability in menstrual cyclicity (>7 days) in women with elevated FSH levels. This stage ends with the final menstrual period, which cannot be recognized until after 12 months of amenorrhea. Early postmenopause is defined as the first 5 years following the final menstrual period. Late postmenopause is variable in length, beginning 5 years after the final menstrual period and continuing until death.

This system is said to include endocrinologic aspects of ovarian aging, but it still depends largely on menstrual cyclicity as a key indicator of ovarian age. The system includes measurement of FSH; however, by the time FSH is elevated, even in the face of cyclic menstrual cycles, oocyte depletion has already proceeded to such an extent that fertility (as a marker of reproductive aging) is significantly diminished. Evidence suggests that genetic and environmental factors influence both age at menopause and the decline in fertility, although the specific nature of these relationships is poorly characterized. Premature menopause can be due to failure to attain adequate follicle numbers in utero or to accelerated depletion thereafter. Potentially, either of these causes could be affected by genetic and environmental factors. The timing of menopause has a consistent impact on overall health with respect to osteoporosis, cardiovascular disease, and cancer risk. Over the next decade, it is estimated that more than 40 million women in the United States will enter menopause.

OOCYTE DEPLETION

As discussed earlier, the leading theory regarding the onset of menopause relates to a critical threshold in oocyte number. The theory that menopause is primarily triggered by ovarian aging is supported by the coincident occurrence of follicular depletion, elevation of gonadotropins, and menstrual irregularity with ultimate cessation.

In 1992 Faddy and colleagues developed a mathematical model to predict the rate of follicular decline. They utilized data from

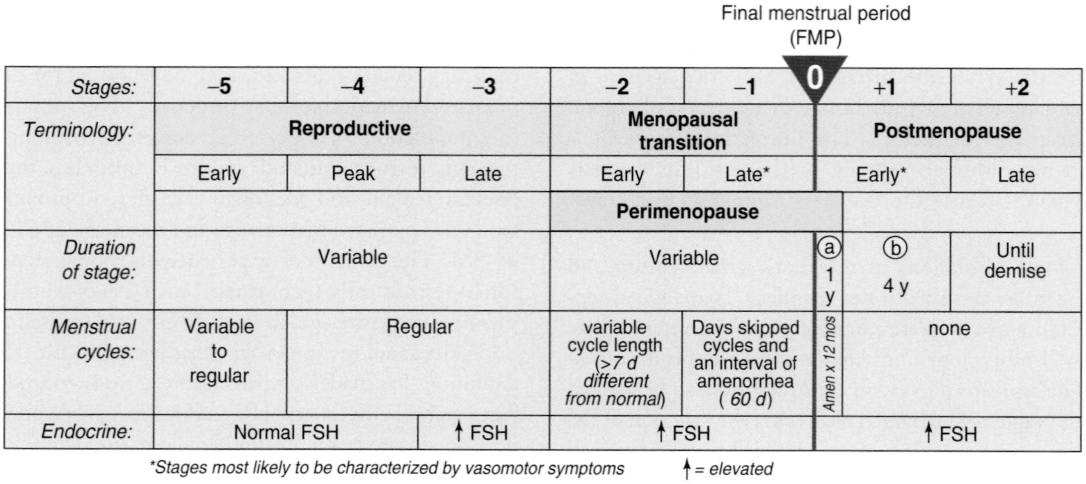

Final menstrual period
(FMP)

Stages:	−5	−4	−3	−2	−1	0	+1	+2
Terminology:	**Reproductive**			**Menopausal transition**			**Postmenopause**	
	Early	Peak	Late	Early	Late*		Early*	Late
				Perimenopause				
Duration of stage:	Variable			Variable		ⓐ 1 y	ⓑ 4 y	Until demise
Menstrual cycles:	Variable to regular	Regular		variable cycle length (>7 d different from normal)	Days skipped cycles and an interval of amenorrhea (≥60 d)	Amen x 12 mos	none	
Endocrine:	Normal FSH		↑ FSH	↑ FSH			↑ FSH	

*Stages most likely to be characterized by vasomotor symptoms   ↑ = elevated

FIGURE 13–14 Stages of reproductive aging. (Reproduced, with permission, from Soules MR, et al. Stages of Reproductive Aging Workshop [STRAW]. *J Women's Health Gend Based Med*. 2001;10:843.)

multiple sources to construct a model that ultimately showed a biexponential decline with an acceleration in oocyte loss beginning in the late thirties. More recently, Hansen et al utilized newer technology and a single population of specimens. They fit the data to multiple models and found that a pattern of gradually increasing atresia fit the decline in nongrowing follicles (Figure 13–15). This same model most closely follows the decline in the antral follicles—small (2-10 mm) growing follicles seen on ultrasound—seen across the reproductive-age span (Figure 13–16). As noted earlier, the loss of follicles (oocytes) is a constant process beginning in utero and continuing throughout reproductive life, even during

pregnancy and in the absence of ovulation, until approximately 1000 follicles/oocytes remain and menopause ensues.

ENDOCRINE SYSTEM CHANGES WITH AGING

The entire endocrine system changes with advancing age. The somatotrophic axis begins to decline in the fourth decade, prior to the decline in ovarian function. This decline is accelerated in the face of ovarian failure and may act to accelerate the decline in

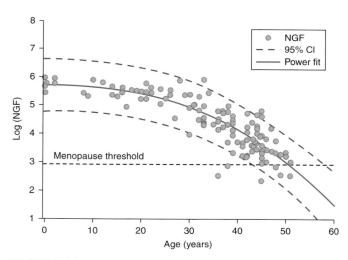

FIGURE 13–15 A new model of reproductive aging: the decline in ovarian nongrowing follicle number (primordial follicles) from birth to menopause. (Reproduced with permission from Hansen KR, et al. A new model of reproductive aging: the decline in ovarian nongrowing follicle number from birth to menopause. *Hum Reprod*. 2008;23:699-708.)

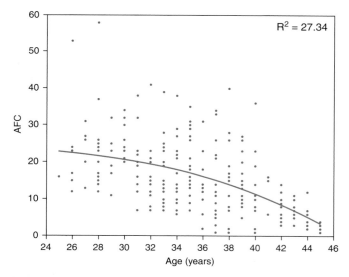

FIGURE 13–16 The antral follicle count (AFC) which declines with age in a Caucasian population is best described as a gradual acceleration in decline with age. Relationship of total AFC and chronological age. (Reproduced with permission from Rosen M, et al. Antral follicle count—absence of significant midlife decline. *Fertil Steril*. 2010: in press.)

ovarian function. However, pituitary concentrations of GH as well as ACTH and TSH remain constant into the ninth decade. While the thyroid gland undergoes progressive fibrosis with age and concentrations of T_3 decline by 25% to 40%, elderly patients still remain euthyroid. Beta cell function also undergoes degeneration with aging such that by age 65 years, 50% of subjects have abnormal glucose tolerance tests. Frank diabetes is less frequent, however, occurring in approximately 7% of the population. The female reproductive system, on the other hand, undergoes complete failure at a relatively early age.

Secretion of reproductive hormones during the menopausal transition (MT) was previously thought to decline progressively in a linear fashion, but hormone levels have since been shown to fluctuate widely. Studies in large cohorts of women have demonstrated that circulating FSH concentrations rise progressively during the MT. The initial monotropic rise in FSH is attributed to a decrease in ovarian inhibin secretion rather than to a decrease in estradiol production.

Inhibin and activin are proteins produced by the granulosa cells and have been shown to play major roles during the MT. Inhibin consists of a covalently bound dimer with an α subunit and one of two different β subunits, designated as β_A and β_B; the resulting heterodimers are known as inhibin A and inhibin B. Inhibin A is secreted by the corpus luteum and inhibin B by antral and dominant follicles. Consequently, inhibin A levels increase during the luteal phase, and inhibin B concentrations rise during the follicular phase. Both inhibins inhibit pituitary FSH secretion. Activins are a related class of proteins that stimulate pituitary FSH release. The activin molecule is a homodimer composed of two covalently linked inhibin β subunits, designated as activin A ($\beta_A\beta_A$) and activin B ($\beta_B\beta_B$).

AMH is also secreted by the granulosa cells of secondary and preantral follicles. Circulating concentrations remain relatively stable across the menstrual cycle and correlate with the number of early antral follicles. Levels of AMH decrease markedly and progressively across the MT to a time point approximately 5 years prior to the final period when levels are below the limit of detection.

During the late reproductive stage (stage –3), follicular phase inhibin B levels decrease as FSH concentrations rise. As the MT progresses, luteal phase inhibin A levels also decline. Activin A concentrations also are elevated in perimenopausal women. Whereas activins clearly play a local role in regulating pituitary FSH secretion, their ability to act as endocrine factors to influence the production of FSH has not been established. Thus, a decrease in secretion of inhibin A and inhibin B, and a corresponding increase in activin production may favor increased FSH secretion in the absence of any decrease (and perhaps an increase) in estradiol production.

Estrogens/Progesterone

The main circulating estrogen during the premenopausal years is 17β-estradiol. Levels of this hormone are controlled by the developing follicle and resultant corpus luteum. The fact that oophorectomy reduces peripheral estradiol levels from 120 to 18 pg/mL confirms that over 85% of circulating estradiol is derived from

the ovary. In perimenopausal women, estradiol production fluctuates with FSH levels and can reach higher concentrations than those observed in young women under age 35. Estradiol levels generally do not decrease significantly until late in the MT. Estradiol levels may be quite variable, with chaotic patterns and occasionally very high or very low levels. This dramatic variability may lead to an increase in symptomatology during the perimenopausal years (stages –2 to –1). As peripheral gonadotropins rise, LH pulsatile patterns become abnormal. There is an increase in pulse frequency, with a decrease in GnRH inhibition by opioids. Despite continuing regular cyclic menstruation, progesterone levels during the early MT are lower than in women of mid-reproductive-age and vary inversely with body mass index. Women in the late MT exhibit impaired folliculogenesis and an increasing incidence of anovulation, compared to mid-reproductive-aged women. Essentially all estradiol in postmenopausal women is derived from peripheral conversion from estrone.

The predominant estrogen in the postmenopausal woman is estrone, with a biologic potency approximately one-third that of estradiol. The circulating levels of estrone (and estrone sulfate) in older women are approximately one-third to one-half of the concentration observed in women of reproductive age (Table 13–6). This is due to estrone production, resulting largely from peripheral aromatization of androstenedione (see earlier). This aromatase activity increases with aging by two- to fourfold and is further amplified by the increased adiposity that typically accompanies the aging process (see earlier). Estrone and estradiol production rates during the postmenopausal years are 40 and 6 μg/d, respectively. This compares with 80 to 500 μg/d for estradiol during the reproductive years.

Androgens

In contrast to estrogens, circulating androgens (DHEAS, androstenedione, and testosterone) decrease less dramatically after physiologic menopause. DHEAS undergoes a linear reduction with aging in both men and women (~2% per year starting at age 30), but there is no specific decline associated with menopause. Changes in DHEAS levels have been associated with alterations in body composition with aging. Androstenedione production

TABLE 13–6 Plasma concentrations of sex steroids in premenopausal and postmenopausal women.

Steroid (concentration)	Premenopausal	Postmenopausal
Estrone (pg/mL)	50->125[a]	30-35
Estrone sulfate (pg/mL)	1000-1800[a]	350
Estradiol (pg/mL)	50->250[a]	10-20
DHEAS (ng/mL)	1-3	0.1-2.7
Testosterone (ng/mL)	<1	<1

[a]Plasma concentration depends on the phase of menstrual cycle.
DHEAS = dehydroepiandrosterone sulfate.

similarly decreases with aging, but the circulating levels are affected less because ovarian secretion is maintained, albeit at a reduced rate (see Table 13–6). Testosterone levels do not vary appreciably during the MT. Testosterone levels decrease after menopause. Historically it was believed the postmenopausal ovary produced a larger percentage of testosterone (50%) than did the premenopausal ovary. However, the literature is conflicting on the origin of androgens in postmenopausal women. The conventional view was that the adrenals, ovaries, and periphery all contributed to circulating androgen levels in postmenopausal women. Contemporary data suggest that androgen production after menopause is largely derived from adrenal precursors. This is supported by studies that have shown that postmenopausal women receiving dexamethasone suppression, or who have endogenous adrenal insufficiency, have undetectable levels of circulating androgens. Investigators have also demonstrated that the postmenopausal ovary has no appreciable enzymatic activities capable of generating sex steroids. The fact that women of reproductive age who undergo a bilateral oophorectomy have less testosterone and androstenedione than menopausal women with intact ovaries challenges this concept. However, the conflict may be explained by the hypothesis that the postmenopausal ovary produces androgens for a limited time.

Hypothalamic/Pituitary

Significant additional information regarding the hormonal changes during the menopausal transition is being developed in the multiethnic, community-based, longitudinal study of perimenopausal women at seven sites throughout the United States, The Study of Women's Health Across the Nation (SWAN). While most attention has been devoted to the role of the ovarian and oocyte decline in the onset of menopause, new evidence suggests potential alterations in the hypothalamic-pituitary feedback system. In evaluating the ability of estradiol to stimulate an effective LH surge, data from SWAN suggest the MT is characterized by three distinct hormonal patterns: (1) estrogen rise with rise in LH but anovulation; (2) estrogen rise without a concomitant rise in LH; or (3) failure of rise in either estradiol or FSH. Additionally, there may be ethnic differences in the sensitivity of the pituitary to negative feedback.

MENOPAUSAL CONSEQUENCES

Given the endocrinologic changes associated with aging, many symptoms appearing in the aging female may be due to estrogen deficiency or diminished androgen or GH secretion. Disorders that are definitely due to estrogen deprivation include vasomotor symptoms and urogenital atrophy. Osteoporosis is also thought to be due largely to estrogen deficiency, and it may be exacerbated by the relative decline in GH levels. The same may be said for the hormone-related increase in the prevalence of atherosclerotic cardiovascular disease and psychosocial symptoms, including insomnia, fatigue, short-term memory changes, and possibly depression. Both DHEAS and GH may impact these phenomena as well. Most women who are symptomatic during the MT present with

frequent or excessive bleeding or with hot flashes and other symptoms of estrogen deficiency. Other common symptoms during the MT include decreased libido, forgetfulness, vaginal dryness, and urinary incontinence.

Mood disorders also are increased during the MT. Community-based surveys have shown that perimenopausal women report significantly more psychological distress and have an increased risk for significant depression, compared with premenopausal or postmenopausal women. In an 8-year longitudinal study of premenopausal women having no prior history of depression, a depressive disorder was more likely to be diagnosed during the MT than in the premenopausal years (OR, 2.5; 95% CI, 1.25-5.02, $p = 0.01$).

Vasomotor Symptoms

Vasomotor symptoms (hot flushes) are experienced with greatest frequency during stages –1 and +1, with about 75% to 85% of women complaining of this symptom. Although 80% of US women have symptoms lasting for at least 1 year, only 25% of women are still symptomatic at 5 years after the final menstrual period. Studies of hot flushes with external monitoring of skin temperature and resistance have shown a frequency of approximately 54 ± 10 minutes. In sleep studies, hot flush frequency has been shown to interrupt rapid eye movement sleep and may contribute to some of the psychosocial complaints. Hot flushes are temporarily correlated with pulses of LH, but exogenous LH does not induce a flush, suggesting that there is some central mediator leading to both the flush and the elevation in LH.

Sleep disturbances, most likely the result of vasomotor activity, also are very common during the MT. In longitudinal studies of perimenopausal women, the prevalence of sleep disturbances has ranged from 32% to 40% in the early MT and from 38% to 46% in the late MT.

Vasomotor symptoms during the MT can be treated with hormone therapy (HT) using estrogen or progestin alone or in combination, neuroactive agents, or other nonhormonal alternatives. Estrogen therapy provides the best treatment for severe vasomotor symptoms, reducing their frequency and severity in 80% to 85% of women over 12 weeks compared with 30% of women receiving placebo. Hormone therapy also may help in the management of depression associated with the MT. In a randomized, placebo-controlled, 12-week trial involving perimenopausal women ages 40 to 55, symptoms of depression were improved in 68% of women receiving unopposed estrogen treatment (0.1 mg transdermal estradiol patch), compared with 20% of those receiving placebo ($p = 0.001$).

Other drugs have been tried in women for whom estrogen is contraindicated, although none have the efficacy associated with ERT. These alternatives include transdermal clonidine, ergot alkaloids, and, more recently, selective serotonin reuptake inhibitors and gabapentin. High-dose progestins may also produce some relief.

Genital Atrophy

The vagina, vulva, urethra, and bladder trigone not only share embryonic proximity but all contain estrogen receptors. Atrophy begins in stage –2 to –1. The most common symptoms include itching and vaginal thinning, with decreased distensibility and reduced secretions, leading to vaginal dryness and pain with intercourse. This and the change in pH with resultant changes in vaginal flora increase the incidence of vaginal and urinary tract infections. Estrogen is the treatment of choice, and treatment must continue for at least 1 to 3 months for symptomatic improvement to be noted. The systemic dosage necessary for vaginal protection is somewhat higher than that needed for bone protection (see later), and local therapy by means of creams or vaginal rings may thus be advisable to limit systemic absorption. It should be noted, however, that vaginal absorption of steroids is quite efficient once estrogenization and revascularization have occurred. If the goal is to limit systemic absorption, slow-release rings may be superior to estrogen creams.

Vaginal estrogen frequently improves symptoms of urinary frequency, dysuria, urgency, and postvoid dribbling. Its direct effect to improve stress incontinence is less clear.

Osteoporosis

Osteoporosis is a condition in which bone loss is sufficient to allow fracture with minimal trauma. Major risk factors for the development of osteoporosis are the peak bone density attained in the late teens and early twenties (stressing the importance of bone building in the young) and the rate of loss (accelerated with estrogen deficiency). Primary or *senile* osteoporosis usually affects women between the ages of 55 and 70 years. The most common sites include the vertebrae and the long bones of the arms and legs. Secondary osteoporosis is caused by a specific disease (such as hyperparathyroidism) or medication usage (such as glucocorticoids) (see Chapter 8).

Menopausal bone loss begins before the final menstrual period during stage –1. Postmenopausal osteoporosis causes over 1.3 million fractures annually in the United States. Most of the more than 250,000 hip fractures are due to primary osteoporosis, and—given that 15% of patients die within a year after a hip fracture and 75% of patients lose their independence—the social costs, not to mention the financial costs, are great.

Bone loss following natural menopause is approximately 1% to 2% per year compared with 3.9% per year following oophorectomy. A woman's genetic background, lifestyle, dietary habits, and coexisting disease also influence the development of osteoporosis. Cigarette smoking, caffeine usage, and alcohol consumption also negatively affect bone loss, whereas weight-bearing activity appears to have a positive influence. See Chapter 8 for a detailed discussion of bone and mineral metabolism and osteoporosis.

A. Osteoporosis treatment

1. **Estrogen therapy**—Estrogen therapy acts via the inhibition of bone resorption. Both BMD and fracture rate are improved with estrogen therapy. However, with cessation of estrogen therapy, there is a rapid and progressive loss of bone mineral content. By 4 years after therapy, bone density is no different from that of patients who were never treated with estrogen. Estrogen is approved for prevention of osteoporosis, and there is also some support for its usage as a treatment modality in established disease. Dosages of 0.625 mg of conjugated estrogens orally daily—and, more recently, as low as 0.3 mg—have been shown to slow bone loss and provide adequate protection against the development of osteoporosis. Higher dosages may be required to treat existing disease.

2. **Alternative therapies for osteoporosis**

   a. **Calcitonin**—Calcitonin is a hormone normally secreted by the thyroid gland. Calcitonin (salmon) is available as a nasal spray specifically developed to decrease local side effects caused by subcutaneous injection. Although few studies have been performed and no data are available regarding reduction in hip fracture, it does seem to be especially beneficial for women with a recent and still painful vertebral fracture. Intranasal calcitonin has also been shown to improve spinal bone density and decrease the vertebral fracture rate in established osteoporosis. The increase in bone density appears to peak in as little as 12 to 18 months. The waning effects of calcitonin therapy over time may be due to downregulation of calcitonin receptors on osteoclasts and/or the development of neutralizing antibodies.

   b. **Bisphosphonates**—These compounds are analogs of pyrophosphates and have a high affinity for hydroxyapatite in bone matrix. The basic structure of bisphosphonates allows a large number of manipulations of the basic molecule, producing different types of bisphosphonates that vary considerably in their potency on bone. In order of increasing potency are pamidronate, alendronate, risedronate, ibandronate, and zoledronic acid.

   Alendronate has been evaluated extensively in patients with osteoporosis. Alendronate has been shown to inhibit markers of bone remodeling and increase BMD at the lumbar spine, hip, and total body and reduces fracture risk. Alendronate is taken orally; the recommended doses are 70 mg once weekly or 10 mg daily; alendronate must be taken according to a strict dosing schedule (in the morning on an empty stomach, with the patient required to remain upright for 30 minutes thereafter). The medication has very poor bioavailability (approximately 1%), and for that reason these instructions must be meticulously obeyed. Alendronate also has a propensity for causing irritation of the esophagus and stomach, especially in women with preexisting esophageal reflux, gastric or duodenal disease. Risedronate is similarly effective in the dosage of 35 mg weekly or 5 mg once daily, and the same dosing regimen is recommended. Ibandronate has the easiest schedule for administration 150 mg once monthly.

   Increases in bone density with alendronate, risedronate, and ibandronate are greater than what is seen with calcitonin and similar to what is seen with HRT. The escape phenomenon seen with calcitonin is not seen with these oral bisphosphonates.

   The final issue concerning long-term administration of bisphosphonates relates to their long half-lives in bone and their incorporation into the bone matrix. Although short-term fracture data appear favorable, the long-term effects of these agents on fracture incidence have never been assessed.

   c. **SERMs**—Raloxifene is the first selective estrogen receptor modulator (SERM) approved for prevention and treatment of osteoporosis and for the prevention of breast cancer. SERMS act selectively as estrogen receptor agonists in some tissues (bone and heart) and antagonists in others (breast and uterus and possibly brain). Data with raloxifene show preservation of BMD, albeit less well than that seen with alendronate, risedronate, ibandronate, or HRT, and spinal fracture data support a protective effect.

It is believed that the differential effects of estrogens and antiestrogens are related to the transcriptional activation of specific estrogen response elements. Two different domains of the estrogen receptor (AF-1 and AF-2) are responsible for this transcriptional activation. Estrogens and antiestrogens appear to act via different domains, leading to their differential effects. Both act to maintain bone density—at least partially—via regulation of the gene for TGF-β.

d. Calcium and vitamin D—These are critical adjuvants for any type of antiresorptive therapy. Decreased ability to absorb calcium among older women is due in part to impaired vitamin D activation and effect. Older women may have limited exposure to sunlight, and their dietary vitamin D intake may be lower than that of younger women.

Daily intakes of 1000 to 1500 mg of calcium and 800 to 1200 IU of vitamin D are probably sufficient to reduce the risk of fragility fractures by 10% or more.

e. Anabolic therapy—The first anabolic therapy for the treatment of severe osteoporosis parathyroid hormone (1-34) or teriparatide has been approved for clinical use. Details about its efficacy and use in advanced postmenopausal osteoporosis are described in Chapter 8.

Atherosclerotic Cardiovascular Disease

Cardiovascular disease is the number one cause of mortality in both men and women in Western societies. This is largely attributed to age and lifestyle. Lifestyle modifications are known to decrease the incidence of atherosclerotic cardiovascular disease. For women, cardiovascular disease is largely a disease of the postmenopause. Women now spend more than a third of their lives in the postmenopausal years, and preventive measures are thus of paramount importance. Although a large body of observational evidence supported a protective effect of ERT on cardiovascular disease, observational data are limited by the confounding variables of patient self-selection. Animal and in vitro studies, as well as assessment of surrogate markers in women, have also shown a positive effect of ERT and HRT against cardiovascular disease development. However, several large randomized, controlled studies have failed to support a protective role for HRT in preventing cardiovascular events.

One of the first such trials was the Heart and Estrogen-Progestin Replacement Study (HERS), a secondary prevention trial that evaluated the use of daily HRT (0.625 mg conjugated estrogens plus 2.5 mg medroxyprogesterone acetate [MPA]) in 2763 postmenopausal women with a mean age of 66.7 years and preexisting vascular disease. The study failed to demonstrate any overall difference in vascular events. This occurred despite improvements in lipid parameters in those patients receiving HRT. The Estrogen Replacement and Atherosclerosis (ERA) Trial compared 3.2 years of treatment with estrogen, combined estrogen and progestin, and placebo in postmenopausal women aged 42 to 80 years. It also failed to demonstrate a significant difference in the rate of progression of coronary atherosclerosis between the three groups. The importance of this study was the inclusion of an estrogen-only arm.

The Women's Health Initiative (WHI) was the first large randomized study to look at primary prevention of cardiovascular disease. This study compared (1) the combination of conjugated equine estrogen (CEE) and MPA with placebo and (2) CEE to placebo. It was designed to assess the overall risks and benefits of HRT in a prospective randomized fashion.

The WHI demonstrated that there was an unacceptable risk profile for the combination HRT arm of the trial. There was an increase in the incidence in breast cancer (an increase of 8 cases per 10,000 women) with no cardiovascular protection (and potentially increased cardiovascular risk). There was, in fact, an increase in venous thromboembolism, strokes, and coronary heart disease. The risk of stroke and thromboembolism continued for the 5 years of study, whereas most of the coronary heart disease was limited to the first year of treatment. There were, however, documented decreases in the risk of fracture and colon cancer.

In the CEE-only arm, there was an increased risk of stroke and a decreased risk in hip fractures compared to placebo. This study showed that the use of ERT had no protective effect on coronary heart disease. Interestingly, there appeared to be a trend toward a reduction in breast cancer (0.77, CI 0.59-1.01) with use of ERT. More recent studies and reevaluation of large datasets have suggested that combined estrogen/progestin has a more profound increased risk on breast cancer, than estrogen alone or cyclic progestins, consistent with increase in mitogenic activity of the breast during the normal luteal phase when progesterone levels are high.

Treatment—Summary

As noted earlier, long-term use of HT in older menopausal women has been associated with increased risks for venous thromboembolism, coronary events, stroke, and breast cancer. Although short-term treatment of symptomatic women during the MT likely poses significantly fewer risks, HT generally should be used in the lowest effective dose and for the shortest time required. Data suggest the use of HT does not increase the risk of breast cancer, on a yearly basis, more than would continuing spontaneous cycles for any given age. This suggests treatment of symptomatic women in their forties may not increase breast cancer risk over normal cycling. Low-dose estrogen regimens (conjugated equine estrogens, 0.3 mg daily, or its equivalent) can achieve as much as a 75% reduction in vasomotor symptoms over 12 weeks, approaching the efficacy of standard-dose HT regimens, and may be associated with fewer risks and side-effects. The decision to use HT should be made only after first carefully reviewing its risks and benefits for the individual.

The relative safety of HT during the MT has not been thoroughly investigated. The results of one observational study have suggested that women who start HT near menopause had a decreased risk of coronary heart disease when taking estrogen alone (relative risk [RR] = 0.66; 95% CI, 0.54-0.80) or in combination with progestin (RR = 0.72; 95% CI, 0.56-0.92). A secondary analysis conducted by the investigators involved in the WHI revealed that risk for coronary heart disease was not significantly increased in women under age 60 years of age or within 10 years of menopause. Further studies to evaluate the safety and efficacy of HT during the MT and the early post-menopausal years are ongoing.

Concerns about the risks of HT have increased interest in non-hormonal alternatives for the treatment of symptoms in the MT. In some women, vasomotor symptoms during the MT can be reduced by wearing layered clothing, avoiding caffeine and alcohol, and by keeping the ambient temperature a few degrees cooler. Herbal treatments such as black cohosh (Remifemin Menopause; Enzymatic Therapy, Green Bay, WI) have been shown to have marginal or no benefit in placebo controlled trials. Neuroactive agents, including selective serotonin reuptake inhibitors (SSRIs), serotonin-norepinephrine reuptake inhibitors (SNRIs), alpha adrenergic agents, and others all have some efficacy in the treatment of vasomotor symptoms (Table 13–7). Both SSRIs and SNRIs may be effective because norepinephrine and serotonin appear to be involved in the hypothalamic regulation of temperature homeostasis and to play a role in the development of hot flashes. Randomized placebo-controlled trials have shown that SSRIs (citalopram, sertraline, paroxetine) and SNRIs (venlafaxine) can help to reduce the severity and frequency of hot flushes. Clonidine (an alpha adrenergic agonist) and gabapentin also have some efficacy. Gabapentin is the only agent compared head-to-head with estrogen suggesting equivalent efficacy when used in high doses.

The WHI study did not address the effect of hormone treatment on hot flushes and vaginal atrophy. Clearly, there are alternatives for the treatment of osteoporosis and cardiovascular disease that are superior if prevention of both conditions is the sole reason for HRT. Every woman should discuss with her caregiver the optimal management for her as an individual. This should take into account medical and family history as well as symptomatology. It can be uniformly recommended, however, that menopausal women maintain appropriate nutrition, weight reduction, and exercise along with moderation in alcohol and caffeine intake and cessation of smoking.

INFERTILITY

Infertility is defined as the inability of a couple to conceive after 1 year of frequent unprotected intercourse without contraception. This definition is based on observational data showing that approximately 85% of couples achieve pregnancy after 1 year of unprotected coitus. Using this definition, approximately 15% of reproductive-age couples experience infertility. However, the diagnosis of infertility does not mean that they cannot conceive—a more precise diagnosis term would be **subfertility**, or a diminished capacity to conceive. The actual probability of the fertility potential of a population may be better assessed with variables that can quantify a monthly cycle rate. The concepts that have been used for quantitative analysis are **fecundability** and **fecundity**. Fecundability is defined as the probability of achieving a pregnancy within one menstrual cycle, and in normal couples the chance of conception after 1 month is approximately 25%. Fecundity is a related concept that is defined as the ability to achieve a live birth within one menstrual cycle.

In the United States, demands for infertility treatment have dramatically increased. The 1995 National Survey of Family Growth reported that 9.3 million women received infertility treatment in their lifetime compared with 6.8 million in 1988. This rise in treatment is due not only to increased public awareness—it also reflects the significant demographic, societal, and economic changes in our society. These include the aging of the baby boom generation, which has increased the size of the reproductive-age population. Perhaps more important is the increased use of contraception and postponement of childbearing until the last two decades of a woman's reproductive life. Approximately 20% of women in the United States now have their first child after 35 years of age.

Age alone has a significant impact on fertility and affects a woman many years before the onset of menopause. One factor is the age-dependent loss of ovarian follicles (see later). A 38-year-old woman has 25% of the fecundability of a woman under 30 years of age. Another age-related subfertility factor is that the spontaneous abortion rate increases with advancing age. The overall incidence of clinical abortion increases from 10% in women under age 30 to more than 40% in women over 40. The increased pregnancy loss can be largely attributed to abnormalities in the aging oocyte; older follicles have an increased rate of meiotic dysfunction, resulting in higher rates of chromosomal abnormalities.

The main causes of female subfertility can be classified in the following way: (1) ovulatory defects, (2) pelvic disorders, and (3) male factors. These factors account for 80% to 85% of couples diagnosed with infertility. They are not mutually exclusive—about 15% of couples have more than one cause of subfertility. In approximately 20% of couples, the cause remains unknown and is classified as unexplained infertility. This section will briefly discuss the causes of subfertility and review the diagnosis and management.

DIAGNOSIS OF INFERTILITY

Ovulatory Defects

Ovulatory disorders are responsible for 25% of cases of infertility. Ovulatory status can be obtained from the history. If a woman experiences cyclic, predictable menses at monthly intervals, ovulation can be predicted 98% of the time. This is not an invariable rule, however, and irregular menstrual cycles are not a sure sign of anovulation.

TABLE 13-7 Treatment for hot flashes.

Drug	Name	Dose (mg/day)
SSRI	Citalopram	10-20
	Fluoxetine	10-20
	Sertraline	25-50
	Paroxetine	10-20
SNRI	Venlafaxine	37.5-150
	Desvenlafaxine	50-100
Alpha adrenergic agents	Clonidine	0.1
Gamma aminobutyric acid	Gabapentin	300-900

The only way to confirm ovulation is by achieving pregnancy. However, a variety of methods can indicate that ovulation has occurred. For example, a thermal shift occurs around the time of ovulation. Prior to ovulation, morning basal body temperature (BBT) is below 98°F (36.7°C), and after ovulation the temperature increases at least 0.4°F (0.2°C) for at least 1 to 3 days. This rise in temperature reflects the progesterone that is secreted from the corpus luteum, which consequently raises the hypothalamic set point for BBT. The temperature rise occurs approximately 2 days after ovulation because of the time and dose required for the progesterone effect at the hypothalamus. BBT can therefore not be utilized to prospectively predict ovulation. Measurements of midluteal serum progesterone concentration can also be performed to document the occurrence of ovulation. If this level is greater than 3 µg/L (9.5 nmol/L), it is a strong indication that ovulation has occurred. An endometrial biopsy can confirm ovulation. It is performed during the luteal phase and gives a qualitative assessment of ovulation, because the duration of progesterone exposure produces predictable endometrial histology. Lastly, a sonographic examination documenting a decrease in follicle size—or disappearance altogether of the previously developed follicle—is suggestive of ovulation. All of these methods indicate that ovulation has occurred.

There are only a few ways to predict that ovulation is going to occur. The most common way is to detect the LH surge. Ovulation typically occurs 34 to 36 hours after the onset of the LH surge.

Although ovulation may occur, some women may have a luteal-phase defect. This is characterized by an inadequate quantity or duration of progesterone secretion by the corpus luteum. There is a distinct window of time for implantation. The theory is that the progesterone deficiency desynchronizes ovulation (egg) and implantation (endometrium). However, the incidence of luteal phase defects is difficult to assess because the definition is not standardized. Typically, the diagnosis is established by luteal phase endometrial dating; if the histologic development of the endometrium lags more than 2 days beyond the day of the cycle, it is diagnostic of a luteal phase defect. However, up to 30% of women with normal cycles meet this criterion. Another method involves measuring midluteal progesterone levels. If progesterone is less than 10 ng/mL, it suggests a luteal phase defect. This is not reliable because progesterone is intermittently secreted, and the serum progesterone level can change from 1 hour to the next in the same individual. Furthermore, the lack of properly validated tests places the existence of luteal phase defects and their association with subfertility in question. Lastly, as empiric treatment for unexplained infertility has developed, delaying treatment (see later: superovulation with IUI) for exact diagnoses has less importance. More sophisticated testing of endometrial proteins required for implantation (eg, integrins, glycodelin) may revive enthusiasm for making a specific diagnosis in the future.

The cause of ovulatory dysfunction has been previously discussed. All anovulatory patients should have determination of PRL and TSH levels—and, if necessary, androgen levels—to identify the cause of the ovulatory disturbance. Treatment should be directed toward the cause, which is discussed in greater detail later. It could be argued that all patients should have evaluation of early follicular cycle (days 2-4) FSH, LH, and estradiol to assess ovarian reserve (age).

Pelvic Disorders

Pelvic disorders account for more than 30% of couples with the diagnosis of infertility. Uterine tube damage and adhesion formation are responsible for most pelvic pathologic processes causing infertility, whereas endometriosis is the primary pelvic disorder causing subfertility. The causes of tubal damage and adhesions include postinfectious state (pelvic inflammatory disease [PID]), endometriosis, and a history of pelvic surgery (especially surgery for ruptured appendicitis).

PID is defined as infection of upper genital tract structures and is usually caused by a sexually transmitted disease. The known initiating organisms are chlamydiae and *Neisseria gonorrhoeae*. The symptoms are variable but usually include lower abdominal pain, nausea, and vaginal discharge. However, in up to 30% of chlamydial infections, PID may be clinically inapparent and may remain undiagnosed until presenting with subfertility.

Endometriosis is the presence of endometrial glands and stroma outside of the uterus. There may be no manifestations other than infertility, or symptoms may progress to include severe pelvic pain, dysmenorrhea, and dyspareunia. The diagnosis is suspected if findings on surgical exploration show characteristic lesions. Lesions can be staged according to published criteria. Diagnosis is confirmed with biopsy of the peritoneal lesions. The disease occurs in approximately 3% to 10% of reproductive-age women and may be responsible for up to 25% to 35% of the female factors responsible for subfertility.

The pathogenesis of endometriosis is not completely known. A prominent theory (Sampson) involves retrograde menstruation. It is well established that menses can flow through the uterine tubes into the abdominal cavity. In fact, this phenomenon is thought to occur in almost all menstruating women. There is good evidence that the endometrial tissue subsequently invades and proliferates into the peritoneum. It is theorized that the immune system should normally dispose of the tissue and that altered immunity may result in implantation of this endometrial tissue outside the uterus in those women who subsequently develop endometriosis.

There is a strong association between adhesive disease and endometriosis. In these cases, the cause of subfertility is a result of distorted anatomy and consequently altered function. However, in mild cases of endometriosis, where only peritoneal lesions are identified and no anatomic distortion exists, the cause of infertility remains uncertain and controversial. There is evidence that the peritoneal fluid is altered in the presence of endometrial tissue with increased macrophages and inflammatory mediators. Several studies suggest that inflammatory changes result in adverse effects on folliculogenesis, ovum transport, fertilization, and implantation.

Tubal damage can be diagnosed with a hysterosalpingogram or surgical exploration. Hysterosalpingography involves the introduction of radiopaque contrast media into the pelvis through the cervix and then fluoroscopy, revealing an outline of contrast in the uterine cavity, uterine tubes, and peritoneal cavity. The diagnosis of pelvic endometriosis can only be made by surgery, and most often the surgical procedure is laparoscopy. Diagnostic laparoscopy is usually done when there is a high suspicion of endometriosis based on the clinical history or adhesive disease based on a history of PID or pelvic surgery. Laparoscopy may also be performed, if all other tests are normal and the couple continues not to achieve a pregnancy.

Male Factor Causes

The male factor contributes in 40% to 50% of cases of diagnosed infertility, and all evaluations should include the male partner. The diagnostic test for male factor infertility is the semen analysis. Although this is a largely descriptive test (volume, sperm count, motility, and morphology), there is some correlation with pregnancy outcome. This should be used solely as a screening test. To understand the pathophysiology of male factors, it is important to review the physiology of spermatogenesis and the anatomy of the male reproductive tract as described in Chapter 12.

Unexplained Infertility

Approximately 15% to 20% of the couples diagnosed with infertility have no identifiable cause after a full investigation. The workup should include documentation of ovulation (regular menstrual cycles, progesterone levels, or LH testing), hysterosalpingography to verify patent fallopian tubes, and a semen analysis. The term *unexplained* implies that there is a potential explanation for the subfertility, but the cause has yet to be identified. The cause may be subtle abnormalities in folliculogenesis, sperm-ovum interactions, or defective implantation.

Several studies have evaluated the natural history of unexplained infertility. It is estimated that fecundity in younger couples (female partner under the age of 40) with unexplained infertility is 3% to 5% compared with 20% to 25% in the age-matched couples with normal fertility. Treatment involves methods that increase fecundability and are discussed later.

MANAGEMENT OF THE INFERTILE COUPLE

It is important to remember that in most couples, there is a chance for spontaneous conception. Recent studies estimate that the average probability for live birth without treatment is 25% to 40% during the 3 years after the first infertility consultation. This translates into a cycle fecundity rate of 0.7% to 1% per month. The presence of endometriosis, abnormal sperm, or tubal disease independently reduces the chance of spontaneous pregnancy and live birth by approximately 50% for each variable. Infertility for more than 3 years, female age over 30 years, and primary infertility were important negative prognostic factors.

Evaluation should focus on known causes of infertility or subfertility: ovulatory defects, pelvic disorders (tubal disease, endometriosis), and male factor issues.

Ovulatory Disorders

Treatment should be diagnosis-specific, if possible. For the female, this means that the cause of any ovulatory defect should be determined and specific treatment then instituted. This enhances outcome and decreases the risk of complications (spontaneous abortion and multiple gestation). This treatment may include the use of dopamine agonists (hyperprolactinemia), thyroid replacement (hypothyroidism), pulsatile GnRH (hypogonadotropic hypogonadism), or clomiphene citrate (for PCOS). The most common cause of anovulation is inappropriate feedback such as in PCOS. Ovulation in patients with PCOS can be induced with clomiphene citrate, a nonsteroidal agonist-antagonist of estrogen that blocks the hypothalamic-pituitary axis from feedback by circulating estrogens. As a result, there is increased gonadotropin release to stimulate follicular recruitment and ovulation. In addition, because PCOS is associated with insulin resistance, and elevated insulin directly has an impact on the ovary, insulin sensitizers such as metformin have been used to enhance ovulatory response in women with PCOS. Recently, a large multicenter randomized trial compared clomiphene to metformin and found clomiphene to be significantly more effective for ovulation induction and achieving a live birth.

Pelvic Disorders

In general, adhesive tubal lesions should be treated surgically. The location and extent of disease should, however, be evaluated. Patients with distal tubal occlusion—unless it is very mild—are most often better served by assisted reproduction (in vitro fertilization [IVF]). Other possible causes of infertility should also be examined. If a patient has a history of documented tubal disease, in addition to other abnormalities (ovulatory dysfunction or male factor infertility), or if they are over 35, the likelihood for successful surgical management decreases by approximately 50%, and consideration for avoiding surgery and moving directly to assisted reproduction is paramount. The exception to this rule is documentation of hydrosalpinges on ultrasound. The presence of hydrosalpinges that retain fluid when nondistended (ie, not seen only with hysterosalpingography) leads to a significant reduction in outcome with assisted reproductive therapy (ART). Prior removal or proximal occlusion of the tube to prevent contamination of the uterine cavity should be performed before ART is offered.

There are conflicting data in the literature concerning the appropriate treatment for mild endometriosis. A well-designed randomized trial from Canada evaluated the effect of surgical treatment on pregnancy outcome for patients diagnosed with mild endometriosis without anatomic distortion. It showed that pregnancy rates at 9 months postlaparoscopy were 27% in the surgically treated group compared with 18% in the untreated group. Severe endometriosis (disease that alters the pelvic anatomy or involves the ovary with endometriomas) should be surgically treated to restore normal pelvic anatomy. There appears to be no advantage to medical therapy for endometriosis in women seeking fertility.

Male Factor Infertility

Male factor infertility is discussed in Chapter 12. Like female partner treatment, therapy should be targeted, if possible, toward the cause of subfertility. Obstructive disease may be treated surgically. A prominent varicocele with a stress pattern on semen analysis (decreased motility with an increase in abnormal morphology) may suggest a need for surgical repair. Any endocrinologic abnormalities (while less common in the male) should be treated (eg, prolactinoma). Unfortunately, beyond this point, most treatments require a combined approach very similar to that discussed below for unexplained infertility.

Unexplained Infertility

The treatment of unexplained infertility can be frustrating for the physician and the patients because the recommendations for therapy are not targeted toward a specific diagnosis. Although there are very limited evidence-based data to guide treatment, therapy should be directed toward increasing the fecundability rate. The two main treatments are superovulation plus intrauterine insemination (IUI) and IVF.

Superovulation methods are designed to qualitatively improve the cycle and to hyperstimulate the ovary with rescue of more follicles (quantitative improvement). Administration of clomiphene citrate or of gonadotropins alone can be used for superovulation. However, higher success rates are observed when superovulation is combined with IUI of washed sperm (Table 13–8). IVF provides a higher fecundability rate. However, these procedures are significantly more costly and more invasive, and they should only be used after a trial (three or four cycles) of superovulation and IUI has failed. With older patients, aggressive therapy should be considered earlier in the treatment effort.

CONTRACEPTION

Approximately 50% of all pregnancies in the United States are unplanned. In adolescents and in women of older reproductive age, the unplanned pregnancy rate is higher, approaching 82% and 77%, respectively. This equates to 3.5 million unplanned pregnancies in the United States per year. The advent of oral contraceptives has meant that women have been able to postpone childbearing. However, approximately 50% of unplanned pregnancies are due to contraceptive failures. Possible causes of failure include lack of education, poor compliance, and side-effect profiles. In this section, we discuss the different methods of hormonal contraception. We shall discuss also the target population for the various modalities of contraception and their mechanisms, side-effects, and ways to decrease failure rates. At the end of the section, emergency contraception will be discussed briefly.

ORAL CONTRACEPTIVES

Combination Pills

In the United States, oral contraceptive pills are the most widely used method for contraception. There are two types of oral contraception: combination pills and progestin-only pills. The various hormones used in birth control pills are illustrated in Figure 13–17.

The development of oral contraceptive agents began with the isolation of progesterone. However, progesterone was very expensive and difficult to isolate. Ethisterone, a derivative of an androgen, was found to have progestin activity and was much easier to isolate than progesterone. With removal of carbon 19, the progestational activity was increased, and the new compound was termed norethindrone. When this hormone was administered to women, ovulation was inhibited. During the process of norethindrone purification, an estrogen contaminant was found. When this contaminant was removed, women would experience breakthrough bleeding. The estrogen was added back, thereby creating the first-generation combination birth control pill, which was approved by the Food and Drug Administration (FDA) in 1960.

Oral contraceptives can be divided into generations based on dose and type of hormone. The first-generation birth control pills contained more than 50 µg of ethinyl estradiol or mestranol and a progestin. The adverse events associated with high-dose estrogen, such as coronary thrombosis, led to development of the second-generation pill, which contained less than 50 µg of

TABLE 13–8 Pregnancy rates after treatment for unexplained infertility. Aggregate data for each treatment.

Treatment	No. of Studies	No. (%) of Pregnancies per Initiated Cycle	Percent of Quality-Adjusted Pregnancies per Initiated Cycle
Control groups	11	64/3,539 (1.8)	1.3
Control groups, randomized studies	6	23/597 (3.8)	4.1
IUI	9	15/378 (4)	3.8
Clomiphene citrate	3	37/617 (6)	5.6
Clomiphene citrate + IUI	5	21/315 (6.7)	8.3
hMG	13	139/1806 (7.7)	7.7
hMG + IUI	14	207/1133 (18)	17.1
IVF	9	378/683 (22.5)	20.7
GIFT	9	158/607 (26.0)	27.0

Reproduced, with permission, from Guzick DS, et al. Efficacy of treatment of unexplained infertility. *Fertil Steril.* 1998;70:207.
GIFT, gamete intrafollicular transfer; hMG, human menopausal gonadotrophin; IVF, in vitro fertilization; IUI, intrauterine insemination.

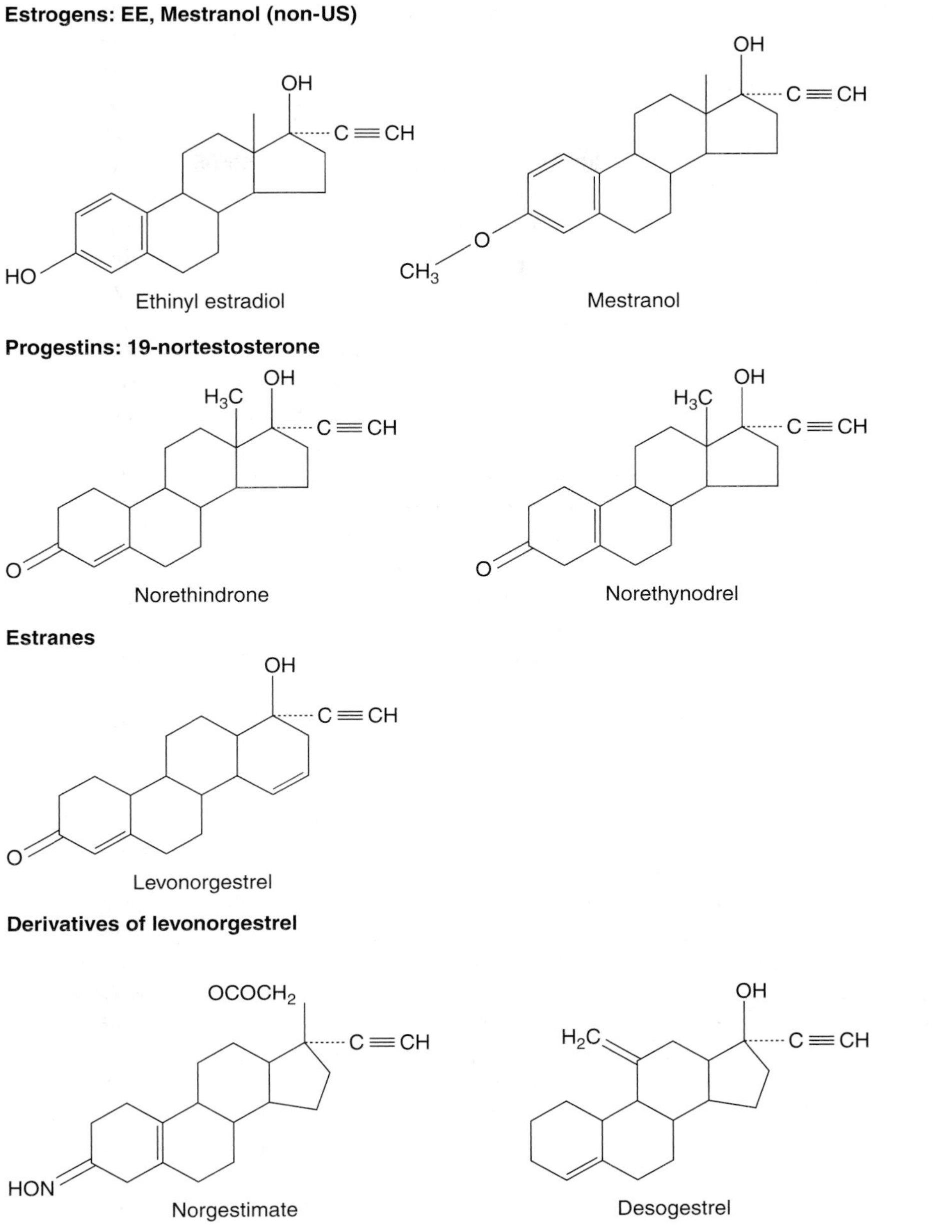

Estrogens: EE, Mestranol (non-US)

Ethinyl estradiol

Mestranol

Progestins: 19-nortestosterone

Norethindrone

Norethynodrel

Estranes

Levonorgestrel

Derivatives of levonorgestrel

Norgestimate

Desogestrel

FIGURE 13–17 Oral contraceptive pill hormonal components. All except endogenous hormones are synthetic steroids.

ethinyl estradiol and progestins other than levonorgestrel derivatives. Next, attention was directed toward the progestin, which was thought to have adverse androgenic effects such as affecting lipid profiles and glucose tolerance. This led to the development of third-generation pills that contained both a lower dose of estrogen (20-30 μg of ethinyl estradiol) and newer progestins (gonanes: desogestrel or norgestimate). Indeed, studies have demonstrated a reduction in metabolic changes associated with these progestins, but limited data are available to show any actual reduction of cardiovascular events. Another recently developed progestin, drospirenone, has antimineralocorticoid and antiandrogenic activity in addition to its pharmacologic

progestational effects. As an analog of spironolactone rather than androgen, it competitively binds to aldosterone receptors, and it may counteract the estrogen stimulation of the renin-angiotensin system, resulting in more weight stability and less water retention. A new combination oral contraceptive, Yasmin, which contains 3 mg drospirenone and 30 μg ethinyl estradiol, has been approved by the FDA and is prescribed for women with hyperandrogenism or other side-effects attributable to oral contraceptives. However, the relative antiandrogenic activity of drospirenone is small compared with cyproterone acetate or the therapeutic dose of spironolactone used for the treatment of hirsutism.

Pregnanes

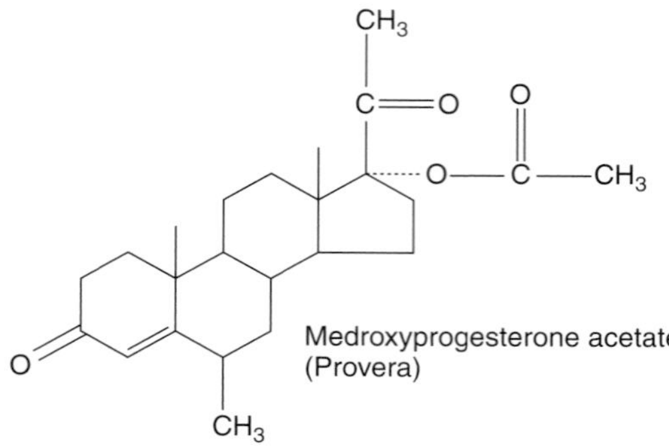

Medroxyprogesterone acetate
(Provera)

Endogenous hormones

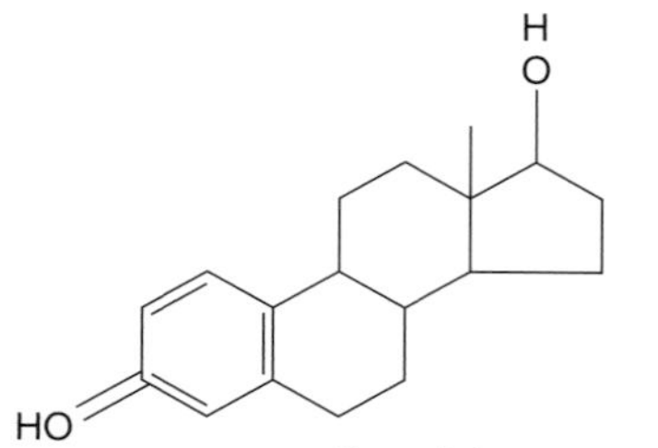

Estradiol

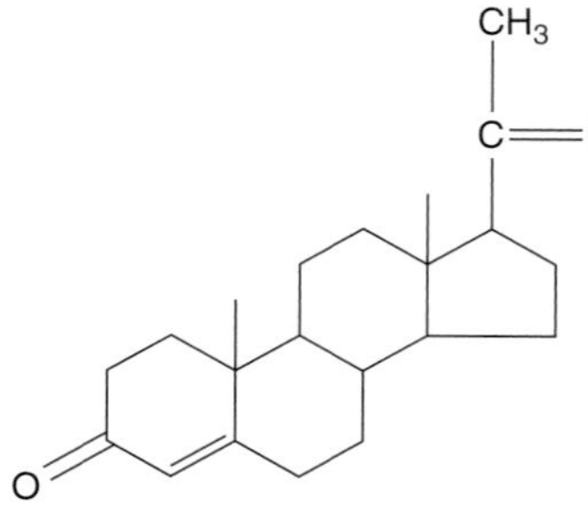

Progesterone

FIGURE 13–17 (*continued*)

Contraceptives can be classified also based on formulas or schedules of administration. The theory behind phasic preparations was to further decrease the amount of total progestin administered in an attempt to reduce metabolic changes attributed to the progestin, thereby decreasing adverse effects. The traditional monophasic pill (eg, Loestrin) contains 30 µg of ethinyl estradiol and 1.5 mg of norethindrone. This dose is given every day for 3 weeks with a 1-week hormone-free interval. The progestin dose remains constant throughout the cycle. The second type is the biphasic pill (eg, Ortho-Novum 10/11), which contains 35 µg of ethinyl estradiol and either 0.5 or 1 mg of norethindrone. The 0.5 mg of norethindrone is administered in the first 10 days of the month, and the 1 mg is administered for the following 11 days. The last 7 days of the cycle are free of hormone. With this combination, there was a theoretical increase in breakthrough bleeding and an increased pregnancy rate. A meta-analysis revealed no difference, but limited data were available.

Because of concerns that this regimen might result in both breakthrough bleeding and pregnancies, another phasic formulation was developed. The triphasic pills (eg, Triphasil, Ortho-Novum 7/7/7) contain 0.5, 0.75, and 1 mg norethindrone combined with 35 µg ethinyl estradiol. Theoretically, this formulation improves cycle control. There are several other regimens, some of which alter estrogen doses to simulate the estrogen cyclic rhythm (Triphasil-30, Triphasil-40, Triphasil-30 µg ethinyl estradiol) and possibly decrease breakthrough bleeding. A meta-analysis comparing biphasic versus triphasic pills revealed that triphasic pills significantly improved cycle control. However, the progestins in each pill tested were different, and this could account for better cycle control rather than the phasic formulation. An additional meta-analysis was performed on triphasic versus monophasic pills to assess cycle control and metabolic effects. This analysis revealed no difference between the formulations. Therefore, there is little scientific rationale for prescribing phasic preparations in preference to the monophasic pill.

The pharmacologic activity of progestins is based on the progestational activity and bioavailability of each progestin as well as the dose. The relative potencies of the different progestins are levonorgestrel greater than norgestrel greater than norethindrone. The active estrogen component of oral contraceptives is ethinyl estradiol (even if mestranol is administered).

When the hormones are administered for 21 days of the cycle, there is enough progestin to inhibit rapid follicle growth for about 7 more days. Figure 13–18 demonstrates that during the steroid-free interval there is no rise in estrogen, indicating no follicular maturation. It is likely that pills missed after this time are responsible for some of the unintended pregnancies. Therefore, it is important that this interval not be extended.

Pharmacologic doses of progestin inhibit ovulation by suppressing GnRH pulsatility and possibly inhibiting release of pituitary LH. Progestins also impair implantation and produce thick, scanty cervical mucus that retards sperm penetration. These latter methods play a minor role in the mechanism of oral contraception.

Ethinyl estradiol helps prevent the selection of a dominant follicle by suppressing pituitary FSH. In addition to FSH suppression, ethinyl estradiol provides stability to the endometrium,

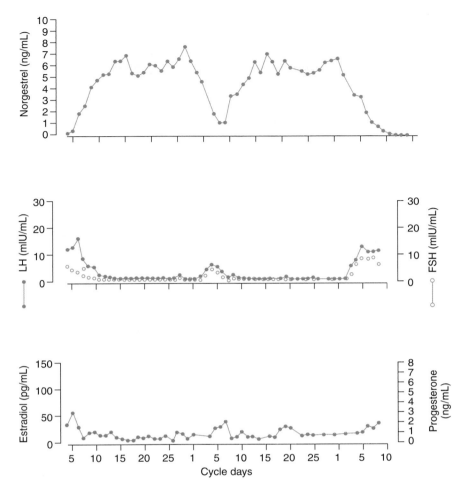

FIGURE 13–18 Progestin effects on steroidogenesis and ovulation. (Reproduced, with permission, from Brenner PF, et al. Serum levels of d-norgestrel, luteinizing hormone, follicle-stimulating hormone, estradiol and progesterone in women during and following ingestion of combination oral contraceptives containing dl-norgestrel. *Am J Obstet Gynecol.* 1997;129:133.)

decreasing breakthrough bleeding. It also upregulates the progesterone receptor and decreases clearance, thereby potentiating the activity of the progestin.

Traditionally, a pill is administered daily for 3 weeks out of 4, preferably at the same time each day (more critical with progestin-only pills). This regimen was designed to mimic the menstrual cycle with monthly withdrawal bleeding. The conventional start date is on the first Sunday after menses (first day of menses for triphasics). An alternative method is to start at the time of the clinic visit, regardless of the day of the menstrual cycle, with a backup method for 7 days (*Quick-Start*). This method has the advantage of immediate contraception without adverse bleeding events. In addition, with the Quick-Start method, women are more likely to start the second pack of oral contraceptives, suggesting increased compliance. During the 28-day regimen, there is a 1-week steroid-free interval. If the steroid-free interval is prolonged beyond the 7-day window, ovulation is possible. Therefore, this is a critical time not to neglect taking pills. On the other hand, a woman may continue to take the hormone pills and skip the steroid-free interval to avoid monthly bleeding.

A randomized trial comparing continuous oral contraception with the traditional cyclic method revealed a significantly greater incidence of erratic bleeding with (overall) the same number of days of bleeding, albeit with a reduced volume of bleeding. New formulations have been developed for those who do not desire cyclic bleeding. This regimen involves 84 days of continuous hormone administration followed by a steroid-free interval of 1 week. This can easily be done with the traditionally packaged oral contraceptive pills.

A routine for daily administration improves compliance and contraceptive efficacy. Failure to take the pill at the same time every day and not understanding the package insert are associated with missing two or more pills during the cycle. To decrease failure rates, women should understand that if they forget to take the pill, they must use barrier prophylaxis.

Postpartum women who are not breast-feeding may begin combination oral contraceptives 3 weeks after delivery. For women who are breast-feeding, it is advised that institution of combination oral contraceptives be delayed until 3 months postpartum. The recommendation for this delay is due to decreased milk letdown secondary to estrogen but may be waived once lactation is well established.

Noncompliance increases the incidence of unwanted pregnancies. Appropriate use of birth control is achieved 32% to 85% of the time in the general population. Teenagers have at most a 50% continuation rate, and 25% of pill users discontinue the practice in the first year. The efficacy of the oral contraceptive under conditions of perfect use is 0.1 failures per 100 woman-years (0.1 per 100 users). With typical use, the failure rate is 3%, with first-year failure rates approaching 7.3% to 8.5%. Side-effects contribute to noncompliance. The most common side-effect is breakthrough bleeding. Other unwanted symptoms include bloating, breast tenderness, nausea, and possibly headaches, weight gain, and depression. Some studies suggest that altering estrogen doses may improve symptoms. Failure rates may also be associated with concomitant use of drugs (eg, rifampin, hydantoins) that accelerate hormone metabolism.

A. Other benefits

There are noncontraceptive benefits to the pill. These include reduced monthly blood loss (less iron deficiency) and less dysmenorrhea as well as reduced benign breast disease and mastalgia. Oral contraceptives also reduce the incidence of PID and ectopic pregnancies. Other significant benefits include a reduction in risk of ovarian cancer, endometrial cancer, and colorectal cancer. Oral contraceptive use also has cosmetic benefits; it can improve excess hair growth and acne (see PCOS). It is not unusual for the pill to be administered for noncontraceptive problems.

B. Potential risks

In general, oral contraceptives have proved to be safe for most women, but the possibility of adverse effects has received much attention. Unfortunately, the literature is full of conflicting reports. Data concerning controversial adverse effects will be discussed in the following section.

Although the estrogen in combination oral contraceptives tends to increase triglycerides and total cholesterol, these levels are still within the normal range, and the contraceptives appear to increase HDL and decrease LDL. Progestins attenuate these effects, which suggest an adverse metabolic milieu. Although it is known that low HDL-LDL ratios are associated with cardiovascular events, the importance of lipid changes associated with birth control pills is unknown. To date there is no strong evidence of an increased incidence of myocardial infarctions in healthy nonsmoking oral contraceptive users. In patients with other cardiovascular risk factors such as hypertension—at least in Europe—there is an up to 12-fold increased risk of cardiovascular events. Women who are over 35 years of age and who smoke are at increased risk of cardiovascular events. This risk is amplified with use of the birth control pills. If more than 15 cigarettes per day are smoked, there is a relative risk (RR) of 3.3 for a cardiovascular event, compared with an RR of 20.8 with concomitant use of oral contraceptives. However, if a woman smokes fewer than 15 cigarettes per day, there is an RR of 2.0 for a cardiovascular event, compared with an RR of 3.5 with concomitant contraceptive use. Former smokers after 1 year have no significant increased risk. First-generation oral contraceptives (>50 μg ethinyl estradiol) imposed an RR for stroke (ischemic or

hemorrhagic) of 5.8. With low-dose agents (<50 μg ethinyl estradiol), there appears to be no significant increased risk of stroke among healthy normotensive nonsmoking women. The RR associated with hemorrhagic stroke for hypertensive women is 10.2 to 14.2. Because the potential exists for adverse outcomes, women taking oral contraceptives should be screened regularly for cardiovascular risk factors to ensure safe administration.

The risk of deep vein thrombosis and pulmonary embolism is increased twofold to threefold with administration of the pill. The mechanism by which oral contraceptives enhance venous thrombosis is unknown, but there may be estrogen-related changes in coagulation parameters. These include increased clotting factors and activation of platelets and a decrease in protein S and fibrinolytic activity. However, these changes in measured serum clotting factors do not predict the occurrence of deep vein thrombosis. Genetic thrombophilias increase the risk of venous thrombosis. The prevalence of factor V Leiden in the general population is 5%. The incidence of deep vein thrombosis among this population is 60 per 100,000 per year, and with use of oral contraceptives, the incidence approaches 280 to 300 per 100,000 per year. The baseline incidence of deep vein thrombosis in women is approximately 3 per 100,000 per year, and with current oral contraceptive uses it is 9.6 to 21.1 per 100,000 per year. For comparison, during pregnancy, the incidence of deep vein thrombosis is 60 per 100,000 per year. Older age (>40-44) increases the incidence two- to three-fold but does not affect the RR. There is no evidence that smoking has an effect on the incidence of deep vein thrombosis with oral contraceptive use. At this time, universal screening for thrombophilias is not cost effective. However, any history of deep vein thrombosis warrants a workup for thrombophilia.

The association of oral contraceptives and cancer risk has been evaluated for breast, cervical, and liver cancer. Observational studies investigating a possible association between oral contraceptive use and breast cancer have reported conflicting results. The most recent information is that oral contraceptive usage (current or past use) has no impact on the incidence of breast cancer—RR 1.0 (CI 95% 0.8-1.3)—among women 35 to 64 years of age. Several observational studies have linked oral contraceptive use with invasive cervical cancer, although it is not clear if this association is causally related. A recent study investigating the association between oral contraception use and cervical cancer revealed a nearly threefold increased risk among human papillomavirus carriers with 5 to 9 years of oral contraceptive use (RR 2.82; 95% CI 1.46-5.42). This evidence suggests that women taking oral contraceptives should be screened yearly with Pap smears to prevent cervical cancer. In the 1980s, there was an association between hepatocellular carcinoma in women under 50 years of age and oral contraceptive use. With further investigation there appears to be no increased risk of hepatic cancer with the use of oral contraceptives.

After discontinuation of oral contraceptives, the activity of the HPO axis gradually returns to a precontraceptive state. After a 2- to 4-week prolongation of the follicular phase, the LH peak is observed, which suggests that the suppressive effects of the oral contraceptive have dissipated and that cyclic menses will resume.

Contraindications to oral contraceptive administration are summarized in Table 13–9.

TABLE 13–9 Contraindications to combination oral contraceptive use.

Pregnancy
History of thromboembolic disease
Smoking and age ≥ 35 y
Hepatoma
Breast cancer
Endometrial cancer
History of cerebrovascular or cardiovascular disease
Undiagnosed vaginal bleeding
First-degree relative with history of thromboembolic disease
Uncontrolled hypertension

Progestin Only

Progestin-only pills (Ortho Micronor, Nor-QD, 0.35 mg norethindrone; Ovrette, 0.075 mg levonorgestrel) are also available for contraception. The target population for administration of progestin-only contraception includes women with contraindications to estrogen, breast-feeding mothers, and older women.

The circulating levels of progestin following ingestion of progestin-only pills (minipill) are 25% to 50% of that following ingestion of estrogen-progestin oral contraceptive pills. Serum levels that peak 2 hours after administration are followed by rapid elimination (Figure 13–19). The peak levels of norethindrone and levonorgestrel vary (4-14 and 0.9-2 ng/mL, respectively), but 24 hours after pill ingestion, serum levels are 0.2 to 1.6 ng/mL and 0.2 to 0.5 ng/mL, respectively. Thus, there is no accumulation of progestin over time. Progestin-only administration results in lower steady state levels and a shorter half-life compared with concomitant administration with estrogen.

Owing to the lower levels of progestin in the progestin-only pill, there is less influence on the inhibition of ovulation and more impact of thickening cervical mucus (*hostile environment*) inhibiting sperm penetration. Sperm that are able to penetrate have decreased mobility. Progestins also alter the endometrial lining (inhibition of progesterone receptor synthesis and reduction in endometrial glandular development, preventing implantation) and perhaps inhibit the motility (number and motility of the cilia) of the uterine tube. LH peaks—as well as FSH peaks—are suppressed compared with pretreatment levels. The change in cervical mucus takes place 2 to 4 hours after the first dose. However, after 24 hours, thinning of the cervical mucus is evident, allowing

A. Norethindrone

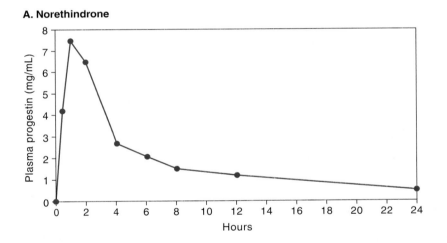

B. Levonorgestrel

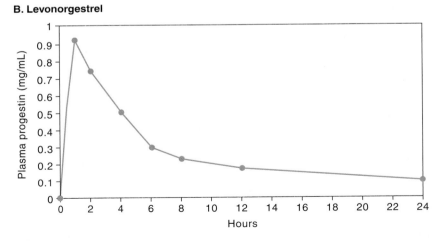

FIGURE 13–19 Serum levels attained with progestin-only pills. [Reproduced, with permission, from McCann MF, Potter LS. Progestin-only oral contraception: a comprehensive review. *Contraception*. 1994;50(6 suppl 1):S1.]

unimpaired sperm penetration, which is why it is critical to take the progestin-only pills at the same time every day.

The progestin-only pill should be started on the first day of menses. This pill should be taken at the same time every day. If administration is 3 hours late, a backup method should be used for 48 hours. If a pill is missed, a backup method should be used for 48 hours, and if two or more pills are missed, a backup method should be used for 48 hours due to rapid resumption of the cervical mucus effect. If no menses occur in 4 weeks, a pregnancy test is necessary. Progestin-only pills may be administered immediately postpartum.

The efficacy of progestin-only pills under conditions of perfect use is 0.3 to 3.1 failures per 100 woman-years (failure rates of 1.1%-9.6% in the first year) or 0.5 per 100 users. This efficacy rate is achieved only with careful compliance. The typical use is associated with a greater than 5% failure rate. Failure rates were lowest in women over 38½ years of age and those who were breast-feeding. The efficacy may also be influenced by body weight and by concomitant use of anticonvulsants. The major disadvantage is that the pill must be administered at the same time every day. As a result of even slight flexibility in the schedule, there is increased contraceptive failure.

The risks associated with progestin-only pills are minimal. Various studies have revealed no significant impact on lipids, carbohydrate metabolism, blood pressure, or the incidence of myocardial infarction and stroke. Furthermore, no adverse coagulation parameters have been associated with its use. There are almost no data on the association of progestin-only pills and endometrial, ovarian, cervical, or breast cancer. The major side-effect is breakthrough bleeding (40%-60%). Other side-effects include acne and persistent ovarian cysts. With discontinuation of the pill, menses resume with no impact on subsequent pregnancy rates or future fertility.

CONTRACEPTION: LONG-ACTING CONTRACEPTIVES

The high rate of unintended pregnancies has led to the development of long-acting reversible contraceptive modalities. Interest in long-acting methods is increasing because they offer convenience, obviate problems of compliance, and thus offer higher efficacy. Most long-acting systems contain either combination or progestin-only hormones. The effectiveness of these hormones is prolonged, mostly due to the sustained system that results in a gradual release. The modes of administration include injectables, transdermal patches, subdermal rods, vaginal rings, and intrauterine devices. The various types of long-acting contraceptives are discussed below.

Injectable Contraceptives

A. Progestin only Injectable progestins that contain medroxyprogesterone acetate (MPA, Depo-Provera) are beneficial when women have contraindications to estrogen, use antiepileptics, are mentally handicapped, or have poor compliance.

Furthermore, there is good evidence that its use is safe in the presence of coronary artery disease, congestive heart failure, diabetes, tobacco use, and a history of venous thromboembolism. Other uses of MPA include treatment of metastatic endometrial or renal carcinoma.

Although most other long-acting contraceptives are sustained-release formulations, Depo-Provera (150 mg MPA) is provided as an aqueous microcrystalline suspension that gradually declines throughout the cycle (Figure 13–20). Pharmacologic levels (>0.5 ng/mL) are achieved within the first 24 hours and peak (at 2 ng/mL) within the first week after the injection. Serum concentrations are maintained at 1 ng/mL for approximately 3 months. Interestingly, estrogen concentration is in the early to midfollicular level (below 100 pg/mL) and persists for 4 months after the last injection. The serum concentration of MPA decreases to 0.2 ng/mL during the last 5 to 6 months (ovulation occurs when levels are <0.1 ng/mL). However, one study observed progesterone levels to rise after 3½ months.

The mechanism of action depends mainly on the ability of higher peaks of hormone to inhibit ovulation (LH surge). Like other progestins, MPA increases cervical mucus viscosity, alters the endometrium, and decreases the motility of the uterine tubes and uterus. FSH levels are minimally suppressed with Depo-Provera.

The manufacturer's recommendation is to administer the agent every 3 months, starting within 5 days of the onset of menses and not to exceed 1 week. The agent is injected deeply into the upper-outer quadrant of the buttock or deltoid without massage to ensure slow release. If the subject is postpartum and not breast-feeding, Depo-Provera should be given within 3 weeks after delivery and if lactating within 6 weeks (Table 13–10).

Because compliance is not an issue, the failure rate is minimal at 0 to 0.7 per 100 woman-years (0.3 per 100 users). Weight and use of concurrent medications do not affect the efficacy. However, continuation rates are poor at 50% to 60% because of the side-effect profile. The major dissatisfaction that leads to discontinuation is breakthrough bleeding, which approaches 50% to 70% in the first year of use. Other side-effects include weight gain (2.1 kg/y), dizziness, abdominal pain, anxiety, and possibly depression. Another disadvantage with the use of Depo-Provera is a delay in fertility after discontinuation. Ovulation returns when serum levels are less than 0.1 ng/mL. The time from discontinuation to ovulation is prolonged. Only 50% of patients ovulate at 6 months after discontinuing the medication, and although the agent does not cause infertility, achieving pregnancy may be delayed for more than 1 year. (The length of time for release at the injection site is unpredictable.) After the first year, 60% of women become amenorrheic, and at 5 years, the incidence of amenorrhea approaches 80%, which can be considered a potential benefit. Other benefits with use of MPA include prevention of iron deficiency anemia, ectopic pregnancy, PID, and endometrial cancer. In addition, Depo-Provera is a recommended contraceptive for women with sickle cell disease (decreased crisis) and seizure disorders (raises seizure threshold). Other therapeutic uses include dysmenorrhea and endometrial hyperplasia or cancer.

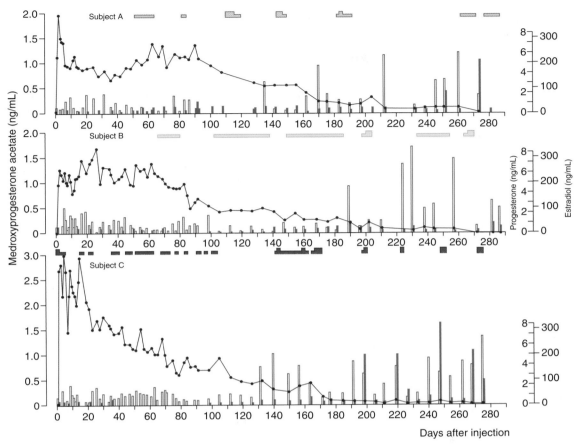

FIGURE 13–20 MPA levels following injection of Depo-Provera. Open bars represent serum estradiol; closed bars represent serum progesterone concentrations. (Reproduced, with permission, from Ortiz A, et al. Serum medroxyprogesterone acetate [MPA] and ovarian function following intramuscular injection of depo-MPA. *J Clin Endocrinol Metab.* 1977;44:32.)

One major concern with use of Depo-Provera is the development of osteopenia, with possible advancement to osteoporosis later in life. Several observational studies have evaluated the potential impact on bone. A prospective trial revealed that current users, after 12 months of use, experience a mean BMD loss of 2.74%. However, on examining former users 30 months later, it was found that mean BMD was similar to that of nonusers, indicating that the loss is reversible and of minimal clinical importance. An ongoing multicenter study assessing BMD in users versus nonusers should clarify the impact of Depo-Provera on bone. BMD in adolescents has also been investigated because adolescence is a critical time in bone mineralization. A small prospective study revealed that BMD was decreased by 1.5% to 3.1% after 1 and 2 years of use in Norplant users compared to increases in BMD of 9.3% and 9.5% in controls. This is a potential concern and has also led to a prospective multicenter study investigating the use of Depo-Provera in adolescents. Although one possible cause is less exposure to estrogen, an alternative and perhaps not exclusive theory involves MPA-dependent glucocorticoid activity that impairs osteoblast differentiation. Other potential risks include an adverse lipid profile (increase in LDL, decrease in HDL) and a slightly increased risk of breast cancer.

The association of breast cancer with use of Depo-Provera is minimal within the first 4 years of use, with no risk after 5 years of use. Paradoxically, MPA has been used for treatment of metastatic breast cancer.

B. Combination The development of monthly combination injectables (Lunelle) has responded to the erratic bleeding associated with Depo-Provera (Figure 13–21). The cycle control is similar to what is achieved with combined oral contraceptives. The monthly withdrawal bleeding occurs 2 weeks after the injection. The target populations are adolescents and women who have difficulty with compliance. Lunelle is an aqueous solution containing 25 mg of MPA and 5 mg of estradiol cypionate per 0.5 mL. In women who receive repeated administration of Lunelle, peak estradiol levels occur approximately 2 days after the third injection and are 247 pg/mL (similar to peak ovulatory levels). The estradiol level returns to baseline 14 days after the last injection (100 pg/mL); the drop in estradiol is associated with menstrual bleeding (2-3 weeks after the last injection). Peak MPA levels (2.17 ng/mL) occur 3½ days after the third monthly injection. The mean MPA level is 1.25 ng/mL. The level at day 28 of the cycle is 0.44 to 0.47 ng/mL (level needed for contraceptive

TABLE 13–10 Scheduling for injectable contraceptives.

Method	DMPA	MPA/E₂C
First injection		
Spontaneous menstrual cycle	Within 5 d of menses onset	Within 5 d of menses onset
Spontaneous or elective first-trimester abortion	Within 7 d	Within 7 d
Term delivery	Within 3 wk postpartum if not lactating; within 6 wk postpartum if lactating	Between 21 and 28 d postpartum if not lactating
Switching from combination OCs	With administered active pills or within 7 d after administering the pill pack's last active tablet	With administered active pills or within 7 d after administering the pill pack's last active tablet
Switching from DMPA	—	Within 13 wk after last DMPA injection
Switching from MPA/E₂C	Within 33 d after previous injection	—
Switching from levonorgestrel implant	Any time within 5 y of implant insertion; use of a condom back-up is recommended for 1 wk	Any time within 5 y of implant insertion; use of a condom backup is recommended for 1 wk
Switching from Copper T 380A IUD	First injection should occur before IUD removal and within 10 y after IUD insertion; a condom should be used as a back-up if the first injection is not administered within 5 d of menses onset	First injection should occur before IUD removal and within 10 y after IUD insertion condom should be used as a back-up if the first injection is not administered within 5 d of menses onset
Subsequent injections		
Injection interval	Every 12 wk or 3 mo; earlier reinjections are acceptable	Every 28 d or 4 wK or monthly; reinjection earlier than 23 d may impair cycle
Grace period	2 wk (14 wk from last injection); after 1 wk manufacturer recommends pregnancy testing before repeat injection	Control ± 5 d (23-33 d from last injection); thereafter, pregnancy testing needed before repeat injection

DMPA, depot medroxyprogesterone acetate; IUD, intrauterine device; MPA/E₂C, medroxyprogesterone acetate and estradiol cypionate; OCs , oral contraceptives.

Reproduced, with permission, from Kaunitz AM. Injectable long-acting contraceptives. *Clin Obstet Gynecol.* 2001;44:73.

effect is 0.1-0.2 ng/mL). The earliest return of ovulation seen in women with multiple injections has been 60 days after the last dose. The mechanism of action is similar to that of combined oral contraceptives.

Lunelle is administered intramuscularly in the buttock or deltoid every month. The first injection should be given within the first 5 days of the menstrual cycle (Table 13–10). Even though pharmacokinetic analysis reveals a delay in ovulation, the manufacturer recommends a 5-day grace period. The failure rate is 0.1 per 100 woman-years. Neither body weight nor use of concomitant drugs appears to affect the efficacy. Although this contraceptive has the advantages of the oral contraceptives and is associated with better compliance, the continuation rate is only 55%. This may be due to its side-effect profile, which is similar to that of the combined oral contraceptives with the addition of monthly injections.

There are limited data on potential risks. The risk potential is probably similar to that of the combined oral contraceptives, with a potentially lower incidence of deep vein thrombosis secondary to the absence of the first-pass effect. On discontinuation of Lunelle, achieving pregnancy may be delayed for as long as to 3 to 10 months after the last injection.

Lunelle was approved for use in the United States in 2000. However, in October 2002, Lunelle was recalled from the market, due to plant manufacturing problems. Alternatives to Lunelle that

are administered outside the United States are: Mesigyna, Perlutal, Yectames, and Chinese Injectable No 1.

Subdermal Implants

The Norplant package consists of six capsules (34 mm in length, 2.4 mm in diameter), with each capsule providing 36 mg of levonorgestrel (total 216 mg). The target population is women who have contraindications to or adverse side-effects from estrogen, women who are postpartum or breast-feeding, and adolescent mothers. This method provides long-term continuous contraception (approved for 5 years) that is rapidly reversible. The advantages, side-effects, risks, and contraindications are similar to those of oral progestins. The major disadvantage—not present with use of oral progestins—is the surgical insertion and removal of the rods. A newer system, Norplant II, contains two rods (4 cm in length, 3.4 cm in diameter) and releases 50 µg/d of norgestrel (approved for 3 years). The two-rod system has the same mechanism of action and side-effect profile as its predecessor. However, the rods are much easier and faster to insert and remove than the capsules.

Within the first 24 hours, serum concentrations of levonorgestrel are 0.4 to 0.5 ng/mL. The capsules release 85 µg of levonorgestrel per 24 hours for the first year (equivalent to the daily dose of progestin-only pills) and then 50 µg for the remaining 5 years. The

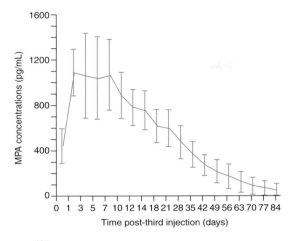

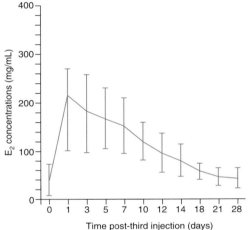

FIGURE 13-21 Serum MPA and estradiol levels following Lunelle injection. [Reproduced, with permission, from Rahimy MH, Ryan KK, Hopkins NK. Lunelle monthly contraceptive injection (medroxyprogesterone acetate and estradiol cypionate injectable suspension): steady-state pharmacokinetics of MPA and E_2 in surgically sterile women. *Contraception*. 1999;60:209.]

mean serum levels of progestin after the first 6 months are 0.25 to 0.6 ng/mL, slightly decreased at 5 years to 0.17 to 0.35 ng/mL. A levonorgestrel concentration below 0.2 ng/mL is associated with increased pregnancy rates. The site of implantation (leg, forearm, and arm) does not affect circulating progestin levels. Even though progestin levels are sufficient to prevent ovulation within the first 24 hours, the manufacturer recommends use of a backup method for 3 days after insertion. On removal, the progestin levels rapidly decline and undetectable serum levels are achieved after 96 hours. As a result, most women ovulate within 1 month after removal of the implants.

Norplant provides contraception in several ways. In the first 2 years, the levonorgestrel concentration is high enough to suppress the LH surge—most likely at the hypothalamic level—and thereby inhibits ovulation. However, given the low concentrations of progestin, there is no real effect on FSH. The estradiol levels approximate those in ovulatory women. In addition, there are irregular serum peaks (often prolonged) and declines in serum estrogen levels that may contribute to erratic bleeding. By 5 years, more than 50% of the cycles are ovulatory. However, ovulatory cycles while using Norplant have been associated with luteal phase insufficiency. Other mechanisms of contraception are similar to oral progestins and include thickening of the cervical mucus, alterations of the endometrium, and changes in tubal and uterine motility.

The failure rate is 0.2 to 2.1 failures per 100 woman-years (0.9 per 100 users). Like oral progestins, body weight affects circulating levels and may result in more failures in the fourth or fifth year of use. Similar to oral progestins, the incidence of ectopic pregnancy among failures is increased to 20% (overall incidence is 0.28-1.3 per 1000 woman-years). The continuation rate (discontinuation rate of 10%-15% per year) is age-dependent and ranges from 33% to 78%. Menstrual disturbances are the most frequent side-effect; they approach 40% to 80%, especially in the first 2 years. Although the incidence of abnormal uterine bleeding is similar to that of Depo-Provera, a significant difference between these methods is that Norplant provides only a 10% amenorrhea rate at 5 years. Other reported side-effects include headache (30% indication for removal) and possibly weight gain, mood changes, anxiety, and depression—as well as ovarian cyst formation (eightfold increase), breast tenderness, acne, galactorrhea (if insertion occurs on discontinuation of lactation), possible hair loss, and pain or other adverse reactions at the insertion site (0.8% of cases at discontinuation).

Transdermal Patch

The transdermal patch (Ortho Evra) is another approach to contraception. The thin 20-cm^2 patch is composed of a protective layer, a middle (medicated) layer, and a release liner that is removed prior to application. The system delivers 150 μg of norelgestromin (active metabolite of norgestimate) and 20 μg of ethinyl estradiol per day to the systemic circulation. The target population is similar to that described above for Lunelle. One advantage of this system over Lunelle is that there are no monthly injections, and as a result, there is greater autonomy for the patient. The patch is applied once a week for 3 consecutive weeks, followed by a patch-free week for monthly withdrawal bleeding. The patch should be changed on the same day each week. The mechanism of action, contraindications, and side effects are similar to what has been described in the section on oral contraceptives.

With use of the transdermal patch, the peak ethinyl estradiol and norelgestromin levels are 50 to 60 pg/mL and 0.7 to 0.8 ng/mL, respectively. Because of this unique delivery system, hormone levels achieve a steady state condition throughout the cycle (see later and Figure 13–22). After the seventh day of application, there are adequate hormone levels to inhibit ovulation for 2 more days. With each consecutive patch, there is minimal accumulation of norelgestromin or ethinyl estradiol. The amount of hormone delivered is not affected by the environment, activity, or site of application (abdomen, buttock, arm, torso). The adhesive is very reliable in a variety of conditions, including exercise, swimming,

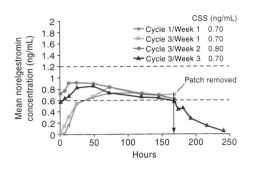

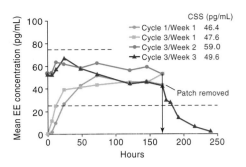

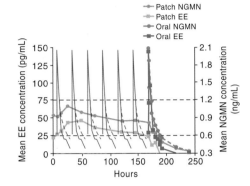

FIGURE 13–22 Comparative serum steroid (CSS) levels of norelgestromin (NGMN) and ethinyl estradiol (EE) following patch administration. (Reproduced, with permission, from Abrams LS, et al. Multiple-dose pharmacokinetics of a contraceptive patch in healthy women participants. *Contraception*. 2001;64:287.)

humidity, saunas, and bathing. Complete detachment occurs in 1.8% of cases and partial detachment in 2.9% of cases.

The failure rate is 0.7 per 100 woman-years under conditions of perfect use. Body weight has not been shown to affect the efficacy. The compliance with perfect use ranges from 88.1% to 91% among all age groups. This is significantly different from what is achieved with oral contraceptives (67%-85%), especially with women under 20 years of age. The side-effect profile is similar to that of oral contraceptives, except that there is slightly more breakthrough bleeding with the transdermal patch in the first 1 to 2 months (up to 12.2% vs 8.1%) and less breast tenderness (6.1% vs 18.8%). The incidence of skin reaction was 17.4%, characterized as mild in 92%, resulting in discontinuation in under 2%.

Vaginal Rings

Since the early 1900s, it has been recognized that the vagina is a place where steroids can be rapidly absorbed into the circulation. A study in the 1960s revealed that silicone rubber pessaries containing sex steroids would release the drug at a continuous rate. These studies led to the development of contraceptive vaginal rings.

As with oral contraceptives, there are combination and progestin-only formulations. Several progestin-only rings have been introduced since the 1970s. However, they were associated with significant menstrual disturbances. More recently, combination types have been developed. The most recent (2002) FDA-approved vaginal ring is a combination type called the NuvaRing.

The NuvaRing is made of ethylene vinyl acetate that provides 0.015 mg of ethinyl estradiol and 0.120 mg of etonogestrel per day. Maximum serum concentrations are achieved within 1 week after placement. The ring is designed to be used for 21 days and then removed for 1 full week to permit withdrawal bleeding. This device is capable of inhibiting ovulation within 3 days after insertion. After removal, the time to ovulation is 19 days. The mechanism of action, contraindications, and risks are similar to those of oral contraceptives. However, when assessing systemic exposure, use of the vaginal ring allows for 50% of the total exposure to ethinyl estradiol (15 μg in the ring compared with a 30-μg ethinyl estradiol-containing oral contraceptive).

The failure rate is similar to that reported with oral contraceptives. The continuation rate is 85.6% to 90%. Irregular bleeding is minimal (5.5%), and overall, the device is well tolerated, with an associated 2.5% discontinuation rate. Side-effects are similar to those of oral contraceptives, but cycle control appears to be improved. The reported incidence of vaginal discharge is 23% versus 14.5% with oral contraceptives. The ring does not appear to interfere with intercourse (1%-2% of partners reported discomfort); however, the device can be removed for 2 to 3 hours during intercourse without changing efficacy.

Intrauterine Devices

Intrauterine devices (IUDs) are another modality of contraception that has been used clinically since the 1960s. Historically, these devices were made of plastic (polyethylene) impregnated with barium sulfate to make them radiopaque. Several other devices were subsequently developed, including the Dalkon Shield. After the introduction of the Dalkon Shield, an increase in pelvic infections was observed secondary to its multifilament tail. Furthermore, tubal infertility and septic abortions were increasing, and massive litigation occurred as a result. Consequently, even though the modern IUD has negligible associated risk, the use of IUDs in the United States is minimal—less than 1% of married women.

Currently, two types of IUDs are used in the United States: the copper- and the hormone-containing devices. The most recent FDA-approved intrauterine system contains levonorgestrel (Mirena) and is approved for 5 years of use. Several studies have demonstrated that these devices are unlike the Dalkon Shield and are very safe and efficacious. The target population is women who desire highly effective contraception that is long-term and rapidly reversible.

The copper (TCu-380A) IUD is a T-shaped device. The mechanism of action is mostly spermicidal due to the sterile inflammatory reaction that is created secondary to a foreign body in the uterus. The abundance of white blood cells that are present as a result kills the spermatozoa by phagocytosis. The amount of dissolution of copper is less than the daily amount ingested in the diet. However, with release of copper, salts are created that alter the endometrium and cervical mucus. Sperm transport is significantly impaired, limiting access to the oviducts.

There are two hormone-containing intrauterine devices: the progesterone-releasing device (Progestasert) and the levonorgestrel-releasing device (Mirena). The Progestasert contains progesterone, which is released at a rate of 65 mg/d (approved for 1 year). This diffuses into the endometrial cavity, resulting in decidualization and atrophy of the endometrium. Serum progesterone levels do not change with the use of Progestasert. The main mechanism of action is to impair implantation. Mirena contains 52 mg of levonorgestrel, which is gradually released at a rate of 20 μg/d (approved for 5 years). Unlike Progestasert, systemic absorption of levonorgestrel inhibits ovulation about half the time. Although women may continue to have cyclic menses, over 40% have impaired follicular growth, with up to 23% developing luteinized unruptured follicles. Other mechanisms of action are similar to those described for Progestasert and the progestin-only pills. Mirena has the added advantage of significantly decreasing menstrual flow and has been used to treat menorrhagia.

The IUD should be placed within 7 days after onset of the menstrual cycle or at any time postpartum. Protection begins immediately after insertion. The failure rates after the first year of use are 0.5% to 0.8% for the TCu-380A, 1.3% to 1.6% for Progestasert, and 0.1% to 0.2% for Mirena. The expulsion rate is approximately 10%.

If a woman becomes pregnant with an IUD in place, the incidence of an ectopic pregnancy is 4.5% to 25%. The incidence of ectopic pregnancies with IUDs varies depending on the type of device. With Progestasert, the ectopic rate is slightly higher (6.80 per 1000 woman-years), most likely because its mechanism of action is limited to inhibiting implantation in the endometrium—in contrast to the copper or levonorgestrel IUD (0.2-0.4 per 1000 woman-years), both of which also interfere with conception.

The continuation rate range for the current IUDs is 40% to 66.2% (Mirena). The side-effects of the copper IUD include dysmenorrhea and menorrhagia. The most common adverse effect associated with the hormone-containing devices is erratic, albeit significantly less, bleeding. In fact, 40% of women experienced amenorrhea at 6 months and 50% at 12 months. The incidence of spotting in the first 6 months was 25% but decreased to 11% after 2 years. Other reported side-effects of levonorgestrel include depression, headaches, and acne. There is a tendency to develop ovarian cysts early after insertion with the levonorgestrel-containing device that resolves after 4 months of use.

The nominal risks associated with IUD use include pelvic infection (within 1 month after insertion), lost IUD (ie, perforation into the abdominal cavity; 1:3000), and miscarriage. There is no association between IUD use and uterine or cervical cancer. Contraindications to IUD use are active genital infection and unexplained bleeding.

EMERGENCY CONTRACEPTION

Postcoital contraception is a method that may be used by a woman who believes her contraceptive method has failed or who has had unprotected intercourse and feels that she may be at risk for an unintended pregnancy. The first study to evaluate the efficacy of emergency contraception with hormones was in 1963. Subsequently, several studies have been performed with various contraceptives that paved the way for more widespread use. In 1997, the FDA approved the use of high-dose oral contraceptives for postcoital contraception. Since then, pharmaceutical companies have marketed specific packaging for the use of emergency contraception. Other methods, including mifepristone (RU-486) and the IUD have also been effective for postcoital contraception.

Similar to the formulas of oral contraception, there are both combination and progestin-only types of emergency contraception. The combination method (Yuzpe regimen) entails administration of two doses of two tablets (Ovral: 50 μg ethinyl estradiol, 0.5 mg norgestrel) 12 hours apart (total: 200 μg ethinyl estradiol, 2 mg norgestrel). Other oral contraceptives may be used with adjustment in the number of pills for equivalence (ie, two doses of four tablets: any second-generation oral contraceptive 12 hours apart). The specific medication (Preven) that is FDA approved and marketed for postcoital contraception contains two doses of four tablets (ethinyl estradiol 50 μg, levonorgestrel 0.25 mg) 12 hours apart. The progestin-only method involves two doses of 10 pills (Ovrette 0.075 mg) 12 hours apart (Plan A). The marketed form (Plan B) contains two doses of one tablet (levonorgestrel 0.75 mg) 12 hours apart.

Following a single oral dose of 0.75 mg of levonorgestrel, the serum concentration peak (5-10 ng/mL) was at 2 hours with a rapid decline during the first 24 hours. The mechanism of action is uncertain, but levonorgestrel most likely inhibits ovulation and alters the endometrium to prevent implantation. Studies have shown decreased sperm recovery from the uterine cavity, possibly due to thickened cervical mucus, or the alkalinization of the intrauterine environment. Others have shown that changes in other factors, such as integrins, can alter endometrial receptivity. The mode of action likely depends on the timing of intercourse relative to ovulation and to the administration of emergency contraception.

Maximum efficacy is achieved if the first dose is administered within 72 hours after intercourse and repeated in 12 hours. Combination formulas have a failure rate of 2% to 3%, and progestin-only preparations have a failure rate of 1%. Emergency contraception effectively reduces the rate of unintended pregnancies from 8% to 2%, a 75% reduction. However, with increasing time since unprotected intercourse, the efficacy changes from 0.4% to 1.2% to 2.7% for the first, second, or third 24-hour period after unprotected intercourse. For maximum efficacy, emergency contraception may be prescribed in advance so women will already have the correct dosing. No increase in risk-taking behavior has been noted with this strategy.

Significant nausea or emesis (51.7%) is associated with use of emergency contraception, although it is substantially less with progestin-only formulations. An antiemetic should be administered 1 hour before each treatment. If a patient vomits within 1 hour after ingestion, additional pills need to be administered.

Contraindications to emergency contraception with the combination regimen are possibly the same as those described for oral contraceptives; for progestin-only pills, there are no contraindications. Emergency contraception should be an optional function of the rape management protocol.

REFERENCES

Embryology and Anatomy

Ahmed SF, Hughes IA. The genetics of male under-masculinization. *Clin Endocrinol (Oxf)*. 2002;56:1. [PMID: 11849240]

McElreavey K, Fellous M. Sex determination and the Y chromosome. *Am J Med Genet*. 1999;89:76. [PMID: 10727993]

Oocyte Development

Braw-Tal R. The initiation of follicle growth: the oocyte or the somatic cells? *Mol Cell Endocrinol*. 2002;18:18. [PMID: 11988306]

Erickson GF. The ovary: basic principles and concepts. In: Felig P, Frohman LA, eds. *Endocrinology and Metabolism*. 4th ed. New York: McGraw-Hill; 2001.

Findlay JK, Drummond AE, Dyson ML, Baillie AJ, Robertson DM, Ethier JF. Recruitment and development of the follicle: the roles of the transforming growth factor-beta superfamily. *Mol Cell Endocrinol*. 2002;191:35. [PMID: 12044917]

Suh CS, Sonntag B, Erickson GF. The ovarian life cycle: a contemporary view. *Rev Endocr Metab Disord*. 2002;3:5. [PMID: 11883105]

Teixeira J, Maheswaran S, Donahoe PK. Müllerian inhibiting substance: an instructive developmental hormone with diagnostic and possible therapeutic applications. *Endocr Rev*. 2001;22:657. [PMID: 11588147]

Ovarian Steroidogenesis

Bulun SE, Adashi EY. The physiology and pathology of the female reproductive axis. In: Larsen et al, ed. *Williams Textbook of Endocrinology*. 10th ed. Philadelphia, PA: WB Saunders; 2003.

Strauss JF, Hsueh AJ. Ovarian hormone synthesis. In: DeGroot LJ, et al, ed. *Endocrinology*. 4th ed. Philadelphia, PA: WB Saunders; 2001.

Menstrual Cycle

Chabbert-Buffet N, Bouchard P. The normal human menstrual cycle. *Rev Endocr Metab Disord*. 2002;3:173. [PMID: 12215712]

McGee EA, Hsueh AJW. Initial and cyclic recruitment of ovarian follicles. *Endocr Rev*. 2000;21:200. [PMID: 10782364]

Amenorrhea

Marcus MD, Loucks TL, Berga SL. Psychological correlates of functional hypothalamic amenorrhea. *Fertil Steril*. 2001;76:310. [PMID: 11476768]

Marshall JC, Eagleson CA, McCartney CR. Hypothalamic dysfunction. *Mol Cell Endocrinol*. 2001;183:29. [PMID: 11604221]

Seminara SB, Hayes FJ, Crowley WF, Jr. Gonadotropin-releasing hormone deficiency in the human (idiopathic hypogonadotropic hypogonadism and Kallmann's syndrome): pathophysiological and genetic considerations. *Endocr Rev*. 1998;19:521. [PMID: 9793755]

Ovarian Failure

Bakalov VK, Vanderhoof VH, Bondy CA, Nelson LM. Adrenal antibodies detect asymptomatic auto-immune adrenal insufficiency in young women with spontaneous premature ovarian failure. *Hum Reprod*. 2002;17:2096. [PMID:12151443]

Christin-Maitre S, Vasseur C, Portnoi M-F, Bouchard P. Genes and premature ovarian failure. *Mol Cell Endocrinol*. 1998;145:75. [PMID: 9933102]

Davison RM, Davis CJ, Conway GS. The X chromosome and ovarian failure. *Clin Endocrinol*. 1999;51:573. [PMID: 10619970]

Layman LC. Human gene mutations causing infertility. *J Med Genet*. 2002;3:153. [PMID: 11897813]

Minton SE, Munster PN. Chemotherapy-induced amenorrhea and fertility in women undergoing adjuvant treatment for breast cancer. *Cancer Control*. 2002;9:466. [PMID:12514564]

Anovulation Due to Polycystic Ovarian Syndrome

Abbott DH, Dumesic DA, Franks S. Developmental origin of polycystic ovary syndrome—a hypothesis. *J Endocrinol*. 2002;174:1. [PMID: 12098657]

Azziz R, Carmina E, Dewailly D, et al; Task Force on the Phenotype of the Polycystic Ovary Syndrome of the Androgen Excess and PCOS Society. The Androgen Excess and PCOS Society criteria for the polycystic ovary syndrome: the complete task force report. *Fertil Steril*. 2009;91(2):456-488. [PMID: 18950759]

Ibanez L, Dimartino-Nardi J, Potau N, Saenger P. Premature adrenarche—normal variant or forerunner of adult disease? *Endocr Rev*. 2000;21:671. [PMID: 11133068]

Legro RS. Polycystic ovary syndrome: the new millennium. *Mol Cell Endocrinol*. 2001;184:87. [PMID: 11694344]

Poretsky L, Cataldo NA, Rosenwaks Z, Giudice LC. The insulin-related ovarian regulatory system in health and disease. *Endocr Rev*. 1999;20:535. [PMID: 10453357]

Rotterdam ESHRE/ASRM-sponsored PCOS Consensus Workshop Group. Revised 2003 consensus on diagnostic criteria and long-term health risks related to polycystic ovary syndrome. *Fertil Steril*. 2004;81:19. [PMID: 14688154]

Anovulation Due to Adrenal Disorders

Betterle C, Dal Pra C, Mantero F, Zanchetta R. Autoimmune adrenal insufficiency and autoimmune polyendocrine syndromes: autoantibodies, autoantigens, and their applicability in diagnosis and disease prediction. *Endocr Rev*. 2002;23:327. [PMID: 12050123]

White PC, Speiser PW. Congenital adrenal hyperplasia due to 21-hydroxylase deficiency. *Endocr Rev*. 2000;21:245. [PMID: 10857554]

Müllerian Anomalies

Homer HA, Li T-C, Cooke ID. The septate uterus: a review of management and reproductive outcome. *Fertil Steril.* 2000;73:1. [PMID: 10632403]

Raga F, Bauset C, Remohi J, Bonilla-Musoles F, Simón C, Pellicer A. Reproductive impact of congenital Müllerian anomalies. *Hum Reprod.* 1997;12(10):2277-2281. [PMID: 9402295]

Menopause: General

Collaborative Group on Hormonal Factors in Breast Cancer. Breast cancer and hormone replacement therapy: collaborative reanalysis of data from 51 epidemiological studies of 52,705 women with breast cancer and 108,411 women without breast cancer. *Lancet.* 1997;350:1047. [PMID: 10213546]

Couzinet B, Meduri G, Lecce MG, et al. The postmenopausal ovary is not a major androgen-producing gland. *J Clin Endocrinol Metab.* 2001;86(10):5060-5066. [PMID: 11600585]

Faddy MJ, Gosden RG, Gougeon A, Richardson SJ, Nelson JF. Accelerated disappearance of ovarian follicles in mid-life: implications for forecasting menopause. *Hum Reprod.* 1992;7(10):1342-1346. [PMID: 1291557]

Hansen KR, Knowlton NS, Thyer AC, et al. A new model of reproductive aging: the decline in ovarian non-growing follicle number from birth to menopause. *Hum Reprod.* 2008;23:699. [PMID: 18192670]

Nair GV, Herrington DM. The ERA trial: findings and implications for the future. *Climacteric.* 2000;3:227. [PMID: 11910581]

Nelson HD, Humphrey LL, Nygren P, Teutsch SM, Allan JD. Postmenopausal hormone replacement therapy: scientific review. *JAMA.* 2002;288(7):872-881. [PMID: 12186605]

Randolph JF, Jr, Sowers M, Bondarenko IV, Harlow SD, Luborsky JL, Little RJ. Change in estradiol and follicle-stimulating hormone across the early menopausal transition: effects of ethnicity and age. *J Clin Endocrinol Metab.* 2004;89(4):1555-1561. [PMID: 15070912]

Reddy SY, Warner H, Guttuso T, et al. Gabapentin, estrogen, and placebo for treating hot flushes: a randomized controlled trial. *Obstet Gynecol.* 2006;108(1):41-48. [PMID: 16816054]

Rosen M, Sternfeld B, Schuh-Huerta SM, Reijo Pera RA, McCulloch CE, Cedars MI. Antral follicle count: absence of significant midlife decline. *Fertil Steril.* 2010; 94(6):2182-2185. [PMID: 20149366]

Soules MR, Sherman S, Parrott E, et al. Executive summary: Stages of Reproductive Aging Workshop (STRAW). *J Womens Health Gend Based Med.* 2001;10(9):843-848. [PMID: 11747678]

Sowers MR, Eyvazzadeh AD, McConnell D, et al. Anti-Mullerian hormone and inhibin B in the definition of ovarian aging and the menopause transition. *J Clin Endocrinol Metab.* 2008;93(9):3478-3483. [PMID: 18593767]

Weiss G, Skurnick JH, Goldsmith LT, Santoro NF, Park SJ. Menopause and hypothalamic-pituitary sensitivity to estrogen. *JAMA.* 2004;292(24): 2991-2996. [PMID: 15613667]

Menopause and Cardiovascular Disease

Anderson GL, Limacher M, Assaf AR, et al. Women's Health Initiative Steering Committee. Effects of conjugated equine estrogen in postmenopausal women with hysterectomy: the Women's Health Initiative randomized controlled trial. *JAMA.* 2004;291(14):1701-1712. [PMID: 15082697]

Barrett-Connor E, Grady D, Sashegyi A, et al. Raloxifene and cardiovascular events in osteoporotic postmenopausal women: four-year results from the MORE (Multiple Outcomes of Raloxifene Evaluation) randomized trial. *JAMA.* 2002;287(7):847-857. [PMID: 11851576]

Rossouw JE, Anderson GL, Prentice RL, et al. Risks and benefits of estrogen plus progestin in healthy postmenopausal women: principal results from the Women's Health Initiative randomized controlled trial. *JAMA.* 2002;288(3):321-333. [PMID: 12117397]

U.S. Preventive Services Task Force. Postmenopausal hormone replacement therapy for primary prevention of chronic conditions: recommendations and rationale. *Ann Intern Med.* 2002;137:834. [PMID: 12435221]

Menopause: Osteoporosis

Cranney A, Tugwell P, Wells G, Guyatt G. Meta-analyses of therapies for postmenopausal osteoporosis. *Endocr Rev.* 2002;23:496. [PMID: 12202464]

Menopause: Selective Estrogen Receptor Modulators

Miller CP. SERMs: evolutionary chemistry, revolutionary biology. *Curr Phar Des.* 2002;8:2089. [PMID: 12171520]

Hormone Replacement and Alzheimer Disease

Fillit HM. The role of hormone replacement therapy in the prevention of Alzheimer's disease. *Arch Intern Med.* 2002;162:1934. [PMID: 12230415]

Infertility

Cedars MI. Infertility in obstetrics and gynecology: a longitudinal approach. In: Moore TR et al, eds. *Gynecology and Obstetrics: A Longitudinal Approach.* New York: Churchill Livingstone; 1993.

Legro RS, Barnhart HX, Schlaff WD, et al. Clomiphene, metformin, or both for infertility in the polycystic ovary syndrome. *N Engl J Med.* 2007 Feb 8;356(6):551-566. [PMID: 17287476]

Te Velde ER, Dorland M, Broekmans FJ. Age at menopause as a marker of reproductive ageing. *Maturitas.* 1998;30:119. [PMID: 9871906]

Contraception

Abma JC, Chandra A, Mosher WD, Peterson LS, Piccinino LJ. Centers for Disease Control and Prevention, National Center for Health Statistics. Fertility, family planning, and women's health: new data from the 1995 National Survey of Family Growth, Report No. 19, Series 23, 1997.

Archer DF. New contraceptive options. *Clin Obstet Gynecol.* 2001;44:122. [PMID: 11219241]

Brenner PF, Mishell DR Jr, Stanczyk FZ, Goebelsmann U. Serum levels of d-norgestrel, luteinizing hormone, follicle-stimulating hormone, estradiol, and progesterone in women during and following ingestion of combination oral contraceptives containing dl-norgestrel. *Am J Obstet Gynecol.* 1977;129:133. [PMID: 900174]

Burkman RT, Collins JA, Shulman LP, Williams JK. Current perspectives on oral contraceptive use. *Am J Obstet Gynecol.* 2001;185(2 suppl):S4. [PMID: 11521117]

Croxatto HB, Devoto L, Durand M, et al. Mechanism of action of hormonal preparations used for emergency contraception: a review of the literature. *Contraception.* 2001;63:(3)111. [PMID: 11368982]

Kaunitz AM. Injectable long-acting contraceptives. *Clin Obstet Gynecol.* 2001;44:73. [PMID: 11219248]

Marchbanks PA, McDonald JA, Wilson HG, et al. Oral contraceptives and the risk of breast cancer. *N Engl J Med.* 2002;346(26):2025-2032. [PMID: 12087137]

McCann MF, Potter LS. Progestin-only oral contraception: a comprehensive review. *Contraception.* 1994;50(6 suppl):S1. [PMID: 10226677]

Ortiz A, Hirol M, Stanczyk FZ, Goebelsmann U, Mishell DR. Serum medroxyprogesterone acetate (MPA) and ovarian function following intramuscular injection of depo-MPA. *J Clin Endocrinol Metab.* 1977;44:32. [PMID: 833262]

Rahimy MH, Ryan KK, Hopkins NK. Lunelle monthly contraceptive injection (medroxyprogesterone acetate and estradiol cypionate injectable suspension): steady-state pharmacokinetics of MPA and E2 in surgically sterile women. *Contraception.* 1999;60;209. [PMID: 10640167]

Disorders of Sex Determination and Differentiation

Felix A. Conte, MD and Melvin M. Grumbach, MD

ACTH	Adrenocorticotropic hormone	**hCG**	Human chorionic gonadotropin
AKR1C2	3α-Hydroxysteroid dehydrogenase-3 (3α-HSD-3)	**HMG**	High mobility group
AMH	Anti-Müllerian hormone	**17β-HSD-3**	17β-Hydroxysteroid dehydrogenase-3
BPES	Blepharophimosis-ptosis-epicanthus inversus syndrome	**ICSI**	Intracytoplasmic sperm injection
		IGF	Insulin-like growth factor
CAH	Congenital adrenal hyperplasia	**LH**	Luteinizing hormone
CIS	Carcinoma in situ	**MAMLD1**	Mastermind-like domain containing 1
CBX2	Chromobox homolog 2, homolog of mouse m33	**MAP3K4**	Mitogen-activated protein kinase kinase kinase 4
CMPD1	Campomelic dysplasia	**Ovotesticular DSD**	Previously designated *true hermaphrodism*
DAX1	DSS-AHC-critical region on the X chromosome gene 1	**PAR**	Pseudoautosomal region
DHEA	Dehydroepiandrosterone	**POR**	P450 oxidoreductase
DHH	Desert hedgehog	**PRKX**	Protein kinase X linked
DHT	Dihydrotestosterone	**PRKY**	Protein kinase Y linked
DMRT1	*Double sex Mab3-related transcription factor gene 1*	**RFLP**	Testriction fragment length polymorphism
DSS	Dosage-sensitive sex reversal	**RSPO1**	R-spondin1
DSD	Disorders of sexual development—congenital conditions in which development of chromosomal, gonadal, or anatomic sex is atypical	**SF-1**	Steroidogenic factor-1
		SHOX	Short stature homeobox gene on the X chromosome
		SOX3	SRY-like HMG box-3
		SOX9	SRY-like HMG box-9
46,XX DSD	Previously designated *female pseudohermaphrodite*	*SRY*	Sex-determining region Y gene
46,XY DSD	Previously designated *male pseudohermaphrodite*	**StAR**	Steroidogenic acute regulatory protein
		TSPY	Testes-specific protein-Y encoded
FISH	Fluorescent in situ hybridization	*WAGR*	Wilms tumor-aniridia-genital anomalies-mental retardation syndrome
FGF-9	Fibroblast growth factor-9		
FOXL2	Forkhead box L2		
FSH	Follicle-stimulating hormone	*WNT4*	Human homolog of Drosophila wingless gene
GATA-4	Member of the GATA family of zinc finger transcription factors	*WT1*	Wilms tumor gene
GH	Growth hormone	*XIST*	X-inactive specific transcript gene
GnRH	Gonadotropin-releasing hormone		

Lowercase letters for genes, for example, *Sry, Sox9, Fgf 9* are used to indicate the mouse homologue of the human gene where a particular function has not yet been demonstrated in humans.

Advances in developmental and cell biology, molecular genetics, experimental embryology, steroid biochemistry, and methods of evaluation of the interaction between the hypothalamus, pituitary, and gonads as well as behavioral science have helped clarify problems of sexual determination and differentiation. Anomalies may occur at any stage of intrauterine development of the hypothalamus, pituitary, gonads, and genitalia and lead to gross ambisexual development or to subtle abnormalities that do not become manifest until sexual maturity is achieved.

HUMAN SEX DIFFERENTIATION

Chromosomal Sex

The normal human diploid cell contains 22 autosomal pairs of chromosomes and two sex chromosomes (two Xs, or one X and one Y). When arranged serially and numbered according to size and centromeric position, they are known as a karyotype. Advances in the techniques of staining chromosomes permit positive identification of each chromosome by its unique *banding* pattern. A technique called fluorescence in situ hybridization (FISH) is particularly useful in identifying quickly both sex chromosomes, mosaicism and structural abnormalities involving the sex chromosomes, the presence or absence of SRY (the testes determining gene on the Y chromosome), and other deleted genes (Figure 14–1). High-resolution chromosome banding and painting techniques provide precise identification of each chromosome.

Studies in animals as well as humans with abnormalities of sexual differentiation indicate that the sex chromosomes (the X and Y chromosomes) and the autosomes harbor genes that influence sex determination and differentiation by causing the bipotential gonad to develop either as a testis or as an ovary. Two intact and normally functioning X chromosomes, in the absence of a Y chromosome or its *SRY* gene, lead to the formation of an ovary under normal circumstances, whereas a Y chromosome (whose *SRY* gene is intact) or the translocation of *SRY*, the testis-determining gene on the short arm of the Y chromosome, to an X chromosome or autosome leads to testicular organogenesis.

In humans, there is a marked discrepancy in size between the X and Y chromosomes. Gene dosage compensation is achieved in all persons with two or more X chromosomes in their genetic constitution by partial inactivation of all X chromosomes except one. This phenomenon is thought to be a random process (except when a structurally abnormal X chromosome is present) that occurs in each cell in the late blastocyst stage of embryonic development, during which either the maternally or the paternally derived X chromosome undergoes heterochromatinization. A result of this epigenetic process is formation of an X chromatin body (Barr body) in the interphase cells of persons having two or more X chromosomes. In patients with two or more X chromosomes, the maximum number of Barr bodies (partially inactivated X chromosomes) seen in interphase cells will be one less than the number of X chromosomes in the karyotype. A gene termed *XIST* (*X-inactive specific transcripts*) is located in the X inactivation center at Xq13.2 on the paracentromeric region of the long arm of the

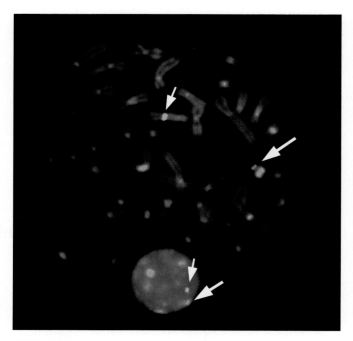

FIGURE 14–1 FISH (fluorescent in situ hybridization) for SRY in metaphase and interphase cells. Image illustrates localization of the SRY probe on the distal short arm of the Y chromosome (Yp11.3) in spectrum orange. The probe for the centromere region of the X chromosome is shown in spectrum green. Note the presence of both probes in the interphase cell below. (Reproduced, with permission, from Grumbach MM, Hughes IA, Conte FA. Disorders of sex differentiation. In: Larsen PR, et al, eds. *Williams Textbook of Endocrinology.* 10th ed. WB Saunders; 2003.)

X chromosome. *XIST* is expressed only by the inactive X chromosome. The *XIST* gene encodes a large RNA that appears to coat the X chromosome and facilitates inactivation of selective genes on the X chromosome.

The distal portion of the short arm of the X chromosome escapes inactivation and has a short (2.5-megabase [mb]) segment homologous to a segment on the distal portion of the short arm of the Y chromosome (Figures 14–2 and 14–3). This segment is called the **pseudoautosomal region (PAR)**; it is these two limited regions of the X and Y that pair during meiosis, undergo obligatory chiasm formation, and allow for exchange of DNA between these specific regions of the X and Y chromosomes. At least 10 genes have been localized to the pseudoautosomal region on the short arm of the X and Y chromosomes. Among these are a gene whose deletion results in the neurocognitive defects observed in Turner syndrome and a gene for short stature, *SHOX* (short stature homeobox gene), which is expressed in bone. A mutation or deletion of SHOX on either the X or Y chromosome is associated with "idiopathic" short stature as well as dyschondrosteosis (Leri-Weill syndrome). Homozygous mutations of this gene are associated with a more severe form of short stature, Langer mesomelic dwarfism. A pseudoautosomal region has also been described for the distal ends of the long arms of the X and Y

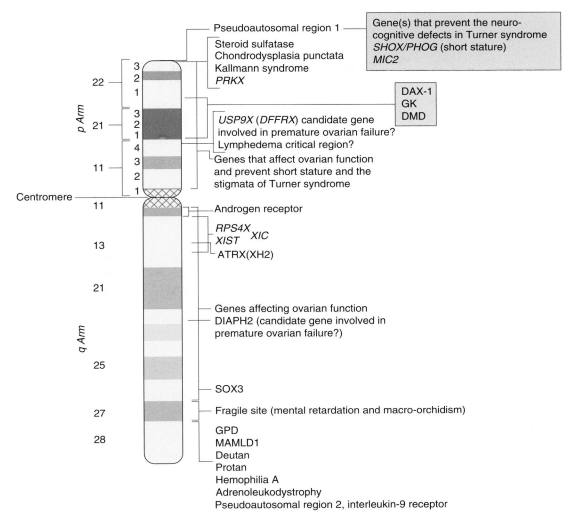

FIGURE 14–2 Diagrammatic representation of G-banded X chromosome. Selected X-linked genes are shown (ATRX, α-thalassemia, X-linked mental retardation; DAX1, DSS-AHC-critical region on the X chromosome gene 1; *DIAPH2*, human homolog of the Drosophila diaphanous gene; DMD, duchenne muscular dystrophy; GK, glycerol kinase; GPD, glucose-6-phosphate dehydrogenase; MAMLD1, mastermind-like domain-containing 1; MIC2, a cell surface antigen recognized by monoclonal antibody 12E7; PRKX, a member of the cAMP-dependent serine-threonine protein kinase gene family [illegitimate X-Y interchange occurs most frequently between PRKX and PRKY]; RPS4X, ribosomal protein S4; *SHOX, short-stature homeobox* gene; SOX3, SRY-like HMG box-3; USP9X, human x-linked homolog of the drosophila fat facets-related gene [DFFRX]; XIC, X-inactivation center; XIST, Xi-specific transcripts). (Reproduced, with permission, from Grumbach MM, Hughes IA, Conte FA. Disorders of sex differentiation. In: Larsen PR, et al, eds. *Williams Textbook of Endocrinology.* 10th ed. WB Saunders; 2003.)

chromosomes (see Figures 14–2 and 14–3). The pseudoautosomal region of the long arms of the X and Y chromosomes contains genes that are mostly growth factors and signaling molecules. The Y chromosome (see Figure 14–3) represents only 2% of the human genomic DNA and is about 60 mb in length. It is unique in that it contains few active genes compared to the X and autosomal chromosomes and has a large apparently noncoding heterochromatic region. It contains at least two genes affecting growth, the *SHOX* gene in the PAR and the **g**rowth **c**ontrol gene on the **Y** chromosome (GCY). The euchromatic region of the short arm of the Y chromosome contains the *SRY* gene (the male determining factor) distal to the PAR region at Yp11.3. The short arm of the Y chromosome contains genes that when deleted produce

the phenotype stigma of Turner syndrome. The pericentromeric region of the Y is the locus for the *TSPY* (*testes-specific protein Y encoded*) genes which predispose to gonadoblastoma formation in the presence of dysgenetic testicular development. The *PRKY* gene is homologous to a gene *PRKX* (*protein kinase X linked*) on the X chromosome and is the locus for Y to X translocation observed in 46,XX SRY-positive males. The euchromatic region of the long arm of the Y chromosome has genes that when deleted result in azoospermia.

Genes involved in organogenesis of the bipotential gonad

WT1   Heterozygous mutations and deletions of the *Wilms tumor* gene *(WT1)* located on 11p13 result in urogenital malformations

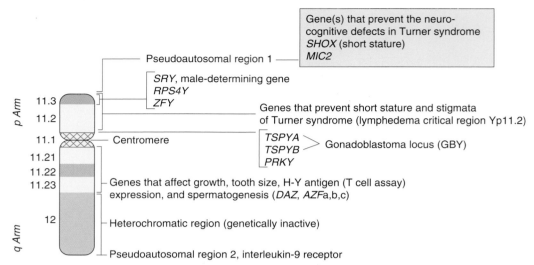

FIGURE 14–3 Diagrammatic representation of a G-banded Y chromosome (AZF, azoospermic factor; DAZ, deleted in azoospermia; *MIC2*, gene for a cell surface antigen recognized by monoclonal antibody 12E7; PRKY, a member of the cAMP-dependent serine-threonine protein kinase gene family; RPS4Y, ribosomal protein S4; *SHOX, short stature homeobox* gene; SRY, sex-determining region Y; TSPYA,B, members of the testes-specific factor gene family; ZFY, zinc finger Y). (Reproduced with permission from Grumbach MM, Hughes IA, Conte FA. Disorders of sex differentiation. In: Larsen PR, et al, eds. *Williams Textbook of Endocrinology*. 10th ed. WB Saunders; 2003.)

as well as Wilms tumor. Knockout of the *Wt1* gene in mice results in apoptosis of the metanephric blastema and as a consequence, absence of the kidneys and gonads. Thus, *WT1*, a transcriptional regulator, appears to act on metanephric blastema early in urogenital development (Figure 14–4A). Dominant-negative point mutations of WT1 in human beings results in the Denys-Drash and Frasier syndromes, whereas a contiguous deletion

of the gene and surrounding DNA results in **W**ilms tumor, **a**niridia, ambiguous **g**enitalia, and mental **r**etardation—the WAGR syndrome.

SF-1   Steroidogenic factor-1 (*SF-1*) is a nuclear receptor involved in transcriptional regulation of many genes, including those that are involved in gonadal development, adrenal development, steroid

Major Genes Involved in Sex Determination

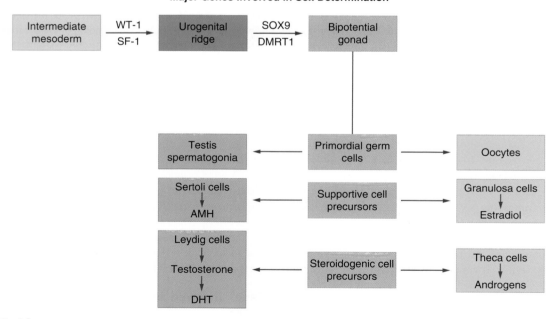

FIGURE 14–4A Major genes involved in sex determination from the intermediate mesoderm to the bipotential gonad. (DMRT1, doublesex and mab-3-related transcription factor 1; PGC, primordial germ cell [arise from an extragonadal site]; SF-1, steroidogenic factor 1; SOX9, SRY-like HMG-box 9; WT1, Wilms tumor suppressor gene-1) The bipotential gonad contains the precursor cells which differentiate into the supporting cells, steroid hormone-producing cells, and germ cells as shown.

synthesis, and reproduction (see Figure 14–4A). SF-1 is located on 9q33 and is expressed in the urogenital ridge as well as in steroidogenic organs. SF-1 is required for the synthesis of testosterone in Leydig cells; in Sertoli cells it regulates the *anti-Müllerian hormone* (*AMH*) gene. Homozygous knockout of the gene encoding *Sf-1* (*Sf-1* is the mouse homologue of mammalian *SF-1*) in mice results in apoptosis of the cells of the genital ridge that give rise to the adrenals and gonads and thus absence of gonadal and adrenal gland morphogenesis in both males and females. This gene has a critical role in the formation of all steroid-secreting glands (ie, adrenals, testes, and ovaries). Initial studies in humans with SF-1 mutations identified individuals with adrenal insufficiency, a 46,XY karyotype, complete gonadal dysgenesis, and the presence of müllerian derivatives, similar to the mouse phenotype. Subsequently, the spectrum of affected patients has included a range of 46,XY disorders of sexual development without adrenal insufficiency including hypospadias, anorchia, micropenis, complete gonadal dysgenesis, infertility in otherwise normal males, and ovarian failure in 46,XX females.

DMRT1   Haploinsufficiency of *DMRT1* (*double sex Mab3-related transcription factor gene 1*)—a gene related to double sex in drosophila and *Mab3* in *Caenorhabditis elegans* is a candidate for the abnormality in testis organogenesis in patients with 9p deletions (see Figure 14–4A). 46,XY patients invariably have the stigmata of the 9p syndrome (mental retardation, trigonocephaly, upslanting palpebral fissures, etc), as well as female or ambiguous external genitalia and Müllerian structures associated with streak gonads or dysgenetic testes. Recent data suggest that ovarian function may either be compromised or normal in 46,XX females with the 9p syndrome.

Ambiguous genitalia has also been reported in 46,XY patients with deletions of 10q. However, as yet a specific mutant gene(s) causing this DSD has not been identified on the 10q region.

Genes involved in testicular determination (Figure 14–4B)

SRY   In studies of 46,XX males with very small Y-to-X translocations, a gene was localized to the region just proximal to the pseudoautosomal boundary of the Y chromosome (Yp11.3) (see Figure 14–3) which has been named *SRY*. Deletions or mutations of the human *SRY* gene occur in about 15% to 20% of 46,XY females with complete XY gonadal dysgenesis and 90% of 46,XX males have a Y to X translocation which includes the *SRY* gene.

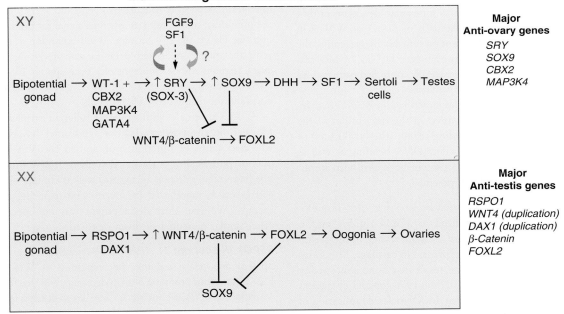

Postulated representation of the cascade of genes involved in mammalian gonadal determination

FIGURE 14–4B Opposing gene signals (differential activation) determines fate of primordial gonad as a testis or ovary. RSPO1, respondin 1; *WNT4*, human homolog of Drosophila wingless gene; FOXL-2, forkhead box L2; β-catenin, key-regulated effector of the WNT-signaling pathway. DAX-1 (DSS-AHC-critical region on the X chromosome gene 1) RSPO1 activates the WNT4/β-catenin canonical-signaling pathway which inhibits SOX9 expression and promotes ovarian differentiation. SRY upregulates SOX9 by binding to testicular enhancing elements in the *SOX9* gene (TESCO), and both SRY and SOX9 (in mice) inhibit the β-catenin canonical-signaling pathway and promote Sertoli cell and consequent testicular development. A feed-forward loop involving SF-1 and FGF-9 has been demonstrated in mice which maintains SOX9 expression. FOXL2 "knockout" in mice causes gonadal sex reversal, i.e., ovary to testes suggesting that FOXL2 inhibits SOX9 expression. No human homozygous FOXL2 null mutations have been reported as yet. Duplication of DAX1 or WNT4 results in inhibition of testicular development and atypical genitalia—dysgenetic 46,XY DSD. MAP3K4, mitogen-activated protein kinase 4; CBX2, chromobox homologue 2. It has been suggested that CBX2 is upstream of SRY. More complete understanding of the exact function of MAP3K4 remains to be elucidated.

Compelling evidence that *SRY* is the testis-determining factor is the observation that transfection of the *Sry* gene into 46,XX mouse embryos results in transgenic 46,XX mice with testes and male sex differentiation.

The *SRY* gene encodes a DNA-binding protein that has an 80 amino acid domain similar to that found in high-mobility group (HMG) proteins. This domain binds to DNA in a sequence-specific manner (A/TAACAAT). It bends the DNA and thus is thought to facilitate interaction between DNA-bound proteins to affect the transcription of downstream genes. The human *SRY* gene has no intron; two nuclear localization sites, calmodulin and importin B are critical for the function of the gene. In mice, *Sry* facilitates the upregulation of *Sox9* by binding to multiple enhancing elements in the *Sox9* gene and along with Sf-1 establishes a feed-forward pathway resulting in upregulation of *Sox9* and its continued expression in Sertoli cells. A feed-forward loop involving Sox9 and Fgf9 has also been demonstrated in the mouse but not yet in the human gonad. Both Sry and Sox9 in mice appear to inhibit the Rspo1 (R-spondin 1)-Wnt4-β-catenin-FOXL2 signaling pathway, facilitating Sertoli cell induction and testicular organogenesis and inhibiting ovarian development (see Figure 14–4B). In the absence of Sry, the Wnt4-β-catenin canonical pathway is stabilized and Sox9 is suppressed which results in ovarian development. Hence, it appears that Sry and Sox9 are repressors of a major ovarian determining pathway—Rspo1-Wnt4-β-catenin—which induces ovarian development along with the downstream gene—*Fox L2* and other genes yet to be defined, as well as germ cells which are essential for ovarian development (but not testicular differentiation). Duplications of DAX1 or WNT4 in humans repress testicular development presumably by preventing the repression of β-catenin on its downstream gene FOXL2 by SRY and SOX9. Ovarian determination is a genetically controlled pathway and not, as previously thought, a *default pathway.*

Most of the mutations thus far described in 46,XY females with gonadal dysgenesis have occurred in the nucleotides of the *SRY* gene encoding the DNA-binding region (the HMG box) of the SRY protein. Mutations that affect DNA bending as well as nuclear transportation of the SRY protein have also been implicated in defective testicular development.

SOX9   SOX9 has an HMG box that is more than 60% homologous to that of SRY. It is localized to 17q24.3-q25.1 and is expressed in the developing sex cords and, thereafter, in the Sertoli cells (see Figure 14–4B). It is also expressed in cartilage. Mutations in one allele of the *SOX9* gene can result in a bone abnormality called campomelic dysplasia (CMPD) and XY gonadal dysgenesis with ambiguous genitalia in affected 46,XY males. Duplication of the *SOX9* gene both in humans and mice results in sex reversal in XX individuals who are *SRY* negative. It appears that *SOX9* is the critical gene acting downstream of *SRY* for Sertoli cell differentiation and consequent testicular development.

DHH   Desert hedgehog (DHH), a gene that codes for a signaling molecule located on chromosome 12q13.1 in humans, is an important gene in mammalian testes organogenesis and function. Mutations in DHH have been reported in individuals with 46,XY gonadal dysgenesis.

GATA4   GATA4 is a transcription factor which interacts with other proteins including SF-1 and FOG2 to regulate the expression of SRY. Recently, a heterozygous missense mutation has been described affecting three male siblings and resulting in 46,XY DSD and congenital heart disease.

Genes involved in ovarian determination

DAX1   A mutation or deletion of *DAX1*, which encodes a transcription factor, results in X-linked adrenal hypoplasia congenita and hypogonadotropic hypogonadism in 46,XY males (see Figures 14–2, 14–4B). Deletion or mutation of the *DAX1* gene in 46,XY individuals has not resulted in an abnormality of testicular differentiation in humans. However, XY gonadal dysgenesis has been reported in individuals with duplications of Xp21, a locus that contains the *DAX1* gene on the X chromosome. Duplication of the *DAX1* gene appears not to affect ovarian morphogenesis and function in 46,XX females. Thus, *DAX1* dosage plays a critical role in testicular development and function (see Figure 14–4B).

WNT4   WNT4 is a signaling molecule encoded by a gene located on the short arm of chromosome region 1 (1p35). Duplication of WNT4 has been associated with dysgenetic testicular development and ambiguous genitalia in 46,XY, SRY, positive individuals. Testis development is inhibited likely as a result of upregulation of *DAX1* and stabilization of β-catenin-FOXL2 which would inhibit SOX9 expression in the developing gonad. 46,XY patients who have duplications of WNT4 exhibit a heterogenous phenotype varying from cryptorchidism alone to female external genitalia. *WNT4* is expressed in the primordial ovary and is an essential signal for ovarian determination (see Figure 14–4B). In mice, *Wnt4* expression in the ovary prevents the migration of steroid (androgen)-producing cells into the ovary, restrains the development of a testis-specific blood vessel (the coelomic vessel), and is critical for the development of the Müllerian ducts and the maintenance of germ cells.

A 46,XX female with absent Müllerian structures (atypical Mayer-Rokitansky-Küster-Hauser syndrome) has been reported who had a loss of function mutation in the *WNT4* gene. Her phenotype was similar to that described in *Wnt4*-mutated mice. She had unilateral renal agenesis as well as clinical signs of androgen excess as manifested by severe acne requiring antiandrogen therapy. Wolffian duct development was not ascertained. Two other similar patients have been reported.

RSPO1 (R-spondin 1)   *RSPO1 (R-spondin 1)*, a gene located in 1p34.3, appears to stabilize the expression of WNT4-β-catenin-FOXL2 and thus promotes ovarian determination (see Figure 14–4B). Mutations in *RSPO1* cause 46,XX females to develop testes and male sexual development, as well as palmoplantar hyperkeratosis and a predisposition to squamous cell carcinoma of the skin. The fact that a mutation in RSPO1 can redirect gonadal development in a 46,XX individual from an ovary to a testes suggests that it is a critical determinant in ovarian determination in humans.

FOXL2 is a putative forkhead transcription factor, which does not cause a DSD in human. Heterozygous FOXL2 mutations in affected 46,XX human females causes premature ovarian failure with or without blepharophimosis. However, induced FoxL2 deletions in the ovary of the mouse lead to transdifferentiation of the ovary into testes.

A 46,XY phenotypic female with normal ovaries and a mutation in the *CBX2* (*chromobox homolog 2*) gene, the human homolog of mouse *m33*, an ortholog of the Drosophila *Polycomb* gene, has recently been reported. It was postulated that this gene is upstream of SRY and that mutations in this gene prevent the repression of the ovarian gene pathway presumably by decreasing SRY/SOX9 expression enabling the expression of RSPO1-WNT4-β-catenin-FOXL2 and other ovarian determining genes.

Our lack of complete understanding of ovarian and testicular determination is illustrated in the study by Dumic et al who reported a familial cohort of 46,XY females. A 46,XY female was reported to have undergone spontaneous menarche and given birth to a 46,XY daughter with gonadal dysgenesis. Studies in this cohort have uncovered a mutation in a gene not previously known to be involved in the sex determination cascade—*mitogen-activated protein kinase kinase kinase 4* (*MAP3K4*). Mutations in this gene involved in the mitogen-activated protein kinase signaling pathway cause a striking decrease in the expression of Sry and Sox9 in the developing mouse gonad resulting in sex reversal. Recently, mutations in *MAP3K1* have been reported to 46,XY DSD leading to either partial or complete gonadal dysgenesis. Further studies in humans will be necessary to elucidate the exact mechanism which allows for repression of testicular development and the genesis of an apparently normal functioning ovary in SRY positive 46,XY individuals.

TESTICULAR AND OVARIAN DIFFERENTIATION (FIGURE 14–5)

The mammalian gonad forms on the surface of the mesonephros within the genital ridge as a result of proliferation of the coelomic epithelium. Until the 12-mm stage (~42 days of gestation), the embryonic gonads of males and females are indistinguishable. By 42 days, 300 to 1300 primordial germ cells have seeded the undifferentiated gonad from their extragonadal origin in the yolk sac dorsal endoderm. These large cells are the progenitors of oogonia and spermatogonia; lack of these cells is incompatible with further ovarian differentiation but not testicular differentiation. The undifferentiated gonad also contains supporting cells and steroidogenic cells. Under the influence of *SRY/SOX9* and other genes that encode male sex determination, the gonad begins to differentiate as a testis at 43 to 50 days of gestation. The supporting cells differentiate into pre-Sertoli cells which organize into seminiferous tubules and surround the germ cells which undergo mitotic arrest. Leydig cells derived from steroidogenic cells are apparent by about 60 days, and differentiation of male external genitalia occurs by 65 to 77 days of gestation.

In the undifferentiated gonad destined to be an ovary, lack of further differentiation persists. At 77 to 84 days—long after differentiation of the testis in the male fetus—a significant number of germ cells enter meiotic prophase to characterize the transition of oogonia into oocytes, which marks the onset of ovarian differentiation from the undifferentiated gonads. The supporting cells become granulosa cells and steroidogenic cells become theca cells. Germ cell meiosis in the developing ovary is induced by retinoic acid signaling. Sry induces an enzyme which metabolizes retinoic acid to an inactive product and prevents meiosis of germ cells in the developing testis. Primordial follicles (small oocytes surrounded by a single layer of flat granulosa cells and a basement membrane) are evident after 90 days. Preantral follicles are seen after 6 months, and a population of fully developed oocytes with fluid-filled cavities and multiple layers of granulosa cells are

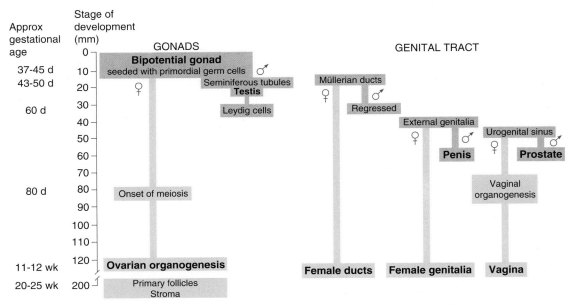

FIGURE 14–5 Schematic sequence of sexual differentiation in the human fetus. Note that testicular differentiation precedes ovarian differentiation. (Reproduced, with permission, from Grumbach MM, Hughes IA, Conte FA. Disorders of sex differentiation. In: Larsen PR, et al, eds. *Williams Textbook of Endocrinology.* 10th ed. WB Saunders; 2003. Modified from Jost A. Hormone factors in sex differentiation of the mammalian fetus. *Philo Trans R Soc Lond Biol.* 1970;259:119.)

present at birth. As opposed to the testes, there is little evidence of hormone production by the fetal ovary.

Differentiation of Genital Ducts (Figure 14–6)

By the seventh week of intrauterine life, the fetus is equipped with the primordia of both male and female genital ducts. The Müllerian ducts, if allowed to persist, form the uterine (fallopian) tubes, the corpus and cervix of the uterus, and the upper third of the vagina. The Wolffian ducts, on the other hand, have the potential for differentiating into the epididymis, vas deferens, seminal vesicles, and ejaculatory ducts of the male. In the presence of a functional testis, the Müllerian ducts undergo apoptosis under the influence of AMH, a dimeric glycoprotein secreted by fetal Sertoli cells. AMH acts locally to cause Müllerian duct repression ipsilaterally. Müllerian duct regression is the earliest indicator of male sex differentiation.

The gene for AMH encodes a 560 amino acid protein, whose carboxyl terminal domain shows marked homology with transforming growth factor-β (TGF-β) and the B chain of inhibin and activin. The gene is localized to the short arm of chromosome 19. AMH is secreted by human fetal and postnatal Sertoli cells and is used as a marker for the presence of these cells. SF-1 (an orphan nuclear receptor) in combination with WT1, SOX9, and GATA4 (Figure 14–7), regulates *AMH* gene expression. The human AMH receptor gene maps to the q13 band of chromosome 12. The receptor is similar to other type II receptors of the TGF-β family.

The differentiation of the Wolffian duct is mediated by testosterone (T) secretion from the testis. SF-1 regulates steroidogenesis by the Leydig cell in the testes by binding to the promoter of the genes encoding P450 side chain cleavage enzyme (P450scc) and 17α-hydroxylase (P450c17). In the presence of an ovary or in the absence of a functional fetal testis, Müllerian duct differentiation occurs, and the Wolffian ducts involute (see Figure 14–6).

Differentiation of External Genitalia (Figure 14–8)

Up to the eighth week of fetal life, the external genitalia of both sexes are identical and have the capacity to differentiate into the genitalia of either sex. Female sex differentiation occurs in the presence of an ovary or streak gonads or if no gonad is present (see Figure 14–8). The fetal ovary does not secrete sex steroids during gestation or AMH during the critical period of female differentiation of the genital ducts and external genitalia. Studies in the past have indicated that the fetal adrenal gland is 3β-HSD-2 (3 beta-hydroxysteroid dehydrogenase-2) deficient and secretes primarily DHEA-S (dehydroepiandrosterone sulfate) until late in gestation. DHEA-S is converted by the placenta to DHEA which is metabolized to T. T is aromatized to estrogen, thereby preventing the exposure of the female external genitalia to high levels of T/dihydrotestosterone (DHT). Placental aromatase activity is low from 8 to 12 weeks of gestation but increases markedly after the first trimester (Figure 14–9). Recent studies indicate that the normal

female genitalia are protected from androgen exposure early in gestation (8-12 weeks), a stage when placental aromatase activity is relatively low. Sex differentiation of the external genitalia is occurring by the transient expression of 3β-HSD-2 in the fetal adrenal, resulting in cortisol secretion, and consequently relative suppression of both adrenocorticotropin (ACTH) and DHEA-S secretion with a resultant decrease in placental testosterone synthesis and secretion. Adrenally derived androgen levels appear to be the same during this period in both males and females. After 12 weeks of gestation, 3β-HSD-2 activity diminishes in the fetal adrenal which leads to an increase in ACTH and DHEA-S secretion. Testosterone is now converted by the increased placental aromatase to estrogen. In addition, androgen receptor activity diminishes in the labioscrotal folds, and excess androgen exposure after 12 to 14 weeks gestation results in only clitoromegaly, but not labioscrotal fusion. Thus, the transient expression of 3β-HSD-2 and the consequent ability of the fetal adrenal gland to transiently synthesize cortisol, as well as the decrease in androgen receptor activity in genital skin protects the female external genitalia from masculinization during the window of dimorphic differentiation of the external genitalia.

Differentiation of the external genitalia along male lines depends on the action of DHT, the 5α-reduced metabolite of T. In the male fetus, T is secreted by the Leydig cells, autonomously at first and later under the influence of human chorionic gonadotropin (hCG), and later fetal pituitary luteinizing hormone (LH). Masculinization of the external genitalia and urogenital sinus of the fetus results from the action of DHT, which is synthesized from T in the target cells by the enzyme 5α-reductase-2 as well as possibly secreted by the testes via the *backdoor pathway* (Figure 14–10). This pathway was first found in marsipials and then implicated in patients with P450 oxidoreductase (POR) deficiency. This backdoor pathway synthesizes DHT, a nonaromatized androgen, without utilizing T as a precursor. This pathway may play a signifcant role in male differentiation; however, further studies are necessary to define this.

DHT (as well as T) is bound to a specific protein receptor in the nucleus of the target cell (Figure 14–11). The transformed steroid-receptor complex dimerizes and binds with high affinity to specific DNA domains, initiating DNA-directed, RNA-mediated transcription. This results in androgen-induced proteins that lead to differentiation and growth of the cell. The gene that encodes the intracellular androgen-binding protein has been localized to the paracentromeric portion of the long arm of the X chromosome (see Figure 14–2). Of note, an X-linked gene controls the androgen response of all somatic cell types by specifying the androgen receptor protein. As noted previously, there is a decrease in androgen receptor activity in the labioscrotal folds after 12 to 14 weeks so that even with intense T/DHT stimulation, labioscrotal fusion does not occur although growth of the genital tubercle can continue resulting in clitoromegaly in females and penile enlargement in males.

Incomplete masculinization of the male fetus results from (1) impairment in the synthesis or secretion of fetal T and/or DHT (3α-HSD-3 deficiency) or the conversion of T to DHT

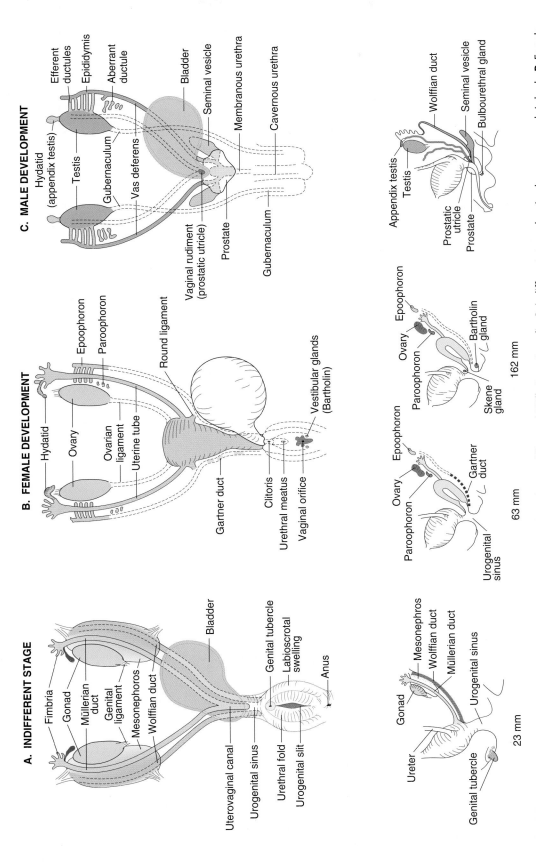

FIGURE 14–6 Embryonic differentiation of male and female genital ducts from Wolffian and Müllerian primordia. **A.** Indifferent stage showing large mesonephric body. **B.** Female ducts. Remnants of the mesonephros and Wolffian ducts are now termed the epoophoron, paroophoron, and Gartner duct. **C.** Male ducts before descent into the scrotum. The only Müllerian remnant is the testicular appendix. The prostatic utricle (vagina masculina) is derived from the urogenital sinus. (Modified from Corning HK, Lehrbuch der Entwicklungsgeschichte des Menschen, JF Bergmann, Munich, 1921; and Wilkins L. The diagnosis and treatment of endocrine disorders. In: Charles C, ed. *Childhood and Adolescence.* 3rd ed. Thomas Publishers; 1965.)

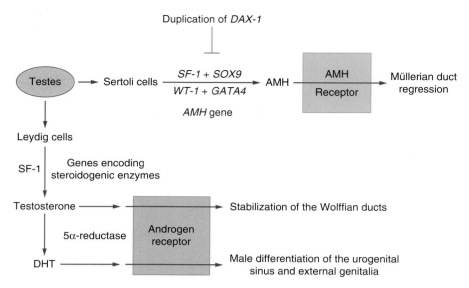

FIGURE 14–7 Hypothetical diagrammatic cascade of major genes involved in male sex differentiation (*DAX1*, DSS-AHC-critical on the X chromosome gene 1; GATA4, transcription factor; SF-1, steroidogenic factor 1; *SOX9*, *SRY homeobox gene 9*; *WT1*, *Wilms tumor suppressor gene*). (Modified from Grumbach MM, Hughes IA, Conte FA. Disorders of sex differentiation. In: Larsen PR, et al, eds. *Williams Textbook of Endocrinology*. 10th ed. WB Saunders; 2003: 842-1002.)

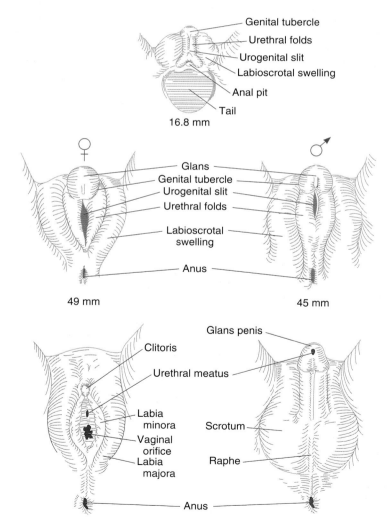

FIGURE 14–8 Differentiation of male and female external genitalia from bipotential primordia. (Adapted from Spaulding MH. The development of the external genitalia in the human embryo. *Contrib Embryol*. [Carnegie Institute of Washington] 1921;13:69-88,. Reproduced with permission from Grumbach MM, Hughes IA, Conte FA. Disorders of sex differentiation. In: Larsen PR, et al, eds. *Williams Textbook of Endocrinology*. 10th ed. WB Saunders, 2003.)

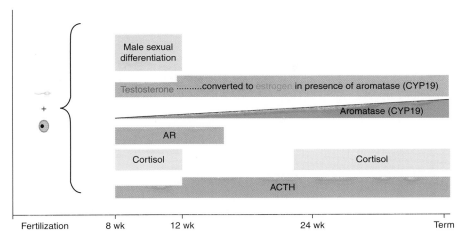

FIGURE 14–9 Sex differentiation of the external genitalia of males is induced by dihydrotestosterone (DHT) which is synthesized in the cells of the external genitalia from fetal testicular testosterone by the enzyme 5alpha-reductase-2. DHT may also be produced via the "back door pathway". Male differentiation of the external genitalia occurs from 8 to 12 weeks of gestation when aromatase activity of the liver and placenta is relatively low. During this *critical window* of dimorphic sexual differentiation, the fetal adrenal transiently expresses 3β-HSD-2, resulting in adrenal secretion of cortisol and a consequent downregulation of fetal ACTH and T precursor (DHEA-S) secretion from the fetal adrenal as well as putative adrenal testosterone secretion. Thus, the female external genitalia are protected from T/DHT exposure and virilization during this period when aromatase activity is low. After 12 weeks of gestation, 3β-HSD-2 activity in the adrenal is extinguished until 24 weeks of gestation resulting in an increase in DHEA-S (T precursor) from the fetal adrenal. However, increased placental aromatase activity and a decrease in androgen receptor activity in the labioscrotal folds of 46,XX females occurs so that excess T/DHT exposure after 12 weeks of gestation results only in clitoromegaly. (Modified from Hanley NA, Arlt W. The human fetal adrenal cortex and the window of sexual differentiation. *Trends Endocrinol Metab.* 2006;17:391.)

(5α-reductase-2 deficiency, (2) deficient or defective androgen receptor activity, or (3) defective production and local action of AMH.

PSYCHOSEXUAL DIFFERENTIATION

Psychosexual differentiation can be classified into four broad categories: (1) gender identity, defined as the identification of self as either male or female; (2) gender role (ie, those aspects of behavior in which males and females differ from one another in one's culture at this time); (3) gender orientation, the choice of sexual partner; and (4) cognitive differences.

For much of the past 50 years, the prevailing dogma has been that newborns are born psychosexually neutral and that gender identity is imprinted postnatally by words, attitudes, family dynamics, and comparisons of one's body with that of others. Gender identity had been hypothesized to be neutral at birth and not established until 12 to 18 months of age. During the last decade, this hypothesis has been rigorously challenged. It has become evident that prenatal exposure to T/DHT and possibly genes on the Y chromosome can influence gender identity in the individual with a DSD. A growing body of evidence indicates that gender identity is more plastic than previously thought. If, at puberty, discordant secondary sexual characteristics are allowed to mature, some individuals, especially those with 5α-reductase deficiency, 45,X/46,XY mosaicism, or 17β-HSD-3 deficiency, have had doubts about their gender identity and have chosen to change their assigned sex from female to male . However, in general, it has been demonstrated that most patients with DSD (except for those mentioned above) will accept their gender assignment even when it is not concordant with their sex chromosome constitution—a phenomenon which underscores both the complexity and plasticity of the processes that determine gender identity. This suggests that androgens have a *facultative* and not a *deterministic* role in gender identity. Androgens have a significant effect on childhood play behavior, maternal interest, and sexual orientation. It is apparent that both genes and hormones (nature) and environment and experience (nurture) are critical factors in the development and maintenance of gender identity. Further studies on patients with ambiguous genitalia, including long-term outcomes of the factors influencing gender identity, gender role, and sexual activity in DSD patients, are critical to furthering our understanding of the multifaceted complexities of the differentiation of gender identity and to support more evidence-based guidelines for decisions about sex assignment.

CLASSIFICATION AND NOMENCLATURE OF DISORDERS OF SEX DETERMINATION (AND DIFFERENTIATION) (TABLE 14–1)

An International Conference on Management of Intersex was held in Chicago, Illinois, in 2005 because of ethical issues and patient

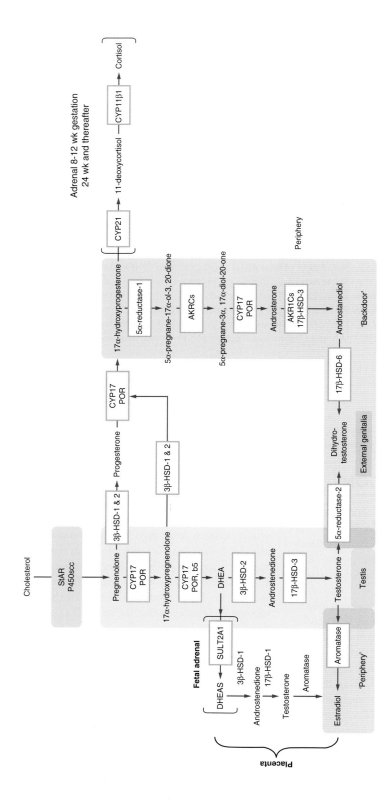

FIGURE 14–10 The enzymatic pathway of testosterone synthesis in the adrenal and testes is shown in blue on the left. A backdoor pathway first described by Wilson and Auchus from studies in marsupials is shown on the right. This pathway utilizes 17-OH progesterone to synthesize dihydrotestosterone independent of testosterone synthesis. The backdoor pathway as well as traditional testosterone synthesis by the fetal testis may be essential for normal male external genitalia differentiation. It has been suggested that virilization in 46,XX individuals with CAH (such as 21-hydroxylase, 11-hydroxylase, P450 oxidoreductase, and possibly 3β-HSD-2 deficiency) who have elevated levels of 17-OH progesterone in utero may involve DHT synthesis via the backdoor pathway. The fetal adrenal is relatively 3β-HSD-2 deficient from 12 to 24 weeks of gestation and DHEA-S is primarily secreted and converted in the liver to 16-OH DHEAS. DHEA-S is converted by placental sulfatase to DHEA which then is metabolized to T and subsequently to estradiol by placental aromatase. Similarly, 16OH-DHEAS is aromatized to estriol. Androstenedione can be directly converted to estrone by (3α-HSD-3 (AKRCs), 3-alpha-hydroxysteroid dehydrogenase-3; b5, cytochrome b5; 3β-HSD-1, 3-beta-hydroxysteroid dehydrogenase type 1; 3β-HSD-2, 3-beta-hydroxysteroid dehydrogenase type 2; 17β-HSD-1, 17-beta hydroxysteroid dehydrogenase type 1; 17β-HSD-3, 17-beta-hydroxysteroid dehydrogenase type 3; CY17, CYP21, 21 hydroxylase; CYP11B1, 11 hydroxylase;17hydroxylase;17hydroxylase; DHEA, dehydroepiandrosterone; P450scc, P450 side chain cleavage; POR, P450 oxidoreductase; StAR, steroidogenic acute regulatory protein; Sulf2A1, sulfatase).

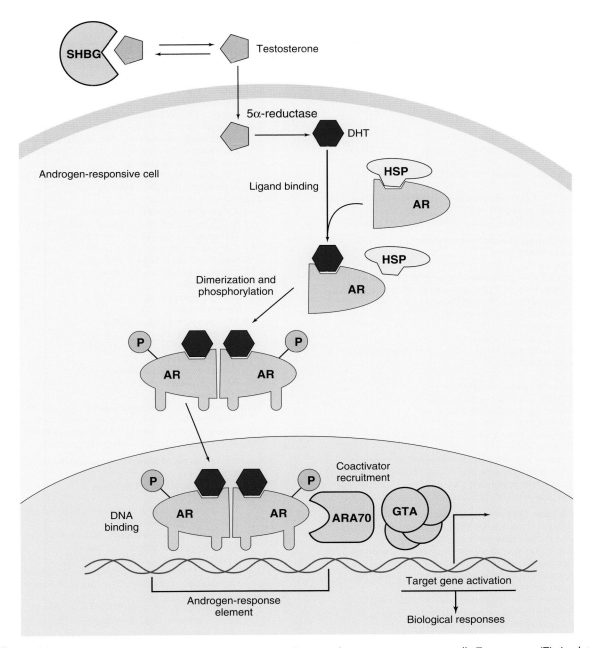

FIGURE 14–11 Diagrammatic representation of the mechanism of action of testosterone on target cells. Testosterone (T) circulates in association with sex hormone–binding globulin (SHBG) but dissociates to enter the cells, where it is either 5α-reduced to dihydrotestosterone (DHT) or aromatized to estradiol (E2). Dihydrotestosterone binds to the androgen receptor (AR) in the cytoplasm and activates it with the release of heat shock proteins (HSP). The activated AR complex is then translocated to the nucleus, where it binds as a dimer to specific hormone response elements of the DNA and, along with coactivators (eg, ARA), initiates transcription, leading to protein synthesis with consequent androgenic effects. (Redrawn and modified from Feldman BJ, Feldman D. The development of androgen-independent prostate cancer. *Nat Rev Cancer.* 2001;1:34.)

concerns about the venerable but antiquated terms *intersex, pseudohermaphrodite, true hermaphrodite,* and so forth, which were perceived by patients as pejorative. A new nomenclature was proposed and accepted. The term, disorders of sexual development (DSD), connoting all conditions in which chromosomal, gonadal, or anatomic sex are atypical, was coined. (See Lee PA et al for the complete consensus statement.)

DSDs are the result of abnormalities in complex processes that originate in genetic information on the X and Y chromosomes as well as on the autosomes. A 46,XY DSD (previously male hermaphrodite) is one whose gonads are exclusively testes in origin but whose genital ducts or external genitalia (or both) exhibit incomplete masculinization. A 46,XX DSD (previously female hermaphrodite) is a person whose gonadal tissue is exclusively

TABLE 14–1   Classification of disorders of sex development.

I. Sex chromosome DSD (disorders of gonadal differentiation)
- A. Seminiferous tubule dysgenesis and its variants (Klinefelter syndrome) : 46,XX testicular DSD
  1. 46,XX males, SRY positive
  2. 46,XX males, SRY negative
  3. SOX9 duplication
  4. RSPO1 mutation
  5. SOX3 mutation
- B. Syndrome of gonadal dysgenesis and its variants (Turner syndrome)
- C. Complete and incomplete forms of XX and XY gonadal dysgenesis
- D. Individuals with both testicular and ovarian tissue: ovotesticular DSD (true hermaphroditism[a])
- E. 46,XY ovarian DSD–Fertile 46,XY female; MAP3K4 mutation

II. 46,XX DSD (female pseudohermaphrodism[a])
- A. Androgen induced
  1. Fetal source
     a. Congenital virilizing adrenal hyperplasia (defective 21-hydroxylation, 11β-hydroxylation, 3β-hydroxysteroid dehydrogenase-2, P450 oxidoreductase (POR))
     b. Glucocorticoid receptor mutation
  2. Fetoplacental source
     a. P450 aromatase deficiency
     b. P450 oxidoreductase deficiency (affecting aromatase)
  3. Maternal source
     a. Iatrogenic
        i. Testosterone and related steroids
        ii. Certain synthetic oral progestagens
     b. Virilizing ovarian or adrenal tumor
     c. Virilizing luteoma of pregnancy
     d. Congenital virilizing adrenal hyperplasia in mother[b]
- B. Non–androgen-induced
  1. Disturbances in differentiation of urogenital structures associated with malformations of intestine and lower urinary tract (non–androgen-induced XX, DSD) (eg, cloacal anomalies, Müllerian agenesis [MURCS], vaginal atresia, labial adhesions)

III. 46, XY DSD (male pseudohermaphrodism[a])
- A. hCG/LH receptor mutation (Leydig cell agenesis or hypoplasia)
- B. Inborn errors of testosterone biosynthesis
  1. Enzyme deficits affecting synthesis of both corticosteroids and testosterone (variants of congenital adrenal hyperplasia)
     a. StAR deficiency (congenital lipoid adrenal hyperplasia): side chain (P450scc) cleavage deficiency
     b. 3β-Hydroxysteroid dehydrogenase-2 deficiency
     c. P450c17 (17α-hydroxylase) deficiency
     d. P450 oxidoreductase deficiency
     e. 7-dehydrocholesterol reductase deficiency (Smith-Lemli-Opitz syndrome)
  2. Enzyme defects primarily affecting testosterone biosynthesis by the testes
     a. P450c17 (17,20-lyase) deficiency
     b. 17β-Hydroxysteroid dehydrogenase-3 deficiency

3. Enzyme defects affecting DHT synthesis
   a. 5α-Reductase-2 deficiency (pseudovaginal perineoscrotal hypospadias) (peripheral)
- C. Defects in androgen-dependent target tissues
  1. End-organ resistance to androgenic hormones (androgen receptor and postreceptor defects)
     a. Syndrome of complete androgen resistance and its variants (testicular feminization and its variant forms)
     b. Syndrome of partial androgen resistance and its variants (Reifenstein syndrome)
     c. Androgen resistance in infertile men
     d. Androgen resistance in fertile men
- D. Dysgenetic 46,XY DSD
  1. XY gonadal dysgenesis (incomplete)
  2. XO/XY mosaicism, SRY mutation structurally abnormal Y chromosome, Xp+ (DAX-1 dupl.), 9p–, 10q–
  3. Denys-Drash, Frasier syndrome (WT-1 mutation)
  4. WAGR syndrome (WT-1 deletion)
  5. Campomelic dysplasia (SOX9 mutation)
  6. SF-1 mutation
  7. WNT-4 duplication
  8. DHH (mutation)
  9. ATRX syndrome (XH2 mutation)
  10. ARX mutation
  11. CBX2 mutation[c]
  12. MAP3K4 mutation
  13. Testicular regression syndrome
  14. GATA4 mutation
  15. FOG2 mutation
- E. Defects in synthesis, secretion, or response to AMH
  1. Female genital ducts in otherwise normal men—*herniae uteri inguinale*; persistent Müllerian duct syndrome
- F. Environmental chemicals (endocrine disrupters)

IV. Unclassified forms of disorders of sexual development
- A. In males
  1. Hypospadias: MAMLD-1 mutation
  2. Aphallia
  3. Ambiguous external genitalia in 46,XY males with multiple congenital anomalies
  4. Intrauterine growth retardation with incomplete masculinization of external genitalia
  5. Cloacal exstrophy
  6. Panoply of syndromes associated with incomplete masculinization of external genitalia (Robinow, Aarskog, hand-foot-genital, etc)
- B. In females
  1. Absence or anomalous development of the vagina, uterus, and Müllerian ducts (Mayer-Rokitansky-Küster-Hauser [MRKH] syndrome) (WNT-4 mutation rare)

[a]These terms are previous terminology and are no longer recommended; they should be abandoned. They are listed in parentheses during this transition period.

[b]In pregnant patient with CAH whose disorder is poorly controlled or who is noncompliant especially during the first trimester.

[c]The patient reported had strikingly elevated gonadotropins in infancy and only sparse primordial follicles on biopsy at 4 years of age suggesting gonadal dysgenesis.

Modified from Grumbach MM, Conte FA. Disorders of sex differentiation. In: Wilson JD, Foster DW, Kronenberg HM, Larsen PR, eds. *Williams Textbook of Endocrinology*. 9th ed. WB Saunders; 1998: 1303-1425.

ovarian in origin but whose genital development exhibits ambiguous or even a male appearance. Persons who possess both ovarian and testicular tissue were previously referred to as true hermaphrodites and now called ovotesticular DSD.

KLINEFELTER SYNDROME AND ITS VARIANTS: SEMINIFEROUS TUBULE DYSGENESIS—SEX CHROMOSOME DSD (SEE ALSO CHAPTER 12)

Klinefelter syndrome is one of the most common forms of primary hypogonadism and infertility in males. Surveys of the prevalence of 47,XXY fetuses by karyotype analysis of unselected newborn infants indicate a prevalence of about 1:700 newborn males. However, there is a striking disparity between the prevalence diagnosed at birth by karyotype screening and the frequency of Klinefelter syndrome identified in adults. It has been estimated that only 25% of individuals with Klinefelter syndrome are diagnosed during life and less than 10% in childhood. This most likely is due to the broad spectrum of phenotypes, testicular function, and psychosocial status found in patients with this syndrome. Ninety percent of affected patients have a 47,XXY sex chromosome constitution and an X chromatin-positive buccal smear, the rest demonstrate a variety of sex chromosome constitutions, including mosaicism. Virtually all of these variants have at least two X chromosomes and a Y chromosome in common, except for the rare group that has only an XX sex chromosome complement (3%-4%).

Hormonal levels are variable, and T levels may be in the low-normal to normal range. In addition, variability in phenotype can result in part from sex chromosome mosaicism with a normal XY cell line as well as variability in androgen sensitivity. The androgen receptor is a ligand-dependent transcription factor that has a polymorphism involving CAG (glutamine) trinucleotide repeats. The longer the length of the CAG repeat, the less the transactivation activity of the ligand-bound receptor. In a study of 35 patients with Klinefelter syndrome, the one genetic factor affecting phenotype was the CAG repeat length of the functional androgen receptor. The repeat lengths correlated inversely with penile length, a T-sensitive organ. Neither an effect of parental origin of the X chromosome (imprinting) nor evidence of skewed X chromosome inactivation affected the phenotype. In a study of 77 patients with Klinefelter syndrome, preferential inactivation of the shorter CAG allele was detected.

The most consistent feature of Klinefelter syndrome is small atrophic testes due to seminiferous tubule dysgenesis and consequent azoospermia. Tall stature is common in Klinefelter syndrome, reflecting the presence of three *SHOX* genes. Adult males with a 47, XXY karyotype tend to be taller than average, with adult height close to the 75th percentile, mainly because of the disproportionate length of their legs, which is present prepubertally. Untreated adult males, especially those with subnormal sex steroid levels, are at increased risk of osteoporosis. In addition, individuals with Klinefelter syndrome have an increased prevalence of

mild diabetes mellitus, autoimmune thyroid disorders, early tooth decay, varicose veins, stasis dermatitis, cerebrovascular disease, chronic pulmonary disease, deep vein thrombosis, carcinoma of the breast, midline germ cell tumors, and Hodgkin lymphoma. The data on carcinoma of the breast are controversial. There were no cases in a cohort of 696 men with Klinefelter syndrome from the Danish cytogenetic register; however, 7 of 93 men with breast cancer in a Swedish study had Klinefelter syndrome. Life expectancy is reduced by about 2.1 years over controls, with a lower death rate than expected from ischemic heart disease and prostate cancer.

Prepubertally, Klinefelter syndrome is characterized by small undescended testes (> 25% of patients), relatively reduced penile length, clinodactyly, hypotonia, disproportionately long legs, personality and behavioral disorders, and a lower mean verbal IQ score. There is no significant difference in full-scale IQ. Deficits are found primarily in specific areas of cognition such as language and problem solving. Severe mental retardation requiring special schooling is uncommon. Gynecomastia and signs of androgen deficiency such as diminished facial and body hair, a small phallus, and poor muscular development occur postpubertally in affected patients.

Patients with Klinefelter syndrome may have delayed adolescence although a recent study suggested that the onset of puberty and early progression were relatively normal. There is an increased risk of malignant extragonadal germ cell tumors in the central nervous system, mediastinum, and sacral region. The germ cell tumors often secrete hCG and cause sexual precocity in the affected prepubertal individual. Accordingly, we recommend that boys with hCG-secreting midline germ cell tumors have a karyotype analysis.

The testicular lesion is progressive and gonadotropin dependent. Gonadal germ cells become depleted at an accelerated rate after the onset of puberty, and there appears to be a maturation arrest of spermatogenesis. The testes are characterized in the adult by extensive seminiferous tubular hyalinization and fibrosis, absent or severely deficient spermatogenesis, and pseudoadenomatous clumping of the Leydig cells. Although hyalinization of the tubules is usually extensive, it varies considerably from patient to patient and even between testes in the same patient. Azoospermia is the rule; patients reported to be spontaneously fertile invariably have been 46,XY/47,XXY mosaics. Using surgical techniques, sperm has been found in 50% of the *nonmosaic* patients with Klinefelter syndrome. In biopsied testes of patients with 47,XXY Klinefelter syndrome, only a minor fraction of tubules contain germ cells. FISH analysis revealed that the spermatocytes were euploid, suggesting that the spermatogonia that undergo mitosis have only one X chromosome thus allowing for progression in cell differentiation and the ability to engage in meiosis. Intracytoplasmic sperm injection (ICSI) with sperm retrieved surgically from testes (TESE) of patients with Klinefelter syndrome has been used with success for ovum fertilization. Using ICSI, most infants born to fathers with Klinefelter syndrome have had normal karyotypes. However, there is an increased incidence of sex chromosome and autosomal aneuploidy, possibly related to the assisted fertility technique (ART). Preimplantation genetic diagnosis (PGD) is recommended. However, the potential risk to the embryo of PGD must be weighed against the risk of chorionic villus biopsy or amniocentesis in the event of a successful pregnancy.

Nondisjunction during the first or second meiotic division of gametogenesis plays an important role in the genesis of a 47,XXY karyotype. Fifty-three percent of cases appear to result from paternal nondisjunction at the first meiotic division, 34% from meiotic nondisjunction during the first maternal meiotic division, and 9% from nondisjunction at the second meiotic division. Only 3% of patients appear to have arisen from postzygotic mitotic nondisjunction. Early studies suggested that parental age was a factor in the etiology of Klinefelter syndrome, but in a study of 228 patients, no association with advanced parental age was found.

Diagnosis: Klinefelter syndrome is suggested by the classic phenotype and hormonal changes. It is confirmed by the finding of an X chromatin-positive buccal smear or an FISH analysis which demonstrates an XXY constitution or the demonstration of a 47,XXY karyotype in blood, skin, or gonads. After puberty, levels of serum gonadotropins especially follicle-stimulating hormone (FSH) are raised. The T production rate, the total and free levels of T, and the metabolic clearance rates of T and estradiol tend to be low, whereas plasma estradiol levels are relatively normal or high for a male. Testicular biopsy reveals the classic findings of hyalinization of the seminiferous tubules, severe deficiency of spermatogonia, and pseudoadenomatous clumping of Leydig cells.

Hormonal evaluation in the newly diagnosed patient with Klinefelter syndrome should include plasma LH and FSH by immunochemiluminescence (ICMA). These levels are usually in the normal range prior to the onset of puberty. Thereafter, a rise in FSH and subsequently LH is usually observed. A plasma estradiol and T by liquid chromatography-tandem mass spectrometry (LCMSMS) should be obtained. In the adolescent or postadolescent patient, a bone density is indicated to determine whether the patient has osteopenia/osteoporosis and requires therapy for this.

Treatment: Treatment in adolescents and adults with Klinefelter syndrome should be directed toward health maintenance and the options for fertility (eg, cryopreservation of sperm from ejaculate in adolescence or TESE in older patients, T replacement if necessary, and prevention of osteopenia/osteoporosis and deep vein thrombosis). Klinefelter patients are born with spermatogonia, and testicular failure is progressive beginning at puberty. Obtaining ejaculated sperm in early adolescence for cryopreservation, if possible, might obviate the need for TESE at a later time. Although several studies have reported that sperm have been found in 8% of ejaculated serum sample fron nonmosaic 47,XXY patients, a recent study reported lack of sperm in samples from 13 patients less than 20 years of age. Because of the progressive nature of testicular failure which occurs after the onset of puberty, surgical sperm retrieval is less successful with advancing age. T therapy in the hypogonadal patient will enhance secondary sexual characteristics and sexual performance, increase muscle mass, prevent or help ameliorate osteopenia/osteoporosis and possibly prevent the development of gynecomastia. If T deficiency is evident in adolescence, therapy with T enanthate in oil at a dose of 50 mg intramuscularly monthly may be initiated. Alternatively, testosterone by patch or gel may be used. The plasma concentration of T can be assessed midway between injections, and

the doses gradually increased to attain a level in the mid-normal range for stage of development and/or age.

In the adult patient, transdermal T by patch or gel can be used for replacement therapy. T levels can be assessed 1 week after the start of therapy and adjusted to maintain levels in the mid-normal range for age. Patients should be informed of the possibility of deep vein thrombosis and the T discontinued if the hematocrit rises above 54% because of the risk of hypercoagulability associated with elevated hematocrit levels. If gynecomastia is present and is not ameliorated by T therapy, surgical reduction is required if it is psychologically disturbing to the patient.

Early diagnosis with remedial therapy for speech and behavior problems, counseling for the patient and parents, as well as support group services appears to improve the well being and overall quality of life in patients diagnosed with Klinefelter syndrome.

Variants of Chromatin-Positive Seminiferous Tubule Dysgenesis

Variants of Klinefelter syndrome   Variants of Klinefelter syndrome include 46,XY/47,XXY mosaics as well as patients with multiple X and Y chromosomes. With increasing numbers of X chromosomes in the genome, both mental retardation and other developmental anomalies such as radioulnar synostosis become prevalent.

46,XX males (46,XX testicular DSD)   Phenotypic males with a 46,XX karyotype have been described since 1964; the incidence of 46,XX males is approximately 1:20,000 births. In general, these individuals have a male phenotype, male psychosocial gender identity, and testes with histologic features similar to those observed in patients with a 47,XXY karyotype. At least 10% of patients have hypospadias or ambiguous external genitalia, primarily those patients who are SRY negative. 46,XX males have normal body proportions and a mean final height that is shorter than that of patients with a 47,XXY sex chromosome constitution or normal males but taller than that of normal females. There is a higher incidence of undescended testes in 46,XX males than in 47,XXY patients. As in 47,XXY individuals, T levels are low or low-normal, gonadotropins are elevated, and spermatogenesis is impaired postpubertally. Gynecomastia is more frequent than that observed in 47,XXY males.

Males with a 46,XX karyotype have acquired one X chromosome from each of their parents. Approximately 90% of XX males have a Y chromosome–specific DNA segment from the distal portion of the Y short arm translocated to the distal portion of the short arm of the paternal X chromosome. This translocated segment is variable in length but always includes the *SRY* gene, which encodes testis-determining factor as well as the pseudoautosomal region of the Y chromosome. Thus, in at least 90% of XX males, an abnormal X-Y terminal exchange during paternal meiosis has resulted in two products: an X chromosome with an *SRY* gene and a Y chromosome deficient in this gene (the latter would result in a female with XY gonadal dysgenesis). Fewer than 10% of XX males tested have lacked Y chromosome–specific DNA sequences (including the *SRY* gene) and the pseudoautosomal region of the Y chromosome. These XX, SRY-negative males tend to have hypospadias and may have relatives with ovotesticular DSD.

The finding of XX males who lack any evidence of Y chromosome–specific genes suggests that testicular determination—and, thus, male differentiation—can occur in the absence of a gene or genes from the Y chromosome. This could be a result of (1) mutation (upregulation) or duplication of a *downstream* autosomal gene involved in male sex determination (eg, SOX9 which if duplicated in a 46,XX individual causes sex reversal both in mice and humans); or (2) mutation, deletion, or aberrant inactivation of a gene sequence, which causes repression of testis determination. Two families with multiple 46,XX phenotypically normal males who had palmoplantar hyperkeratosis and a predisposition to squamous cell carcinomas have been reported. All affected males had a homozygous deletion of 2700 base pairs of the *R-spondin1* gene. *RSPO1*, an ovary-determining gene, has no role in testes determination as evidenced by the description of a 46,XY male with a homozygous mutation of *RSPO1* who had normal testicular function; or (3) circumscribed Y chromosome mosaicism (eg, occurring only in the gonads); (4) A 46,XX SRY negative male has recently been described with a mutation in SOX3. SOX3 is a member of the SRY HMG box family of genes and is found on the X chromosome at Xp26-27. This mutation is postulated to cause aberrant expression of SOX3 in gonadal primordia and thereby upregulating SOX9 expression resulting in testicular determination.

SYNDROME OF GONADAL DYSGENESIS: TURNER SYNDROME AND ITS VARIANTS

Turner Syndrome: 45,X Gonadal Dysgenesis

One in 2000 to 2500 newborn females have an absence of a second sex chromosome (either an X or Y), a structural rearrangement of the X chromosome, and/or mosaicism. Patients with a 45,X karyotype represent approximately 50% of all patients with X chromosome abnormalities. It has been estimated that 99% of 45,X fetuses do not survive beyond 28 weeks of gestation probably related to congenital heart anomalies, and 15% of all first-trimester abortuses have a 45,X karyotype. In about 70% to 80% of 45,X individuals, the X chromosome is of maternal origin.

The cardinal features of 45,X gonadal dysgenesis are a variety of somatic anomalies, sexual infantilism at puberty secondary to gonadal dysgenesis, and short stature. Patients with a 45,X karyotype can be recognized in infancy, usually because of lymphedema of the extremities and loose skin folds over the nape of the neck. In later life, the typical patient is often recognizable by her distinctive facies in which micrognathia, epicanthal folds, prominent low-set ears, a fish-like mouth, and ptosis are present to varying degrees. The chest is shield-like, and the neck is short, broad, and webbed (40% of patients). Additional anomalies associated with Turner syndrome include renal abnormalities (30%), pigmented nevi, cubitus valgus, congenital hip subluxation, a tendency to keloid formation, lymphedema of the lower extremities or puffiness of the dorsum of the hands and feet, short fourth metacarpals and metatarsals, Madelung deformity of the wrist, scoliosis, and

recurrent otitis media, which may lead to conductive hearing loss. The high prevalence of otitis media is a consequence of an abnormal relationship between the Eustachian tube and the middle ear. Sensorineural hearing loss increases with age and is present in 61% of women with Turner syndrome over 35 years of age. All patients should have routine periodic auditory screening.

Patients with Turner syndrome have an increased prevalence of cardiovascular anomalies. The incidence of bicuspid aortic valves diagnosed by echocardiography has varied between 9% and 34%. A bicuspid aortic valve is a risk factor for subacute bacterial endocarditis. With age there is an increased tendency for a stenotic and/or insufficient aortic valve. Coarctation of the aorta is present in 10% of patients, especially individuals with a webbed neck. Bicuspid aortic valves, coarctation, aortic dilation, and hypertension are critical risk factors for aneurysm formation and death due to aortic rupture. Thus, all patients with Turner syndrome should have a complete cardiac evaluation by a cardiologist at diagnosis as well as periodic follow-up echocardiography or magnetic resonance imaging (MRI) as necessary to monitor aortic diameter and cardiovascular status. Routine intravenous urography or renal sonography is indicated to detect a surgically correctable renal abnormality. The most common renal anomalies are a horseshoe kidney, duplication of the renal pelvis and ureter, and hydronephrosis secondary to uteropelvic obstruction. Complete absence of a kidney and gross renal ectopia have been reported. The internal ducts as well as the external genitalia of these patients are invariably female except in rare patients with a 45,X karyotype, in whom a Y-to-autosome or Y-to-X chromosome translocation or cryptic mosaicism for a Y-containing cell line has been found.

Short stature is an invariable feature of the syndrome of gonadal dysgenesis. Mean final height in 45,X patients is 143 cm, with a range of 133 to 153 cm. Short stature found in patients with the syndrome of gonadal dysgenesis is not due to a deficiency of growth hormone (GH), insulin-like growth factor I (IGF-I), sex steroids, or thyroid hormone. It is related, at least in part, to haploinsufficiency of the *SHOX* gene in the pseudoautosomal region of the X and Y chromosome (see earlier sections). The administration of high-dose recombinant human GH leads to an increase in final height.

Gonadal dysgenesis is a cardinal feature of patients with a 45,X chromosome constitution. The gonads at adolescence are typically streak-like and usually contain only fibrous stroma arranged in whorls. Longitudinal studies of both basal and gonadotropin-releasing hormone (GnRH)-evoked gonadotropin secretion in patients with gonadal dysgenesis indicate a lack of feedback inhibition of the hypothalamic-pituitary axis by the dysgenetic gonads in affected infants and adolescents (Figure 14–12). Plasma and urinary gonadotropin levels, particularly FSH levels, are high during early infancy and after 9 to 10 years of age. Because ovarian function is impaired, puberty does not usually ensue spontaneously; sexual infantilism is a hallmark of this syndrome. Rarely, patients with a 45,X karyotype may undergo spontaneous pubertal maturation, menarche, and even pregnancy. It has been suggested that measurable levels of inhibin B may indicate the presence of functional follicles and the possibility of spontaneous pubertal development while low levels of AMH might herald ovarian failure. A variety of other disorders are associated with this

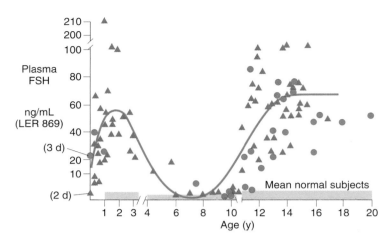

FIGURE 14-12 Diphasic variation in basal levels of plasma follicle-stimulating hormone (FSH) (ng/mL-LER 869) in patients with a 45,X karyotype (solid triangles) and patients with structural abnormalities of the X chromosome and mosaics (solid circles). Note that mean basal levels of plasma FSH in patients with gonadal dysgenesis are in the castrate range before 4 years and after 10 years of age. (Reproduced with permission from Conte FA, Grumbach MM, Kaplan SL. A diphasic pattern of gonadotropin secretion in patients with the syndrome of gonadal dysgenesis. *J Clin Endocrinol Metab*. 1975;40:670.)

syndrome, including obesity, nonosteoporotic fractures in childhood and osteoporotic fractures in adulthood, congenital dislocation of the hip, type 2 diabetes mellitus, an increased number of melanocytic nevi but no increase in melanoma, orthodontic problems, Hashimoto thyroiditis, rheumatoid arthritis, inflammatory bowel disease, intestinal telangiectasia with bleeding, hypertension, coeliac disease, ischemic heart disease, stroke, and anorexia nervosa. Abnormal liver enzymes with elevation of transaminases, alkaline phosphatase, and gamma-glutaryl transferase have been reported in more than 50% of adults. Most patients with Turner syndrome have normal intelligence. Only a small percentage of patients have significant developmental delay. However, 70% have learning disabilities involving spatial relationships, nonverbal problem-solving, and attention. Early testing and remediation is recommended, as well as psychologic support.

Diagnosis: Phenotypic females with the following features should have a karyotype analysis: (1) short stature (>2.5 standard deviations [SDs] below the mean value for age) with or without somatic anomalies associated with the syndrome of gonadal dysgenesis; and (2) delayed adolescence with an increased concentration of plasma FSH; (3) patients with clinical findings suggestive of Turner syndrome (eg, lymphedema of hands or feet, left-sided cardiac anomalies, characteristic facies, short fourth metacarpals, etc).

The initial evaluation of a patient with Turner syndrome should include karyotype analysis as well as FISH of 200 cells to rule out mosaicism or the presence of a Y chromosome in individuals with a 45,X karyotype and in those in whom a small nonidentifiable marker chromosome is present. A renal ultrasound is indicated to rule out surgically correctable anomalies. A cardiac evaluation with echocardiogram or MRI should be done to evaluate aortic size and rule out coarctation of the aorta and an anomaly of the aortic valve. Besides routine chemistries, gonadotropins, AMH (provides an estimate of the number of antral follicles), and inhibin B should be assessed in order to determine the status of the gonads. Periodic assessment of the cardiac status, especially in those with bicuspid aortic valves and/or

hypertension, is indicated throughout the lifetime of the patient. Other systems which need periodic evaluation include: (1) thyroid function studies, (2) assessment of tissue transglutaminase activity for celiac disease, (3) hearing evaluation, (4) orthodontics, and (5) psychosocial and school performance issues. In view of the increased incidence of specific learning defects involving spatial relationships, executive skills, and so forth, it is prudent to evaluate these functions at 4 to 5 years of age so that appropriate remedial therapy can be undertaken as early as possible if warranted.

At adolescence, in addition to the continuing above assessments, lipids, fasting glucose and insulin, and liver function should be assessed. Psychosocial and educational issues should continue to be addressed with the patient and the parents.

Treatment: Maximizing growth and hormone replacement at puberty in order to engender an orderly progressive development of secondary characteristics at a time concordant with peers are two of the main goals of therapy in patients with Turner syndrome.

Individuals with Turner syndrome treated with recombinant GH (0.375 mg/kg/wk divided into seven once-daily doses (maximum dose 15-18 mg/wk), with or without oxandrolone (0.0625 mg/kg/d by mouth), have an increase in the rate of growth that is sustained and results in a mean increase in height of 7 to 10 cm after 3 to 7 years of therapy. The serum IGF-1 level should be followed and the dose titered to maintain the IGF-1 level below the upper limit of normal for age. Beginning GH therapy earlier (as soon as growth failure is evident) in childhood allows for a longer duration of therapy which results in a greater gain in height and fosters initiation of estrogen replacement at an age commensurate with normal puberty. Before initiation of GH therapy, a thorough analysis of the costs, benefits, and possible side-effects must be discussed with the parents and the child. Significant side effects include: (1) the accelerated onset of diabetes mellitus in the prediabetic, (2) pseudotumor cerebri, (3) slipped femoral epiphysis, and (4) unknown long-term side effects. The influence of the gain in height on any of the quality of life parameters in individuals with Turner syndrome treated with GH has been questioned by some. There is no synergistic effect of combined estrogen replacement and GH therapy on final height in this disorder. However, in a recent study, percutaneous estrogen administration for pubertal induction was associated with a 2.1 cm greater adult height than oral estrogen administration. These data suggest that, as observed in adult women, oral estrogens decrease the plasma concentrations of IGF-1 and suppress IGF-1's metabolic effects. In patients who have been treated with GH and have achieved an acceptable height and in those who have refused GH therapy and have evidence of gonadal dysgenesis, estrogen replacement therapy is usually initiated after 11 to 13 years of age.

Increasingly, transcutaneous estrogen administration by patch or gel, which avoids first pass through the liver, is the treatment of choice to induce female secondary sexual characteristics in hypogonadal girls. In a study of 15 patients, an estradiol patch was placed nocturnally for 12 hours to simulate the diurnal pattern of estradiol secretion in early puberty. By cutting the 25-μg patch (Vivelle-Dot) when necessary and measuring serum estradiol concentrations, it was concluded that 0.08 to 0.12 μg/kg of body weight was an appropriate starting dose of estradiol transcutaneously. Plasma concentrations of estradiol were measured in the morning and maintained in a range appropriate for Tanner stage by adjusting the dose. The starting dose was usually maintained for 9 months before increasing the dose. The aim was to achieve midpuberty estradiol levels by 15 months. A progestin was added to the estradiol within 2 years after the start of estradiol.

Conjugated estrogens (0.3 mg or less) or ethinyl estradiol (3-5 μg) can be given orally for the first 21 days of the calendar month. Thereafter, the dose of estrogen is gradually increased over the next several years to 1.25 mg of conjugated estrogens or 10 μg of ethinyl estradiol daily for the first 21 days of the month. The minimum dose of estrogen necessary to initiate and maximize uterine development, secondary sexual characteristics, and menses, as well as to prevent osteoporosis should be administered. After the first 18 to 24 months of estrogen therapy, medroxyprogesterone acetate (5 mg) or a comparable progestin is given on the tenth to twenty-first days of the month to ensure physiologic menses and to reduce the risk of endometrial carcinoma, which is associated with unopposed estrogen stimulation.

We recommend a transition program when transferring adolescent or young adult patients to an adult caregiver. Ideally, this program will introduce the patient to the physicians who will be involved in her future care which may include an internist, endocrinologist, reproductive endocrinologist, ENT specialist, adult cardiologist, and psychologist.

Many of the morbidities that contribute to the decrease in lifespan are detectable with comprehensive medical surveillance and are amenable to medical and/or surgical therapy. Protocols for the management of the adult Turner syndrome patient have been published (see Gravholt et al; Bondy et al; Conway in reference list at the end of this chapter). Individuals with Turner syndrome by nature are very maternal. They should be reassured about their sexual function and informed about their potential for maternity with donor eggs and in vitro fertilization in an age-appropriate manner. The success rate of ovum donation is 40% per treatment cycle, and only 50% of pregnancies achieve a live birth due to a high miscarriage rate. In one study, 38% of patients had pregnancy associated hypertensive problems. There is an increased risk of aortic dissections during pregnancy. Thus, all women with Turner syndrome who desire a pregnancy should have a careful, complete cardiac evaluation prior to egg implantation and close continued monitoring if pregnancy ensues. We recommend caesarian delivery to avoid the increased stress to the cardiovascular system associated with labor and because of the risk of cephalopelvic dystocia in these women.

X Chromatin–Positive Variants of the Syndrome of Gonadal Dysgenesis

Patients with structural abnormalities of the X chromosome (deletions and additions) and sex chromosome mosaicism with a 45,X cell line may manifest the somatic as well as the gonadal features of the syndrome of gonadal dysgenesis . Evidence suggests that genes on both the long and short arms of the X chromosome control gonadal differentiation, whereas genes primarily on the short arms of the X prevent the short stature and somatic anomalies that are seen in 45,X patients (see Figure 14–2). In general, 45,X/46,XX mosaicism modifies the 45,X phenotype toward normal and can even result in normal gonadal function and fertility. Patients with duplication of the long arms of the X chromosome and deletion of the short arm—the so-called Xq isochromosome—appear to have an increased prevalence of autoimmune thyroiditis, type 2 diabetes, and inflammatory bowel disease in comparison to those with a 45,X karyotype. Patients with a 46,XrX (ring) cell line in their karyotype may manifest mental retardation and congenital anomalies not usually associated with Turner syndrome. These abnormalities are related to lack of inactivation of small ring X chromosomes and, hence, functional disomy for genes on the ring X chromosome and the normal X chromosome.

X Chromatin–Negative Variants of the Syndrome of Gonadal Dysgenesis

These patients usually have mosaicism with a 45,X and a Y-bearing cell line—45,X/46,XY; 45,X/47,XXY; 45,X/46,XY/47,XYY—or perhaps a structurally abnormal Y chromosome. They range from phenotypic females with the features of Turner syndrome to patients with ambiguous genitalia to completely normal-appearing males with few stigmas of Turner syndrome and short stature. The variations in gonadal differentiation range from bilateral streaks to bilateral dysgenetic testes to apparently normal testes, and there may be asymmetric development (eg, a streak on one side and a dysgenetic testis or, rarely, a normal testis on the other side)—sometimes called mixed gonadal dysgenesis. The development of the external genitalia and of the internal ducts correlates with the degree of testicular differentiation and the capacity of the fetal testes to secrete AMH and T.

The risk of gonadal tumors is greatly increased in patients with 45,X/46,XY mosaicism and streak or dysgenetic gonads; hence, prophylactic removal of streak gonads or dysgenetic undescended testes in this syndrome is indicated. Breast development at or after the age of puberty in these patients is commonly associated with a gonadal neoplasm, usually a gonadoblastoma. Pelvic sonography, computed tomography (CT), or MRI may be useful in screening for neoplasms in these patients. Gonadoblastomas are calcified and so may be visible even on a plain film of the abdomen.

Diagnosis: The diagnosis of 45,X/46,XY mosaicism can be established by the demonstration of both 45,X and 46,XY cells in blood, skin, or gonadal tissue. In some mosaics, a marker chromosome is found that is cytogenetically indistinguishable as X or Y. In these cases, either FISH or molecular analyses with X- and Y-specific probes is indicated to definitively determine the origin of the marker chromosome, because gonadoblastomas have been reported in patients with deleted Y chromosomes—even those with deletions of the *SRY* gene. Ninety percent of patients with 45,X/46,XY mosaicism ascertained by amniocentesis have normal male genitalia and normal testicular histology. Thus, the ambiguity of the genitalia invariably described in patients with 45,X/46,XY mosaicism is due to ascertainment bias. We have observed a short 30-year-old male with documented 45,X/46,XY mosaicism who has normal male genitalia and is fertile.

Treatment: The decision regarding the sex of rearing in this variant of the syndrome of gonadal dysgenesis should be based on the age at diagnosis and the potential for normal function of the external genitalia. In phenotypic females with 45,X/46,XY mosaicism assigned a female gender role, the dysgenetic gonads should be removed because of the risk of malignancy. Estrogen therapy should be initiated at the age of puberty, as in patients with a 45,X karyotype (see earlier). In affected infants who are assigned a male gender role, all gonadal tissue except that which appears functionally and histologically normal and is in the scrotum should be removed. An excellent phallic response to T can be anticipated. Repair of hypospadias is also indicated. At puberty, depending on the functional integrity of the retained gonads, T replacement therapy may be indicated in doses similar to those prescribed for patients with the incomplete form of XY gonadal dysgenesis. In patients with retained scrotal testes, frequent clinical examinations and ultrasonography is indicated. A gonadal biopsy postpubertally to rule out the possibility of carcinoma in situ (CIS), a premalignant lesion, should be performed. If CIS is present, low-dose radiation therapy or gonadectomy after sperm retrieval is indicated.

In infants and children with 45,X/46,XY mosaicism who have normal genitalia and normal testicular integrity as assessed by AMH, inhibin B, gonadotropin levels, and ultrasonography, the gonads should be retained and followed closely both hormonally and by ultrasound. In those 45,X/46,XY individuals with presumably "normal" testes, a gonadal biopsy should be performed, post-pubertally. If biopsy and sonography show no evidence of CIS, a second biopsy at 20 years of age is recommended. The risk of gonadal malignancies in males with 45,X/46,XY mosaicism, who have normal male genitalia and histologically and functionally normal testes in the scrotum, remains to be ascertained, although we hypothesize it may be no higher than that seen in 46,XY males.

Dysgenetic 46,XX and 46,XY DSD (46,XX and 46,XY Gonadal Dysgenesis)

The terms complete XX and XY gonadal dysgenesis have been applied to 46,XX or 46,XY patients who have bilateral streak gonads, a female phenotype, and no somatic stigmas of Turner syndrome. After the age of puberty, these patients exhibit sexual infantilism, castrate levels of plasma and urinary gonadotropins, normal or tall stature, and eunuchoid proportions.

Dysgenetic 46,XX DSD (46,XX Gonadal Dysgenesis)

Normal ovarian determination is dependent on X chromosomal genes as well as autosomal genes. Unlike the testes, the ovary requires the presence of germ cells in order to develop and function. Therefore, mutations in genes on the autosomes and X chromosome that affect gonadal determination (eg, DMRT1 and SF-1) as well as those that affect germ cell differentiation and development, migration into the gonadal ridge, and maturation into oocytes can cause XX gonadal dysgenesis. Expansion of the CAG repeat region of the fragile X locus can cause accelerated oocyte depletion and premature ovarian failure. Haploinsufficiency of *FOXL2*, a gene on chromosome 3q23, is a cause of autosomal dominant blepharophimosis-ptosis-epicanthus inversus syndrome (BPES type 1) and XX gonadal dysgenesis. A woman with a FOXL2 mutation, but without the BPES phenotype, has been described. Recently, SF-1 mutations in members of four families as well as 2/25 subjects with isolated ovarian insufficiency have extended the spectrum of phenotypes associated with SF-1 mutations. A multiplicity of genes involved in meiosis, DNA repair and folliculogenesis have recently been implicated as a cause of ovarian dysgenesis.

Familial and sporadic cases of XX gonadal dysgenesis are reported with an estimated incidence as high as 1:8300 females in Finland. Pedigree analysis of familial cases is consistent with autosomal recessive inheritance. Analysis of familial cases in Finland linked a locus on chromosome 2p to XX gonadal dysgenesis in females; the gene for the FSH receptor resides on chromosome 2p. A mutation in exon 7 of the gene encoding the FSH receptor segregates with XX gonadal dysgenesis. This mutation is in the extracellular ligand-binding domain of the FSH receptor and reduces the binding capacity and, consequently, signal transduction of the receptor. At puberty, this resulted in variable ovarian function, including streak ovaries and hypergonadotropic hypogonadism in some girls. Several studies of females with 46,XX gonadal dysgenesis in Western Europe and the United States were negative for *FSH receptor* gene mutations, suggesting that a mutation in this gene is a rare cause of XX gonadal dysgenesis outside of Finland. Males homozygous for this mutation are phenotypically normal, with spermatogenesis varying from normal to absent.

Studies of familial cohorts have supported heterogeneity in the pathogenesis of this syndrome. Siblings, one with a 46,XX karyotype and the other with a 46,XY karyotype, both with gonadal agenesis, have been reported, supporting the involvement of an autosomal gene in this family. However, in view of the normal phenotype in XY males observed with a mutation in the FSH receptor, it seems unlikely that these patients have an FSH receptor defect. In one family, four affected women had an inherited interstitial deletion of the long arm of the X chromosome involving the q21-q27 region (see Figure 14–2). This region apparently contains a gene or genes critical to ovarian development and function. In several affected families, XX gonadal dysgenesis was associated with deafness of the sensorineural type as well as other neurologic dysfunction.

Diagnosis: 46,XX gonadal dysgenesis should be suspected in phenotypic females with sexual infantilism and normal Müllerian structures who lack the somatic stigmas of the syndrome of gonadal dysgenesis (Turner syndrome). Karyotype analysis reveals only 46,XX cells. As in Turner syndrome, gonadotropin levels are high, inhibin A and B and AMH levels as well as estrogen levels are low. Ultrasound or MRI reveals a streak or dysgenetic ovary, and treatment consists of cyclic estrogen and progesterone replacement as previously discussed for patients with Turner syndrome.

Sporadic cases of XX gonadal dysgenesis, similar to familial cases, may represent a heterogeneous group of patients from a pathogenetic point of view. XX gonadal dysgenesis should be distinguished from ovarian failure due to radiation and chemotherapy for childhood malignancies, infections such as mumps, antibodies to gonadotropin receptors, biologically inactive FSH, gonadotropin-insensitive ovaries, and galactosemia.

46,XY DSD (Complete or Partial Gonadal Dysgenesis)

46,XY gonadal dysgenesis occurs both sporadically and in familial aggregates. Patients with the complete form of this syndrome have female external genitalia, normal or tall stature, bilateral streak gonads, Müllerian duct development, sexual infantilism, eunuchoid habitus, and a 46,XY karyotype. Clitoromegaly is common and, in familial cases as well as sporadic cases, a continuum of involvement ranging from the complete syndrome to ambiguity of the external genitalia has been described. The phenotypic difference between the complete and incomplete forms of XY gonadal dysgenesis is related to the degree of differentiation of testicular tissue and the functional capacity of the fetal testis to produce T and AMH. Early in infancy and after the age of puberty, plasma gonadotropin levels are markedly elevated.

Analyses of familial and sporadic cases of 46,XY gonadal dysgenesis indicate that about 15% to 20% of patients have a mutation of the *SRY* gene that affects DNA binding or bending by the SRY protein or a mutation in the calmodulin or importin domains of the *SRY* gene that affects the nuclear localization signals. Most patients in whom mutations have been detected have had complete gonadal dysgenesis. Patients with deletions of the short arm of the Y chromosome may have, in addition to gonadal dysgenesis, stigmas of Turner syndrome. A mutation in the HMG box of the *SRY* gene has been described in normal 46,XY fathers of daughters who had 46,XY gonadal dysgenesis. These familial cohorts suggest the possibility of germ cell mosaicism in the father or that a mutation or modifier genes may affect either the level or the timing of *SRY* expression and in this manner result in either normal or abnormal testicular differentiation. Mutations outside the HMG box region of the *SRY* gene or in X-linked or autosomal genes involved in testicular determination and function may be responsible for those individuals in

whom no molecular abnormality in the *SRY* gene has been found. Three of six 46,XY patients with complete gonadal dysgenesis in one study had homozygous mutations of the gene encoding DHH (Desert Hedgehog).

A number of patients with 46,XY gonadal dysgenesis has been reported with a duplication of the Xp21.2 → p22.11 region of the X chromosome. This region contains the *DAX1* gene. Deletion or mutation of *DAX1* in males causes adrenal hypoplasia congenita and hypogonadotropic hypogonadism. The finding that 46,XY males with adrenal hypoplasia and hypogonadotropic hypogonadism have normal sex differentiation suggests that *DAX1* is not required for testicular differentiation in the human; duplication of *DAX1*, however, impairs testis differentiation possibly by upregulating B-catenin/WNT4, which downregulates SOX9 preventing testicular development.

XY gonadal dysgenesis associated with campomelic dysplasia is due to a mutation of one allele of an *SRY*-related gene, *SOX9* on chromosome 17. Sometimes the mutation occurs in upstream regulatory elements of the gene. In addition, XY gonadal dysgenesis has been associated with 9p–(DMRT1) and 10q–deletions, mutations in, as well as duplication of, 1p31-35 (WNT4).

Steroidogenic factor-1 (SF-1) is a transcriptional regulator of adrenal and gonadal development, hormone synthesis, and functions with other genes in the sex determination and differentiation cascade. The phenotype is variable and depends on whether the individual has a heterozygous or homozygous mutation as well as the functional deficiency in SF-1 activity as a result of the specific mutation. The phenotype is also most likely affected by background genetic factors and cofactors. Mutations in the gene encoding SF-1 are associated with 46,XY DSD. Similar to the mouse knockout, the severely affected XY individual presents with gonadal streaks with female sex differentiation and neonatal onset adrenal insufficiency. Recently, 46,XY patients with ambiguous genitalia (and in one case, female external genitalia) with or without Müllerian ducts and normal adrenal function have been reported, which suggests that adrenal development and function are less sensitive to SF-1 dosage levels than gonadal development and function. The phenotypic spectrum of SF-1 deficiency includes 46,XY males with micropenis and in one case normal male external genitalia and anorchia as well as infertile males and 46,XX females with primary or secondary ovarian failure. The phenotypic spectrum was recently expanded to include a 46,XY newborn with hypospadias and micropenis who virilized normally at puberty but had evidence of progressive Sertoli cell deficiency as evidenced by elevated FSH levels and low inhibin B levels. Thus, as with other genes in the sex determination cascade, gene dosage and cofactors play a critical role in phenotypic expression. Both heterozygous and homozygous mutations in SF-1 have been described in 46,XX females with isolated primary ovarian insufficiency.

Mutations and deletions of the Wilms tumor repressor gene *WT1* are a cause of XY gonadal dysgenesis and renal disease (eg, Denys-Drash syndrome, Frasier syndrome, and the WAGR syndrome). Denys-Drash syndrome is due to a mutation in a coding exon of the *WT1* gene. These mutations act in a dominant-negative fashion to produce the Denys-Drash phenotype, which is characterized by testicular dysgenesis, early renal failure due to mesangial sclerosis, and a predisposition to the development of Wilms tumor. Müllerian ducts may be present or absent depending on the degree of Sertoli cell dysfunction. The external genitalia are undervirilized. Frasier syndrome is due to a mutation in the donor splice site of exon 9, resulting in loss of three amino acids—lysine, threonine, and serine (KTS), thus changing the ratio of KTS+ to KTS− isoforms of this protein. The resultant phenotype is characterized by streak gonads, the presence of Müllerian structures, female external genitalia, late-onset nephropathy due to segmental glomerulosclerosis, and an increased risk of gonadoblastoma. WAGR syndrome is due to a deletion of a segment of 11p13, which contains the *WT1* gene and the *PAX6* gene causing haploinsufficiency of these genes. The resultant phenotype includes **W**ilms tumor, **a**niridia **g**enitourinary abnormalities, and mental **r**etardation.

A 46,XY patient with normal female genitalia and Müllerian structures had a homozygous mutation of CBX2—the human homologue of *m33*, a gene that when mutated causes sex reversal in mice. This gene is postulated to be upstream of SRY in the ever-expanding gene cascade of sex development. The patient had elevated FSH levels in infancy and the presence of "bilateral ovaries" with sparse primordial follicles on biopsy at 4½ years of age suggesting gonadal dysgenesis.

Mutations in the Map3k1 have been recently demonstrated to cause sex reversal in mice as well as 46,XY humans. Recently, mutations in this gene have been described in patients with partial and complete gonadal dysgenesis. In two families, the mutation was inherited as a sex limited autosomal dominant. Interestingly, in these families the mutation resulted in activation of the MAPK pathway as opposed to inactivation as observed in the mouse and in a 46,XY fertile female. A resolution to this apparent discrepancy in action is still to be clarified.

Therapy: Therapy for phenotypic females with 46,XY gonadal dysgenesis involves prophylactic gonadectomy at diagnosis, due to the high risk of malignancy in these gonads, and estrogen substitution at puberty. In the incomplete form of XY gonadal dysgenesis, assignment of a male gender is possible and treatment with testosterone to augment phallic size in infancy is recommended. Prophylactic gonadectomy must be considered, because fertility is unlikely (gonadotropins are invariably elevated, and AMH and inhibin B levels are low or unmeasurable). In addition, there is an increased risk of malignant transformation of the dysgenetic gonads in these patients, especially those who are SRY-positive and have intra-abdominal dysgenetic gonads and those with Frasier and Denys-Drash syndrome. If a gonad is preserved in the scrotum because it is histologically normal and hormonally functional, it should be followed closely by physical examination and ultrasound and biopsied postpubertally to rule out CIS, a premalignant lesion. In affected individuals raised as males, we recommend that prosthetic testes be implanted at the time of gonadectomy and androgen substitution therapy instituted at the age of puberty. Testosterone enanthate in oil (or another long-acting T ester) is used, beginning with 50 mg intramuscularly every 4 weeks and gradually increasing after a bone age of 14½ years to a full replacement

dose of 200 mg intramuscularly every 2 weeks. Alternatively T patches or gels may be used.

OVOTESTICULAR DSD (INDIVIDUALS WITH BOTH OVARIAN AND TESTICULAR TISSUE)

In these individuals, both ovarian and testicular tissues are present in one or both gonads. Differentiation of the internal and external genitalia is highly variable. The external genitalia may simulate those of a male or female, but most often they are atypical. Cryptorchidism and hypospadias are common. A testis or ovotestis, if present, is located in the labioscrotal folds in one-third of patients, in the inguinal canal in one-third, and in the abdomen in the remainder. A uterus is usually present, although it may be hypoplastic or unicornuate. The differentiation of the genital ducts usually follows that of the ipsilateral gonad. The ovotestis is the most common gonad found in these individuals (60%), followed by an ovary and, least commonly, by a testis. At puberty, breast development is usual in untreated patients, and menses occur in over 50% of cases. Whereas the ovary or the ovarian portion of an ovotestis may function normally, the testis or testicular portion of an ovotestis is invariably dysgenetic and should be removed in 46,XX patients raised as females.

Sixty percent have a 46,XX karyotype, 20% are 46,XY, and about 20% have sex chromosome mosaicism or 46,XX/46,XY chimerism. Those with a 46,XX karyotype are genetically heterogeneous. Only a small proportion, including some in family cohorts with 46,XX males, are *SRY* positive. In these individuals, Y-to-X and Y-to-autosome translocations, hidden sex chromosome mosaicism, or chimerism may explain the pathogenesis. A number of families have been reported in which both *SRY*-negative 46,XX males and 46,XX ovotesticular DSDs occurred. This latter observation suggests a common genetic pathogenesis in these patients. Possible genetic mechanisms to explain *SRY*-negative individuals include (1) mutation of a downstream autosomal gene or modifier gene involved in testicular determination; (2) mutation, deletion, or anomalous inactivation of an X- or autosome-linked locus involved in repression of testis determination. A 46,XX ovotesticular DSD with palmoplantar keratoderma, congenital bilateral corneal opacification, onychodystrophy, and hearing impairment has been reported. This patient had a homozygous splice site mutation in the *RSPO1* gene. This is the first demonstration of a mutation in a single gene (in the ovarian determining pathway) causing ovotesticular DSD; or (3) circumscribed chimerism or mosaicism that occurred only in the gonads. Studies of eight ovotestes from 46,XX individuals detected low levels of the *SRY* gene. Immunohistochemistry has identified SRY protein localized predominantly in Sertoli and germ cells.

Diagnosis: Ovotesticular DSD should be considered in all patients with ambiguous genitalia. The finding of a 46,XX/46,XY karyotype or a bilobulate gonad compatible with an ovotestis in the inguinal region or labioscrotal folds suggests the diagnosis. Basal plasma T levels are elevated above 40 ng/dL in affected patients under 6 months of age, and T levels increase after hCG stimulation. The estradiol and inhibin A response to human menopausal gonadotropins or recombinant human FSH is a reliable test for the presence of ovarian tissue. This test, when coupled with the hCG-induced rise in T, differentiates infants with both ovarian and testicular tissue from those with other disorders of sexual differentiation.

If all other forms of 46,XY and 46,XX DSD have been excluded and hormonal studies are nondiagnostic, laparotomy and histologic confirmation of both ovarian and testicular tissue establish the diagnosis. The management of these individuals is contingent on both the age at diagnosis and of a careful assessment of the functional capacity of the gonads, the genital duct differentiation, and the appearance of the external genitalia. In general, 46,XX individuals are raised as females, with the possible exception of the well-virilized patient in whom no uterus is found. Preservation of the ovarian tissue and removal of all testicular tissue are sometimes possible in patients who have an ovary on one side or an ovotestis with distinct margins of separation (bilobate). Fertility has been reported in 46,XX individuals with functional ovarian gonadal tissue.

Gonadal Neoplasms in Dysgenetic Gonads

Gonadal tumors are rare in patients with 47,XXY Klinefelter syndrome and 45,X gonadal dysgenesis. However, the prevalence of gonadal neoplasms is greatly increased in patients with 46,XY DSDs with dysgenetic testes (Table 14–2). The frequency is increased in 45,X/46,XY mosaics who have female or ambiguous genitalia; in those with a structurally abnormal Y chromosome; and in those with XY gonadal dysgenesis, either with a female phenotype or with ambiguous genitalia (eg, Frasier [60%], Denys-Drash syndrome [40%]) (see Table 14–2). Gonadoblastomas, germinomas, seminomas, and teratomas are found most frequently. Prophylactic gonadectomy is indicated in these patients as well as in those with Turner syndrome who manifest signs of virilization, regardless of karyotype. The significance of hidden mosaicism for Y chromosomal DNA determined by polymerase chain reaction analysis in patients with 45,X Turner syndrome is controversial with respect to the risk of gonadal neoplasms. Registry studies in Denmark indicate that the incidence of gonadoblastoma in patients with Turner syndrome without a cytogenetically identified Y chromosome is rare. Thus, routine use of polymerase chain reaction studies of all patients with 45,X Turner syndrome is not indicated. Gonadoblastomas have been reported in patients with marker chromosomes of Y origin lacking the SRY gene. Thus, screening by FISH for Y chromosomal DNA in blood seems prudent in these patients, as well as other patients with Turner syndrome, as it enables one to count a large number of cells with a minimum of effort and time. The testis should be preserved in patients who are to be raised as males, only if it is histologically and functionally normal, and it is or can be situated in the scrotum. The fact that a testis is palpable in the scrotum does not preclude malignant degeneration and tumor dissemination, because seminomas tend to metastasize at an early stage before a mass is obvious.

Malignant testicular germ cell tumors including seminomas, embryonal carcinomas, teratomas, and yolk sac tumors appear to develop from CIS. These cells are thought to arise in utero from fetal gonocytes and to metamorphose with time in the dysgenetic

TABLE 14–2 Risk of germ cell malignancy in various forms of 46,XY DSD.

Risk	Condition	Risk (%)	Proposed Management	Number of Studies	Number of Patients
High	GD (Y+), intra-abd[a]	15-35	Gonadectomy	12	>350
	PAIS, nonscrotal[a]	15	Gonadectomy	3	80
	Frasier syndrome (Y+)[a]	60	Gonadectomy	1	15
	Denys-Drash (Y+)[a]	40	Gonadectomy	1	5
Intermediate	Turner (Y+)	12	Gonadectomy	11	43
	17β-HSD	28	Strict follow-up; biopsy if raised as males. Gonadectomy if female GID	2	7
Low	CAIS[b]	0.8	Biopsy/in case of CIS: irradiation or gonadectomy	3	120
	Ovotesticular (DSD)	3	Removal of testicular tissue in case of female sex assignment	3	426
	Turner (Y–)	1	None	11	557
Unknown	5α reductase deficiency	0	Unknown	1	3
	Leydig cell hypoplasia	0	Unknown	1	2
	GD (Y+), scrotal	?	Biopsy; in case of CIS: irradiation?	0	0
	PAIS, scrotal gonads	?	Biopsy, in case of CIS: irradiation?	0	0

[a]Gonadectomy is recommended in these patients at diagnosis because germ cell tumors in these patients may occur in infancy and childhood.

[b]Patients with CAIS should be allowed to feminize spontaneously at puberty. In CAIS patients who refuse prophylactic gonadectomy, a biopsy of the gonads to rule out CIS is recommended. In XO/XY males with scrotal testes being raised as males, careful follow-up with ultrasound prepubertally and biopsy postpubertally to rule out CIS is indicated.

CAIS, complete androgen insensitivity syndrome; CIS, carcinoma in situ; GD, gonadal dysgenesis; GID, gender identity; intra-abd, intra-abdominal gonads; PAIS, partial androgen insensitivity syndrome.

Modified from Cools M, Drop SL, Wolffenbuttel KP, et al. Germ cell tumors in the intersex gonad: old paths, new directions, moving frontiers. *Endocr Rev.* 2006;27:468.

environment into testicular malignancies. The incidence of CIS and seminomas is low in patients with complete androgen insensitivity but significantly higher in patients with partial androgen insensitivity with intra-abdominal gonads (see Table 14–2). Clues to the presence of CIS are the presence of an inhomogeneous testicular parenchyma and testicular microlithiasis, as well as a low inhibin B level. It has been suggested that immunohistochemistry for *Oct 3/4* is mandatory when evaluating testicular biopsies for CIS, since *Oct 3/4* is a gene that may be involved in germ cell tumors and is not normally expressed in postpubertal testes. An increased prevalence of low sperm counts, cryptorchidism, hypospadias, and testicular cancer has been reported in Denmark compared to Finland. This has been called the **testicular dysgenesis syndrome** and ascribed to both genetic and environmental factors such as exposure to endocrine disrupters.

46,XX DSD ANDROGEN INDUCED (FEMALE PSEUDOHERMAPHRODITISM)

Affected individuals have normal ovaries and Müllerian derivatives associated with ambiguous external genitalia. In the absence of testes, a female fetus is masculinized if subjected to increased circulating levels of androgens derived from a fetal or maternal source. The degree of masculinization depends on the stage of differentiation at the time of exposure (Figure 14–13). After 12 weeks of gestation, androgens produce only clitoral hypertrophy. Rarely, ambiguous genitalia that superficially resemble those produced by androgens are the result of other teratogenic factors.

Fetal Source: Congenital Adrenal Hyperplasia (Figure 14–14, Table 14–3)

Congenital adrenal hyperplasia (CAH) is responsible for most cases of 46,XX DSD and about 50% of all cases of ambiguous genitalia. There are six major types of CAH, all transmitted as autosomal recessive disorders. The common denominator of all six types is a defect in the synthesis of cortisol that results in an

increase in ACTH and consequently adrenal hyperplasia and the secretion of steroids synthesized prior to the enzymatic block. Both males and females can be affected, but males are rarely diagnosed at birth unless they have ambiguous genitalia, are salt-losers and manifest adrenal crises, are identified during newborn screening, or are known to be at risk because they have an affected sibling. Defects in 21-hydroxylation and 11β-hydroxylation are confined to the adrenal gland and produce virilization.

A new form of CAH has been described due to mutations in the gene encoding P450 oxidoreductase (POR), a single flavoprotein that donates electrons to all microsomal cytochrome P450 enzymes, including 17α-hydroxylase/17,20-lyase, 21-hydroxylase, and aromatase. The mothers of affected fetuses are at risk for virilization during pregnancy if aromatase activity is significantly affected by the mutation. 46,XX patients with this defect in adrenal and ovarian steroidogenesis have ambiguous genitalia, whereas those with a 46,XY karyotype have incomplete masculinization of the external genitalia.

P450c21 Hydroxylase Deficiency

21-Hydroxylase activity is mediated by P450c21, a microsomal cytochrome P450 enzyme that is expressed as an autosomal recessive. A deficiency of this enzyme results in the most common type of adrenal hyperplasia, with an overall prevalence of 1:14,000 live births in Caucasians. More than 90% of patients with CAH in North America and Europe have 21-hydroxylase deficiency. The locus for the gene that encodes 21-hydroxylation is on the short arm of chromosome 6, close to the locus for C4 (complement) between HLA-B and HLA-D. DNA analysis has detected two genes, designated *P450c21A (CYP21p)* and *P450c21B (CYP21)*, in this region in tandem with the two genes for complement, *C4A* and *C4B*, as well as two genes *Xa* and *Xb*, which overlap one another on the opposite strands of DNA from *P450c21A* and *P450c21B*. *Xa* and *Xb* code for an extracellular matrix protein called Tenascin-X. *P450c21A* is a nonfunctional pseudogene (ie, it is missing critical structural sequences and does not encode a functional 21-hydroxylase). Seventy-five to eighty percent of patients

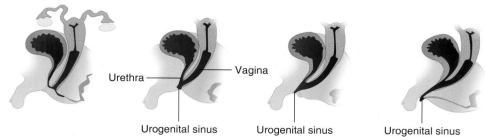

FIGURE 14–13 46,XX DSD (female pseudohermaphroditism) induced by prenatal exposure to androgens. Exposure after the 12th fetal week leads only to clitoral hypertrophy (diagram at left). Exposure at progressively earlier stages of differentiation (depicted from left to right in drawings) leads to retention of the urogenital sinus and labioscrotal fusion. If exposure occurs sufficiently early, the labia will fuse to form a penile urethra. (Reproduced, with permission, from Grumbach MM, Ducharme J. The effects of androgens on fetal sexual development: androgen-induced female pseudohermaphroditism. *Fertil Steril.* 1960;11:757.)

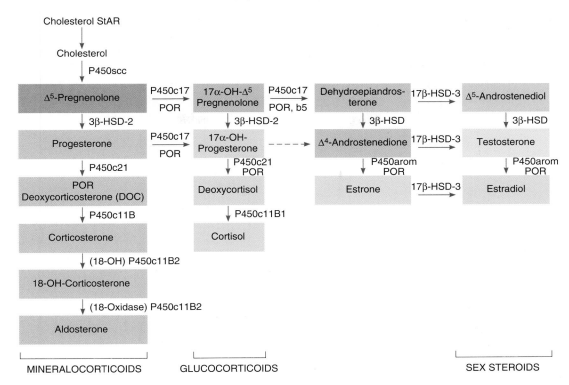

FIGURE 14–14 A diagrammatic representation of the steroid biosynthetic pathways in the adrenals and gonads. (OH, hydroxy or hydroxylase; StAR, steroidogenic regulatory protein; P450scc, cholesterol side-chain cleavage, previously termed 20,22 desmolase; 3β-HSD-2, 3β-hydroxysteroid dehydrogenase and Δ^5-isomerase type 2; P450c17, 17-hydroxylase; POR, P450 oxidoreductase—the flavoprotein that contributes electrons to microsomal cytochrome P450; P450c21, 21-hydroxylase; P450c17, 17-hydroxylase also mediates 17,20-lyase activity; b5, cytochrome b5; P450arom, aromatase; 17β-HSD-3, 17β-hydroxysteroid dehydrogenase type 3; P450c11B2 (aldosterone synthase) mediates 18-hydroxylase and 18-oxidase reactions; P450c11B1 mediates 11-hydroxylation of deoxycortisol to cortisol and deoxycorticosterone to corticosterone). The dashed arrow indicates that this reaction occurs at a low rate in humans. (Modified and reproduced, with permission, from Conte FA, Grumbach MM. Pathogenesis, classification, diagnosis, and treatment of anomalies of sex. In: DeGroot L, ed. *Endocrinology*. Grune & Stratton; 1989.)

with classic P450c21 deficiency have point mutations that change a portion of the *P450c21B* to a sequence similar to that in the nonfunctional *P450c21A* gene—hence a microgene conversion. Approximately 15% of severely affected *21-OH* genes have a deletion extending from a position between exon 3 and exon 8 of the *P450c21A* pseudogene to a similar region of the *21-OHB* gene, resulting in a nonfunctional fusion *21-OHA/21-OHB* gene. This is the result of misalignment and unequal crossing over. The remainder have de novo point mutations and macrogene conversions.

Classic salt-wasting 21-hydroxylase deficiency is associated with point mutations, deletions, or gene conversions that abolish or severely reduce 21-hydroxylase activity. Most patients with 21-hydroxylase deficiency are compound heterozygotes (ie, they have a different genetic mutation on each of their *P450c21B* allelic genes) having inherited a mutant gene from each of their parents. A spontaneous mutation in the *21-hydroxylase* gene occurs in 1% to 2% of patients.

The phenotypic spectrum—salt loss with severe virilization, simple virilization, or late onset of virilization—is a consequence of the degree of enzymatic deficiency. The phenotype is determined

in patients with compound heterozygosity by the functionally less severely mutated *P450c21B* allele. In rare cases, there is variability between genotype and phenotype. The gene for P450c21 (21-hydroxylase) deficiency is not only closely linked to the HLA supergene complex, but certain specific HLA subtypes are found to be statistically increased in patients with 21-hydroxylase deficiency.

P450c21 hydroxylase deficiency with virilization and salt loss The salt-losing variant of P450c21 hydroxylase deficiency accounts for about 80% of patients with classic 21-hydroxylase deficiency and involves a severe reduction (98%) in P450c21-hydroxylase activity, leading to impaired secretion of both cortisol and aldosterone. This results in electrolyte and fluid losses after the fifth day of life and, as a consequence, hyponatremia, hyperkalemia, acidosis, dehydration, and vascular collapse. Rarely, this can occur as late as 6 to 12 weeks, usually associated with a concomitant physiologic stress. In the female fetus before 12 weeks' gestation, high fetal DHT levels result from increased T and DHEA-S secreted from the 21-hydroxylase-deficient adrenal gland which cannot synthesize cortisol when aromatase activity is

TABLE 14–3 Clinical manifestations of the various types of congenital adrenal hyperplasia.

Enzymatic Defect	StAR[a] (Defect in Cholesterol Transport)		3β-Hydroxysteroid Dehydrogenase		P450c17 (17α-Hydroxylase)		P450c11 (11β-Hydroxylase)		P450c21 (21α-Hydroxylase)		P450scc[b]		POR[c]	
Chromosomal	XX	XY	XX	XY	XX	XY	XX	XY	XX	XY	XX	XY	XX	XY
External genitalia (at birth)	Female	Female (classic), Male (nonclassic form)	Female, w/wo clitoromegaly	Ambiguous (hypospadias)	Female	Female or ambiguous	Ambiguous[d]	Male	Ambiguous[d] Female (nonclassic form)	Male	Female	Ambiguous male (mild form)	Ambiguous →normal female	Ambiguous → micro penis normal male
Postnatal virilization	Normal female puberty, later primary ovarian failure	Sexual infantilism at puberty (classic), normal pubertal development (nonclassic form)	+ or –	Mild to moderate	(Sexual infantilism at puberty)		+		+		Normal female	Sexual infantilism at puberty	–	
Addisonian crises	+		+ or –		–		–		+ in 80% (classic)[e] – (nonclassic)		+[f]		±	
Hypertension	–		–		+		+		–		–		–	

[a] StAR, steroidogenic acute regulatory protein. StAR deficiency leads to secondary P450scc deficiency.

[b] A nonclassic form has been reported.

[c] Patients may manifest dysmorphic features (Antley-Bixler syndrome). Virilization is not progressive in females. Males with mild mutations may have normal genitalia and infertility.

[d] Normal female genitalia in nonclassic late-onset and cryptic form. These forms do not manifest clinical or biochemical evidence of aldosterone deficiency.

[e] The 20% of patients who appear to be non-salt losers may manifest classic adrenal crises with severe illness and will develop hyponatremia when challenged with a low sodium diet.

[f] Late-onset form with ambiguous or hypospadiac male genitalia and cortisol insufficiency in childhood.

Reproduced, with permission, from Grumbach MM, Hughes IA, Conte FA. Disorders of sex differentiation. In: Larson PR, et al, ed. *Williams Textbook of Endocrinology*. 10th ed. WB Saunders; 2003.

relatively low. In addition, P450c21-21-hydroxylase deficiency results in an elevated level of 17OH progesterone which is not readily converted to androstenedione in humans but may be converted via a backdoor steroid pathway to DHT, a nonaromatizable androgen (see Figure 14–10). It has been suggested that DHT synthesis from elevated 17OH progesterone levels may contribute to the fetal masculinization of the external genitalia and the post-natal virilization of patients with P450c21-hydroxylase deficiency. Elevated DHT levels from 8 to 12 weeks of gestation results in varying degrees of labioscrotal fusion and clitoromegaly in affected 46,XX females. After 12 weeks, androgen receptor activity in the labioscrotal folds diminishes, and only clitoromegaly ensues from the elevated DHT levels.

Masculinization of the external genitalia of affected females who are salt-losers tends to be more severe than individuals with apparent non–salt-losing P450c21-hydroxylase deficiency. Affected males may have macrogenitosomia. Recently, patients with 21-hydroxylase and 11β-hydroxylase deficiency have been shown to have adrenomedullary hypofunction secondary to low intra-adrenal concentrations of cortisol and developmental defects in formation of the adrenal medulla. This defect in catecholamine synthesis may predispose these patients to hypoglycemia with stress in infancy.

P450c21 hydroxylase deficiency with virilization alone The simple virilizing form of P450c21 (21-hydroxylase) deficiency results in impaired cortisol synthesis, increased ACTH levels, and increased adrenal androgen precursor and androgen secretion. It accounts for about 20% of individuals with classic P450c21 hydroxylase deficiency and is primarily due to missense mutations such as I172N, which retain enough P450c21-hydroxylase activity to produce sufficient aldosterone to prevent hyponatremia/hyperkalemia under normal circumstances. In general, affected females have a less severe degree of masculinization of their external genitalia than those with the salt-wasting form of P450c21 hydroxylase deficiency. In the male fetus, no abnormalities in the external genitalia are evident at birth, but the phallus may be enlarged. These patients produce sufficient amounts of aldosterone to prevent the signs and symptoms of mineralocorticoid deficiency except when they are salt-deprived. They may also manifest a defect in mineralocorticoid synthesis as evidenced by an elevated plasma renin level. Virilization continues after birth in untreated patients. This results in rapid growth and bone maturation as well as the physical signs of excess androgen secretion (eg, acne, seborrhea, increased muscular development, premature development of pubic or axillary hair, and phallic enlargement). True (central) precocious puberty can occur following initiation of glucocorticoid therapy in affected children with advanced bone ages.

Nonclassic P450c21 hydroxylase deficiency Mild defects in P450c21 (21-hydroxylase) activity not causing a DSD have been reported. Patients can be symptomatic (late-onset or nonclassic) or asymptomatic (cryptic form). These mild forms of P450c21 hydroxylase deficiency are HLA-linked, as is classic P450c21 hydroxylase deficiency; however, they occur much more frequently than the classic form of the disease in certain ethnic populations. It has been postulated that nonclassic P450c21 hydroxylase deficiency is the most common autosomal recessive disorder. The frequency of nonclassic P450c21 hydroxylase deficiency is thought to be as high as 1 in 27 for Ashkenazi Jews, 1 in 53 for Hispanics, 1 in 333 for Italians, and 1 in 1000 for other Caucasians. The prevalence of heterozygosity for a nonclassic allele has varied from 1.2 to 6%. Affected patients with nonclassical 21-hydroxylase deficiency are either homozygous for a mild mutation (eg, V281L) or are compound heterozygotes with the other allele harboring a severe mutation (27%-76% of the time). Thus, it is prudent to genotype the partners of a nonclassic patient who is carrying a severe mutation, in order to offer genetic counseling and, if necessary, prenatal diagnosis. The clinical expression of nonclassical congenital adrenal hyperplasia is very variable in individuals with the same genotypes within families with some being asymptomatic (cryptic). Females with late-onset P450c21 hydroxylase deficiency have normal female genitalia at birth. Mild virilization occurs later in childhood and adolescence manifesting primarily as hirsutism. Other signs of excess androgen secretion, such as the premature development of pubic or axillary hair (premature pubarche), slight clitoral enlargement, advanced bone age, menstrual irregularities acne, polycystic ovary syndrome, decreased fertility, may also occur. Affected males have normal male genitalia at birth. Later in childhood, some become symptomatic and exhibit premature growth of pubic or axillary hair, and advancement of their bone age. Although they are tall as children, they end up short as adults due to advanced bone maturation and premature epiphysial fusion unless they are treated.

Diagnosis: The diagnosis of P450c21 hydroxylase deficiency should always be considered in the following: (1) patients with ambiguous genitalia who have a 46,XX karyotype with a uterus and ovaries on ultrasonography; (2) apparent cryptorchid males; (3) infants who present with shock, hypoglycemia, and serum chemistries compatible with adrenal insufficiency; and (4) males or females with signs of virilization before puberty, including premature pubarche. In the past, the diagnosis of P450c21 hydroxylase deficiency was based on the finding of elevated levels of 17-ketosteroids and pregnanetriol in the urine. Although urinary steroid determinations are still useful, they have been replaced by the simpler and more cost-effective measurement of plasma 17-hydroxyprogesterone, androstenedione, and T levels by liquid chromatography and tandem mass spectroscopy (LCMSMS).

The concentration of plasma 17-hydroxyprogesterone is elevated in umbilical cord blood but rapidly decreases into the range of 100 to 200 ng/dL (3-6 nmol/L) by 48 hours after delivery. In premature infants and in stressed full-term newborns, the levels of 17-hydroxyprogesterone are higher than those observed in non-stressed full-term infants. In patients with P450c21 hydroxylase deficiency, the 17-hydroxyprogesterone values usually are greater than 5000 ng/dL (150 nmol/L) on baseline samples drawn after 48 hours, depending on the age of the patient and the severity of P450c21 hydroxylase deficiency. Patients with mild P450c21 hydroxylase deficiency (eg, late-onset and cryptic forms) may have borderline basal 17-hydroxyprogesterone values, but they can be distinguished from heterozygotes by the magnitude of the

17-hydroxyprogesterone response to the parenteral administration of ACTH as well as by genotyping. Patients with baseline 17-OH progesterone levels over 10,000 µg/dL after 2 days of age or those with ACTH-induced responses that are over 10,000 µg/dL have classic 21-hydroxylase deficiency. Those who have levels at baseline which are above the normal range and who respond to ACTH with levels at 1500 to 10,000 ng/dL probably have nonclassic 21-hydroxylase deficiency. Those who are unaffected or heterozygotes respond to ACTH with a rise to less than 1500 ng/dL. Patients with borderline 17-OH progesterone responses can be genotyped to ascertain their status. As 17-OH progesterone levels are elevated in patients with 11-hydroxylase deficiency, 3-beta-dehydrogenase, 17,20-lyase, and P450 oxidoreductase deficiencies, it is prudent to do an ACTH stimulation test measuring 17-OH progesterone, 11-deoxycortisol, 17-OH pregnenolone, DOC, progesterone, T, and cortisol at baseline and at 1 hour before reaching a definitive diagnosis. Elevated 21-deoxycortisol levels are a specific and sensitive indicator of 21-hydroxylase deficiency. 21-deoxycortisol measurements can be used to differentiate between patients with elevated 17-hydroxyprogesterone levels, who have 21-hydroxylase deficiency and sick newborns and premature infants who have false positive 17-hydroxyprogesterone levels on screening.

In patients with the salt-losing form of 21-hydroxylase deficiency, aldosterone levels in both plasma and urine are low in relation to the serum sodium concentration, while plasma renin activity is markedly elevated. The plasma aldosterone-renin ratio will be low. Breast milk and infant formulas have a low concentration of sodium which usually unmasks the diagnosis of salt loss by 7 to 14 days. The salt-losing episode is heralded by a rise in serum potassium with a subsequent fall in sodium and bicarbonate. The diagnosis of nonclassic (late-onset 21-hydroxylase deficiency) can be made in the symptomatic patient (eg, one with early development of pubic hair, acne, and other signs of androgen excess) by measuring a plasma 17-OH progesterone level between 7 to 9 AM. Levels below 200 ng/dL rule out late-onset CAH. Higher levels should be evaluated by an ACTH test which will distinguish 21-hydroxylase deficiency from other causes of elevated 17-OH progesterone levels.

The diagnosis of 21-hydroxylase deficiency in newborn males has been facilitated by routine neonatal screening or 17-OH progesterone by filter paper (Guthrie cards) at 2 to 3 days of life. Screening reduces the morbidity and mortality associated with late or nondiagnosis especially in male infants with the salt-losing form of 21-hydroxylase deficiency. Males with simple virilization may not be diagnosed until later in infancy when virilization and advanced bone maturation associated with prepubertal testes are evident. Prematurity and illness are confounding factors since both are associated with elevated levels of 17-OH progesterone. If the patient is reported positive by the laboratory and the levels are borderline or moderately elevated, it is prudent to examine the patient, review the history (especially confounders such as prematurity, concomitant stress, day of life specimen obtained, etc.), and repeat the 17-OH progesterone screen by LCMSMS (liquid chromatography, tandem mass spectrometry) from a venous sample. The parents should be counseled about possible symptomatology until the results return. If the screening value is a lot higher than

the cutoffs, then examination, electrolytes, plasma 17-OH progesterone, androstenedione, and T levels by LCMSMS should be obtained. Depending on the age and clinical status of the infant, hospitalization, an ACTH test and therapy should be considered. A karyotype and pelvic ultrasound are always indicated in any infant with atypical genitalia and in apparent males with undescended testes especially those with evidence of salt loss.

P450c11 hydroxylase deficiency   Classic P450c11 hydroxylase deficiency (virilization with hypertension) is rare. It occurs in 1:100,000 births in persons of European ancestry. However, in the Middle Eastern population, it is much more common. In the patient with classic disease, a defect in 11-hydroxylation leads to decreased cortisol levels with a consequent increase in ACTH and the hypersecretion of DOC (deoxycorticosterone) and 11-deoxycortisol in addition to adrenal androgens. Marked heterogeneity in the clinical and hormonal manifestations of this defect has been described, including mild, late-onset, and even cryptic forms. Patients with this form of adrenal hyperplasia classically exhibit virilization, secondary to increased androgen production, and hypertension, related to increased DOC secretion. Plasma renin activity is either normal or suppressed. The hypertension is variable; it occurs in approximately two-thirds of patients and may be associated with hypokalemic alkalosis. Newborns with 11-hydroxylase deficiency may manifest transient salt loss probably related to their salt-restricted diet and relative resistance to mineralocorticoids.

Two P450c11 hydroxylase genes have been localized to the long arm of chromosome 8: P450c11b1 and P450c11b2. Similar to 21-hydroxylase, these two genes are 95% homologous. P450c11b1 encodes the enzyme for 11-hydroxylation and is expressed in the zona fasciculata and zona reticularis and is ACTH dependent. It primarily mediates 11-hydroxylation of 11-deoxycortisol to cortisol and DOC to corticosterone. It has about one-twelfth the capacity of P450c11b2 for 18-hydroxylation and does not oxidize 18-hydroxycorticosterone to aldosterone. P450c11b2 encodes the angiotensin-dependent isozyme aldosterone synthase and is only expressed in the zona glomerulosa, where it mediates 11-hydroxylation, 18-hydroxylation, and 18-oxidation. Mutations, deletions, and gene duplications of these genes can produce a wide variety of clinical manifestations from virilization and hypertension (P450c11b1 deficiency) to isolated salt-wasting (P450c11b2 [aldosterone synthase] deficiency) to glucocorticoid-remedial hypertension (due to fusion of the ACTH-dependent regulatory region of the 11-hydroxylase gene with the coding region of aldosterone synthase). Both genes encoding P450c11b1 and P450c11b2 are located on chromosome 8 and thus are not linked to HLA. ACTH stimulation tests have thus far failed to demonstrate a consistent biochemical abnormality in obligate heterozygotes.

Diagnosis: The diagnosis of P450c11b1-hydroxylase deficiency can be confirmed by demonstration of elevated basal or ACTH-induced plasma levels of 11-deoxycortisol and DOC, at least three times higher than the 95th percentile for age, and increased excretion of their metabolites in urine (mainly tetrahydro-11-deoxycortisol). As previously noted, these patients have elevated 17-OH progesterone levels and need to be distinguished from those with other forms of CAH by measuring the steroid levels at baseline or after ACTH stimulation.

StAR, P450scc, 17α-hydroxylase (17,20-lyase), 3β-HSD

Defects in steroidogenic acute regulatory protein (StAR), P450scc (side chain cleavage), 17α-hydroxylase (17,20-lyase), and 3β-HSD type II have in common blocks in cortisol and sex steroid synthesis in both the adrenals and the gonads. The latter types produce chiefly incomplete masculinization in the male and little or no virilization in the female (Table 14–3). Consequently, these are discussed primarily as forms of 46,XY DSD (disorders of androgen synthesis).

Treatment

Treatment of patients with salt-losing adrenal hyperplasia may be divided into acute and chronic phases. In acute adrenal crises, a deficiency of both cortisol and aldosterone results in hypoglycemia, hyponatremia, hyperkalemia, hypovolemia, acidosis, and shock. If the patient is hypoglycemic, an intravenous bolus of glucose (0.25-0.5 g/kg; maximum 25 g), should be administered. If the patient is in shock, an infusion of normal saline (20 mL/kg) may be given over the first hour; thereafter, replacement of glucose, fluid, and electrolytes is calculated on the basis of deficits and standard maintenance requirements. Hydrocortisone sodium succinate (50 mg/m^2) should be given as a bolus and another 50 to 100 mg/m^2 over 24 hours, divided into every 6 hour doses. If hyponatremia and hyperkalemia are present, fludrocortisone (0.05-0.1 mg) by mouth may be given along with the intravenous saline and hydrocortisone. Because hydrocortisone has mineralocorticoid activity, it may suffice to correct the electrolyte abnormality along with the saline. In extreme cases of hyponatremia, hyperkalemia, and acidosis, sodium bicarbonate and a cation exchange resin (eg, sodium polystyrene sulfonate) may be needed. In patients with presumed chronic hyponatremia, it is always prudent to raise the sodium cautiously and slowly to avoid the possibility of central pontine myelinolysis. Initially, in newly diagnosed patients and newborns in the first few days of treatment, hydrocortisone in doses of 25 to 50 mg/m^2/d are commonly used to facilitate suppression of the CRH-ACTH-adrenal axis. This dose should be reduced as soon as the steroid levels are suppressed to the desired range, usually after 5 to 7 days.

Once the patient is stabilized and a definitive diagnosis has been arrived at by means of appropriate steroid studies, the patient should receive suppressive doses of glucocorticoids to permit normal growth, development, and bone maturation (hydrocortisone, ~10-15 mg/m^2/d by mouth in three divided doses). The dose of hydrocortisone must be titrated in each patient depending on steroid hormone levels in plasma and urine, linear growth, bone maturation, and clinical signs of steroid overdose or of virilization. Therapy can be monitored by consistently timed (in relation to dose administration) steroid determinations, for example, the measurement of 17-OH progesterone, androstenedione, and T at 8 AM before the morning dose of hydrocortisone. A target concentration for 17-OH progesterone (400-1200 ng/dL) with

androstenedione and T levels in the normal range has been suggested. However, these levels will vary depending on when the evening dose of hydrocortisone is administered. Salt-losers need treatment with mineralocorticoid (fludrocortisone, 0.05-0.2 mg/d by mouth) and added dietary salt (1-3 g/d) in infancy. The dose of mineralocorticoid should be adjusted so that the electrolytes and blood pressure, as well as the plasma renin activity, are in the normal range.

Recently, as a result of the difficulty of optimally treating these patients, several novel therapies have been proposed. These include adrenalectomy in patients with null mutations of P450c21, GH to augment final height, and the use of physiologic doses of hydrocortisone (8 mg/m^2), fludrocortisone, flutamide (an androgen receptor blocker), and an aromatase inhibitor in combination.

The parents need to be presented the *whole picture* diagnosis, natural history, possible medical and surgical therapy, risks, complications, and unknowns. It is critical that they have the knowledge and time to make an informed decision about any surgical procedures on their child. Only patients with markedly ambiguous external genitalia (Prader III-V) should be considered for surgery. Vaginoplasty and clitoral recession or clitoroplasty for markedly enlarged clitori—*not clitoridectomy*—is indicated. Surgical reconstruction done in infancy may need refinement at puberty. Surgery, if done, must emphasize function rather than cosmesis. It should be performed by a surgeon who is experienced in the operative procedure and is cognizant of the importance of preserving the functional integrity of the genital area. The variability of *normalcy* in relationship to size and appearance of the external genitalia of adult women has recently been quantified. These data can serve as a reference with respect to the need for surgery in older patients with CAH. The timing of any surgery remains controversial. This is a decision that needs to be made after careful discussion with the parents. It should be noted that there are no outcome data for delaying functionally cosmetic surgery on an infant with ambiguous genitalia until an age of consent as suggested by some psychologists and patient advocates.

The dose of glucocorticoid needs to be increased in response to stress, for example, temperature above 100°F orally, gastroenteritis with dehydration, trauma, and surgery. The daily maintenance hydrocortisone dose should be tripled and divided into every 6 hour doses around the clock until the fever or gastroenteritis has abated for 12 hours. Thereafter, the child may resume his/her maintenance dose. In the event that the oral dose cannot be administered, hydrocortisone (50 mg/m^2) or its equivalent can be given intramuscularly and the child maintained on a dose of 50 to 100 mg/m^2/d in divided doses until he/she is able to take medication by mouth. It is prudent to check electrolytes in any patient who is a salt-loser, manifests vomiting, and is a candidate for parenteral hydrocortisone. Even if electrolytes are normal, patients who are unable to take medication and fluid orally for longer than 6 to 8 hours usually require hospitalization for parenteral fluids, especially if they are salt-losers. All caregivers should be prepared to administer hydrocortisone in an emergency, and all patients should have a medi-alert notification with them.

Prenatal therapy of pregnant women who are at risk of carrying a female fetus with atypical genitalia due to 21-hydroxylase deficiency is controversial. Therapy with oral dexamethasone given to the mother beginning at 6 to 7 weeks of gestation has been advocated to reduce or eliminate virilization of the affected female genitalia. Statistically, only one in eight fetuses will be a female with CAH. Although this therapy is effective, in diminishing genital ambiguity, more long-term studies are needed to ascertain the long-term morbidities, both physical and psychological.

In postpubertal patients who have reached their final height, glucocorticoid replacement can be implemented with more potent glucocorticoids that have longer half-lives than hydrocortisone such as prednisone (5-7 mg/d divided into two doses) or methylprednisolone (4-6 mg/d in two doses). As with children, the lowest dose of medication required to optimally suppress adrenal androgen secretion and prevent glucocorticoid side-effects should be used. The dose needs to be titrated to the plasma steroid values, or better yet, the urinary 17 ketosteroids—an integrated 24-hour assessment of androgen secretion. Similar to hydrocortisone, the dose is a function of absorption, metabolism, and sensitivity and varies from patient to patient.

A host of studies indicate that the vast majority of 46,XX females with 21-hydroxylase deficiency and consequent virilization of their external genitalia have a female gender identity. Gender dysphoria, although rare, is more prevalent in these patients than in the general population. Behavior characterized as masculinization/defeminization occurs in affected females who play more with traditionally boys' toys, are more aggressive, and show less interest in infants than their unaffected female siblings.

Treatment of adults with CAH should be directed toward preventing and remediating the morbidities of long-term glucocorticoid therapy and optimizing sexual, reproductive, and bone health (see Auchus PMID 20613954). Continued monitoring of serum 17-OH progesterone, androstenedione, and T levels (in females) and/or 24-hour urinary 17-ketosteroids is indicated in order to prevent further virilization or the morbidity of excess glucocorticoid therapy. While many salt-losers appear not to need mineralocorticoid due to increased salt intake or extra adrenal 21-hydroxylation, it is prudent to follow plasma renin activity, since elevated plasma renin levels are a marker of mineralocorticoid deficiency and are associated with the need for higher doses of glucocorticoids to suppress adrenal androgen secretion. Multiple factors play a role in the decreased fertility rate seen in women with CAH. These include decreased sexual activity due to vaginal stenosis which results in painful intercourse, poor surgical repairs resulting in lack of sensation, lack of desire for maternity, and poor self-image. In males, spermatogenesis and Leydig cell function may be compromised by poor hormonal control or testicular adrenal rest tumors which can be readily identified by ultrasound.

Dual energy x-ray absorptiometry (DXA) scans have shown that osteopenia is present in 40% to 50% of patients less than 30 years and 70% of patients over 30 years old. The severity of the osteopenia/osteoporosis is related to the severity of the CAH, the age of the patient, and dose of glucocorticoid given. Thus, periodic DXA scans and vitamin D and calcium supplementation are indicated, both prophylactically and therapeutically. Quality of life issues need to be addressed. These include physical and psychological status as well as social and sexual relationships.

Glucocorticoid Receptor Gene Mutation

Glucocorticoid resistance due to a homozygous mutation in the gene encoding the glucocorticoid receptor reportedly induces 46,XX DSD. Glucocorticoid resistance results in an increase in ACTH levels with a consequent increase in cortisol, mineralocorticoids, and adrenal androgens. The latter steroids induce virilization, which in the female infant results in 46,XX DSD.

Feto-Placental Source

P450 oxidoreductase   P450 oxidoreductase (POR) is a flavoprotein that transfers electrons from nicotinamide adenine dinucleotide to all microsomal P450s. These include P450c21, P450 17-hydroxylase/17,20-lyase and P450 aromatase which are involved in steroidogenesis, lanosterol 14-alpha-demethylase (P45014DM), and squalene monooxidase (SQLE), which are involved in cholesterol synthesis. POR deficiency is inherited as an autosomal recessive, and affected individuals are either homozygous or compound heterozygotes, predominantly for an A287P mutation in Caucasians and an R487H mutation in Japanese. More than 50 different mutations have been described. A broad range of phenotypes has been reported related to the degree of enzymatic function determined by the mutation and the specificity of the mutation for each one of the enzymes involved. Most, but not all patients reported with this condition, have skeletal abnormalities such as craniosynostosis, midfacial hypoplasia, and radioulnar synostosis. The phenotype of the skeletal dysmorphism has been termed the Antley-Bixler syndrome and appears to correlate with the degree of decrease in enzyme activity resulting from the mutations. The skeletal abnormalities of Antley-Bixler syndrome are digenic in origin. Individuals with normal genitalia and the Antley-Bixler phenotype have a mutation in the gene encoding fibroblast growth factor receptor-2 (FGFR-2) and no abnormality in steroidogenesis, whereas those with one or more of the above-mentioned skeletal abnormalities and ambiguous genitalia are found to have mutations in POR.

POR deficiency can cause ambiguous genitalia in both males and females, and micropenis, hypospadias, and infertility in males with mild mutations. The spectrum of patients reported includes females with normal genitalia who present with PCOS-like symptoms and have primary amenorrhea. There is evidence to suggest that virilization of the external genitalia in females with POR deficiency results from the synthesis of DHT in utero via the "backdoor" pathway (see Figure 14–10). Androgen excess can also result from a decrease in P450 aromatase activity in the placenta, which can cause maternal and fetal virilization during pregnancy. In patients with mild mutations, maternal virilization is not present, and males may have normal genitalia and rarely micropenis. The virilization in females is not progressive. After birth, however, in a Japanese cohort, pubertal maturation was definitely affected in females.

Diagnosis: POR deficiency should be suspected in males and females with ambiguous genitalia and the Antley-Bixler phenotype, in females whose virilization does not progress postnatally, and in patients with modestly elevated 17-OH progesterone levels. The diagnosis can be suspected from ACTH-induced steroid levels. Cortisol levels are normal at baseline, but there is a blunted response to ACTH. Both serum progesterone and 17-OH progesterone values in response to ACTH are higher than normal suggesting a defect in both 17- and 21-hydroxylation, whereas DHEA and androstenedione levels may be low. Genotyping will verify the diagnosis. Depending on the baseline concentration and ACTH-induced cortisol level, cortisol replacement may be indicated in some patients. In view of the blunted cortisol responses observed, it is prudent to give stress steroid coverage for illness, surgical procedures, and severe trauma.

P450 AROMATASE DEFICIENCY

Another form of androgen-induced 46,XX DSD is due to aromatase deficiency. Mutations in the gene *CYP19*, encoding P450 aromatase, result in defective placental conversion of C_{19} steroids to estrogens (C_{18}), leading to exposure of the fetus to excessive amounts of T and to masculinization of the external genitalia of the female fetus. Virilization of the mother during gestation occurs commonly. The female fetus is virilized, due to the inability of the placenta to aromatize testosterone produced by the placenta from the conversion of fetal adrenal DHEA. At puberty, defective aromatase activity in the ovary leads to pubertal failure, hypergonadotropic hypogonadism, polycystic ovaries, mild virilization, tall stature, and osteopenia. A striking delay in bone age with continuing growth occurs in both affected males and females, despite increased concentrations of plasma T, supporting the concept that estrogens, rather than androgens, are the major sex steroids affecting bone maturation, bone turnover, and epiphyseal fusion in males as well as females. A nonclassic phenotype has been described in two females with sufficient aromatase activity to result in the development of Tanner stage 2 and 4 breast development.

Diagnosis: The diagnosis of aromatase deficiency is suggested by the above clinical picture as well as elevated plasma androstenedione and T levels in the face of low estrogen levels, elevated gonadotropins, and ovarian cysts in females. Gonadotropin levels are elevated due to lack of estrogen feedback. There is striking osteopenia. Low plasma concentrations of maternal estriol during pregnancy associated with maternal virilization can facilitate the prenatal diagnosis. Affected males have normal genitalia, normal pubertal development, osteoporosis, and tall stature due to lack of epiphyseal fusion as a result of estrogen deficiency.

MATERNAL SOURCE ANDROGENS AND PROGESTOGENS

Masculinization of the external genitalia of a female infant can occur, if the mother is given T, other androgenic steroids, or certain synthetic progestational agents during pregnancy. Norethindrone, ethisterone, norethynodrel, and medroxyprogesterone acetate have all been implicated in masculinization of the female fetus. These drugs were given in the past in an effort to control threatened or habitual abortions. Nonadrenal 46,XX DSD can occur as a consequence of maternal ingestion of danazol, the 2,3-D-isoxazol derivative of 17α-ethinyl T. In rare instances, masculinization of a female fetus is due to a virilizing maternal ovarian or adrenal tumor, congenital virilizing adrenal hyperplasia in the mother, or a luteoma of pregnancy. The fetus is protected from excess T exposure by the ability of the fetal-placental unit to aromatize T to estrogens, especially after the first trimester. The diagnosis of 46,XX DSD arising from transplacental passage of androgenic steroids is based on exclusion of other forms of female pseudohermaphrodism and a history of drug exposure. Surgical correction of the genitalia, if needed, is the only therapy necessary.

Nonadrenal 46,XX DSD can be associated with imperforate anus, renal anomalies, and other malformations of the lower intestine and urinary tract and in some affected individuals. There may be anomalies of the ovaries and Müllerian structures. Sporadic as well as familial cases have been reported.

46,XY DSD (Male Pseudohermaphrodism)

Patients with 46,XY DSD have gonads that are testes, but the genital ducts or external genitalia, or both, that are not completely masculinized. 46,XY DSD can result from deficient T secretion as a consequence of (1) defective testicular differentiation (testicular dysgenesis); (2) failure of T secretion by Leydig cell due to a mutation in the Leydig cell hCG/LH receptor which is associated with Leydig cell hypoplasia as well as an inability to respond to hCG/LH stimulation; (3) impaired secretion of T; (4) failure of conversion of T to DHT; (5) failure of target tissue response to T and DHT; (6) impaired secretion of AMH or defective AMH receptors; and (7) environmental influences.

Testicular Unresponsiveness to hCG and LH (Leydig Cell Hypoplasia)

Male sexual differentiation is dependent on the production of T by fetal Leydig cells. Leydig cell T secretion is initially autonomous and then later hCG dependent during the critical period of male sexual development in the latter part of the first trimester. After the first trimester, Leydig cell T secretion is dependent on stimulation by pituitary LH, as evidenced by the finding of micropenis in 46,XY patients associated with anencephaly, apituitarism, or congenital hypothalamic hypopituitarism.

Absence, hypoplasia, or unresponsiveness of Leydig cells to hCG-LH results in deficient T production and, consequently, ambiguous male genitalia. The extent of the genital ambiguity is a function of the degree of T deficiency. The phenotype ranges from complete forms with female external genitalia, undescended testes, absent Müllerian ducts, rudimentary Wolffian ducts, and hypergonadotropic hypogonadism to milder forms with micropenis or males with normal male genitalia and hypergonadotropic hypogonadism at puberty. Testes are small postpubertally and have decreased or absent Leydig cells, normal-appearing Sertoli cells, and seminiferous tubules with spermatogenic arrest. A number of patients with absent, hypoplastic, or unresponsive Leydig cells due to a mutation in the gene encoding the LH-hCG receptor have been reported. Studies in patients with the clinical and chemical features of Leydig cell hypoplasia indicate that 50% of the patients with this phenotype have had no identifiable mutation in the LH-hCG receptor. Recently a mutation in a previously unrecognized exon has been described in some of these patients. 46,XX females with mutations in the LH beta subunit of LH receptor have female external genitalia, feminization at puberty, oligoamenorrhea, and infertility.

Diagnosis: Plasma 17α-hydroxyprogesterone, androstenedione, and T levels are low, and hCG elicits little or no response in T or its precursors in the complete form and a blunted T response in the partial form, in which partial virilization can occur at puberty. Adrenal steroidogenesis is normal in these patients.

Treatment depends on the age at diagnosis and the extent of masculinization. A female sex assignment has usually been chosen in patients with female external genitalia. In patients with predominantly male external genitalia, T augments penile development in infancy and childhood and virilizes the patient at puberty.

Inborn Errors of Testosterone Biosynthesis

Figure 14–15 demonstrates the major pathway in T biosynthesis in the testes; each step is associated with an inherited defect that results in T deficiency and, consequently, 46,XY DSD. Steps 1, 2, and 3 are enzymatic deficiencies that occur in both the adrenals and gonads and result in defective synthesis of both corticosteroids and T. Thus, they represent forms of CAH, whereas steps 4 and 5 in T synthesis are confined to the testes.

Star deficiency (congenital lipoid adrenal hyperplasia), P450scc

46,XY DSD with female or ambiguous genitalia, sexual infantilism, and adrenal insufficiency are consequences of very early defects in the synthesis of all steroids affecting the conversion of cholesterol to Δ⁵-pregnenolone and result in severe adrenal and gonadal deficiency. Recessive mutations in the gene encoding StAR, a protein that effects transport of cholesterol from the outer to the inner mitochondrial membrane (where it is converted to pregnenolone), have been identified in almost all patients with the clinical syndrome of congenital lipoid adrenal hyperplasia. Mutations in this gene located on chromosome 8 are prevalent in Japan and Korea where patients with lipoid adrenal hyperplasia represent the second most common form of CAH

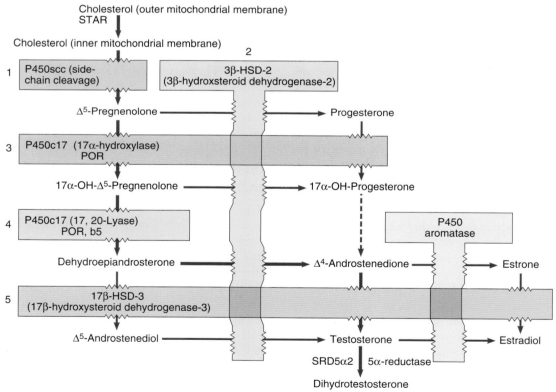

FIGURE 14–15 Enzymatic defects in the biosynthetic pathway for testosterone. All five of the enzymatic defects cause 46,XY DSD (male pseudohermaphroditism) in affected males. Although all of the blocks affect gonadal steroidogenesis, those at steps 1, 2, and 3 are associated with major abnormalities in the biosynthesis of glucocorticoids and mineralocorticoids in the adrenal. Chemical names for enzymes are shown with traditional names in parentheses. (Modified and reproduced, with permission, from Conte FA, Grumbach MM. Pathogenesis, classification, diagnosis, and treatment of anomalies of sex. In: DeGroot L, ed. *Endocrinology.* Grune & Stratton; 1989.)

after 21-hydroxylase deficiency. StAR is expressed in the adrenals and gonads but not in the placenta. Hence, placental synthesis of progesterone, which is required to maintain pregnancy after midgestation, is not affected by mutations in StAR. Affected males usually have female or, less commonly, ambiguous external genitalia with a blind vaginal pouch and hypoplastic male genital ducts, no Müllerian derivatives, adrenal insufficiency, and hypergonadotropic hypogonadism. Many infants with StAR deficiency do not manifest evidence of salt wasting until after several weeks of life. The accumulation of cholesterol in steroidogenic organs that are functioning in utero (adrenals and testes) destroys the function of these organs resulting in the phenotype, for example, adrenal insufficiency and impaired differentiation of the genitalia in males. Death in early infancy from adrenal insufficiency is not uncommon. Affected females have normal genitalia and go into puberty as the ovaries are relatively quiescent until puberty and roughly 14% of steroidogenesis is not StAR-dependent, apparently allowing for estrogen production until cholesterol engorgement destroys the function of the ovary and results in hypergonadotropic hypogonadism and large polycystic ovaries filled with cholesterol. The absence of Müllerian anlage distinguishes StAR/P450scc deficiency from patients with a similar phenotype due to SF-1 deficiency. As in other genetic defects, phenotypic variability results from the magnitude of the functional activity of the mutation. A nonclassic late-onset form of this condition has been described. Affected males have normal external genitalia; they develop, usually in the first decade of life, cortisol deficiency with or without mineralocorticoid deficiency. Those individuals with only cortisol deficiency need to be distinguished from those with isolated familial glucocorticoid deficiency due to mutations in the ACTH receptor (MC2R) and the melanocortin-2 receptor accessory protein (MRAP).

Diagnosis: The diagnosis is confirmed by the lack of or low levels of all C_{21}, C_{19}, and C_{18} steroids in plasma and urine and an absent response to ACTH and hCG stimulation. Large lipid-laden adrenals, that displace the kidneys downward, may be demonstrated by intravenous urography, abdominal ultrasonography, or CT scan. Treatment involves replacement with appropriate doses of glucocorticoids and mineralocorticoids, prophylactic orchiectomy in affected 46,XY patients raised as females, and estrogen replacement at puberty. Since the adrenals are not functionally hyperplastic, the glucocorticoid dose needed in these patients is less than is the case of P450c21-hydroxylase deficiency. A nonclassic late-onset form of this condition has been described.

P450scc The *P450scc* gene has been cloned and localized to chromosome 15. It codes for the enzyme scc, which is the first step in the conversion of cholesterol to pregnenolone in all steroidogenic organs. Seven patients with mutations in the *P450scc* gene(s) have been reported. All seven cases reported have had a 46,XY karyotype. Female genitalia were present in five of seven, clitoromegaly in one patient, and midshaft hypospadias in another. The onset of adrenal insufficiency varied from the neonatal period to as late as 9 years of age in the patient with hypospadias. The latter patient and two more recently described patients with compound heterozygosity for P450scc mutations had residual P450scc activity.

These patients had later onset of adrenal insufficiency than seen in classic patients and the males had hypospadias. These patients are similar to the non-classic form of StAR deficiency, both clinically and hormonally, except none had normal or enlarged adrenals on MRI or ultrasound. It has been suggested that patients with P450scc deficiency survive gestation due to either residual P450scc activity or due to continuing progesterone secretion beyond midgestation by the maternal corpus luteum.

Diagnosis: P450scc deficiency is suggested by the finding of a 46,XY DSD with undervirilization of the external genitalia, absent Müllerian ducts, adrenal insufficiency, and low baseline and deficient steroid responses to ACTH and hCG. The absence of adrenal enlargement on MRI or ultrasound distinguishes P450scc deficiency from a StAR deficiency.

3β-Hydroxysteroid dehydrogenase type 2 Δ^5-isomerase deficiency

3β-HSD type 2 Δ^5-isomerase deficiency is an early defect in steroid synthesis that results in inability of the adrenals and gonads to convert 3β-hydroxy-Δ^5 steroids to 3-keto-Δ^4 steroids. Deficiency leads to 46,XY or 46,XX DSD and adrenal insufficiency. This enzyme is encoded for by a recessive gene on the short arm of chromosome number 1. There are two highly homologous genes encoding 3β-HSDs on chromosome 1. The type 1 *3β-HSD* gene is expressed in the placenta, liver, skin, and other peripheral tissues, whereas type 2 is expressed in the adrenals and gonads. 3β-HSD is not a cytochrome P450 enzyme, and it requires NAD^+ as a cofactor.

Mutations causing frame-shifts, stops, and missense have been reported in the *type 2* gene in affected patients. Mutations which decrease enzymatic activity of the type 2 enzyme significantly result in a severe deficiency of aldosterone, cortisol, T, and estradiol secretion (see Figure 14–15). Males with this defect are incompletely masculinized due to the defect in 3β-hydroxysteroid dehydrogenase in the testes. They have a small penis, hypospadias, a blind vaginal pouch, and absent Müllerian structures. Females have normal female genitalia or mild clitoromegaly.

The undervirilization in males is readily explainable by the block in T synthesis in the testes during the critical period of male genital differentiation. However, the mild virilization observed in some females is still not readily explained. It has been suggested that the conversion of Δ^5-17-OH pregnenolone to 17-hydroxyprogesterone in utero by peripheral 3β-HSD-1 facilitates the production of low levels of DHT via the backdoor pathway (see Figure 14–10). Alternatively, the conversion of excess DHEA-S to T by 3β-HSD-1 in the placenta during the critical window of sex differentiation, when aromatase activity is relatively low, may be implicated. Further studies of steroidogenesis in affected patients with null mutations may shed light on this question.

Adrenal crises with salt loss usually occurs in early infancy in affected patients. Affected males may experience normal male puberty but often have prominent gynecomastia. Rare cases with normal puberty and fertility have been reported. Individuals with a mild non-salt-losing form of 3β-HSD type 2 deficiency are reported as well as a late-onset form in individuals presenting with premature pubarche alone. These patients had elevated Δ^5 steroids as well as mutations in the *3β-HSD type 2* gene.

Diagnosis: The diagnosis of 3β-HSD deficiency type 2 is based on finding elevated concentrations of Δ^5-pregnenolone, Δ^5-17α-hydroxypregnenolone, DHEA and its sulfate, and other 3β-hydroxy-Δ^5 steroids in the plasma and urine. 3-Keto-Δ^4 steroids (ie, 17-hydroxyprogesterone and androstenedione) may be elevated due to peripheral conversion of 3β-hydroxy-Δ^5 to 3-keto-Δ^4 steroids by the enzyme encoded by the *type 1* gene. The diagnosis of 3β-HSD-2 deficiency may be facilitated by detecting abnormal levels of serum Δ^5-17α-hydroxypregnenolone and DHEA and its sulfates as well as abnormal ratios of Δ^5 to Δ^4 steroids after intravenous administration of ACTH. For example, after ACTH stimulation, 17-hydroxypregnenolone levels are more than 5.3 SD above the mean for normal individuals in affected infants, more than 35 SD above the mean in prepubertal children, and more than 21 SD above the mean in adults. The 17-hydroxypregnenolone-cortisol ratio is more than 6.4 SD above the mean in infants, more than 23 SD above the mean in prepubertal children, and more than 221 SD above the mean in adults. The diagnosis is confirmed by detecting mutations in the *type 2 3β-HSD-Δ^5 isomerase* gene. Suppression of the increased plasma and urinary 3β-hydroxy-Δ^5 steroids by the administration of dexamethasone distinguishes 3β-HSD deficiency from a virilizing adrenal tumor.

Treatment of this condition is similar to that of other forms of adrenal hyperplasia.

P450c17 deficiency, 17α-hydroxylase deficiency

A single gene on chromosome 10 encodes both adrenal and testicular P450c17 hydroxylase as well as 17,20-lyase activity. This enzyme catalyzes the 17-hydroxylation of pregnenolone and progesterone to 17-hydroxypregnenolone and 17-hydroxyprogesterone as well as the scission (lyase) of 17-hydroxypregnenolone to the C_{19} steroid (DHEA) in the adrenal cortex and gonads. Mutations affecting 17-hydroxylase activity have included stop codons, frame-shifts, deletions, and missense substitutions. P450c17 deficiency is transmitted in a manner similar to other enzymatic defects in steroidogenesis as an autosomal recessive trait.

A defect in 17α-hydroxylation in the zona fasciculata of the adrenal and in the gonads results in impaired synthesis of 17-hydroxyprogesterone and 17-hydroxypregnenolone and, consequently, cortisol and sex steroids. The secretion of large amounts of corticosterone and DOC leads to hypertension, hypokalemia, and alkalosis. Although these patients are cortisol-deficient, the excess mineralocorticoid secretion, as well as elevated levels of corticosterone, prevents symptomatic adrenal insufficiency except during stress. Increased DOC secretion from the zona fasciculata results in hypertension and hypokalemia, and suppression of renin (low renin hypertension) and, decreased aldosterone secretion. Affected 46,XY individuals with less than 25% enzymatic activity present with female genitalia with a blind vaginal pouch or hypoplastic male genitalia, hypertension, and hypokalemic alkalosis with hypergonadotropic hypogonadism at puberty. Müllerian structures are absent; Wolffian structures are hypoplastic. Partial forms of 17-hydroxylase deficiency have been described with hypospadias, with or without hypertension.

Affected 46,XX females have normal development of the internal ducts and external genitalia but manifest sexual infantilism

with elevated gonadotropin concentrations at puberty and low renin hypertension. Affected females with 5% or greater activity of the enzyme can make estrogen at puberty and feminize, although menses are usually irregular.

Diagnosis: 17α-Hydroxylase deficiency should be suspected in a 46,XY DSD with hypokalemic alkalosis and hypertension, as well as a 46,XX female with the above findings and sexual infantilism at puberty. ACTH stimulation testing will reveal elevated levels of DOC, corticosterone, and 18-hydroxycorticosterone as well as progesterone and Δ^5 pregnenolone, but low levels of 17-hydroxyprogesterone, 17-hydroxypregnenolone, sex steroids, and cortisol. Glucocorticoid therapy, as given for 21-hydroxylase deficiency, suppresses ACTH and hence deoxycorticosterone production. This decreases the blood pressure and returns the potassium and aldosterone levels to normal. These patients usually require sex steroid replacement at puberty.

Smith-Lemli-Opitz syndrome

The phenotypic spectrum of this syndrome typically includes microcephaly, mental retardation, ptosis, micrognathia, severe hypospadias, micropenis, growth failure, and, rarely, adrenal insufficiency. The genitalia in affected 46,XY males may range from normal male to female. The syndrome is caused by a mutation in the gene encoding sterol Δ-7-reductase, *DHCR7*, causing defective cholesterol synthesis. The diagnosis is made by the clinical features and confirmed by demonstration of low levels of cholesterol and increased levels of 7-dehydrocholesterol.

Enzyme Defects Primarily Affecting Testosterone Biosynthesis by the Testes

7,20-lyase deficiency

The enzyme encoded by the *P450c17* gene mediates both the 17-hydroxylation of pregnenolone and progesterone to 17-hydroxypregnenolone and 17-hydroxyprogesterone and the scission of the $C_{17,20}$ bond of 17-hydroxypregnenolone to yield DHEA in the adrenals and gonads (see Figure 14-15). In humans, the scission of 17-hydroxyprogesterone to androstenedione occurs at a low level. In this rare autosomal recessive disorder, the defect involves only the scission of the C_{21} steroids to C_{19} steroids. This results in a defect in T synthesis and, as a consequence, 46,XY DSD in the male and affected females with estradiol deficiency, hypergonadotropic hypogonadism, and giant ovarian cysts. The initially reported 46,XY DSD individuals both had micropenis, perineal hypospadias, a bifid scrotum, a blind vaginal pouch, and cryptorchidism. The administration of hCG resulted in a marked rise in plasma 17-hydroxyprogesterone with a poor response in plasma DHEA, androstenedione, and T consistent with a diagnosis of isolated 17,20-lyase deficiency. Analyses of the *P450c17* gene in affected individuals has revealed mutations that result in a specific decrease in 17,20-lyase activity encoded by the *P450c17* gene, but not 17-hydroxylase activity.

Affected 46,XY males with 17,20-lyase deficiency may present with female external genitalia. Patients with 17,20-lyase deficiency have low circulating levels of T, androstenedione, DHEA, and estradiol in the face of markedly elevated levels of progesterone and 17-hydroxyprogesterone. At puberty, poor virilization occurs with elevated gonadotropins in affected 46,XY patients.

Cytochrome b5 reductase is a cofactor for 17,20-lyase. Mutations in this gene cause methemoglobinemia as well as a defect on 17,20-lyase. Two patients have been reported with mutations in b5 reductase causing 46,XY DSD.

Diagnosis: The diagnosis of 17,20-lyase deficiency can be confirmed by demonstration of an increased ratio of 17-hydroxy C_{21} steroids to C_{19} steroids (T, DHEA, Δ^5-androstenediol, and androstenedione) after stimulation with ACTH or hCG and by DNA analysis of the *P450c17* gene. Patients require sex steroid replacement at puberty.

17β-Hydroxysteroid dehydrogenase-3 (17β-HSD-3) deficiency

At least six isoenzymes of 17β-HSD mediate steroidogenesis in humans. The last step in T biosynthesis by the testes involves the reduction of androstenedione to T, and estrone to estradiol by 17-hydroxysteroid dehydrogenase-3, an NADPH-dependent microsomal enzyme. This gene is located on chromosome 9q22 and is expressed primarily in the testes. As with other genes which code for enzymes, it is autosomal recessive. 17β-HSD-3 is not expressed in the ovary. The conversion of estrone to estradiol is mediated by 17β-HSD-1 expressed in the granulosa cells of the ovary.

Mutations in 17β-HSD-3 are a cause of 46,XY DSD. At birth, males with a deficiency of the enzyme 17β-HSD-3 have predominantly female or mildly ambiguous external genitalia resulting from T deficiency during the critical period of male differentiation. They have male duct development, absent Müllerian structures with a blind vaginal pouch, and inguinal or intra-abdominal testes. Affected infants with female genitalia are invariably raised as females, and the phenotypic appearance of the genitalia, along with the absence of Müllerian duct derivatives, can be confused with complete androgen insensitivity. The finding of Wolffian ducts, associated with female external genitalia in these patients, is not yet well explained. At puberty, progressive virilization with clitoral hypertrophy occurs as a result of peripheral extraglandular conversion of androstenedione to T by 17β-HSD-5. This is often associated with the concurrent development of gynecomastia related to increased estrone levels. Plasma gonadotropin, androstenedione, and estrone levels are elevated, whereas T and estradiol concentration are relatively low.

Analysis of a cohort of 17 patients with classic 17β-HSD-3 deficiency revealed 14 mutations in the *17β-HSD-3* gene. Twelve patients had homozygous mutations, four were compound heterozygotes, and one was a presumed heterozygote. In a large cohort from the Gaza Strip, an Arg[80] → Gln mutation was found with partial (15%-20%) enzymatic activity. In this isolate, virilization at puberty generally resulted in a change of gender identity from female to male.

Diagnosis: 17-HSD-3 deficiency should be included in the differential diagnosis of (1) 46,XY DSDs with absent Müllerian derivatives who have no abnormality in glucocorticoid or mineralocorticoid synthesis; and (2) 46,XY DSDs who virilize at puberty, especially if they also exhibit gynecomastia. The diagnosis of 17β-HSD-3 deficiency is confirmed by the demonstration of

inappropriately high plasma levels of estrone and androstenedione and increased ratios of plasma androstenedione to T and estrone to estradiol after prolonged stimulation with hCG in infants and children.

Management of affected individuals depends on the age at diagnosis, the degree of ambiguity of the external genitalia, surgical options, and family and cultural views, as it does with those with other forms of 46,XY DSD. In the patient assigned a male sex identity, plastic repair of the genitalia and T augmentation of phallic growth prepubertally, as well as T replacement therapy at puberty, is necessary to suppress the pituitary gonadotropin levels and, consequently, the elevated estrone levels that result in gynecomastia in untreated pubertal patients. Retained testes must be observed closely by palpation and ultrasound because an increased incidence of malignancy has been reported in a small cohort of patients. In patients reared as females, the appropriate treatment is castration or prevention of virilization with GnRH agonist at puberty until the individual's gender identity can be confirmed. Affected 46,XX females have no abnormalities in phenotype or gonadal function because 17β-HSD-3 is not expressed in the ovary.

The prevalence of a female-to-male gender role change in patients with 17β-HSD-3 deficiency appears to approximate that found in patients with 5α-reductase-2 deficiency. Both these conditions are associated with spontaneous virilization at puberty in patients whose testes were not removed. However, a number of the large cohorts of patients with 17β-HSD-3 deficiency summarized in the literature are from areas where a primacy is placed on a male role by the cultural advantages of the society. In individuals diagnosed in infancy, the information on the change in sex makes discussion of this issue with the parents mandatory before they make an informed decision about sex assignment.

Enzyme Defects Affecting DHT Synthesis; 5α-Reductase-2 Deficiency (Pseudovaginal Perineoscrotal Hypospadias, Peripheral)

The products of two genes catalyze the conversion of T to DHT. They are termed type 1 and type 2 5α-reductase. The type 1 enzyme is expressed in skin postnatally until 2 to 3 years of age and thereafter remains low until puberty. No instances of mutation in the *type 1* gene as yet have been reported. The type 2 isoenzyme is found in fetal genital skin, male accessory glands, and the prostate. 5α-Reductase-2 deficiency is transmitted as an autosomal recessive trait, and the enzymatic defect exhibits genetic heterogeneity. In patients with 5α-reductase deficiency, the isozyme with a pH 5.5 optimum is deficient (type 2). The gene encoding this enzyme contains five exons and is located on chromosome 2, band p23. A variety of mutations are reported, including deletions, nonsense, splicing defects, and the more common missense mutations. Two-thirds of patients are homozygous for a single mutation, and the remainder are compound heterozygotes.

The defective conversion of T to DHT produces a unique form of 46,XY DSD. Phenotypically, these individuals may vary from those with a microphallus to individuals with pseudovaginal perineoscrotal hypospadias. At birth, in the most severely affected individuals, ambiguous external genitalia are characterized by a small hypospadiac phallus bound down in chordee, a bifid scrotum, and a urogenital sinus that opens onto the perineum. A blind vaginal pouch is present, opening either into a urogenital sinus or directly into the urethra. The testes are either inguinal or labial. Müllerian structures are absent, and the Wolffian structures are well differentiated. At puberty, affected males virilize; the voice deepens, muscle mass increases, and the phallus enlarges. The bifid scrotum becomes rugose and pigmented. The testes enlarge and descend into the labioscrotal folds, and spermatogenesis may ensue. Gynecomastia is notably absent in these patients. Of note is the absence of acne, temporal hair recession, and hirsutism. The striking virilization noted at puberty, as opposed to its absence in utero, is attributed to the expression and function of the *type 1* gene at puberty and, as a consequence, the generation of sufficient amounts of DHT by peripheral conversion to induce phallic growth and other signs of masculinization. A remarkable feature of this form of 46,XY DSD is the change in gender identity by many from female to male at puberty.

In the first 1 to 3 months of life after the onset of puberty, patients with 5α-reductase-2 deficiency have normal to elevated T concentrations and slightly elevated plasma concentrations of LH. As expected, plasma DHT is low, and the T/DHT ratio is abnormally high. Apparently, lack of 5α reduction of T to DHT in utero, during the critical phases of male sex differentiation, results in incomplete masculinization of the urogenital sinus and external genitalia. However, T-dependent Wolffian structures are normally developed. Partial and mild forms of 5α-reductase deficiency have been described, in which affected individuals can present with hypospadias and/or microphallus. Compound heterozygotes for 5α-reductase-2 deficiency are described who had a hypospadias repair in infancy and, as adults, were fertile.

Diagnosis: 5α-Reductase-2 deficiency should be suspected in 46,XY DSDs with a blind vaginal pouch and in males with hypospadias and microphallus. The diagnosis can be confirmed by demonstration of an abnormally high plasma T/DHT ratio, either under basal conditions (>10.5) or after hCG stimulation (>8.5). The T-DHT levels need to be measured accurately, preferably by LCMSMS. Other confirmatory findings, especially in newborns, include an increased 5β/5α ratio of urinary C_{19} and C_{21} steroid metabolites. 5α-reductase deficiency should be ruled out in all 46,XY DSDs who have a normal or elevated T response to hCG. In the event that the T/DHT ratio in blood or the 5β/5α ratio of urinary steroids is not diagnostic, genotyping should be performed.

The early diagnosis of this condition is particularly critical. In view of the natural history of this disorder, a male gender assignment is indicated, and DHT or high-dose T therapy should be initiated in order to augment phallic size. Repair of hypospadias should be performed in infancy or early childhood. In patients who are diagnosed after infancy in whom gender identity is unequivocally female after the age of informed consent, genitoplasty, prophylactic orchiectomy, and estrogen substitution therapy are still the treatments of choice.

Disorders of Androgen Action (Androgen Receptor and Postreceptor Defects)

Syndrome of complete androgen resistance (insensitivity) and its variants
The androgen receptor gene is located on the X chromosome between Xq11 and Xq13. Androgen resistance is transmitted as an X-linked recessive trait. Of note about 30% of mutations occur spontaneously. The gene is composed of eight exons. Exon 1 encodes the amino terminal end of the androgen receptor protein and is involved in the regulation of transcription. Exons 2 and 3 encode the DNA-binding zinc finger. The 5′ portion of exon 4 is called the hinge region and plays a role in nuclear targeting. Exons 5 to 8 specify the carboxyl terminal portion of the androgen receptor—the androgen-binding domain. The gene has eight serine residues that can be phosphorylated, three lysine residues that can be acetylated, and two lysine residues that can be sumoylated. More than 600 mutations in the androgen receptor are described.

The syndrome of complete androgen resistance (insensitivity) is characterized by a 46,XY karyotype, bilateral testes, absent or hypoplastic Wolffian ducts, female-appearing external genitalia with a hypoplastic clitoris and labia minora, a blind vaginal pouch, and absent or rudimentary Müllerian derivatives. Testes are present in the labial folds, inguinal canal or intra-abdominally. At puberty, female secondary sexual characteristics develop, but menarche does not ensue. Pubic and axillary hair is usually sparse and in one-third of patients is totally absent. Affected patients are taller than average females (mean height 162.3 cm). Some patients have a variant form of this syndrome and exhibit slight clitoral enlargement. These patients may exhibit mild virilization in addition to the development of breasts and a female habitus at puberty.

Androgen resistance during embryogenesis prevents masculinization of the external genitalia and complete differentiation of the Wolffian ducts. The finding of Wolffian duct derivatives in some patients with apparent complete androgen resistance has been attributed to mutant receptors that have some residual activity and can respond to high local levels of T in vivo or to cofactors which modulate androgen sensitivity. Secretion of AMH by the fetal Sertoli cells leads to regression of the Müllerian derivatives—the ducts, uterus, and upper one-third of the vagina. At puberty, androgen resistance results in augmented LH secretion with increases in T secretion and estradiol production due to lack of T feedback on the hypothalamus. FSH levels are normal because of inhibin B and estradiol feedback. Estradiol arises mainly from peripheral conversion of T and androstenedione as well as from direct secretion by the testes. Androgen resistance, coupled with increased testicular estradiol secretion and conversion of T to estradiol, results in the development of female secondary sexual characteristics at puberty. The timing of the onset of the pubertal growth spurt is similar to that in normal females.

Patients with complete androgen resistance exhibit heterogeneity in DHT binding to the androgen receptor. Receptor-negative and receptor-positive individuals with qualitative defects such as thermolability, instability, and impaired binding affinity as well as individuals with presumed normal binding are reported. Analysis of the androgen receptor gene in individuals with androgen resistance has shed light on the heterogeneity of DHT binding. Patients with the receptor-negative form of complete androgen resistance usually have point mutations or substitutions in exons 5 to 8, which encode the androgen-binding domain of the receptor; a striking number of missense mutations occur in the ligand-binding region of the androgen receptor.

Other genetic defects such as deletions, mutations in a splice donor site, and nonsense mutations causing premature termination codons are less common in this group of patients. Mutations in exon 1 commonly cause complete androgen resistance; almost all code for a premature stop codon that results in a truncated nonfunctional androgen receptor. Mutations in exon 3 (which encodes the DNA-binding segment of the androgen receptor) are associated with normal binding of DHT to the receptor but the inability of the ligand-receptor complex to bind to DNA and initiate mRNA transcription. These mutations result in receptor-positive complete androgen resistance. The phenotype of the affected patient correlates better with the transcriptional activity of the ligand-androgen receptor complex than with in vitro studies of the androgen receptor–binding activity.

Other factors that play a role in genotype-phenotype variations include somatic mosaicism, transcriptional coregulatory proteins, and other *modifier* genes. Somatic mutations—mutations that occur after zygote formation—result in the presence of both wild-type and mutant androgen receptor. Individuals with a somatic mutation may exhibit virilization at puberty owing to the presence of the wild-type receptor, even though some of these patients may present in infancy with the clinical picture of apparent complete androgen resistance.

Diagnosis: In the absence of a family history, the presence of a testis-like mass in the inguinal canal or labia majora may be the only clue to the diagnosis. Approximately 1% to 2% of females with inguinal herniae have androgen resistance. Postpubertally, the patients present with primary amenorrhea, normal breast development, and absent or sparse pubic or axillary hair. Pelvic examination or ultrasound confirms the absence of a cervix and uterus.

The complete and incomplete forms of androgen resistance must be distinguished from other forms of 46,XY DSD due to androgen deficiency, such as biosynthetic defects in T synthesis and 5α-reductase deficiency. There is no readily available, rapid, in vivo or in vitro assay to determine androgen sensitivity. The diagnosis is suggested by the clinical picture, the family history, and the presence of elevated basal and hCG-induced T levels with normal levels of DHT. Neonates with complete androgen resistance do not have elevated basal LH and T levels and do not experience a postnatal rise in these values, as is observed in normal infants and in those with incomplete androgen resistance. It has been suggested that an elevated AMH concentration is a marker of androgen resistance and androgen deficiency. It is not specific, as it may be elevated in other causes of 46,XY DSD. Defective or absent androgen receptor expression in Sertoli cells is responsible for the absence of AMH suppression. Determination of abnormalities in androgen binding as well as transactivation studies are diagnostic, but they are labor intensive and not universally available, whereas mutational analysis of the androgen receptor gene is commercially available.

Management: The of patients with complete androgen resistance, as with most other patients with DSD, is complex. It requires a team of experienced physicians—an endocrinologist, psychologist and/or psychiatrist, a surgeon, and a social worker, as well as a primary care physician. When the diagnosis is definitive, the parents need to be fully informed about the karyotype, genetics, pathophysiology, medical and surgical options, and the natural history of complete androgen resistance. They should be informed that so far, except for very rare patients, gender identity, role, and behavior are female. Inguinal herniae, if present, need to be repaired. A gonadal malignancy rate of 1% to 2% is present after 14 years of age. Thus, it is prudent to allow these girls to feminize spontaneously at puberty and after full disclosure, discuss the question of prophylactic gonadectomy with them and their parents (who have been previously informed of this possibility). Spontaneous feminization at puberty may help to reinforce their sense of being a normal although infertile female. Allowing them to make an informed decision about gonadectomy reinforces their sense of autonomy. Hormonal replacement will be necessary postgonadectomy.

Postpubertally, the functional adequacy of the vagina should be assessed. Vaginoplasty is rarely necessary. Vaginal dilation with plastic molds is invariably successful in augmenting vaginal size and should be initiated if necessary postpubertally with the patient's informed consent.

The continuing involvement of the psychologist or psychiatrist will facilitate the question of when, how, and by whom the patients should be fully informed of their karyotype, infertility, and therapeutic options. There is no mandated guideline for this, and the approach needs to be individualized for each patient and family. In general, information is given in an age-appropriate way, taking into consideration the patient's age, cognitive abilities, and psychologic development. It is a gradual process, done in an understandable, caring way, which culminates in full disclosure. Continuing psychologic/psychiatric counseling should be available concerning sexual relationships and psychosocial issues. The Androgen Insensitivity Society (http://www.aissg.org) is a valuable support group for patients as well as parents and provides information, experiences from older, affected patients and parents, and the ability to meet and talk with females who have similar DSDs.

Syndrome of partial androgen resistance (insensitivity) and its variants (Reifenstein syndrome)

Patients with partial androgen resistance manifest a wide spectrum of phenotypes as far as the degree of masculinization is concerned. The external genitalia at birth are classically characterized by perinoscrotal hypospadias, micropenis, and a bifid scrotum. The testes may be undescended. Isolated hypospadias may occur in the mildest form of partial androgen resistance. There is variability of masculinization of affected males even within kinships. Müllerian duct derivatives are absent and Wolffian duct derivatives are present, but they are usually hypoplastic. At puberty, virilization usually recapitulates that seen in utero and is generally poor; pubic and axillary hair as well as gynecomastia are usually present. The most common phenotype postpubertally is the male posthypospadial repair with a small phallus and gynecomastia. Axillary and pubic hairs are normal. The testes remain small and exhibit azoospermia as a consequence of germinal cell arrest. Unlike patients with complete androgen resistance, in infancy the levels of plasma LH and T are elevated. Postpubertally, as in individuals with complete androgen resistance, LH, T, and estradiol are elevated. However, the degree of feminization in these individuals, despite increased estradiol levels, is less than that found in those with the syndrome of complete androgen resistance.

Androgen receptor studies in these patients have usually shown quantitative or qualitative abnormalities in androgen binding. Mutations leading to partial reduction of androgen action result in incomplete virilization. As previously noted, the best correlation with the phenotype is the degree of impairment of transcriptional activity of the ligand-androgen receptor complex. A wide variety of androgen receptor gene mutations may result in the same phenotype, and a specific mutation is not always associated with the same phenotype. In general, point mutations that result in more conservative amino acid substitutions are more likely to result in partial rather than complete androgen resistance. In 111 individuals with partial androgen resistance in which DNA was sequenced, only 27 (24%) had an identifiable mutation. The majority of the patients with mutations had abnormal DHT binding to the androgen receptor.

Diagnosis: The differential diagnosis of patients with ambiguous genitalia and absent Müllerian structures includes partial androgen resistance, all the forms of dysgenetic 46,XY DSD, Leydig cells unresponsive to hCG/LH, biosynthetic errors in T synthesis, 5α-reductase deficiency, and SF-1 mutations. These entities may be parsed by steroid analysis in response to ACTH and hCG stimulation. A protocol frequently used for hCG stimulation is as follows: (1) a baseline LH, FSH by ICMA, AMH, inhibin B, androstenedione, T/DHT; (2) 2000 U/m^2 hCG × 3 days; (3) serum androstenedione, T/DHT, and urine for steroid analysis 24 hours after the third dose of hCG. hCG will elicit an augmented T response in patients with partial androgen resistance and 5α-reductase deficiency. 5α-Reductase deficiency can be generally ruled out by a T/DHT ratio <8.5 after hCG or by the ratio of 5β/5α steroid metabolites in urine. However, in some reported cases with mild mutations, only genotyping was diagnostic. All the above entities, except for partial androgen resistance, will result in a "normal" penile response to a trial of administration of T enanthate in oil, 25 mg intramuscularly × 3 months in infants. We have utilized this test to diagnose partial androgen insensitivity syndrome (PAIS) before assigning a definitive sex of rearing.

Follow-up data have indicated dissatisfaction in many patients with PAIS, whether they are raised as males or females. The prevalence of gender dysphoria in partial androgen resistance is estimated at 10%. In individuals reared as males, a major decrease in all aspects of sexual function has been documented. If a decision is made to raise the infant in a female sex role, then gonadectomy prior to puberty or GnRH therapy pending definitive ascertainment of gender identity is indicated to avoid the possible risk of signs of virilization at puberty. In view of the incidence of gender dysphoria and the apparent unhappiness about their assigned sex in individuals with partial androgen resistance, a male sex of rearing is a judicious choice in individuals with Prader III or greater ambiguous genitalia or hypoplastic male genitalia because it preserves a choice. In some patients, high doses of T has engendered penile enlargement. Psychologic/psychiatric consultation is important in these individuals whether raised as males or females, since available follow-up studies indicate dissatisfaction with the outcome when they are assigned a male or female sex of rearing.

Androgen resistance in men with normal male genitalia   Partial androgen resistance has been described in a group of infertile men who have a normal male phenotype but may exhibit gynecomastia. Unlike other patients with androgen resistance, some of these patients have normal plasma LH and T levels. Infertility in otherwise normal men may be the only clinical manifestation of androgen resistance. Infertility, however, is always associated with androgen resistance. Five phenotypic males in one affected family had gynecomastia and a small penis. Plasma LH and T levels were elevated, and a subtle qualitative abnormality in ligand binding was found. Fertility was documented in four of the five males. This is the mildest form of androgen resistance.

Dysgenetic 46,XY DSD (Ambiguous Genitalia due to Dysgenetic Gonads)

See previous discussions of sex determination, XY gonadal dysgenesis, XO/XY mosaicism, Denys Drash/Frasier/WAGR syndromes, etc.

Testicular Regression Syndrome (Vanishing Testes Syndrome; XY Agonadism; Rudimentary Testes Syndrome; Congenital Anorchia)

Cessation of testicular function during the critical phases of male sex differentiation can lead to various clinical syndromes depending on when testicular function ceases. At one end of the clinical spectrum of these heterogeneous conditions are the XY patients in whom testicular deficiency occurred before 8 weeks of gestation, which results in female differentiation of the internal and external genitalia—so-called XY gonadal dysgenesis. At the other end of the spectrum are the patients with anorchia or vanishing testes in which the testes are lost later in gestation after the critical period of male genital differentiation from 8 to 12 weeks. These patients have normal male differentiation of their internal and external structures, but gonadal tissue is absent. The phallus varies in size dependent upon when Leydig cell failure occurs. Testicular regression may occur unilaterally especially on the left side or bilaterally, and the condition is seen in family cohorts. The latter suggests a genetic etiology, but only one individual with a mutation in the gene (*SF-1*) has been reported.

Diagnosis: Bilateral anorchia should be suspected in all 46,XY phenotypic males with undescended testes especially those with micropenis. MRI usually reveals absence of the gonads in the inguinal canal and no Müllerian duct derivatives. Plasma gonadotropins, especially FSH are elevated under 4 years of age and after

10 years of age. Inhibin B and AMH levels, measures of Sertoli cell integrity, are unmeasurable and a lack of rise in T at 1 to 3 months—"the window of opportunity"—will be evident. The absence of Leydig cell function is documented by the failure of the administration of hCG to elicit a rise in T. Finally, laparoscopic exploration, if necessary, indicates that 90% of patients lack testicular tissue, and in 10%, a testicular remnant without germ cells is present. Treatment of these males includes T therapy in childhood for microphallus, and at 12 to 13 years administration of T to induce male secondary sex characteristics and, thereafter, as replacement therapy.

Persistent Müllerian Duct Syndrome (Defects in the Synthesis, Secretion, or Response to Antimüllerian Hormone)

This male-limited autosomal recessive syndrome is associated with normal male development of the external genitalia but with Müllerian duct derivatives. The retention of Müllerian structures is either due to failure of the Sertoli cells to synthesize and secrete AMH or to an end-organ defect in the response of the Müllerian duct to AMH. The gene for AMH maps to chromosome 19; a variety of mutations in the *AMH* gene cause the syndrome as well as mutations in the gene encoding the AMH receptor. Individuals with mutations in the AMH receptor have Müllerian ducts, despite the normal to high concentrations of plasma AMH. Therapy involves removal of the Müllerian structures.

Environmental Chemicals

An increase in disorders of development and function of the urogenital tract in males has been noted over the past 50 years. It has been hypothesized that this increased incidence of reproductive abnormalities observed in human males is related to increasing exposure in utero to endocrine disrupters especially estrogens and androgen receptor blockers found in the diet both naturally and as a result of chemical contamination. It has been demonstrated that p,p′-DDE (dichlorodiphenyldichloroethylene)—the major and persistent DDT metabolite—binds to the androgen receptor and inhibits androgen action in developing rodents. Other chemicals such as phthalates, herbicides, and fungicides inhibit androgen actions. The term **testicular dysgenesis syndrome** describes a phenotype that has been attributed to endocrine disrupters. Further studies on the levels as well as the risks to humans of environmental chemicals and other endocrine disruptors are necessary before abnormalities of the reproductive tract can be confidently ascribed to these agents.

UNCLASSIFIED FORMS OF ABNORMAL SEXUAL DEVELOPMENT IN MALES

Hypospadias

Hypospadias is one of the most common genital abnormalities. It has an incidence of 1 in 125 live male births in the United States.

It is often associated with ventral curvature of the penis, a condition called chordee. The aberrant urethral meatus can open anywhere along the shaft of the penis, penoscrotally (at the base of the shaft), or even on the perineum.

The etiology of hypospadias is multifactorial, and both genetic and environmental factors appear to play a role in its pathogenesis. Deficient virilization of the male genitalia implies subnormal fetal testosterone production or action at the end organ. Hence, mutations in genes such as *WT1, SF-1, SRY, SOX9,* and *DHH* can result in dysgenetic 46,XY DSD with varying degrees of hypospadias and other genital abnormalities. Mutations in genes that encode steroidogenic enzymes (eg, *3β-HSD, 17α-hydroxylase, 17,20-lyase, POR,* and *SF-1*) or those that affect androgen action and lead to partial androgen resistance as well as 5α-reductase-2 deficiency are all uncommon causes of hypospadias. In the majority of cases of isolated hypospadias with no other genital abnormality, the etiology is uncertain. Hypospadias is also a component of a number of dysmorphic syndromes, including Smith-Lemli-Opitz syndrome (a defect in cholesterol synthesis), as well as hand, foot, and genital syndrome due to a mutation in *HOX13*.

Several paternal and maternal risk factors have been associated with the occurrence of hypospadias in a fetus. These include subfertility and/or genital anomalies in the father, maternal age, IUGR, and fetal exposure to oral progestins or combined progestins and estrogens. These all are associated with an increased risk of hypospadias. Ten percent of hypospadias cases occur in familial cohorts. An increase in hypospadias has also been noted in infants conceived by in vitro fertilization. However, advanced maternal age and subfertility, as well as the administration of progestational agents to the mother, may play a role in these patients.

There is a 15% risk of hypospadias in the sibling of a child with hypospadias and a 7% risk if the father has hypospadias, suggesting a genetic etiology. A mutation in a gene called *MAMLD1* (mastermind-like domain containing 1, previously known as CXorf6 (chromosome X open reading frame 6), which appears to impair T secretion during the critical period (8-12 weeks) of male external genital differentiation, results in hypospadias.

Analysis of international demographic trends for hypospadias indicates that it is highly variable in different countries worldwide. The prevalence of hypospadias in Denmark is 1.1%, which is significantly higher than the prevalence in other Scandinavian countries, especially Finland. Hypospadias was associated with fetal growth retardation (small for gestational age), lower placental weight, and elevated plasma FSH levels at 3 months. Androgen receptor mutations were not found, and the CAG repeats in the androgen receptors were normal for the Danish population. It was suggested that environmental exposure is a likely explanation, but data of environmental exposure including demographic differences in endocrine disruptors (eg, organochloride, phalathes, xenoestrogens) are lacking.

Patients with severe hypospadias (perineoscrotal) especially those with micropenis and/or cryptorchidism should be evaluated. The evaluation should include gonadotropin, AMH, inhibin B, and an assessment of testosterone secretion either during the "window of opportunity" at 1-3 months of age or in response to hCG stimulation.

Micropenis

Micropenis without hypospadias results from a heterogeneous group of disorders; the most common cause is fetal T deficiency. Micropenis is rarely associated with 5α-reductase deficiency or mild defects in the androgen receptor (Table 14–4). In the human male fetus, T synthesis by the fetal Leydig cell during the critical period of male differentiation (8-12 weeks) appears to be autonomous at first, then influenced by hCG. After midgestation, fetal pituitary LH modulates fetal T synthesis by the Leydig cell and, consequently, affects the growth of the differentiated penis. Thus, males with congenital hypopituitarism or isolated gonadotropin deficiency and late fetal testicular failure (after 8-12 weeks) present with normal male differentiation and micropenis at term birth (by definition a penis length <2.5 cm) (Table 14–5).

Evaluation of the infant with micropenis should include anterior pituitary functions (ie, determination of the plasma concentration of GH, prolactin, ACTH, cortisol, thyroid-stimulating hormone, thyroxine, and gonadotropins), to rule out multiple pituitary hormone deficiencies. In infancy, there is a "window of opportunity" at 1 to 3 months of age when the perinatal rise in gonadotropin and T/DHT occurs. A lack of rise in T/DHT and

TABLE 14–5 Normal values for stretched penile length.

Age	Length (cm) (mean ± SD)
Newborn: 30 wk[a]	2.5 ± 0.4
Newborn: full-term[a]	3.5 ± 0.4
0-5 mo[b]	3.9 ± 0.8
6-12 mo[b]	4.3 ± 0.8
1-2 y[b]	4.7 ± 0.8
2-3 y[b]	5.1 ± 0.9
3-4 y[b]	5.5 ± 0.9
5-6 y[b]	6.0 ± 0.9
10-11 y	6.4 ± 1.1
Adult[c]	12.4 ± 2.7

[a]Data from Feldman and Smith (1975); see Tuladhar et al (1998) for the normal range of penile length in preterm infants between 24 and 36 weeks of gestational age.

[b]Data from Schonfeld and Beebe (1942).

[c]Data from Wessels et al (1996).

From Bin-Abbas B, Conte FA, Grumbach MM, et al. Congenital hypogonadotropic hypogonadism and micropenis: effect of testosterone treatment on adult penile size—why sex reversal is not indicated. *J Pediatr.* 1999;134:579.

TABLE 14–4 Etiology of micropenis.

I. Deficient testosterone secretion
  A. Hypogonadotropic hypogonadism
    1. Isolated, including Kallmann syndrome
    2. Associated with other pituitary hormone deficiencies
    3. Prader-Willi syndrome
    4. Laurence-Moon-Biedl syndrome
    5. Bardet-Biedl syndrome
    6. Rudd syndrome
  B. Primary hypogonadism
    1. Anorchia
    2. Klinefelter and poly X syndromes
    3. Gonadal dysgenesis (incomplete form)
    4. LH receptor defects (incomplete forms)
    5. Genetic defects in testosterone steroidogenesis (incomplete forms)
    6. Noonan syndrome
    7. Testicular dysgenesis syndrome
    8. Trisomy 21
    9. Robinow syndrome

II. Defects in testosterone synthesis and action
  A. P450 oxidoreductase deficiency (mild enzymatic defect)
  B. 5α-Reductase deficiency (incomplete forms)
  C. Androgen receptor defects (incomplete forms)
  D. GH/IGF-1 deficiency
  E. Fetal hydantoin syndrome

III. Developmental anomalies
  A. Aphallia
  B. Cloacal exstrophy

IV. Idiopathic

V. Associated with other congenital malformation

From Bin-Abbas B, Conte FA, Grumbach MM, et al. Congenital hypogonadotropic hypogonadism and micropenis: effect of testosterone treatment on adult penile size—why sex reversal is not indicated. *J Pediatr.* 1999;134:579. [PMID: 10228293]

LH and FSH suggests hypogonadotropic hypogonadism, while an abnormally high (>10.5 on unstimulated sample) T/DHT ratio suggests 5α-reductase-type 2 deficiency. All patients with micropenis should receive a trial of T therapy to ascertain the phallic response and to augment its length into the normal range for age. Infants with fetal T deficiency as a cause of micropenis—whether due to gonadotropin deficiency or to a primary testicular disorder—respond to 25 mg of T enanthate in oil intramuscularly monthly for 3 months with a mean increase of 2 cm in penile length. Older children require higher doses—50 mg intramuscularly monthly × 3 doses. A long-term study of eight males with micropenis, due to congenital hypogonadotropic hypogonadism who were followed in our clinic, revealed that fetal deficiency of gonadotropins and T did not prevent the penis from responding to T in infancy and at the age of puberty. Final penile length for all patients who were treated with one or more short courses of repository T in infancy or childhood and with replacement doses of T in adolescence was in the normal adult range. Furthermore, these patients had a male gender identity, erections, ejaculation, and orgasm. No clinical, psychologic, or physiologic indication supports conversion of males with micropenis, due to diminished fetal T secretion, to females.

Aphallia

Complete absence of the phallus is a rare anomaly. The urethra may open on the perineum or into the rectum. Assignment of a female sex of rearing, castration, and plastic repair of the genitalia and urethra has been the approach followed in the past; however, this policy is currently questioned by some investigators because of concern about the action of normal male fetal levels of circulating T on the fetal brain and its potential effect on postnatal psychosexual development and gender identity. There are no long-term follow-up studies of gender identity in patients with aphallia. A study investigated 46,XY patients with cloacal extrophy who were castrated in the neonatal period and assigned a female gender role. Fifty percent of this cohort announced their gender identity as male in childhood or adolescence. These data suggest that prenatal exposure to normal amounts of T during gestation is probabilistic but not deterministic in the establishment of gender identity.

UNCLASSIFIED FORMS OF ABNORMAL SEXUAL DEVELOPMENT IN FEMALES

Müllerian duct agenesis is characterized by congenital absence of the uterus and the upper one-third of the vagina and is termed the Mayer-Rokitansky-Küster-Hauser (MRKH) syndrome. Ovarian function is usually normal. If Müllerian agenesis is associated with renal abnormalities and cervicothoracic dysplasia, it is referred to as the MURCS syndrome. Patients with the MRKH syndrome or the MURCS syndrome have not as yet had genetic mutations identified, although familial cases have been reported. Recently, an atypical form of the MRKH syndrome has been described in three patients who had primary amenorrhea with normal breasts and pubic hair development, lack of Müllerian duct development, and clinical and biochemical evidence of androgen excess. All three patients had a heterozygous mutation of the WNT4 gene. These patients illustrate the role of WNT4 in Müllerian duct development in humans as well as in inhibiting Leydig cell development and androgen synthesis by the ovary.

Features Which Suggest a DSD

A DSD should be suspected in apparent females with clitoromegaly (>0.9 cm) at birth in those with a mass in the labia, inguinal canal or with an inguinal herniae, and in those with edema of the distal extremities and/or loose skin folds over the nape of the neck. A DSD should be suspected in infants with truly ambiguous genitalia, in putative males with cryptorchidism, micropenis (<2.5 cm), and hypospadias, especially perineal, siblings or relatives of patients with DSDs, and in infants whose prenatal genital appearance by sonography is not congruent with their karyotype on amniocentesis.

MANAGEMENT OF PATIENTS WITH DSD

The evaluation and management of the patient with atypical genitalia is complex and best undertaken by a team consisting of a pediatric endocrinologist, psychiatrist or psychologist, pediatric surgeon or urologist, social worker, religious counselor if appropriate, and an informed primary care physician at a center of excellence. The goal of management of patients with atypical genitalia is to establish an etiologic diagnosis promptly and with the informed consent of the parents, assign a sex of rearing which is

most compatible with the prospect for a stable gender identity, well-adjusted life, sexual adequacy, and fertility if possible. Steps in the diagnosis of the infant with a DSD are set forth in Figures 14-16 and 14-17.

Before any decision about sex assignment is made, a thorough, comprehensive evaluation must be undertaken. The diagnostic evaluation should include a karyotype, pelvic sonography and determination of gonadotropins, and adrenal and gonadal steroids, AMH, and inhibin B levels. Depending on the karyotype and ultrasound, further analysis of steroids after hCG and ACTH stimulation may be indicated (see Figure 14-17). In all 46,XY DSDs with a micropenis (Tables 14-4 and 14-5), it is prudent to assess the phallic response to T to exclude partial androgen resistance before the decision about definitive sex assignment is made by the parents. Clitoral enlargement (Table 14-6) in 46,XX females suggests either an endogenous or exogenous source of androgens.

Gender identity—the identification of oneself as either male or female—is a complex and incompletely understood dimorphic phenomenon. During the last 20 years, it has been increasingly evident that both *nature* (eg, prenatal exposure to T) as well as genes on the X and Y chromosome, and *nurture* (sex assignment, psychosocial and experiential factors) play a role in determining one's gender identity. In any given infant, one can never be sure whether nature or nurture will be deterministic or prevail. Thus, physicians are faced with the daunting task of helping parents to make a critical decision about the sex of rearing of their child in the face of incomplete understanding of the complexity of gender identity. The task is further complicated by the limited ability to make a definitive etiologic diagnosis in many 46,XY DSDs, as well as by the lack of outcome data that incorporate modern guidelines, recent surgical advances, and advances in psychologic/psychiatric support for both the child and the parents.

It is the physician's and consultant's tasks to evaluate the patient thoroughly and to fully inform the parents. The ultimate decision of sex of rearing is made by the completely well-informed parents. It must be clearly stated which anatomic abnormalities can be surgically repaired, that hormone therapy can be given at an appropriate time and that continuing psychosocial support will be available both from the physicians involved and from community-based support groups. Repeated, lucid, simple, comprehensive discussions about the cause of their child's atypical genitalia and what is known about the long-term follow-up of similar patients with DSD, as well as the results of reconstructive surgery in terms of sexual gratification and fertility, must be discussed. The discussion needs to take into account parental concerns, religious views, cultural factors, social mores, and the parents' level of understanding. The parents need to be assured that an expeditous, definitive diagnosis can be made, but that naming the baby, sending out birth announcements, and filing the birth certificate may need to be delayed. They will need support, reassurance, and counseling as to how to deal with relatives and others.

In the individual with atypical genitalia, the option of assigning a sex of rearing but deferring surgery unless it is medically

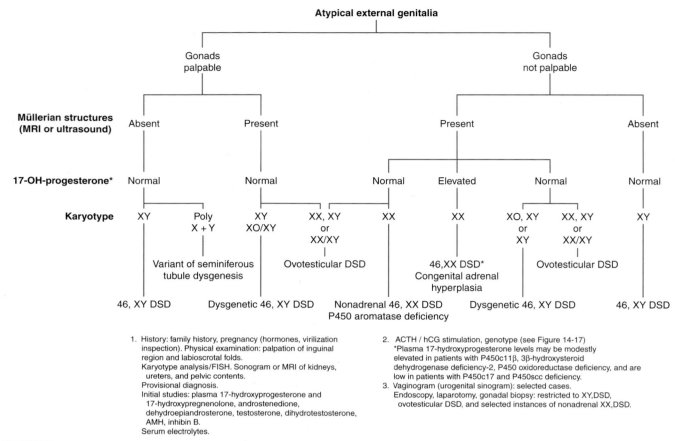

FIGURE 14–16 Steps in the diagnosis of intersexuality in infancy and childhood. Step 1 involves evaluation and provisional diagnosis. Step 2 is used in selected cases, and step 3 can be used for specific disorders.

necessary until the patient has the opportunity to give his or her informed consent, has been proposed by advocacy groups and espoused by some DSD clinics. However, it should be noted that there are no data on patients with DSD and atypical genitalia to support the efficacy of this approach. On the other hand, a long-term study of 41 patients with DSD suggested that early surgical intervention accompanied by endocrinologic and psychologic/psychiatric support for the patient and parents resulted in positive outcomes in terms of cosmesis, minimal impairment in quality of life and appropriate gender identity. We concur with this position and feel that it is desirable to initiate plastic repair of the external genitalia as soon as is feasible with the informed consent of the parents. Surgeons experienced in genital repair recommend a one-stage repair by 4 to 6 months of age. In children raised as females, clitoroplasty should be performed only by experienced surgeons with the emphasis being on function rather than cosmesis. We do not recommend routine clitoroplasty for mild to moderate clitoromegaly (Prader II or III). Vaginoplasty can be deferred until adolescence when the patient may participate in the decision for surgery. Each patient is unique and must be treated as such. There

is no rubric that can be applied to the management of all patients. However, the following are a few guidelines.

Male sex assignment is recommended in 46,XY DSDs, with the exception of those with complete androgen resistance syndrome; those who have completely female external genitalia; those with partial androgen resistance, who have less than Prader III ambiguity; or those who have a compelling reason for female sex assignment, including the parents' informed decision. In the latter case, extensive discussion with the family is especially warranted, particularly in the 46,XY infant whose ambiguous genitalia is evidence of significant fetal T exposure. The parents need to be aware of the effect of T during gestation on gender identity and counseled about the possibility of gender dysphoria if the child is assigned a female sex of rearing. In this case, it may be prudent to do no surgery unless medically indicated, until the child's gender identity can be verified, and informed consent for surgery obtained from the patient. In patients with XO/XY mosaicism, 17β-HSD-3 deficiency, and 5α-reductase deficiency diagnosed in infancy, the significant occurrence of female to male gender role change should be discussed with the parents. In some societies, the

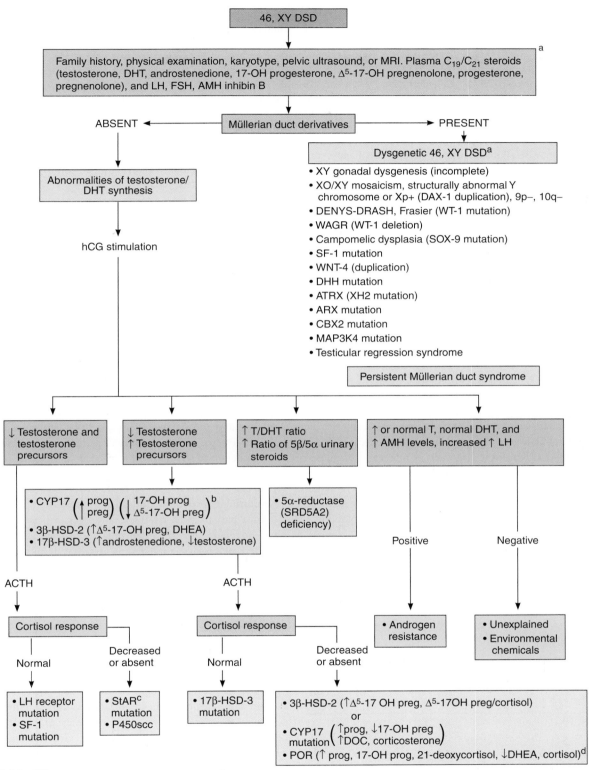

FIGURE 14–17 Steps in the differential diagnosis of 46,XY DSD.

[a]The phenotype and comorbidities of any mutation causing a 46,XY DSD are variable and depend on the degree of enzymatic activity resulting from the particular mutation. Thus, in these patients, the degree of ambiguity of the external genitalia varies, and the Müllerian structures may or may not be present.

[b]CYP17 (P450c17) catalyzes the 17-hydroxylation of progesterone and pregnenolone to 17-hydroxyprogesterone and 17-hydroxypregnenolone, as well as the scission (lyase) of 17-hydroxypregnenolone to DHEA. Patients with 17,20-lyase have elevated basal and hCG-induced levels of

17-hydroxyprogesterone and 17-hydroxypregnenolone and low levels of androstenedione and DHEA. Cytochrome b5 is a cofactor for 17,20 lyase activity of 17α-hydroxylase. Mutations result in ambiguous genitalia and methhemoglobinuria.

[c]The StAR (steroidogenic acute regulatory) protein is involved in the transport of cholesterol from the outer to the inner mitochondrial membrane, where the enzyme CYP11A1 (P450scc) resides. StAR mutations result in a markedly diminished ability to convert cholesterol to Δ^5 pregnenolone, although side chain cleavage (CYP11A1) activity is intact. WAGR, Wilms tumor, aniridia, genital anomalies, and mental retardation; SF-1, steroidogenic factor-1; CYP17, 17α-hydroxylase/17,20-lyase; 3β-HSD 2, 3β-hydroxysteroid dehydrogenase/Δ^5-isomerase; 17β-HSD 3, 17β-hydroxysteroid dehydrogenase (oxidoreductase) type 3; T, testosterone; DHT, dihydrotestosterone; AMH, anti-Müllerian hormone; DHEA, dehydroepiandrosterone; POR, P450 oxidoredutase; b5, cytochrome b5.

[d]POR, P450 oxidoreductase, the definitive steroid pattern for POR is variable depending on the severity of the POR mutation and its specificity for one of the three P450s it interacts with. However, 17OH progesterone levels are invariably elevated at baseline and after ACTH. Cortisol levels are blunted on ACTH stimulation. Many patients also manifest the Antley-Bixler phenotype; virilization in the affected female is not progressive postnatally; in utero it is due to deficient placental aromatase activity. (Modified from Grumbach MM, Hughes IA, Conte FA. Disorders of sex differentiation. In: Larsen PR, et al, ed. *Williams Textbook of Endocrinology*. 10th ed. W.B. Saunders, 2003.)

---

social, cultural, and economic benefits of a male sex assignment are more compelling than phallic adequacy and are a prevailing—if not the most important—factor in the parents' sex of rearing decision. Male sex assignment in 46,XY DSD individuals, especially those who can respond to T allows for a choice later in adolescence, by not removing functional genital structures which cannot be replaced.

All 46,XX DSDs with Prader I to IV (see Figure 14–13) external genitalia should be raised as females. 46,XX DSDs with Prader V genitalia (penile urethra) represent a management dilemma. As with other forms of DSD, there are at present insufficient long-term outcome data on these patients. Raising the child as male would require gonadectomy of a potentially fertile female. These infants are raised as females if diagnosed in infancy. If diagnosed after infancy and a male gender assignment has been made, a full discussion with the parents and psychologic/psychiatric evaluation of the child should ensue before any definitive decisions are made regarding gender assignment. Reassignment of sex in childhood is always a difficult psychosocial problem for the patient, the parents, and the physicians involved. Although easier in the infant under 1 year of age, it should only be undertaken after much deliberation and with provision for long-term medical and psychiatric supervision and counseling. 46,XX males and 46,XX ovotes-

ticular DSDs with male genitalia and absent Müllerian ducts are exceptions to the suggestion that a female sex assignment be considered in 46,XX DSDs.

Psychologic studies in 46,XX DSD secondary to CAH suggests that the vast majority of 46,XX DSDs with CAH have a female gender identity. In some individuals, sex-specific behavior may be more masculine. The incidence of bisexuality and homosexuality is increased. In one study, the prevalence of bisexuality and homosexuality correlated modestly with the degree of masculinization of nonsexual behavior and the genitalia.

Removal of rudimentary gonads in children with Y-containing cell lines and gonadal dysgenesis should be performed at the time of initial repair of the external genitalia; gonadoblastomas, seminomas, and germinomas can occur during the first decade (see Table 14–2). Histologically and functionally normal scrotal testes can be retained in 45,X/46,XY males and others with regular monitoring as previously discussed.

In a patient with complete androgen resistance, the testes may be left in situ (provided they are not situated in the labia majora) to provide endogenous estradiol at puberty. There is one possible exception that of the rare somatic mosaics for the androgen receptor who are at risk of virilization at puberty, due to the presence of a population of cells with normal androgen receptors. Having had the female identity reinforced by normal feminization at puberty, prophylactic castration can then be performed, if informed consent by the patient and parents is obtained.

In patients with partial androgen resistance reared as females or in patients with errors of T biosynthesis reared as females in whom some degree of masculinization occurs at puberty, orchidectomy should be performed before the age of puberty or later if doubt exists about the gender identity. GnRH agonists can be given to prevent androgen secretion and virilization until the gender identity is confirmed. Cyclic estrogen and progestin replacement therapy are used in individuals reared as females in whom a uterus is present. In males, masculinization is achieved by the administration of repository or topical preparations of T.

Continuing endocrinologic and psychologic support are critical aspects of follow-up and should be available throughout infancy, childhood, adolescence, and adulthood for the patient

TABLE 14–6 Clitoral size.

Clitoral Size		
Newborn, full-term	Length[a] 0.4 ± 0.12 cm	Width 0.33 ± 0.078 cm
Adult women Nulliparous	Length[b] 1.6 ± 0.45 cm[b] 1.9 ± 0.87 cm (range 0.5-3.5 cm)[c]	

[a]Data from Oberfield SE, Mondok A, Shahrivar F, et al. Clitoral size in full-term infants. *Am J Perinatol*. 1989;6:453-454. [PMID: 2789544]

[b]Data from Verkauf BS, Von Thron J, O'Brien WF. Clitoral size in normal women. *Obstet Gynecol*. 1992;80:41-44. [PMID: 1603495]

[c]Data from Lloyd J, Crouch NS, Minto CL, et al. Female genital appearance: "normality" unfolds. *BJOG*. 2005;112:643-646. [PMID:15842291]

as well as for the parents. Patients should have progressive, step-by-step, age-appropriate discussions about their diagnosis, its pathophysiology, their quality of life, and the potential for fertility. Disclosure is critical! However, in those mature adult DSD patients who are well-adjusted and happy with their lives and their assigned sex and who in the past have not had the opportunity of having full disclosure, disclosure may be on a *need to know* basis. Patients have access to their medical records. It is infinitely better to proceed with full disclosure if the patient has expressed a desire to know more about their diagnosis and management. Full disclosure should be approached in a similar manner as that carried out with parents and with the cooperation and help of a psychologist or psychiatrist familiar with the patient and issues of gender identity. The patient (when possible) and the parents should always be involved in decisions about surgery and sex hormone replacement.

In sum, the physician and the medical team concerned with the diagnosis, selection of sex of rearing, and management of the infant with DSD must be prepared to address the complex ethical, cultural, social, religious, clinical, legal, and surgical issues presented by the DSD patient in order to maximize the patient's potential for a well-adjusted, normal life. This task remains complicated by deficiencies in the availability of long-term outcome data as well as the inability to diagnose specifically many patients with a DSD especially those with a 46,XY karyotype.

REFERENCES

Ankarberg-Lindgren C, Elfving M, Wikland KA, Norjavaara E. Nocturnal application of transdermal estradiol patches produces levels of estradiol that mimic those seen at the onset of spontaneous puberty in girls. *J Clin Endocrinol Metab.* 2001;86:3039. [PMID: 11443165]

Arnhold IJ, Lofrano-Porto A, Latronico AC. Inactivating mutations of luteinizing hormone beta-subunit or luteinizing hormone receptor cause oligo-amenorrhea and infertility in women. *Horm Res.* 2009;71:75. [PMID: 19129711]

Asklund C, Jørgensen N, Kold Jensen T, Skakkebaek NE. Biology and epidemiology of testicular dysgenesis syndrome. *BJU Int.* 2004;93:6. [PMID: 15086436]

Auchus RJ. The backdoor pathway to dihydrotestosterone. *Trends Endocrinol Metab.* 2004;15:432. [PMID: 15519890]

Auchus RJ. Management of the adult with congenital adrenal hyperplasia. *Int J Pediatr Endocrinol.* 2010;2010:614107. [PMID: 20613954]

Berenbaum SA, Bailey JM. Effects on gender identity of prenatal androgens and genital appearance: evidence from girls with congenital adrenal hyperplasia. *J Clin Endocrinol Metab.* 2003;88:1102. [PMID: 12629091]

Berenbaum SA, Korman Bryk K, Duck SC, Resnick SM. Psychological adjustment in children and adults with congenital adrenal hyperplasia. *J Pediatr.* 2004; 144:741, 2004. [PMID: 15192620]

Bernard P, Sim H, Knower K, Vilain E, Harley V. Human SRY inhibits beta-catenin-mediated transcription. *Int J Biochem Cell Biol.* 2008;40:2889. [PMID: 18598779]

Berra M, Liao LM, Creighton SM, Conway GS. Long-term health issues of women with XY karyotype. *Maturitas.* 2010;65:172. [PMID: 20079588]

Biason-Lauber A, Konrad D, Meyer M, DeBeaufort C, Schoenle EJ. Ovaries and female phenotype in a girl with 46,XY karyotype and mutations in the CBX2 gene. *Am J Hum Genet.* 2009;84:658. [PMID: 19361780]

Biason-Lauber A, Konrad D, Navratil F, Schoenle EJ. A WNT4 mutation associated with Müllerian-duct regression and virilization in a 46,XX woman. *N Engl J Med.* 2004;351:792, 2004. [PMID: 15317892]

Bidet M, Bellanné-Chantelot C, Galand-Portier MB, et al. Clinical and molecular characterization of a cohort of 161 unrelated women with nonclassical congenital adrenal hyperplasia due to 21-hydroxylase deficiency and 330 family members. *J Clin Endocrinol Metab.* 2009;94:1570. [PMID: 19208730]

Bin-Abbas B, Conte FA, Grumbach MM, Kaplan SL. Congenital hypogonadotropic hypogonadism and micropenis: effect of testosterone treatment on adult penile size—why sex reversal is not indicated. *J Pediatr.* 1999;134:579. [PMID: 10228293]

Bogani D, Siggers P, Brixey R, et al. Loss of mitogen-activated protein kinase kinase kinase 4 (MAP3K4) reveals a requirement for MAPK signalling in mouse sex determination. *PLoS Biol.* 2009;7:e1000196. [PMID: 19753101]

Boisen KA, Chellakooty M, Schmidt IM, et al. Hypospadias in a cohort of 1072 Danish newborn boys: prevalence and relationship to placental weight, anthropometrical measurements at birth, and reproductive hormone levels at three months of age. *J Clin Endocrinol Metab.* 2005;90:4041. [PMID: 15870122]

Bondy CA; Turner Syndrome Study Group. Care of girls and women with Turner syndrome: a guideline of the Turner Syndrome Study Group. *J Clin Endocrinol Metab.* 2007;92:10. [PMID: 17047017]

Boukari K, Meduri G, Brailly-Tabard S, et al. Lack of androgen receptor expression in Sertoli cells accounts for the absence of anti-Müllerian hormone repression during early human testis development. *J Clin Endocrinol Metab.* 2009;94:1818. [PMID: 19276236]

Bouvattier C, Carel JC, Lecointre C, et al. Postnatal changes of T, LH, and FSH in 46,XY infants with mutations in the AR gene. *J Clin Endocrinol Metab.* 2002;87:29. [PMID: 11788616]

Bouvattier C, Mignot B, Lefèvre H, Morel Y, Bougnères P. Impaired sexual activity in male adults with partial androgen insensitivity. *J Clin Endocrinol Metab.* 2006;91:3310. [PMID: 16757528]

Canto P, Söderlund D, Reyes E, Méndez JP. Mutations in the desert hedgehog (DHH) gene in patients with 46,XY complete pure gonadal dysgenesis. *J Clin Endocrinol Metab.* 2004;89:4480. [PMID: 15356051]

Capel B. R-spondin1 tips the balance in sex determination. *Nat Genet.* 2006;38:1233. [PMID: 17072299]

Carel JC. Growth hormone in Turner syndrome: twenty years after, what can we tell our patients? *J Clin Endocrinol Metab.* 2005;90:3793. [PMID: 15917486]

Carel JC, Ecosse E, Bastie-Sigeac I, et al. Quality of life determinants in young women with Turner's syndrome after growth hormone treatment: results of the StaTur population-based cohort study. *J Clin Endocrinol Metab.* 2005;90:1992. [PMID: 15644402]

Chassot AA, Gregoire EP, Magliano M, Lavery R, Chaboissier MC Genetics of ovarian differentiation: Rspo1, a major player. *Sex Dev.* 2008;2:219. [PMID: 18987496]

Chassot AA, Ranc F, Gregoire EP, et al. Activation of beta-catenin signaling by Rspo1 controls differentiation of the mammalian ovary. *Hum Mol Genet.* 2008;17:1264. [PMID: 18250098]

Chevalier N, Letur H, Lelannou D, et al. Materno-Fetal cardiovascular complications in Turner Syndrome after oocyte donation: insufficient prepregnancy screening and pregnancy follow-up are associated with poor outcome. *J Clin Endocrinol Metab.* 2010 Dec 8. [Epub ahead of print] [PMID: 21147890]

Clayton PE, Miller WL, Oberfield SE, Ritzen EM, Sippell WG, Speiser PW. Joint LWPES/ESPE CAH Working Group. Consensus statement on 21-hydroxylase deficiency from the Lawson Wilkins Pediatric Endocrine Society and the European Society for Paediatric Endocrinology. *J Clin Endocrinol Metab.* 2002;87:4048. [PMID: 12213842]

Cohen-Kettenis PT. Gender change in 46,XY persons with 5-alpha-reductase-2 deficiency and 17-beta-hydroxysteroid dehydrogenase-3 deficiency. *Arch Sex Behav.* 2005;34:399. [PMID: 16010463]

Cohen-Kettenis P. Psychological long-term outcome in intersex conditions. *Horm Res.* 2005;64:27. [PMID: 16286767]

Conte FA, Grumbach MM. Diagnosis and management of ambiguous external genitalia. *Endocrinologist.* 2003;13:260.

Conte FA, Grumbach MM, Ito Y, Fisher CR, Simpson ER. A syndrome of female pseudohermaphrodism, hypergonadotropic hypogonadism, and multicystic ovaries associated with missense mutations in the gene encoding aromatase (P450arom). *J Clin Endocrinol Metab.* 1994;78:1287. [PMID: 8200927]

Conway GS. Adult care of pediatric conditions: lessons from Turner's syndrome. *J Clin Endocrinol Metab.* 2009;94:3185. [PMID: 19734446]

Cools M, Drop SL, Wolffenbuttel KP, Oosterhuis JW, Looijenga LH. Germ cell tumors in the intersex gonad: old paths, new directions, moving frontiers. *Endocr Rev.* 2006;27:468-484. [PMID: 16735607]

Coutant R, Mallet D, Lahlou N, et al. Heterozygous mutation of steroidogenic factor-1 in 46,XY subjects may mimic partial androgen insensitivity syndrome. *J Clin Endocrinol Metab.* 2007;92:2868. [PMID: 17488792]

Crawford JM, Warne G, Grover S, Southwell BR, Hutson JM. Results from a pediatric surgical centre justify early intervention in disorders of sex development. *J Pediatr Surg.* 2009;44:413. [PMID:19231546]

Davenport ML, Crowe BJ, Travers SH, et al. Growth hormone treatment of early growth failure in toddlers with Turner syndrome: a randomized, controlled, multicenter trial. *J Clin Endocrinol Metab.* 2007;92:3406-3416. [PMID: 17595258]

Deeb A, Mason C, Lee YS, Hughes IA. Correlation between genotype, phenotype and sex of rearing in 111 patients with partial androgen insensitivity syndrome. *Clin Endocrinol.* 2005;63:56. [PMID: 15963062]

Dessens AB, Slijper FM, Drop SL. Gender dysphoria and gender change in chromosomal females with congenital adrenal hyperplasia. *Arch Sex Behav.* 2005;34:389. [PMID: 16010462]

DiNapoli L, Capel B. SRY and the standoff in sex determination. *Mol Endocrinol.* 2008;22:1. [PMID: 17666585]

Dumic M, Lin-Su K, Leibel NI, et al. Report of fertility in a woman with a predominantly 46,XY karyotype in a family with multiple disorders of sexual development. *J Clin Endocrinol Metab.* 2008;93:182. [PMID: 18000096]

Elzinga-Tinke JE, Sirre ME, Looijenga LH, van Casteren N, Wildhagen MF, Dohle GR. The predictive value of testicular ultrasound abnormalities for carcinoma in situ of the testis in men at risk for testicular cancer. *Int J Androl.* 2009. [Epub ahead of print] [PMID: 19845800]

Feldman KW, Smith DW. Fetal phallic growth and penile standards for newborn male infants. *J Pediatr.* 1975;86:395. [PMID: 1113226]

Ferraz-de-Souza B, Lin L, Achermann JC. Steroidogenic factor-1 (SF-1, NR5A1) and human disease. *Mol Cell Endocrinol.* 2010 Nov 13. [Epub ahead of print] [PMID: 21078366]

Flück CE, Tajima T, Pandey AV, et al. Mutant P450 oxidoreductase causes disordered steroidogenesis with and without Antley-Bixler syndrome. *Nat Genet.* 2004;36:228. [PMID: 14758361]

Fukami M, Nishimura G, Homma K, et al. Cytochrome P450 oxidoreductase deficiency: identification and characterization of biallelic mutations and genotype-phenotype correlations in 35 Japanese patients. *J Clin Endocrinol Metab.* 2009;94:1723. [PMID: 19258400]

Goto M, Piper Hanley K, Marcos J, et al. In humans, early cortisol biosynthesis provides a mechanism to safeguard female sexual development. *J Clin Invest.* 2006;116:953. [PMID: 16585961]

Gravholt CH. Clinical practice in Turner syndrome. *Nat Clin Pract Endocrinol Metab.* 2005;1:41. [PMID: 16929365]

Gravholt CH, Fedder J, Naeraa RW, Müller J. Occurrence of gonadoblastoma in females with Turner syndrome and Y chromosome material: a population study. *J Clin Endocrinol Metab.* 2000;85:3199. [PMID: 10999808]

Grumbach MM. Commentary. A window of opportunity: the diagnosis of gonadotropin deficiency in the male infant. *J Clin Endocrinol Metab.* 2005;90:3122. [PMID: 15728198]

Grumbach MM, Hughes IA, Conte FA. Disorders of sex differentiation. In: Larsen PR, Kronenberg HM, Melmed S, Polonsky KS, eds. *Williams Textbook of Endocrinology.* 10th ed. Philadelphia, PA: WB Saunders; 2003.

Handelsman DJ, Liu PY. Klinefelter's syndrome—a microcosm of male reproductive health. *J Clin Endocrinol Metab.* 2006;91:1220. [PMID: 16601196]

Hanley NA, Arlt W. The human fetal adrenal cortex and the window of sexual differentiation. *Trends Endocrinol Metab.* 2006;17:391. [PMID: 17046275]

Hines M, Ahmed SF, Hughes IA. Psychological outcomes and gender-related development in complete androgen insensitivity syndrome. *Arch Sex Behav.* 2003;32:93. [PMID: 12710824]

Hines M, Brook C, Conway GS. Androgen and psychosexual development: core gender identity, sexual orientation and recalled childhood gender role behavior in women and men with congenital adrenal hyperplasia (CAH). *J Sex Res.* 2004; 41:75. [PMID: 15216426]

Hiort O, Holterhus PM, Werner R, et al. Homozygous disruption of P450 side-chain cleavage (CYP11A1) is associated with prematurity, complete 46,XY sex reversal, and severe adrenal failure. *J Clin Endocrinol Metab.* 2005;90:538. [PMID: 15507506]

Jameson JL. Of mice and men: the tale of steroidogenic factor-1. *J Clin Endocrinol Metab.* 2004;89:5927. [PMID: 15579738]

Kalfa N, Philibert P, Sultan C. Is hypospadias a genetic, endocrine or environmental disease, or still an unexplained malformation? *Int J Androl.* 2009;32:187. [PMID: 18637150]

Kim CJ, Lin L, Huang N, et al. Severe combined adrenal and gonadal deficiency caused by novel mutations in the cholesterol side chain cleavage enzyme, P450scc. *J Clin Endocrinol Metab.* 2008;93:696. [PMID: 18182448]

Köhler B, Lin L, Mazen I, et al. The spectrum of phenotypes associated with mutations in steroidogenic factor 1 (SF-1, NR5A1, Ad4BP) includes severe penoscrotal hypospadias in 46,XY males without adrenal insufficiency. *Eur J Endocrinol.* 2009;161:237. [PMID: 19439508]

Köhler B, Lumbroso S, Leger J, et al. Androgen insensitivity syndrome: somatic mosaicism of the androgen receptor in seven families and consequences for sex assignment and genetic counseling. *J Clin Endocrinol Metab.* 2005;90:106. [PMID: 15522944]

Kok RC, Timmerman MA, Wolffenbuttel KP, Drop SL, de Jong FH. Isolated 17,20-lyase deficiency due to the cytochrome b5 mutation W27X. *J Clin Endocrinol Metab.* 2010;95:994. [PMID: 20080843]

Lanfranco F, Kamischke A, Zitzmann M, Nieschlag E. Klinefelter's syndrome. *Lancet.* 2004;364:273. [PMID: 15262106]

Lau YF, Li Y. The human and mouse sex-determining SRY genes repress the Rspol/beta-catenin signaling. *J Genet Genomics.* 2009;36:193. [PMID: 19376480]

Dumic M, Lin-Su K, Leibel NI, et al. Consensus statement on management of intersex disorders. International Consensus Conference on Intersex. *Pediatrics.* 2006;118:e488-500 [PMID: 16882788]

Lin L, Ercan O, Raza J, et al. Variable phenotypes associated with aromatase (CYP19) insufficiency in humans. *J Clin Endocrinol Metab.* 2007;92:982. [PMID: 17164303]

Liu CF, Bingham N, Parker K, Yao HH. Sex-specific roles of beta-catenin in mouse gonadal development. *Hum Mol Genet.* 2009;18:405 [PMID: 18981061]

Lloyd J, Crouch NS, Minto CL, Liao LM, Creighton SM. Female genital appearance: "normality" unfolds. *BJOG.* 2005;112:643. [PMID: 15842291]

Lourenço D, Brauner R, Lin L, et al. Mutations in NR5A1 associated with ovarian insufficiency. *N Engl J Med.* 2009;360:1200, 2009. [PMID: 19246354]

Lourenço D, Brauner R, Rybczynska M, Nihoul-Fékété C, McElreavey K, Bashamboo A. Loss-of-function mutation in GATA4 causes anomalies of human testicular development. *Proc Natl Acad Sci U S A.* 2011. [PMID: 21220346]

Lutfallah C, Wang W, Mason JI, et al. Newly proposed hormonal criteria via genotypic proof for type II 3 beta-hydroxysteroid dehydrogenase deficiency. *J Clin Endocrinol Metab.* 2002;87:2611. [PMID: 12050224]

Maatouk DM, DiNapoli L, Alvers A, Parker KL, Taketo MM, Capel B. Stabilization of beta-catenin in XY gonads causes male-to-female sex-reversal. *Hum Mol Genet.* 2008;17:2949. [PMID: 18617533]

Matura LA, Ho VB, Rosing DR, Bondy CA. Aortic dilatation and dissection in Turner syndrome. *Circulation.* 2007;116:1663. [PMID: 17875973]

Mazur T. Gender dysphoria and gender change in androgen insensitivity or micropenis. *Arch Sex Behav.* 2005;34:411. [PMID: 16010464]

McElreavey K. Genetic disorders of sex differentiation. Proceedings of the 2nd World Conference: *Hormonal and Genetic Basis of Sexual Differentiation Disorders,* January 15-17, 2010, Miami Beach, FL.

Mendez JP, Schiavon R, Diaz-Cueto L, et al. A reliable endocrine test with human menopausal gonadotropins for diagnosis of true hermaphroditism in early infancy. *J Clin Endocrinol Metab.* 1998;83:3523. [PMID: 9768658]

Mendonca BB, Domenice S, Arnhold IJ, Costa EM. 46,XY disorders of sex development (DSD). *Clin Endocrinol.* 2009;70:173. [PMID: 18811725]

Mendonca BB, Leite MV, de Castro M, et al. Female pseudohermaphrodism caused by a novel homozygous missense mutation of the GR gene. *J Clin Endocrinol Metab.* 2002;87:1805. [PMID: 11932321]

Merke DP. Approach to the adult with congenital adrenal hyperplasia due to 21-hydroxylase deficiency. *J Clin Endocrinol Metab.* 2008;93:653. [PMID: 18326005]

Metherell LA, Naville D, Halaby G, et al. Nonclassic lipoid congenital adrenal hyperplasia masquerading as familial glucocorticoid deficiency. *J Clin Endocrinol Metab.* 2009;94:3865. [PMID: 19773404]

Meyer-Bahlburg HF. Attitudes of adult 46,XY intersex persons to clinical management policies. *J Urol.* 2004;171:1615. [PMID: 15017234]

Meyer-Bahlburg HF. Gender identity outcome in female-raised 46,XY persons with penile agenesis, cloacal exstrophy of the bladder, or penile ablation. *Arch Sex Behav.* 2005;34:423. [PMID: 16010465]

Meyer-Bahlburg HF, Dolezal C, Baker SW, Carlson AD, Obeid JS, New MI. Prenatal androgenization affects gender-related behavior but not gender identity in 5-12-year-old girls with congenital adrenal hyperplasia. *Arch Sex Behav.* 2004;33:97. [PMID: 15146142]

Meyer-Bahlburg HF, Dolezal C, Baker SW, Ehrhardt AA, New MI. Gender development in women with congenital adrenal hyperplasia as a function of disorder severity. *Arch Sex Behav.* 2006;35:667. [PMID: 16902816]

Meyer-Bahlburg HF, Dolezal C, Baker SW, New MI. Sexual orientation in women with classical or non-classical congenital adrenal hyperplasia as a function of degree of prenatal androgen excess. *Arch Sex Behav.* 2008;37:85. [PMID: 18157628]

Miller WL, Auchus RJ. The molecular biology, biochemistry, and physiology of human steroidogenesis and its disorders. *Endocr Rev.* 2010 Nov 4 [Epub ahead of print] [PMID: 21051590].

Morel Y, Rey R, Teinturier C, et al. Aetiological diagnosis of male sex ambiguity: a collaborative study. *Eur J Pediatr.* 2002; 161:49. [PMID: 11808880]

Morishima A, Grumbach MM, Simpson ER, Fisher C, Qin K. Aromatase deficiency in male and female siblings caused by a novel mutation and the physiological role of estrogens. *J Clin Endocrinol Metab.* 1995;80:3689. [PMID: 8530621]

Nef S, Vassalli JD. Complementary pathways in mammalian female sex determination. *J Biol.* 2009;8:74. [PMID: 19735582]

Oberfield SE, Mondok A, Shahrivar F, Klein JF, Levine LS. Clitoral size in full-term infants. *Am J Perinatol.* 1989;6:453. [PMID: 2789544]

Ogata T, Laporte J, Fukami M. MAMLD1 (CXorf6): a new gene involved in hypospadias. *Horm Res.* 2009;71:245. [PMID: 19339788]

Ortenberg J, Oddoux C, Craver R, et al. SRY gene expression in the ovotestes of XX true hermaphrodites. *J Urol.* 2002;167:1828. [PMID: 11912443]

Ottolenghi C, Omari S, Garcia-Ortiz JE, et al. FoxL2 is required for commitment to ovary differentiation. *Hum Mol Genet.* 2005;14:2053. [PMID: 15944199]

Paduch DA, Bolyakov A, Cohen P, Travis A. Reproduction in men with Klinefelter syndrome: the past, the present, and the future. *Semin Reprod Med.* 2009;27:137. [PMID: 19247915]

Parma P, Radi O, Vidal V, et al. R-spondin1 is essential in sex determination, skin differentiation and malignancy. *Nat Genet.* 2006;38:1304. [PMID: 17041600]

Pearlman A, Loke J, Le Caignec C, et al. Mutations in MAP3K1 cause 46,XY disorders of sex development and implicate a common signal transduction pathway in human testis determination. *Am J Hum Genet.* 2010; 87:898-904. [PMID: 21129722]

Philibert P, Biason-Lauber A, Rouzier R, et al. Identification and functional analysis of a new WNT4 gene mutation among 28 adolescent girls with primary amenorrhea and Müllerian duct abnormalities: a French collaborative study. *J Clin Endocrinol Metab.* 2008;93:895. [PMID: 18182450]

Philibert P, Polak M, Colmenares A, et al. Predominant Sertoli cell deficiency in a 46,XY disorders of sex development patient with a new NR5A1/SF-1 mutation transmitted by his unaffected father. *Fertil Steril.* 2010 Dec 14. [PMID: 21163476]

Practice Committee, American Society for Reproductive Medicine. Increased maternal cardiovascular mortality associated with pregnancy in women with Turner syndrome. *Fertil Steril.* 2005;83:1074. [PMID: 15820837]

Ravel C, Lakhal B, Elghezal H, et al. Novel human pathological mutations. Gene symbol: SRY. Disease: XY sex reversal. *Hum Genet.* 2009;126:333. [PMID: 19694000]

Reiner WG, Gearhart JP. Discordant sexual identity in some genetic males with cloacal exstrophy assigned to female sex at birth. *N Engl J Med.* 2004;350:333. [PMID: 14736925]

Reiner WG. Gender identity and sex-of-rearing in children with disorders of sexual differentiation. *J Pediatr Endocrinol Metab.* 2005;18:549. [PMID: 16042322]

Richards JS, Pangas SA. The ovary: basic biology and clinical implications. *J Clin Invest.* 2010;120:963. [PMID: 20364094]

Rosler A. 17 beta-hydroxysteroid dehydrogenase 3 deficiency in the Mediterranean population. *Pediatr Endocrinol Rev.* 2006;3:455. [PMID: 17551466]

Rubtsov P, Karmanov M, Sverdlova P, Spirin P, Tiulpakov A. A novel homozygous mutation in CYP11A1 gene is associated with late-onset adrenal insufficiency and hypospadias in a 46,XY patient. *J Clin Endocrinol Metab.* 2009;94:936, 2009. [PMID: 19116240]

Safe S. Clinical correlates of environmental endocrine disruptors. *Trends Endocrinol Metab.* 2005;16:139. [PMID: 15860409]

Sahakitrungruang T, Huang N, Tee MK, et al. Clinical, genetic, and enzymatic characterization of P450 oxidoreductase deficiency in four patients. *J Clin Endocrinol Metab.* 2009;94:4992. [PMID: 19837910]

Sahakitrungruang T, Soccio RE, Lang-Muritano M, Walker JM, Achermann JC, Miller WL. Clinical, genetic, and functional characterization of four patients carrying partial loss-of-function mutations in the steroidogenic acute regulatory protein (StAR). *J Clin Endocrinol Metab.* 2010;95:3352. [PMID: 20444910]

Sahakitrungruang T, Tee MK, Blackett PR, Miller WL. Partial defect in the cholesterol side-chain cleavage enzyme P450scc (CYP11A1) resembling nonclassic congenital lipoid adrenal hyperplasia. *J Clin Endocrinol Metab.* Dec 15 [Epub ahead of print][PMID: 21159840]

Schoemaker MJ, Swerdlow AJ, Higgins CD, Wright AF, Jacobs PA; United Kingdom Clinical Cytogenetics Group. Mortality in women with Turner syndrome in Great Britain: a national cohort study. *J Clin Endocrinol Metab.* 2008;93:4735. [PMID: 18812477]

Schlessinger D, Garcia-Ortiz JE, Forabosco A, Uda M, Crisponi L, Pelosi E. Determination and stability of gonadal sex. *J Androl.* 2010;31:16. [PMID: 19875493]

Schonfeld WA, Beebe GW. Normal growth and variation in male genitalia from birth to maturity. *J Urol.* 1942;64:759.

Sciurano RB, Luna Hisano CV, Rahn MI, et al. Focal spermatogenesis originates in euploid germ cells in classical Klinefelter patients. *Hum Reprod.* 2009;24:2353. [PMID: 19443454]

Scott RR, Miller WL. Genetic and clinical features of p450 oxidoreductase deficiency. *Horm Res.* 2008;69:266. [PMID: 18259105]

Sekido R. SRY: a transcriptional activator of mammalian testis determination. *Int J Biochem Cell Biol.* 2010;42:417. [PMID: 20005972]

Sekido R, Lovell-Badge R. Sex determination and SRY: down to a wink and a nudge? *Trends Genet.* 2009;25:19. [PMID: 19027189]

Simard J, Ricketts ML, Gingras S, Soucy P, Feltus FA, Melner MH. Molecular biology of the 3beta-hydroxysteroid dehydrogenase/delta5-delta4 isomerase gene family. *Endocr Rev.* 2005;26:525. [PMID: 15632317]

Sinclair A, Smith C. Females battle to suppress their inner male. *Cell.* 2009;139:1051. [PMID: 20005799]

Slijper FM, Drop SL, Molenaar JC, de Muinck Keizer-Schrama SM. Long-term psychological evaluation of intersex children. *Arch Sex Behav.* 1998;27:125. [PMID: 9562897]

Speiser PW, White PC. Congenital adrenal hyperplasia. *N Engl J Med.* 2003;349:776. [PMID: 12930931]

Speiser PW, Azziz R, Baskin LS, et al. Congenital adrenal hyperplasia due to steroid 21-hydroxylase deficiency: an Endocrine Society clinical practice guideline. *J Clin Endocrinol Metab.* 2010;95:4133. [PMID: 20823466]

Sutton E, Hughes J, White S, et al. Identification of SOX3 as an XX male sex reversal gene in mice and humans. *J Clin Invest.* 2011;121:328. [PMID: 21183788]

Swain A. Sex determination: time for meiosis? The gonad decides. *Curr Biol.* 2006;16:R507. [PMID: 16824913]

Szarras-Czapnik M, Lew-Starowicz Z, Zucker KJ. A psychosexual follow-up study of patients with mixed or partial gonadal dysgenesis. *J Pediatr Adolesc Gynecol.* 2007;20:333. [PMID: 18082854]

Tang P, Park DJ, Marshall Graves JA, Harley VR. ATRX and sex differentiation. *Trends Endocrinol Metab.* 2004;15:339. [PMID: 15350606]

Tomaselli S, Megiorni F, De Bernardo C, et al. Syndromic true hermaphroditism due to an R-spondin1 (RSPO1) homozygous mutation. *Hum Mutat.* 2008;29:220. [PMID: 18085567]

Tomizuka K, Horikoshi K, Kitada R, et al. R-spondin1 plays an essential role in ovarian development through positively regulating Wnt-4 signaling. *Hum Mol Genet.* 2008;17:1278. [PMID: 18250097]

Tuladhar R, Davis PG, Batch J, Doyle LW. Establishment of a normal range of penile length in preterm infants. *J Paediatr Child Health.* 1998;34:471. [PMID: 9767514]

Uhlenhaut NH, Jakob S, Anlag K, et al. Somatic sex reprogramming of adult ovaries to testes by FOXL2 ablation. *Cell.* 2009;139:1130. [PMID: 20005806]

van Casteren NJ, de Jong J, Stoop H, et al. Evaluation of testicular biopsies for carcinoma in situ: immunohistochemistry is mandatory. *Int J Androl.* 2008;32:666. [PMID: 18798762]

Veitia RA. FOXL2 versus SOX9: a lifelong "battle of the sexes". *Bioessays.* 2010;32:375. [PMID: 20414895]

Virtanen HE, Rajpert-De Meyts E, Main KM, Skakkebaek NE, Toppari J. Testicular dysgenesis syndrome and the development and occurrence of male reproductive disorders. *Toxicol Appl Pharmacol.* 2005;207:501. [PMID: 16005920]

Warne GL. Long-term outcome of disorders of sex development. *Sex Dev.* 2008;2:268. [PMID: 18987501]

White PC. Ontogeny of adrenal steroid biosynthesis: why girls will be girls. *J Clin Invest.* 2006;116:872. [PMID: 16585958]

Wilhelm D, Palmer S, Koopman P. Sex determination and gonadal development in mammals. *Physiol Rev.* 2007;87:1. [PMID: 17237341]

Wisniewski AB, Mazur T. 46,XY DSD with female or ambiguous external genitalia at birth due to androgen insensitivity syndrome, 5alpha-reductase-2 deficiency, or 17beta-hydroxysteroid dehydrogenase deficiency: a review of quality of life outcomes. *Int J Pediatr Endocrinol.* 2009:567430. [PMID: 19956704]

Wisniewski AB, Migeon CJ, Malouf MA, Gearhart JP. Psychosexual outcome in women affected by congenital adrenal hyperplasia due to 21-hydroxylase deficiency. *J Urol.* 2004;171:2497. [PMID: 15126884]

Zitzmann M, Depenbusch M, Gromoll J, Nieschlag E. X-chromosome inactivation patterns and androgen receptor functionality influence phenotype and social characteristics as well as pharmacogenetics of testosterone therapy in Klinefelter patients. *J Clin Endocrinol Metab.* 2004;89:6208. [PMID: 15579779]

Puberty

Dennis Styne, MD

ACTH	Adrenocorticotropin	**IGF-1**	Insulin-like growth factor 1
AZF	Azoospermia factor	**KAL1**	Kallmann syndrome
cAMP	Cyclic adenosine monophosphate	**LDL**	Low-density lipoprotein
DHEA	Dehydroepiandrosterone	**LH**	Luteinizing hormone
DHEAS	Dehydroepiandrosterone sulfate	**LHX3**	*LIM homeobox gene 3*
FSH	Follicle-stimulating hormone	**PROP-1**	*Prophet of PIT 1*
GH	Growth hormone	**PROK1**	Prokineticin receptor 2
GnRH	Gonadotropin-releasing hormone	**PRL**	Prolactin
hCG	Human chorionic gonadotropin	**PSA**	Prostate-specific antigen
HESX-1	Hesx-1 homeodomain	**SHBG**	Sex hormone–binding globulin
HDL	High-density lipoprotein	**SF-1**	*Steroidogenic factor 1*
HPLC MS/MS	High performance liquid chromatography tandem mass spectroscopy	**SHOX**	*Short stature homeobox*
hGH	Human growth hormone	**SRIF**	Somatostatin
ICMA	Immunochemiluminometric assay	**TGF-α**	Transforming growth factor alpha

Puberty is best considered as one stage in the continuing process of growth and development that begins during gestation and continues until the end of reproductive life. After an interval of childhood quiescence—the juvenile pause—the hypothalamic pulse generator increases activity in the peripubertal period, just before the physical changes of puberty commence. This leads to increased secretion of pituitary gonadotropins and, subsequently, gonadal sex steroids that bring about secondary sexual development, the pubertal growth spurt, and fertility. Historical records show that the age at onset of particular stages of puberty in boys and girls in Western countries has steadily declined over the last several hundred years; this is probably due to improvements in socioeconomic conditions, nutrition, and, therefore, the general state of health during that period. This trend appears to be continuing but now due more to the effects of the obesity epidemic than the improvement in general health.

Many endogenous and exogenous factors can alter age at onset of puberty. While obesity may decrease the age of onset of puberty, chronic illness and malnutrition often delay puberty.

There is a significant concordance of age at menarche between mother-daughter pairs and within ethnic populations, indicating the influence of genetic factors. Recent study of genetic loci associated with the age of onset of puberty suggests the existence of several genes that are likely involved in the regulation of menarche and puberty.

PHYSIOLOGY OF PUBERTY

Physical Changes Associated with Puberty

Descriptive standards proposed by Tanner for assessing pubertal development in males and females are in wide use (denoted as Sexual Maturation stages or, often, Tanner stages). They focus attention on specific details of the examination and make it possible to objectively record subtle progression of secondary sexual development that may otherwise be overlooked. Self-assessment of pubertal development by subjects using reference pictures is used in clinical studies but reliability is less than that achieved by physical examination.

A. Female changes The first sign of puberty in the female, as noted in longitudinal studies, is an increase in height velocity that heralds the beginning of the pubertal growth spurt; girls are not usually examined frequently enough to demonstrate this change in clinical practice, so breast development is the first sign of puberty noted by most examiners. Breast development (Figure 15–1) is stimulated chiefly by ovarian estrogen secretion, although other hormones also play a part. The size and shape of the breasts may be determined by genetic and nutritional factors, but the characteristics of the stages in Figure 15–1 are similar in all females. Standards are available for the change in areolar (nipple) plateau diameter during puberty: nipple diameter changes little from stages B1 to B3 (mean of 3-4 mm) but enlarges substantially in subsequent stages (mean of 7.4 mm at stage B4 to 10 mm at stage B5), presumably as a result of increased estrogen secretion at the time of menarche. Areolae become more pigmented and erectile as development progresses. Other features reflecting estrogen action include enlargement of the labia minora

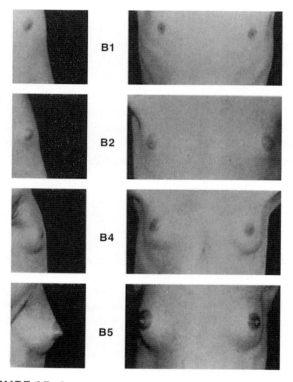

FIGURE 15–1 Stages of breast development, according to Marshall and Tanner. (Photographs from Van Wieringen JC, et al. *Growth Diagrams 1965 Netherlands: Second National Survey on 0 -24 Year Olds.* Institute for Preventive Medicine NO Leiden, Wolters-Noordhoff Publishing; 1971; with permission.) **Stage B1:** Preadolescent; elevation of papilla only. **Stage B2:** Breast bud stage; elevation of breast and papilla as a small mound, and enlargement of areolar diameter. **Stage B3 (not shown):** Further enlargement of breast and areola with no separation of their contours. **Stage B4:** Projection of areola and papilla to form a secondary mound above the level of the breast (not shown). **Stage B5:** Mature stage; projection of papilla only, due to recession of the areola to the general contour of the breast.

and majora, dulling of the vaginal mucosa from its prepubertal reddish hue to more of a pink color (due to cornification of the vaginal epithelium), and production of a clear or slightly whitish vaginal secretion prior to menarche. Pubic hair development (Figure 15–2) is determined chiefly by adrenal and ovarian androgen secretion. Breast development and growth of pubic hair usually proceed at similar rates, but because discrepancies in rates of advancement are possible, it is best to stage breast development separately from pubic hair progression.

Uterine size and shape change with pubertal development as reflected by ultrasonographic studies. With prolonged estrogen stimulation, the fundus-cervix ratio increases, leading to a bulbous form, and the uterus elongates. An endometrial stripe appears with the onset of puberty that is not found in premature thelarche. Ovaries enlarge with pubertal progression. Small cysts are normally present in prepubertal girls and a multicystic appearance develops during puberty, but the polycystic appearance seen in abnormalities of puberty or during the reproductive years in normal girls is not present. Experienced ultrasonographers can determine the developmental stage of the uterus and ovaries by comparing the results with established standards.

It is important to note that girls achieve reproductive maturity prior to physical maturity and certainly prior to psychologic maturity.

B. Male changes The first sign of normal puberty in boys is usually an increase in the size of the testes to more than 2.5 cm in the longest diameter, excluding the epididymis: this is equivalent to a testicular volume of 4 mL or more. Most of the increase in testicular size is due to seminiferous tubular development secondary to stimulation by follicle-stimulating hormone (FSH), with a smaller component due to Leydig cell stimulation by luteinizing hormone (LH). Thus, if only Leydig cells are stimulated, as with a human chorionic gonadotropin (hCG)-secreting tumor, the testis does not grow as large as in normal puberty. Pubic hair development is brought about by adrenal and testicular androgen secretion and is classified separately from genital development, as noted in Figure 15–3. A longitudinal study of more than 500 boys suggests adding a stage 2a (absence of pubic hair in the presence of a testicular volume of 3 mL or more) to the classic five stages of pubertal development. Further pubertal development occurred in 82% of the subjects in stage 2a after the passage of 6 months: thus, reaching stage 2a would allow the examiner to reassure a patient that further spontaneous development is likely soon. The appearance of spermatozoa in early morning urinary specimens (spermarche) occurs at a mean chronologic age of 13.4 years or a similar mean bone age; this usually occurs at gonadal stage 3 to 4 and pubic hair stage 2 to 4. Remarkably, spermaturia is more common earlier in puberty than later, suggesting that sperm are directly released into the urine early in puberty while ejaculation may be required for the presence of sperm in the urines of older children. However, boys are reported with spermaturia and no secondary sexual development.

It is important to note that boys achieve reproductive maturity prior to physical maturity and certainly prior to psychologic maturity.

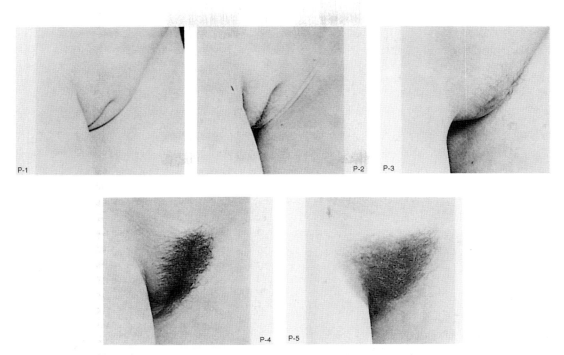

FIGURE 15–2 Stages of female pubic hair development, according to Marshall and Tanner. (Photographs from Van Wieringen JC, et al. *Growth Diagrams 1965 Netherlands: Second National Survey on 0 -24 Year Olds.* Institute for Preventive Medicine NO Leiden, Wolters-Noordhoff Publishing; 1971; with permission.) **Stage P1:** Preadolescent; the vellus over the area is no further developed than that over the anterior abdominal wall (ie, no pubic hair). **Stage P2:** Sparse growth of long, slightly pigmented, downy hair, straight or only slightly curled, appearing chiefly along the labia. This stage is difficult to see on photographs and is subtle. **Stage P3:** Hair is considerably darker, coarser, and curlier. The hair spreads sparsely over the superior junction of the labia majora. **Stage P4:** Hair is now adult in type, but the area covered by it is still considerably smaller than in most adults. There is no spread to the medial surface of the thighs. **Stage P5:** Hair is adult in quantity and type, distributed as an inverse triangle of the classic feminine pattern. Spread is to the medial surface of the thighs but not up the linea alba or elsewhere above the base of the inverse triangle.

C. Age at onset Ideally, the upper and lower boundaries encompassing the age at onset of puberty should be set at 2.5 standard deviations (SDs) above and below the mean (encompassing 98.8% of the normal population). Previously, there was no comprehensive study of the start of secondary sexual development adequate to determine the lower limits of normal in US children, as national studies began reporting children who were already 12 years of age or older. Thus, European standards, primarily those of Tanner, were modified for use in the United States. However, a study conducted in medical offices by specially trained pediatricians studying 17,070 girls brought in for routine visits provided information on girls in the United States as young as 3 years. The study revealed that 3% of white girls reach stage 2 breast development by 6 years of age and 5% by 7 years, whereas 6.4% of black girls had stage 2 breast development by 6 years and 15.4% by 7 years. Although this was not a randomly chosen population sampled by longitudinal study (and this led to controversy), it is the largest study available. These data led to the Lawson Wilkins Pediatric Endocrine Society statement that the diagnosis of precocious puberty could be defined as secondary sexual development starting prior to 6 years in black girls and prior to 7 years in white girls who are otherwise healthy. Recent analysis of data from NHANES III demonstrated that children of normal BMI values rarely have breast or pubic hair development before 8 years, although increased BMI in a subset of girls or

Hispanic and African American ethnicity led to earlier development. *It is essential to use any such guidelines only in healthy girls with absolutely no signs of neurologic or other disease that might pathologically advance puberty or a grave diagnosis may be missed.*

Recent data indicate that boys with elevated body mass indices have earlier onset of puberty. However, there has been no change in the age at onset of puberty in boys in the general population, so 9 years is taken as the lower limit of normal pubertal development in males, whereas 13½ years is the upper limit of normal development (although 14 years is often used as a simplified limit). The mean age at menarche in the United States is 12.8 years since the last government study was published in 1974. White girls have menarche later (12.9 years) than black girls (12.3 years), but this 6-month difference is less than the 1-year difference in the age at onset of puberty between the two groups. A compensation occurs in pubertal development so that those girls who enter puberty at the earliest ages of the normal range take more time to reach menarche, and those who enter at older ages of the normal range progress faster to menarche.

There is frequent discussion about an earlier age of puberty in children in the United States, which is demonstrated in some longitudinal studies in the US and abroad. The Bogalusa Heart Study shows that the gap between the age of menarche in Blacks and Whites has widened in the past decades, and this may be due to differing patterns of weight (and fat) gain. However longitudinal

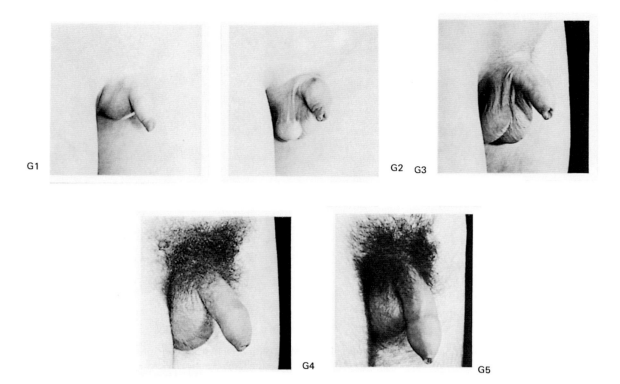

FIGURE 15–3 Stages of male genital development and pubic hair development, according to Marshall and Tanner. Genital: **Stage G1:** Preadolescent. Testes, scrotum, and penis are about the same size and proportion as in early childhood. **Stage G2:** The scrotum and testes have enlarged, and there is a change in the texture and some reddening of the scrotal skin. There is no enlargement of the penis. **Stage G3:** Growth of the penis has occurred, at first mainly in length but with some increase in breadth; further growth of testes and scrotum. **Stage G4:** Penis further enlarged in length and girth with development of glans. Testes and scrotum further enlarged. The scrotal skin has further darkened. **Stage G5:** Genitalia adult in size and shape. No further enlargement takes place after stage G5 is reached. Pubic hair: Stage P1: Preadolescent. The vellus is no further developed than that over the abdominal wall (ie, no pubic hair). Stage P2: Sparse growth of long, slightly pigmented, downy hair, straight or only slightly curled, appearing chiefly at the base of the penis. This is subtle. Stage P3: Hair is considerably darker, coarser, and curlier and spreads sparsely. Stage P4: Hair is now adult in type, but the area it covers is still considerably smaller than in most adults. There is no spread to the medial surface of the thighs. Stage P5: Hair is adult in quantity and type, distributed as an inverse triangle. Spread is to the medial surface of the thighs but not up the linea alba or elsewhere above the base of the inverse triangle. Most men have further spread of pubic hair. (Photographs from Van Wieringen JC, et al. *Growth Diagrams 1965 Netherlands: Second National Survey on 0-24 Year Olds.* Institute for Preventive Medicine NO Leiden, Wolters-Noordhoff Publishing; 1971; with permission.)

study from the Fells Institute shows that those girls who develop early have a tendency to increase their body mass index values after more than those who start puberty later. The presence or absence of menarche however, does not affect the interpretation of a BMI value. Late onset of pubertal development above the upper age limit of normal may indicate hypothalamic, pituitary, or gonadal failure or, alternatively, normal variation (constitutional delay). The time from onset of puberty until adult development is complete is also of importance; significant delays in reaching subsequent stages may indicate any type of hypogonadism.

D. Growth spurt   The striking increase in growth velocity in puberty (pubertal growth spurt) is under complex endocrine control involving thyroid hormone, growth hormone (GH), and estrogen. Hypothyroidism decreases or eliminates the pubertal growth spurt. The amplitude of GH secretion increases in puberty, as does production of insulin-like growth factor (IGF-I); peak serum IGF-I concentrations are reached about 1 year after peak

growth velocity, and serum IGF-I levels remain above normal adult levels for up to 4 years thereafter. GH and estrogen are important in the pubertal growth spurt; when either or both are deficient, the growth spurt is decreased or absent. Estrogen indirectly stimulate IGF-I production by increasing the secretion of GH. It also directly stimulates IGF-I production in cartilage. Estrogen is the most important factor in stimulating maturation of the chondrocytes and osteoblasts, ultimately leading to epiphysial fusion. A patient reported with estrogen receptor deficiency was tall, with continued growth past the age of 20 years with a remarkable retardation of skeletal maturation (and decreased bone density). Patients with aromatase deficiency, and therefore, impaired conversion of testosterone to estrogen, also demonstrate diminished advancement of bone age and decreased bone density, as well as continued growth extending into the third decade. With exogenous estrogen administration, the bone age advanced, and the bone density increased. Such patients demonstrate the key role played by estrogen in advancing bone age and bringing about the cessation of growth by epiphysial fusion as well as the importance of estrogen in increasing bone density.

In girls, the pubertal growth spurt begins in early puberty and is mostly completed by menarche. In boys, the pubertal growth spurt occurs toward the end of puberty, at an average age 2 years older than in girls. Total height attained during the growth spurt in girls is about 25 cm; in boys, it is about 28 cm. The mean adult height differential of 12 cm between men and women is due in part to heights already attained before onset of the pubertal growth spurt and in part to the height gained during the spurt.

Twin studies from Finland demonstrate that the heritability estimate (*proportion of variance of age of onset of puberty attributable to genetic variance*) for age at onset of pubertal growth spurt was 0.91, 0.93 for age at peak height velocity, and 0.97 for adult height. In addition, the age at onset of the pubertal growth spurt was negatively associated with BMI in childhood.

Precocious puberty may coexist with GH deficiency: this situation may occur, for example, in a child with a brain tumor causing central precocious puberty, who is treated with central nervous system radiation that subsequently causes GH deficiency. The precocious puberty may raise the growth rate to the normal range, cloaking the GH deficiency but the child does not grow at the excessive rate characteristic of precocious puberty with GH sufficiency.

E. Changes in body composition   Changes in body composition are also prominent during pubertal development. Prepubertal boys and girls start with equal lean body mass, skeletal mass, and body fat, but at maturity men have approximately 1½ times the lean body mass, skeletal mass, and muscle mass of women, whereas women have twice as much body fat as men. Attainment of peak values of percentage of body fat, lean body mass, and bone mineral density is earlier by several years in girls than in boys, as is the earlier peak of height velocity and velocity of weight gain in girls.

The most important phases of bone accretion occur during infancy and during puberty. Girls reach peak mineralization between 14 and 16 years of age, whereas boys reach a later peak at 17.5 years; both milestones occur after peak height velocity (Figure 15–4). The density of bone is determined by genetic factors; decreased bone mass is found in familial patterns even if subjects are studied before puberty. Patients with delay in puberty for any reason have a significant decrease in bone accretion and a delay in reaching peak bone mineral density, although bone density may later reach normal values in those with constitutional delay in puberty. Moderate exercise increases bone mass, but excessive exercise itself delays puberty; the ultimate outcome of excessive exercise in girls is the combination of exercise-induced amenorrhea, premature osteoporosis, and disordered eating, which is known as the female athletic triad.

Unfortunately, in the United States, only a minority of adolescents receive the recommended daily allowance of calcium (>1000 mg/d depending on age) and vitamin D, and a future epidemic of osteopenia or even osteoporosis in normal subjects who have this deficiency is a possibility although genetic influences are prominent in later adult bone density. It is especially important to ensure adequate calcium intake and vitamin D in patients with delayed or

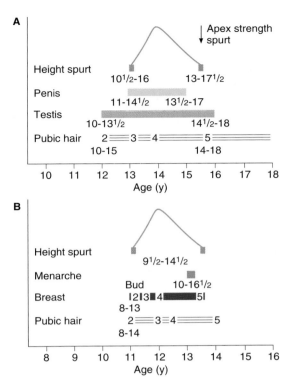

FIGURE 15–4 Sequence of secondary sexual development in British males **(A)** and females **(B)**. The range of ages in Britain is indicated. American boys and girls start pubertal stages earlier than British children (see text) but the sequence is the same. (Reproduced, with permission, from Marshall WA, Tanner JM. Variations in the pattern of pubertal changes in boys. *Arch Dis Child.* 1970;45:13.)

absent puberty and in patients treated with gonadotropin-releasing hormone (GnRH) agonists.

F. Other changes of puberty   Other changes that are characteristic of puberty are mediated either directly or indirectly by the change in sex steroids. For example, seborrheic dermatitis may appear, the mouth flora changes, and periodontal disease, rare in childhood, may occur. Insulin resistance intensifies in normal adolescents as well as those with type 1 diabetes mellitus.

Endocrine Changes from Fetal Life to Puberty

Pituitary gonadotropin secretion is controlled by the hypothalamus, which releases pulses of GnRH into the pituitary-portal system to reach the anterior pituitary gland by 20 weeks of gestation. Control of GnRH secretion is exerted by a *hypothalamic pulse generator* in the arcuate nucleus. It is sensitive to feedback control from sex steroids and inhibin, a gonadal protein product that controls the frequency and amplitude of gonadotropin secretion during development in both sexes and during the progression of the menstrual cycle in females (see Chapter 13).

In males, LH stimulates the Leydig cells to secrete testosterone, and FSH stimulates the Sertoli cells to produce inhibin. Inhibin feeds back on the hypothalamic-pituitary axis to inhibit FSH. Inhibin is also released in a pulsatile pattern, but concentrations do not change with pubertal progression.

In females, FSH stimulates the granulosa cells to produce estrogen and the follicles to secrete inhibin, and LH appears to play a minor role in the endocrine milieu until menarche. Then LH triggers ovulation and later stimulates the theca cells to secrete androgens (see Chapter 13).

A. Fetal life   The concept of the continuum of development between the fetus and the adult is well illustrated by the changes that occur in the hypothalamic-pituitary-gonadal axis. Gonadotropins are demonstrable in fetal pituitary glands and serum during the first trimester. The pituitary content of gonadotropins rises to a plateau at midgestation. Fetal serum concentrations of LH and FSH rise to a peak at midgestation and then gradually decrease until term. During the first half of gestation, hypothalamic GnRH content also increases, and the hypophyseal-portal circulation achieves anatomic maturity. These data are compatible with a theory of early unrestrained GnRH secretion stimulating pituitary gonadotropin secretion, followed by the appearance of central nervous system factors that inhibit GnRH release and decrease gonadotropin secretion after midgestation. Because the male fetus has measurable serum testosterone concentrations but lower serum gonadotropin concentrations than the female fetus, negative feedback inhibition of gonadotropin secretion by testosterone appears to operate after midgestation.

B. Changes at birth   At term, serum gonadotropin concentrations are suppressed in the neonate, but with postnatal clearance of high circulating estrogen concentrations, negative inhibition is reduced and postnatal peaks of serum LH and FSH are measurable for several months to up to a few years after birth. Serum testosterone concentrations may be increased to midpubertal levels during the several months after birth in normal males, and serum estradiol rises in pulses for the first 2 years in infant girls. These peaks of gonadotropins and sex steroids in normal infants complicate the diagnosis of central precocious puberty at these youngest ages, because it is difficult to decide whether to attribute the gonadotropin and sex steroid peaks to central precocious puberty or to normal physiology (the mini-puberty of infancy). While episodic peaks of serum gonadotropins may occur until 2 years of age, serum gonadotropin concentrations are low during later years in normal childhood.

C. The juvenile pause or the midchildhood nadir of gonadotropin secretion   While serum gonadotropin concentrations are low in midchildhood, sensitive assays indicate that pulsatile secretion occurs and that the onset of puberty is heralded more by an increase in amplitude of secretory events than a change in frequency. Twenty-four-hour mean concentrations of LH, FSH, and testosterone rise measurably within 1 year before the development of physical pubertal changes. Patients with gonadal failure—such as those with the syndrome of gonadal dysgenesis (Turner syndrome)—demonstrate an exaggeration of the normal

pattern of gonadotropin secretion, with exceedingly high concentrations of serum LH and FSH during the first several years of life. Such patients show that negative feedback inhibition is active during childhood; without sex steroid or inhibin secretion to exert inhibition, serum gonadotropin values are greatly elevated. During midchildhood, normal individuals and patients with primary hypogonadism have lower serum gonadotropin levels than they do in the neonatal period, but the range of serum gonadotropin concentrations in hypogonadal patients during midchildhood is still higher than that found in healthy children of the same age. The decrease in serum gonadotropin concentrations in primary agonadal children during midchildhood is incompletely understood, but has been attributed to an increase in the central nervous system inhibition of gonadotropin secretion during these years. Thus, the juvenile pause in normal children and those with primary gonadal failure appears to be due to central nervous system restraint of GnRH secretion.

D. Peripubertal gonadotropin increase   Prepubertal children demonstrate a circadian rhythm of LH and FSH secretion of low amplitude with a pattern of low levels of sex steroid secretion lagging behind the gonadotropin rhythm. The delay is presumably due to the time necessary for biosynthesis and secretion of sex steroids. Thus, the changes that are described later and that occur at puberty do not arise de novo but are based on preexisting patterns of endocrine secretion. In the peripubertal period, endogenous GnRH secretion increases in amplitude and frequency during the early hours of sleep and serum testosterone and estrogen concentrations rise several hours later, suggesting that biosynthesis or aromatization occurs during the period of delay—a pattern that differs from the prepubertal period mainly in the increased amplitude of the secretion encountered in puberty. As puberty progresses in both sexes, the peaks of serum LH and FSH occur more often during waking hours; and, finally, in late puberty, the peaks occur at all times, eliminating the diurnal variation.

During the peripubertal period of endocrine change prior to secondary sexual development, gonadotropin secretion becomes less sensitive to negative feedback inhibition. Before this time, a small dose of exogenous sex steroids virtually eliminates gonadotropin secretion, whereas afterward a far larger dose is required to suppress serum FSH and LH. Thus, an equilibrium of pubertal concentrations of gonadotropins and sex steroids is reached.

The switch that triggers the onset of puberty is unknown, but several neurotransmitters are invoked in the process, including gamma-aminobutyric acid and *N*-methyl-D-aspartate. Most recently, KISS1, a human metastasis suppressor gene at locus 19p13.3, which codes for metastin (or kisspeptin), a 145 amino acid peptide, has been implicated. Metastin is the endogenous agonist for GPR54, a Gq/11-coupled receptor of the rhodopsin family (metastin receptor), which is found in the brain, mainly in the hypothalamus and basal ganglia, as well as in the placenta. KISS1 mRNA levels increase with puberty in intact male and female monkeys from the juvenile to midpubertal stages. Furthermore, administration of KISS1 via intracerebral catheters to GnRH-primed juvenile female rhesus monkeys stimulates GnRH release, release that is abolished by infusion of GnRH antagonist. Thus, it is postulated that KISS1 signaling through the GPR54 receptor of primate hypothalamus may be activated at the end of the juvenile pause and contribute to the pubertal resurgence of pulsatile GnRH release of puberty, serving as a trigger for the onset of puberty.

Highly sensitive *sandwich* assays (immunoradiometric [IRMA]) and immunochemiluminometric assays (ICMA) are available for gonadotropin determination. They can be used to indicate the onset of pubertal development solely with basal samples usually without the necessity for GnRH testing (see GnRH and GnRH agonist testing in the Central Precocious Puberty section). Elevated basal LH values (>0.3 IU/L) determined by third-generation assays in random blood samples are highly predictive of elevated peak GnRH-stimulated LH and therefore indicate the onset of central precocious puberty or normal puberty. These third-generation assays further reflect the remarkable logarithmic increase in spontaneous LH secretion in the latest stages of prepuberty and earliest stages of puberty as the testicular volume increases from 1 mL to 10 mL; these increases in serum LH are far greater proportionately than those found in the last stages of pubertal development. The magnitude of increase in serum testosterone is also greater in the early stages of puberty and correlates with the increase in serum LH during this same period of early pubertal development. Note that standard LH and FSH assays are not sensitive enough to detect the changes seen with the ultrasensitive assays. Furthermore, the laboratory must have pubertal standard values available to permit accurate interpretation of the measurements. Since both types of assays are available commercially, care in ordering is needed.

E. Sex steroid secretion Sex steroid secretion is correlated with the development of gonadotropin secretion. During the postnatal period of increased episodic gonadotropin secretion, plasma concentrations of gonadal steroids are episodically elevated. This indicates the potential for secretory activity in the neonatal gonad. Later, when gonadotropin secretion decreases in midchildhood, gonadal activity decreases, but the testes can still be stimulated by LH or hCG and the ovaries by FSH, with resulting secretion of gonadal steroids. An ultrasensitive estradiol assay demonstrates higher values of serum estradiol in prepubertal girls than prepubertal boys, indicating definite basal ovarian activity during the juvenile pause. With the onset of puberty, serum gonadal steroid concentrations progressively increase. While sex steroids are secreted in a diurnal rhythm in early puberty, as are gonadotropins, sex steroids are bound to sex hormone–binding globulin (SHBG), so that the half-life of sex steroids is longer than that of gonadotropins. Thus, random daytime measurements of serum sex steroids are more helpful in determining pubertal status than random measurements of serum gonadotropins but still are not infallible.

Most (97%-99%) of the circulating estradiol and testosterone is associated with SHBG. The free hormone is the active fraction, but SHBG modulates the activity of the total testosterone and estradiol. Prepubertal boys and girls have equal concentrations of SHBG, but because testosterone decreases SHBG and estrogen increases SHBG, adult males have only half the concentration of SHBG compared with adult females. Thus, lower SHBG levels amplify androgen effects in men. While adult men have 20 times the amount of plasma testosterone that adult women have, adult men have 40 times the amount of free testosterone that adult women have.

F. GnRH stimulation The use of intravenous, exogenous GnRH has further clarified the pattern of pubertal development. When GnRH is administered to children less than 2 years of age, pituitary secretion of LH and FSH increases markedly. During the juvenile pause, the period of low basal gonadotropin secretion (after age 2 until the peripubertal period), exogenous GnRH has less effect on LH release. By the peripubertal period, intravenous GnRH or GnRH agonist induces a greater rise in LH concentrations in boys and girls, and this response continues until adulthood. There is no significant change in the magnitude of FSH secretion after GnRH with the onset of puberty, though females at all ages release more FSH than males.

Gonadotropins are released in secretory spurts in response to endogenous GnRH, which itself is secreted episodically about every 90 to 120 minutes in response to a central nervous system *pulse generator*. GnRH can be administered to patients in episodic boluses by a programmable pump that mimics the natural secretory episodes. A prepubertal subject without significant gonadotropin peaks demonstrates the normal pubertal pattern of episodic secretion of gonadotropins after only a few days of exogenously administered GnRH boluses. Hypogonadotropic patients, who in the basal state do not have normal secretory episodes of gonadotropin release, may be converted to a pattern of normal adult episodic gonadotropin secretion by this method of pulsatile GnRH administration.

This phenomenon is used in clinical practice to bring about ovulation or spermatogenesis to foster fertility. Varying the timing of pulsatile GnRH administration can regulate the ratio of FSH to LH just as the frequency of endogenous hypothalamic GnRH release shifts during the menstrual cycle and puberty to alter this ratio naturally. Increasing the frequency of GnRH pulses increases the LH-FSH ratio; an increased ratio is characteristic of midcycle and peripubertal dynamics. Alternatively, if GnRH is administered continuously rather than in pulses or if long-acting superactive analogs of GnRH are given, a brief period of increased gonadotropin secretion is followed by LH and FSH suppression (see later). This phenomenon is responsible for the therapeutic effects of GnRH analogs in conditions such as central precocious puberty.

G. Leptin and puberty Leptin is a hormone produced in adipose cells that suppresses appetite through interaction with its receptor in the hypothalamus. Leptin plays a major role in pubertal development in mice and rats. Genetically leptin-deficient mice (ob/ob) do not initiate puberty. Leptin replacement promotes pubertal development in this mouse, and leptin administration causes an immature normal mouse to progress through puberty. A leptin-deficient girl at 9 years of age was remarkably obese and had a bone age of 13 years (usually appropriate for the onset of normal puberty) but no significant gonadotropin pulses and no physical evidence of pubertal development. With leptin treatment, gonadotropin peaks appeared, and pubertal development followed. Individuals with leptin receptor deficiency also have disordered puberty. While these and other data suggested that leptin might be the elusive factor that triggers the onset of puberty, clinical data proved otherwise. Longitudinal studies demonstrate that leptin increases in girls during puberty in synchrony with the increase in fat mass, while leptin decreases in boys, with increased lean body mass and decreased fat mass in relation to testosterone production. While leptin does not appear to trigger the onset of puberty in normal adolescents, leptin may accompany pubertal changes rather than cause them. Leptin is a necessary component of pubertal development in human beings but not a major stimulant to this development.

Ovulation and Menarche

The last stage in hypothalamic-pituitary development is the onset of positive feedback, leading to ovulation and menarche. The ovary contains a paracrine system that regulates follicular atresia or development; it is only in the last stages of puberty that gonadotropins come into play in the maturation of the follicle. After midpuberty, estrogen in the appropriate amount at the appropriate time can stimulate gonadotropin release, whereas higher doses of estrogen can suppress gonadotropin secretion. The frequency of pulsatile GnRH release increases during the late follicular phase of the normal menstrual cycle and raises the ratio of LH to FSH secretion. This stimulates the ovary to produce more estrogen and leads to the midcycle LH surge that causes ovulation. Administration of pulsatile GnRH by programmable pump can be used to bring about fertility in patients with hypothalamic GnRH deficiency by mimicking this natural pattern as noted earlier.

However, even if the midcycle surge of gonadotropins is present, ovulation may not occur during the first menstrual cycles; 90% of menstrual cycles are anovulatory in the first year after menarche, and it is not until 4 to 5 years after menarche that the percentage of anovulatory cycles decreases to less than 20%. This high prevalence of anovulatory periods may be due to unrecognized PCOS in the young rather than a normal developmental phenomenon in some individuals. However, some of the first cycles after menarche may be ovulatory, and fertility is possible in the first cycle.

Just as boys are reproductively mature prior to physical maturity, girls may become fertile and even pregnant prior to physical or emotional maturity.

Adrenarche

Although the hypothalamic-pituitary axis has been well characterized in recent years, our understanding of the mechanism of control of adrenal androgen secretion is still somewhat rudimentary. The adrenal cortex normally secretes the weak androgens dehydroepiandrosterone (DHEA), its sulfate, dehydroepiandrosterone sulfate (DHEAS), and androstenedione in increasing amounts beginning at about 6 to 7 years of age in girls and 7 to 8 years of age in boys (Table 15–1). A continued rise in adrenal androgen secretion persists until late puberty. Thus, adrenarche (the secretion of adrenal androgens) occurs years before gonadarche (the secretion of gonadal sex steroids). The observation that patients with Addison disease, who do not secrete adrenal androgens, and patients with premature adrenarche, who secrete increased amounts of adrenal

TABLE 15–1 Pubertal gonadotropin and adrenal and gonadal sex steroid values.

Tanner Stage	Boys				Girls			
	LH (IU/L)	FSH (IU/L)	Testosterone (ng/d L)	DHEAS (µg/d L)	LH (IU/L)	FSH (IU/L)	Estradiol (pg/mL)	DHEAS (µg/dL)
I	≤0.52	≤3.0	≤5	≤89	≤0.15	0.50-4.50	≤16	≤46
II	≤1.76	0.30-4.00	≤167	≤81	≤2.91	0.40-6.50	≤65	15-113
III	≤4.06	0.30-4.00	21-719	22-126	≤7.01	0.40-6.50	≤142	42-162
IV	0.06-4.77	0.40-7.40	25-912	33-177	0.10-14.7	0.80-8.50	≤283	42-241
V	0.06-4.77	0.40-7.40	110-975	110-510	0.10-14.7	0.80-8.50	[a]See below	45-320

[a]Estradiol, ultrasensitive by HPLC MS/MS, in cycling females:

Follicular stage 39-375 pg/mL

Midcycle stage 94-762 pg/mL

Luteal stage 48-440 pg/mL

LH-pediatric is an immunometric (sandwich) electrochemiluminescent (ECL) ultrasensitive assay. FSH-pediatric is a immunometric (sandwich) chemiluminescent ultrasensitive ELISA (C-ELISA) assay.

Testosterone by HPLC MS/MS.

Estradiol, ultrasensitive is a tandem mass spectrometry by HPLC MS/MS as say.

DHEA-S is a competitive chemiluminescent immunoassay.

Values according to Quest Diagnostics, 2010; other laboratories will return other standards.

androgens at an early age, usually enter gonadarche at a normal age. This suggests that age at adrenarche does not significantly influence age at gonadarche. Furthermore, patients treated with a GnRH agonist to suppress gonadotropin secretion progress through adrenarche despite their suppressed gonadarche.

Miscellaneous Metabolic Changes

The onset of puberty is associated with many changes in laboratory values that are either directly or indirectly caused by the rise of sex steroid concentrations. Thus, in boys, hematocrit rises, and high-density lipoprotein (HDL) concentrations fall as a consequence of increasing testosterone. In both boys and girls, alkaline phosphatase rises normally during the pubertal growth spurt (often this rise is incorrectly interpreted as evidence for a tumor or liver abnormality). Serum IGF-I concentrations rise with the growth spurt, but IGF-I is more closely correlated with sex steroid concentration than with growth rate. IGF-I levels peak 1 year after peak growth velocity is reached and remain elevated for 4 years thereafter, even though growth rate is decreasing. Prostate-specific antigen (PSA) is measurable after the onset of puberty in boys and provides another biochemical indication of pubertal onset.

DELAYED PUBERTY OR ABSENT PUBERTY (SEXUAL INFANTILISM)

Any girl of 13 or boy of 14 years of age without signs of pubertal development falls more than 2.5 SD above the mean and is considered to have delayed puberty (Table 15–2). By this definition, 0.6% of the healthy population is classified as having delay in growth and adolescence. These normal patients need reassurance rather than treatment and ultimately progress through the normal stages of puberty, albeit later than their peers. The examining physician must make the sometimes difficult decision about which patients older than these guidelines are constitutionally delayed and which have organic disease.

Constitutional Delay in Growth and Adolescence

A patient with delayed onset of secondary sexual development, whose stature is shorter than that of age-matched peers but who consistently maintains a normal growth velocity for bone age and whose skeletal development is delayed more than 2 SD from the mean, is likely to have constitutional delay in puberty (Figure 15–5). These patients are at the older end of the normal distribution curve describing the age at onset of puberty. A family history of a similar pattern of development in a parent or sibling supports the diagnosis. The subject is usually thin as well. In many cases, even if they show no physical signs of puberty at the time of examination, the initial elevation of gonadal sex steroids has already begun, and their basal LH concentrations measured by ultrasensitive third-generation assays or their plasma LH response to intravenous GnRH or GnRH agonist is pubertal. In boys, an 8 AM serum testosterone value above 20 ng/dL (0.7 mmol/L) also indicates

TABLE 15–2 Classification of delayed puberty.

Constitutional delay in growth and adolescence
Hypogonadotropic hypogonadism
Central nervous system disorders
Congenital disorders of the hypothalamus or pituitary
Tumors
Other acquired disorders
Infection
Trauma
Irradiation
Defects of the hypothalamic-pituitary axis
Isolated gonadotropin deficiency
Kallmann syndrome
Gonadotropin deficiency with normal sense of smell
Multiple pituitary hormonal deficiencies
Miscellaneous disorders
Prader-Willi syndrome
Laurence-Moon, Bardet-Biedl syndromes
Chronic disease
Weight loss
Anorexia nervosa
Increased physical activity in female athletes
Hypothyroidism
Hypergonadotropic hypogonadism
Male phenotype
Klinefelter syndrome
Other forms of primary testicular failure (including chemotherapy)
Enzymatic defects of androgen production
Anorchia or cryptorchism
Female phenotype
Turner syndrome
Other forms of primary ovarian failure (including chemotherapy)
Pseudo–Turner syndrome
Noonan syndrome
XX and XY gonadal dysgenesis

that secondary sexual development will commence within a period of months.

In some cases, observation for endocrine or physical signs of puberty must continue for a period of months or years before the diagnosis is made. Generally, signs of puberty appear after the patient reaches a skeletal age of 11 years (girls) or 12 years (boys), but there is great variation. Patients with constitutional delay in adolescence almost always manifest secondary sexual development by 18 years of chronologic age, although there is one reported case of spontaneous puberty occurring at 25 years of age. Reports of patients with Kallmann syndrome and others with constitutional delay in puberty within one family suggest a possible relationship between the two conditions (see later and Chapter 4). Adrenarche is characteristically delayed—along with gonadarche—in constitutional delay in puberty.

Hypogonadotropic Hypogonadism

The absent or decreased ability of the hypothalamus to secrete GnRH or of the pituitary gland to secrete LH and FSH leads to hypogonadotropic hypogonadism. This classification suggests an irreversible condition requiring replacement therapy. If the pituitary deficiency is limited to gonadotropins, patients are usually

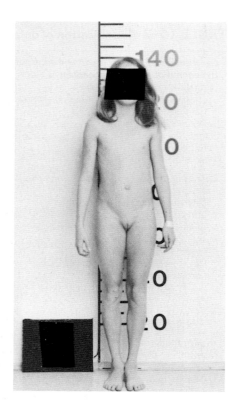 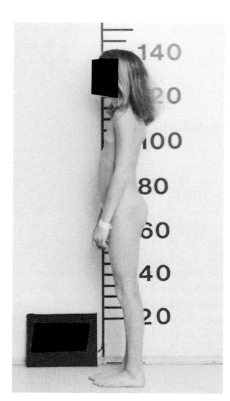

FIGURE 15–5 Girl, 13-4/12 years old, with constitutional delay in growth and puberty. History revealed a normal growth rate but short stature at all ages. Physical examination revealed a height of 138 cm (−4.5 SD) and a weight of 28.6 kg (−3 SD). The patient recently had early stage 2 breast development, with 1 cm of glandular tissue on the right breast and 2 cm on the left breast. The vaginal mucosa was dulled, and there was no pubic hair. Karyotype was 46,XX. Bone age was 10 years. After administration of GnRH, LH, and FSH rose in a pubertal pattern. Estradiol was 40 pg/mL. She has since spontaneously progressed through further pubertal development. (Reproduced, with permission, from Styne DM, Kaplan SL. *Pediatr Clin North Am.* 1979;26:123.)

close to normal height for age until the age of the pubertal growth spurt, in contrast to the shorter patients with constitutional delay. Bone age is usually not delayed in childhood but does not progress normally after the patient reaches the age at which sex steroid secretion ordinarily stimulates maturation of the skeleton. Patients may reach taller stature than expected. However, if GH deficiency accompanies gonadotropin deficiency, severe short stature will result.

A. Central nervous system disorders

1. Tumors—A tumor involving the hypothalamus or pituitary gland can interfere with hypothalamic-pituitary-gonadal function as well as control of GH, adrenocorticotropic hormone (ACTH), thyrotropin (TSH), prolactin (PRL), and vasopressin secretion. Thus, delayed puberty may be a manifestation of a central nervous system tumor accompanied by any or all of the following: GH deficiency, secondary hypothyroidism, secondary adrenal insufficiency, hyperprolactinemia, and diabetes insipidus. The combination of anterior and posterior pituitary deficiencies acquired after birth makes it imperative that a hypothalamic-pituitary tumor be considered as the cause.

Craniopharyngioma is the most common type of hypothalamic-pituitary tumor leading to delay or absence of pubertal development. This neoplasm originates in Rathke

pouch but may develop into a suprasellar tumor. The peak age incidence of craniopharyngioma is between 6 and 14 years. Presenting symptoms may include headache, visual deficiency, growth failure, polyuria, and polydipsia; presenting signs may include visual defects (bitemporal hemianopsia is classic), optic atrophy, or papilledema. Clinical manifestations and laboratory evaluation may reflect endocrinopathies (found in 70%-75% including GH, axis abnormalities in 75%, hyperprolactinemia 48%, hypothyroidism in 25%, adrenal insufficiency in 25%, diabetes insipidus (DI) in 4.%, as well as gonadotropin deficiency in 40% in one series. Bone age is often retarded at the time of presentation.

Calcification in the suprasellar region is the hallmark of craniopharyngiomas; 80% of cases have calcifications on lateral skull x-ray, and a higher percentage show this on computed tomography (CT); however, calcifications cannot be seen on magnetic resonance imaging (MRI). The tumor often presents a cystic appearance on CT or MRI scan and at the time of surgery may contain dark, cholesterol-laden fluid. The rate of growth of craniopharyngiomas is quite variable—some are indolent and some are quite aggressive. Small intrasellar tumors may be resected by transsphenoidal surgery; larger ones require partial resection and radiation therapy (see Chapter 4). Recurrence of this tumor after apparent complete removal is noted and lends support to the use of radiation therapy in addition to surgery.

Extrasellar tumors that involve the hypothalamus and produce sexual infantilism include germinomas, gliomas (sometimes with neurofibromatosis), and astrocytomas (see Chapter 4). However, depending on endocrine secretory activity or location, these tumors may alternatively produce central precocious puberty. Intrasellar tumors such as chromophobe adenomas are quite rare in children compared with adults. Hyperprolactinemia—with or without a diagnosed microadenoma or galactorrhea—may delay the onset or progression of puberty; with therapy to decrease PRL concentrations, puberty progresses.

2. **Other acquired central nervous system disorders**—These disorders may lead to hypothalamic-pituitary dysfunction. Granulomatous diseases such as Hand-Schüller-Christian disease or histiocytosis X, when involving the hypothalamus, most frequently lead to diabetes insipidus, but any other hypothalamic defect may also occur, including gonadotropin deficiency. Tuberculous or sarcoid granulomas, other postinfectious inflammatory lesions, vascular lesions, and trauma more rarely cause hypogonadotropic hypogonadism.

3. **Developmental defects**—Developmental defects of the central nervous system may cause hypogonadotropic hypogonadism or other types of hypothalamic dysfunction. Cleft palate or other midline anomalies may also be associated with hypothalamic dysfunction. Optic dysplasia is associated with small, hypoplastic optic disks and, in some patients, absence of the septum pellucidum on CT or MRI (septo-optic dysplasia); associated hypothalamic deficiencies are often present (see Chapters 4 and 6) (Hesx-1 homeodomain, HESX-1 *601802. *Homeobox* gene expressed in ES cells; HESX-1 #182230, septooptic dysplasia).

Optic hypoplasia or dysplasia must be differentiated from optic atrophy; optic atrophy implies an acquired condition and may indicate a hypothalamic-pituitary tumor. Both anterior and/or posterior pituitary deficiencies may occur with either congenital midline defects or acquired hypothalamic-pituitary defects. **Early-onset GH deficiency or early onset of a combination of anterior and posterior pituitary deficiencies suggests a congenital defect.** Patients who have isolated deficiency of gonadotropins tend to be of normal height until the teenage years but lack a pubertal spurt. They have eunuchoid proportions of increased span for height and decreased upper to lower segment ratios. Their skeletal development is delayed for chronologic age during the teenage years, they continue to grow after an age when normal adolescents stop growing. Adult height is often increased in hypogonadotropic hypogonadal individuals.

4. **Radiation therapy**—Central nervous system radiation therapy involving the hypothalamic-pituitary area can lead to hypogonadotropic hypogonadism with onset at 6 to 18 months (or longer) after treatment. GH is more frequently affected than gonadotropin secretion, and GH deficiency occurs with exposure to as little as an 18-Gy dose. Other hypothalamic deficiencies such as gonadotropin deficiency, hypothyroidism, and hyperprolactinemia occur more often with higher doses of radiation.

B. Isolated gonadotropin deficiency

Kallmann syndrome 1 is the most common genetic form of isolated gonadotropin deficiency (Figure 15–6). Gonadotropin deficiency in these patients is associated with hypoplasia or aplasia of the olfactory lobes and olfactory bulb causing hyposmia or anosmia. Remarkably, patients may not notice that they have no sense of smell, although olfactory testing reveals the finding. GnRH-containing neurons fail to migrate from the olfactory placode (where they originate) to the medial basal hypothalamus in Kallmann syndrome. This is a familial syndrome of variable manifestations in which anosmia may occur with or without hypogonadism in a given member of a kindred. **X-linked Kallmann syndrome** is due to gene deletions in the region of Xp22.3 (+308700.KAL1), causing the absence of the *KAL1* gene which codes for anosmin, which appears to code for an adhesion molecule that plays a key role in the migration of GnRH neurons and olfactory nerves to the hypothalamus. There is an association of Kallmann syndrome 1 with X-linked ichthyosis due to steroid sulfatase deficiency, developmental delay, and chondrodysplasia punctata, probably due to a microdeletion. Associated abnormalities in Kallmann syndrome 1 may affect the kidneys and bones, and patients may have undescended testes, gynecomastia, and obesity. Mirror hand movements (bimanual synkinesia) are reported, with MRI evidence of abnormal development of the corticospinal tract. Adult height is normal, although patients are delayed in reaching adult height. **Kallmann syndrome 2** is inherited in an autosomal dominant pattern and is due to a mutation in the *FGFR1* (*fibroblast growth factor receptor 1* [*136350]) gene. **Kallmann syndrome 3** (*607002) exhibits an autosomal recessive pattern and appears to be related to mutations in PROKR2 (*607123) and PROK2 (PROK2 *607002), encoding pokineticin receptor-2 and prokineticin-2. FGF8 may also be involved.

While kisspeptin and GRP54 (G protein–coupled receptor 54) play roles of importance in the onset of puberty, only rare patients have been reported with defects in the kisspeptin-GPR54 axis due to a mutation in the gene for the GRP54 receptor. The first human beings with defects in these molecules were reported in several kindreds, some consanguineous, presenting with hypogonadotropic hypogonadism. Other cases of hypogonadotropic hypogonadism may occur sporadically or in an autosomal recessive pattern without anosmia. The *GnRH* gene would seem a likely candidate for the cause of the condition, but while mutations of the *GnRH receptor* gene, *GnRHR*, were noted years ago, not until 2009 were mutations in the *GnRH1* gene demonstrated. Other mutations causing hypogonadotropic hypogonadism without anosmia include the *GPR56*, *SF-1* (*steroidogenic factor 1*), *HESX-1* (*Hesx-1 homeodomain*), 3 *LHX3* (*600577) (*LIM homeobox gene 3*) *PROP-1* (*prophet of PIT1*) (*601538) genes. X-linked congenital adrenal hypoplasia is associated with hypogonadotropic hypogonadism (*DAX1* #300200). Adrenal hypoplasia, congenital AHC, glycerol kinase deficiency, and muscular dystrophy have also been linked to this syndrome. The gene locus is at Xp21.3-p21.2 and involves a mutation in the *DAX1* gene in many but not all patients. An autosomal recessive form of congenital adrenal hypoplasia is reported. Some hypogonadal patients lack only LH secretion and have spermatogenesis without testosterone production (fertile eunuch syndrome); others lack only FSH (see Chapters 12 and 13). While a specific genetic diagnosis for hypogonadotropic hypogonadism suggests a permanent defect,

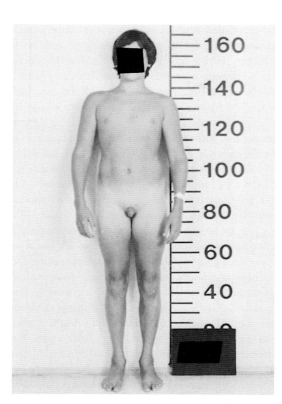 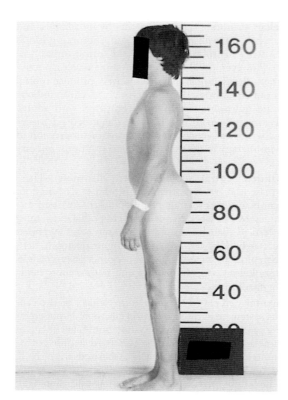

FIGURE 15–6 Boy, 15-10/12 years old, with Kallmann syndrome. His testes were originally undescended, but they descended into the scrotum after human chorionic gonadotropin treatment was given. His height was 163.9 cm (−1.5 SD), and the US-LS ratio was 0.86 (eunuchoid). The penis prepubertal measurement was 6.3 cm × 1.8 cm. Each testis was 1 cm × 2 cm, prepubertal. Plasma LH was not detectable and rose little after administration of 100 μg of GnRH; FSH rose minimally. Testosterone did not change from 17 ng/dL. He had no ability to smell standard odors. (Reproduced, with permission, from Styne DM, Grumbach MM. In: Yen SSC, Jaffe RB, eds. *Reproductive Endocrinology.* WB Saunders; 1978.)

long-term studies do not bear this out. Men with a variety of mutations followed for years are reported to revert to normal or near-normal gonadotropin function in some cases. Thus, long-term follow-up is indicated.

C. Idiopathic hypopituitary dwarfism (growth hormone deficiency in the absence of defined anatomic or organic defects)
Patients with congenital GH deficiency have early onset of growth failure (Figure 15–7); this feature distinguishes them from patients with GH deficiency due to hypothalamic tumors, who usually have late onset of growth failure. Even without associated gonadotropin deficiency, untreated GH-deficient patients often have delayed onset of puberty associated with their delayed bone ages. With appropriate human growth hormone (hGH) therapy; however, onset of puberty occurs at a normal age. Patients who have combined GH and gonadotropin deficiency do not undergo puberty even when bone age reaches the pubertal stage. Idiopathic hypopituitarism is usually sporadic, but may follow an autosomal recessive or X-linked inheritance pattern due to one of the gene defects listed earlier.

The syndrome of microphallus (penile length <2 cm at birth due to congenital gonadotropin or GH deficiency) and neonatal hypoglycemic seizures (due to congenital ACTH deficiency or GH deficiency) must be diagnosed and treated early to avoid

central nervous system damage due to hypoglycemia (these findings may occur in septo-optic dysplasia). Patients with this syndrome do not undergo spontaneous pubertal development. Testosterone in low doses (testosterone enanthate, 25 mg intramuscularly every month for three doses) can increase the size of the penis in infants diagnosed with congenital hypopituitarism without significantly advancing the bone age. Males with isolated GH deficiency can also have microphallus; the penis enlarges with hGH therapy in these patients. It is important to note that microphallus due to hypopituitarism may be successfully treated with testosterone leading to adult male sexual function, and sex reversal should not be considered (see Chapter 14).

Birth injury, asphyxia, or breech delivery is more common in the neonatal history of patients with idiopathic hypopituitarism, especially affected males. While some subjects with breech delivery have central nervous system MRI abnormalities including interrupted pituitary stalk and ectopic posterior pituitary gland, cause and effect is not established as some individuals with breech delivery and hypopituitarism have no such MRI findings.

D. Miscellaneous disorders
1. Prader-Willi syndrome—Prader-Willi syndrome (#176270) occurs sporadically and is associated with fetal and infantile hypotonia, short stature, poor feeding in infancy but insatiable

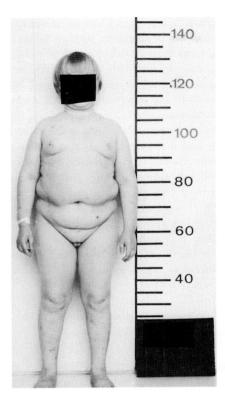

FIGURE 15–7 Twenty-year-old male with congenital deficiency of GRF, GnRH, TRF, and CRF. Height was 8 SD below the mean, and the phallus was 2 cm × 1 cm. Bone age was 10 years, and the sella turcica was small on lateral skull x-ray. LH rose minimally from a low basal value after administration of 100 μg of GnRH. Testosterone was virtually undetectable and did not rise after administration of GnRH. (Reproduced, with permission, from Styne DM, Grumbach MM. In: Yen SSC, Jaffe RB, eds. *Reproductive Endocrinology*. WB Saunders; 1978.)

hunger later, leading to remarkable obesity, characteristic facies with almond-shaped eyes, small hands and feet after infancy, mental retardation, and emotional instability in patients of either sex. Delayed menarche in females and micropenis and cryptorchism in males is common; while there is hypothalamic hypogonadism, there is also testicular dysfunction in males. Osteoporosis is common in these patients during the teenage years, but sex steroid replacement, when indicated, may increase bone density, although the effects are not proven to be long lasting if sex steroids administration cease. Behavioral modification may improve the usual pattern of rampant weight gain, but the constant vigilance of caregivers is necessary. Patients have deletion or translocation of chromosome 15q11-13 derived from their fathers. If an abnormality in this area derives from the mother, Angelman syndrome results. Fluorescent in situ hybridization for this area of the chromosome is available commercially for diagnosis.

2. **Laurence-Moon and Bardet-Biedl syndromes**—These autosomal recessive conditions are characterized by obesity, short stature, mental retardation, and retinitis pigmentosa. Hypogonadotropic hypogonadism and primary hypogonadism have variously been reported in affected patients. A distinction between Bardet-Biedl syndrome (#209900) a disorder thought to be linked to a defect in the basal body of ciliated cells) and

Laurence-Moon syndrome has been made, with the latter demonstrating polydactyly and obesity and the former being characterized by paraplegia. Recently it has been suggested that these two syndromes really represent a single entity, as was the case in the past.

3. **Chronic disease and malnutrition**—A delay in sexual maturation may be due to chronic disease or malnutrition. For example, children with intractable asthma have delayed pubertal development leading to short stature during the teenage years, although they ultimately reach an appropriate adult height for family. Children with other chronic diseases may not fare so well in long-term follow-up; for example, HIV infection in adolescence causes poor growth and pubertal progression. Weight loss to less than 80% of ideal body weight, caused by disease or voluntary dieting, may result in gonadotropin deficiency; weight gain toward the ideal usually restores gonadotropin function.

   Chronic disease may have effects on sexual maturation separate from nutritional state. For example, there is a high incidence of hypothalamic hypogonadism in thalassemia major, even with regular transfusion and chelation therapy.

4. **Anorexia nervosa**—Anorexia nervosa involves weight loss associated with a significant psychologic disorder. This condition usually affects girls who develop a disturbed body image and exhibit typical behavior such as avoidance of food and induction of regurgitation after ingestion. Weight loss may be so severe as to cause fatal complications such as immune dysfunction, fluid and electrolyte imbalance, or circulatory collapse. Primary or secondary amenorrhea is a classic finding in these patients and has been correlated with the degree of weight loss, although there is evidence that patients with anorexia nervosa may cease to menstruate before their substantial weight loss is exhibited. Other endocrine abnormalities in anorexia nervosa include elevated serum GH and decreased IGF-I (these are characteristic of other types of starvation), decreased serum triiodothyronine, decreased serum 1,25-dihydroxyvitamin D and elevated 24,25-hydroxyvitamin D levels. Weight gain to the normal range for height, however, does not ensure immediate resumption of menses. There is an increased incidence of anorexia nervosa in ballet dancers or ballet students; the incidence of scoliosis and mitral valve insufficiency is also increased in these patients. Functional amenorrhea may also occur in women of normal weight, some of whom demonstrate evidence of psychologic stress. Decreased LH response to GnRH administration, impaired monthly cycles of gonadotropin secretion, and retention of a diurnal rhythm of gonadotropin secretion are found in anorexia nervosa patients, patterns that indicate a reversion to an earlier stage of the endocrine changes of puberty.

5. **Increased physical activity**—Girls who regularly participate in activities such as strenuous athletics and ballet dancing may have delayed thelarche, delayed menarche, and irregular or absent menstrual periods. Increased physical activity and not decreased weight appears to be the cause of the amenorrhea in some girls; such amenorrheic patients may resume menses while temporarily bedridden even though weight does not yet change. Statistical analysis of mothers' ages at menarche and the type of sport pursued by their daughters indicates that late maturation of some gymnasts may be referable to a familial tendency to late menarche, suggesting that gymnastic activity may not be the primary cause of late menarche. On the other hand, there are studies indicating that intensive gymnastics training at an early age leads to a decrease in ultimate stature.

6. **Hypothyroidism**—Hypothyroidism can delay all aspects of growth and maturation, including puberty and menarche. Galactorrhea may occur in severe primary hypothyroidism due to concomitant elevation of serum PRL due to TSH stimulation. With thyroxine therapy, catch-up growth and resumed pubertal development and menses occur. Conversely, severe primary hypothyroidism may be associated with precocious puberty and galactorrhea (due to elevated serum PRL) in some patients (Van Wyk-Grumbach syndrome). There is evidence that excessive TSH can stimulate FSH receptors, leading to estrogen secretion and breast development.

Hypergonadotropic Hypogonadism

Primary gonadal failure is heralded by elevated gonadotropin concentrations due to the absence of negative feedback effects of gonadal sex steroids and inhibin. The most common causes of hypergonadotropic hypogonadism are associated with chromosomal and somatic abnormalities (see Chapter 14), but isolated gonadal failure can also present with delayed puberty without other physical findings. When hypergonadotropic hypogonadism is present in patients with a Y chromosome or a fragment of a Y chromosome (genetic males or conditions noted later), testicular dysgenesis must be considered in the differential diagnosis. The risk of testicular cancer rises in testicular dysgenesis (testicular cancer in normal boys is rare; eg, the incidence in Scandinavia is rising but still 0.5 per 100,000 in childhood).

A. Syndrome of seminiferous tubule dysgenesis (Klinefelter syndrome)
A common form of primary testicular failure is Klinefelter syndrome (47,XXY karyotype), with an incidence of 1:1000 males. Before puberty, patients with Klinefelter syndrome have decreased upper segment-lower segment ratios, small testes, and an increased incidence of developmental delay and personality disorders. Onset of puberty is not usually delayed, because Leydig cell function is characteristically less affected than seminiferous tubule function in this condition and testosterone is adequate to stimulate pubertal development. Serum gonadotropin levels rise to castrate concentrations after the onset of puberty; the testes become firm and are rarely larger than 3.5 cm in diameter. After the onset of puberty, there are histologic changes of seminiferous tubule hyalinization and fibrosis, adenomatous changes of the Leydig cells, and impaired spermatogenesis. Gynecomastia is common, and variable degrees of male secondary sexual development are found. Surviving sperm have been found by microdissection of some seminiferous tubules in a few patients leading to successful fertilization of a partner's ovum. Other forms of male hypergonadotropic hypogonadism are found with 46,XX/47,XXY, 48,XXYY, 48,XXXY, and 49,XXXXY karyotypes. Phenotypic males are described with 46,XX karyotypes and some physical features of Klinefelter syndrome; they may have the *SRY* gene translocated to an X chromosome (see Chapter 14).

B. Other forms of primary testicular failure
Patients surviving treatment for malignant diseases form a growing category of testicular failure. Chemotherapy—primarily with alkylating agents—or radiation therapy directed to the gonads may lead to gonadal failure. Injury is more likely if treatment is given during puberty than if it occurs in the prepubertal period, but even prepubertal therapy leads to risk. Normal pubertal development may occur in boys treated with chemotherapy before puberty, although they demonstrate elevated peak serum LH and elevated basal and peak serum FSH after GnRH, as well as a high incidence of decreased or absent sperm counts. This indicates that prepubertal status does not protect a child against testicular damage from chemotherapy and that normal physical development may hide significant endocrine and reproductive damage.

The **Sertoli cell only syndrome** (germinal cell aplasia) is a congenital form of testicular failure manifested by azoospermia and elevated FSH concentrations but generally normal secondary sexual characteristics, normal testosterone concentrations, and no other anomalies. A mutation in a gene at Yq11.23, the azoospermia factor *(AZF)* (#415000 spermatogenic failure, nonobstructive, Y-linked) appears to play a role in the lack of production of spermatocytes.

Patients with Down syndrome may have elevated LH and FSH levels even in the presence of normal testosterone levels, suggesting some element of primary gonadal failure.

C. Cryptorchism or anorchia
Phenotypic males with a 46,XY karyotype but no palpable testes have either cryptorchism or anorchia. Cryptorchid males should produce a rise in testosterone levels greater than 2 ng/mL 72 hours after intramuscular administration of hCG (3000 U/m^2) in the newborn period, although repeated doses are required after the first postnatal months. Testes may also descend during 2 weeks of treatment with hCG given three times a week.

Patients with increased plasma testosterone levels in response to hCG administration, but without testicular descent, have cryptorchism. Their testes should be brought into the scrotum by surgery to decrease the likelihood of further testicular damage due to the elevated intra-abdominal temperature and to guard against the possibility of undetected tumor formation. Cryptorchid testes may demonstrate congenital abnormalities and may not function normally even if brought into the scrotum early in life. Furthermore, the descended testis in a unilaterally cryptorchid boy may itself show abnormal histologic features; such patients have a 69% incidence of decreased sperm counts. Thus, unilateral cryptorchid patients can be infertile even if they received early treatment of their unilateral cryptorchism. Since both the descended and the undescended testes may be affected, there may be preexisting disease that is manifested by the lack of descent of one testis. Lack of normal descent of the testes is hypothesized to cause the testicular dysgenesis syndrome (TDS), which explains the late occurrence of testicular disease. In addition, patients undergoing orchiopexy may sustain subtle damage to the vas deferens, leading to the later production of antibodies to sperm that may result in infertility. This finding may depend on the surgical technique used.

It is important to determine if any testicular tissue is present in a boy with no palpable testes, because unnoticed malignant degeneration of the tissue is a possibility. The diagnosis of anorchia due to the testicular regression syndrome may be pursued by ultrasound,

MRI, laparotomy, or laparoscopic examination. There are other endocrine evaluations besides the hCG test that may help in diagnosis. The presence of anti-Müllerian factor in a young child indicates the presence of testicular tissue, although during puberty anti-Müllerian factor becomes undetectable, and this test cannot be employed at that stage. Inhibin may be measured as an indication of functioning testicular tissue. Except for the absence of testes, 46 XY patients who are otherwise normal and have the *vanishing testes* syndrome of late fetal loss of the testes have normal infantile male genital development, including Wolffian duct formation and Müllerian duct regression. The testes were presumably present in these patients early in fetal life during sexual differentiation, but degenerated after the 13th week of gestation for unknown reasons (see Chapter 14). When these boys reach adulthood, they are reported to establish a normal male gender identity. The presence of normal basal gonadotropin levels in a prepubertal boy without palpable testes at least suggests the presence of testicular tissue even if the testosterone response to hCG is low, whereas the presence of elevated gonadotropin levels without any testosterone response to hCG suggests anorchia.

D. Syndrome of gonadal dysgenesis (Turner syndrome)

45,XO gonadal dysgenesis is associated with short stature, female phenotype with sexual infantilism, and a chromatin-negative buccal smear. We do not recommend routinely ordering a buccal smear; it is now difficult for laboratories to perform the test reliably, and it has been replaced with modern karyotyping procedures. Patients have streak gonads consisting of fibrous tissue without germ cells. Other classic but variable phenotypic features include micrognathia, *fish* mouth (downturned corners of the mouth), ptosis, low-set or deformed ears, a broad shield-like chest with the appearance of widely spaced nipples, hypoplastic areolae, a short neck with low hairline and webbing of the neck (pterygium colli), short fourth metacarpals, cubitus valgus, structural anomalies of the kidney, extensive nevi, hypoplastic nails, and vascular anomalies of the left side of the heart (most commonly coarctation of the aorta associated with hypertension proximal to the coarctation). However, some affected girls can have almost normal female phenotypes. The medical history of patients with the syndrome of gonadal dysgenesis often reveals small size at birth, lymphedema of the extremities most prominent in the newborn period, and loose posterior cervical skin folds. (The terms *Bonnevie-Ullrich syndrome* and *infant Turner syndrome* are applied to this neonatal appearance.) Affected patients often have a history of frequent otitis media with conductive hearing loss. There may be frequent urinary tract infections associated with a horseshoe-shaped kidney, duplication of ureters, or other anatomic defects. Intelligence is normal, but there is often impaired spatial orientation, which may lead to difficulty in mathematics, especially geometry. Patients have no pubertal growth spurt, and reach a mean final height of 143 cm. Short stature is a classic feature of Turner syndrome, but not of other forms of hypergonadotropic hypogonadism that occur without karyotype abnormalities. The short stature is linked to the absence of the (*short stature homeobox*) *SHOX* homeobox gene of the pseudoautosomal region of the X

chromosome (Xpter-p22.32) (OMIM*312865). GH function is usually normal in Turner syndrome. However, exogenous hGH treatment improves growth rate and increases adult stature toward the normal range in affected girls. It improves lipid profiles and decreases diastolic blood pressure (see Chapter 6). Pubic hair may appear late and is usually sparse in distribution owing to the absence of any ovarian secretions; thus, adrenarche progresses in Turner syndrome even in the absence of gonadarche. Autoimmune thyroid disease (usually hypothyroidism) is common in Turner syndrome, and determination of thyroid function and thyroid antibody levels is important in evaluation of these patients.

Serum gonadotropin concentrations in Turner syndrome are extremely high between birth and about age 4 years. They decrease toward the normal range in prepubertal patients in the juvenile pause and then rise again to castrate levels after age 10 years (see Chapter 14).

Sex chromatin–positive variants of gonadal dysgenesis include 45,X/46,XX, 45,X/47,XXX, and 45,X/46,XX/47,XXX mosaicism with chromatin-positive buccal smears. Patients with these karyotypes may resemble patients with the classic syndrome of gonadal dysgenesis, or they may have fewer manifestations and normal or nearly normal female phenotypes. Streak gonad formation is not invariable; some patients have had secondary sexual development, and menarche and rare pregnancies have been reported.

Sex chromatin–negative variants of the syndrome of gonadal dysgenesis have karyotypes with 45,X/46,XY mosaicism. Physical features vary; some patients have the features of classic Turner syndrome, whereas others may have ambiguous genitalia or even the features of phenotypic males. Gonads are usually dysgenetic but vary from streak gonads to functioning testes. These patients are at risk for gonadoblastoma formation; this is a benign tumor that has the potential for malignant transformation and then may metastatize. Because gonadoblastomas may secrete androgens or estrogens, patients with gonadoblastoma may virilize or feminize as though they had functioning gonads, confusing the clinical picture. Gonadoblastomas may demonstrate calcification on abdominal x-ray. Malignant germ cell tumors may arise in dysgenetic testes, and orchiectomy is generally indicated. In some mosaic patients with one intact X chromosome and one chromosomal fragment, it is difficult to determine whether the fragment is derived from an X chromosome or a Y chromosome. Polymerase chain reaction techniques to search for specific Y chromosome sequences may be helpful if a karyotype reveals no Y chromosomal material.

Patients with Turner syndrome who desire fertility can be treated with in vitro fertilization techniques. After exogenous hormonal preparation, a fertilized ovum (possibly a sister's ovum fertilized by the patient's male partner, or an extra fertilized ovum from another couple undergoing in vitro fertilization) can be introduced into the patient's uterus, and the pregnancy is then brought to term by support with exogenous hormone administration. A serious possible complication is uterine rupture.

E. Other forms of primary ovarian failure

Ovaries appear to be more resistant to damage from the chemotherapy used in the treatment of malignant disease than are testes. Nonetheless, ovarian failure can occur with medical therapy. Damage is common if the ovaries are not surgically *tacked* out of the path of the beam or shielded by lead in abdominal radiation therapy. Normal gonadal function after chemotherapy does not guarantee normal function later. Late-onset gonadal failure has been described after chemotherapy. Bone marrow transplantation with whole-body irradiation for acute lymphoblastic leukemia or non–Hodgkin lymphoma appear to cause the most damage to endocrine function.

Premature menopause has also been described in otherwise healthy girls owing to the presence of anti-ovarian antibodies. Patients with Addison disease may have autoimmune oophoritis as well as adrenal failure. A sex steroid biosynthetic defect due to 17α-hydroxylase deficiency (P450c17) manifests as sexual infantilism and primary amenorrhea in a phenotypic female (regardless of genotype) with hypokalemia and hypertension (see Chapter 14). A patient with 17α-hydroxylase deficiency may have ovaries or testes and still present as a phenotypic female.

F. Noonan syndrome (pseudo–Turner syndrome, Ullrich syndrome, male Turner syndrome (OMIM#163950 Noonan syndrome 1; NS1)

Noonan syndrome is associated with phenotypic manifestations of Turner syndrome such as webbed neck, ptosis, short stature, cubitus valgus, and lymphedema, but other additional clinical findings such as a normal karyotype, triangular facies, pectus excavatum, right-sided heart disease, and an increased incidence of developmental delay differentiate these patients from those with Turner syndrome. Males may have undescended testes and variable degrees of germinal cell and Leydig cell dysfunction. Noonan syndrome follows an autosomal dominant pattern of inheritance with incomplete penetrance (gene locus 12q24). hGH is approved by the FDA to increase stature in these patients.

G. Familial and sporadic forms of 46,xx or 46,xy gonadal dysgenesis

These forms of gonadal dysgenesis are characterized by structurally normal chromosomes and streak gonads or partially functioning gonads. They do not have the physical features of Turner syndrome. If there is some gonadal function, 46,XY gonadal dysgenesis may present with ambiguous genitalia or virilization at puberty. If no gonadal function is present, patients appear as phenotypic sexually infantile females. Patients with 46,XY gonadal dysgenesis and dysgenetic testes should undergo gonadectomy to eliminate the possibility of malignant germ cell tumor formation.

H. Primary amenorrhea associated with normal secondary sexual development

If a structural anomaly of the uterus or vagina interferes with the onset of menses but the endocrine milieu remains normal, the patient presents with primary amenorrhea in the presence of normal breast and pubic hair development. A transverse vaginal septum may seal the uterine cavity from the vaginal orifice, leading to the retention of menstrual flow—as may an imperforate hymen. The Rokitansky-Küster-Hauser syndrome (OMIM #277000) combines congenital absence of the vagina with abnormal development of the uterus, ranging from a rudimentary bicornuate uterus that may not open into the vaginal canal to a virtually normal uterus; surgical repair may be possible in patients with minimal anatomic abnormalities, and fertility has been reported. Associated abnormalities include major urinary tract anomalies and spinal or other skeletal disorders. The rarest anatomic abnormality in this group is absence of the uterine cervix in the presence of a functional uterus.

46,XY disorder of sexual development (DSD), previously called male pseudohermaphroditism, is an alternative cause of primary amenorrhea if a patient has achieved thelarche. The syndrome of complete androgen resistance leads to female external genitalia and phenotype without axillary or pubic hair development in the presence of pubertal breast development (syndrome of testicular feminization; see Chapter 14).

Differential Diagnosis of Delayed Puberty (Table 15–3)

Patients who do not begin secondary sexual development by age 13 (girls) or age 14 (boys) and patients who do not progress through development on a timely basis (girls should menstruate within 5 years

TABLE 15–3 Differential diagnosis of delayed puberty.

	Serum Gonadotropins	Serum Gonadal Steroids[a]	Miscellaneous
Constitutional delay in growth and adolescence	Prepubertal (low)	Low	Patient usually has short stature for chronologic age but appropriate height and growth rate for bone age. Both adrenarche and gonadarche are delayed.
Hypogonadotropic hypogonadism	Prepubertal (low)	Low	Patient may have anosmia (Kallmann syndrome) or other associated pituitary hormone deficiencies. If gonadotropin deficiency is isolated, the patient usually has normal height and growth rate but lacks a pubertal growth spurt. Adrenarche may occur at a normal stage in spite of absent gonadarche (serum DHEAS may be pubertal).
Hypergonadotropic hypogonadism	Elevated	Low	Patient may have abnormal karyotype and stigmatas of Turner syndrome or Klinefelter syndrome.

[a]In a pediatric specific assay.

after breast budding; boys should reach stage 5 pubertal development 4½ years after onset) should be evaluated for hypogonadism. The yield of diagnosable conditions is quite low in children younger than these ages, but many patients and families request evaluation well before these limits. Without significant signs or symptoms of disorders discussed above, it is best to resist evaluation and offer support until these ages in most cases.

A patient with constitutional delay may have a characteristic history of short stature for age with normal growth velocity for bone age and a family history of delayed but spontaneous puberty. The patient's mother may have had late onset of menses, or the father may have begun to shave late or continued growing after high school. Not all patients with constitutional delay are so classic, and gonadotropin-deficient patients may have some features similar to those of constitutional delay in adolescence. Indeed, patients with Kallmann syndrome and others with constitutional delay are occasionally found in the same kindred.

If the diagnosis is not obvious on the basis of physical or historical features, the differential diagnostic process begins with determination of whether plasma gonadotropins are (1) elevated due to primary gonadal failure or (2) decreased due to secondary or tertiary hypogonadism or constitutional delayed puberty. Gonadotropins must be measured in a third generation assay with pediatric standards as the customary gonadotropin determinations are too insensitive to reveal the small changes of puberty. A single ultrasensitive, third-generation determination of serum LH concentration in the pubertal range suggests that puberty is progressing. Determination of the rise in LH after administration of GnRH or GnRH agonist is helpful in differential diagnosis; secondary sexual development usually follows within months after conversion to a pubertal LH response to GnRH. Because it is difficult, if not impossible, to obtain GnRH presently, GnRH agonists are more frequently used for diagnosis with serum LH values measured 2 hours after administration. Frequent nighttime sampling (every 20 minutes through an indwelling catheter) to determine the amplitude of peaks of LH secretion during sleep is an alternative to GnRH or GnRH agonist testing but is too cumbersome for most clinical settings. Unfortunately, the results of GnRH infusions or nighttime sampling are not always straightforward. Patients may have pubertal responses to exogenous GnRH but may not spontaneously secrete adequate gonadotropins to allow secondary sexual development. In females with amenorrhea, the frequency and amplitude of gonadotropin secretion may not change to allow monthly menstrual cycles. The retention of a diurnal rhythm of gonadotropin secretion (normal in early puberty) into late puberty is a pattern linked to inadequate pubertal progression. In males, a morning serum testosterone concentration over 20 ng/dL (0.7 mmol/L) indicates the likelihood of pubertal development within 6 months. Measurement of testosterone or estradiol must be done in an ultrasensitvie assay with pediatric standards or, as with gonadotropin assays, the small changes of pubertal development will be missed. Presently highly sensitive high performance liquid chromatography tandem mass spectroscopy (HPLC MS/MS) assays are available at national laboratories for this purpose.

Other methods of differential diagnosis between constitutional delay and hypogonadotropic hypogonadism have been proposed but are complex or are not definitive. Clinical observation for signs of pubertal development and laboratory evaluation for the onset of rising levels of sex steroids may have to continue until the patient is 18 years of age before the diagnosis is definite. In most cases, if spontaneous pubertal development is not noted by 18 years of age, the diagnosis is gonadotropin deficiency. Of course, the presence of neurologic impairment or other endocrine deficiencies should immediately lead to investigation for central nervous system tumor or congenital defect in a patient with delayed puberty. CT or MRI scanning is helpful in this situation.

Treatment of Delayed Puberty

A. Constitutional delay in growth and adolescence

Psychologic support.   Teenagers who are so embarrassed about short stature and lack of secondary sexual development that they have significant psychologic problems may require psychological evaluation and therapy if they have passed the ages of 13 years for girls or 14 years for boys. Patients with constitutional delay in growth and adolescence should be counseled that normal pubertal development will occur spontaneously. Peer pressure and teasing can be oppressive. Although the majority of these patients do quite well, severe depression must be treated appropriately, because short patients with pubertal delay have become suicidal. In some cases, it helps to excuse the patient from physical education class, because the lack of development is most apparent in the locker room. In general, boys feel more stress than girls when puberty is delayed.

Sex steroids.   New preparations of topical sex steroids, that have different systemic effects and length of action than parenteral or oral sex steroids, have enlarged the therapeutic armamentarium for delayed puberty. The classic recommendation for girls has been a 3-month course of conjugated estrogen (0.3 mg) or ethinyl estradiol (5-10 µg) given orally each day. Topical estrogen is said to carry less risk of hypertension, gallstones, increased fat mass, decreased insulin sensitivity, and increased triglycerides (topical estrogen does not, however, increase HDL cholesterol and decrease low-density lipoprotein [LDL] cholesterol, as does oral estrogen). Estrogen-impregnated patches are available and might be used to initiate puberty, but the lowest dose available leads to serum estrogen values higher than physiologic levels found in early puberty. They might be used for only a few days each week to reduce the delivered dose. Alternatively, 17-beta estradiol patches (0.025 mg/patch; Vivelle Dot matrix patch) may be cut into fragments the size of one-eighth to one-fourth of a patch fragments to initiate pubertal development with more physiologic estrogen values. However, the use of such topical estrogen preparations is not approved by the Food and Drug Administration (FDA).

The classic recommendation for boys is a 3-month course of testosterone enanthate or cypionate (50 mg) given intramuscularly once every 28 days for three doses. The possibility that a higher dose will cause priapism limits the initial dose to 50 mg. New patch or testosterone gel preparations could be used to initiate puberty, but the dose in manufactured packets is too high to mimic the physiologic levels found in early puberty. These preparations are made for full replacement in adult males. The entire gel packet or lowest-dose patch could be used every other day over the 3-month period of treatment, although this leads to variable daily dosage. The gel is available in a pump but even one pump dose is too high for the initial therapy. The testosterone patches are not impregnated like the estrogen patches and cannot be cut down in size. Thus, to date, the low-dosage injection of testosterone or the use of an estimated one-half or less of the 5 mg testosterone gel packet are the only methods of reaching appropriate dosage. The topical use of testosterone is not approved by the FDA for such purposes. Therapy with oxandrolone has been suggested as a method of increasing secondary sexual development and increasing growth without advancing skeletal development. This method is not widely preferred. Furthermore, testosterone, which can be aromatized, increases the generally low endogenous GH secretion in constitutional delayed puberty to normal, whereas oxandrolone, which cannot be aromatized, does not increase GH secretion.

Hormonal treatment of boys or girls elicits noticeable secondary sexual development and a slight temporary increase in stature. The low doses recommended do not advance bone age substantially and do not significantly change adult height if used for 3 months. Low-dose sex steroid treatment has been reported to promote spontaneous pubertal development after sex steroid therapy is discontinued, although responding individuals may include those boys who are on the brink of further pubertal development and are, therefore, most likely to achieve a growth response to androgen therapy. However, a short course of therapy may improve patients' psychologic outlook and allow them to await spontaneous pubertal development with greater confidence. Continuous gonadal steroid replacement in these patients is not indicated, because it advances bone age and leads to epiphyseal fusion and a decrease in ultimate stature. After a 3- to 6-month break to observe spontaneous development, a second course of therapy may be offered if no spontaneous pubertal progression occurs during observation.

B. Permanent hypogonadism

Once a patient has been diagnosed as having delayed puberty due to permanent primary or secondary hypogonadism, replacement therapy must be considered at the average age of onset of puberty, in most cases when the diagnosis is made in childhood.

Males with hypogonadism may be treated with testosterone gel, testosterone patches, or testosterone enanthate or cypionate given intramuscularly every month, as described earlier for temporary conditions. Treatment as for constitutional delay should be started and gradually increased to the adult range over months to years to mimic the normal progression of puberty and to avoid abrupt exposure to high-dose androgen and the possibility of frequent erections or priapism. Oral halogenated testosterone and methylated testosterone are never recommended because of the risk of hepatocellular carcinoma or cholestatic jaundice. Testosterone therapy may not cause adequate pubic hair development, but patients with secondary or tertiary hypogonadism may benefit from hCG administration with increased pubic hair growth resulting from endogenous testicular androgen secretion in addition to the exogenous testosterone.

Testosterone gel or patches, as described earlier, are used for permanent replacement but are not FDA-approved for individuals less than 16 years. Girls may be treated with oral ethinyl estradiol

(increasing from 5 μg/d to 10 to 20 μg/d depending on clinical results), or conjugated estrogens (0.3 or 0.625 mg/d). One may start with daily doses with eventual conversion to treatment on days 1 to 21 of the month after several months of daily ingestion. Five to ten milligrams of medroxyprogesterone acetate are then added on days 12 to 21 after physical signs of estrogen effect are noted and breakthrough bleeding occurs (and always within 6 months after initiating estrogen). Neither hormone is administered from day 22 to the end of the month to allow regular withdrawal bleeding (see Chapter 13). Later, the patient may be switched to sequential oral contraceptives to simplify treatment. As described earlier, estrogen patch therapy may have benefits (but these are not proven) over oral estrogen and may be preferable (but these are not FDA-approved for individuals under 16 years of age). Gynecologic examinations should be performed yearly for those on replacement therapy.

Hypothalamic hypogonadism may be treated with GnRH pulses by programmable pumps to achieve fertility or to promote pubertal development. Likewise, in the absence of a functional pituitary gland, hCG and menotropins (human postmenopausal gonadotropin) may be administered in pulses. These techniques are cumbersome and best reserved for the time when fertility is desired.

C. Coexisting GH deficiency

The treatment of patients with coexisting GH deficiency requires consideration of their bone age and amount of growth left before epiphyseal fusion. If such a patient has not yet received adequate treatment with GH, sex steroid therapy may be kept at the lower dosage or even delayed to optimize adult height. The goal is to allow appropriate pubertal changes to support psychologic development and to allow the synergistic effects of combined sex steroids and GH without fusing the epiphyses prematurely.

Constitutional delayed puberty may be associated with decreased GH secretion in 24-hour profiles of spontaneous secretion or in stimulated testing. GH secretion increases when pubertal gonadal steroid secretion rises due to the effects of estrogen, so decreased GH secretion in this condition should be considered temporary. Nonetheless, true GH-deficient patients may have delayed puberty due to the GH deficiency or to coexisting gonadotropin deficiency. Therefore, deciding whether a pubertal patient has temporary or a permanent GH deficiency can be difficult; previous observation may indicate a long history characteristic of constitutional delay in adolescence, whereas a recent decrease in growth rate may suggest the onset of a brain tumor or other cause of hypopituitarism.

D. The syndrome of gonadal dysgenesis

In the past, patients with the syndrome of gonadal dysgenesis were frequently not given estrogen replacement until after age 13 years, for fear of compromising adult height. However, low-dose estrogen therapy (5-10 μg of ethinyl estradiol orally) can be administered to allow feminization and improve psychologic status at 12 to 13 years of age without decreasing final height, as shown in several studies. Low-dose estrogen increases growth velocity, whereas high-dose estrogen suppresses it. Even if growth velocity is increased, however, adult height is not increased with such estrogen treatment.

Treatment of Turner syndrome with GH successfully increases adult stature (see Chapters 6 and 14). During childhood these girls must be regularly screened for strabismus, hearing loss, and autoimmune thyroid disease as well as learning difficulties. There are several recommendations for the preparation of these girls to transition to adult care and necessary follow-up for issues that will affect their later life, including monitoring for the development of aortic dilation at 5- to 10-year intervals since this defect may progress to aortic aneurysms. The induction of fertility was described earlier in this chapter.

E. Bone mass   After infancy, most bone mass accrual takes place during the second decade of life, and disorders of puberty may affect this process. Delayed puberty in boys causes decreased cross-sectional bone density, when the subjects are tested as young adults, because they have not yet reached peak bone acquisition. Although there is some controversy, it appears likely that normalization of volumetric bone density occurs with maturity and exposure to a normal androgen milieu. A range of defects in girls such as anorexia nervosa, athletics-induced delayed puberty, and Turner syndrome also cause decreased bone density. The use of testosterone in boys and estrogen and progesterone in girls with hypogonadotropic hypogonadism is helpful in increasing bone mass but has not been demonstrated to result in normal adult bone mass. Appropriate ingestion of dairy products containing calcium or calcium supplementation and vitamin D should be encouraged in hypogonadal or constitutionally delayed patients as well as in normal children at least as a common sense measure. No long-term follow-up is yet available, however, to prove the efficacy of this therapy in susceptible subjects.

PRECOCIOUS PUBERTY (SEXUAL PRECOCITY)

All sources agree that the appearance of secondary sexual development before the age of 9 years in boys is precocious puberty. However, there remains controversy over the lower limits of normal in girls. There is acceptance by the Pediatric Endocrine Society that the appearance of secondary sexual development before the age of 7 years in Caucasian girls and 6 years in African-American girls constitutes precocious sexual development but others remain concerned that pubertal development between 7 and 8 years for Caucasian and 6 and 8 for African American girls indicate a pathological state (Table 15–4). However, if a girl has the onset of puberty before 8 years, one must have a high index of suspicion for pathology. The child must have absolutely no sign of central nervous system disorder or other possible cause that might trigger pathologic precocious puberty. A careful search for historical or physical features of organic disease must occur before a girl with precocious puberty between 6 or 7 and 8 is considered normal. When the cause of precocious puberty is premature activation of the hypothalamic-pituitary axis and the condition is gonadotropin dependent, the diagnosis is **central (complete or true) precocious puberty;** if ectopic gonadotropin secretion occurs in boys or autonomous sex steroid secretion occurs in either

TABLE 15–4   Classification of precocious puberty.

Central (complete or true) GnRH-dependent isosexual precocious puberty
Constitutional
Idiopathic
Central nervous system disorders (including congenital defects)
Tumors
Infection
Trauma
Radiation
Following androgen exposure
Incomplete GnRH-independent isosexual precocious puberty
Males
Gonadotropin-secreting tumors
Excessive androgen production
Testicular or adrenal tumors
Virilizing congenital adrenal hyperplasia
Premature Leydig and germinal cell maturation
Females
Ovarian cysts
Estrogen-secreting neoplasms
Severe hypothyroidism
Males and females
McCune-Albright syndrome
Incomplete contrasexual precocity
Males
Estrogen-secreting tumor
Females
Androgen-secreting tumor
Virilizing congenital adrenal hyperplasia
Iatrogenic sexual precocity due to gonadotropin or sex Steroid exposure
Variation in pubertal development
Premature thelarche
Premature menarche
Premature pubarche
Adolescent gynecomastia

sex, the condition is not gonadotropin-dependent, and the diagnosis is **incomplete precocious puberty**. If feminization occurs in girls and virilization occurs in boys, the condition is **isosexual precocity**, but if the feminization occurs in boys and virilization in girls, the condition is **contrasexual precocity**. In all forms of sexual precocity, there is an increase in growth velocity, somatic development, and skeletal maturation. When unchecked, this rapid skeletal development may lead to tall stature during the early phases of the disorder but to short final stature because of early epiphysial fusion. This is the paradox of the tall child growing up to become a short adult. Plasma IGF-I values may be elevated for age but are appropriate for pubertal stage in untreated precocious puberty.

Central (Complete or True) Precocious Puberty (Figure 15–8)

A. Constitutional or familial central (complete or true) precocious puberty
Otherwise normal children who demonstrate isosexual precocity at an age slightly more than 2.5 SD below the mean may simply represent the lower reaches of the distribution

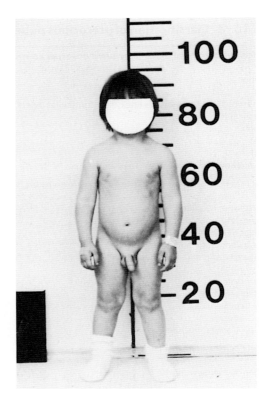

FIGURE 15–8 Boy 2-5/12 years of age with idiopathic true precocious puberty. By 10 months of age, he had pubic hair and phallic and testicular enlargement. At 1 year of age, his height was 4 SD above the mean; the phallus was 10 cm × 3.5 cm; each testis was 2.5 cm × 1.5 cm. Plasma LH was pubertal and rose in an adult pattern after administration of 100 μg of GnRH. Plasma testosterone was 416 ng/dL. At the time of the photograph, he had been treated with medroxyprogesterone acetate (to suppress LH and FSH secretion) for 1½ years, with reduction of his rapid growth rate and decreased gonadotropin and testosterone secretion. At that point his height was 95.2 cm (>2 SD above mean height for his age); plasma testosterone was 7 ng/dL, and after 100 μg of GnRH, plasma LH rose only slightly, demonstrating suppression. (Reproduced, with permission, from Styne DM, Grumbach MM. In: Yen SSC, Jaffe RB, eds. *Reproductive Endocrinology*. WB Saunders; 1978.)

curve describing the age of onset of puberty; often there is a familial tendency toward early puberty. True precocious puberty is reported, rarely, to be due to an autosomal dominant or (in males) X-linked dominant trait.

B. Idiopathic central (complete or true) isosexual precocious puberty Affected children, with no familial tendency toward early development and no organic disease, may be considered to have idiopathic central isosexual precocious puberty. Epilepsy and developmental delay are associated with central precocious puberty in the absence of a central nervous system anatomic abnormality, indicating a central nervous system process is responsible for the condition.

Pubertal development may follow the normal course or may wax and wane. Serum gonadotropin and sex steroid concentrations and response to GnRH or GnRH agonists are similar to those found in normal pubertal subjects. In idiopathic central precocious puberty, as in all forms of true isosexual precocity, testicular enlargement in boys should be the first sign; in girls, breast development or, rarely, pubic hair appearance may be first. Girls present with idiopathic central precocious puberty more commonly than boys. Children with precocious puberty have a tendency toward obesity based on elevated body mass index in the untreated state. While families with inactivating mutations of the *GRP54* gene experience absent or delayed puberty, a patient presented with isosexual precocious puberty and demonstrated a mutation of *GRP54* that led to prolonged activation of intracellular signaling pathways in response to kisspeptin. This further emphasizes the importance of the GRP54 Kisspepetin axis in the control of puberty.

C. Central nervous system disorders

1. **Tumors**—Central nervous system tumors are more common causes of central precocious puberty in boys than in girls but may occur in either, so a high index of suspicion is essential. Optic gliomas or hypothalamic gliomas, astrocytomas, ependymomas, germinomas, and other central nervous system tumors may cause precocious puberty by interfering with neural pathways that inhibit GnRH secretion, thus releasing the central nervous system restraint of gonadotropin secretion. Patients with optic gliomas and neurofibromatosis type 1 may have precocious puberty, but no patients with isolated neurofibromatosis (that did not have optic gliomas) are reported with precocious puberty. Remarkably, craniopharyngiomas, which are known to cause delayed puberty, can also trigger precocious pubertal development. Radiation therapy is often indicated in radiosensitive tumors such as germinomas and craniopharyngiomas, where complete surgical extirpation is impossible. Reportedly, complete removal of craniopharyngiomas is associated with unexpected recurrence; radiation therapy appears to be a key therapy for this tumor in addition to surgery.

   Hamartomas of the tuber cinereum contain GnRH and neurosecretory cells similar to those found in the median eminence; they may cause precocious puberty by secreting GnRH. Some hypothalamic hamartomas associated with central precocious puberty do not elaborate GnRH but instead contain transforming growth factor (TGF)-α, which stimulates GnRH secretion itself. With improved methods of imaging the central nervous system, hamartomas, with their characteristic radiographic appearance, are now more frequently diagnosed in patients who were previously thought to have idiopathic precocious puberty. These tumors do not enlarge and so pose no additional threat to the patients in the absence of intractable seizures. These seizures are rare in patients with the pedunculated hamartomas causing central precocious puberty. Because of the location of the hamartoma, surgery is a dangerous alternative to GnRH analog therapy.

   Tumors or other abnormalities of the central nervous system may cause GH deficiency in association with central precocious puberty. GH deficiency may also occur after irradiation therapy for such tumors, even if precocious puberty was the sole endocrine finding before irradiation. Such patients grow much faster than isolated GH-deficient patients but slower than children with classic precocious puberty and adequate GH secretion. Often, the GH deficiency is unmasked after successful treatment of precocious puberty. This combination must be considered during the diagnostic process (see also Chapter 6).

2. **Other causes of true precocious puberty**—Infectious or granulomatous conditions such as encephalitis, brain abscess, postinfectious (or postsurgical or congenital) suprasellar cysts, sarcoidosis, and tuberculous granulomas of the hypothalamus cause central precocious puberty. Suprasellar cysts and hydrocephalus cause central precocious puberty that is particularly amenable to surgical correction. Brain trauma may be followed by either precocious or delayed puberty. Radiation therapy for acute lymphoblastic leukemia of the central nervous system, or prior to bone marrow transplantation, is characteristically associated with hormonal deficiency, but there are increasing reports of precocious puberty occurring after such therapy. Higher doses of radiation may be more likely to cause GnRH deficiency, and lower doses down to 18 Gy may lead to central precocious puberty.

D. Virilizing syndromes Patients with long-untreated virilizing adrenal hyperplasia who have advanced bone ages may manifest precocious puberty after treatment with glucocorticoid suppression. Children with virilizing tumors or those given long-term androgen therapy may follow the same pattern when the androgen source is removed. Advanced maturation of the hypothalamic-pituitary-gonadal axis appears to occur with any condition causing excessive androgen secretion and advanced skeletal age.

Incomplete Isosexual Precocious Puberty in Boys

Males may manifest premature sexual development in the absence of hypothalamic-pituitary maturation from either of two causes: (1) ectopic or autonomous endogenous secretion of hCG or LH or iatrogenic administration of hCG, which can stimulate Leydig cell production of testosterone; or (2) autonomous endogenous secretion of androgens from the testes or adrenal glands or from iatrogenic exogenous administration of androgens. (In females, secretion of hCG does not by itself cause secondary sexual development.)

A. Gonadotropin-secreting tumors These include hepatomas or hepatoblastomas of the liver as well as teratomas or choriocarcinoma of the mediastinum, gonads, retroperitoneum, or pineal gland and germinomas of the central nervous system. The testes are definitely enlarged but not to the degree found in central precocious puberty since only Leydig cells are stimulated by hCG.

B. Autonomous androgen secretion Secretion of androgens can occur because of inborn errors of adrenal enzyme function, as in 21-hydroxylase deficiency (P450c21 OMIM#201910 adrenal hyperplasia, congenital, caused by 21-hydroxylase) or 11β-hydroxylase deficiency (P450c11β OMIM#202010). Adrenal hyperplasia, congenital, caused by steroid 11-beta-hydroxylase deficiency), virilizing adrenal carcinomas, interstitial cell tumors of the testes, or premature Leydig and germinal cell maturation. Late-onset congenital adrenal hyperplasia, generally of the 21-hydroxylase

deficiency form, may occur years after birth with no congenital or neonatal manifestations of virilization. Adrenal rest tissue may be found in the testes as a vestige of the common embryonic origin of the adrenal glands and the testes; in states of ACTH excess—primarily congenital adrenal hyperplasia—adrenal rests can enlarge (sometimes to remarkable size) and secrete adrenal androgens (see Chapter 14).

In boys with familial gonadotropin-independent premature Leydig and germinal cell maturation (#176410. precocious puberty, male-limited), plasma testosterone levels are in the pubertal range, but plasma gonadotropin levels and the LH response to exogenous GnRH are in the prepubertal range or lower because autonomous testosterone secretion suppresses endogenous GnRH release. The cause of this sex-limited dominant condition lies in a constitutive activation of the LH receptor (leaving the LH receptor *on*), causing increased cyclic adenosine monophosphate (cAMP) production in the absence of LH. Several mutations have been reported in the LH receptor gene in different families (eg, Asp^{578} to Gly or Met^{571} to Ile). The differential diagnosis rests between testosterone-secreting tumor of the adrenal, testosterone-secreting Leydig cell neoplasm, and premature Leydig and germinal cell maturation.

If hCG secretion causes incomplete male isosexual precocity, FSH is not elevated. As only the Leydig cells are stimulated and because the seminiferous tubules are not stimulated, the testes do not enlarge as much as in complete sexual precocity. If incomplete sexual precocity is due to a testicular tumor, the testes may be large, asymmetric, and irregular in contour. Symmetric bilateral moderate enlargement of the testes suggests familial gonadotropin-independent premature maturation of Leydig and germinal cells, which is a sex-limited dominant condition. The testes are somewhat smaller in this condition than in true precocious puberty but are still over 2.5 cm in diameter.

Incomplete Contrasexual Precocity in Boys

Estrogen may be secreted by rare adrenal tumors leading to feminization in boys. Sertoli cell tumors associated with Peutz-Jeghers syndrome is another possible etiology.

Incomplete Isosexual Precocious Puberty in Girls

Females with incomplete isosexual precocity have a source of excessive estrogens. In all cases of autonomous endogenous estrogen secretion or exogenous estrogen administration, serum LH and FSH levels are low.

A. Follicular cysts If follicular cysts are large enough, they can secrete sufficient estrogen to cause breast development and even vaginal withdrawal bleeding; some girls have recurrent cysts that lead to several episodes of vaginal bleeding. Patients with cysts may have levels of serum estrogen high enough to mimic a tumor. Larger follicular cysts can twist on their pedicles and become infarcted, causing symptoms of acute abdomen in addition to the precocious estrogen effects.

B. Other ovarian tumors　Granulosa or theca cell tumors of the ovaries secrete estrogen and are palpable in 80% of cases. Gonadoblastomas are found in streak gonads, lipoid tumors, and cystadenomas. Ovarian carcinomas are rare ovarian sources of estrogens or androgens.

C. Adrenal rest tissue　Adrenal rest tissue has long been known to cause testicular enlargement and androgen secretion in boys, particularly with the increased ACTH secretion of untreated or incompletely congenital adrenal hyperplasia. While the hyperplastic tissue is not a neoplasm by itself, neoplastic transformation may follow.

D. Exogenous estrogen administration　Ingestion of estrogen-containing substances or even cutaneous absorption of estrogen can cause feminization in children. Epidemics of gynecomastia and precocious thelarche in Puerto Rico and Italy have variously been attributed to ingestion of estrogen-contaminated food, estrogens in the environment, soy formula, or undetermined causes. One outbreak of gynecomastia in boys and precocious thelarche in girls in Bahrain was traced to ingestion of milk from a cow which was given continuous estrogen treatment by its owner to ensure uninterrupted milk production. Tea tree and lavender oils have estrogenic effects in children and exposure can cause thelarche.

E. Hypothyroidism　Severe untreated hypothyroidism can be associated with sexual precocity and galactorrhea (Van Wyk-Grumbach syndrome); treatment with thyroxine corrects hypothyroidism, halts precocious puberty and galactorrhea, and lowers PRL levels. The cause of this syndrome was initially postulated to be increased gonadotropin secretion associated with the massive increase in TSH secretion. However, it appears that TSH, at high concentrations, can activate FSH receptors.

F. McCune-Albright syndrome　McCune-Albright syndrome (#174800. McCune-Albright syndrome; MAS) is classically manifested as a triad of irregular café au lait spots, fibrous dysplasia of long bones with cysts, and precocious puberty. However, hyperthyroidism, adrenal nodules with Cushing syndrome, acromegaly, hyperprolactinemia, hyperparathyroidism, hypophosphatemic hyperphosphaturic rickets, or autonomous endogenous-functioning ovarian cysts (in girls) also occur. Precocious puberty may be central or incomplete; longitudinal studies demonstrate that some patients start with incomplete precocious puberty and progress to central precocious puberty. Long-term follow-up of patients with McCune-Albright syndrome reveals a high incidence of pathologic fractures and orthopedic deformities due to the bone cysts, as well as hearing impairment due to the thickening of the temporal area of the skull. Thickening of the skull base can impinge on local brain structures with fatal consequences. Bone growth may be partly mediated by elevated GH secretion and may cease with somatostatin analogue therapy. Patients may have a mutation of Arg_{201} in exon 8 of the gene encoding the Gs alpha subunit that stimulates cAMP formation; this mutation impairs GTPase activity of the alpha subunit and increases adenylate cyclase activity leading to the endocrine abnormalities described earlier. This defect originates in somatic rather than germ cells, leading to genetic mosaicism wherever the defective gene product is expressed; thus, a wide variety of tissues can be affected.

Incomplete Contrasexual Precocity in Girls

Excess androgen effect can be caused by premature adrenarche or more significant pathologic conditions such as congenital or nonclassic adrenal hyperplasia or adrenal or ovarian tumors. P450c21 adrenal hyperplasia can be diagnosed on the basis of elevated serum 17-hydroxyprogesterone concentrations in the basal or ACTH-stimulated state (other adrenal metabolites may be elevated depending on the defect under investigation) (see Chapter 14). Both adrenal and ovarian tumors are associated with elevation of serum testosterone; adrenal tumors secrete DHEA. Thus, the source of the tumor may be difficult to differentiate if it produces only testosterone. MRI or CT scanning may be inadequate to diagnose the tumor's organ of origin, and selective venous sampling may be needed. The rare families reported with aromatase deficiency had contrasexual development although not precocious puberty per se. One affected 46,XX individual had virilized genitalia at birth and further virilization at a pubertal age with the additional feature of polycystic ovaries. The patient, in spite of high serum testosterone concentrations, had elevated FSH and LH in the absence of estrogen production.

Variations in Pubertal Development

A. Premature thelarche　The term **premature thelarche** denotes unilateral or bilateral breast enlargement without other signs of androgen or estrogen secretion. Patients are usually younger than 3 years of age; the breast enlargement may regress within months or remain until actual pubertal development occurs at a normal age. Areolar development and vaginal mucosal signs of estrogen effect are usually absent or minimal. Premature thelarche may be caused by brief episodes of estrogen secretion from ovarian cysts. Plasma estrogen levels are usually low in this disorder, perhaps because blood samples are characteristically drawn after the initiating secretory event. However, ultrasensitive estradiol assays show a difference in estrogen production between control girls and those with premature thelarche. Classically, premature thelarche is self-limited and does not lead to central precocious puberty. However, there are reports of progression to central precocious puberty in a minority of cases, and follow-up for such progression is indicated. Other abnormalities in ovulation and menstruation have been reported following premature thelarche. Recently, girls with fluctuating thelarche were reported as having mutations in the *GNAS1* gene, though without other signs of McCune-Albright syndrome.

B. Premature menarche　In rare cases, girls may begin to menstruate at an early age without showing other signs of estrogen effect. An unproved theory suggests that they may be manifesting increased uterine sensitivity to estrogen. In most subjects, menses stop within 1 to 6 years, and normal pubertal progression occurs thereafter.

C. Premature Adrenarche   The term **premature adrenarche** denotes the early appearance of pubic or axillary hair without other signs of virilization or puberty. This nonprogressive disorder is compatible with then the occurrence of other signs of puberty at the normal age for puberty. Prematue adrenarche is more common in girls than in boys, and premature adrenarche is usually found in children over 6 years of age. Sometimes premature adrenarche can overlap with the new age limits of puberty in girls. Plasma and urinary DHEAS levels are elevated to stage 2 pubertal levels, higher than normally found in this age group but well below those seen with. Bone and height ages may be slightly advanced for chronologic age. Patients may have abnormal electroencephalographic tracings without other signs of neurologic dysfunction.

The presenting symptoms of late-onset adrenal hyperplasia may be similar to those of premature adrenarche, and the differential diagnosis may require ACTH stimulation testing (see Chapter 14). This condition may also present in a manner similar to polycystic ovarian syndrome (see Chapter 13). Infants born small for gestational age (SGA) have a predilection to develop premature adrenarche. These girls may also progress to polycystic ovarian syndrome. Daughters of women with PCOS demonstrate elevated androgen concentrations before the age of puberty, and these daughters may progress themselves to develop PCOS.

D. Adolescent gynecomastia   Up to 75% of boys have transient unilateral or bilateral gynecomastia, usually beginning in stage 2 or 3 of puberty and regressing about 2 years later. Serum estrogen and testosterone concentrations are normal, but the estradiol-testosterone ratio may be elevated and SHBG concentrations may be high. Reassurance is usually all that is required, but some severely affected patients with extremely prominent breast development require reduction mammoplasty if psychologic distress is extreme. After 2 years of gynecomastia, the likelihood of spontaneous regression decreases due to the formation of scar tissue. Early studies of aromatase inhibitors in the medical treatment of gynecomastia were disappointing, but more recent evaluation of anastrazole demonstrate promise.

Some pathologic conditions such as Klinefelter and the syndromes of incomplete androgen resistance are also associated with gynecomastia; these disorders should be clearly differentiated from the gynecomastia of normal puberty in males.

Differential Diagnosis of Precocious Puberty

The history and physical examination should be directed toward one of the diagnostic possibilities discussed earlier. Serum gonadotropin and sex steroid concentrations are determined in order to distinguish gonadotropin-mediated secondary sexual development (serum gonadotropin and sex steroid levels elevated to pubertal levels) from autonomous endogenous secretion or exogenous administration of gonadal steroids (serum gonadotropin levels suppressed and sex steroid levels elevated). Gonadotropins must be measured in a third generation assay with pediatric standards as the customary gonadotropin determinations are too insensitive to reveal the small changes of puberty.

Measurement of testosterone or estradiol must be done in an ultrasensitive assay with pediatric standards or, as with gonadotropin assays, the small changes of pubertal development will be missed. Presently highly sensitive high performance liquid chromatography tandem mass spectroscopy (HPLC MS/MS) assays are available at national laboratories for this purpose. Third-generation ultrasensitive immunoassays can identify the onset of increased gonadotropin secretion with a single basal unstimulated serum sample. In the past, a GnRH test was required to confirm an increase in LH secretion at puberty because of the overlap of pubertal and prepubertal values of LH in the basal state. These third-generation gonadotropin assays can be applied to urine as well as serum samples; this may someday eliminate the need for GnRH agonist testing or serial serum sampling.

If serum LH concentrations, measured in an assay that cross-reacts with hCG, are quite high in a boy or if a pregnancy screening test (β-hCG) is positive, the likely diagnosis is an extra-pituitary, hCG-secreting tumor. β-LH values are suppressed, so no confusion with hCG levels is possible. If no abdominal or thoracic source of hCG is found, MRI of the brain with particular attention to the hypothalamic-pituitary area is indicated to evaluate the possibility of a germinoma of the pineal gland.

If serum sex steroid levels are very high and gonadotropin levels are low in third-generation assays, an autonomous source of gonadal steroid secretion must be assumed. If plasma gonadotropin and sex steroid levels are in the pubertal range, the most likely diagnosis is complete precocious puberty (Table 15–5).

Differentiation between premature thelarche and central precocious puberty is usually accomplished by physical examination, but determination of serum estradiol or gonadotropins may be required. The evaluation of uterine size by ultrasound may also be useful, because premature thelarche causes no increase in uterine volume while central precocious puberty does and also is associated with an "endometrial stripe." Ovarian size determination is a less useful method of distinguishing between the two possibilities but may reveal pubertal ovarian cysts. As noted earlier, some girls initially thought to have precocious thelarche progress to complete precocious puberty, but there is no way presently to distinguish girls who will progress from those who will not.

The onset of true or complete precocious puberty may indicate the presence of a hypothalamic tumor. Boys more often than girls have central nervous system tumors associated with complete precocious puberty. Skull x-rays are not usually helpful, but CT or MRI scanning is indicated in children with true precocious puberty. The present generation of CT and MRI scanners can make thin cuts through the hypothalamic-pituitary area with good resolution; small hypothalamic hamartomas are now being diagnosed more frequently. Generally, MRI is preferable to CT because of better resolution; the use of contrast may help evaluate possible central nervous system lesions.

Treatment of Precocious Puberty

A. Central precocious puberty   In the past, medical treatment of true precocious puberty involved medroxyprogesterone

TABLE 15–5 Differential diagnosis of precocious puberty.

	Serum Gonadotropin Concentrations	LR Response to GnRH or GnRH Agonist	Serum Sex Steroid Concentrations	Gonadal Size	Miscellaneous
Central (complete or true) precocious puberty	Pubertal	Pubertal pattern	Pubertal values	Normal pubertal enlargement of gonads in males	MRI scan of head to rule out a central nervous system tumor, hamartoma, or other central nervous system lesion
Incomplete precocious puberty _Males_ Chorionic gonadotropin secreting tumor	High hCG (or LH in cross-reactive assay), positive pregnancy test, but β-LH (specific assay) is low	High basal hCG or LH that does not rise with GnRH, but β-LH is low and does not rise	High or pubertal values	Slight to moderate enlargement of gonads	Hepatic tumor must be considered. MRI scan of head if hCG-secreting central nervous system tumor suspected. If the LH assay measures hCG, both results may be high while β-hCG is high and β-LH, in an assay which does not detect hCG, is low
Leydig cell tumor	Prepubertal (low)	Prepubertal or suppressed pattern	Extremely high testosterone	Irregular asymmetric enlargement of testes	
Familial gonadotropin-indepen-dent sexual precocity with premature Leydig and germ cell maturation	Prepubertal (low)	Prepubertal or suppressed pattern	Pubertal or higher values	Testes longer than 2.5 cm but smaller than expected for stage of pubertal development	Found in sex-limited dominant patterns
Females Granulosa cell tumor (follicular cysts may have similar presentation)	Prepubertal (low)	Prepubertal or suppressed pattern	Extremely high estradiol	Ovarian enlargement on physical, CT, MRI, or sonographic examination	Granulosa cell tumor is usually palpable on rectal examination
Follicular cyst	Prepubertal (low)	Prepubertal or suppressed pattern of LH secretion. FSH secretion may rise above normal range	High to extremely high estradiol	Cysts may be visible on sonogram	Withdrawal bleeding may occur when estrogen levels decrease. Cysts may recur

acetate or cyproterone acetate—progestational agents that reduce gonadotropin secretion by negative feedback.

However, current treatment for precocious puberty due to a central nervous system lesion involves the use of GnRH agonists that suppress sexual maturation and decrease growth rate and skeletal maturation. Chronic administration of highly potent and long-acting analogs of GnRH has been shown to downregulate GnRH receptors and reduce pituitary gland response to GnRH, thereby causing decreased secretion of gonadotropin and sex steroids and rapidly stopping the progression of sexual precocity. In girls, pubertal enlargement of the ovaries and uterus reverts toward the prepubertal state, and the multicystic appearance of the pubertal ovary regresses as well. This suppressive effect is reversed after

therapy is discontinued and puberty progresses. GnRH agonist treatment has been successful for idiopathic precocious puberty and precocious puberty caused by hamartomas of the tuber cinereum, neoplasms of the central nervous system, or long-term androgen exposure. The GnRH agonists were originally given by daily subcutaneous injection or intranasal insufflation. Injection of these agents every 4 weeks in depot preparations has now made treatment much easier and has improved compliance.

Complete suppression of gonadotropin secretion is necessary because an incompletely suppressed patient may appear to have arrested pubertal development while actually secreting low but significant levels of sex steroids. Under these conditions, bone age advances while the growth rate is decreased, leading to even shorter adult stature. Side effects of these agonists have generally been limited to allergic skin reactions and elevation of immunoglobulins directed against GnRH. Significant anaphylactic reactions to an injection have rarely been reported. Decrease in bone mineral density is a potential side effect of GnRH agonists; increased dietary calcium and recommended vitamin D intake supplementation is wise especially in the era of frequent deficiencies of these in all children. The FDA has approved histrelin, a GnRH agonist administered on a daily basis, and leuprolide acetate, a long-acting GnRH agonist, administered every 28 days, for the management of precocious puberty. A daily dose form of leuprolide is also approved for precocious puberty but a 3-month preparation is presently only approved for adults. Individual monitoring is essential to ascertain gonadotropin suppression. A new implantable depot preparation of GnRH agonist may be left in for 1 year without the requirement for frequent monitoring.

Growth velocity decreases within 5 months after the start of therapy, and rapid bone age advancement decreases to a rate below the increase in chronologic age. Without therapy, height in patients with central precocious puberty approaches 152 cm in girls and 155 to 164 cm in boys. The first patients treated with GnRH agonists have now reached adult height: the girls have a mean height of 157 cm and the boys a mean height of 164 cm—a definite improvement over the untreated state. The worst height prognosis is found in children with an early diagnosis of precocious puberty who are not treated. The best outcomes of therapy are noted when diagnosis and therapy are achieved early, and as earlier diagnosis is now made in children with central precocious puberty and earlier therapy is offered, better results are expected in the future. Menarche and even pregnancy are reported after the discontinuation of therapy in girls, indicating a reversion to normal pubertal endocrine function following GnRH agonist treatment. The new lower age limits of normal pubertal development in girls have led clinicians to reassess the criteria used to identify appropriate candidates for therapy. Patients without significant elevation of serum estrogen, who have a predicted height appropriate for family, and who have slowly progressing variants without early menarche will likely achieve an appropriate adult height without therapy. Psychologic support is important for patients with sexual precocity. The somatic changes or menses frighten some children and may make them the object of ridicule. These patients do not experience social maturation to match their physical development, although their peers, teachers, and relatives tend to treat them as if they were older because of their large size. Thus, supportive counseling must be offered to both patient and family. Children with precocious puberty are more often sexually abused, so appropriate precautions are necessary.

B. Incomplete precocious puberty Treatment of the disorders discussed earlier under incomplete precocious puberty is directed toward the underlying tumor or abnormality rather than toward the signs of precocious puberty. If the primary cause is controlled, signs of sexual development are halted in progression or may even regress.

Males with familial Leydig and germ cell maturation do not initially respond to GnRH agonist therapy, but some have improved with medroxyprogesterone acetate. Affected boys were successfully treated with ketoconazole, an antifungal agent that can block 17,20-lyase and therefore decrease testosterone production. Ketoconazole also suppresses adrenal function as a significant side effect. After initial control with ketoconazole, the boys developed central precocious puberty, because prolonged exposure to androgens led to maturation of their hypothalamic-pituitary axis; treatment with a GnRH agonist then effectively halted this pubertal progression.

Newer therapy for McCune-Albright syndrome in girls is a combination of testolactone (an aromatase inhibitor) and spironolactone (which acts as an antiandrogen). Long-term follow-up demonstrated some decrease in menses, improvement in growth patterns and bone age advancement. Some escaped from control, necessitating the addition of a GnRH agonist, which then suppressed pubertal development. Tamoxifen, an estrogen agonist and antagonist, combined with aromatase inhibitors (such as anastrazole or newer agents such as letrazole) has been successfully used to decrease uterine bleeding and advancement in bone age in clinical trials. Girls with recurrent estrogen-secreting ovarian cyst formation may have a decreased incidence of cysts with medroxyprogesterone acetate therapy. A GnRH agonist may also be effective in such cases. Surgical removal of ovarian cysts may be unnecessary if such medical therapy is first utilized.

Precocious thelarche or adrenarche requires no treatment, as both are self-limited benign conditions. No therapy has been reported for premature menarche. Severe, persistent cases of adolescent gynecomastia have been reportedly treated successfully by testolactone and dihydrotestosterone heptanoate, although surgical removal of breast tissue is often necessary, as noted earlier.

REFERENCES

General

Greulich WW, Pyle SI. *Radiographic Atlas of Skeletal Development of the Hand and Wrist.* 2nd ed. Stanford. CA: Stanford University Press; 1959.

Grumbach MM, Auchus RJ. Estrogen: consequences and implications of human mutations in synthesis and action. *J Clin Endocrinol Metab.* 1999;84:4677. [PMID: 10599737]

Herman-Giddens ME, Slora EJ, Wasserman RC, et al. Secondary sexual characteristics and menses in young girls seen in office practice: a study from the Pediatric Research in Office Settings network. *Pediatrics.* 1997;99:505. [PMID: 9093289]

Himes JH, Park K, Styne D. Menarche and assessment of body mass index in adolescent girls. *J Pediatr.* 2009;155:393. [PMID: 199559445]

Kaiser UB, Kuohung W. KiSS-1 and GPR54 as new players in gonadotropin regulation and puberty. *Endocrine.* 2005;26:277. [PMID:12944565]

Rosenfeld RL, Lipton RB, Drum ML. Thelarche, pubarche, and menarche attainment in children with normal and elevated body mass index. *Pediatrics.* 2009;123;84. [PMID: 19117864]

Seminara SB, Messager S, Chatzidaki EE, et al. The GPR54 gene as a regulator of puberty. *N Engl J Med.* 2003;349:1614. [PMID:14573733]

Shahab M, Mastronardi C, Seminara SB, Crowley WF, Ojeda SR, Plant TM. Increased hypothalamic GPR54 signaling: a potential mechanism for initiation of puberty in primates. *Proc Natl Acad Sci USA.* 2005;102:2129. [PMID:15684075]

Smith EP, Boyd J, Frank GR, et al. Estrogen resistance caused by a mutation in the estrogen-receptor gene in a man. *N Engl J Med.* 1994;331:1056. [PMID: 8090165]

Styne DM, Cuttler L. Normal pubertal development. In: Rudolph C, Rudolph A, eds. *Rudolphs Textbook of Pediatrics.* 2008.

Styne DM. Puberty, obesity and ethnicity. *Trends Endocrinol Metab.* 2004;15:472. [PMID: 15541646]

Styne DM, Grumbach MM. Puberty, ontogeny, neuroendocrinology, physiology, and disorders. In: Larsen PR, et al, eds. *Williams Textbook of Endocrinology.* 11th ed. Philadelphia, PA: WB Saunders; 2002.

Physical Changes Associated with Puberty

Bayley N, Pinneau SF. Tables for predicting adult height from skeletal age: revised for use with the Greulich-Pyle standards. *J Pediatr.* 1952;40:423. [PMID: 14918032]

Marshall WA, Tanner JM. Variations in the pattern of pubertal changes in girls. *Arch Dis Child.* 1969;44:291. [PMID: 5785179]

Marshall WA, Tanner JM. Variations in the pattern of pubertal changes in boys. *Arch Dis Child.* 1970;45:13. [PMID: 5440182]

Van Wieringen JC, et al. *Growth Diagrams 1965 Netherlands: Second National Survey on 0–24 Year Olds.* Groningen, Netherlands: Institute for Preventive Medicine NO Leiden, Wolters-Noordhoff Publishing; 1971.

Delayed Puberty and Sexual Infantilism

Barrio R, de Luis D, Alonso M, Lamas A, Moreno JC. Induction of puberty with human chorionic gonadotropin and follicle-stimulating hormone in adolescent males with hypogonadotropic hypogonadism. *Fertil Steril.* 1999;71:244. [PMID: 9988392]

Davenport ML. Approach to the patient with Turner syndrome. *J Clin Endocrinol Metab.* 2010;95:1487. [PMID: 20375216]

Grumbach MM, Conte FA. Disorders of sexual differentiation. In: Larsen PR, et al, eds. *Williams Textbook of Endocrinology.* 10th ed. Philadelphia, PA: WB Saunders; 2002.

Johansson T, Ritzen EM. Very long-term follow-up of girls with early and late menarche. *Endocr Dev.* 2005;8:126. [PMID: 15722621]

Massa G, Heinrichs C, Verlinde S, et al. Late or delayed induced or spontaneous puberty in girls with Turner syndrome treated with growth hormone does not affect final height. *J Clin Endocrinol Metab.* 2003;88:4168. [PMID: 12970282]

Nabhan ZM, Dimeglio LA, Qi R, Perkins SM, Eugster EA. Conjugated oral versus transdermal estrogen replacement in girls with Turner syndrome: a pilot comparative study. *J Clin Endocrinol Metab.* 2009;94:2009. [PMID: 19318455]

Sedlmeyer IL, Palmert MR. Delayed puberty: analysis of a large case series from an academic center. *J Clin Endocrinol Metab.* 2002;87:1613. [PMID: 11932291]

Seminara SB, Hayes FJ, Crowley WFJ. Gonadotropin-releasing hormone deficiency in the human (idiopathic hypogonadotropic hypogonadism and Kallmann's syndrome): pathophysiological and genetic considerations. *Endocr Rev.* 1999;19:521. [PMID: 9793755]

Sexual Precocity

Bar A, 7776106. Bayley-Pinneau method of height prediction in girls with central precocious puberty: correlation with adult height. *J Pediatr.* 1995;126:955. [PMID: 7776106]

Carel JC, Eugster EA, Rogol A. Consensus statement on the use of gonadotropin-releasing hormone analogs in children. *Pediatrics.* 2009;123:e752. [PMID: 19332438]

Eugster EA, Rubin SD, Reiter EO, et al. Tamoxifen treatment for precocious puberty in McCune-Albright syndrome: a multicenter trial. *J Pediatr.* 2003;143:60. [PMID: 12915825]

Fahmy JL, Kaminsky CK, Kaufman F, Nelson MD Jr, Parisi MT. The radiological approach to precocious puberty. *Br J Radiol.* 2000;73:560. [PMID: 10884758]

Ibáñez L, Dimartino-Nardi J, Potau N, Saenger P. Premature adrenarche—normal variant or forerunner of adult disease? *Endocr Rev.* 2000;21:671. [PMID: 11133068]

Klein KO, Barnes KM, Jones JV, Feuillan PP, Cutler GB Jr. Increased final height in precocious puberty after long-term treatment with LHRH agonists: the National Institutes of Health experience. *J Clin Endocrinol Metab.* 2001;86:4711. [PMID: 11600530]

Leschek EW, Jones J, Barnes KM, Hill SC, Cutler GB Jr. Six-year results of spironolactone and testolactone treatment of familial male-limited precocious puberty with addition of deslorelin after central puberty onset. *J Clin Endocrinol Metab.* 1999;84:175. [PMID: 9920079]

Mul D, Bertelloni S, Carel JC, Saggese G, Chaussain JL, Oostdijk W. Effect of gonadotropin-releasing hormone agonist treatment in boys with central precocious puberty: final height results. *Horm Res.* 2002;58:1. [PMID: 12169774]

Palmert MR, Malin HV, Boepple PA. Unsustained or slowly progressive puberty in young girls: initial presentation and long-term follow-up of 20 untreated patients. *J Clin Endocrinol Metab.* 1999;84:415. [PMID: 10022394]

Reiter EO, Lindberg A, Ranke MB, et al. The KIGS experience with the addition of gonadotropin-releasing hormone agonists to growth hormone (GH) treatment of children with idiopathic GH deficiency. *Horm Res.* 2003;60(suppl 1):68. [PMID: 12955021]

Salardi S, Cacciari E, Mainetti B, Mazzanti L, Pirazzoli P. Outcome of premature thelarche: relation to puberty and final height. *Arch Dis Child.* 1998;79:173. [PMID: 9797603]

Tanaka T, Niimi H, Matsuo N, et al. Results of long-term follow-up after treatment of central precocious puberty with leuprorelin acetate: evaluation of effectiveness of treatment and recovery of gonadal function. The TAP-144-SR Japanese Study Group on Central Precocious Puberty. *J Clin Endocrinol Metab.* 2005;90:1371. [PMID: 15598675]

Teilmann G, Petersen JH, Gormsen M, Damgaard K, Skakkebaek NE, Jensen TK. Early puberty in internationally adopted girls: hormonal and clinical markers of puberty in 276 girls examined biannually over two years. *Horm Res.* 2009;72(4):236-246.

Volta C, Bernasconi S, Cisternino M, et al. Isolated premature thelarche and thelarche variant: clinical and auxological follow-up of 119 girls. *J Endocrinol Invest.* 1998;21:180. [PMID: 9591214]

Weise M, Flor A, Barnes KM, Cutler GB Jr, Baron J. Determinants of growth during gonadotropin-releasing hormone analog therapy for precocious puberty. *J Clin Endocrinol Metab.* 2004;89:103. [PMID: 14715835]

16

The Endocrinology of Pregnancy

Robert N. Taylor, MD, PhD and Martina L. Badell, MD

ACTH	Adrenocorticotropin hormone	**HELLP syndrome**	Hemolysis, elevated liver enzymes, and low platelets
AFP	Alph-afetoprotein	**hPL**	Human placental lactogen
AMH	Anti-Müllerian hormone	**IGF**	Insulin-like growth factor
BMI	Body mass index	**LH**	Luteinizing hormone
BV	Bacterial vaginosis	**NSAID**	Nonsteroidal anti-inflammatory drug
CRH	Corticotropin-releasing hormone	**PDGF**	Platelet-derived growth factor
DHEA	Dehydroepiandrosterone	**PIGF**	Placental growth factor
EGF	Epidermal growth factor	**PRL**	Prolactin
fFN	Fetal fibronectin	**PROM**	Premature rupture of membranes
FGF	Fibroblast growth factor	**PTB**	Preterm birth
GDM	Gestational diabetes mellitus	**sEng**	Soluble endoglin
GH	Growth hormone	**sFlt-1**	Soluble fms-like tyrosine kinase 1
GnRH	Gonadotropin-releasing hormone	**SHBG**	Sex hormone–binding globulin
GTN	Gestational trophoblastic neoplasia	**TRH**	Thyrotropin-releasing hormone
		TSH	Thyroid-stimulating hormone
hCG	human chorionic gonadotropin	**VEGF**	Vascular endothelial growth factor

Throughout pregnancy, the fetal-placental unit secretes protein and steroid hormones that alter the function of every endocrine gland in the mother's body. Both clinically and in the laboratory, pregnancy can mimic hyperthyroidism, Cushing disease, pituitary adenoma, diabetes mellitus, polycystic ovary syndrome, and more.

The endocrine changes associated with pregnancy are adaptive, allowing the mother to nurture the developing fetus. Although maternal reserves are usually adequate, in cases of gestational diabetes or hypertensive disease of pregnancy, a woman may develop overt signs of disease as a direct result of pregnancy.

Aside from creating a satisfactory nutritive environment for fetal development, the placenta serves as an endocrine, respiratory, alimentary, and excretory organ. Measurements of fetal-placental products in the maternal serum provide one means of assessing fetal well being. This chapter will consider the changes in maternal endocrine function in pregnancy and during parturition as well as fetal endocrine development. The chapter concludes with a discussion of some endocrine disorders complicating pregnancy.

CONCEPTION AND IMPLANTATION

Fertilization

In fertile women, ovulation occurs approximately 12 to 16 days after the onset of the previous menses. The ovum must be fertilized within 24 to 48 hours if conception is to result. For about 48 hours around ovulation, cervical mucus is copious, nonviscous, slightly alkaline, and forms a gel matrix that acts as a filter and conduit for sperm. Sperm begin appearing in the outer third of the fallopian tube (the ampulla) 5 to 10 minutes after coitus and continue to migrate to this location from the cervix for about 24 to 48 hours. Of the 200×10^6 sperm that are deposited in the vaginal fornices, only approximately 200 reach the distal tube. Fertilization normally occurs in the ampulla.

Implantation and hCG Production

Embryonic invasion of the uterus occurs during a specific window of implantation 8 to 10 days after ovulation and fertilization, when the conceptus is a blastocyst. Vitronectin, an alpha-v-beta-3 integrin receptor ligand, serves as one of several links between the maternal and embryonic epithelia. The two layers of placental epithelial cells, cytotrophoblasts and syncytiotrophoblasts, develop after the blastocyst invades the endometrium (Figure 16–1). Columns of invading cytotrophoblasts anchor the placenta to the endometrium. The differentiated syncytiotrophoblast, derived from fusion of cytotrophoblasts, is in direct contact with the maternal circulation. The syncytiotrophoblast is the

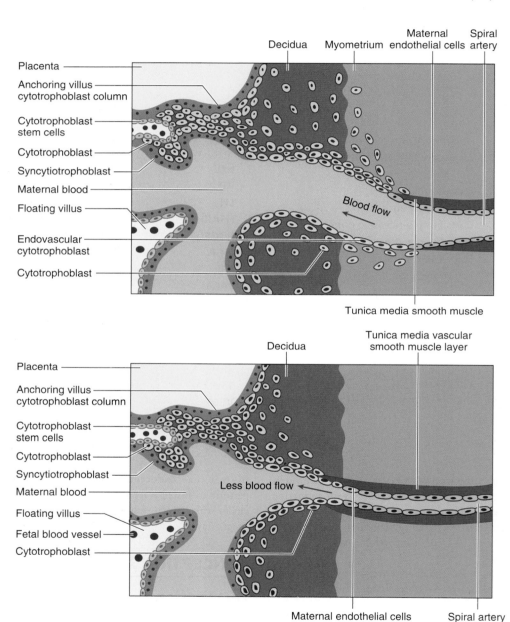

FIGURE 16–1 Microanatomy of the human placental bed. Oxygen, nutrients, and waste products are exchanged between the fetus and the mother across this interface. In normal placental development (upper panel), invasive cytotrophoblasts of fetal origin invade the maternal spiral arteries, displacing maternal endothelial cells and transforming the vessels from small-caliber resistance vessels to high-caliber capacitance vessels capable of placental perfusion adequate to sustain fetal growth. In preeclampsia and some cases of fetal growth restriction, cytotrophoblasts fail to adopt an invasive endothelial phenotype. Instead, invasion of the spiral arteries is shallow and they remain small-caliber resistance vessels (lower panel). This can lead to placental ischemia. (Adapted, with permission, from Karumanchi SA, et al. Preeclampsia: a renal perspective. *Kidney Int.* 2005;67:2101.)

major source of hormone production, containing the cellular machinery needed for synthesis and secretion of both steroid and polypeptide hormones.

In most spontaneously conceived pregnancies, the dates of ovulation and implantation are not known. Weeks of gestation (*gestational age*) are by convention calculated from the first day of the last menstrual period. Within 24 hours after implantation, or at about 3 weeks of gestation, human chorionic gonadotropin (hCG), produced by syncytiotrophoblasts (see Figure 16–1), is detectable in maternal serum. Under the influence of increasing hCG production, the corpus luteum secretes progesterone and estradiol in increasing quantities.

Ovarian Hormones of Pregnancy

The hormones produced by the corpus luteum include progesterone, 17-hydroxyprogesterone, relaxin, and estradiol. The indispensability of the corpus luteum in early pregnancy has been demonstrated by ablation studies, in which luteectomy or oophorectomy before 42 days of gestation results in precipitous decreases in levels of serum progesterone and estradiol, followed by abortion. Exogenous progesterone will prevent abortion, proving that progesterone alone is required for maintenance of early pregnancy. After about the seventh gestational week, the corpus luteum can be removed without subsequent abortion owing to compensatory progesterone production by the placenta.

Because the placenta does not express the 17α-hydroxylase enzyme (P450C17), it cannot produce appreciable amounts of 17-hydroxyprogesterone; thus, this steroid provides a marker of corpus luteum function. As shown in Figure 16–2, the serum concentrations of estrogens and total progesterone exhibit a steady increase, but the concentration of 17-hydroxyprogesterone rises and then declines to low levels that persist for the duration of the pregnancy. Another marker of corpus luteum function is the polypeptide hormone relaxin, a protein with a molecular mass of about 6000. Pharmacologically, relaxin ripens the cervix, softens the pubic symphysis, promotes decidual angiogenesis, and acts synergistically with progesterone to inhibit uterine contractions.

Symptoms and Signs of Pregnancy

Breast tenderness, fatigue, nausea, absence of menstruation, softening of the uterus, and a sustained elevation of basal body temperature are mostly attributable to hormone production by the corpus luteum and developing placenta.

FETAL-PLACENTAL-DECIDUAL UNIT

The function of the placenta is to establish effective communication between the mother and the developing fetus while maintaining the immune and genetic integrity of both individuals. Initially, the placenta functions autonomously. By the end of the first trimester, however, the fetal endocrine system is sufficiently developed to complement placental function and to provide some hormone precursors to the placenta. From this time, it is useful to consider the endocrine conceptus as the fetal-placental unit.

The decidua is the endometrium of pregnancy. Decidual cells are capable of synthesizing a variety of polypeptide hormones, including relaxin, prolactin (PRL), and a variety of paracrine factors, in particular insulin-like growth factor (IGF)-binding protein 1. The precise function of the decidua as an endocrine organ has not been established, but its role as a source of prostaglandins during labor is certain (see "Endocrine Control of Parturition," later).

POLYPEPTIDE HORMONES

Human Chorionic Gonadotropin

The first marker of trophoblast differentiation and the first measurable product of the placenta is hCG, a glycoprotein consisting of 237 amino acids. It is similar in structure to the pituitary glycoprotein hormones in that it consists of two chains: a common alpha chain and a specific beta chain, which determines receptor interaction and ultimate biologic specificity. The alpha chain is identical in sequence to the alpha chains of thyroid-stimulating hormone (TSH), follicle-stimulating hormone (FSH), and luteinizing hormone (LH). The beta chain has 67% sequence homology with LH and an additional 30 amino acids not found in LH beta.

In early pregnancy (up to 6 weeks), the concentration of hCG doubles every 1.7 to 2 days, and serial measurements provide a sensitive index of early trophoblast function and viability. Maternal plasma hCG peaks during the 10th gestational week and then declines gradually in the third trimester. Peak concentrations correlate temporally with the establishment of maternal blood flow in the intervillous space (see Figure 16–1, upper panel).

The long plasma half-life of hCG (24 hours) allows the tiny mass of cells comprising the blastocyst to produce sufficient hormone to be detected in the peripheral circulation within 24 hours of implantation. Thus, pregnancy can be diagnosed several days before symptoms occur or a menstrual period has been missed. Antibodies to the unique beta-carboxyl terminal segment of hCG do not cross-react significantly with any of the pituitary glycoproteins.

hCG is also produced in gestational trophoblastic neoplasia (GTN) by hydatidiform mole and choriocarcinoma, and the concentration of hCG-beta is used as a tumor marker for diagnosis and for monitoring the success of chemotherapy in these disorders. Women with very high hCG levels due to GTN may become clinically hyperthyroid due to the action of hCG on TSH receptors; they can revert to euthyroidism as hCG is reduced during chemotherapy.

Human Placental Lactogen

A second placental polypeptide hormone, this one with homology to pituitary growth hormone (GH), is human placental lactogen (hPL). hPL is produced by early trophoblasts, but detectable serum concentrations are not reached until 4 to 5 gestational

SYSTEM	HORMONE	PATTERN	AVERAGE PEAK CONCENTRATION (TIME)
Placenta and corpus luteum	Progesterone	Rises to term	190 ng/mL (552 nmol/L) (term)
	17-Hydroxy-progester-one	Peaks at 5 wk, then declines	6 ng/mL (19 nmol/L) (5 wk)
Adrenal	Cortisol	Increases to 3 times prepregnancy values at term	300 ng/mL (0.83 μmol/L) (term)
	Aldosterone	Plateaus at 34 wk with small rise near term	100 ng/mL (277 nmol/L) (term)
	DOC	Increases to 10 times prepregnancy value at term	1200 pg/mL (3.48 nmol/L) (term)
Thyroid	Total T₄	Increases during first trimester, then plateaus	150 ng/mL (193 pmol/L)
	Free T₄	Unchanged	30 pg/mL (38.6 pmol/L)
	Total T₃	Increases during first trimester, then plateaus	2 ng/mL (3.1 nmol/L)
	Free T₃	Unchanged	4 pg/mL (5.1 pmol/L)

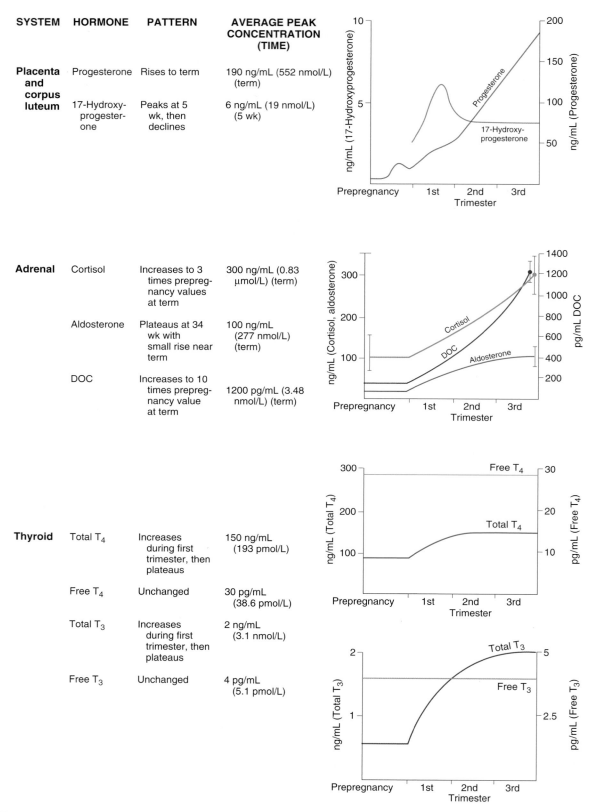

FIGURE 16–2 Maternal serum hormone changes during pregnancy.

SYSTEM	HORMONE	PATTERN	AVERAGE PEAK CONCENTRATION (TIME)
Anterior pituitary	GH	Unchanged	
	LH, FSH	Low, basal levels	
	ACTH	Unchanged	
	TSH	Reaches nadir during first trimester, then plateaus	
	PRL	Rise to term	200 ng/mL (9 nmol/L) (term)
Placental proteins	hCG	Peaks at 10 wk, then decreases to a lower plateau	5 µg/mL (0.2 µmol/L) (end of first trimester)
	hPL	Rises with placental weight	5-25 µg/mL (term) (0.2-1.0 µmol/L)
	CRH	Rises acutely about 20 d before delivery	1-3 ng/mL (2-6 nmol/L) at term
Fetopla-cental estrogens	Estriol	Increases to term	15-17 ng/mL (55-62 nmol/L) (term)
	Estradiol	Increases to term	12-15 ng/mL (42-52 nmol/L) (term)
	Estrone	Increases to term	5-7 ng/mL (18.5-26 nmol/L) (term)
Fetopla-cental androgens	Testos-terone	Rises to 10 times pre-pregnancy values	2000 pg/mL (6.9 nmol/L) (term)
	DHEA	Falls during pregnancy	5 ng/mL (17.3 nmol/L) (pre-pregnancy)
	Andro-stenedione	Small increase	2.6 ng/mL (9.0 nmol/L) (term)

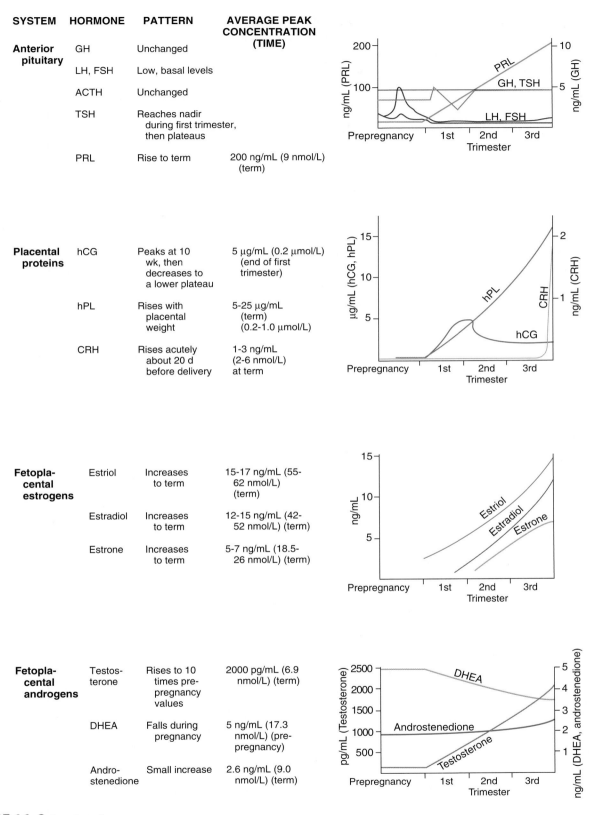

FIGURE 16-2 *(continued)*

weeks (see Figure 16–2). hPL is a protein of 190 amino acids whose primary, secondary, and tertiary structures are similar to those of GH and PRL. hPL is diabetogenic and lactogenic, but it has minimal growth-promoting activity as measured by standard GH bioassays.

The physiologic role of hPL during pregnancy remains controversial, and normal pregnancy without detectable hPL production has been reported. Although not clearly shown to be a mammotropic agent, hPL contributes to altered maternal glucose metabolism and mobilization of free fatty acids; causes a hyperinsulinemic response to glucose loads; appears to directly stimulate pancreatic islet insulin secretion; and contributes to the peripheral insulin resistance characteristic of pregnancy. Along with prolonged fasting and insulin-induced hypoglycemia, pre-beta-HDL and apoprotein A-I are two factors that stimulate release of hPL. hPL production is roughly proportionate to placental mass. Actual production rates may reach as much as 1 to 1.5 g/d at term.

Serum hPL concentrations were used historically as a clinical indicator of the health of the placenta, but the range of normal values was wide, and serial determinations were necessary; it is therefore no longer used clinically.

Other Chorionic Peptide Hormones and Growth Factors

Other chorionic peptides have been identified, but their functions remain poorly defined. Activin, inhibin, corticotropin-releasing hormone, and multiple peptide growth factors, including fibroblast growth factor (FGF), epidermal growth factor (EGF), platelet-derived growth factor (PDGF), and the IGFs all have been isolated from placental tissue. Placental growth factor (PlGF) and the related vascular endothelial growth factor (VEGF) are suggested to play a role in placental angiogenesis, preeclampsia, and fetal growth.

STEROID HORMONES

In contrast to the impressive synthetic capability exhibited in the production of placental proteins, the placenta does not have the ability to synthesize steroids de novo. However, the trophoblasts have remarkable capacity to efficiently interconvert steroids derived from maternal or fetal precursors. This activity is demonstrable even in the early blastocyst, and by the seventh gestational week, when the corpus luteum undergoes involution, the placenta becomes the dominant source of steroid hormones.

Progesterone

The placenta relies on maternal cholesterol as its substrate for progesterone production. Fetal death has no immediate influence on progesterone production, suggesting that the fetus is a negligible source of substrate. Enzymes in the placenta cleave the cholesterol side chain, yielding pregnenolone, which in turn is isomerized to progesterone; 250 to 350 mg of progesterone are produced daily by the third-trimester placenta, and most enters the maternal circulation

(see Figure 16–2). Whereas exogenous hCG stimulates progesterone production in early pregnancy, hypophysectomy, adrenalectomy, or oophorectomy have no effect on progesterone levels after the luteoplacental shift at 7 to 9 weeks' gestation. Likewise, the administration of adrenocorticotropin (ACTH) or cortisol does not influence placental progesterone secretion.

Progesterone is necessary for establishment and maintenance of pregnancy. Insufficient production of progesterone may contribute to failure of implantation, recurrent pregnancy loss, and preterm delivery. Progesterone, along with relaxin and nitric oxide, maintains uterine quiescence during pregnancy. Clinical trials have indicated that the administration of 17α-hydroxyprogesterone caproate can reliably prevent preterm delivery in high-risk pregnancies. Progesterone also inhibits T cell–mediated allograft rejection. Thus, high local concentrations of progesterone may contribute to immunologic tolerance by the uterus of invading trophoblast tissue from the semiallogeneic fetus.

Estrogens

Estrogen production by the placenta also depends on circulating precursors, but in this case both fetal and maternal steroids are important sources. Most of the placental estrogens are derived from fetal androgens, primarily dehydroepiandrosterone (DHEA) sulfate. Fetal DHEA sulfate, produced mainly by the fetal adrenal, is converted by placental sulfatase to free DHEA and then, through enzymatic pathways common to steroid-producing tissues, to androstenedione and testosterone. These androgens are finally aromatized by the placenta to estrone and estradiol, respectively. 17α-Hydroxysteroid dehydrogenase type II prevents fetal exposure to potent estrogens by catalyzing the conversion of estradiol to less potent estrone.

Most fetal DHEA sulfate is metabolized to produce a third estrogen: estriol. Estriol is a weak estrogen with 1/10 the potency of estrone and 1/100 the potency of estradiol. Serum estrone and estradiol concentrations are increased during pregnancy about 50-fold over their maximal prepregnancy values, but estriol increases approximately 1000-fold. The substrate for the reaction is 16α-hydroxy-DHEA sulfate produced in the fetal adrenal and liver, not in maternal or placental tissues. The final steps of desulfation and aromatization to estriol occur in the placenta. Maternal serum or urinary estriol measurements, unlike measurements of progesterone or hPL, reflect fetal as well as placental function. Rising serum or urinary estriol concentrations were once used as biochemical indicators of fetal well-being (see Figure 16–2). Decreased estriol production can result from congenital derangements or iatrogenic intervention. Maternal estriol remains low in pregnancies with placental sulfatase deficiency and in cases of fetal anencephaly. In the first case, DHEA sulfate cannot be hydrolyzed; in the second, little fetal DHEA is produced because fetal adrenal growth stimulation by ACTH is lacking. Maternal administration of glucocorticoids also inhibits fetal ACTH and lowers maternal estriol. Administration of DHEA to the mother during a healthy pregnancy increases estriol production. Placental corticotropin-releasing hormone (CRH) also may be an important regulator of fetal adrenal DHEA sulfate secretion.

Modern methods of screening for fetal chromosomal aneuploidy, particularly trisomy 21 (Down syndrome), utilize circulating biochemical markers. Screening by maternal age alone (>35 years) led to the prenatal identification of only about 25% of aneuploid fetuses. As an aneuploid chromosome complement affects both fetal and placental tissues, their protein and steroid products have been evaluated. A combination of alpha-fetoprotein (AFP), hCG, inhibin-A and unconjugated estriol concentrations, measured in maternal serum between 15 and 18 weeks' gestation, can be used to identify fetal Down syndrome and trisomy 18 with a detection rate of 80% over all age groups.

MATERNAL ADAPTATION TO PREGNANCY

As a successful *parasite*, the fetal-placental unit manipulates the maternal *host* for its own gain but normally avoids imposing excessive stress that would jeopardize the pregnancy. The prodigious production of polypeptide and steroid hormones by the fetal-placental unit directly or indirectly results in physiologic adaptations of virtually every maternal organ system. These alterations are summarized in Figure 16–3. Most of the commonly measured maternal endocrine function tests are radically changed. In some cases, true physiologic alteration has occurred; in others, the changes are due to increased production of hormone-binding proteins by the liver or to decreased serum levels of albumin due to the mild dilutional anemia of pregnancy. In addition, some endocrine changes are mediated by altered clearance rates due to increased glomerular filtration, decreased hepatic excretion, or metabolic clearance of steroid and protein hormones by the placenta. The changes in endocrine function tests are summarized in Table 16–1. Failure to recognize normal pregnancy-induced alterations in endocrine function tests can lead to unnecessary diagnostic tests and therapy that may be seriously detrimental to mother and fetus.

Maternal Pituitary Gland

The mother's anterior pituitary gland hormones have little influence on pregnancy after implantation has occurred. The gland itself enlarges by about one-third, with the major component of this increase being hyperplasia of the lactotrophs in response to the high plasma estrogens. PRL, the product of the lactotrophs, is the only anterior pituitary hormone that rises progressively during pregnancy and peaks at the time of delivery. In spite of its high serum concentrations, pulsatile release of PRL and food-induced and nocturnal increases persist. Hence, the normal neuroendocrine regulatory mechanisms appear to be intact in the maternal adenohypophysis. In nonlactating women, maternal PRL decreases to pregestational levels within 3 months of delivery. Pituitary ACTH and TSH secretion remain unchanged. Serum FSH and LH fall to the lower limits of detectability and are unresponsive to GnRH stimulation during pregnancy. GH concentrations are not significantly different from nonpregnant levels, but pituitary response to provocative testing is markedly altered. GH response to hypoglycemia and arginine infusion is enhanced in early pregnancy but thereafter becomes depressed. Established pregnancy can continue in the face of hypophysectomy, and in women hypophysectomized prior to pregnancy, induction of ovulation and normal pregnancy can be achieved with appropriate gonadotropin replacement therapy. In cases of primary pituitary hyperfunction, the fetus is not affected.

Maternal Thyroid Gland

The thyroid becomes palpably enlarged during the first trimester, and a subtle bruit may be present. Thyroid iodide clearance and thyroidal ^{131}I uptake, which are clinically contraindicated in pregnancy, have been shown to be increased. These changes are due in large part to the increased renal clearance of iodide, which causes a relative iodine deficiency. Although total serum thyroxine is elevated as a result of estrogen-stimulated increased thyroid hormone–binding globulin (TBG), free thyroxine and triiodothyronine are normal (see Figure 16–2). High circulating concentrations of hCG, particularly asialo-hCG, which has weak TSH-like activity, contribute to the thyrotropic action of the placenta in early pregnancy. In fact, there is significant, though transient, biochemical hyperthyroidism associated with hCG stimulation in early gestation.

Maternal Parathyroid Gland

The net calcium requirement imposed by fetal skeletal development is estimated to be about 30 g by term. This is met by hyperplasia of the maternal parathyroid glands and elevated serum levels of parathyroid hormone. The maternal serum calcium concentration declines to a nadir at 28 to 32 weeks, largely due to the mild hypoalbuminemia of pregnancy but also to fetal bone formation. Ionized calcium is maintained at normal concentrations throughout pregnancy.

Maternal Pancreas

The nutritional demands of the fetus require alteration of maternal metabolic homeostatic control, which results in both structural and functional changes in the maternal pancreas. The size of pancreatic islets increases, and insulin-secreting beta cells undergo hyperplasia. Basal levels of insulin are lower or unchanged in early pregnancy but increase during the second trimester as a result of increased secretion rather than decreased metabolic clearance. Thereafter, pregnancy is a hyperinsulinemic state, with resistance to its peripheral metabolic effects. Pancreatic production of glucagon remains responsive to the usual endocrine stimuli and is suppressed by glucose loading, although the degree of responsiveness has not been well evaluated in pregnancy.

The major roles of insulin and glucagon involve the intracellular transport of nutrients, specifically glucose, amino acids, and fatty acids. Insulin is not transported across the placenta, but rather exerts its effects on transportable metabolites. During pregnancy, peak insulin secretion in response to meals is accelerated, and glucose tolerance curves are characteristically altered. Fasting glucose levels are maintained at low-normal levels. Excess

SYSTEM	PARAMETER	PATTERN
Cardiovascular	Heart rate	Gradually increases 20%
	Blood pressure	Gradually decreases 10% by 34 wk, then increases to prepregnancy values
	Stroke volume	Increases to maximum at 19 wk, then plateaus
	Cardiac output	Rises rapidly by 20%, then gradually increases an additional 10% by 28 wk
	Peripheral venous distention	Progressive increase to term
	Peripheral vascular resistance	Progressive decrease to term
Pulmonary	Respiratory rate	Unchanged
	Tidal volume	Increases by 30%-40%
	Expiratory reserve	Gradual decrease
	Vital capacity	Unchanged
	Respiratory minute volume	Increases by 40%
Blood	Volume	Increases by 50% in second trimester
	Hematocrit	Decreases slightly
	Fibrinogen	Increases
	Electrolytes	Unchanged
Gastrointestinal	Sphincter tone	Decreases
	Gastric emptying time	Increases

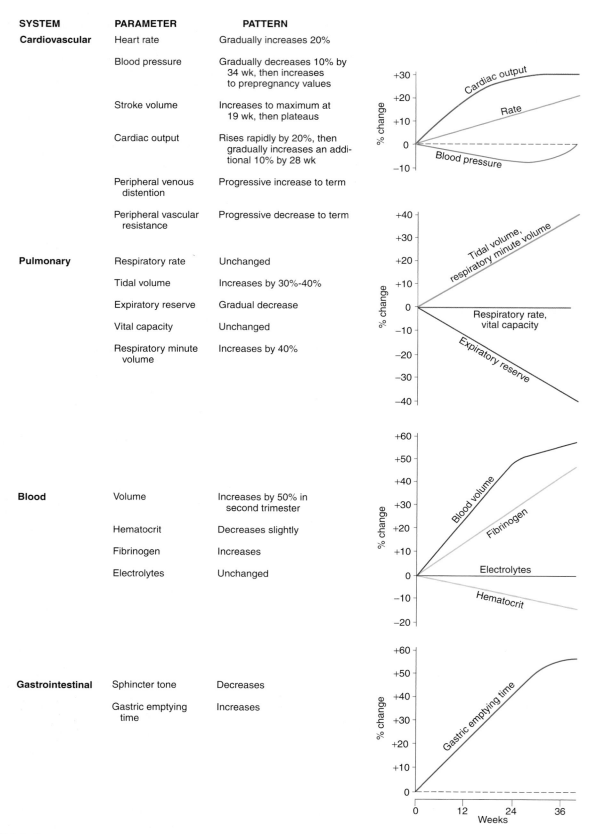

FIGURE 16-3 Maternal physiologic changes during pregnancy.

SYSTEM	PARAMETER	PATTERN
Renal	Renal flow	Increases 25%-50%
	Glomular filtration rate	Increases early, then plateaus
Weight	Uterine weight	Increases from about 60-70 g to about 900-1200 g
	Body weight	Average 11-kg (25-lb) increase

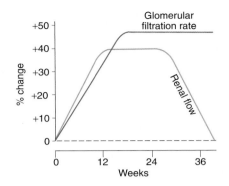

FIGURE 16–3 (continued)

carbohydrate is converted to fat, and fat is readily mobilized during decreased caloric intake.

Maternal Adrenal Cortex

Total plasma cortisol concentrations increase to three times nonpregnant levels by the third trimester. Most of the changes can be explained by increased estrogens causing higher corticosteroid-binding globulin (CBG) production. The actual production of cortisol by the zona fasciculata also is increased in pregnancy. The net effect of these changes increases plasma-free cortisol, which is approximately doubled by late pregnancy. In spite of cortisol concentrations approaching those found in Cushing syndrome, diurnal variation in plasma cortisol is maintained. The elevated free cortisol concentration probably contributes to the insulin resistance of pregnancy and possibly to the appearance of striae, but most signs of hypercortisolism do not occur in pregnancy. It is suggested that high progesterone levels act to antagonize glucocorticoid effects.

Serum aldosterone also is markedly elevated in pregnancy, due to an eight fold increased production rate by the zona glomerulosa. Renin substrate is increased due to the influence of estrogen on hepatic synthesis, and renin also is elevated, leading to increased angiotensin. In spite of these dramatic changes, normal pregnant women show few signs of hyperaldosteronism. There is no tendency toward hypokalemia or hypernatremia, and blood pressure at midpregnancy—when changes in the renin-angiotensin-aldosterone system are maximal—actually tends to be lower than in the nonpregnant state. Progesterone is an effective competitive inhibitor of mineralocorticoids in the distal renal tubules. Thus, increases in renin and aldosterone may simply be an appropriate response to the high gestational levels of progesterone. Elevated angiotensin II does not normally result in hypertension, because of diminished sensitivity of the maternal vascular system to angiotensin. Exogenous angiotensin provokes a smaller increase in blood pressure than in the nonpregnant state. Finally, in patients with preeclampsia, the most common form of pregnancy-related hypertension, serum renin, aldosterone, and angiotensin levels are unchanged or even lower than in normal pregnancy, thus ruling out a primary role for the renin-angiotensin system in this disorder.

In normal pregnancy, the maternal production of androgens is slightly increased but these are buffered by sex hormone–binding globulin (SHBG). Levels of SHBG are increased by estrogens. Testosterone, which binds avidly to SHBG, increases to the normal male range by the end of the first trimester, but free testosterone levels are actually lower than in the nonpregnant state. DHEA sulfate does not bind significantly to SHBG, and plasma concentrations of DHEA sulfate actually decrease during pregnancy.

TABLE 16–1   Effect of pregnancy on endocrine function tests.

	Test	Result
Pituitary FSH, LH	GnRH stimulation	Unresponsive from third gestational week until puerperium
GH	Insulin tolerance test	Response increases during the first half of pregnancy and then is blunted until the puerperium
	Arginine stimulation	Hyperstimulation during the first and second trimesters, then suppression
TSH	TRH stimulation	Response unchanged
Pancreas Insulin	Glucose tolerance	Peak glucose increases, and glucose concentration remains elevated longer
	Glucose challenge	Insulin concentration increases to higher peak levels
	Arginine infusion	Insulin response is blunted in mid to late pregnancy
Adrenal Cortisol	ACTH infusion	Exaggerated cortisol and aldosterone responses
	Metyrapone	Diminished response
Mineralocorticoids	ACTH infusion	No DOC response
	Dexamethasone suppression	No DOC response

The desulfation of DHEA sulfate by the placenta and the conversion of DHEA to estrogens by the fetal-placental unit are important factors in its increased metabolic clearance.

FETAL ENDOCRINOLOGY

Because of the physical inaccessibility of the human fetus, much of our information about fetal endocrinology is derived indirectly. Most early studies of fetal endocrinology relied on observations of infants with congenital disorders or inferences from ablation studies or acute manipulation in experimental animals. The development of effective cell culture methods and sensitive immunoassays, as well as the ability to achieve stable preparations of chronically catheterized monkey fetuses, have increased our understanding of the dynamics of intrauterine endocrine events. The endocrine system is among the first to develop in fetal life, but its study is complicated by its relative physical isolation as well as the multiplicity of sources of the various hormones. Dating of events in fetal development is usually given in *fetal weeks*, which begin at the time of fertilization. Thus, fetal age is always 2 weeks less than gestational age.

Fetal Pituitary Hormones

The characteristic anterior pituitary cell types are discernible as early as 8 to 10 fetal weeks, and all of the hormones of the adult anterior pituitary are extractable from the fetal adenohypophysis by 12 weeks. Similarly, the hypothalamic hormones thyrotropin-releasing hormone (TRH), gonadotropin-releasing hormone (GnRH), and somatostatin are present by 8 to 10 weeks. The direct circulatory connection between hypothalamus and pituitary develops later, with capillary invasion initially visible at about 16 fetal weeks.

The role of the fetal pituitary in organogenesis during the first trimester appears to be negligible. None of the pituitary hormones are released into the fetal circulation in large quantities until after 20 fetal weeks. Even GH appears not to be influential, and in fact total absence of GH is consistent with normal development at birth. Development of the gonads and adrenals during the first trimester appears to be directed by hCG rather than by fetal pituitary hormones, so that these organs initially develop even in the face of anencephaly.

During the second trimester, there is a marked increase in secretion of all of the anterior pituitary hormones, which coincides with maturation of the hypophysial portal system. Female fetuses exhibit higher FSH levels in both pituitary and serum than do males. Differentiation of the gonads is crucial for normal male sexual development and reproductive potential in both sexes. ACTH rises significantly during the second trimester and assumes an increasing role in directing the maturation of the differentiated adrenal, as shown by the anencephalic fetus, in which the fetal zone of the adrenal undergoes atrophy after 20 weeks. Fetal PRL secretion also increases after the 20th fetal week, but its functional significance is unknown. Vasopressin and oxytocin are demonstrable by 12 to 18 weeks in the fetal posterior pituitary gland and correlate with the development of their sites of production, the supraoptic and paraventricular nuclei, respectively.

Fetal Thyroid Gland

The fetal thyroid gland develops initially in the absence of detectable TSH. By 12 weeks the thyroid is capable of iodine-concentrating activity and thyroid hormone synthesis, but prior to this time the maternal thyroid appears to be the primary source for T_4. This has implications in that infants born to even mildly hypothyroid mothers are reported to have lower IQs and other health problems. The function of the fetal thyroid hormones appears crucial to somatic growth and for successful neonatal adaptation. In particular, auditory maturational events are regulated by thyroid hormones.

During the second trimester, TRH, TSH, and free T_4 all begin to rise. The maturation of feedback mechanisms is suggested by the subsequent plateau of TSH at about 20 fetal weeks. Fetal T_3 and reverse T_3 do not become detectable until the third trimester. The hormone produced in largest amount throughout fetal life is T_4, with the metabolically active T_3 and its inactive derivative, reverse T_3, rising in parallel to T_4 during the third trimester. At birth, conversion of T_4 to T_3 is demonstrable. Goitrogenic agents such as propylthiouracil are transferred across the placenta and may induce fetal hypothyroidism and goiter.

Fetal Adrenal Cortex

The fetal adrenal cortex is identifiable as early as 4 weeks of fetal age, and by the seventh week, steroidogenic activity can be detected in the inner zone layers.

During gestation, the adrenal cortex differs anatomically and functionally from the adult gland and occupies as much as 0.5% of total body volume. Most of this tissue is composed of a unique fetal zone that subsequently is transformed into the definitive (adult) zone during the early neonatal period. The inner fetal zone is responsible for the majority of steroids produced during fetal life and comprises 80% of the mass of the adrenal. During the second trimester, the inner fetal zone continues to grow, while the outer zone remains relatively undifferentiated. At about 25 weeks, the definitive (adult) zone develops, ultimately assuming the principal role in steroid synthesis during the early postnatal weeks.

Fetal Gonads

The testis is histologically identifiable by about 6 fetal weeks. Primary testis differentiation begins with development of the Sertoli cells at 8 weeks' gestation. SRY, the sex-determining locus on the Y chromosome directs the differentiation of the Sertoli cells, the sites of anti-Müllerian hormone (AMH) synthesis. AMH, a member of the transforming growth factor-beta family of growth factors, specifically triggers the ipsilateral resorption of the Müllerian tract in males and prevents development of female internal structures. Embryonic androgen production begins in the developing Leydig cells at about 10 weeks, coincident with the peak production of placental hCG. Binding of hCG to fetal testes with stimulation of testosterone release has been demonstrated in the laboratory. Other fetal testicular products of importance are inhibin and the 5α-reduced testosterone metabolite dihydrotestosterone. Dihydrotestosterone is responsible for development of the male external genital structures.

Little is known about early fetal ovarian function, but by 7 to 8 weeks of intrauterine life the ovaries become morphologically recognizable. Oogonia mitosis is active and steroid-producing theca cell precursors are identifiable at 20 weeks. This corresponds with peak gonadotropin levels from the fetal pituitary. Activin and inhibin peptide subunits are expressed in the midtrimester human testis but not in the midtrimester human ovary. In contrast to the male fetus, ovarian steroid production by the fetus is not essential for female phenotypic development (see Chapter 13).

ENDOCRINE CONTROL OF PARTURITION

During the last few weeks of normal pregnancy, two processes herald approaching labor. Sporadic uterine contractions, usually painless, become increasingly frequent, and the lower uterine segment and cervix become softer and thinner, a process known as effacement, or ripening. Although false alarms are not uncommon, the onset of true labor is usually fairly abrupt, with the establishment of regular contractions every 2 to 5 minutes, leading to delivery in less than 24 hours. An extensive literature describes the physiologic and biochemical events that occur during human labor, but the key inciting event has eluded detection. In sheep, the fetus controls the onset of labor. The initial measurable event is an increase in fetal plasma cortisol, which, in turn, alters placental steroid production, resulting in a drop in progesterone. Cortisol reliably induces labor in sheep, but in humans, glucocorticoids do not induce labor and there is no clear drop in plasma progesterone concentrations prior to labor.

Sex Steroids

Progesterone is essential for maintenance of early pregnancy, and withdrawal of progesterone leads to termination of pregnancy. Progesterone causes hyperpolarization of myometrial cells decreasing the amplitude of action potentials and preventing effective contractions. In various experimental systems, progesterone decreases alpha-adrenergic receptors, stimulates cAMP production, and inhibits oxytocin receptor synthesis. Progesterone also inhibits estrogen receptor synthesis, promotes the storage of prostaglandin precursors in the decidua and fetal membranes, and stabilizes lysosomes containing prostaglandin-synthesizing enzymes. Estrogen opposes progesterone in many of these actions and may have an independent role in ripening the uterine cervix and promoting uterine contractility. It has been shown that an increase in the estrogen-progesterone ratio increases the number of oxytocin receptors and myometrial gap junctions; this finding may explain the coordinated, effective contractions that characterize true labor as opposed to the nonpainful, ineffective contractions of false labor.

Oxytocin

Oxytocin infusion is commonly used to induce or augment labor. Both maternal and fetal oxytocin levels increase spontaneously during labor, but neither has been convincingly shown to increase prior to labor. Data in animals suggest that oxytocin's role in initiation of labor is due to increased sensitivity of the uterus to oxytocin rather than increased plasma concentrations of the hormone. Even women with posterior pituitary failure, manifested as diabetes insipidus, are able to deliver without oxytocin augmentation; thus a maternal source of the hormone is not indispensable. Clinical studies using the oxytocin receptor inhibitor, atosiban, have demonstrated a delay of delivery for 24 to 48 hours but meta-analyses do not show an improvement in fetal outcome.

Prostaglandins

Prostaglandin $F_{2\alpha}$ administered intra-amniotically, vaginally, or intravenously is an effective abortifacient as early as 14 weeks of gestation. Prostaglandin E_2 administered vaginally induces labor in most women in the third trimester. The amnion and chorion contain high concentrations of arachidonic acid, and the decidua contains active prostaglandin synthetase. Prostaglandins are almost certainly involved in maintenance of labor once it is established. They also probably are important in initiating labor in some circumstances, such as in amnionitis or when the membranes are *stripped* by the physician. Prostaglandins are believed to be the *final common pathway* of labor.

PRETERM LABOR/BIRTH

Preterm birth (PTB) is one of the most important problems in obstetrics today as it complicates approximately 12% of all births in the United States and accounts for over 70% of perinatal morbidity and mortality. Approximately 45% to 50% of PTB is idiopathic or spontaneous, defined as regular uterine contractions leading to cervical change prior to 37 weeks of gestation, 30% is related to preterm rupture of membranes and the other 15% to 20% is attributed to medically indicated or elective preterm delivery, typically due to worsening maternal disease or fetal compromise. PTB is a complex disorder with heterogeneous risk factors, genetic and environmental susceptibilities, and pathophysiologic pathways. Risk factors for preterm labor are varied and include history of prior preterm labor, uterine anomalies, multiple gestation, maternal medical complications, low prepregnancy body mass index, gestational bleeding, low socioeconomic status, minority race, behavioral habits such as smoking, alcohol, drug abuse, stressful events, limited or no prenatal care, and infection. The pathophysiology of preterm labor is not well understood but may result from mechanical factors, hormonal changes, infection, or interruption of normal mechanisms responsible for sustaining uterine quiescence. Unfortunately the rate of PTBs continues to increase slightly each year. Despite this, survival rates have improved due to the use of antenatal corticosteroids and improvements in neonatal resuscitation and care.

There is a well-documented racial disparity in rates of PTB with African Americans at 17% versus only 11% in Caucasians. Further, the infant mortality rate for African American babies is 2.5 times higher than Caucasians. Population-based studies indicate that this disparity cannot be explained by socioeconomic status, maternal behavior, marital status, or education alone and likely point to true genetic differences.

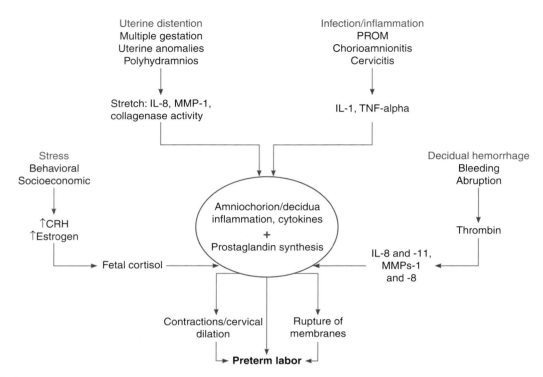

FIGURE 16–4 Major mechanistic pathways leading to preterm birth.

Four major mechanistic pathways leading to PTB have been proposed: (1) stress or activation of maternal or fetal hypothalamic-pituitary-adrenal axis, (2) pathologic uterine distention, (3) inflammation/infection, and (4) decidual hemorrhage and coagulation. These are summarized in Figure 16–4. Each of these pathways has different epidemiologic, clinical, and biochemical features, but all are likely to initiate labor via prostaglandin production, myometrial activation, and degradation of extracellular matrix components leading to premature rupture of membranes and cervical dilation. The fetoplacental endocrine unit can trigger labor prematurely, activating CRH release in cases of a hostile intrauterine environment such as stress and chorioamnionitis.

Maternal/Fetal Stress

Both exogenous and endogenous maternal stress, ranging from heavy workload to depression, is associated with PTB. The exact mechanism is not well understood, but CRH is thought to play an important role. Maternal CRH levels are elevated in both preterm and term labor and appear to activate the parturition pathway by increasing prostaglandins, inhibiting progesterone, and stimulating fetal cortisol and DHEA production.

Pathologic Uterine Distention

Myometrial stretching due to multiple gestations, polyhydramnios, and Mullerian anomalies has been associated with an increased risk of preterm labor. This is thought to occur as distension can induce myometrial contractility, prostaglandin release, collagenase activity, and increased oxytocin receptor expression.

Infection/Inflammation

Infection is the only pathologic process for which there is a clear causal link to preterm birth exhibited by the fact that: (1) intrauterine and extrauterine infections are associated with preterm birth; (2) antibiotics for intrauterine infection can prevent preterm birth; and (3) treatment of asymptomatic bacteruria prevents preterm birth. Microbiology studies suggest that infection may account for 25% to 40% of preterm births. Ascending infection is believed to be the most common source of microbial invasion of the amniotic cavity. Endotoxins from bacteria induce proinflammatory mediators such as IL-1 and TNF-alpha from the decidua, which stimulates prostaglandin production. Double knockout mice for IL-1 and TNF-alpha had decreased rates of PTB after administration of microorganisms. Other inflammatory cytokines and chemokines also have been implicated in infection-induced preterm labor.

Decidual Hemorrhage and Coagulation

Any vaginal bleeding during pregnancy is a known risk factor for preterm birth. Decidual hemorrhage and uteroplacental ischemia are thought to contribute to preterm labor via generation of thrombin. Thrombin stimulates myometrial contractility in a dose-dependent manner and also binds to protease-activated receptor type 1, which increases expression of metalloproteniases leading to cervical ripening and possible subsequent preterm delivery.

A. Predictors/prevention of preterm labor Unfortunately, clinical symptoms to identify women at risk for PTB have been shown to be inaccurate and unreliable. Given the clinical, emotional, and financial gravity of preterm birth, multiple tests have been developed over the years to attempt to identify women at risk for preterm delivery. Home uterine activity monitors are not currently recommended as they have not been shown to improve outcome. The presence of bacterial vaginosis (BV) has been associated with preterm delivery independent of other known risk factors, however, there is insufficient data to support screening and treating women with positive cultures. Maternal estradiol and estriol levels have been used to predict activation of the fetal hypothalamic-pituitary-adrenal axis, but trials have failed to establish their clinical usefulness in accurately predicting preterm labor.

Numerous studies have confirmed the association between cervical shortening and subsequent preterm delivery. Transvaginal cervical ultrasonography has been shown to be a reliable and reproducible way to assess the length of the cervix. Despite the usefulness of cervical length determination as a predictor of preterm labor, routine use is not recommended because of the lack of proven treatments affecting outcome.

Fetal fibronectin (fFN) is a basement membrane protein of placental membranes and decidua. Numerous trials have shown that the risk of PTB is increased in the presence of fFN and decreased in its absence. The relationship among fFN, short cervix, BV, and traditional historical risk factors for spontaneous preterm birth suggest the highest associations of preterm birth with positive fFN, followed by cervical length less than 25 mm and a history of preterm birth. A negative fFN test indicates a 95% likelihood of not delivering within 14 days; therefore it is particularly useful in ruling out preterm delivery.

Supplemental progesterone therapy has been shown to reduce the rate of preterm delivery in high-risk populations. Weekly injections of 17α-hydroxyprogesterone caproate from 16 to 20 weeks until 36 weeks of gestation has been found to significantly reduce recurrent preterm birth in women with history of preterm delivery. A recent meta-analysis of 10 placebo-controlled trials found progesterone therapy to significantly reduce the frequency of recurrent preterm birth from 36% to 26%. Given the lack of other available treatments, many providers are using progesterone as preventative therapy in high-risk patients, but progesterone does not reverse established labor.

B. Management of preterm labor Once preterm labor has been diagnosed, care should be taken to determine if patient warrants tocolysis, expectant management, or delivery. It is important to confirm an accurate gestational age because if less than 34 weeks, glucocorticoids should be administered as they clearly decrease neonatal morbidity and mortality in this population.

Tocolytic therapy is used to attempt to prolong pregnancy to allow time for corticosteroid administration. However, both tocolytic and steroid therapy may result in untoward maternal and fetal consequences and, therefore, their use should be limited to women in true preterm labor at high risk for spontaneous PTB.

In general, tocolytic drugs may prolong pregnancy for 2 to 7 days. There is no first-line tocolytic drug and the choices include beta-mimetics, magnesium sulfate, calcium channel blockers, and NSAIDs (nonsteroidal anti-inflammatory drugs). The tocolytic chosen should be based on maternal/fetal conditions, side effects, and gestational age. Prolonged use of any tocolytic drug is generally not indicated as it may increase maternal-fetal risk. Serious adverse events are rare but potentially life-threatening. Beta-mimetics, magnesium sulfate, and calcium channel blockers are all associated with an increased risk of pulmonary edema. Specifically, beta-mimetics are potent cardiovascular stimulants and can cause maternal myocardial ischemia, metabolic derangements (eg, hyperglycemia and hypokalemia), and fetal cardiac effects. Magnesium sulfate may cause maternal lethargy, drowsiness, double vision, nausea, and vomiting. NSAIDs can cause fetal oligohydramnios and premature closure of the ductus arteriosus. Calcium channel blockers used as a single agent appear to have a good maternal and fetal safety profile. Combining tocolytic drugs potentially increases maternal morbidity and should be used with caution.

POSTTERM PREGNANCY

Postterm pregnancy refers to gestation that has extended to or beyond 42 weeks and is associated with significant risks to the fetus. Most importantly, the perinatal mortality rate (stillbirths plus early neonatal deaths) beyond 42 weeks is twice that at term (4-7 deaths vs 2-3 deaths per 1000 deliveries) and is six fold higher after 43 weeks or more. Potential causes include uteroplacental insufficiency, meconium aspiration, and intrauterine infection. Postterm pregnancy is also a risk factor for low Apgar scores, oligohydramnios, and neonatal complications such as hypoglycemia, seizures, respiratory insufficiency, and increased risk of death within the first year of life. Postterm pregnancy is associated with some complications for the mother including a twofold increased risk of severe perineal injury and cesarean delivery. Because pregnancy past 41 weeks is associated with high costs of antenatal testing and induction of labor, as well as a source of significant anxiety for pregnant women, there has been a movement in obstetrics to effect delivery before 41 completed weeks. The most common cause of a prolonged gestation is incorrect dating; other risk factors include primiparity, prior postterm pregnancy, and male sex of the fetus. Recently, obesity has been identified as a modifiable risk factor. The mechanism for this association is unclear but it is likely due to a derangement in endocrine factors that initiate labor. In rare cases, postterm pregnancy has been associated with placental sulfatase deficiency or fetal anencephaly.

Management of Postterm Pregnancy

Standard management of postterm pregnancy focuses on antenatal fetal surveillance and timely initiation of delivery if spontaneous labor does not occur. Although antepartum testing for postterm pregnancies is universally accepted, it has not been validated in prospective trials to decrease perinatal mortality. Given the ethical and medicolegal concerns for a control group, randomized studies to prove benefit will likely never be done. Timing of delivery is generally recommended when risks to continuing the pregnancy are greater than the benefit to mother or fetus after or during birth. In high-risk cases such as diabetics and, hypertensives, pregnancy should not be allowed to progress beyond 41 weeks. However, management of low-risk postterm pregnancy is more controversial. Because delivery cannot always be induced readily, maternal risks and considerations complicate this decision. Factors to consider include gestational age, results of antepartum fetal testing, cervical exam, and maternal preference after counseling regarding the risks, benefits, and alternatives to expectant management with antepartum monitoring versus labor induction.

ENDOCRINOLOGY OF THE PUERPERIUM

Extirpation of any active endocrine organ leads to compensatory changes in other organs and systems. Delivery of the infant and placenta causes both immediate and long-term adjustment to loss of the pregnancy hormones. The sudden withdrawal of fetal-placental hormones at delivery permits determination of their serum half-lives and some evaluation of their effects on maternal systems.

Physiologic and Anatomic Changes

Some physiologic and anatomic adjustments that take place after delivery are both hormone dependent and independent. For example, major readjustments of the cardiovascular system occur in response to the normal blood losses associated with delivery and to loss of the low-resistance placental shunt. By the third postpartum day, blood volume is estimated to decline to about 80% of predelivery values. These cardiovascular changes influence renal and liver function, including clearance of pregnancy hormones.

Uterine Changes

The uterus involutes progressively at the rate of about 500 g/wk and continues to be palpable abdominally until about 2 weeks postpartum, after which it reoccupies its position entirely within the pelvis. Nonpregnant size and weight (60-70 g) are reached by 6 weeks postpartum. The reversal of myometrial hypertrophy occurs with a decrease in size of individual myometrial cells rather than by reduction in number. The endometrium, which is sloughed at the time of delivery, regenerates rapidly; by the seventh postpartum day there is restoration of surface epithelium. These rapid regenerative changes do not apply to the area of placental implantation, which requires much longer for restoration and retains pathognomonic histologic evidence of placentation indefinitely.

Endocrine Changes

A. Steroids   With expulsion of the placenta, many steroid levels decline precipitously, with half-lives of minutes. Plasma progesterone falls to luteal-phase levels within 24 hours after delivery and to follicular-phase levels within several days. Removal of the corpus luteum results in a fall to follicular levels within 24 hours. Estradiol reaches follicular phase levels within 1 to 3 days after delivery.

B. Pituitary hormones   The pituitary gland, which enlarges during pregnancy owing primarily to an increase in lactotrophs, does not diminish in size until after lactation ceases. Secretion of FSH and LH continues to be suppressed during the early weeks of the puerperium, and stimulus with bolus doses of GnRH results in subnormal release of LH and FSH. Over the ensuing weeks, responsiveness to GnRH gradually returns to normal and most women exhibit follicular-phase serum levels of LH and FSH by the third or fourth postpartum week.

C. Prolactin   Serum PRL, which rises throughout pregnancy, falls with the onset of labor and then exhibits variable patterns of secretion depending on whether breast-feeding occurs. Delivery is associated with a surge in PRL, which is followed by a rapid fall in serum concentrations over 7 to 14 days in the nonlactating mother. In nonlactating women, the return of normal cyclic function and ovulation may be expected within 3 months, with the initial ovulation occurring at an average of 9 to 10 weeks postpartum. In actively lactating women, PRL can cause a persistence of anovulation. Surges of PRL are believed to act on the hypothalamus to inhibit GnRH secretion. Administration of exogenous GnRH during this time induces normal pituitary responsiveness, and occasional ovulation may occur spontaneously even during lactation.

LACTATION

Development of the breast alveolar lobules occurs throughout pregnancy. This period of mammogenesis requires the concerted participation of estrogen, progesterone, PRL, GH, and glucocorticoids. hPL may also play a role but is not indispensable. Lactation requires PRL, insulin, and adrenal steroids and is associated with further enlargement of the lobules, followed by synthesis of milk constituents such as lactose and casein. Lactopoiesis does not occur until unconjugated estrogens fall to nonpregnant levels at about 36 to 48 hours postpartum. Evidence from GH-deficient and hypothyroid patients suggests that GH and thyroid hormone are not required.

PRL is essential to milk production. Its action involves induced synthesis of large numbers of PRL receptors. These receptors appear to be autoregulated because PRL increases receptor levels in cell culture and bromocriptine, an inhibitor of PRL release, causes a decrease in both PRL and its receptors. In the absence of PRL, milk secretion does not take place. However, even in the presence of high levels of PRL during the third trimester, milk secretion does not take place until after delivery, due to the blocking effect of high levels of estrogen.

Milk secretion requires the additional stimulus of suckling, which activates a neural arc. Milk ejection occurs in response to a surge of oxytocin, which induces a contractile response in the smooth muscle surrounding the gland ductules. Oxytocin release is occasioned by stimuli of a visual, psychologic, or physical nature that prepare the mother for breast-feeding; whereas PRL release is limited to the suckling reflex arc.

ENDOCRINE DISORDERS AND PREGNANCY

Hyperthyroidism in Pregnancy

Pregnancy mimics hyperthyroidism because it causes thyroid enlargement, increased cardiac output, and peripheral vasodilation. Owing to the increase in TBG in pregnancy, total serum thyroxine is in the range expected for hyperthyroidism. Free thyroxine, the free thyroxine index, and TSH levels, however, remain in the normal range (see Chapter 7).

True hyperthyroidism complicates 1 to 2 per 1000 pregnancies. The most common form of hyperthyroidism during pregnancy is Graves disease. Hyperthyroidism is associated with an increased risk of preterm delivery (11%-25%) and may modestly increase the risk of early abortion. In Graves disease, thyroid-stimulating immunoglobulin, a 7S immune gamma globulin, crosses the placenta and may cause fetal goiter and transient neonatal hyperthyroidism.

A. Management of the mother The treatment of maternal hyperthyroidism is complicated in pregnancy. Radioiodine is strictly contraindicated. Iodide therapy can lead to huge fetal goiter and is contraindicated except as acute therapy to prevent thyroid storm before thyroid surgery. All antithyroid drugs cross the placenta and may cause fetal hypothyroidism and goiter or cretinism in the newborn. However, propylthiouracil in doses of 300 mg/d or less has been shown to be reasonably safe, although even at low doses about 10% of newborns will have a detectable goiter. A reasonable plan of management is to begin therapy with propylthiouracil in doses high enough to bring the free T_4 index into the mildly hyperthyroid range and then to taper the dose gradually. Propranolol has been used to control maternal cardiovascular symptoms but may result in fetal bradycardia, growth restriction, preterm labor, and neonatal respiratory depression. Partial or total thyroidectomy, especially in the second trimester, is a reasonably safe procedure except for the risk of preterm labor.

B. Management of the newborn Newborns should be observed carefully. In infants of mothers given propylthiouracil, even equivocal evidence of hypothyroidism is an indication for thyroxine replacement therapy. Neonatal Graves disease, which may present as late as 2 weeks after delivery, requires intensive therapy (see Chapter 7).

Hypothyroidism in Pregnancy

Hypothyroidism is uncommon in pregnancy because most women with the untreated disorder are anovulatory. As a practical matter, women taking thyroid medication at the time of conception should be maintained on the same or a slightly higher dose throughout pregnancy, whether or not the obstetrician believes thyroid replacement was originally indicated. Physiologic doses of thyroid hormone replacement are innocuous, but maternal hypothyroidism is hazardous to the developing fetus. Women with a personal or family history of thyroid disease or with symptoms suggestive of hypothyroidism should have TSH tested prior to conception. The correlation between maternal and fetal thyroid status is poor, and hypothyroid mothers frequently deliver euthyroid infants. The strongest correlation between maternal and newborn hypothyroidism occurs in areas where endemic goiter due to iodide deficiency is common. In an iodine-deficient population, treatment with iodine in the first and second trimesters of pregnancy significantly reduces the incidence of cretinism (growth failure, mental retardation, and other neuropsychologic deficits). Overt maternal hypothyroidism has been associated with fetal neurodevelopmental damage and low IQs in the offspring. This is thought to be due to inadequate transplacental supply of thyroxine T_4 in early pregnancy as the mother is the only source of T_4 for the early developing fetal brain.

Pituitary Disorders in Pregnancy

In women of reproductive age, small tumors of the anterior pituitary are not uncommon (see also Chapter 4). Although many are nonfunctional and asymptomatic, the most common symptom of pituitary microadenomas is amenorrhea, frequently accompanied by galactorrhea. In the past, few affected women became pregnant, but now most can be made to ovulate and to conceive with the aid of clomiphene citrate, recombinant gonadotropins and hCG, or bromocriptine. Before ovulation is induced in any patient, serum PRL should be determined. Modest elevations of PRL warrant checking IGF-I levels, because hyperprolactinemia occurs in 25% of patients with GH-producing adenomas. If PRL or IGF-1 is elevated, the sella turcica should be evaluated by magnetic resonance imaging. About 10% of women with secondary amenorrhea are found to have adenomas, and 20% to 50% of women with amenorrhea and galactorrhea have detectable tumors.

The effect of pregnancy on pituitary adenomas depends on their size. Microadenomas rarely (1%) lead to visual field defects. However, approximately 20% of macroadenomas may lead to abnormalities in visual fields or other neurologic signs, usually in the first half of pregnancy. These changes almost always revert to normal after delivery, so aggressive therapy for known pituitary adenomas is not indicated except in cases of rapidly progressive visual loss. Monitoring of patients with known PRL-secreting adenomas during pregnancy is primarily based on clinical examination. The normal gestational increase in PRL may obscure an increase attributable to the adenoma, and radiographic procedures are undesirable in pregnancy.

A. Management Management of the pregnant woman with a pituitary adenoma includes early ophthalmologic consultation for formal visual field mapping and repeat examinations every other month throughout pregnancy. If visual field disturbances are minimal, pregnancy may be allowed to proceed to term. If symptoms become progressively more severe and the fetus is mature, labor should be induced. If symptoms are severe and the fetus is immature, management may consist of transsphenoidal resection of the adenoma or medical treatment with bromocriptine. Although bromocriptine inhibits both fetal and maternal pituitary PRL secretion, it does not affect decidual PRL secretion. Bromocriptine appears not to be teratogenic, and no adverse fetal effects have been reported. In most cases, it is probably preferable to surgery. The newer, selective dopamine D_2 receptor agonist cabergoline has shown excellent results in normalizing PRL levels, inducing tumor shrinkage, and minimizing side effects. The data available on pregnancies in which cabergoline was used do not show adverse effects; however, because the data are limited compared with the large numbers for bromocriptine safety, the latter is recommended. Both have category B classification for pregnancy. Radiation therapy should not be used in pregnancy, however, focused gamma knife pituitary radiation, with abdominal shielding, is gaining popularity in this setting with less than 0.01% of the radiation dose reaching the uterus.

Lymphocytic hypophysitis is an autoimmune inflammation of the pituitary that classically occurs in women in late pregnancy or during the puerperium. The clinical presentation is difficult to distinguish from that of a large PRL-secreting adenoma. Expectant conservative medical management with corticosteroids is sometimes possible, with vigilant postpartum observation to prevent consequences of pituitary insufficiency.

A. Prognosis and follow-up   There appears to be no increase in obstetric complications associated with pituitary adenomas, and no fetal jeopardy. The rate of prematurity increases in women with tumors requiring therapy, but this is probably due to aggressive intervention rather than to direct effects on spontaneous preterm labor. The postpartum period is characterized by rapid relief of even severe symptoms, with less than 4% of untreated tumors developing permanent sequelae. In some cases, tumors improve following pregnancy, with normalization or lowering of PRL relative to prepregnancy values. Management should include imaging and assessment of PRL levels 4 to 6 weeks after delivery. There are no contraindications to breast-feeding.

Obesity and Pregnancy

Obesity is a complicated metabolic and endocrine condition that has been implicated in a number of pregnancy-related complications. Its prevalence has dramatically increased in the United States over the last 20 years. Currently approximately one-third of adult women are obese (body mass index [BMI] >30). This is a particular problem for non-Hispanic black women (49%) and Mexican American women (38%). Obese women are at increased risk for a number of adverse outcomes during pregnancy, including spontaneous abortion, stillbirth, preeclampsia, gestational diabetes, congenital anomalies, cesarean section, venous thromboembolism, and increased surgical morbidity. Complications in pregnancy are generally related to maternal pregravid obesity rather than excessive weight gain during pregnancy. In 1990, the Institute of Medicine published guidelines recommending weight gain of 25 to 35 lb for pregnant women with a normal BMI, 15 to 25 lb for overweight women, and no more than 15 lb for obese women. These were initially designed to help prevent fetal growth restriction. However, most overweight/obese women have mean weight gain exceeding these guidelines. Because of the risks to the fetus, it is recommended that women attempt to lose weight prior to conception.

A. Early pregnancy risks associated with obesity   There is a well-documented increased risk of early miscarriage in obese women in both spontaneous pregnancies and after infertility treatments. Maternal obesity is also associated with an increased risk of a range of structural anomalies particularly neural tube defects, heart defects, and omphalocele. As these types of anomalies are also associated with diabetes, it has been suggested that some of these women may be undiagnosed diabetics. To complicate this further, obesity can affect accuracy of diagnostic testing for congenital anomalies. Heavier women have lower AFP levels likely from greater plasma volume and therefore adjustments have to be made for serum screening based on maternal weight. Ultrasound is the primary diagnostic tool for identifying structural abnormalities. Increasing maternal weight is associated with increasing impairment of adequate ultrasound visualization particularly of cardiac and craniospinal abnormalities. For these reasons, it is important to encourage preconception weight loss and perform early screening for diabetes.

B. Late pregnancy risks associated with obesity   Maternal obesity in pregnancy is associated with a significantly increased rate of gestational diabetes (GDM), preeclampsia, and stillbirths. In a large prospective study of 16,102 women, obese women and morbidly obese women were 2.5 and 3.2 more likely, respectively, to develop gestational hypertension, and 1.6 and 3.3 times more likely to develop preeclampsia. Given the potential increase in oxidative stress from maternal adipose tissue, antioxidants such as vitamin C and E have been studied in the prevention of preeclampsia in obese women; however, they have yet to show any benefit. Gestational diabetes occurs due to decreased insulin sensitivity and inadequate insulin secretory response. Obese women, in general, are more insulin resistant at baseline; therefore, it is not surprising that they are at higher risk of developing GDM. Overweight and obese women have a 2.0- to 2.4-fold increased risk of unexplained fetal death, respectively. The exact pathophysiology of unexplained intrauterine fetal death in obese women is currently unknown.

C. Peripartum risks associated with obesity   Overweight and obese women also have an increased rate of cesarean section and surgical complications, including risks of anesthesia, wound infection, excessive blood loss, endometritis, and deep venous thrombosis. In a recent report, the rate of cesarean section in overweight women was 33.8% and 47% in obese women, compared to only 20.7% in normal weight controls.

D. Long-term risks associated with obesity   Maternal obesity is a risk factor for fetal macrosomia. Accumulating evidence indicates fetal macrosomia is associated with adolescent and adult obesity and metabolic syndrome. A large retrospective study recently found that children born to obese mothers were twice as likely to be obese at 2 years of age. Both maternal obesity and maternal diabetes may independently affect the risk of adolescent obesity in children. Macrosomic infants are also at increased risk of subsequent development of diabetes. Thus, the epidemics of obesity and diabetes may continue to increase further as a result of fetal overgrowth and adiposity in utero.

Parathyroid Disease and Pregnancy

Pregnancy is associated with an approximately 25 to 30 g accumulation of calcium in the mother by term. Most of this calcium is used for fetal skeletal development. Elevated levels of 1,25-hydroxyvitamin D from the decidua leads to increased calcium absorption by the maternal gastrointestinal tract. The kidneys also work to conserve calcium during pregnancy by increasing reabsorption. Overall PTH levels are slightly lower throughout pregnancy and calcium is actively transported across the placenta to the fetus against a concentration gradient. The fetus is relatively hypercalcemic, hypercalcitonemic, and hypoparathyroid in comparison to the mother, but this resolves shortly after birth.

A. Hyperparathyroidism Hyperparathyroidism can be either primary, from an overactive parathyroid gland(s), or a secondary physiologic response to low calcium or vitamin D deficiency. Primary hyperparathyroidism in pregnancy is rare and is due to a solitary or multiple parathyroid adenomas, hyperplasia, or carcinoma. Symptoms of hyperparathyroidism are nonspecific including fatigue, anorexia, nausea, vomiting, constipation, mental status changes, and depression and are generally present when serum calcium levels are over 12 mg/dL. Complications during pregnancy from uncontrolled hyperparathyroidism include nephrolithiasis, pancreatitis, hyperemesis gravidarum, and hypercalcemic crisis. There is an increased incidence of these complications during the postpartum period when the fetal/placental drain of calcium has been removed if the hyperparathyroidism persists after birth of the infant. Fetal complications have been reported to be as high as 80% and include increased risk of spontaneous abortions, intrauterine growth restriction, low birth weight, intrauterine demise, and postpartum neonatal hypocalcemia/tetany due to suppression of the fetal parathyroid glands. In general, neonates do well if supplemental calcium and vitamin D are started promptly and serum biochemistries are closely monitored. If possible, delivery should be delayed until eucalcemia is achieved in order to allow for normal development of the fetal parathyroid glands. Surgical excision of a symptomatic adenoma is generally recommended in pregnancy during the second trimester. Conservative management throughout pregnancy is, however, possible with close maternal and fetal surveillance, if the patient is asymptomatic and only mild elevations in serum calcium are present.

B. Hypoparathyroidism Hypoparathyroidism in pregnancy is even rarer than hyperparathyroidism and is most commonly due to incidental resection of or damage to the parathyroid glands during thyroidectomy. Symptoms from hypocalcemia include numbness and tingling of fingers and perioral area. If serum calcium levels are maintained within normal limits, pregnancy outcome should not be negatively affected. If not treated, maternal hypocalcemia can lead to hyperparathyroidism in the fetus causing bone demineralization, and labor may be complicated by tetany. Treatment of hypoparathyroidism involves administration of supplemental calcium and vitamin D or its metabolite 1,25-dihydroxyvitamin D.

PREECLAMPSIA/ECLAMPSIA

Preeclampsia is an idiopathic multisystem disease seen only in pregnancy and during the peripartum period. The incidence of preeclampsia is approximately 7%. Risk factors include nulliparity, African American race, extremes of age, chronic hypertension, multiple gestation, prior history of preeclampsia, family history of preeclampsia, chronic renal disease, antiphospholipid antibody syndrome, hydramnios, diabetes, and obesity. Preeclampsia is characterized by onset of hypertension and proteinuria after 20 weeks' gestation. Other signs and symptoms include headache, visual disturbances, epigastric pain, nausea/vomiting, thrombocytopenia, abnormal liver and kidney function tests. Eclampsia is the occurrence of seizures that cannot be attributed to other causes in women with preeclampsia and is associated with a maternal mortality rate as high as 10%. Preeclampsia accounts for approximately 15% of maternal deaths in the United States. Deaths occur most frequently from cerebral hemorrhage, renal failure, disseminated intravascular coagulopathy, acute pulmonary edema, or hepatic failure. Preeclampsia is also associated with perinatal fetal death and morbidity, due most commonly to iatrogenic prematurity.

Pathophysiology

The exact pathogenesis of preeclampsia remains poorly understood despite a significant amount of research in the field. It likely involves both maternal and placental factors as it is also seen in molar pregnancies with only trophoblastic and no fetal tissue. Abnormalities in placental vasculature development are postulated to result in placental hypoxia, which leads to factors being released that cause hypertension and microangiopathy of target organs. Both epidemiologic and experimental data support the role of the placenta in the etiology of preeclampsia as placental tissue is necessary for the development of the disease and once the placenta is removed its signs and symptoms begin to abate.

In preeclampsia, cytotrophoblast invasion is shallow and only the decidual portion of the spiral arteries is remodeled. In contrast, in normal pregnancies the cytotrophoblasts infiltrate deeper into the muscular tunica media of the spiral arteries, transforming these small muscular arterioles into large vessels with low resistance that facilitate placental blow flow (see Figure 16–1). It is likely that environmental, immunologic, and genetic factors all play a role in this important process.

Hypoperfusion and hypoxia are likely both a cause and effect of abnormal placental vascularization and subsequent preeclampsia. Animal models support this theory as induced preeclampsia generally requires mechanically reduced uteroplacental perfusion.

In addition, maternal medical conditions associated with vascular dysfunction such as hypertension, lupus, and renal disease increase the risk of preeclampsia, as do obstetric conditions that increase placental volume without increasing placental blood flow, such as twins and hydatidiform moles.

Generalized endothelial dysfunction may explain many of the multiple clinical features of preeclampsia. Evidence to support this includes enhanced vascular reactivity to angiotensin II, impaired flow-mediated vasodilation, decreased production of endothelial-derived vasodilators such as nitric oxide and prostacyclin, and increased production of vasoconstrictors like endothelins and thromboxanes.

Extensive placental angiogenesis is required to supply the necessary nutrients and oxygen to the fetus. Normal placental vessel development relies on a balance between proangiogenic factors such as VEGF and placental growth factor (PlGF) and antiangiogenic factors such as soluble fms-like tyrosine kinase 1 (sFlt-1) and soluble endoglin (sEng). It is proposed that free sFlt-1 in the maternal circulation antagonizes the angiogenic activities of VEGF and PlGF, leading to ischemia and vasospasm. sEng from the placenta is elevated in preeclamptic women, and appears to inhibit TGF-beta-1-mediated vasodilation.

Despite extensive research and multiple hypotheses regarding its etiology and pathophysiology, there is still no unifying theory that explains all the features of preeclampsia. It is generally accepted that the basis for the development of preeclampsia occurs early in pregnancy. While the roles of antiangiogenic factors such as sFlt-1 and sEng are convincing with regard to the pathogenesis of preeclampsia, the clinical utility of these biomarkers to predict, diagnose, prevent, or treat this disease remains unknown.

Clinical Features

Preeclampsia is classified as mild or severe, the latter designation being applied if any of the following signs or symptoms are present: headache, blurred vision, scotomata, altered mental status, right upper quadrant or epigastric pain, severe hypertension (160/110 mm Hg), pulmonary edema, oliguria (<500 cc/24 h), massive proteinuria (>5 g/24 h), renal failure (creatinine >1 mg/dL over baseline), elevated liver function tests (>2× normal), thrombocytopenia (platelets <100,000), coagulopathy or HELLP syndrome (hemolysis, elevated liver enzymes, low platelets). Despite knowledge of the many risk factors described above, it is still not possible to determine which mothers will ultimately develop preeclampsia and there are no effective preventative treatments. Large clinical trials using low-dose aspirin, calcium, and antioxidant vitamin supplementation revealed minimal to no benefit in preventing the development of preeclampsia. Instead, the current focus of management is for regular prenatal care with screening of blood pressure and proteinuria in hopes of early identification and aggressive monitoring.

Treatment/Management of Preeclampsia

The only definitive therapy for preeclampsia is delivery of fetus and placenta. This is straightforward for pregnancies near term.

However, pregnancies between 24 to 34 weeks are more complicated as the obstetrician must balance the significant perinatal morbidity and mortality associated with preterm delivery versus the maternal and fetal risk of prolonging these high-risk pregnancies. Antihypertensive medications should be used in setting of severe hypertension to prevent a maternal stroke; however, their use in mild to moderate hypertension has not been shown to improve maternal or fetal outcome. Magnesium sulfate therapy is initiated as the anticonvulsant of choice for preeclamptics during labor, while administering corticosteroids prior to a planned preterm delivery, and for 24 hours postpartum.

REFERENCES

General

Haig D. Evolutionary conflicts in pregnancy and calcium metabolism—a review. *Placenta.* 2004;25(suppl A):S10. [PMID: 15033301]

Thung SF, Norwitz ER. Endocrine diseases of pregnancy. In: Strauss JF, Barbieri RL, eds. *Yen and Jaffe's Reproductive Endocrinology. Physiology, Pathophysiology and Clinical Management.* 6th ed. Philadelphia, PA: Elsevier Saunders; 2009.

Chorionic Proteins and Pregnancy Tests

Cole LA. New discoveries on the biology and detection of human chorionic gonadotropin. *Reprod Biol Endocrinol.* 2009;7:8. [PMID: 19171054]

Driscoll DA, Gross S. Clinical practice. Prenatal screening for aneuploidy. *N Engl J Med.* 2009;360:2556. [PMID: 19516035]

Ovarian Proteins

Goldsmith LT, Weiss G. Relaxin in human pregnancy. *Ann N Y Acad Sci.* 2009;1160:130. [PMID: 19416173]

Tsigkou A, Luisi S, Reis FM, Petraglia F. Inhibins as diagnostic markers in human reproduction. *Adv Clin Chem.* 2008;45:1. [PMID: 18429491]

Steroid Hormones

Chang K, Zhang L. Review article: steroid hormones and uterine vascular adaptation to pregnancy. *Reprod Sci.* 2008;15:336. [PMID: 18497342]

Kallen CB. Steroid hormone synthesis in pregnancy. *Obstet Gynecol Clin North Am.* 2004;31:795. [PMID: 15550336]

Miller WL. Steroidogenic enzymes. *Endocr Dev.* 2008;13:1. [PMID: 18493130]

Fetal Endocrinology

de Escobar GM, Ares S, Berbel P, Obregón MJ, del Rey FE. The changing role of maternal thyroid hormone in fetal brain development. *Semin Perinatol.* 2008;32:380. [PMID: 19007674]

Grattan DR. Fetal programming from maternal obesity: eating too much for two? *Endocrinology.* 2008;149:5345. [PMID: 18936494]

MacLaughlin DT, Donahoe PK. Sex determination and differentiation. *N Engl J Med.* 2004;350:367. [PMID: 14736929]

Parturition

Florio P, Romero R, Chaiworapongsa T, et al. Amniotic fluid and umbilical cord plasma corticotropin-releasing factor (CRF), CRF-binding protein, adrenocorticotropin, and cortisol concentrations in intraamniotic infection and inflammation at term. *J Clin Endocrinol Metab.* 2008;93:3604. [PMID: 18559919]

Meis PJ, Aleman A. Progesterone treatment to prevent preterm birth. *Drugs.* 2004;64:2463. [PMID: 15482003]

Mesiano S, Welsh TN. Steroid hormone control of myometrial contractility and parturition. *Semin Cell Dev Biol.* 2007;18:321. [PMID: 17613262]

Smith R, Smith JI, Shen X, et al. Patterns of plasma corticotropin-releasing hormone, progesterone, estradiol, and estriol change and the onset of human labor. *J Clin Endocrinol Metab.* 2009;94:2066. [PMID: 19258402]

Preterm Labor

de Heus R, Mol BW, Erwich JJ, et al. Adverse drug reactions to tocolytic treatment for preterm labour: prospective cohort study. *BMJ.* 2009;5:338. [PMID: 19264820]

Iams JD, Creasy RK. Preterm labor and delivery. In: Creasy RK, Resnick R, eds. Maternal-Fetal Medicine: Principles and Practice. 6th ed. Philadelphia, PA: WB Saunders; 2008.

Menon R, Pearce B, Velez DR, et al. Racial disparity in pathophysiologic pathways of preterm birth based on genetic variants. *Reprod Biol Endocrinol.* 2009;7:62. [PMID: 19527514]

Postterm Pregnancy

Caughey AB, Stotland NE, Washington AE, Escobar GJ. Who is at risk for prolonged and postterm pregnancy? *Am J Obstet Gynecol.* 2009;200:683. [PMID: 19380120]

Puerperium and Lactation

Buhimschi CS. Endocrinology of lactation. *Obstet Gynecol Clin North Am.* 2004;31:963. [PMID: 15550345]

Henderson JJ, Hartmann PE, Newnham JP, Simmer K. Effect of preterm birth and antenatal corticosteroid treatment on lactogenesis II in women. *Pediatrics.* 2008;121:e92. [PMID: 18166549]

Thyroid Disease in Pregnancy

Gyamfi C, Wapner RJ, D'Alton ME. Thyroid dysfunction in pregnancy: the basic science and clinical evidence surrounding the controversy in management. *Obstet Gynecol.* 2009;113:702. [PMID: 19300337]

Patil-Sisodia K, Mestman JH. Graves' hyperthyroidism and pregnancy: a clinical update. *Endocr Pract.* 2009;15:1. [PMID: 19833580]

Toft A. Increased levothyroxine requirements in pregnancy—why, when, and how much? *New Engl J Med.* 2004;351:292. [PMID: 15254288]

Pituitary Adenomas

Christin-Maître S, Delemer B, Touraine P, Young J. Prolactinoma and estrogens: pregnancy, contraception and hormonal replacement therapy. *Ann Endocrinol (Paris).* 2007;68:106. [PMID: 17540335]

Obesity

Catalano PM. Management of obesity in pregnancy. *Obstet Gynecol.* 2007;109:419. [PMID:17267845]

Parathyroid Disease

Sato K. Hypercalcemia during pregnancy, puerperium, and lactation: review and a case report of hypercalcemic crisis after delivery due to excessive production of PTH-related protein (PTHrP) without malignancy (humoral hypercalcemia of pregnancy). *Endocr J.* 2008;55:959. [PMID: 18614854]

Hypertensive Disorders

Karumanchi SA, Maynard SE, Stillman IE, Epstein FH, Sukhatme VP. Preeclampsia: a renal perspective. *Kidney Int.* 2005;67:2101. [PMID: 15882253]

Redman CW, Sargent IL. Placental stress and pre-eclampsia: a revised view. *Placenta.* 2009;30 (suppl A):S38. [PMID: 19138798]

Roberts JM. Pregnancy-related hypertension. In: Creasy RK, Resnick R, eds. *Maternal-Fetal Medicine: Principles and Practice.* 6th ed. Philadelphia, PA: WB Saunders; 2008.

Sibai BM. Maternal and uteroplacental hemodynamics for the classification and prediction of preeclampsia. *Hypertension.* 2008;52:805. [PMID: 18824659]

Pancreatic Hormones and Diabetes Mellitus

Umesh Masharani, MB, BS, MRCP (UK)
and Michael S. German, MD

ABCC8	ATP-binding cassette transporter sub-family C member 8		**FFA**	Free fatty acid
ACE	Angiotensin-converting enzyme		**FHR**	Fetal heart rate
ADA	American Diabetes Association		**Foxo1**	Forkhead box, subfamily O, member 1
ADH	Antidiuretic hormone (vasopressin)		**FOXP3**	Forkhead box, subfamily P, member 3
AGE	Advanced glycation end product		**GABA**	Gamma-aminobutyric acid
AGPAT	1-acylglycerol-3-phosphate-O-acyltransferase 2		**GAD**	Glutamic acid decarboxylase
AKT/PKB	AKR mouse tumor 8 kinase/protein kinase B		**GCK**	Glucokinase
			GH	Growth hormone
AIRE	Autoimmune regulator		**GHb**	Glycohemoglobin
ALT	Alanine aminotransferase		**GHSR**	Growth hormone-secretagogue receptor
AMPK	Adenosine monophosphate-activated protein kinase		**GI**	Glycemic index
APS1	Autoimmune polyendocrinopathy syndrome type 1		**GIP**	Gastric inhibitory polypeptide
			GLIS3	Glioma-associated oncogene homolog—similar 3
ATF6	Activating transcription factor 6		**GLP-1**	Glucagon-like peptide-1
BMI	Body mass index		**GLP-2**	Glucagon-like peptide-2
cAMP	Cyclic adenosine monophosphate		**GLUT**	Glucose transporter
CCK	Cholecystokinin		**GPCR**	G protein–coupled receptor
CEL	Carboxyl-ester lipase		**GRPP**	Glicentin-related polypeptide
cGMP	Cyclic 3′,5′-guanosine monophosphate		**GWAS**	Genome-wide association study
CIDEC	Cell death-inducing DFFA-like effector C		**HDL**	High-density lipoprotein
CSII	Continuous subcutaneous insulin infusion		**HLA**	Human leukocyte antigen
CST	Contraction stress test		**HNF**	Hepatocyte nuclear factor
DCCT	Diabetes Control and Complications Trial		**hPL**	Human placental lactogen
DIDMOAD	Diabetes insipidus, diabetes mellitus, optic atrophy, deafness (Wolfram syndrome)		**IA2**	Insulinoma antigen 2
			IAA	Insulin autoantibody
DPP	Diabetes Prevention Program		**IAPP**	Islet amyloid polypeptide
DPP-4	Dipeptidyl peptidase 4		**ICA**	Islet cell antibody
DPT-1	Diabetes Prevention Trial-1		**IFG**	Impaired fasting glucose
EIF2AK3	Eukaryotic translation initiation factor 2-α kinase 3		**IGF-1**	Insulin-like growth factor 1
			IGT	Impaired glucose tolerance
ER	Endoplasmic reticulum		**IL-6**	Interleukin-6
FDA	Food and Drug Administration		**INS**	Insulin

IP3	Inositol 1,4,5-triphosphate	**PGC1α**	PPAR gamma coactivator-1α
IPEX	Immunodysregulation polyendocrinopathy enteropathy, X-linked	**PNDM**	Permanent neonatal diabetes mellitus
IPF-1	Insulin promoter factor-1	**POEMS**	Polyneuropathy, organomegaly, endocrinopathy, monoclonal gammopathy, and skin changes
IRE1	Inositol-requiring enzyme 1		
IRS	Insulin receptor substrate	**PP**	Pancreatic polypeptide
ISL1	Islet transcription factor 1	**PPAR**	Peroxisome proliferator-activated receptor
IUGR	Intrauterine growth restriction	**PTF1A**	Pancreatic transcription factor 1α
KPD	Ketosis-prone diabetes	**PTP1b**	Protein tyrosine phosphatase 1b
KCNJ11	Potassium inwardly-rectifying channel, subfamily J, member 11	**RFX6**	Regulatory factor X-6
		RXR	9-*cis*-retinoic acid receptor
Kir6.2	Potassium channel, inwardly-rectifying 6.2	**SCL19A2**	Solute carrier family 19 (thiamine transporter), member 2
LADA	Latent autoimmune diabetes of adulthood	**SOCS**	Suppressor of cytokine signaling
		SREBP1c	Sterol regulatory element-binding protein 1c
LBK1	Liver kinase B1	**SSTR**	Somatostatin receptor
LDL	Low-density lipoprotein	**SUR1**	Sulfonylurea receptor 1
MAPK	Mitogen-activated protein kinase	**TCF7L2**	Transcription factor 7-like 2
MODY	Maturity-onset diabetes of the young	**TGF-β**	Transforming growth factor-β
MHC	Major histocompatibility complex	**TNDM**	Transient neonatal diabetes mellitus
mTOR	Mammalian target of rapamycin	**TNF-α**	Tumor necrosis factor-α
NeuroD1	Neural differentiation factor 1	**UGDP**	University Group Diabetes Program
Neurog3	Neural genesis factor 3	**UKPDS**	United Kingdom Prospective Diabetes Study
NIH	National Institutes of Health		
NPH	Neutral protamine hagedorn	**VEGF**	Vascular endothelial growth factor
NST	Nonstress test	**VLDL**	Very low density lipoprotein
PAI-1	Plasminogen activator inhibitor-1	**VNTR**	Variable number of tandem repeats
PAX4	Paired homeobox 4	**WFS1**	Wolfram syndrome protein 1
PCSK	Proprotein convertase, subtilisin/kexin	**ZAC**	Zinc finger protein-inducing apoptosis and cell cycle arrest
PDE5	Phosphodiesterase type 5		
PDX1	Pancreatic duodenal homeobox-1	**ZnT8**	Zinc transporter 8
PERK	Protein kinase R-like endoplasmic reticulum kinase	**ZFP57**	Zinc finger protein 57

THE ENDOCRINE PANCREAS

The pancreas comprises two functionally distinct organs: the **exocrine pancreas**, the major digestive gland of the body; and the **endocrine pancreas,** the source of insulin, glucagon, somatostatin, pancreatic polypeptide (PP), and ghrelin. Whereas the major role of the products of the exocrine pancreas (the digestive enzymes) is the processing of ingested foodstuffs so that they become available for absorption, the hormones of the endocrine pancreas modulate every other aspect of cellular nutrition from rate of adsorption of foodstuffs to cellular storage or metabolism of nutrients. Dysfunction of the endocrine pancreas or abnormal responses to its hormones by target tissues cause serious disturbances in nutrient homeostasis, including the important clinical syndromes grouped under the name **diabetes mellitus.**

ANATOMY AND HISTOLOGY

The endocrine pancreas consists of approximately 1 million small endocrine glands—the islets of Langerhans—scattered throughout the glandular substance of the exocrine pancreas. The exocrine pancreas consists of the enzyme-producing cells organized into acini, and the duct system that delivers those enzymes to the lumen of the duodenum. The islet volume comprises 1% to 1.5% of the total mass of the pancreas and weighs about 1 to 2 g in adult humans. At least five cell types—α, β, δ, ε, and PP—have been identified in the islets (Table 17–1). Each of these islet cell types produces a distinguishing peptide hormone: glucagon, insulin, somatostatin, ghrelin, and PP, respectively. Within individual islets, the different cell types are scattered throughout. A typical human islet is depicted in Figure 17–1.

TABLE 17–1 Cell types in adult human pancreatic islets of Langerhans.

Cell Types	Approximate Percentage of Islet Volume	Secretory Products
α Cell	25%	Glucagon, proglucagon
β Cell	55%	Insulin, C peptide, proinsulin, IAPP, γ-aminobutyric acid (GABA)
δ Cell	10%	Somatostatin-14
ε Cell	3%	Ghrelin
PP cell	5%	Pancreatic polypeptide

These cell types are not distributed uniformly throughout the pancreas. The PP cells reside primarily in islets in the posterior portion (posterior lobe) of the head, a discrete lobe of the pancreas separated from the anterior portion by a fascial partition. This lobe originates in the primordial ventral bud as opposed to the dorsal bud. The posterior lobe receives its blood supply from the superior mesenteric artery; the remainder of

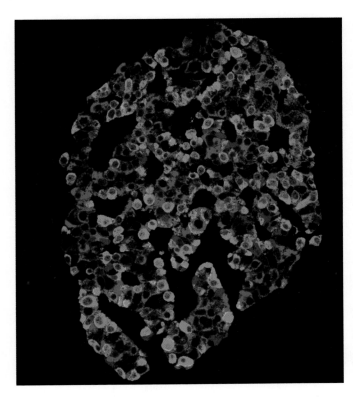

FIGURE 17–1 Human islet of Langerhans. Staining for insulin (red), glucagon (green), and somatostatin (blue) was performed by immunofluorescence and imaged by confocal microscopy. (Reproduced, with permission, from Cabrera O, Berman DM, Kenyon NS, Ricordi C, Berggren PO, Caicedo A. The unique cytoarchitecture of human pancreatic islets has implications for islet cell function. *Proc Natl Acad Sci.* 2006;103(7):2334.)

the pancreas derives most of its blood flow from the celiac artery. The islets themselves are richly vascularized, receiving five to ten times the blood flow of the surrounding exocrine pancreatic tissue. Each islet is surrounded by a lattice of astroglial cells and innervated by sympathetic, parasympathetic, and sensory neurons.

HORMONES OF THE ENDOCRINE PANCREAS

1. INSULIN

Biosynthesis

The human insulin gene resides on the short arm of chromosome 11. A unique set of transcription factors found in the β cell nucleus activates the transcription of the preproinsulin mRNA from the *insulin* gene (Figure 17–2). A precursor molecule, **preproinsulin**, a peptide of MW 11,500, is translated from the preproinsulin messenger RNA in the rough endoplasmic reticulum of pancreatic β cells (see Figure 17–2). Microsomal enzymes cleave preproinsulin to proinsulin (MW ~9000) almost immediately after synthesis. Proinsulin is transported to the Golgi apparatus, where packaging into clathrin-coated secretory granules takes place. Maturation of the secretory granule is associated with loss of the clathrin coating and conversion of proinsulin into insulin and a smaller connecting peptide, or C peptide, by proteolytic cleavage at two sites along the peptide chain. Mature secretory granules contain insulin and C peptide in equimolar amounts and only small quantities of proinsulin, a small portion of which consists of partially cleaved intermediates.

Biochemistry

Proinsulin (Figure 17–3) consists of a single chain of 86 amino acids, which includes the A and B chains of the insulin molecule plus a connecting segment of 35 amino acids. Two proteins—the prohormone-converting enzymes type 1 and 2 (PCSK1 and PCSK2)—are packaged with proinsulin in the immature secretory granules. These enzymes recognize and cut at pairs of basic amino acids, thereby removing the intervening sequence. After the two pairs of basic amino acids are removed by carboxypeptidase E, the result is a 51 amino acid insulin molecule and a 31 amino acid residue, the C peptide, as shown in Figure 17–3.

A small amount of proinsulin produced by the pancreas escapes cleavage and is secreted intact into the bloodstream, along with insulin and C peptide. Most anti-insulin sera used in the standard immunoassay for insulin cross-react with proinsulin; about 3% to 5% of immunoreactive insulin extracted from human pancreas is actually proinsulin. Because proinsulin is not removed by the liver, it has a half-life three to four times that of insulin. Its long half-life allows proinsulin to accumulate in the blood, where it accounts for 12% to 20% of the circulating immunoreactive insulin in the basal state in humans. Human proinsulin has about 7% to 8% of the biologic activity of insulin. The kidney is the principal site of proinsulin degradation.

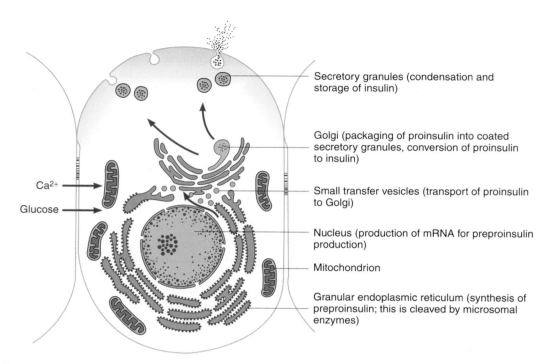

FIGURE 17–2 Structural components of the pancreatic β cell involved in glucose-induced biosynthesis and release of insulin. (Modified and reproduced, with permission, from Junqueira LC, Carneiro J, Long JA. *Basic Histology*. 5th ed. McGraw-Hill; 1986.)

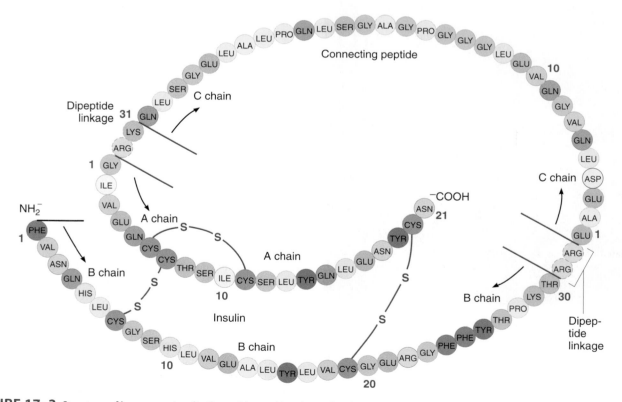

FIGURE 17–3 Structure of human proinsulin C peptides and insulin molecules connected at two sites by dipeptide links.

Of the two major proinsulin split products present in plasma, the one split at arginine 32-33 far exceeds in amount the barely detectable 65-66 split product. In control subjects, concentrations of proinsulin and 32-33 split proinsulin after an overnight fast averaged 2.3 and 2.2 pmol/L, respectively, with corresponding postprandial rises to 10 and 20 pmol/L.

C peptide, the 31 amino acid peptide (MW 3000) released during cleavage of insulin from proinsulin, has no known biologic activity. β Cells release C peptide in equimolar amounts with insulin. It is not removed by the liver but is degraded or excreted chiefly by the kidney. It has a half-life three to four times that of insulin. In the basal state after an overnight fast, the average concentration of C peptide may remain as high as 1000 pmol/L.

Insulin is a protein consisting of 51 amino acids contained within two peptide chains: an A chain, with 21 amino acids; and a B chain, with 30 amino acids. The chains are connected by two disulfide bridges as shown in Figure 17–3. In addition, an intra-chain disulfide bridge links positions 6 and 11 in the A chain. Human insulin has a molecular weight of 5808.

Endogenous insulin has a circulatory half-life of 3 to 5 minutes. It is degraded chiefly by insulinases in liver, kidney, and placenta. A single pass through the liver removes approximately 50% of the plasma insulin.

Secretion

The human pancreas secretes about 30 units of insulin per day into the portal circulation of normal adults in distinct pulses with a period of approximately 5 minutes. The basal concentration of insulin in the peripheral blood of fasting humans averages 10 μU/mL (0.4 ng/mL, or 61 pmol/L). In normal control subjects, insulin seldom rises above 100 μU/mL (610 pmol/L) after standard meals. After ingestion of food, peripheral insulin concentration increases within 8 to 10 minutes, reaches peak concentrations by 30 to 45 minutes, and then rapidly declines to baseline values by 90 to 120 minutes postprandially.

Basal insulin secretion occurs in the absence of exogenous stimuli, in the fasting state. Plasma glucose levels below 80 to 100 mg/dL (4.4-5.6 mmol/L) do not stimulate insulin release, and most other physiologic regulators of insulin secretion only function in the presence of stimulatory levels of glucose. Stimulated insulin secretion occurs in response to exogenous stimuli. In vivo, ingested meals provide the major stimuli for insulin secretion. Glucose is the most potent stimulant of insulin release. The perfused pancreas releases insulin in two phases in response to glucose stimulation (Figure 17–4). When the glucose concentration increases suddenly, an initial short-lived burst of insulin release occurs (the **first phase**); if the glucose elevation persists, the insulin release gradually falls off and then begins to rise again to a steady level (the **second phase**). However, sustained levels of high glucose stimulation (~4 hours in vitro or >24 hours in vivo) result in a reversible desensitization of the β cell response to glucose but not to other stimuli.

The β cell senses glucose through its metabolism (Figure 17–5). Indeed, agents such as 2-deoxyglucose that inhibit the metabolism of glucose block the release of insulin. Glucose enters the pancreatic β cell by passive diffusion, facilitated by membrane proteins termed glucose transporters (see later). Because the transporters function in both directions, and the β cell has an excess of glucose transporters, the glucose concentration inside the β cell is

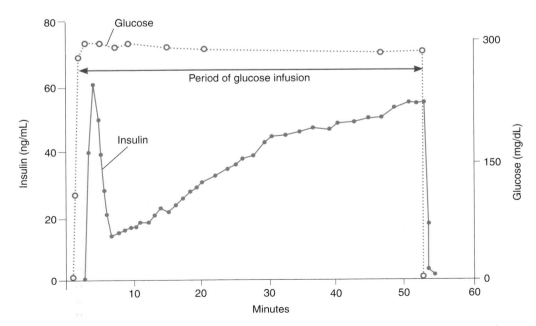

FIGURE 17–4 Multiphasic response of the in vitro perfused rat pancreas during constant stimulation with glucose. (Modified from Grodsky GM, et al. Further studies on the dynamic aspects of insulin release *in vitro* with evidence for a two-compartment storage system. *Acta Diabetol Lat.* 1969;6[suppl 1]:554.)

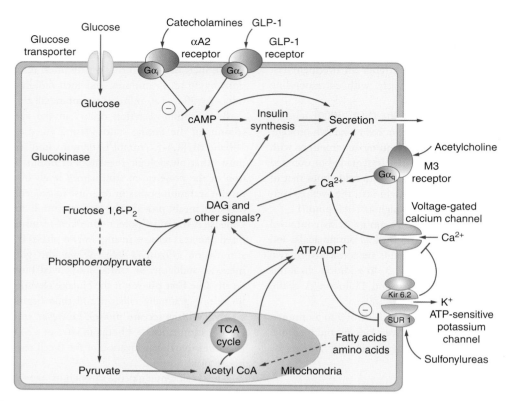

FIGURE 17–5 A simplified outline of glucose-sensing and regulated insulin secretion from the β cell. The blue arrows indicate stimulation, and the red lines indicate inhibition. Glucose enters the β cell through facultative glucose transporters, is phosphorylated to glucose-6-phosphate by glucokinse, and enters glycolysis. This results in the production of pyruvate, which enters the mitochondria, is converted to acetyl-CoA, and feeds the tricarboxylic acid (TCA) cycle and oxidative phosphorylation to produce ATP. When ATP levels rise or sulfonylureas bind to the regulatory subunit (SUR1/ABCC8) of the ATP-sensitive K$^+$ channels, the channel subunit (Kir6.2/KCNJ11) closes. This block of the K$^+$ current depolarizes the cell, allowing the voltage-gated calcium channels to open. The entry of calcium drives the fusion of insulin granules with the cell surface membrane and exocytosis of insulin. Glucose metabolism and extracellular signals modulate this pathway through release of Ca^{2+} from intracellular stores and changes in diacylglycerol (DAG), cAMP, and other intracellular signaling pathways.

in equilibrium with the extracellular glucose concentration. The low-affinity enzyme glucokinase catalyzes the subsequent, and rate-limiting, step in glucose metabolism by the pancreatic β cell, the phosphorylation of glucose to glucose-6-phosphate. Glucose catabolism in the β cell causes a rise in the intracellular ATP-ADP ratio. Acting through the sulfonylurea receptor (SUR1), the nucleotide-sensing subunit of the ATP-sensitive potassium channels on the surface of the β cell, the rise in ATP-ADP ratio closes the potassium channels and depolarizes the cell, thereby activating the voltage-sensitive calcium channels and allowing the entry of calcium ions into the cell.

Insulin release requires calcium ion signaling. In addition to the voltage-dependent entry of extracellular Ca^{2+} into the β cell as described earlier, glucose also retards Ca^{2+} efflux from the β cell and releases Ca^{2+} from intracellular compartments (predominantly the endoplasmic reticulum) into the cytosol. Some nonglucose stimuli of insulin release also function through increases in cytoplasmic Ca^{2+}. The sulfonylurea and meglitinide (such as repaglinide) medications act by closing the ATP-sensitive potassium channels. Secretagogues such as acetylcholine that act through G protein–coupled receptors of the Gα$_q$ class stimulate the release of

intracellular Ca^{2+} stored in the endoplasmic reticulum by activating phospholipase C and releasing the intracellular signaling molecule inositol 1,4,5-triphosphate (IP3).

Glucose metabolism in the β cell also generates additional signals that amplify the secretory response to elevations in cytoplasmic Ca^{2+} concentration. The exact mechanisms of these amplifying signals remains unknown but involve multiple pathways and include increases in the intracellular signaling molecules diacylglycerol and cAMP. Secretagogues such as the gut hormones glucagon-like peptide-1 (GLP-1) and gastric inhibitory polypeptide (also known as glucose-dependent insulinotropic peptide, GIP) that act via G protein–coupled receptors of the Gα$_s$ class also stimulate insulin secretion through elevations in cAMP.

Other factors involved in the regulation of insulin secretion are summarized in Table 17–2. These factors can be divided into three categories: **direct stimulants**, which directly raise cytoplasmic calcium ion concentrations and thus can act in the absence of stimulatory glucose concentrations; **amplifiers**, which potentiate the response of the β cell to glucose; and **inhibitors**. Many of the amplifiers are **incretins**: gastrointestinal hormones that are released in response to the ingestion of meals and stimulate insulin secretion.

TABLE 17–2 Regulation of insulin release.

Stimulants of insulin release	Glucose Amino acids: Leucine Neural: Vagal stimulation, acetylcholine Drugs: Sulfonylureas, meglitinides

Amplifiers of glucose-induced insulin release	Enteric hormones:
	  Glucagon-like peptide 1 (7–37) (GLP1)
	  Gastric inhibitory peptide (GIP)
	  Cholecystokinin, gastrin
	  Secretin
	Neural: β-adrenergic effect of
	  catecholamines
	Amino acids: arginine
	Drugs: GLP1 agonists

Inhibitors of insulin release	Neural: α-adrenergic effect of
	  catecholamines
	Humoral: somatostatin
	Drugs: diazoxide, thiazides, β-blockers,
	  clonidine, phenytoin, vinblastine,
	  colchicine

The action of the incretins explains the observation that orally ingested glucose provokes a greater insulin secretory response than does the same amount of intravenously administered glucose.

Insulin Receptors and Insulin Action

Insulin action begins with the binding of insulin to a receptor on the surface of the target cell membrane. Most cells of the body have specific cell surface insulin receptors. In fat, liver, and muscle cells, binding of insulin to these receptors is associated with the biologic response of these tissues to the hormone. These receptors bind insulin rapidly, with high specificity and with an affinity high enough to bind picomolar amounts.

Insulin receptors, members of the growth factor receptor family (see Chapter 1), are membrane glycoproteins composed of two protein subunits encoded by a single gene. The larger alpha subunit (MW 135,000) resides entirely extracellularly, where it binds the insulin molecule. The alpha subunit is tethered by disulfide linkage to the smaller beta subunit (MW 95,000). The beta subunit crosses the membrane, and its cytoplasmic domain contains a tyrosine kinase activity that initiates specific intracellular signaling pathways.

Downstream signaling.   On binding of insulin to the alpha subunit, the beta subunit activates itself by autophosphorylation. The activated beta subunit then recruits additional proteins to the complex and phosphorylates a network of intracellular substrates, including insulin receptor substrate-1 (IRS-1), insulin receptor substrate-2 (IRS-2), and others (Figure 17–6). These activated substrates each lead to subsequent recruitment and activation of additional kinases, phosphatases, and other signaling molecules in a complex pathway that generally contains two arms: the mitogenic pathway, which mediates the growth effects of insulin and the metabolic pathway, which regulates nutrient metabolism.

In the metabolic signaling pathway, activation of phosphatidylinositol-3-kinase leads to the activation of serine/threonine kinase AKT/PKB. AKT activation drives the movement of glucose transporter (GLUT) 4–containing vesicles to the cell membrane, increases glycogen and lipid synthesis, and stimulates protein synthesis through the activation of mTOR. In the mitogenic signaling pathway, activation of Ras initiates a cascade of activating phosphorylations via the MAP kinase pathway, leading to cell growth and proliferation.

Transcriptional regulation.   In addition, the insulin-signaling pathway regulates the activity of several nuclear transcription factors that in turn control the expression of genes involved in metabolism and growth. These include members of the forkedhead family of transcription factors, including Foxo1, which is inactivated by phosphorylation by AKT downstream of insulin signaling. Foxo1 coordinates the expression of gene networks involved in nutrient metabolism in multiple tissues, generally activating genes involved in the response to fasting. In this process, Foxo1 works with several other transcriptional regulators including the lipogenic transcription factor SREBP1c, members of the PPAR family of nuclear receptors and the PPAR coactivator PGC1α (Figure 17–7). Foxo1 also inhibits β cell proliferation and survival.

The three members of the PPAR family of nuclear hormone receptors play pleiotropic roles in regulating genes involved in metabolism in many tissues. They may function as targets of insulin signaling, modulators of insulin signaling, or both. Despite overlap in the tissue expression and gene targets of the three PPARs, some general conclusions can be drawn about the function of each. PPARα regulates genes involved in fatty acid catabolism and gluconeogenesis and is most highly expressed in brown fat, heart, liver, kidney, and intestine. PPARβ/δ is broadly expressed and activates gene programs involved in fatty acid oxidation. PPARγ is most highly expressed in adipose tissue, intestine, and immune cells, but also at lower levels in many other tissues. PPARγ drives white adipocyte differentiation and lipid storage and inhibits production of many of the pro-resistance adipokines and pro-inflammatory cytokines in adipose tissue (see section on insulin resistance later). In macrophages, PPARγ acts to promote their alternative activation to the anti-inflammatory M2 state, rather than the pro-inflammatory M1 state.

The PPARs bind to DNA as heterodimers with the 9-*cis*-retinoic acid receptor (RXR), and recruit a variety of coactivators and corepressors. PGC1α was originally identified as a coactivator interacting with PPARγ, but the interaction is not exclusive. On different genes PPARγ works with different coactivators, and PGC1α interacts with the other PPARs and many other transcription factors. In collaboration with a variety of different transcription factors in various tissues, PGC1α orchestrates the expression of a set of genes involved in metabolism. PGC1α itself is highly regulated by several signaling pathways including insulin signaling, which inhibits PGC1α activity via phosphorylation by AKT.

A number of natural and synthetic lipids and related compounds can act as PPAR ligands, but the endogenous ligands acting in vivo remain a mystery. The fibrate class of lipid-lowering drugs, used clinically to lower circulating triglyceride levels, act as PPARα ligands. The thiazolidinedione class of insulin-sensitizing

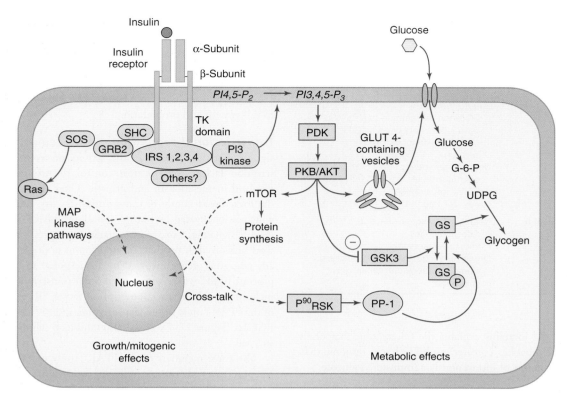

FIGURE 17-6 A simplified outline of insulin signaling. A minimal diagram of the mitogenic and metabolic arms of the insulin-signaling pathway is shown. GLUT 4, glucose transporter 4; Grb-2, growth factor receptor–binding protein 2; GS, glycogen synthase (P indicates the inactive phosphorylated form); GSK-3, glycogen synthase kinase 3; IRS, insulin receptor substrate (four different proteins); MAP kinase, mitogen-activated protein kinase; mTOR, mammalian target of rapamycin; PDK, phospholipid-dependent kinase; PI3 kinase, phosphatidylinositol 3 kinase; PKB/AKT, protein kinase B/AKR mouse tumor 8 kinase; PP-1, glycogen-associated protein phosphatase-1; Ras, rat sarcoma protein; SHC, Src and collagen homology protein; SOS, son-of-sevenless related protein; TK, tyrosine kinase).

drugs, used for the treatment of type 2 diabetes (see later), act as PPARγ ligands.

Deactivation of insulin signaling. Once activated by binding to insulin, the insulin receptor and downstream signaling cascades rapidly deactivate again by several mechanisms. Insulin can simply disengage from the receptor, or the receptor can be internalized and degraded. The receptor and its tyrosine-phosphorylated substrates can be deactivated by specific protein tyrosine phosphatases such as PTP1b. In addition, inhibitory SOCS (suppressor of cytokine signaling) proteins block interactions between the phosphorylated receptor and interacting IRS proteins, direct the ubiquitination and degradation of the IRS proteins, and terminate the activation of downstream components of the signaling pathway. Finally, serine phosphorylation of the insulin receptor and its active substrates by several different serine/threonine kinases, including components of the insulin-signaling pathway such as AKT, blocks insulin signaling. Many of these mechanisms may play a role in the development of insulin resistance (see later).

Metabolic Effects of Insulin

The major function of insulin is to promote storage of ingested nutrients. Although insulin directly or indirectly affects the function of almost every tissue in the body, the discussion here will be limited to a brief overview of the effects of insulin on the major tissues specialized for energy metabolism: liver, muscle, adipose tissue, and brain. In addition, the paracrine effects of insulin will be discussed briefly.

A. Paracrine effects The effects of the products of endocrine cells on surrounding cells are termed **paracrine effects,** in contrast to actions that take place at sites distant from the secreting cells, which are termed **endocrine effects** (see Chapter 1). Paracrine effects of the β and δ cells on the nearby α cells (see Figure 17–1) are of considerable importance in the endocrine pancreas. Insulin directly inhibits α cell secretion of glucagon. In addition, somatostatin, which δ cells release in response to most of the same stimuli that provoke insulin release, also inhibits glucagon secretion.

Because glucose stimulates only β and δ cells (whose products then inhibit α cells) whereas amino acids stimulate glucagon as well as insulin, the type and amounts of islet hormones released during a meal depend on the ratio of ingested carbohydrate to protein. The higher the carbohydrate content of a meal, the lower the amount of glucagon released by any amino acids absorbed. In contrast, a predominantly protein meal results in relatively greater glucagon secretion, because amino acids are less effective at stimulating insulin release in the absence of concurrent hyperglycemia but are potent stimulators of α cells.

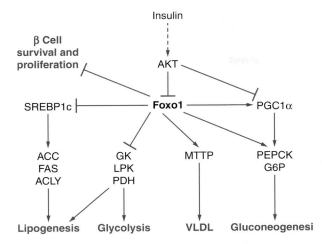

FIGURE 17–7 Regulation and function of Foxo1. The blue arrows indicate stimulation, and the red lines indicate inhibition. Processes activated by Foxo1 are labeled in blue, while the processes inhibited by Foxo1 are shown in red. (ACC, acetyl-CoA carboxylase; ACLY, ATP-citrate lyase; AKT, AKR mouse tumor 8 kinase; FAS, fatty acid synthase; G6P, glucose-6-phosphatase; GK, glucokinase; LPK, liver pyruvate kinase; MTTP, microsomal triglyceride transfer protein; PDH, pyruvate dehydrogenase; PEPCK, phosphoenolpyruvate carboxykinase; PGC1α, peroxisome proliferator-activated receptor gamma coactivator-1; SREBP1c, sterol regulatory element-binding protein 1c).

TABLE 17–3 Endocrine effects of insulin.

Tissue	Effect of Insulin
Liver	**Catabolic Pathways** Inhibits glycogenolysis Inhibits conversion of fatty acids and amino acids to keto acids Inhibits conversion of amino acids to glucose **Anabolic Pathways** Promotes glucose storage as glycogen (induces glucokinase and glycogen synthase, inhibits phosphorylase) Increases triglyceride synthesis and VLDL formation
Muscle	**Protein Synthesis** Increases amino acid transport Increases ribosomal protein synthesis **Glycogen Synthesis** Increases glucose transport Induces glycogen synthethase Inhibits phosphorylase
Adipose Tissue	**Triglyceride Storage** Lipoprotein lipase is induced by insulin to hydrolyze triglycerides in circulating lipoproteins for delivery of fatty acids to the adipocytes Glucose transport into cell provides glycerol phosphate to permit esterification of fatty acids supplied by lipoprotein transport Intracellular lipase is inhibited by insulin
Brain	**Decreased appetite** **Increased energy expenditure**

B. Endocrine effects (Table 17–3)

1. **Liver**—The first major organ reached by insulin via the bloodstream is the liver. Insulin exerts its action on the liver in two major ways:

   a. **Insulin promotes anabolism**—Insulin promotes glycogen synthesis and storage while inhibiting glycogen breakdown. These effects are mediated by changes in the activity of enzymes in the glycogen synthesis pathway (see below). The liver has a maximum storage capacity of 100 to 110 g of glycogen, or approximately 440 kcal of energy.

   Insulin increases both protein and triglyceride synthesis and very low density lipoprotein (VLDL) formation by the liver. It also inhibits gluconeogenesis and promotes glycolysis through its effects on the function and expression of key enzymes of both pathways.

   b. **Insulin inhibits catabolism**—Insulin acts to reverse the catabolic events of the postabsorptive state by inhibiting hepatic glycogenolysis, ketogenesis, and gluconeogenesis.

2. **Muscle**—Insulin promotes protein synthesis in muscle by increasing amino acid transport, as well as by stimulating ribosomal protein synthesis. In addition, insulin promotes glycogen synthesis to replace glycogen stores expended by muscle activity. This is accomplished by increasing glucose transport into the muscle cell, enhancing the activity of glycogen synthase, and inhibiting the activity of glycogen phosphorylase. Approximately 500 to 600 g of glycogen are stored in the muscle tissue of a 70-kg man, but because of the lack of glucose 6-phosphatase in this tissue, it cannot be used as a source of blood glucose, except for a small amount produced when the debranching enzyme releases unphosphorylated glucose from branch points in the glycogen polymer, and the glucose indirectly produced via the liver from lactate generated by muscle.

3. **Adipose tissue**—Fat, in the form of triglyceride, is the most efficient means of storing energy. It provides 9 kcal/g of stored substrate, as opposed to the 4 kcal/g generally provided by protein or carbohydrate. In the typical 70-kg man, the energy content of adipose tissue is about 100,000 kcal.

   Insulin acts to promote triglyceride storage in adipocytes by a number of mechanisms. (1) It induces the production of lipoprotein lipase in adipose tissue (this is the lipoprotein lipase that is bound to endothelial cells in adipose tissue and other vascular beds), which leads to hydrolysis of triglycerides from circulating lipoproteins, thereby yielding fatty acids for uptake by adipocytes. (2) By increasing glucose transport into fat cells, insulin increases the availability of α-glycerol phosphate, a substance used in the esterification of free fatty acids into triglycerides. (3) Insulin inhibits intracellular lipolysis of stored triglyceride by inhibiting intracellular lipase (also called **hormone-sensitive lipase**). This reduction of fatty acid flux to the liver is a key regulatory factor in the action of insulin to lower hepatic gluconeogenesis and ketogenesis.

4. **Central nervous system**—Although the brain is traditionally not considered an insulin-sensitive tissue, and overall glucose utilization by the brain is not acutely regulated by insulin, key regions of the brain can respond to insulin. Insulin signaling via PI3 kinase in key cells in the hypothalamus functions with leptin signaling to decrease appetite and increase energy expenditure (see Chapter 20).

C. AMPK and insulin-independent regulation of nutrient metabolism

Insulin, along with the counter-regulatory hormones and other circulating enhancers and inhibitors of their actions, coordinates nutrient metabolism in response to the overall needs of the organism. At the level of the individual cell, however, additional mechanisms sense and respond to the local energy state. Among these mechanisms, adenosine monophosphate protein kinase (AMPK) plays a central role. When energy availability falls, the drop in cellular ATP concentration and rise in AMP trigger a conformational change in the trimeric AMPK complex and the subsequent activation of the catalytic domain by the serine/threonine kinase LBK1/STK11. AMPK then drives the production of ATP by activating catabolic pathways and inhibiting synthetic pathways in the cell (Figure 17–8). In muscle, in response to the rise in AMP during exercise, AMPK increases fatty acid oxidation and insulin-independent glucose uptake while inhibiting mTOR and protein synthesis. In the long term, AMPK also drives mitochondrial biogenesis. In liver cells, AMPK blocks fatty acid and triglyceride synthesis while activating fatty acid oxidation, and also inhibits the gluconeogenic program by blocking cAMP activation of gene expression and inhibiting Foxo1/PGC1α-driven expression of the gluconeogenic genes. In brain, AMPK also functions as an energy sensor and plays a role in the regulation of appetite and energy expenditure by the hypothalamus. AMPK has also been implicated in the regulation of insulin secretion by β cells.

While predominantly an intracellular energy sensor, AMPK increases the sensitivity of cells to insulin, although the mechanisms remain uncertain. AMPK also responds to extracellular signals, and

contributes to the regulation of metabolism by many of the adipokines and cytokines (see later) as well as cannabinoids. The biguanide drugs, including metformin, which is used in the treatment of type 2 diabetes, activate AMPK by reducing mitochondrial production of ATP and raising intracellular levels of AMP, and thereby lower blood glucose levels by inhibiting gluconeogenesis.

Glucose Transporter Proteins

Glucose oxidation provides energy for most cells and is critical for brain function. Because cell membranes are impermeable to hydrophilic molecules such as glucose, all cells require carrier proteins to transport glucose across the lipid bilayers into the cytosol. Whereas the intestine and kidney have an energy-dependent Na^+-glucose cotransporter, all other cells utilize non-energy-dependent transporters that facilitate diffusion of glucose from a higher concentration to a lower concentration across cell membranes. Facilitative glucose transporters (GLUTs) comprise a large family including at least 13 members, although some of the recently identified members of the family have not yet been shown to transport glucose. The first four members of the family are the best characterized, and they have distinct affinities for glucose and distinct patterns of expression.

GLUT 1 is present in all human tissues. It mediates basal glucose uptake, because it has a very high affinity for glucose and,

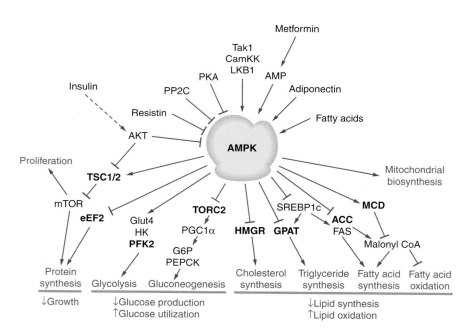

FIGURE 17–8 Regulation and function of AMPK. Proteins that are directly phosphorylated by AMPK are shown in bold font. The blue arrows indicate stimulation, and the red lines indicate inhibition. Processes activated by AMPK are labeled in blue, while the processes inhibited by AMPK are shown in red. (ACC, acetyl-CoA carboxylase; AKT, AKR mouse tumor 8 kinase; CamKK, calcium/calmodulin-dependent protein kinase kinase; eEF2, eukaryotic translation elongation factor 2; FAS, fatty acid synthase; G6P, glucose-6-phosphatase; GPAT, glycerol-3-phosphate acyltransferase, mitochondrial; HK, hexokinase; HMGR, HMG-CoA reductase; LKB1, liver kinase B1; MCD, malonyl-CoA decarboxylase; mTOR, mammalian target of rapamycin; PEPCK, phosphoenolpyruvate carboxykinase; PFK2, 6-phosphofructo-2-kinase/fructose-2,6-bisphosphatase; PGC1α, peroxisome proliferator-activated receptor gamma coactivator-1; PKA, protein kinase A; PP2C, protein phosphatase 2C; SREBP1c, sterol regulatory element–binding protein 1c; Tak1, TGF-beta-activated kinase 1; transducer of regulated cAMP response element-binding protein 2; TSC1/2, tuberous sclerosis 1).

therefore, can transport glucose at the relatively low concentrations found in the fasted state. For this reason, its presence on the surface of the endothelial cells of the brain vascular system (blood–brain barrier) ensures adequate transport of plasma glucose into the central nervous system.

GLUT 3, which is also found in all tissues, is the major glucose transporter on neurons. It also has a very high affinity for glucose and is responsible for transferring glucose into neuronal cells at the lower concentrations found in the central nervous system.

In contrast, GLUT 2 has a lower affinity for glucose and thus increases glucose transport when plasma glucose levels rise, such as postprandially. It is a major transporter of glucose in hepatic, intestinal, and renal tubular cells. The low affinity of GLUT 2 for glucose reduces hepatic uptake of glucose during fasting, while its ability to transport glucose equally efficiently in both directions assists in the export of glucose from hepatocytes. GLUT 2 is also expressed on the surface of the β cells in rodents, but it is not detected at significant levels on human β cells.

GLUT 4 is found in two major insulin target tissues: skeletal muscle and adipose tissue. It is sequestered mainly within an intracellular compartment of these cells and thus does not function as a glucose transporter until insulin signaling causes translocation of GLUT 4 to the cell membrane, where it facilitates glucose entry into these tissues after a meal (see Figure 17–6). In muscle, exercise also drives GLUT 4 translocation to the cell surface by activating AMPK.

Islet Amyloid Polypeptide

Islet amyloid polypeptide (IAPP), or amylin, is a 37 amino acid peptide produced and stored with insulin in pancreatic β cells but only at a low ratio of approximately one molecule of IAPP to 100 of insulin. β Cells cosecrete IAPP with insulin in response to glucose and other β cell secretagogues. Although it plays a role in regulating gut physiology by decreasing gastric emptying and gut motility after meals, the full physiologic functions of IAPP remain uncertain. A soluble analog of IAPP called pramlintide has been approved for use in patients with type 1 diabetes and insulin-treated type 2 diabetes (see later).

IAPP produces amyloid deposits in pancreatic islets of most patients with type 2 diabetes of long duration. These amyloid deposits are insoluble fibrillar proteins generated from IAPP oligomers that encroach on and may even occur within pancreatic β cells. Islets of nondiabetic elderly persons may contain less extensive amyloid deposits. Whether amyloid fibrils and deposition contributes to the islet dysfunction and β cell loss seen in type 2 diabetes or is simply a consequence of disordered and hyper-stimulated islet function remains an unresolved question.

2. GLUCAGON

Biochemistry

Pancreatic glucagon, along with several other biologically active peptides, derives from the large proglucagon peptide encoded by the preproglucagon gene located on human chromosome 2. Tissue-specific proteases (the prohormone convertases) cleave different sets of peptide products from the proglucagon molecule in the endocrine L-cells of the gut and the α cells in the islet (Figure 17–9). The activity of prohormone convertase 2 in α cells generates the glucagon peptide, along with the amino-terminal glicentin-related peptide, a small central hexapeptide, and a large carboxyl-terminal fragment.

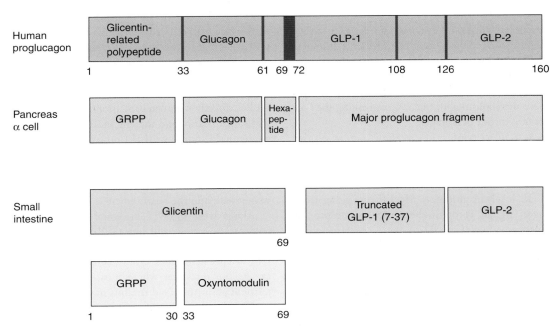

FIGURE 17–9 Tissue-specific secretory products of human proglucagon (GLP-1, glucagon-like peptide-1; GLP-2, glucagon-like peptide-2; GRPP, glicentin-related polypeptide).

Glucagon consists of 29 amino acids in a single-chain polypeptide with a molecular weight of 3485. In healthy humans, the average fasting plasma immunoreactive glucagon level is 75 pg/mL (25 pmol/L). Only 30% to 40% of this is actually pancreatic glucagon, the remainder being a heterogeneous composite of higher-molecular-weight molecules with glucagon immunoreactivity such as proglucagon, glicentin, and oxyntomodulin. Circulating glucagon has a half-life of 3 to 6 minutes due to removal by the liver and kidney.

Secretion

In contrast to its stimulation of insulin secretion, glucose inhibits glucagon secretion. Conflicting data surround the question of whether glucose directly inhibits secretion from the α cell or whether it only acts via release of insulin and somatostatin from the β and δ cells, both of which inhibit the α cell directly. In addition, because β cells release gamma-aminobutyric acid (GABA) and α cells express inhibitory GABA receptors, GABA also may participate in the inhibition of α cells during β cell stimulation.

Many amino acids stimulate glucagon release, although they differ in their ability to do so. Some, such as arginine, release both glucagon and insulin; others (eg, alanine) stimulate primarily glucagon release. Leucine, an effective stimulant of insulin release, does not stimulate glucagon. Other substances that promote glucagon release include catecholamines, gastrointestinal hormones (cholecystokinin [CCK], gastrin, and gastric inhibitory polypeptide [GIP]), and glucocorticoids. Both sympathetic and parasympathetic (vagal) stimulation promote glucagon release, especially in response to hypoglycemia. High levels of circulating fatty acids suppress glucagon secretion.

Action of Glucagon

In contrast to insulin, which promotes energy storage in a variety of tissues in response to feeding, glucagon provides a humoral mechanism for delivering energy from the liver to the other tissues between meals. The ratio of insulin to glucagon affects key target tissues by regulating the expression and activity of key enzymes controlling nutrient metabolism and, thereby, controlling the flux of these nutrients into or out of storage.

The liver, because of its connection to the pancreas via the portal vein, represents the major target organ for glucagon, with portal vein glucagon concentrations reaching as high as 300 to 500 pg/mL (100-166 pmol/L) during fasting. It is unclear whether physiologic levels of glucagon affect tissues other than the liver. Glucagon signals through the glucagon receptor, a G protein–coupled receptor (GPCR) of the $G\alpha_s$ class found predominantly on the surface of hepatocytes. Binding of glucagon to its receptor in the liver activates adenylyl cyclase and the generation of cAMP, which in turn mediates the phosphorylation or dephosphorylation of key enzymes regulating nutrient metabolism. In addition, like insulin, glucagon receptor signaling modifies the activity of a set of cAMP responsive transcriptional regulators that in turn control the expression of the genes encoding these same enzymes.

Glucagon signaling in the liver stimulates the breakdown of stored glycogen, maintains hepatic output of glucose from amino acid precursors (gluconeogenesis), and promotes hepatic output of ketone bodies from fatty acid precursors (ketogenesis). Glucagon facilitates the uptake of the gluconeogenic substrate alanine by liver, and directs fatty acids away from reesterification to triglycerides and toward ketogenic pathways. In sum, glucagon signaling results in the net release of readily available energy stores from the liver in the form of glucose and ketones.

Glucagon-Related Peptides

In the intestinal L-cells, found predominantly in the distal ileum and colon, prohormone convertase 1 generates a different set of peptides from the proglucagon molecule, including glicentin, glicentin-related polypeptide (GRPP), oxyntomodulin, and the two glucagon-like peptides **GLP-1** and **GLP-2** (see Figure 17–9). Several biological activities have been attributed to glicentin and oxyntomodulin based on studies using high concentrations of the peptides, but all these actions can be explained by low-affinity interactions with the receptors for glucagon, GLP-1 and GLP-2. Specific receptors for glicentin and oxyntomodulin have not been identified, and it remains uncertain whether these peptides play any biological role at physiologic concentrations. GRPP also has no clearly established biological activity. The other two gut-derived glucagon-related peptides, GLP-1 and GLP-2, however, play important roles in nutrient metabolism and gastrointestinal physiology (Table 17–4).

There are two active forms of GLP-1: GLP-1(7-36) amide, and GLP-1(7-37). The intestinal L-cells secrete GLP-1 in response to meals, through dietary glucose and lipids and parasympathetic stimulation. The L-cells sense dietary fat in the gut lumen in part through the GPR119 receptor, which binds the long chain fatty acid derivative oleoylethanolamide. GPR119 is also expressed on the surface of the β cells. GLP-1 binds to the GLP-1 receptor, a GPCR similar to the glucagon receptor. The ubiquitous protease dipeptidyl peptidase 4 (**DPP-4**) rapidly inactivates circulating GLP-1 (half-life <2 min) by removing the two amino-terminal amino acids. Pancreatic islets are major targets of GLP-1 action. GLP-1 directly stimulates the production and secretion of insulin and somatostatin, and thereby indirectly inhibits the secretion of glucagon. In addition, GLP-1 protects the β cells from destruction and stimulates β cell growth. Other targets of GLP-1 include the stomach, where the peptide inhibits gastric emptying and gastric acid secretion; the brain, where it inhibits appetite and induces weight loss; and the heart, where it has some protective effects.

Along with GLP-1, intestinal L-cells cosecrete GLP-2 in response to eating; and like GLP-1, GLP-2 binds to a specific GPCR closely related to the glucagon and GLP-1 receptors. DPP-4 also inactivates GLP-2. GLP-2 signaling predominantly targets the intestine, where it stimulates mucosal growth and nutrient absorption and inhibits motility.

The K cells in the duodenum and jejunum produce a related 42 amino acid incretin peptide, **GIP**, that has both functional and sequential similarity to GLP-1, but is the product of a distinct gene and binds to a distinct receptor, GIPR, which also belongs to

TABLE 17–4 Biologic roles of glucagon-related peptides.

Target Tissue	Glucagon	GLP-1	GLP-2	GIP
Islet	**Stimulates** insulin secretion	**Stimulates** insulin and somatostatin secretion **Inhibits** glucagon secretion (indirectly) **Increases** β cell mass by inhibiting β cell death and inducing β cell proliferation		**Stimulates** insulin, somatostatin, and glucagon secretion **Inhibits** glucagon secretion (indirectly) **Increases** β cell mass by inhibiting β cell death and inducing β cell proliferation
Liver	**Stimulates** glycogenolysis, glucogenesis, fatty acid oxidation, and ketogenesis **Inhibits** glycogen synthesis and fatty acid synthesis			
Stomach		**Inhibits** gastric acid secretion **Inhibits** gastric emptying		**Inhibits** gastric acid secretion and gastric emptying
Intestine			**Stimulates** mucosal growth and nutrient absorption **Inhibits** motility	
Adipose tissue				**Stimulates** adipogenesis, lipogenesis, and adipokine production
Brain (hypothalamus)		**Inhibits** appetite		

the family of glucagon-related $G\alpha_s$-linked receptors. The K cells secrete GIP in response to glucose—via the same pathway used by the β cell (see Figure 17–5)—and lipids. Interestingly, the GIP prepropeptide is also expressed in α cells, but prohormone convertase 2 in α cells produces a shorter peptide, GIP_{1-30}, which lacks the 12 carboxyl amino acids present in intestinal GIP_{1-42}. The two forms of GIP appear to function identically. GIP signaling through its receptor has similar effects to those of GLP-1 on the stomach and β cells. α Cells also express the GIP receptor, through which GIP directly stimulates glucagon secretion; but GIP concomitantly suppresses glucagon secretion indirectly through its stimulation of insulin secretion. The GIP receptor is also expressed in adipose tissue and bone. In adipose tissue, GIP plays an important role in the differentiation of new adipocytes, and also drives lipogenesis and adipokine production in mature adipocytes. In bone, GIP stimulates the osteoblasts and increases bone density.

3. SOMATOSTATIN

The pancreatic δ cells transcribe the gene for somatostatin on the long arm of chromosome 3. It codes for a 116 amino acid peptide, preprosomatostatin, from whose carboxyl end is cleaved the hormone somatostatin, a 14 amino acid cyclic polypeptide with a molecular weight of 1640 (Figure 17–10). First identified in the hypothalamus, it owes its name to its ability to inhibit the release of growth hormone (GH; pituitary somatotropin). Since that time, somatostatin has been found in a number of tissues, including many areas of the brain and peripheral nervous system, the endocrine D cells in the epithelial lining of the stomach and

intestine, and the δ cells in the pancreatic islets. In neurons, gastric D cells and the islet, somatostatin-14 predominates, but approximately 5% to 10% of the somatostatin-like immunoreactivity in the brain consists of a 28 amino acid peptide, somatostatin-28. Somatostatin-28 consists of an amino terminal region of 14 amino acids and a carboxyl terminal segment containing somatostatin-14. In small intestine, the larger molecule predominates, with 70% to 75% of the hormone in the 28 amino acid form and only 25% to 30% as somatostatin-14. Somatostatin-28 is 10 times more potent than somatostatin-14 in inhibiting growth hormone and insulin secretion, whereas somatostatin-14 is more effective in inhibiting glucagon release.

Most known stimulators of insulin release also promote somatostatin release from δ cells. This includes glucose, arginine, gastrointestinal hormones, and sulfonylureas. The importance of circulating somatostatin is unclear; the major action of this peptide appears to be paracrine regulation of the pancreatic islet and the gastrointestinal tract. Physiologic levels of somatostatin in humans seldom exceed 80 pg/mL (49 pmol/L). The metabolic clearance of exogenously infused somatostatin in humans is extremely rapid; the half-life of the hormone is less than 3 minutes.

Molecular cloning has identified five somatostatin receptors (SSTR1-5), all of which are GPCRs. They vary in size from 364 to 418 amino acids (with 105 amino acids invariant) and function in the central nervous system and a wide variety of peripheral tissues, including the pituitary gland, the small intestine, and the pancreas. All five receptors belong to the $G\alpha_i$ class and inhibit the activity of adenylate cyclase, thereby lowering intracellular levels

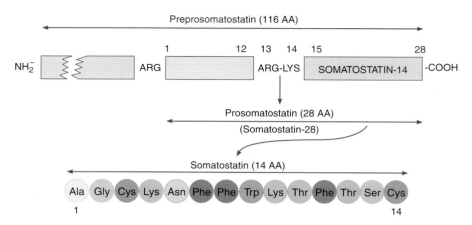

FIGURE 17–10 Amino acid sequence of somatostatin and its cleavage from dibasic amino acid residue in prosomatostatin and preprosomatostatin.

of cAMP and inhibiting cAMP-activated secretion. In addition, however, each of the different somatostatin receptors interacts with additional distinct downstream effectors that modify the cellular consequences of receptor activation. Binding of ligand to SSTR5 on β cells mediates the inhibition of insulin secretion, whereas inhibition of GH release from pituitary somatotrophs as well as glucagon release from α cells of the pancreas works through SSTR2. This explains why an analog of somatostatin, octreotide, which has a much greater affinity for SSTR2 than for SSTR5, is effective in correcting GH excess without having much effect on carbohydrate tolerance when used to treat acromegaly.

Somatostatin acts in several ways to restrain the movement of nutrients from the intestinal tract into the circulation. It prolongs gastric emptying time, decreases gastric acid and gastrin production, diminishes pancreatic exocrine secretion, decreases splanchnic blood flow, and retards xylose absorption.

4. PANCREATIC POLYPEPTIDE

PP is found in PP cells located chiefly in islets in the posterior portion of the head of the pancreas. Similar to the other islet hormones, PP derives from a larger prepropeptide of 85 amino acids that is cleaved to a single 36 amino acid peptide with a molecular weight of 4200. Circulating levels of the peptide increase in response to a mixed meal; however, intravenous infusion of glucose or lipid does not produce such a rise, and intravenous amino acids induce only a small increase. In contrast, vagotomy abolishes the response to an ingested meal, demonstrating that PP secretion responds predominantly to neural, rather than nutrient signals.

In healthy subjects, basal levels of PP average 24 ± 4 pmol/L and may become elevated owing to a variety of factors including old age, alcohol abuse, diarrhea, chronic renal failure, hypoglycemia, or inflammatory disorders. Values above 300 pmol/L are found in most patients with pancreatic endocrine tumors such as glucagonoma or vasoactive intestinal polypeptide-secreting tumor and in all patients with tumors of the pancreatic PP cell. As many as 20% of patients with insulinoma and one-third of those with

gastrinomas also have plasma concentrations of PP that are greater than 300 pmol/L.

Although it has been implicated in the regulation of exocrine pancreatic secretion and gall bladder contraction, the physiologic actions of PP remain uncertain.

5. GHRELIN

The peptide hormone ghrelin was originally identified in extracts from the stomach based on its ability to bind to and activate the growth hormone secretagogue receptor (GHSR) and stimulate growth hormone release from the pituitary. The P/D1 endocrine cells in the gastric mucosa and the ε cells in the islet make ghrelin, as do a few cells in the heart, lung, kidney, immune system, hypothalamus, and pituitary. The human *GHRELIN* gene comprises four exons, and the major splice product encodes the 117 amino acid preproghrelin peptide. Processing in the ε cells yields the active form of ghrelin: a 28 amino acid peptide (amino acids 24-51 of preproghrelin) with the serine in position 3 modified by the attachment of an octanoyl side chain. Full biological activity requires the *n*-octanoyl modification. In addition, protease cleavage generates a second peptide, obestatin (amino acids 76-98 of preproghrelin) of less certain biological function.

Initially identified as a stimulator of growth hormone secretion, ghrelin signals through its receptor, the previously identified GHSR, which is a GPCR found in a variety of tissues, including the hypothalamus, pituitary, intestine, and islet. Ghrelin signaling stimulates growth hormone secretion directly through its receptor on pituitary somatotrophs, and also through its stimulation of hypothalamic GHRH secretion. In addition, Ghrelin induces gastric emptying and acid secretion and regulates appetite and energy balance via neurons in the arcuate nucleus of the hypothalamus (see Chapter 20). The role of ghrelin signaling in the pancreas, and the relative contribution of islet-derived ghrelin to the overall actions of ghrelin remains unresolved.

DIABETES MELLITUS

Clinical diabetes mellitus is a syndrome of disordered metabolism with inappropriate hyperglycemia due to an absolute or relative deficiency of insulin. There may also be a defect in insulin action (insulin resistance).

CLASSIFICATION

Diabetes is classified into four main groups based on known pathological and etiologic mechanisms—type 1, type 2, other specific types, and gestational diabetes (Table 17–5). Type 1 diabetes (previously referred to as juvenile-onset or insulin dependent diabetes mellitus [IDDM]) results from pancreatic islet β cell destruction most commonly by an autoimmune process. These patients are prone to developing ketoacidosis and require insulin replacement. Type 2 diabetes (previously referred to as adult-onset or non-insulin-dependent diabetes mellitus [NIDDM]), the most prevalent form of diabetes, is a heterogeneous disorder most commonly associated with insulin resistance in the presence of an associated impairment in compensatory insulin secretion.

TYPE 1 DIABETES MELLITUS

Type 1 diabetes is immune-mediated in more than 95% of cases (type 1a) and idiopathic in less than 5% (type 1b). The rate of pancreatic β cell destruction may vary, but in most cases the process is prolonged, extending over months or years, since evidence for an immune response can be detected long in advance of hyperglycemia in patients that eventually develop type 1 diabetes. It is a catabolic disorder in which circulating insulin is virtually absent, plasma glucagon is elevated, and the pancreatic β cells fail to respond to all known insulinogenic stimuli. In the absence of insulin, the three main target tissues of insulin (liver, muscle, and

TABLE 17–5 Etiologic classification of diabetes mellitus.

I. Type 1 diabetes[a] (β cell destruction, usually leading to absolute insulin deficiency)
  A. Immune-mediated, type 1a
  B. Idiopathic, type 1b
 	
II. Type 2 diabetes[a] (may range from predominantly insulin resistance with relative insulin deficiency to a predominantly secretory defect with minimal insulin resistance)
 	
III. Other specific types
  A. Autosomal dominant genetic defects of pancreatic β cells
    1. Maturity onset diabetes of the young (MODY)
    2. Insulin gene (*INS*)
    3. ATP-sensitive potassium channel (*KCNJ11* and *ABBC8*)
  B. Other genetic defects of pancreatic β cells
    1. Autosomal recessive genetic defects
    2. Mitochrondrial DNA
    3. Ketosis-prone diabetes (KPD)
  C. Genetic defects in insulin action
    1. Insulin receptor mutations
    2. Lipoatrophic diabetes
  D. Neonatal diabetes
    1. Transient
    2. Permanent
  E. Diseases of the exocrine pancreas
    1. Pancreatitis
    2. Trauma, pancreatectomy
    3. Neoplasia
    4. Cystic fibrosis
    5. Hemochromatosis
    6. Fibrocalculous pancreatopathy
  F. Endocrinopathies
    1. Acromegaly
    2. Cushing syndrome
    3. Glucagonoma
    4. Pheochromocytoma
    5. Hyperthyroidism
    6. Somatostatinoma
    7. Aldosteronoma
	G. Drug- or chemical-induced
	    1. β cell toxicity: vacor, pentamidine, cyclosporine
	    2. β cell autoimmunity: α-interferon
	    3. β cell dysfunction: thiazide and loop diuretics, diazoxide, α agonists, β blockers, phenytoin, opiates
	    4. Insulin resistance: glucocorticoids, progesterone, nicotinic acid, thyroid hormone, β blockers, atypical antipsychotic drugs, antiretroviral protease inhibitors
	  H. Infections
	    1. Congenital rubella
	    2. Other viruses: cytomegalovirus, coxsackievirus B, adenovirus, mumps
	  I. Uncommon forms of immune-mediated diabetes
	    1. Stiff-person syndrome
	    2. Immunodysregulation polyendocrinopathy enteropathy, X-linked (IPEX)
	    3. Autoimmune polyendocrinopathy syndrome type 1
	    4. Anti-insulin receptor antibodies
	    5. Ataxia telangiectasia syndrome (antireceptor antibodies)
	    6. POEMS syndrome
	  J. Other genetic syndromes sometimes associated with diabetes
	    1. Chromosomal defects: Down, Klinefelter, and Turner syndromes
	    2. Neuromuscular syndromes: Friedreich ataxia, Huntington chorea, myotonic dystrophy, porphyria, and others
	    3. Obesity syndromes: Laurence-Moon-Biedl, Bardet-Biedl, Prader-Willi syndromes, and others
	    4. Wolfram syndrome
	
	IV. Gestational diabetes mellitus (GDM)

[a]Patients with any form of diabetes may require insulin treatment at some stage of their disease. Such use of insulin does not, of itself, classify the patient.

Modified from American Diabetes Association: *Diabetes Care*. 2010;33(suppl 1):S65.

fat) not only fail to appropriately take up absorbed nutrients but continue to deliver glucose, amino acids, and fatty acids into the bloodstream from their respective storage depots. Furthermore, alterations in fat metabolism lead to the production and accumulation of ketones. This inappropriate persistence of the fasted state postprandially can be reversed by the administration of insulin.

The incidence of type 1 diabetes varies widely in different populations. Scandinavia and northern Europe have the highest incidence of type 1 diabetes: the yearly incidence per 100,000 youngsters 14 years of age or less is as high as 40 in Finland, 31 in Sweden, 22 in Norway, 27 in Scotland, and 20 in England. The incidence of type 1 diabetes generally decreases across the rest of Europe to 11 in Greece and 9 in France. Surprisingly, the island of Sardinia has as high an incidence as Finland, even though in the rest of Italy, including the island of Sicily, the incidence is only 11 per 100,000 per year. The United States averages 16 per 100,000. The lowest incidence of type 1 diabetes worldwide is less than 1 per 100,000 per year in China and parts of South America.

Worldwide incidence of type 1 diabetes continues to increase steadily. In Finland, the incidence has more than tripled since 1953, when it was 12/100,000/year, with an average increase of 2.4% per year. The EURODIAB study group reported recently 0.6 % to 9.3 % annual increases in incidence of type 1 diabetes in children younger than 15 years in various European countries. The most rapid increases have occurred in low-prevalence countries and in younger patients. Changes in environmental factors most likely explain this increased incidence.

Latent autoimmune diabetes of adulthood (LADA): Type 1 diabetes can present at any age, although peaks in incidence occur before school age and again at around puberty. Older adults often present with a more indolent onset that sometimes leads to misdiagnosis and has led to the use of the term **latent autoimmune diabetes of adulthood (LADA)** to distinguish these patients. These initially unrecognized patients may retain enough β cell function at the outset to avoid ketosis, but develop increasing dependence on insulin therapy over time as their β cell mass diminishes. Islet cell antibody surveys among northern Europeans indicate that up to 15% of patients previously diagnosed with type 2 diabetes may actually have LADA.

Autoimmunity and Type 1 Diabetes

Most patients with type 1 diabetes at diagnosis have circulating antibodies against β cell proteins: islet cell antibodies (ICA), insulin autoantibodies (IAA), and antibodies to glutamic acid decarboxylase 65 (GAD), tyrosine phosphatase IA2 (ICA512), and zinc transporter 8 (ZnT8) (Table 17–6). These autoreative antibodies can often be detected well before the onset of frank hyperglycemia, even decades earlier, providing evidence that the autoimmune process may be prolonged. After diagnosis, autoantibody levels often decline with increasing duration of the disease. Also, once patients are treated with insulin, low levels of IAA develop, even in patients that do not have an autoimmune etiology for their diabetes.

Although useful for diagnosing and predicting type 1 diabetes, antibodies against β cell proteins do not directly cause the destruction of β cells in type 1 diabetes. Instead, it is the cellular immune

TABLE 17–6   Diagnostic sensitivity and specificity of autoimmune markers in newly diagnosed patients with type 1 diabetes mellitus.

	Sensitivity	Specificity
Glutamic acid decarboxylase (GAD65)	70%-90%	99%
Insulin (IAA)	40%-70%	99%
Tyrosine phosphatase IA2 (ICA512)	50%-70%	99%
Zinc transporter 8 (ZnT8)	50%-70%	99%

system, the T lymphocytes, that infiltrate the islets (a process called insulitis) and destroy the β cells. At the time of diagnosis, the islets of patients with type 1 diabetes are extensively infiltrated with both helper and cytotoxic T lymphocytes.

Normally, the thymus deletes autoreactive T cells during development so that the immune system becomes tolerant of self-antigens. In addition, certain specialized T cells, the regulatory T cells, further prevent attacks against healthy tissues by retraining the activity of any autoreactive cytotoxic and helper T cells that escape the thymus. Type 1 diabetes results from a breakdown in these processes of self-tolerance in the immune system.

Type 1b diabetes: Approximately 5% of patients with the clinical features of type 1 diabetes lack serum evidence of autoimmunity. Some of these individuals have high risk HLA haplotypes (see later) and may have T-cell–mediated β cell destruction in the absence of measurable levels of the known autoantibodies. Others in this group have low-risk HLA haplotypes, and appear to have a nonautoimmune cause for loss of β cell function. Such nonautoimmune type 1 diabetes has been referred to as type 1b diabetes, but a variety of terms has been used. This probably represents a heterogeneous group of disorders that lead to profound β cell dysfunction or loss, absolute insulin deficiency and a syndrome clinically similar to autoimmune type 1a diabetes. Under the accepted classification system, as specific disorders within this subgroup become defined and the genetic or environmental causes are identified, these disorders become reclassified within the group of "Other Specific Types of Diabetes."

Included within this group are patients that present with a course of relapsing diabetic ketoacidosis with intervening normoglycemia that eventually progresses to permanent insulin-deficient diabetes. This disorder, ketosis prone diabetes (KPD, see later), has also been referred to as type 1b diabetes, and may result from unknown environmental insults combined with genetic defects in the β cell.

Autoimmune diabetes and stiff person syndrome: GAD antibodies, the first identified in type 1 diabetes, remain among the most clinically useful. Human pancreatic β cells produce GAD65, which functions as an enzyme that catalyzes the synthesis of GABA from glutamate. GAD65 and the closely related isoform GAD67 are also found in central nervous system inhibitory neurons that secrete GABA. Some patients with GAD antibodies develop a rare neurologic condition, **stiff person syndrome**, caused by the depletion of GABA in the central nervous system and characterized by progressive rigidity and fluctuating muscle spasms. Approximately half of the patients with stiff person syndrome develop type 1 diabetes.

The vast majority of patients with type 1 diabetes do not develop symptoms of stiff person syndrome, despite the presence of GAD antibodies. The rare patients that develop the syndrome usually have much higher titers of GAD antibodies than typical patients with type 1 diabetes alone.

Genetics of Type 1 Diabetes

Family members of patients with type1 diabetes have an increased lifetime risk of developing type 1 diabetes. The offspring of a mother with type 1 diabetes have a risk of 3%, whereas the risk is 6% for children of affected fathers. The risk in siblings of affected individuals is related to the number of human leukocyte antigen (HLA) haplotypes (see later) that the sibling shares. If one haplotype is shared, the risk is 6% and if two haplotypes are shared, the risk increases to 12% to 25%. For monozygotic twins, the concordance rate reaches 25% to 50%. Although these data demonstrate a strong genetic contribution to the risk of type 1 diabetes, genetics plays an even larger role in type 2 diabetes, and environment also clearly contributes substantially to the risk of type 1 diabetes.

Genes in the major histocompatibility (MHC) locus on the short arm of chromosome 6 explain at least half of the familial aggregation of type 1 diabetes. Within the MHC locus lie a number of closely packed genes involved in the function and regulation of the immune response. Although a number of genes within the MHC locus have been linked to the risk of developing type 1 diabetes, the most important of these are the genes encoding the HLA class II molecules DQ and DR. The professional antigen-presenting cells—dendritic cells, macrophages and B lymphocytes—use the class II molecules on their cell surface to present peptide antigens to T lymphocytes through the T-cell receptor. T cells activated by antigen-presenting cells carry out the β cell destruction that leads to type 1 diabetes. Although exact mechanisms remain uncertain, the variations in the amino acid sequence of individual HLA class II molecules may impact their ability to present specific self-peptides to T cells either in the process of central or peripheral tolerization or later during the development of the autoimmune response, thereby contributing to the risk of developing type 1 diabetes.

The DR haplotypes DR3 and DR4 are major susceptibility risk factors for type 1 diabetes. As many as 95% of type 1 diabetic patients have a DR3 or a DR4 haplotype—or both—compared with 45% to 50% of Caucasian nondiabetic controls. Individuals who express both a DR3 and a DR4 allele carry the highest risk for type 1 diabetes in the United States.

The high-risk *DR* genes are generally in linkage disequilibrium with *DQ* genes that themselves confer high risk, particularly DQA1*0501, DQB1*0201 (coupled with DR3), and DQA1*0301, DQB1*0302 (coupled with DR4). DQ alleles are associated not only with risk for type 1 diabetes but also with dominant protection, often in linkage with HLA-DR2. The most protective of these—and a quite common allele—is DQA1*0102, DQB1*0602. It occurs in over 20% of individuals in the United States but in less than 1% of children who develop type 1 diabetes.

An independent genetic link to chromosome 11 has also been identified in type 1 diabetes. Studies of a polymorphic DNA locus flanking the 5′ region of the *insulin* gene on chromosome 11 revealed a small but statistically significant linkage between type 1 diabetes and this genetic locus in a Caucasian population with type 1 diabetes. This polymorphic locus, which consists of a variable number of tandem repeats (VNTRs) with two common sizes in Caucasians, small (26-63 repeats) or large (140-243 repeats), does not encode a protein. An intriguing proposal to explain how the VNTR might influence susceptibility to type 1 diabetes was based on findings that *insulin* gene transcription is facilitated in the fetal thymus gland by the presence of the large allele of the VNTR locus flanking the *insulin* gene. The large VNTR allele might produce a dominant protective effect by promoting negative selection (deletion) by the thymus of insulin-specific T lymphocytes that play a critical role in the immune destruction of pancreatic β cells.

The established genetic association with the MHC region of chromosome 6 contributes much more (about 50%) to the genetic susceptibility to type 1 diabetes than does this locus flanking the *insulin* gene on chromosome 11, which contributes about 10%. Both candidate gene studies and genome-wide association studies (GWAS) have identified a number of additional risk loci that make smaller contributions to the genetic risk of type 1 diabetes. Many of the genes linked to these additional loci also play important roles in the function and regulation of the immune response.

Mutations in two genes involved in T-cell tolerance cause rare syndromes of type 1 diabetes together with other autoimmune diseases. In the autosomal recessive disease autoimmune polyglandular syndrome type 1 (APS1; see Chapter 2), homozygous mutations in the gene encoding the autoimmune regulator (*AIRE*) prevent the expression of certain self-proteins in the thymus, thus allowing mature autoreactive T cells to leave the thymus. In addition to other autoimmune diseases and mucocutaneous candidiasis, approximately 20% of patients with APS1 develop type 1 diabetes. The second gene, *FOXP3*, found on the X chromosome, encodes a transcription factor required for the formation of regulatory T cells. Mutations in *FOXP3* cause immunodysregulation polyendocrinopathy enteropathy X-linked (IPEX) syndrome. IPEX presents in male patients with very early onset type 1 diabetes, often neonatal, combined with other autoimmune endocrinopathies, autoimmune skin disorders, diarrhea secondary to autoimmune enteropathy, and frequent severe infections.

Environmental Factors in Type 1 Diabetes

While genetic inheritance may play an important role in causing type 1 diabetes, the monozygotic twin studies demonstrate that other causes, stochastic or environmental, are at least as important. Most individuals with type 1 diabetes do not have other family members with the disease. Environmental factors associated with increased risk of type 1 diabetes include viruses (mumps, congenital rubella, Coxsackie virus B4), toxic chemical agents such as vacor (a nitrophenylurea rat poison), and other destructive cytotoxins such as hydrogen cyanide from spoiled tapioca or cassava root. How these environmental insults lead to type 1 diabetes is unknown; they may directly damage β cells in some cases, or may act as initiators or accelerators of the autoimmune attack on the β cells. In some cases, molecular mimicry, wherein the immune system mistakenly targets β cell proteins that share homologies with certain viral or other foreign peptides may play a role.

Epidemiological studies have demonstrated an association between breast-feeding in the first 6 months of life and protection from type 1 diabetes. While it has been suggested that proteins in cow's milk may be the culprits, the strongest evidence supports the idea that human breast milk may reduce the risk of autoimmune disease.

Accumulating evidence shows that in the process of modernizing and improving public health, the risk of type 1 diabetes has increased, possibly due to the removal of some protective factors. Type 1 diabetes is almost unheard of in many third-world countries, and has its highest incidence in countries with the best public health systems, such as the Scandinavian countries. In addition, the incidence of the disease has been steadily increasing over the past century in western and westernizing countries and is especially high among the more affluent. This has led to the suggestion that a dirty environment, one with more infections (especially more parasitic diseases) and more antigen exposure, may reduce the risk of type 1 disease.

TYPE 2 DIABETES

Type 2 diabetes mellitus—previously called non-insulin-dependent diabetes or adult-onset diabetes mellitus—results from relative insulin deficiency, in contrast to the absolute insulin deficiency of patients with type 1 diabetes. Type 2 diabetes is a heterogeneous disorder and probably represents a large number of different primary genetic and environmental insults leading to relative insulin deficiency—a mismatch between insulin production and insulin requirements. Clinically, patients with type 2 diabetes can range from those with severe insulin resistance and minimal insulin secretory defects to those with a primary defect in insulin secretion.

Type 2 diabetes accounts for 80% to 90% of cases of diabetes in the United States. These patients commonly present as adults with some degree of obesity, although increasing rates of obesity are leading to earlier onset of the disease in adolescents and children. At onset, most patients with type 2 diabetes do not require insulin to survive, but over time their insulin secretory capacity tends to deteriorate, and many eventually need insulin treatment to achieve optimal glucose control. Ketosis seldom occurs spontaneously, and if present, it is a consequence of severe stress from trauma or infection.

Most patients with type 2 diabetes, irrespective of weight, have some degree of tissue insensitivity to insulin attributable to several interrelated factors (Table 17–7). These include putative (mostly

TABLE 17–7 Factors reducing response to insulin.

Pre-receptor	Insulin autoantibodies Reduced transendothelial transit

Primary defect in insulin signaling	Insulin receptor mutations
	  Leprechaunism (complete)
	  Rabson-Mendenhall syndrome (partial)
	  Type A (mild)
	Defects in other genes involved in insulin signaling
	Insulin receptor autoantibodies (Type B)
	Ataxia telangectasia syndrome

Secondary to other endocrine disorders	Cushing syndrome Acromegaly Pheochromocytoma Glucagonoma Hyperthyroidism Insulinoma
Secondary to other disorders	Visceral obesity Stress (infection, surgery, etc) Uremia Hyperglycemia (mild resistance seen in type 1 diabetes) Liver disease Cytogenetic disorders (Down, Turner, Klinefelter) Neuromuscular disorders (muscular dystrophies, ataxias, muscle inactivity) Congenital lipodystrophies/lipoatrophy Acquired lipodystrophy
Secondary to normal physiologic states	Puberty Pregnancy Starvation
Secondary to medications	Glucocorticoids Atypical antipsychotic drugs Antiretroviral protease inhibitors Nicotinic acid Thiazide diuretics Oral contraceptive Progesterone β blockers

as yet undefined) genetic factors, which are aggravated in time by further enhancers of insulin resistance such as aging, a sedentary lifestyle, and abdominal visceral obesity. Not all patients with obesity and insulin resistance develop hyperglycemia, however. An underlying defect in the ability of the β cells to compensate for the increased demand determines which patients will develop diabetes in the setting of insulin resistance. Furthermore, both the tissue resistance to insulin and the impaired β cell response to glucose appear to be further aggravated by sustained hyperglycemia, which may impede both insulin signaling and β cell function. Treatment that reduces the blood glucose levels toward normal reduces this acquired defect in insulin resistance and may also improve glucose-induced insulin release to some degree, although the long-term decline in β cell function continues.

Type 2 diabetes frequently goes undiagnosed for many years because the hyperglycemia may develop quite gradually and without initial symptoms. Despite this mild presentation, these patients develop microvascular, and, especially, macrovascular complications. Furthermore, as noted above, patients with type 2 diabetes suffer from a progressive decline in β cell capacity, leading to worsening hyperglycemia over time.

A. Obesity in type 2 diabetes   The majority of people with type 2 diabetes have excess adiposity, although the prevalence of obesity in association with type 2 diabetes varies among different racial groups. Sixty to eighty percent of North Americans, Europeans, or Africans with type 2 diabetes and close to 100% of individuals with type 2 disease among Pima Indians or Pacific Islanders from Nauru or Samoa have obesity as defined by body mass index (BMI, see Chapter 20), while as few as 30% of Chinese and Japanese patients with type 2 diabetes are obese. However, many of those individuals with type 2 diabetes who do not meet BMI criteria for obesity have a predominantly abdominal distribution of fat, producing an abnormally high waist to hip ratio. Increases in visceral adiposity correlate with increased insulin resistance.

B. Insulin resistance in type 2 diabetes   Insulin resistance can be broadly defined as a decrease in tissue responsiveness to insulin. Clinically it can be assessed directly by measuring the ability of a fixed dose of insulin to promote total body glucose disposal. It can be assessed indirectly by measuring fasting insulin levels. An increase in insulin levels with normal plasma glucose indicates insulin resistance.

As adiposity increases, especially abdominal visceral fat deposits, total body insulin sensitivity decreases. Since adipose tissue only removes a small fraction of plasma glucose, clearly the increased adipose fat stores impact total body insulin sensitivity through effects on other tissues, especially muscle and liver, causing them to decrease insulin-stimulated glucose disposal. The exact means by which fat storage in adipocytes affects the insulin sensitivity of other cells remains uncertain, but experimental evidence suggests several possible mechanisms.

Abnormalities of insulin receptors—in concentration, affinity, or both—affect insulin action. Target tissues downregulate the number of insulin receptors on the cell surface in response to chronically elevated circulating insulin levels, probably by increased intracellular degradation. When insulin levels are low, on the other hand, receptor binding is upregulated. Conditions associated with high insulin levels and lowered insulin binding to the receptor include obesity, high intake of carbohydrates, and chronic exogenous overinsulinization. Conditions associated with low insulin levels and increased insulin binding include exercise and fasting. The insulin receptor itself is probably not the major determinant of insulin sensitivity under most circumstances, however. Clinically relevant insulin resistance most commonly results from defects in postreceptor intracellular signaling pathways.

Adipokines.   Adipose tissue can affect the insulin sensitivity of other tissues through the secretion of signaling molecules, **adipokines**, that inhibit (TNF-α, IL-6, leptin, resistin, and others) or enhance (adiponectin) insulin signaling locally or in distal target tissues (see Chapter 20). Levels of fat storage in adipocytes, along with insulin signaling itself, regulate the production and secretion of many of the adipokines. Some of these mediators of insulin resistance may reduce insulin signaling by blocking access of insulin to target tissues through reduced transendothelial transit. However, most evidence suggests that the secreted adipokines influence insulin signaling in distant tissues through effects on postreceptor intracellular signaling pathways. Potential intracellular effectors include protein tyrosine phosphatases that dephosphorylate the receptor and pathway components, inhibitors such as the SOCS proteins that block receptor–IRS interactions, and serine/threonine kinases that inhibit the receptor and substrates through serine phosphorylation.

Free fatty acids and ectopic lipid storage.   The release of fatty acids by the engorged adipocytes (especially visceral adipocytes, from which fatty acids are more readily mobilized) may play a role in the development of insulin resistance as well. Oxidation of fatty acids by muscle and other tissues could inhibit glycolysis and reduce insulin-stimulated glucose removal (the Randle hypothesis, named after its original proponent). Increased fat storage in adipocytes and release of fatty acids may also eventually cause a shift in lipid storage, increasing lipid uptake and storage in nonadipose tissues such as muscle, liver, and β cells. Ectopic lipid storage in these tissues may lead to a decrease in their insulin sensitivity. In addition, free fatty acids may function directly in a signaling role both locally within the adipose tissue and systemically.

Inflammation.   In addition to adipocytes, adipose tissue contains a variety of other cell types including inflammatory/immune cells, such as macrophages and lymphocytes. Recent evidence implicates these cells in obesity-induced insulin resistance. As adipocyte lipid stores rise, the increased release of free fatty acids and proinflammatory adipokines recruits macrophages to the adipose tissue and activates them. The activated macrophages then release a variety of molecules (TNF-α, IL-6, nitric oxide, and others) that decrease the insulin sensitivity of the adipocytes and further increase their release of proinflammatory fatty acids and peptides, creating a positive feedback loop that maintains a chronic state of local inflammation and insulin resistance. Release of these adipokines and proinflammatory cytokines, along with the increased release of free fatty acids and the development of ectopic lipid accumulation, promotes the development of inflammation and insulin resistance in the other key insulin-target tissues, such as muscle and liver. Similar mechanisms could also lead to inflammation in the islets and contribute to β cell failure.

PPARγ activity in the adipose tissue generally has beneficial effects on systemic insulin signaling through several mechanisms: (1) Promotion of adipose lipid storage, which thereby decreases ectopic lipid storage in nonadipose tissues; (2) Inhibition of the production of adipokines and proinflammatory cytokines, which promote insulin resistance, by adipocytes; (3) Promotion of the alternative activation of macrophages to the anti-inflammatory M2 state, rather than the proinflammatory M1 state; (4) Inhibition of the release of proinflammatory and proresistance cytokines by macrophages. Although it is expressed at much lower levels in muscle than in adipose tissue, PPARγ in myocytes might also have a direct role in controlling muscle insulin sensitivity; however, these findings remain controversial.

Tissue heterogeneity in insulin resistance.   Finally, it must be kept in mind that not all tissues necessarily develop insulin resistance in parallel. The combination of local and systemic contributors to obesity-induced insulin resistance may explain the different levels of insulin resistance in different tissues of the same patient. Even in the same cell, insulin resistance may impact different arms of the insulin-signaling pathway discordantly. This heterogeneity leads to changes in tissue energy storage and insulin sensitivity that could explain unique syndromes associated with insulin resistance like hepatic steatosis and polycystic ovary syndrome.

Other causes of insulin resistance.   Visceral obesity is not the only cause of insulin resistance, although it is by far the most common cause in most populations. Other causes of insulin resistance include a variety of genetic and acquired defects that impact the insulin receptors or postreceptor signaling pathways (see Table 17–7).

Clinical consequences of insulin resistance.   In addition to the impact on glucose metabolism, severe insulin resistance and the resulting elevation in circulating insulin levels can cause other clinical consequences including acanthosis nigricans, pseudoacromegaly, and hyperandrogenism. Acanthosis nigricans appears to be a consequence of very high circulating insulin levels that cross over to bind to IGF receptors on epidermal and melanin-containing cutaneous cells. This leads to local skin hyperplasia with papillomatosis, hyperkeratosis, and hyperpigmentation. The dark, velvety patches of skin most commonly appear on the back of the neck, axillae, and anticubital fossae. In extreme and prolonged cases of insulin resistance, the secondary increase in signaling through the IGF-1 receptor, or possibly residual signaling through the mitogenic arm of the insulin signaling pathway, can cause pseudoacromegaly, a syndrome with all of the bone and soft tissue changes of acromegaly (see Chapter 4), but no elevation in growth hormone or IGF-1. A similar action of extremely high insulin levels on ovarian hilar cells has been implicated in women with insulin resistance who develop hyperandrogenism and hirsutism associated with menstrual irregularities, enlarged cystic ovaries and infertility (polycystic ovary syndrome).

C. β Cell defects in type 2 diabetes

Although the majority of people with type 2 diabetes have insulin resistance, most people with insulin resistance do not have diabetes because their β cells compensate for the insulin resistance by producing and secreting more insulin. Those individuals with insulin resistance who develop type 2 diabetes have a defect in the compensatory response of their β cells to insulin resistance. Functionally, this defect is revealed by a reduction in first phase insulin secretion and the maximal insulin secretion stimulated by glucose.

While increased insulin secretion per β cell may contribute to the compensatory response to insulin resistance, increases in the number of β cells play a role as well. In the setting of obesity, hyperplasia of pancreatic β cells is often present and probably accounts for the normal or exaggerated insulin responses to glucose and other stimuli seen in obese individuals without type 2 diabetes. Assessment of total β cell mass at autopsy has revealed that β cell mass increases in obesity, but the individuals with type 2 diabetes have decreased β cell mass when compared to nondiabetic individuals with the same BMI.

Several possible defects could contribute to the failure of β cell mass compensation in people with type 2 diabetes. Underlying genetic differences in the pathways that drive β cell expansion appear to limit compensation in individuals with high genetic risk of diabetes. In susceptible individuals with obesity, ectopic fat deposition in the islets, local obesity-induced inflammation in the islets, and local and circulating adipokines and inflammatory cytokines may accelerate β cell loss. As β cell failure progresses, levels of glucose and free fatty acids start to rise, which in turn can cause further β cell toxicity. Increased demand on a decreased β cell mass may cause further damage through ER stress and the increased formation of toxic IAPP oligomers. Then, once diabetes is established, all of these mechanisms may further contribute to the progressive decline in β cell function that characterizes type 2 diabetes.

D. Metabolic syndrome

Patients with visceral obesity and insulin resistance often present with a cluster of abnormalities commonly termed the metabolic syndrome. Hyperglycemia in these patients is frequently associated with hyperinsulinemia, dyslipidemia, and hypertension, which together lead to coronary artery disease and stroke. It has been suggested that this aggregation results from a genetic defect producing insulin resistance, particularly when obesity aggravates the degree of insulin resistance. In this model, impaired action of insulin predisposes to hyperglycemia, which in turn induces hyperinsulinemia. If this hyperinsulinemia is of insufficient magnitude to correct the hyperglycemia, type 2 diabetes is manifested. The excessive insulin level could also increase sodium retention by renal tubules, thereby contributing to or causing hypertension. Increased VLDL production in the liver, leading to hypertriglyceridemia (and consequently a decreased high-density lipoprotein [HDL] cholesterol level), has also been attributed to hyperinsulinism. Moreover, it has been proposed that high insulin levels can stimulate endothelial and vascular smooth muscle cell proliferation—by virtue of the hormone's action on growth factor receptors—to promote atherosclerosis.

Although there is full agreement on an association of these disorders, the mechanism of their interrelationship remains speculative and open to experimental investigation. Controversy persists about whether or not hypertension is caused by the hyperinsulinism that results from insulin resistance. Moreover, patients with hyperinsulinism due to an insulinoma are generally normotensive, and there is no reduction of blood pressure after surgical removal of the insulinoma restores normal insulin levels.

An alternative unifying hypothesis could be that visceral obesity directly induces the other components of this syndrome. Visceral obesity is an independent risk factor for all of the other components of the metabolic syndrome. In addition to the metabolic effects of visceral obesity, the adipokines and inflammatory cytokines generated from overloaded and inflamed adipose tissue may contribute to the pathophysiology of the syndrome. Although the full details of the role of these molecules in causation of the metabolic syndrome remain under investigation, the adipocytes and associated macrophages clearly are not just innocent bystanders but play active roles in the development of systemic insulin resistance, hypertension, and hyperlipidemia. Furthermore, thrombi in atheromatous vessels may be more hazardous in patients with visceral obesity because of an associated increase in plasminogen activator inhibitor-1 (PAI-1), a circulating factor produced by omental and visceral adipocytes that inhibits clot lysis. This model emphasizes the importance of measures such as diet and exercise that reduce visceral adiposity in the management of patients with metabolic syndrome and obese type 2 diabetes.

The main value of grouping these disorders as a syndrome, regardless of its nomenclature, is to remind physicians that the therapeutic goals in these patients must not only correct hyperglycemia but also manage the elevated blood pressure and hyperlipidemia that result in considerable cardiovascular morbidity as well as cardiovascular deaths. In addition, it reminds physicians that when choosing antihypertensive agents or lipid-lowering drugs to manage one of the components of this syndrome, their possible untoward effects on other components of the syndrome should be carefully considered. For example, physicians aware of this syndrome are less likely to prescribe antihypertensive drugs that raise lipids (diuretics, beta blockers) or that raise blood glucose (diuretics). Likewise, they may refrain from prescribing drugs that correct hyperlipidemia, but increase insulin resistance with aggravation of hyperglycemia (nicotinic acid).

E. Genetics of type 2 diabetes

Type 2 diabetes has a strong genetic link. Depending on the population studied, monozygotic twins have lifetime concordance rates for type 2 diabetes exceeding 90%. In contrast, concordance rates for type 1 diabetes in monzygotic twins are 25% to 50%. Most individuals with type 2 diabetes have other family members with the disease, but the inheritance rarely fits Mendelian patterns, supporting the conclusion that multiple genes with varying degrees of penetrance contribute. Because of the heterogeneous nature of type 2 diabetes, and its complex inheritance, efforts to identify the genes that contribute to the disease have had very limited success in the vast majority of affected patients. There has been considerable success, however, in identifying small subsets of patients with unique monogenic forms of the disease. When the etiologic defect has been defined, these patients have been reclassified within a group designated "Other Specific Types of Diabetes" (see Table 17–5).

Efforts to identify the genes involved in polygenic type 2 diabetes have focused on two approaches: candidate gene testing and genome-wide association studies (GWAS). To date candidate gene and GWAS approaches have identified 19 loci with common variants linked to type 2 diabetes. Although statistically significant and validated in additional populations, these loci independently make very small contributions to type 2 diabetes risk. The highest risk of these common variants is found at a locus adjacent to the gene encoding TCF7L2, a transcription factor involved in Wnt signaling and implicated in β cell turnover. Inheritance of the high-risk TCF7L2 allele increases the probability of developing diabetes by 1.5-fold.

Among the genes identified so far, most are involved in β cell function and turnover. When combined with the predominance of β cell genes implicated in mongenic forms of diabetes (see Other Specific Types of Diabetes), these results reinforce the critical role of the β cell in controlling blood glucose and its involvement in the pathophysiology of type 2 diabetes. Hopefully, with the advent of high-throughput whole genome sequencing technologies, the identification of rarer, but higher risk, variants will further expand our understanding of the genetics of type 2 diabetes in the near future.

F. Environmental factors in type 2 diabetes

Despite the critical role of genetics in type 2 diabetes, environment contributes as well, especially in determining the age of onset and severity of the disease. There is generally a low incidence of type 2 diabetes in underdeveloped countries, especially in rural areas. Western countries and westernizing countries suffer from a much higher incidence. Over the past half-century, the incidence of type 2 diabetes has increased rapidly in almost all world populations but especially in emerging third-world countries. This increase correlates with increasing rates of obesity in the same populations and reflects increased access to food with high caloric content and decreased physical activity. This combination inevitably leads to increased adiposity, especially in the more readily mobilized fat stores surrounding the viscera in the abdomen.

One of the most dramatic recent changes in the epidemiology of diabetes has been the growing incidence of type 2 diabetes in children. While rarely seen in children a generation ago, type 2 diabetes is now as common as type 1 diabetes in teenagers in the United States and is seen with increasing frequency, even in younger children. Again, this increase is directly related to increasing visceral adiposity.

OTHER SPECIFIC TYPES OF DIABETES

Autosomal Dominant Genetic Defects of Pancreatic β Cells

MODY: This subgroup of monogenic disorders is characterized by the onset of diabetes in late childhood or before the age of 25 years as a result of a partial defect in glucose-induced insulin release and accounts for up to 5% of diabetes in North American and European populations. A strong family history of early-onset diabetes occurring in one parent and in one-half of the parent's offspring suggests autosomal dominant transmission. In contrast to most patients with type 2 diabetes, these patients are generally nonobese and lack associated insulin resistance. Instead they exhibit predominantly a defect in glucose-stimulated insulin secretion. However, because they are not ketosis-prone and may initially achieve good glycemic control without insulin therapy, their disease has been called **maturity-onset diabetes of the young (MODY)**. Several distinct types have been described with single-gene defects, and all have been shown to produce a defect in

TABLE 17–8 Autosomal dominant genetic defects of pancreatic β cell function.

Syndrome	Mutated Protein	Gene	Function
MODY 1	Hepatocyte nuclear factor-4α	HNF4A	Transcription factor
MODY 2	Glucokinase	GCK	Glucose sensor
MODY 3	Hepatocyte nuclear factor-1α	HNF1A	Transcription factor
MODY 4	Pancreatic duodenal homeobox-1	PDX1	Transcription factor
MODY 5	Hepatocyte nuclear factor-1β	HPF1A	Transcription factor
MODY 6	NeuroD1	NEUOROD1	Transcription factor
MODY 7	Kruppel-like factor 11	KLF11	Transcription factor
MODY 8	Carboxyl-ester lipase	CEL	Exocrine enzyme
MODY 9	Paired homeobox 4	PAX4	Transcription factor
Mutant insulin or proinsulin	Preproinsulin	INS	Hormone
KATP mutations	Inward-rectifying K+ channel 6.2	KCNJ11	Ion channel
	Sulfonylurea receptor 1	ABBC8	Ion channel

glucose-induced insulin release. MODY 2 results from an abnormal glucokinase enzyme. Most of the other forms of MODY are due to mutations of nuclear transcription factors that regulate the expression of genes in β cells or β cell precursors (Table 17–8).

MODY 1 includes multiple members of a large pedigree known as the R-W family, descendants of a German couple who immigrated to Michigan in 1861. They were studied prospectively since 1958, and in 1996 the genetic defect was shown to be a nonsense mutation of a nuclear transcription factor found in liver as well as in pancreatic β cells. This gene has been termed *hepatocyte nuclear factor 4α (HNF4α)* and is found on chromosome 20. Mutations of this gene are among the rarest of the MODY groups, with very few reported in families outside the Michigan pedigree. These patients display a progressive decline in β cell function and eventually develop chronic complications of diabetes including microangiopathy at a rate approaching that of people with type 1 diabetes. They often fare better with insulin therapy.

MODY 2 was first described in French families but has now been found in racial groups from most parts of the world. Multiple different mutations of the *glucokinase* gene (*GCK*) on chromosome 7 have been identified and characterized. In pancreatic β cells, glucokinase controls the rate-limiting step in glycolysis and thereby determines the rate of ATP production from glucose and the insulin secretory response to glucose (see Figure 17–5).

Reduced glucokinase activity resets the sensitivity of the β cell to glucose so that it requires higher plasma glucose levels to stimulate insulin secretion, resulting in fasting hyperglycemia and mild diabetes. Although some of these mutations can completely block the enzyme's function, others interfere only slightly with its action. In contrast to all the other forms of MODY, most patients with one mutated *GCK* allele (heterozygotes) have a benign course with few or no chronic complications and respond well to diet therapy or oral antidiabetic drugs without the need for insulin treatment. On the other hand, rare individuals who inherit two mutated *GCK* alleles have permanent neonatal diabetes (see later), a nonimmune form of absolute insulin deficiency that presents at birth.

In contrast to the mutations that reduce glucokinase enzyme activity and cause MODY 2, rare mutations in *GCK* that increase the enzymatic activity of glucokinase can cause increased insulin secretion and hypoglycemia (see Chapter 18), demonstrating the key role of this enzyme in determining the sensitivity of the β cell to glucose.

MODY 3 is caused by mutations of *hepatocyte nuclear factor 1α (HNF1α)*, whose gene is located on chromosome 12. This is the most common form of MODY in European populations, with many different mutations having been reported. Like *HNF4α*, the *HNF1α* transcription factor is expressed in pancreatic β cells as well as in liver. Also similar to *HNF4α*, mutations in *HNF1α* cause a progressive form of diabetes with declining β cell function that often leads to dependence on insulin therapy and high rates of microvascular complications. Noteworthy, early in the course of the disease, these patients may display an exaggerated response to sulfonylureas.

Together, *HNF1α* and *HNF4α*, along with several other β cell transcription factors including *PDX1* (discussed later), form an interacting network of transcription factors. This transcriptional network regulates genes involved in multiple β cell functions, including glucose-sensing and insulin secretion. Target genes include *GCK*, as well as genes implicated in the formation, maturation and expansion of β cells. Impairment in β cell formation and regeneration may explain the progressive nature of the MODY transcription factor syndromes and reinforces the importance of β cell mass in preventing hyperglycemia.

MODY 4 results from mutation of a pancreatic nuclear transcription factor known as *pancreatic and duodenal homeobox-1 (PDX1)*, whose gene is on chromosome 13. It mediates *insulin* gene transcription and regulates expression of other β cell-specific genes including *GCK*. When both alleles of this gene are nonfunctioning, agenesis of the entire pancreas results; but in the presence of a heterozygous mutation of *PDX1*, a mild form of MODY has been described in which affected individuals developed diabetes at a later age (mean onset at 35 years) than occurs with the other forms of MODY, in whom onset generally occurs before the age of 25 years.

MODY 5 was initially reported in a Japanese family with a mutation of *HNF1β*, a hepatic nuclear transcription factor closely related in structure and molecular function to *HNF1α*. The two *HNF1* factors, however, are expressed by different cells. *HNF1β* is expressed early in the development of the liver, pancreas, kidneys, and genitourinary system, and is not found in mature β cells.

Mutations in this gene cause a moderately severe form of MODY with progression to insulin treatment and severe diabetic complications in those affected. Consistent with its expression pattern early in development, *HNF1β* mutations also frequently cause reduction in the overall size of the pancreas, decreased insulin production, and congenital defects in the kidney and urogenital tract. Patients may also suffer from varying degrees of cholestatic jaundice, hyperuricemia, nephropathy, and hypomagnesemia secondary to renal magnesium wasting.

MODY 6, a milder form of MODY similar to MODY 4, results from mutations in the gene encoding the islet transcription factor NeuroD1. Like PDX1, NeuroD1 plays an important role in the expression of insulin and other β cell genes, and in the formation and maintenance of β cells.

Other *MODY* genes: The six MODY genes listed above explain the majority of cases of MODY in patients of European ancestry, but less than half of those in non-European populations. Several rare variants in other genes have been implicated in autosomal dominant diabetes in a few families (see Table 17–8); however, a consensus has not yet been reached that these families fit the criteria for MODY and that the reported variants cause the disorder. The causative genes in most non-Europeans with MODY remain unknown.

The identification of mutations in multiple genes encoding pancreatic transcription factors in patients with MODY has led to the screening of other genes encoding pancreatic transcription factors in patients with diabetes. Heterozygous mutations in genes encoding several transcription factors, including *Isl1*, *Pax6*, and *Pax4*, have been identified in patients with later onset diabetes. The association of diabetes with heterozygous mutations in so many β cell genes highlights the critical importance of optimal β cell function in metabolic regulation. Even modest defects in glucose-induced insulin secretion can result in hyperglycemia.

Insulin mutations: Sequencing of the *insulin* gene more than 30 years ago led to the first descriptions of heterozygous mutations in the coding sequence of the *insulin* gene that produce abnormal circulating forms of insulin. Most of these initial cases presented with high circulating levels of insulin, but normal insulin sensitivity and normal glucose levels. Because the abnormal insulins in these cases bind to receptors poorly, they have very low biologic activity and are cleared at a slower rate, leading to accumulation in the blood at higher levels than normal insulin and a subnormal molar ratio of C peptide to immunoreactive insulin. They typically are not associated with hyperglycemia.

However, a mutation in the insulin B chain in one family was associated with decreased circulating levels of both the mutant and normal insulins, and diabetes. Subsequent extensive sequencing of the *INS* gene has identified several other mutant insulins that produce a similar heterozygous form of diabetes. Modeling of these dominant insulin mutations in mice demonstrates that they lead to the accumulation of aberrantly folded proteins in the endoplasmic reticulum, activation of the unfolded protein response in the ER, and β cell apoptosis. Patients with diabetes secondary to *INS* gene mutations usually present at a younger age than most patients with MODY, often developing the disease as neonates (see later). Because of the profound β cell loss, these patients follow a disease course similar to type 1 diabetes with absolute insulin deficiency and ketosis, and they require insulin therapy.

This syndrome highlights the sensitivity of the β cells to ER stress, which may explain why β cells often fail when presented with the increased insulin demands associated with insulin resistance, the toxicity of IAPP oligomers, or mutations in genes involved in the unfolded protein response pathway (see later).

Mutations in the subunits of the ATP-sensitive potassium channel: β cells sense rising blood glucose concentrations by increasing the production of ATP from glucose. The rising intracellular ATP levels cause the closure of ATP-sensitive potassium channels on the cell surface, which depolarizes the cell and sets off a cascade of events that leads to the secretion of insulin (Figure 17–5). Rare dominant activating mutations in either of the two units of the channel, SUR1 and Kir6.2 (gene names *ABCC8* and *KCNJ11*, respectively), can cause the channels to remain open and prevent glucose-induced depolarization and insulin secretion. Children heterozygous for these mutations present with early-onset diabetes, commonly as neonates, and may have associated neurologic deficits implying a role for these channels in the central nervous system. Depending on the exact mutation, some of these children can still respond to treatment with sulfonylureas, which may also ameliorate the neurologic symptoms.

Other Genetic Defects of Pancreatic β Cells

Autosomal recessive genetic defects: Although less common than the autosomal dominant β cell disorders, mutations in several genes causing autosomal recessive syndromes with defects in β cell function have been identified in patients with diabetes (Table 17–9). Due to the severity of the β cell defect, many of these present with neonatal diabetes. This group of disorders includes homozygous mutations in the MODY genes *GCK* and *PDX1*. Homozygous mutations in *GCK* cause a much more severe syndrome than the mild glucose-sensing defect seen in MODY 2. Patients with homozygous *GCK* mutations present at birth with severe hyperglycemia and require insulin therapy.

In patients with mutations in both alleles of *PDX1*, the pancreas fails to form, and they have pancreatic exocrine deficiency as well as diabetes. Homozygous mutations in several other pancreatic transcription factor genes have been described as well, including *PTF1A*, *NEUROG3*, *RFX6*, and *GLIS3*. Like *PDX1*, homozygous mutation of *PTF1A* causes diabetes and pancreatic agenesis, but it also causes cerebellar atrophy as well. The transcription factor Neurog3 drives the formation of the endocrine cells in both the pancreas and gut. In addition to diabetes onset prior to puberty, infants born with homozygous *NEUROG3* mutations have severe malabsorption associated with a lack of gut endocrine cells from birth.

Homozygous mutations in *RFX6*, which encodes a transcription factor that functions downstream of *NEUROG3* and upstream of *PDX1* in β cell development, cause **Mitchell–Riley syndrome** in which neonates present with diabetes in association with complete absence of all islet cell types except PP cells, hypoplasia of the pancreas and gall bladder, intestinal atresia, and severe malabsorption.

TABLE 17–9 **Autosomal recessive genetic defects of pancreatic β cell function.**

Function	Protein	Gene	Associated Defects
Glucose sensing	Glucokinase	GCK	
Transcription factor	Pancreatic duodenal homeobox-1	PDX1	Pancreatic agenesis
	Pancreatic transcription factor 1a	PTF1A	Pancreatic and cerebellar agenesis
	Neurogenenin3	NEUROG3	Absence of gut endocrine cells, malabsorption
	Regulatory factor X-box 6	RFX6	Mitchell-Riley syndrome: absence of gut endocrine and islet α, β, and δ cells, pancreatic and gall bladder hypoplasia, intestinal atresia, malabsorption
	GLI Similar-3	GLIS3	Hypothyroidism, cholestasis, polycystic kidneys, hypoplastic pancreas
Unfolded protein response	Eukaryotic translation initiation factor 2-α kinase 3/PKR-like ER kinase (PERK)	EIF2AK3	Wolcott-Rallison syndrome: epiphyseal dysplasia and growth retardation; variable hepatic, renal, cardiac, and pancreatic exocrine defects
	Wolfram syndrome protein 1 (WFS1)	WFS1	Wolfram syndrome: diabetes insipidus, diabetes mellitus, optic atrophy and deafness (DIDMOAD)
Thiamine transport	Solute carrier family 19 (thiamine transporter), member 2	SLC19A2	Thiamine-responsive megaloblastic anemia: anemia, deafness

The zinc finger transcription factor GLIS3 is expressed broadly in many tissues and plays a role in the transcription of the *insulin* gene. Homozygous mutations in *GLIS3* cause congenital hypothyroidism in addition to neonatal diabetes.

In the autosomal recessive **Wolcott-Rallison syndrome**, affected children present with neonatal diabetes, epiphyseal dysplasia, and growth retardation together with a variety of progressive hepatic, renal, cardiac, and pancreatic exocrine defects and developmental delay. The causative gene, *EIF2AK3,* encodes a kinase (PKR-like ER kinase [PERK]) activated by the presence of unfolded proteins in the ER. PERK controls one of the three parallel arms of the unfolded protein response; inositol-requiring enzyme 1 (IRE1) and activating transcription factor 6 (ATF6) activate the other two arms. Together these three molecules activate signaling pathways that protect the cell from ER stress but lead to apoptosis when these protective mechanisms fail. Mice lacking PERK have an inadequate response to ER stress, which leads to accelerated β cell apoptosis. With the high load of insulin production in the ER, β cells are uniquely sensitive to ER stress, and this sensitivity probably underlies the damage caused by mutant insulins, IAPP oligomers, and Wolfram syndrome as well.

Wolfram syndrome is an autosomal recessive neurodegenerative disorder first evident in childhood. Patients present with diabetes insipidus, diabetes mellitus, optic atrophy, and deafness—hence the acronym DIDMOAD. Diabetes mellitus usually develops in the first decade together with the optic atrophy, followed by central diabetes insipidus and sensorineural deafness during the second decade in 60% to 75% of patients. Ureterohydronephrosis, neurogenic bladder, cerebellar ataxia, peripheral neuropathy, and psychiatric illness develop later in many patients. The diabetes mellitus is nonimmune and not linked to specific HLA antigens, but on autopsy these patients have selective loss of β cells in the pancreas. Genetic studies mapped the causative mutations to a gene called *WFS1*, which encodes a 100.3-kDa transmembrane protein localized to the endoplasmic reticulum membranes of all cells. *WFS1* is expressed at particularly high levels in β cells. Studies in mice have shown that the WFS1 protein forms part of the unfolded protein

response downstream of PERK and IRE1 and helps protect the β cells from ER stress and apoptosis, especially during periods of high insulin demand.

Children with **thiamine-responsive megaloblastic anemia syndrome** carry mutations in the high-affinity thiamine transporter SLC19A2 found on cell and mitochondrial membranes. They develop megalobastic anemia, diabetes, and sensorineuronal deafness. The diabetes usually presents in the first decade of life. In the absence of SLC19A2, cells and mitochondria can still transport thiamine through lower affinity transporters, and both the anemia and the diabetes respond to pharmacologic treatment with thiamine. However, all patients eventually require insulin replacement despite thiamine therapy. It remains unclear how partial defects in cellular and mitochondrial thiamine transport cause β cell failure.

Mitochondrial DNA mutations: Because sperm do not contain mitochondria, only the mother transmits mitochondrial genes to her offspring. Diabetes due to a mutation of mitochondrial DNA that impairs the transfer of leucine into mitochondrial proteins has now been described in a large number of families, and results from impaired β cell function. The incidence of this disorder is as high as 1% to 3% in patients with diabetes in Japan and Korea, but lower in European populations. Most patients have a mild form of maternally transmitted diabetes with insulin deficiency that responds to oral hypoglycemic agents; however, some patients have a more severe clinical picture similar to type 1a diabetes. As many as 63% of patients with this subtype of diabetes have hearing loss and a smaller proportion (15%) have a syndrome of myopathy, encephalopathy, lactic acidosis, and stroke-like episodes.

Ketosis-Prone Diabetes

First described in young adult African American males from the Flatbush neighborhood in New York City, but since described in a number of populations of both African and non-African ancestry, these patients typically present with diabetic ketoacidosis and absolute insulin deficiency, followed by extended clinical remission off insulin. When tested during remission, however, maximal insulin secretory capacity remains markedly reduced, and these patients follow a relapsing course of DKA and hyperglycemia with eventual permanent insulin-deficient diabetes. These patients do not have islet cell autoantibodies or increased frequencies of HLA haplotypes associated with risk of autoimmune type 1a diabetes. Although there is often a family history of similar diabetes, the inheritance is not clearly Mendelian. Although KPD patients have been distinguished based on the history of relapsing β cell dysfunction, it remains controversial as to whether KPD represents a clinical entity distinct from other forms of nonautoimmune type 1b diabetes.

In a study of KPD patients of West African ancestry, linkage was established with coding variants in the *PAX4* gene. *PAX4* encodes for a transcription factor that functions downstream of *NEUROG3* in the formation of β cells. Fourteen to twenty-one percent of individuals of West African ancestry carry a coding variant that substitutes tryptophan for arginine at position 133 in Pax4 and reduces its ability to repress transcription of target genes. Interestingly, the R133W variant is unique to people of West African ancestry. The R133W allele is approximately twice as frequent in individuals with KPD, and all individuals homozygous for R133W have KPD. An additional Pax4 coding variant with reduced ability to bind to DNA was identified in one patient with KPD. Different coding variants in *PAX4* have also been identified in Thai families with MODY (MODY 9) and in Japanese patients (both heterozygous and homozygous) with early onset insulin-deficient diabetes similar to KPD. Taken together, these data suggest that coding variants in the *PAX4* gene predispose to insulin-deficient diabetes, but the clinical phenotype may depend on the exact nature of the variant and interactions with other genes and environmental factors.

Genetic Defects of Insulin Action

These are rare and unusual causes of diabetes that result from mutations of the insulin receptor or from other genetically determined postreceptor abnormalities of insulin action. Metabolic abnormalities associated with these disorders may range from hyperinsulinemia and modest hyperglycemia to severe diabetes. Many individuals have acanthosis nigricans, polycystic ovaries with hyperandrogenism, and, in exceptional cases, pseudoacromegaly (see earlier).

Familial forms of insulin resistance associated with acanthosis nigricans have been termed type A insulin resistance, and are often associated with heterozygous mutations in the **insulin receptor** or homozygous mutations that retain some insulin-signaling capacity. Because of the capacity of the β cell to compensate for insulin resistance, these patients often do not present with hyperglycemia, but have severely elevated levels of circulating insulin.

If both copies of the insulin receptor gene carry mutations that nearly or completely abrogate signaling, the affected children present at birth with a syndrome known as **Leprechaunism** (or **Donohue syndrome**) that includes growth retardation, multiple developmental defects, lipoatrophy, severely elevated insulin levels, and hyperglycemia that does not respond to insulin therapy. These patients generally do not survive beyond a few weeks.

Patients with **Rabson-Mendenhall syndrome** also have homozygous or compound heterozygous mutations in the insulin receptor, but with some small amount of residual signaling that results in a slightly less severe syndrome associated with abnormalities in the nails, teeth, and pineal gland. They may survive into adolescence.

Familial forms of type A insulin resistance without mutations in the insulin receptor have been described, and some of these may result from mutations in downstream components of the insulin-signaling cascade, although to date few such mutations have been found in humans. Variants in IRS1 have been identified in patients with diabetes, but also occur in people with normal insulin sensitivity. Rare coding mutations in the genes encoding the p85α subunit of PI3 kinase, in AKT2, and in PPARγ have been associated with severe insulin resistance in a very small number of patients. The one patient with homozygous mutation of *AKT2* also had mild atrophy of subcutaneous limb adipose tissue.

Congenital and acquired forms of lipodystrophy can cause severe insulin resistance. Except in newborns with lipoatrophy secondary to complete loss of insulin receptors (Leprechaunism), alterations in the structure and function of the insulin receptor cannot be demonstrated in patients with insulin-resistant lipodystrophic diabetes, suggesting that the cause of the insulin resistance in these patients must reside in postreceptor pathways. Replacement of the adipokines leptin and adiponectin can reverse insulin resistance in mouse models of severe lipoatrophy, and leptin has been helpful in human cases of generalized lipodystrophy, demonstrating the importance of the adipocyte in regulating insulin function. Also, the loss of adipose storage depots in lipoatrophy leads to very high levels of circulating triglyceride-rich lipoprotein particles and increased deposition of fat in nonadipose tissues such as liver and muscle, which may contribute to dysfunction and insulin resistance in these tissues. The increase in ectopic fat deposition leads to profound hepatic steatosis in affected patients and can progress to cirrhosis and liver failure.

The congenital syndromes can be divided into generalized and partial lipodystrophies with or without dystrophic features in other tissues. The generalized syndromes are often identified in neonates, have severe insulin resistance at diagnosis and rapidly develop hyperglycemia, acanthosis nigricans, hyperandrogenism, and pseudoacromegaly. Recessive mutations causing generalized congenital lipodystrophy have been identified in three genes encoding proteins involved in the formation of lipid droplets (seipin and caveolin-1) and triglyceride (1-acylglycerol-3-phosphate-*O*-acyltransferase 2 [AGPAT2]).

Two syndromes of familial partial lipodystrophy without associated dysmorphic defects have been described in which the lipotrophy usually first appears late in childhood, but may be proceeded by evidence of insulin resistance. The type 1 syndrome consists of atrophy of limb, gluteal and subcutaneous abdominal fat with sparing or increases of the abdominal visceral, upper trunk, head, and neck fat. In the type 2 syndrome, truncal and visceral fat are also affected and only vulval and head and neck depots are spared.

To date no genetic causes of the type 1 syndrome have been identified. In the type 2 syndrome, dominant mutations have been found in *LMNA*, the gene encoding the nuclear intermediate filament lamin A/C. In addition, one individual with the type 2 syndrome has been identified with a homozygous nonsense mutation in the gene encoding the lipid droplet protein CIDEC, and one individual was identified with a homozygous truncation of the gene encoding lipase maturation factor 1, a protein required for the maturation of both lipoprotein lipase and hepatic lipase.

Consistent with its known role in adipocytes differentiation, dominant mutations in the gene encoding PPARγ have also been described in patients with familial partial lipodystrophy and insulin resistance. These patients have a pattern of lipoatrophy similar to the type 2 syndrome with *LMNA* mutations, but with less severe subcutaneous fat loss, and have been labeled type 3 familial partial lipodystrophy.

Several syndromes of lipodystrophy associated with other dysmorphic features have been described. Autosomal recessive mutations in *ZMPSTE24*, which encodes a metalloproteinase that cleaves prolamin A to produce mature lamin A, cause generalized lipodystrophy associated with mandibulo-acral dysplasia. In patients with partial lipodystrophy combined with mandibulo-acral dysplasia, autosomal recessive mutations have been identified in *LMNA*, but these mutations are distinct from those that cause familial partial lipodystrophy type 2. Remarkably, yet a different set of mutations in *LMNA* cause the autosomal recessive syndrome Hutchinson–Gilford progeria, which includes severe early onset generalized lipodystrophy. Additional distinct mutations in *LMNA* cause several other congenital dysmorphic syndromes, including muscular dystrophies, familial dilated cardiomyopathy, and Charcot-Marie-Tooth disease.

Acquired forms of partial and generalized lipodystrophy with insulin resistance and diabetes can develop secondary to infections, autoimmunity, paraneoplastic syndromes, collagen vascular disorders, drugs, or unknown causes. One common form is seen in patients with HIV infection following treatment with protease inhibitors.

Neonatal Diabetes

Neonatal diabetes, defined as diabetes diagnosed before 6 months of age, is rare, occurring in fewer than 1 in 200,000 live births. Children with neonatal diabetes often present with decreased birth weight (intrauterine growth retardation, IUGR) and decreased fat stores in addition to hyperglycemia. Most commonly these children have reduced circulating insulin and C-peptide levels caused by inherited β cells defects, although rare inherited defects in insulin signaling can also present in neonates. In approximately half of cases, neonatal diabetes is transient: the diabetes goes into remission (normoglycemia with no therapy) before 18 months of age, although it usually returns at puberty. In the remainder of cases, the diabetes is permanent.

Transient neonatal diabetes (TNDM): Defects in imprinting underlie most cases of TNDM. The most common genetic defect is paternal uniparental isodysomy (replacement of the maternal copy of the region with the paternal copy) of an imprinted region at chromosome 6q24. In this region, the maternal copy of the chromosome is normally silenced by methylation. Simple

duplication of the paternal copy of this region, or mutations in ZFP57, a zinc-finger protein required globally for the methylation of imprinted regions, can give the same TNDM phenotype. The affected region of 6q24 contains two genes of uncertain function, but one of them, *ZAC*, has been identified as a tumor suppressor gene and may activate the expression of an inhibitor of cell proliferation. An increase in hypomethylated copies of *ZAC* may lead to the inhibition of β cell proliferation and inadequate β cell mass.

Some autosomal dominant activating mutations in *KCNJ11* and *ABCC8*, the genes encoding the two subunits of the ATP-sensitive potassium channels in β cells (Figure 17–5) and listed among autosomal dominant forms of heritable diabetes (see earlier) can cause TNDM. Autosomal dominant mutations in the MODY 5 gene, *HNF1B*, can also cause TNDM.

Permanent neonatal diabetes (PNDM): Autosomal dominant activating mutations in *KCNJ11* and *ABCC8* can also cause PNDM. Some of the autosomal dominant insulin mutations that cause rapid β cell apoptosis will result in permanent diabetes in neonates. In addition, most of the syndromes caused by autosomal recessive genetic defects in β cells (see Table 17–9) present in neonates. These include mutations in the MODY genes *GCK* and *PDX1*, the transcription factor genes *PTF1A*, *GLIS3*, and *RFX6*, and the Wolcott–Rallison syndrome gene *EIF2AK3*. The IPEX syndrome (see Genetics of Type 1 Diabetes above), caused by mutations in *FOXP3*, can also present with accelerated autoimmune type 1 diabetes in neonates. Finally, mutations that cause complete, or nearly complete, loss of insulin signaling (Leprechaunism) also present with PNDM.

Several other syndromes of neonatal diabetes of unknown etiology associated with a variety of other developmental defects have been described. With the advent of rapid whole genome sequencing, the genetic defects that cause these syndromes, as well as later onset diabetes, may soon be identified, providing further insights into the pathogenesis of diabetes and identifying potential therapeutic targets.

Diabetes due to Diseases of the Exocrine Pancreas

Any process that diffusely damages or substantially displaces the pancreas can cause diabetes, although individuals with a predisposition to type 2 diabetes are probably more susceptible to developing diabetes with lesser degrees of pancreatic involvement. Because glucagon-secreting α cells are also damaged or removed by these processes, less insulin is usually required for replacement—as compared with most other forms of diabetes that leave α cells intact.

Acquired causes include pancreatitis, trauma, infection, pancreatic carcinoma, and pancreatectomy. Fibrocalculous pancreatopathy, a form of acquired pancreatitis with extensive fibrosis and ductal calculi seen commonly in tropical regions, may result from both dietary and genetic contributors, although the exact cause remains obscure. Like chronic pancreatitis from a variety of causes, fibrocalculous involvement of the pancreas may be accompanied by abdominal pain radiating to the back and associated with pancreatic calcifications on x-ray. When extensive enough, hemochromatosis and cystic fibrosis can also displace β cells and reduce insulin secretion. Autosomal dominant mutations in carboxyl-ester lipase (CEL), an exocrine enzyme, cause accelerated exocrine pancreatic damage and diabetes at a young age, and have been designated as MODY 8 (see Table 17–8).

Endocrinopathies

Excess production of certain hormones—GH (acromegaly), glucocorticoids (Cushing syndrome or disease), catecholamines (pheochromocytoma), thyroid hormone (thyrotoxicosis), glucagon (glucagonoma), or pancreatic somatostatin (somatostatinoma)—can produce relative insulin deficiency and diabetes by a number of mechanisms. In all but the last instance (somatostatinoma), peripheral responsiveness to insulin is impaired. In addition, excess of catecholamines or somatostatin decreases insulin release from β cells. Diabetes mainly occurs in individuals with underlying defects in insulin secretion, and hyperglycemia typically resolves when the hormone excess is corrected.

Drug- or Chemical-Induced Diabetes

Many drugs are associated with carbohydrate intolerance or frank diabetes mellitus. Some act by interfering with insulin release from the β cells (thiazides, phenytoin, cyclosporine), some by inducing insulin resistance (glucocorticoids, oral contraceptive pills, niacin, and antiviral protease inhibitors), and some by causing β cell destruction (intravenous pentamidine). Patients receiving β interferon have been reported to develop diabetes associated with β cell antibodies and in certain instances severe insulin deficiency. Atypical antipsychotic medications can provoke substantial weight gain and insulin resistance, but the high reported incidence of diabetic ketoacidosis in patients on these drugs suggests that they may also impair β cell function.

Adrenergic drugs impact glucose metabolism in complex and often opposing ways because of differing effects on insulin secretion, glucagon secretion, hepatic glucose output, peripheral insulin sensitivity, and weight gain. In clinical practice, the first generation, nonselective β blockers such as propanolol tend to modestly increase glucose levels, at least in part due to increases in insulin resistance, but potentially by decreasing insulin secretion as well. The second generation, selective β1 blockers also tend to increase blood glucose, but the third generation drugs with combined α and β blockade have minimal effects on blood glucose. In contrast, nonselective α agonist and α2 agonists tend to raise blood glucose, probably due to their combined effects on insulin secretion and hepatic glucose output. However, although β blockers and α2 agonists like clonidine, as well as calcium channel blockers, inhibit glucose-induced insulin release from in vitro preparations of pancreatic β cells, these drugs have minimal or modest effects on blood glucose control at the levels used in standard antihypertensive therapy in humans.

Finally it must be kept in mind that the most common toxin causing diabetes is ethanol. Chronic alcoholic pancreatitis with secondary loss of β cells accounts for approximately 1% of diabetes in the United States.

Infections Causing Diabetes

Certain viruses have been associated with direct pancreatic β cell destruction in animals. Diabetes is also known to develop frequently in humans who had congenital rubella, although most of these patients have HLA and immune markers characteristic of type 1 diabetes. In addition, coxsackievirus B, cytomegalovirus, adenovirus, and mumps have been implicated in inducing certain cases of diabetes.

Uncommon Forms of Immune-Mediated Diabetes

A severe form of insulin resistance has been reported in patients who developed high titers of antibodies that bind to the insulin receptor and block the action of insulin in its target tissues. As in other states of extreme insulin resistance, these patients often have acanthosis nigricans. In the past, this form of immune-mediated diabetes was termed type B insulin resistance. Most commonly these antibodies are of idiopathic origin, but they have also been described in monoclonal gamopathies and multiple myeloma and in patients with ataxia telangectasia syndrome.

Several syndromes of altered immune function with multiple endocrine gland involvement have been described. The APS1 and IPEX syndromes are described in the section on the genetics of type 1 diabetes and in Chapter 2. Patients with POEMS, a syndrome of plasma cell dyscrasia associated with polyneuropathy, organomegaly, endocrinopathy, monoclonal gammopathy, and skin changes, have an increased incidence of diabetes as well as other endocrine disorders. The cause of the diabetes in these patients has not been established.

Other Genetic Syndromes Sometimes Associated with Diabetes

More than 50 distinct genetic syndromes involve an increased incidence of diabetes mellitus. These include the chromosomal abnormalities of Down syndrome, Klinefelter syndrome, and Turner syndrome. In addition, a number of complex syndromes associated with neuromuscular pathologies (Freidriech ataxia, Huntington chorea, porphyria, muscular dystrophies) or severe obesity (Laurence-Moon-Biedl, Bardet-Biedl, and Prader-Willi syndromes) have been associated with diabetes.

CLINICAL FEATURES OF DIABETES MELLITUS

The principal clinical features of the two major types of diabetes mellitus are listed for comparison in Table 17–10.

Type 1 Diabetes

Patients with type 1 diabetes present with symptoms and signs related to hyperglycemia and hyperketonemia. The severity of the insulin deficiency and the acuteness with which the catabolic state develops determine the intensity of the osmotic and ketotic excess.

TABLE 17–10   Clinical features of diabetes at diagnosis.

	Diabetes Type 1	Diabetes Type 2
Polyuria and thirst	++	+
Weakness or fatigue	++	+
Polyphagia with weight loss	++	–
Recurrent blurred vision	+	++
Vulvovaginitis or pruritus	+	++
Peripheral neuropathy	+	++
Nocturnal enuresis	++	–
Often asymptomatic	–	++

A. Symptoms   Increased urination is a consequence of osmotic diuresis secondary to sustained hyperglycemia. This results in a loss of glucose as well as free water and electrolytes in the urine. Nocturnal enuresis due to polyuria may signal the onset of diabetes in very young children. Thirst is a consequence of the hyperosmolar state, as is blurred vision, which often develops as the lenses and retinas are exposed to hyperosmolar fluids.

Weight loss, despite normal or increased appetite, is a common feature of type 1 diabetes when it develops subacutely over a period of weeks. The weight loss is initially due to depletion of water, glycogen, and triglyceride stores. Chronic weight loss due to reduced muscle mass occurs as amino acids are diverted to form glucose and ketone bodies.

Lowered plasma volume produces dizziness and weakness due to postural hypotension when sitting or standing. Total body potassium loss and the general catabolism of muscle protein contribute to the weakness.

Paresthesias may be present at the time of diagnosis of type 1 diabetes, particularly when the onset is subacute. They reflect a temporary dysfunction of peripheral sensory nerves and usually clear, as insulin replacement restores glycemic levels closer to normal; thus, their presence suggests neurotoxicity from sustained hyperglycemia.

When insulin deficiency is severe and of acute onset, the above symptoms progress in an accelerated manner. Ketoacidosis exacerbates the dehydration and hyperosmolality by producing anorexia, nausea, and vomiting, thus interfering with oral fluid replacement. As plasma osmolality exceeds 330 mOsm/kg (normal, 285-295 mOsm/kg), impaired consciousness ensues. With progression of acidosis to a pH of 7.1 or less, deep breathing with a rapid ventilatory rate (Kussmaul respiration) occurs as the body attempts to eliminate carbonic acid. With worsening acidosis (to pH 7.0 or less), the cardiovascular system may be unable to maintain compensatory vasoconstriction; severe circulatory collapse may result.

B. Signs   The patient's level of consciousness can vary depending on the degree of hyperosmolality. When insulin deficiency develops relatively slowly and sufficient water intake is maintained to permit renal excretion of glucose and appropriate dilution of extracellular sodium chloride concentration, patients remain relatively alert and physical findings may be minimal. When vomiting occurs in response to worsening ketoacidosis, dehydration

progresses and compensatory mechanisms become inadequate to keep plasma osmolality below 330 mOsm/kg. Under these circumstances, stupor or even coma may occur. Evidence of dehydration in a stuporous patient, with rapid deep breathing and the fruity breath odor of acetone, suggests the diagnosis of diabetic ketoacidosis.

Postural hypotension indicates a depleted plasma volume; hypotension in the recumbent position is a serious prognostic sign. Loss of subcutaneous fat and muscle wasting are features of more slowly developing insulin deficiency. In occasional patients with slow, insidious onset of insulin deficiency, subcutaneous fat may be considerably depleted. An enlarged liver, eruptive xanthomas on the flexor surface of the limbs and on the buttocks, and lipemia retinalis indicate that chronic insulin deficiency has resulted in chylomicronemia, with elevated circulating triglycerides, usually to over 2000 mg/dL (Chapter 19).

Type 2 Diabetes

Patients with type 2 diabetes usually have less severe insulin deficiency than type 1 patients and the symptoms and signs at presentation reflect this difference.

A. Symptoms   Many patients with type 2 diabetes have an insidious onset of hyperglycemia and may be relatively asymptomatic initially. The diagnosis may be made only after glycosuria or hyperglycemia is noted during routine laboratory studies. Chronic skin infections are common. Generalized pruritus and symptoms of candidal vaginitis are frequently the initial complaints of women with type 2 diabetes. Men may complain of an itchy rash of the prepuce. Some patients can remain undiagnosed for many years and the initial presentation may be due to complications such as visual disturbance due to retinopathy or foot pain or infection due to a peripheral neuropathy. Patients with a more severe insulin deficiency have the classical symptoms of polyuria, thirst, blurred vision, paresthesias, and fatigue. This is especially true in individuals who consume large amounts of carbohydrate-rich fluids in response to the thirst.

B. Signs   Many patients are obese or overweight. Even those patients who are not significantly overweight often have a characteristic fat distribution with more fat in the upper part of the body (particularly the abdomen, chest, neck, and face) and relatively less fat on the appendages, which may be quite muscular (the *metabolically obese*). This centripetal fat distribution has been termed **android** and is characterized by a high waist circumference. It differs from the more centrifugal **gynecoid** form of obesity, in which fat is localized more in the hips and thighs and less in the upper parts of the trunk. A larger waist circumference increases the risk for diabetes for any given body mass index (BMI). Thus in patients with the metabolic syndrome, a waist circumference >40 in (102 cm) in men and >35 in (88 cm) in women is associated with an increased risk of diabetes. MRI and CT scans reveal that these patients with increased waist circumference have accumulation of fat in the omental and mesenteric distributions. This visceral fat correlates with insulin resistance, whereas fat predominantly in subcutaneous tissues of the abdomen has little, if any, association with insulin insensitivity.

Some patients, especially the obese, may have acanthosis nigricans—hyperpigmented, hyperkeratotic skin in the axilla, groin, and back of neck. This sign is associated with significant insulin resistance. Hypertension may be present especially in the obese patient. Eruptive xanthomata on the flexor surface of the limbs and on the buttocks and lipemia retinalis due to hyperchylomicronemia can occur in patients with uncontrolled type 2 diabetes who also have a familial form of hypertriglyceridemia. In women, candidal vaginitis with a reddened, inflamed vulvar area and a profuse whitish discharge may herald the presence of diabetes. In men, candidal infection of the penis may lead to reddish appearance of the penis and/or prepuce with eroded white papules and a white discharge. The occasional patient who has had undiagnosed diabetes for some time may present with retinopathy or peripheral neuropathy.

Patients can also present in hyperglycemic hyperosmolar coma—profoundly dehydrated, hypotensive, lethargic, or comatose without Kussmaul respirations.

Laboratory Testing in Diabetes Mellitus

Tests of urine glucose and ketone bodies, as well as whole blood or plasma glucose measured in samples obtained under basal conditions and after glucose administration, are very important in evaluation of the patient with diabetes. Tests for glycosylated hemoglobin have proved useful in both initial evaluation and in assessment of the effectiveness of therapeutic management. In certain circumstances, measurements of insulin or C-peptide levels and levels of other hormones involved in carbohydrate homeostasis (eg, glucagon, GH) may be useful. In view of the increased risk of atherosclerosis in patients with diabetes, determination of serum cholesterol, HDL—cholesterol, triglycerides, and LDL-cholesterol may be helpful.

Urine Glucose

Several problems are associated with using urine glucose as an index of blood glucose, regardless of the method employed. First of all, the glucose concentration in bladder urine reflects the blood glucose at the time the urine was formed. Therefore, the first voided specimen in the morning contains glucose that was excreted throughout the night and does not reflect the morning blood glucose at all. Some improvement in the correlation of urine glucose to blood glucose can be obtained if the patient *double voids*—that is, empties the bladder completely, discards that sample, and then urinates again about one-half hour later, testing only the second specimen for glucose content. However, difficulty in completely emptying the bladder (large residual volumes), problems in understanding the instructions, and the inconvenience impair the usefulness of this test. Self-monitoring of blood glucose has replaced urine glucose testing in most patients with diabetes (particularly those receiving insulin therapy).

Several commercial products are available for determining the presence and amount of glucose in urine. The older and more cumbersome bedside assessment of glycosuria with Clinitest tablets has generally been replaced by the dipstick method, which is rapid, convenient, and glucose specific. This method consists of paper strips (Clinistix, Tes-Tape) impregnated with enzymes (glucose oxidase and hydrogen peroxidase) and a chromogenic dye that is colorless in the reduced state. Enzymatic generation of hydrogen peroxide oxidizes the dye to produce colors whose intensity depends on the glucose concentration. These dipsticks are sensitive to as little as 0.1% glucose (100 mg/dL) but do not react with the smaller amounts of glucose normally present in nondiabetic urine. The strips are subject to deterioration if exposed to air, moisture, and extreme heat and must be kept in tightly closed containers except when in use. False-negative results may be obtained in the presence of alkaptonuria and when certain substances such as salicylic acid or ascorbic acid are ingested in excess. All these false-negative results occur because of the interference of strong reducing agents with oxidation of the chromogen.

Although glycosuria reflects hyperglycemia in more than 90% of patients, two major classes of nondiabetic glycosuria must be considered:

A. Alterations in renal handing of glucose Disorders associated with abnormalities in renal glucose handling include Fanconi syndrome, a group of disorders characterized by combined renal wasting of multiple solutes including amino acids, uric acid, phosphate, and bicarbonate as well as glucose and caused by both genetic and acquired defects of the proximal renal tubule. Familial renal glycosuria, a benign inherited disorder manifest only by persistent glycosuria in the setting of euglycemia is caused by mutations in SGLT2, the sodium-glucose cotransporter responsible for the bulk of glucose reabsorption in the proximal tubule.

In addition, glycosuria is relatively common in pregnancy as a consequence of the increased load of glucose presented to the tubules by the elevated glomerular filtration rate during pregnancy. As many as 50% of pregnant women normally have demonstrable sugar in the urine, especially after the first trimester.

B. Excretion of sugars other than glucose in the urine Occasionally, a sugar other than glucose is excreted in the urine. Lactosuria during the late stages of pregnancy and the period of lactation is the most common example. Much rarer are other conditions in which inborn errors of metabolism allow fructose, galactose, or a pentose (1-xylose) to be excreted in the urine. Testing the urine with glucose-specific strips helps differentiate true glucosuria from other glycosurias.

Microalbuminuria and Proteinuria

Urinary albumin can now be detected in microgram concentrations using high-performance liquid chromatography or immunoassay methodology that is more sensitive than previous available tests. Conventional 24-hour urine collections, in addition to being inconvenient for patients, also show wide variability of albumin excretion, because several factors such as sustained upright posture, dietary protein, and exercise tend to increase albumin excretion rates. For these reasons, it is preferable to measure the albumin-creatinine ratio in an early morning spot urine collected on awakening—prior to breakfast or exercise—and brought in by the patient for laboratory analysis. A ratio of albumin (μg/L) to creatinine (mg/L) of less than 30 is normal, and a ratio of 30 to 300 indicates abnormal microalbuminuria. Values greater than 300 are referred to as macroalbuminuria.

The minimal detection limit of protein on a standard urine dipstick is 10 to 20 mg/dL. If the dipstick is positive then it is likely that the patient has microalbuminuria and this should be specifically tested. The information from a spot urine sample is adequate for diagnosis and treatment and it is not usually necessary to perform a 24-hour urine collection for protein loss and creatinine clearance.

Blood Glucose Testing

A. Venous blood samples

Venous glucose samples should be collected in tubes containing sodium fluoride, which inhibits enolase and prevents glycolysis in the blood sample that would artifactually lower the measured glucose level. In the absence of fluoride, the rate of disappearance of glucose in the presence of blood cells has been reported to average 10 mg/dL/h—the rate increases with glucose concentration, temperature, and white blood cell count. Fluoride takes about 1 hour to effectively stop glycolysis. Therefore, the rate of decline during the first hour is the same in tubes with or without fluoride. A very high white blood cell count will lower glucose levels even in the presence of fluoride. Ideally the blood should be collected in a sodium fluoride/potassium oxalate tube, placed on ice and the plasma separated from the cells within 60 minutes.

Plasma or serum from venous blood samples has the advantage over whole blood of providing values for glucose that are independent of hematocrit and reflect levels in the interstitial spaces to which body tissues are exposed. For these reasons—and because plasma and serum lend themselves to automated analytic procedures—they are used in most laboratories. The glucose concentration is 10% to 15% higher in plasma or serum than in whole blood because structural components of blood cells are absent. Whole blood glucose determinations are seldom used in clinical laboratories, but are used by patients using home blood glucose monitors.

Glucose levels can be measured in the laboratory using enzymatic methods (such as glucose oxidase or hexokinase), condensation methods (such as *o*-toluidine), or reducing methods. The reducing methods take advantage of the reducing properties of glucose to change the redox state of a metal ion; however, the method is nonspecific and any strong reducing agent can cross-react to yield spuriously elevated glucose values. In condensation methods, the aldehyde group of glucose undergoes condensation with aromatic compounds to yield a colored product. In the most commonly used condensation reaction, *o*-toluidine reacts with glucose to form a glucosamine that has an intense green color. The colour is measured spectrophotometrically to estimate the glucose concentration. *o*-Toluidine, however, has the drawback of being highly corrosive and toxic. In the enzymatic method, glucose oxidase reacts with glucose, water, and oxygen to form gluconic acid and hydrogen peroxide. The hydrogen peroxide can then be used

TABLE 17–11   **Criteria for the diagnosis of diabetes.**

	Normal Glucose Tolerance	Prediabetes	Diabetes Mellitus[a]
Fasting plasma glucose (mg/dL)[b]	<100	100-125 (impaired fasting glucose)	≥126
2 h after glucose load (mg/dL)[c]	<140	≥140-199 (impaired glucose tolerance)	≥200
HbA$_{1c}$ (%)[a]	<5.7	5.7-6.4	≥6.5
Symptoms and random glucose level (mg/dL)	–	–	≥200

[a]A fasting plasma glucose or HbA$_{1c}$ is diagnostic of diabetes if confirmed by repeat testing. HbA$_{1c}$ test should be performed using an assay certified by the National Glycohemoglobin Standardization program and standardized to the DCCT assay.

[b]A fasting plasma glucose ≥126 mg/dL is diagnostic of diabetes if confirmed on a subsequent day to be in the diabetic range after an overnight fast.

[c]Give 75 g of glucose dissolved in 300 mL of water after an overnight fast in subjects who have been receiving at least 150 to 200 g of carbohydrate daily for 3 days before the test. In the absence of unequivocal hyperglycemia, the result should be confirmed by repeat testing.

to oxidize a chromogen or the consumption of oxygen measured to estimate the amount of glucose present. Current laboratories use enzymatic methods to determine glucose levels.

The range of normal fasting plasma or serum glucose is 70 to 100 mg/dL (3.9-5.5 mmol/L). A plasma glucose level of 126 mg/dL (7.0 mmol/L) or higher on more than one occasion after at least 8 hours of fasting is diagnostic of diabetes mellitus (Table 17–11). Fasting plasma glucose levels of 100 mg/dL (5.6 mmol/L) to 125 mg/dL (6.9 mmol/L) are associated with increased risk for diabetes (impaired fasting glucose).

B. Capillary blood samples

Capillary blood glucose measurements performed by patients themselves, as outpatients, are extremely useful. In type 1 patients in whom tight metabolic control is attempted, they are indispensable. There are several paper strip (glucose oxidase; hexokinase; glucose dehydrogenase with nicotinamide adenine dinucleotide, glucose dehydrogenase with flavin-adenine dinucleotide, glucose dehydrogenase with pyrroloquinoline quinine) methods for measuring glucose on capillary blood samples. A reflectance photometer or an amperometric system is then used to measure the reaction that takes place on the reagent strip. A large number of blood glucose meters are now available. All are accurate, but they vary with regard to speed, convenience, size of blood samples required, and cost. Popular models include those manufactured by Life-Scan (One Touch), Bayer Corporation (Breeze, Contour), Roche Diagnostics (Accu-Chek), and Abbott Laboratories (Precision, FreeStyle). A Freestyle Flash meter, for example, which requires only 0.3 microliter of blood and gives a result in 5 seconds, is illustrative of the continued progress in this technologic area. Various glucometers appeal to a particular consumer need and are relatively inexpensive, ranging from $50.00 to $100.00 each. Test strips remain a major expense, costing 50 to 75 cents each. The meters have memories and can compute blood glucose averages. The data can be downloaded into a computer. In self-monitoring of blood glucose, patients must prick a finger with 26- to 33-gauge lancets. This can be facilitated by a small plastic trigger device such as an Accu-chek multi-clix (Roche Diagnostics), Microlet (Boehringer-Mannheim), or one touch lancing device (Lifescan, Inc.). Some meters such as the FreeStyle (Abbott Laboratories) have been approved for measuring glucose in blood samples obtained at alternative sites such as the forearm and thigh. There is, however, a 5- to 20-minute lag in the glucose response on the arm with respect to the glucose response on the finger. Forearm blood glucose measurements could therefore result in a delay in detection of rapidly developing hypoglycemia.

The clinician should be aware of the limitations of the self-glucose monitoring systems. First, some meters require input of a code for each batch of strips—failure to enter the code can result in misleading results. Many of the newer meters no longer require this step. Second, increases or decreases in hematocrit can decrease or increase the measured glucose values, respectively. The mechanism underlying this effect is not known, but presumably it is due to the impact of red cells on the diffusion of plasma into the reagent layer. Third, the meters and the test strips are calibrated over glucose concentrations ranging from 60 to 160 mg/dL, and the accuracy is not as good for higher and lower glucose levels. Thus, when the glucose is less than 60 mg/dL, the difference between the meter and the laboratory value may be as much as 20%. Fourth, glucose-oxidase-based amperometric systems underestimate glucose levels in the presence of high oxygen tension. This may be important in critically ill patients who are on supplemental oxygen, and under these circumstances, a glucose dehydrogenase-based system may be preferable. Fifth, glucose-dehydrogenase pyrroloquinoline quinine (GDH-PQQ) systems may report falsely high glucose levels in patients who are receiving parenteral products containing nonglucose sugars such as maltose, galactose, or xylose or their metabolites. Patients have been given insulin based on the falsely high glucose values resulting in life-threatening hypoglycemia. The accuracy of data obtained by glucose monitoring requires education of the patient in sampling and measuring procedures as well as in proper calibration of the instruments. Bedside glucose monitoring in a hospital setting requires rigorous quality control programs and certification of personnel to avoid errors.

Interstitial Fluid Glucose Samples

A number of continuous glucose monitoring (CGM) systems are currently available for clinical use. The systems manufactured by Medtronic MiniMed, Abbott Diagnostics, and Dex Com involve inserting a subcutaneous biosensor (rather like an insulin pump cannula) that measures glucose concentrations in the interstitial fluid for 3 to 7 days. The glucose values are available for review by the patient at time of measurement. The systems also display directional arrows indicating rate and direction of change and alarms can be set for dangerously low or high glucose values. Patients still have to calibrate the devices with periodic fingerstix glucose levels; and since there are concerns about the reliability of the measurements, it is still necessary to perform a confirmatory capillary blood glucose measurement before intervening. The individual glucose levels are not that critical—what matters are the

direction and the rate at which glucose is changing and the low glucose alerts that allow the user to take corrective action. The user also gains insight into the way particular foods or activities affect their glucose levels. Clinical trials with these systems show that they do enable some patients with type 1 diabetes to improve control without increasing the risk for hypoglycemia. The MiniMed insulin pump marketed in Europe can be programmed to automatically suspend insulin delivery for two hours when the glucose levels on their CGM device falls to a preset level. This feature may help reduce the risk for dangerous hypoglycemia especially when the patient is asleep. They are increasingly being approved by insurance companies. The out of pocket cost of the systems is about $4000 annually.

There is great interest in using the data obtained from these CGM systems to automatically deliver insulin by continuous subcutaneous insulin infusion pump. Algorithms have been devised to link CGM to insulin delivery and preliminary clinical studies appear promising.

Urine and Serum Ketone Determinations

In the absence of adequate insulin, three major ketone bodies are formed and excreted into the urine: β-hydroxybutyrate (often the most prevalent in diabetic ketoacidosis), acetoacetate, and acetone. Acetone and acetoacetate react with sodium nitroprusside (nitroferricyanide) in the presence of alkali to produce a purple-colored complex. Acetest tablets, Ketostix, and Keto-Diastix strips utilize this nitroprusside reaction to quantify acetone and acetoacetate levels in urine and plasma. When a few drops of serum are placed on a crushed Acetest tablet, the appearance of a purple color indicates the presence of ketones. A strongly positive reaction in undiluted serum correlates with a serum ketone concentration of at least 4 mmol/L. Although these tests do not detect β-hydroxybutyric acid, which lacks a ketone group, the semiquantitative estimation of the other ketone bodies is nonetheless usually adequate for clinical assessment of ketonuria. Ketostix and Keto-Diastix have short shelf-lives (90 days) once the containers are opened and using expired strips can give false-negative results. It is better therefore to buy individually foil wrapped strips.

Specific enzymatic techniques are available to quantitate each of the ketone acids, but these techniques are cumbersome and are not necessary in most clinical situations. There is also a paper strip method that patients can use to measure capillary blood β-hydroxybutyrate levels (Precision Xtra, Abbott Diagnostics). This technology uses hydroxybutyrate dehydrogenase to catalyse the oxidation of β-hydroxybutyrate to acetoacetate with concomitant reduction of NAD^+ to NADH. The NADH is reoxidized to NAD^+ by a redox mediator and a current is generated that is directly proportional to β-hydroxybutyrate concentration. β-Hydroxybutyrate levels >0.6 nmol/L require evaluation. Levels >3.0 nmol/L, which is equivalent to very large urine ketones, will require hospitalization.

Other conditions besides diabetic ketoacidosis may cause ketone bodies to appear in the urine; these include starvation, high-fat diets, alcoholic ketoacidosis, fever, and other conditions in which metabolic requirements are increased.

Glycated Hemoglobin Assays

Ketoamine reactions between glucose and other sugars and free amino groups on the alpha and beta chain lead to glycated forms of hemoglobin. Only glycation of the *N*-terminal valine of the beta chain imparts sufficient negative charge to the hemoglobin molecule to allow separation by charge-dependent techniques. The charge-separated hemoglobins are collectively referred to as hemoglobin A_1 (HbA$_1$). The major form of HbA$_1$ is hemoglobin A_{1c} (HbA$_{1c}$), where glucose is the carbohydrate. This form comprises 4% to 6% of total hemoglobin. The remaining HbA$_1$ species contain fructose 1,6-diphosphate (HbA$_{1a1}$), glucose 6-phosphate (HbA$_{1a2}$), and an unknown carbohydrate moiety (HbA$_{1b}$). The hemoglobin A_{1C} fraction is abnormally elevated in diabetic patients with chronic hyperglycemia. Some laboratories measure the sum of these glycohemoglobins (GHbs) and report the total as hemoglobin A$_1$, but most laboratories have converted to the highly specific HbA$_{1c}$ assay. Methods for measuring Hb$_{A1c}$ include electrophoresis, cation exchange chromatography, boronate affinity chromatography, and immunoassays.

Office-based immunoassays using capillary blood give a result in about 9 minutes, and this allows for immediate feedback to the patients regarding their glycemic control. Because GHbs circulate within red blood cells whose life span lasts up to 120 days, they generally reflect the state of glycemia over the preceding 8 to 12 weeks, thereby providing an improved method of assessing diabetic control. The HbA$_{1c}$ value, however, is weighted to more recent glucose levels (previous month) and this explains why significant changes in HbA$_{1c}$ are observed with short term (1 month) changes in mean plasma glucose levels. Measurements should be made in patients with either type of diabetes mellitus at 3- to 4-month intervals so that adjustments in therapy can be made if GHb is either subnormal or if it is more than 1% above the upper limits of normal for a particular laboratory. In patients monitoring their own blood glucose levels, GHb values provide a valuable check on the accuracy of monitoring. In patients who do not monitor their own blood glucose levels, GHb values are essential for adjusting therapy.

The various HbA$_{1c}$ assays have been standardized to the assay used in the Diabetes Control and Complications Trial (DCCT) allowing the results to be related to the risks of developing microvascular complications. There is a linear relationship between the HbA$_{1c}$ value and average glucose. A recent study (A1$_c$-Derived Average Glucose Study) collected 3 months of blood glucose data on 507 subjects—normals, type 1 and type 2 diabetics. The estimated average glucose was calculated by combining weighted results from 2 days of continuous glucose monitoring per month and seven point capillary blood glucose profiles (preprandial, postprandial, and bedtime) for at least 3 d/wk. The HbA$_{1c}$ was measured at the end of the 3 months. The relationship between average glucose and HbA$_{1c}$ based on liner regression analysis was:

Average glucose = $(28.7 \times \text{HbA}_{1c}) - 46.7$ (see also Table 17–12)

The accuracy of HbA$_{1c}$ values can be affected by hemoglobin variants or derivatives, the effect depending on the specific hemoglobin variant or derivative and the specific assay used.

TABLE 17–12   Correlations of HbA$_{1c}$ levels with average of capillary glucose measurements (preprandial, postprandial, and bedtime) in the previous 3 months.

HbA$_{1c}$ Value (%) Determined Using DCCT Standardized Assay	Mean Capillary Blood Glucose Levels (mg/dL)
5	97
6	126
7	154
8	183
9	212
10	240
11	269
12	298

Adapted from Nathan, et al. Translating the A$_{1c}$ assay into estimated average glucose values. *Diabetes Care.* 2008 Aug;31(8):1473-1478.

Immunoassays that use an antibody to the glycated amino terminus of β globin do not recognize the terminus of the γ globin of hemoglobin F, and so in patients with high levels of hemoglobin F, immunoassays give falsely low estimates of HbA$_{1c}$. Cation exchange chromatography separates hemoglobin species by charge differences. Therefore, hemoglobin variants that coelute with HbA$_{1c}$ can lead to an overestimation of the HbA$_{1c}$ value. Chemically modified derivatives of hemoglobin such as carbamylated (in renal failure) or acetylated (high-dose aspirin therapy) hemoglobin can, in some methods, coelute with HbA$_{1c}$.

Any condition that shortens erythrocyte survival or decreases mean erythrocyte age (eg, recovery from acute blood loss, hemolytic anemia) falsely lower HbA$_{1c}$ irrespective of the assay method used. Alternative methods such as fructosamine (see later) should be considered for these patients. Vitamins C and E are reported to falsely lower test results, possibly by inhibiting glycation of hemoglobin. The National Glycohemoglobin Standardization Program website (www.ngsp.org) has information on the impact of frequently encountered hemoglobin variants and derivatives on the results obtained with the commonly used HbA$_{1c}$ assays.

The American Diabetes Association (ADA) has now endorsed using the HbA$_{1c}$ as a diagnostic test for diabetes (see Table 17–11). A cutoff value of 6.5% was chosen because the risk for retinopathy increases substantially above this value. The advantages of using the HbA$_{1c}$ to diagnose diabetes is that there is no need to fast; it has lower intra-individual variability than the fasting glucose test and the oral glucose tolerance test; and it gives a better picture of glucose control for 2 to 3 months. People with HbA$_{1c}$ levels of 5.7 % to 6.4% should be considered at high risk for developing diabetes (prediabetes). The diagnosis should be confirmed with a repeat HbA$_{1c}$ test, unless the patient is symptomatic with plasma glucose levels >200 mg/dL. This test would not be appropriate to use in populations with high prevalence of hemoglobinopathies or in conditions with increased red cell turnover. Also, the testing should be performed using a National Glycohemoglobin Standardization Program certified method and standardized to the Diabetes Control and Complications Trial assay.

Serum Fructosamine

Serum fructosamine is formed by nonenzymatic glycosylation of serum proteins (predominantly albumin). Because serum albumin has a much shorter half-life (14-21 days) than hemoglobin, serum fructosamine generally reflects the state of glycemic control for the preceding 2 or 3 weeks. Reductions in serum albumin (eg, nephrotic state or hepatic disease) lower the serum fructosamine value. When abnormal hemoglobins or hemolytic states affect the interpretation of GHb or when a narrower time frame is required, such as for ascertaining glycemic control at the time of conception in a woman with diabetes who has recently become pregnant, serum fructosamine assays offer some advantage. Normal values vary in relation to the serum albumin concentration and are 200 to 285 umol/L when the serum albumin level is 5 g/dL. HbA_{1c} values and fructosamine are highly correlated. The following relationship between fructosamine levels and HbA_{1c} has been reported based on linear regression analysis:

$$HbA_{1c} = 0.017 \times \text{fructosamine level (uM/L)} + 1.61.$$

Thus fructosamine levels of 317, 375, and 435 are equivalent to HbA_{1c} values of 7%, 8%, and 9%, respectively.

In most circumstances, however, glycohemoglobin assays remain the preferred method for assessing long-term glycemic control in patients with diabetes.

Oral Glucose Tolerance Test

It is easy to screen for diabetes using an HbA_{1c} or a fasting plasma glucose level (see Table 17–11). The oral glucose tolerance test, therefore, is mostly performed for research studies or when there is a suspicion of the diagnosis but the fasting plasma glucose is less than 126 mg/dL or the HBA_{1c} level is below 6.5%. The test might be considered, for example, in a woman with a history of delivering an infant above 9 lb (4.1 kg).

In order to optimize insulin secretion and effectiveness, especially when patients have been on a low-carbohydrate diet, a minimum of 150 to 200 g of carbohydrate per day should be included in the diet for 3 days preceding the test. The patient should eat nothing after midnight prior to the test day. Adults are given 75 g of glucose in 300 mL of water; children are given 1.75 g of glucose per kilogram of ideal body weight. The glucose load is consumed within 5 minutes. The test should be performed in the morning because there is some diurnal variation in oral glucose tolerance and patients should not smoke; drink coffee, tea, or alcohol; or be active during the test.

Blood samples for plasma glucose are obtained at 0 and 120 minutes after ingestion of glucose. A fasting plasma glucose value of 126 mg/dL (7 mmol/L) or higher or a 2-hour value of greater than 200 mg/dL (11.1 mmol/L) is diagnostic of diabetes mellitus (see Table 17–11). An oral glucose tolerance test is normal if the fasting venous plasma glucose value is less than 100 mg/dL (5.6 mmol/L)

and the 2-hour value falls below 140 mg/dL (7.8 mmol/L). Patients with 2-hour values of 140 to 199 mg/dL have impaired glucose tolerance. False-positive results may occur in patients who are malnourished at test time, bedridden, or afflicted with an infection or severe emotional stress. Diuretics, oral contraceptives, glucocorticoids, excess thyroxine, phenytoin, nicotinic acid, and some of the psychotropic drugs may also cause false-positive results.

Insulin Levels

Normal immunoreactive insulin levels range from 5 to 20 μU/mL in the fasting state. During an oral glucose tolerance test, they reach 50 to 130 μU/mL at 1 hour, and usually return to levels below 30 μU/mL by 2 hours. Insulin measurements are rarely of clinical usefulness. They are principally used in research studies to determine insulin sensitivity.

The homeostasis model of insulin resistance ($HOMA_{IR}$) estimates insulin sensitivity using the following formula:

$$HOMA_{IR} \text{ (mmol/L} \times \mu U/mL) = \text{(fasting glucose [mmol/L]} \times \text{fasting insulin [}\mu U/mL\text{])}/22.5$$

The higher the $HOMA_{IR}$ value the more resistant the individual. Data from the oral glucose tolerance test can also be used to estimate insulin sensitivity. The Matsuda & DeFronzo Insulin Sensitivity Index is calculated as:

$$\text{Insulin sensitivity index (ISI)} = 10,000/\text{square root of} \\ \text{[fasting glucose} \times \text{fasting insulin]} \times \text{[mean glucose} \times \\ \text{mean insulin during OGTT]}$$

The lower the ISI the more insulin resistant the subject.

Intravenous Glucose Tolerance Test

The intravenous glucose tolerance test (IVGTT) is performed by giving a bolus of 50 g of glucose per 1.7 m^2 body surface area (or 0.5 g/kg of ideal body weight) as a 25% or 50% solution over 2 to 3 minutes after an overnight fast. Timing begins with injection and samples for plasma glucose determination are obtained from an indwelling needle in the opposite arm at 0, 10, 15, 20, and 30 minutes. The plasma glucose values are plotted on semilogarithmic paper against time. K, a rate constant that reflects the rate of fall of blood glucose in percent per minute, is calculated by determining the time necessary for the glucose concentration to fall by one-half ($t_{1/2}$) and using the following equation:

$$K(\text{glucose}) = \frac{0.693}{t_{1/2}} \times 100$$

The average K value for a nondiabetic patient is approximately 1.72% per minute; this value declines with age but remains above 1.3% per minute. Patients with diabetes almost always have a K value of less than 1% per minute. The disappearance rate reflects the patient's ability to dispose of a glucose load. Perhaps its most widespread present use is to screen siblings at risk for type 1 diabetes to determine if autoimmune destruction of β cells has reduced first phase insulin responses (at 1-5 minutes after the glucose bolus) to levels below the normal lower limit of 40 μU/mL.

The IVGTT has been modified by giving a glucose dose of 0.3 g/kg, with more frequent plasma sampling and extending the test to 3 to 4 hours. Also at 20 minutes, a 5-minute infusion of insulin is given (0.03 U/kg for the subject who is likely to be insulin sensitive and 0.06 U/kg for the likely resistant subject). Plasma glucose is sampled at 3, 4, 5, 6, 8, 10, 14, 19, 22, 25, 27, 30, 40, 50, 60, 80, 100, 140, and 180 minutes. Analysis of the time course of glucose and insulin during this frequently sampled IVGTT (FSIVGTT) allows for measurements of insulin sensitivity (Si), that is, fractional glucose clearance per unit insulin concentration; the first phase insulin response ($AIR_{glucose}$); and glucose effectiveness (S_G), the ability of glucose itself to enhance its own disappearance independent of any change in insulin. The data analysis requires use of specific software (Minmod).

Lipoproteins in Diabetes

Levels of circulating lipoproteins are dependent on normal levels and action of insulin, just as is the plasma glucose. In type 1 diabetes, moderately deficient control of hyperglycemia is associated with only a slight elevation of low-density lipoprotein (LDL) cholesterol and serum triglycerides and little if any changes in HDL cholesterol. Once the hyperglycemia is corrected, lipoprotein levels are generally normal. However, patients with type 2 diabetes frequently have a dyslipidemia that is characteristic of the insulin resistance syndrome. Its features are a high serum triglyceride level (300-400 mg/dL), a low HDL cholesterol (<30 mg/dL), and a qualitative change in LDL particles producing a smaller dense LDL whose membrane carries supranormal amounts of free cholesterol. Because *low* HDL cholesterol is a major feature predisposing to macrovascular disease, the term *dyslipidemia* has preempted the previous label of *hyperlipidemia*, which mainly described the elevated triglycerides. Measures designed to correct obesity and hyperglycemia, such as exercise, diet, and hypoglycemic therapy substantially correct the dyslipidemia but most patients require pharmacotherapy. Chapter 19 discusses these matters in detail.

Clinical Trials in Diabetes

Findings of the Diabetes Control and Complications Trial (DCCT) and of the United Kingdom Prospective Diabetes Study (UKPDS) have confirmed the beneficial effects of intensive therapy to achieve improved glycemic control in both type 1 and type 2 diabetes, respectively (see later). In addition, with increased understanding of the pathophysiology of both type 1 and type 2 diabetes, large prospective studies—Diabetes Prevention Trial-1 (DPT-1) and the Diabetes Prevention Program (DPP) have been conducted to identify interventions that prevent the onset of these disorders.

Clinical Trials in Type 1 Diabetes

A. The Diabetes Control and Complications Trial (DCCT)
This long-term randomized prospective study of patients with type 1 diabetes reported that lowering of blood glucose levels with intensive insulin therapy delayed the onset and slowed the progression of microvascular and neuropathic complications of diabetes.

More than 1000 patients from 29 medical centers ranging in age from 13 to 39 were divided into two study groups with equal numbers of subjects. Approximately half of the total group had no detectable diabetic complications (primary prevention group), whereas mild background retinopathy was present in the other half (secondary prevention group). Some patients in the latter group also had slightly elevated microalbuminuria and mild neuropathy, but no one with serious diabetic complications was enrolled in the trial. Multiple insulin injections (66%) or insulin pumps (34%) were used in the intensively treated group, and those subjects were trained to modify their therapy in response to frequent glucose monitoring. The conventionally treated group used no more than two insulin injections, and clinical well-being was the goal with no attempt to modify management based on glycated hemoglobin or glucose results.

In the intensively treated subjects, mean glycated hemoglobin of 7.2% (normal, <6%) and a mean blood glucose of 155 mg/dL were achieved, whereas in the conventionally treated group glycated hemoglobin averaged 8.9% and the average blood glucose was 225 mg/dL. Over the study period, which averaged 6.5 years, there was an approximately 60% reduction in risk of diabetic retinopathy, nephropathy, and neuropathy in the intensively treated group. The benefits were seen in both the primary and secondary prevention groups. The intensively treated group also had a nonsignficant reduction in the risk of macrovascular disease of 41% (95% CI, −10%-68%).

Intensively treated patients had a three fold greater risk of serious hypoglycemia as well as a greater tendency toward weight gain. However, there were no deaths from hypoglycemia in any subjects in the DCCT study, and no evidence of posthypoglycemic neurologic damage was detected.

Subjects participating in the DCCT study were subsequently enrolled in a follow-up observational study (Epidemiology of Diabetes Interventions and Complications [EDIC]). Even though the between group differences in HbA$_{1c}$ narrowed within 4 years, the group assigned to intensive therapy had a lower risk for retinopathy at 4 years and microalbuminuria at 7 to 8 years of post study follow-up. Moreover, by the end of the 11 year follow-up period, the intensive therapy group had significantly reduced risk of any cardiovascular disease events by 42% (95% CI, 9%-23%; $p = 0.02$). Thus it seems that the benefits of good glucose control persist even if control deteriorates at a later date.

The general consensus of the ADA is that intensive insulin therapy associated with comprehensive self-management training should become standard therapy in most patients with type 1 diabetes after the age of puberty. Exceptions include those with advanced renal disease and the elderly, because the detrimental risks of hypoglycemia outweigh the benefit of tight glycemic control in these groups. In children under age 7 years, the risk of developing brain damage from hypoglycemia contraindicates attempts at tight glycemic control, particularly because diabetic complications do not seem to occur until some years after the onset of puberty.

B. Diabetes Prevention Trial-1 (DPT-1) This NIH-sponsored multicenter study was designed to determine whether the development of type 1 diabetes could be prevented or delayed by immune intervention therapy. Daily low-dose insulin injections were administered for up to 8 years in first-degree relatives of individuals with type 1 diabetes who were selected as being at high risk for development of type 1 diabetes because of detectable ICAs and reduced early-insulin release. Unfortunately, this immune intervention failed to affect the onset of type 1 diabetes, which was approximately 15% per year in both the treated and control groups. A related study using oral insulin in lower risk first-degree relatives, who had ICAs but whose early insulin release remained intact also failed to show an effect on the onset of type 1 diabetes. After an average of 4.3 years of observation, type 1 diabetes developed in about 35% of persons in both the oral insulin and the placebo groups.

C. Immune intervention trials in new-onset type 1 diabetes At time of diagnosis of type 1 diabetes, patients still have significant β cell function. This explains why soon after diagnosis, patients go into a partial clinical remission (honeymoon) requiring little or no insulin. This clinical remission is short-lived, however, and eventually patients lose all β cell function and have more labile glucose control. Attempts have been made to prolong this partial clinical remission using drugs such as cyclosporine, azathioprine, prednisone, and antithymocyte globulin. These agents, however, have had limited efficacy, and there were concerns about their toxicity and the need for continuous treatment.

More specific strategies for immunosuppression, such as the use of monoclonal antibodies against particular T-cell products, may reduce the hazards of long-term immunotherapy. Phase I/II clinical trials using humanized monoclonal antibodies against CD3, hOKT3γ1 (Ala-Ala) (teplizumab), and ChAglyCD3 (otelexizumab) showed efficacy in reducing the decline in insulin production in patients newly diagnosed with type 1 diabetes. The CD3 complex is the major signal transducing element of the T-cell receptor. The anti-CD3 antibodies are believed to modulate the autoimmune response by selectively inhibiting pathogenic T cells and/or by inducing regulatory T cells. Patients were treated with the antibody for 14 days within 6 weeks of diagnosis of type 1 diabetes. One year later, the majority of patients in the treated group had maintained or increased insulin production and improved glycemic control relative to the control group. Larger phase II/III clinical trials are currently in progress.

These and other approaches that selectively modulate the autoimmune T-cell response hold the promise that type 1 diabetes may eventually be preventable without prolonged immunosuppression.

Clinical Trials in Type 2 Diabetes

A. Kumamoto study The Kumamoto study involved a relatively small number of patients with type 2 diabetes ($n = 110$) who were nonobese and only slightly insulin resistant, requiring less than 30 units of insulin per day for intensive therapy. Over a 6-year period it was shown that intensive insulin therapy, achieving a

mean HbA$_{1c}$ of 7.1%, significantly reduced microvascular end points compared with conventional insulin therapy, which achieved a mean HbA$_{1c}$ of 9.4%. Cardiovascular events were neither worsened nor improved by intensive therapy, and weight changes were likewise not influenced by either form of treatment.

B. The United Kingdom Prospective Diabetes Study (UKPDS) This multicenter study was designed to determine whether the risk of macrovascular or microvascular complications in patients with type 2 diabetes could be reduced by intensive blood glucose control with oral hypoglycemic agents or insulin and whether any particular therapy was better than the others. Patients aged 25 to 65 years who were newly diagnosed with type 2 diabetes were recruited between 1977 and 1991, and a total of 3867 were studied over 10 years. The median age at baseline was 54 years; 44% were overweight (>20% over ideal weight), and baseline HbA$_{1c}$ was 9.1%. Therapies were randomized to include a control group on diet alone and separate groups intensively treated with insulin, chlorpropamide, glyburide, or glipizide. Metformin was included as a randomization option in a subgroup of 342 overweight patients, and—much later in the study—an additional subgroup of both normal-weight and overweight patients, who were responding unsatisfactorily to sulfonylurea therapy, were randomized to either continue on their sulfonylurea therapy alone or to have metformin combined with it.

After the study was initiated, a further modification was made to evaluate whether tight control of blood pressure with stepwise antihypertensive therapy would prevent macrovascular and microvascular complications in 758 hypertensive patients among this UKPDS population—compared with 390 patients whose blood pressure was treated less intensively. The tight control group was randomly assigned to treatment with either an angiotensin-converting enzyme (ACE) inhibitor (captopril) or a beta blocker (atenolol). Both drugs were stepped up to maximum doses of 100 mg/d, and then, if blood pressure remained higher than the target level of less than 150/85 mm Hg, more drugs were added in the following stepwise sequence—a diuretic, slow-release nifedipine, methyldopa, and prazosin—until the target level of tight control was achieved. In the control group, hypertension was conventionally treated to achieve target levels less than 180/105 mm Hg, but these patients were not given either ACE inhibitors or beta blockers.

Intensive glycemic therapy in the entire group of 3897 patients newly diagnosed with type 2 diabetes patients followed over 10 years showed that intensive treatment with either sulfonylureas, metformin, combinations of these, or insulin achieved mean HbA$_{1c}$ levels of 7.0%. This level of glycemic control decreased the risk of microvascular complications in comparison with conventional therapy (mostly diet alone), which achieved mean levels of HbA$_{1c}$ of 7.9%. Weight gain occurred in intensively treated patients except when metformin was used as monotherapy. There was a trend towards reduction in cardiovascular events (fatal or nonfatal MI; sudden death) with intensive treatment but this did not reach statistical significance (16% reduction, $p = 0.052$). Hypoglycemic reactions occurred in the intensive treatment groups, but only one death from hypoglycemia was documented over 27,000 patient-years of intensive therapy.

When therapeutic subgroups were analyzed, some unexpected and paradoxical results were noted. Among the obese patients, intensive treatment with insulin or sulfonylureas did not reduce microvascular complications compared with diet therapy alone. This was in contrast to the significant benefit of intensive therapy with these drugs in the total group. Furthermore, intensive therapy with metformin was more beneficial in the overweight and obese persons than diet alone with regard to reducing myocardial infarctions, strokes, and diabetes-related deaths, but there was no significant reduction of diabetic microvascular complications with metformin as compared with the diet group. Moreover, in the subgroup of obese and nonobese patients in whom metformin was added to sulfonylurea failures, rather than showing a benefit, there was a 96% increase in diabetes-related deaths compared with the matched cohort of patients with unsatisfactory glycemic control on sulfonylureas who remained on sulfonylurea therapy. Chlorpropamide also came out poorly on subgroup analysis in that those receiving it as intensive therapy did less well as regards progression to retinopathy than those conventionally treated with diet. The University Group Diabetes Program (UGDP) study was designed to evaluate the effects of glucose-lowering therapies on vascular complications in type 2 diabetes and reported that tolbutamide may increase the risk for cardiovascular deaths. The UKPDS study refutes this concern by failing to confirm any cardiovascular hazard with sulfonylurea treatment.

Intensive antihypertensive therapy to a mean of 144/82 mm Hg had beneficial effects on microvascular disease as well as on all diabetes-related end points, including virtually all cardiovascular outcomes, in comparison with looser control at a mean of 154/87 mm Hg. In fact, the advantage of reducing hypertension by this amount was substantially more impressive than the benefit that accrued by improving the degree of glycemic control from a mean HbA_{1c} of 7.9% to 7.0%. More than half of the patients needed two or more drugs for adequate therapy of their hypertension, and there was no demonstrable advantage of ACE inhibitor therapy over beta blockers as regards diabetes end points. Use of a calcium channel blocker added to both treatment groups appeared to be safe over the long term in this population with diabetes, despite some controversy in the literature about its safety in such individuals.

The UKPDS researchers, like the DCCT group, performed posttrial monitoring to determine if there were long-term benefits of having been in the intensively treated glucose and blood pressure arms of the study. The between group differences in HbA_{1c} were lost within the first year of follow-up but the reduced risk of development or progression of microvascular complications in the intensively treated group persisted for 10 years (24%, $p = 0.001$). The intensively treated group also had significantly reduced risk for myocardial infarction (15%, $p = 0.01$) and death from any cause (13%, $p = 0.007$) during the follow-up period. The subgroup of overweight or obese subjects who were initially randomized to metformin therapy showed sustained reduction in risk of myocardial infarction and death from any cause in the follow-up period. The between group blood pressure differences disappeared within 2 years of the end of the trial. Unlike the sustained benefits seen with glucose control, there was no sustained benefit from having been in the more tightly controlled blood pressure group. Both blood pressure groups had similar risks for microvascular events and diabetes related end-points in the follow-up period.

Thus, the follow-up of the UKPDS type 2 diabetes cohort showed that, as in type 1 diabetes, the benefits of good glucose control persist even if control deteriorates at a later date. Blood pressure benefits, however, last only as long as the blood pressure is well controlled.

C. Diabetes Prevention Program (DPP)   This was a randomized clinical trial in 3234 overweight men and women, aged 25 to 85 years, who showed impaired glucose tolerance. Results from this study indicated that intervention with a low-fat diet and 150 minutes of moderate exercise (equivalent to a brisk walk) per week reduces the risk of progression to type 2 diabetes by 58% as compared with a matched control group. Another arm of this trial demonstrated that use of 850 mg of metformin twice daily reduced the risk of developing type 2 diabetes by 31% but was relatively ineffective in those who were either less obese or in the older age group.

D. The Steno-2 Study   This was designed in 1990 to validate the efficacy of targeting multiple concomitant risk factors for both microvascular and macrovascular disorders in type 2 diabetes. A prospective, randomized, open, blinded end-point design was used in which 160 patients with type 2 diabetes and microalbuminuria were assigned to conventional therapy with their general practitioner or to intensive care at the Steno Diabetes Center. In the intensively treated group, stepwise introduction of lifestyle and pharmacologic interventions was aimed at keeping glycated hemoglobin less than 6.5%, blood pressure less than 130/80 mm Hg, total cholesterol less than 175 mg/dL, and triglycerides less than 150 mg/dL. All subjects in the intensively treated group received ACE inhibitors and if intolerant, an angiotensin II receptor blocker. The lifestyle component of intensive intervention included reduction in dietary fat intake to less than 30% of total calories, a smoking cessation program, light to moderate exercise, and a daily vitamin-mineral supplement (vitamins C and E and chromium picolinate). Initially, aspirin was given as secondary prevention to patients with a history of ischemic cardiovascular disease, but later all patients received aspirin.

After a mean follow-up of 7.8 years, 44% of patients in the conventional arm and 24% in the intensive multifactorial arm developed cardiovascular events (myocardial infarction, angioplasties, coronary bypass grafts, strokes, amputations, vascular surgical interventions)—a 53% reduction. Rates of nephropathy, retinopathy, and autonomic neuropathy were also lower in the multifactorial intervention arm—61%, 58%, and 63% of rates in the conventional arm, respectively.

The subjects who participated in this trial were subsequently enrolled in an observational follow-up study for an average of 5.5 years. Even though the significant differences in glycemic control and levels of risk factors for cardiovascular disease between the groups had disappeared by the end of the follow-up period, the interventional group continued to have a lower risk for retinal photocoagulation, renal failure, cardiovascular endpoints, and cardiovascular mortality.

The data from the UKPDS and this study thus provide support for guidelines recommending vigorous treatment of concomitant microvascular and cardiovascular risk factors in patients with type 2 diabetes.

E. Accord, Advance, and VADT studies The ACCORD study was a randomized controlled study designed to determine whether normal HbA_{1c} levels would reduce the risk of cardiovascular events in middle-aged or older individuals with type 2 diabetes. About 35% of the 10,251 recruited subjects had established cardiovascular disease at study entry. The intensive arm of the study was discontinued after 3.5 years of follow-up because of more unexplained deaths in the intensive arm when compared to the conventional treatment arm (22%, $p = 0.020$). Analysis of the data at time of discontinuation showed that the intensively treated group (HbA_{1c} 6.4%) had a 10% reduction in cardiovascular event rate compared to the standard treated group (HbA_{1c} 7.5%), but this difference was not statistically significant. The ADVANCE trial randomly assigned 11,140 patients in their 60s with type 2 diabetes to standard or intensive glucose control. The primary outcomes were major macrovascular (nonfatal myocardial infarction or stroke or death from cardiovascular causes) or microvascular events. Thirty-two percent of the subjects had established cardiovascular disease at study entry. After a median follow-up of 5 years, there was a nonsignificant reduction (6%) in major macrovascular event rate in the intensively treated group (HbA_{1c} 6.5%) compared to the standard therapy group (HbA_{1c} 7.3%).

The Veteran Administration Diabetes Trial (VADT) randomly assigned 1791 patients in their 50s and 60s with type 2 diabetes to standard or intensive glucose control. Ninety seven percent of the subjects were men. The primary outcome was a composite of myocardial infarction, death from cardiovascular causes, congestive heart failure, vascular surgery, inoperable coronary artery disease, and amputation for gangrene. All patients had optimized blood pressure and lipid levels. After a median follow-up of 5.6 years, there was no significant difference in the primary outcome in the intensively treated group (HbA_{1c} 6.9%) compared to the standard therapy (HbA_{1c} 8.4%). Within this larger study, there was an embedded study evaluating the impact of intensive therapy in patients who were categorized as having low, moderate, and high coronary calcium scores on CT scans. Patients with low coronary calcium score showed reduced number of cardiovascular events with intensive therapy.

Thus, the ACCORD, ADVANCE, and VADT results do not provide support for the hypothesis that near-normal glucose control in type 2 diabetes will reduce cardiovascular events. It is, however, important not to over-interpret the results of these three studies. The results do not exclude the possibility that cardiovascular benefits might accrue with longer duration of near-normal glucose control. In the UKPDS, risk reductions for

myocardial infarction and death from any cause were only observed during 10 years of posttrial follow-up. Specific subgroups of type 2 diabetes patients may also have different outcomes. The ACCORD, ADVANCE, and VADT studies recruited patients who had diabetes for 8 to 10 years, and a third of them had established cardiovascular disease. Patients in the UKPDS, in contrast, had newly diagnosed diabetes, and only 7.5% had a history of macrovascular disease. It is possible that the benefits of tight glycemic control on macrovascular events are attenuated in patients with longer duration of diabetes or with established vascular disease. Specific therapies used to lower glucose may also affect cardiovascular event rate or mortality. Severe hypoglycemia occurred more frequently in the intensively treated groups of the ACCORD, ADVANCE, and VADT studies; and the ACCORD investigators were not able to exclude undiagnosed hypoglycemia as a potential cause for the increased death rate in their intensive arm group.

A formal meta-analysis performed on the raw trial data from the ACCORD, ADVANCE, VADT, and UKPDS studies found that allocation to more intensive glucose control reduced the risk of MI by 15% (hazard ratio 0.85, 95% CI 0.76-0.94). The benefit appeared to be in patients who did not have preexisting macrovascular disease.

TREATMENT OF DIABETES MELLITUS

Diet

A well-balanced, nutritious diet remains a fundamental element of therapy for diabetes. However, in more than half of cases, patients with diabetes fail to follow their diets. The American Diabetes Association (ADA) recommends about 45% to 65% of total daily calories in the form of carbohydrates; 25% to 35% in the form of fat (of which less than 7% are from saturated fat), and 10% to 35% in the form of protein. In prescribing a diet, it is important to relate dietary objectives to the type of diabetes. In patients with type 2 diabetes, limiting the carbohydrate intake and substituting some of the calories with monounsaturated fats, such as olive oil, rapeseed (canola) oil, or the oils in nuts and avocados, can lower triglycerides and increase HDL cholesterol. In addition, in those patients with obesity and type 2 diabetes, weight reduction by caloric restriction is an important goal of the diet. Patients with type 1 diabetes or type 2 diabetes who take insulin should be taught *carbohydrate counting*, so they can administer their insulin bolus for each meal based on its carbohydrate content.

The current recommendations for both types of diabetes continue to limit cholesterol to 300 mg daily, and individuals with LDL cholesterol more than 100 mg/dL should limit dietary cholesterol to 200 mg daily. High protein intake may cause progression of renal disease in patients with diabetic nephropathy; for these individuals, a reduction in protein intake to 0.8 kg/d (or about 10% of total calories daily) is recommended.

Exchange lists for meal planning can be obtained from the American Diabetes Association and its affiliate associations or from the American Dietetic Association, 216 W. Jackson Blvd., Chicago, IL 60606 (312-899-0040 or http://www.eatright.org).

Special Considerations in Dietary Control

A. Dietary fiber   Plant components such as cellulose, gum, and pectin are indigestible by humans and are termed **dietary fiber.** Insoluble fibers such as cellulose or hemicellulose increase stool bulk and decrease transit time. Soluble fibers such as gums and pectins, found in beans, oatmeal, or apple skin, can delay glucose absorption and so diminish postprandial hyperglycemia. Although the ADA diet does not require insoluble fiber supplements such as added bran, it recommends foods such as oatmeal, cereals, and beans with relatively high soluble fiber content as stable components of the diet in patients with diabetes. High soluble fiber content in the diet may also have a favorable effect on blood cholesterol levels.

B. Glycemic index   Quantitation of the relative glycemic contribution of different carbohydrate foods has formed the basis of a **glycemic index** in which the area of blood glucose (plotted on a graph) generated over a 3-hour period following ingestion of a test food containing 50 g of carbohydrate is compared with the area plotted after giving a similar quantity of reference food such as glucose or white bread:

$$\frac{\text{Blood glucose area of test food}}{\text{Blood glucose area of reference food}} \times 100$$

White bread is preferred to glucose as a reference standard because it is more palatable and has less tendency to slow gastric emptying by high tonicity, as happens when glucose solution is used. Eating foods with low glycemic index will result in lower glucose levels after meals. Low glycemic index foods have values of 55 or less and include many fruits (apples, oranges) and vegetables, grainy breads, pasta, legumes, milk, and yoghurt. High glycemic index foods have values of 70 and over and include baked potato, white bread, and most white rice. Glycemic index is lowered by the presence of fats and protein when the food is consumed in a mixed meal. Cooking methods can also affect the glycemic index—thus mashed potatoes have a higher glycemic index than baked potato. Since you have to have 50 g of available carbohydrate to measure the glycemic index, you cannot assign glycemic indices to foods which have very little carbohydrate. Even though it may not be possible to accurately predict the impact of the glycemic index of a particular food in the context of a meal, it is still reasonable to choose foods with low glycemic index.

C. Sweeteners   The nonnutritive sweetener **saccharin** is widely used as a sugar substitute (sweet and low). **Aspartame** (NutraSweet) consists of two major amino acids, aspartic acid, and phenylalanine, which combine to produce a nutritive sweetener 180 times as sweet as sucrose. A major limitation is its heat lability, which precludes its use in baking or cooking. Sucralose (Splenda) and acesulfame potassium (Sunett, Sweet One, DiabetiSweet) are two other nonnutritive sweeteners that are heat stable and can be used in cooking and baking.

Fructose represents a *natural* sugar substance that is a highly effective sweetener. It induces only slight increases in plasma glucose levels and does not require insulin for its utilization. However, because of potential adverse effects of large amounts of fructose (up to 20% of total calories) on raising serum cholesterol, triglycerides, and LDL cholesterol, it does not have any advantage as a sweetening agent in the diabetic diet. This does not preclude, however, ingestion of fructose-containing fruits and vegetables or fructose-sweetened foods in moderation.

Sugar alcohols, also known as polyols or polyalcohol, are commonly used as sweeteners and bulking agents. They occur naturally in a variety of fruits and vegetables but are also commercially made from sucrose, glucose, and starch. Examples are sorbitol, xylitol, mannitol, lactitol, isomalt, maltitol, and hydrogenated starch hydrolysates (HSH). They are not as easily absorbed as sugar, so they do not raise blood glucose levels as much as conventional sugars. Therefore, sugar alcohols are often used in food products that are labeled as *sugar free*, such as chewing gum, lozenges, hard candy, and sugar-free ice cream. However, if consumed in large quantities, they will raise blood glucose and can also cause bloating and diarrhea.

D. Fish oils and other oils   Omega-3 fatty acids in high doses have been shown to lower plasma triglycerides and VLDL cholesterol. They may also reduce platelet aggregation. In the Lyon Diet Heart Study in nondiabetic patients, a high intake of α-linolenic acid was beneficial in secondary prevention of coronary heart disease. This diet, which is rich in vegetables and fruits, also supplies a high intake of natural antioxidants. There is limited clinical information on the use of these oils in patients with diabetes.

AGENTS FOR THE TREATMENT OF HYPERGLYCEMIA

The drugs for treating type 2 diabetes (Table 17–13), other than insulin, fall into several categories. (1) Drugs that act on the sulfonylurea receptor complex of the β cell: sulfonylureas remain the most widely prescribed drugs for treating hyperglycemia. The meglitinide analog repaglinide and the D-phenylalanine derivative nateglinide also bind the sulfonylurea receptor and stimulate insulin secretion. (2) Drugs that principally lower glucose levels by their actions on liver, skeletal muscle, or adipose tissue: metformin works primarily in the liver, and the peroxisome proliferator-activated receptor agonists (PPARs) rosiglitazone and pioglitazone appear to have their main effects on skeletal muscle and adipose tissue. (3) Drugs that principally affect absorption of glucose: the α-glucosidase inhibitors acarbose and miglitol are currently available drugs in this class. (4) Drugs that mimic incretin effects or prolong incretin action: the GLP-1 receptor agonists and the DPP-4 inhibitors fall into this category. (5) Other drugs: these include pramlintide, which lowers glucose by suppressing glucagon and slowing gastric emptying.

TABLE 17–13 Drugs for treatment of type 2 diabetes.

Drug	Tablet Size	Daily Dose	Duration of Action (h)
Sulfonylureas			
Tolbutamide (Orinase)	250 and 500 mg	0.5-2 g in two or three divided doses	6-12
Tolazamide (Tolinase)	100, 250, and 500 mg	0.1-1 g as single dose or in two divided doses	Up to 24
Acetohexamide (Dymelor)	250 and 500 mg	0.25-1.5 g as single dose or in two divided doses	8-24
Chlorpropamide (Diabinese)	100 and 250 mg	0.1-0.5 as single dose	24-72
Glyburide (DiaBeta, Micronase)	1.25, 2.5, and 5 mg	1.25-20 mg as single dose or in two divided doses	Up to 24
(Glynase)	1.5, 3, and 6 mg	1.5-18 mg as single dose or in two divided doses	Up to 24
Glipizide (Glucotrol)	5 and 10 mg	2.5-40 mg as single dose or in two divided doses on an empty stomach	6-12
(Glucotrol XL)	2.5, 5, and 10 mg	Up to 20 mg daily as a single dose	Up to 24
Gliclazide (not available in United States)	80 mg	40-80 mg as single dose; 160-320 mg as divided dose	12
Glimepiride (Amaryl)	1, 2, and 4 mg	1-4 mg as single dose	Up to 24
Meglitinide Analogs			
Repaglinide (Prandin)	0.5, 1, and 2 mg	0.5 to 4 mg three times a day before meals	3
Mitiglinide (available in Japan)	5 and 10 mg	5 or 10 mg three times a day before meals	2
D-Phenylalanine			
Nateglinide (Starlix)	60 and 120 mg	60 or 120 mg three times a day before meals	1.5
Biguanides			
Metformin (Glucophage)	500, 850, and 1000 mg	1-2.5 g; one tablet with meals two or thee times daily	7-12
Extended-release metformin (Glucophage XR)	500 and 750 mg	500-2000 mg once a day	Up to 24
Thiazolidinediones			
Rosiglitazone (Avandia)	2, 4, and 8 mg	4-8 mg daily (can be divided)	Up to 24
Pioglitazone (Actos)	15, 30, and 45 mg	15-45 mg daily	Up to 24
α-Glucosidase inhibitors			
Acarbose (Precose)	50 and 100 mg	75-300 mg in three divided doses with first bite of food	4
Miglitol (Glyset)	25, 50, and 100 mg	75-300 mg in three divided doses with first bite of food	4
GLP-1 receptor agonists			
Exenatide	5 and 10 µg	5 µg by subcutaneous injection within 1 hour of breakfast and dinner. Increase to 10 µg twice a day after about a month. Refrigerate between uses.	6
Liraglutide	0.6, 1.2, and 1.8 mg	0.6 mg by subcutaneous injection once a day starting dose. Increase to 1.2 mg after a week if no adverse reactions. Dose can be further increased to 1.8 mg if necessary.	24
DPP-4 inhibitors			
Sitagliptin	25, 50, and 100 mg	100 mg orally once a day. Reduce dose to 50 mg if calculated creatinine clearance is 30 to 50 mL/min. Give 25 mg daily if creatinine clearance less than 30.	24
Saxagliptin	2.5 and 5 mg	2.5 or 5 mg once a day. Use 2.5 mg dose if calculated creatinine clearance is ≤50 mL/min or if also taking strong CYP3A4/5 inhibitors like ketoconazole	24
Vildagliptin (not available in United States)	50 mg	50 mg once or twice a day. Contraindicated in patients with calculated creatinine clearance ≤60 mL/min or AST/ALT three times upper limit of normal	24
Others			
Pramlintide	5-mL vial containing 0.6 mg/mL	For insulin-treated type 2 patients, start at 60-µg dose three times a day (10 U on U100 insulin syringe) and increase to 120 µg three times a day (20 U) if patient has no nausea for 3-7 d. Give immediately before meal. For type 1 patients, start at 15 µg three times a day (2.5 U on U100 insulin syringe) and increase by increments of 15 µg to a maximum of 60 µg three times a day as tolerated. Lower insulin dose by 50% on initiation of therapy to avoid hypoglycemia.	3

1. DRUGS THAT ACT ON THE SULFONYLUREA RECEPTOR COMPLEX

Sulfonylureas

The sulfonylureas contain a sulfonic acid-urea nucleus that can be modified by chemical substitutions to produce agents that have similar qualitative actions but differ widely in potency. They bind the ATP-sensitive potassium channels (K_{ATP}) on the surface of pancreatic β cells, resulting in closure of the channel and depolarization of the β cell. This depolarized state permits calcium to enter the cell and actively promote insulin release (Figure 17–5).

In β cells, the ATP-sensitive channels contain four copies each of two subunits, the regulatory subunit SUR1, which binds ATP, ADP, and sulfonylureas, and the potassium channel subunit Kir6.2. K_{ATP} channels composed of the same subunits are found in α cells, GLP-1 secreting intestinal L-cells, and the brain. The SUR1/Kir6.2 complexes are opened by diazoxide and closed by sulfonylureas at low concentrations (IC_{50} about 1 nM for glyburide). Inactivating mutations in SUR1 or Kir6.2 cause persistent depolarization of the β cells and have been identified in patients with hyperinsulinemic hypoglycemia of infancy (see Chapter 18). Activating mutations in SUR1 or Kir6.2 prevent depolarization of the β cells and have been identified in patients with neonatal diabetes (see section on Neonatal Diabetes earlier).

K_{ATP} channels with different subunit combinations are found in other tissues. The combination of SUR2A/Kir6.2 is found in cardiac and skeletal muscle, and SUR2B/Kir6.1 in vascular smooth muscle. Channel configurations containing SUR2 subunits are insensitive to diazoxide but sensitive to other potassium channel agonists such as pinacidil and cromakalim. Certain channel *closers* have much higher affinity for SUR1-containing channels than SUR2-containing channels (the sulfonylureas tolbutamide and gliclazide and the meglitinides nateglinide and mitiglinide), while others have similar affinities for both of them (glyburide, glimepiride, and repeglinide). It remains uncertain whether the different affinities of these drugs for the two classes of receptors have clinical relevance.

Sulfonylureas are not indicated for use in type 1 diabetes patients since these drugs require functioning pancreatic β cells to produce their effect on blood glucose. These drugs are used in patients with type 2 diabetes, in whom acute administration improves the early phase of insulin release that is refractory to acute glucose stimulation. Sulfonylureas are metabolized by the liver and apart from acetohexamide, whose metabolite is more active than the parent compound, the metabolites of all the other sulfonylureas are weakly active or inactive. The metabolites are excreted by the kidney and, in the case of the second-generation sulfonylureas, partly excreted in the bile. Sulfonylureas are generally contraindicated in patients with severe liver or kidney impairment. Idiosyncratic reactions are rare, with skin rashes or hematologic toxicity (leukopenia, thrombocytopenia) occurring in less than 0.1% of users.

First-generation sulfonylureas (tolbutamide, tolazamide, acetohexamide, and chlorpropamide)—Tolbutamide is supplied in tablets of 500 mg. It is rapidly oxidized in the liver to an inactive form. Because its duration of effect is short (6-10 hours), it is usually administered in divided doses (eg, 500 mg before each meal and at bedtime). The usual daily dose is 1.5 to 3 g; some patients, however, require only 250 to 500 mg daily. Acute toxic reactions such as skin rashes are rare. Because of its short duration of action, which is independent of renal function, tolbutamide is probably the safest agent to use in elderly patients, in whom hypoglycemia would be a particularly serious risk. Prolonged hypoglycemia has been reported rarely, mainly in patients receiving certain drugs (eg, warfarin, phenylbutazone, or sulfonamides) that compete with sulfonylureas for hepatic oxidation, resulting in maintenance of high levels of unmetabolized active sulfonylureas in the circulation.

Tolazamide, acetohexamide, and chlorpropamide are rarely used. Chlorpropamide has a prolonged biologic effect, and severe hypoglycemia can occur especially in the elderly, because their renal clearance declines with aging. Its other side effects include alcohol-induced flushing and hyponatremia due to its effect on vasopressin secretion and action. Tolazamide is comparable to chlorpropamide in potency but is devoid of disulfiram-like or water-retaining effects. Its duration of action may last up to 20 hours, with maximal hypoglycemic effect occurring between the 4th and 14th hours.

Second-generation sulfonylureas: glyburide, glipizide, gliclazide, and glimepiride—these agents have similar chemical structures, with cyclic carbon rings at each end of the sulfonylurea nucleus; this causes them to be highly potent (100- to 200-fold more so than tolbutamide). The drugs should be used with caution in patients with cardiovascular disease as well as in elderly patients, in whom hypoglycemia would be especially dangerous.

a. **Glyburide (glibenclamide)**—Glyburide is supplied in tablets containing 1.25, 2.5, and 5 mg. The usual starting dose is 2.5 mg/d, and the average maintenance dose is 5 to 10 mg/d given as a single morning dose. If patients are going to respond to glyburide, they generally do so at doses of 10 mg/d or less, given once daily. If they fail to respond to 10 mg/d, it is uncommon for an increase in dosage to result in improved glycemic control. Maintenance doses higher than 20 mg/d are not recommended and may even worsen hyperglycemia. Glyburide is metabolized in the liver into products with such low hypoglycemic activity that they are considered clinically unimportant unless renal excretion is compromised. Although assays specific for the unmetabolized compound suggest a plasma half-life of only 1 to 2 hours, the biologic effects of glyburide clearly persist for 24 hours after a single morning dose in diabetic patients. Glyburide is unique among sulfonylureas in that it not only binds to the pancreatic β cell membrane sulfonylurea receptor but also becomes sequestered within the β cell. This may also contribute to its prolonged biologic effect despite its relatively short circulating half-life.

A formulation of micronized glyburide, which apparently increases its bioavailability, is available in easy to divide tablet sizes of 1.5, 3, and 6 mg.

Glyburide has few adverse effects other than its potential for causing hypoglycemia. It should not be used in patients with liver failure and renal failure because of the risk of hypoglycemia. Elderly patients are at particular risk of hypoglycemia even with relatively small daily doses. For this reason, drugs with a shorter half-life (eg, tolbutamide or possibly glipizide) are preferable in the treatment of type 2 diabetes in the elderly patient. Glyburide does not cause water retention, as chlorpropamide does, and even slightly enhances free water clearance.

b. Glipizide (glydiazinamide)—Glipizide is supplied in tablets containing 5 and 10 mg. For maximum effect in reducing postprandial hyperglycemia, this agent should be ingested 30 minutes before breakfast, because rapid absorption is delayed when the drug is taken with food. The recommended starting dose is 5 mg daily but 2.5-mg dose may be sufficient in elderly patients with early diabetes. The dose can gradually be increased by 2.5 or 5-mg increments. Although as much as 15 mg can be given as a single daily dose before breakfast, most patients do better with divided dosing, taking 5 mg before each meal or taking 10 mg before breakfast and before dinner. The maximum recommended dose is 40 mg/d, although doses above 20 mg probably provide little additional benefit in poor responders. Because of its lower potency and shorter half-life, it is preferable to glyburide in elderly patients. At least 90% of glipizide is metabolized in the liver to inactive products, and only a small fraction is excreted unchanged in the urine. Glipizide therapy is contraindicated in patients with liver failure.

Glipizide is also available as a slow-release preparation (Glucotrol-XL, 2.5, 5, and 10-mg tablets). The medication is enclosed in a nonabsorbable shell that contains an osmotic compartment that expands slowly, thereby slowly pumping out the glipizide in a sustained manner. It provides extended release during transit through the gastrointestinal tract, with greater effectiveness in lowering of prebreakfast hyperglycemia than the shorter duration, immediate-release standard glipizide tablets. However, this formulation appears to have sacrificed glipizide's reduced propensity for severe hypoglycemia compared with longer acting glyburide without showing any demonstrable therapeutic advantages over glyburide.

c. Gliclazide (not available in the United States)—This drug is another intermediate duration sulfonylurea with a duration of action of about 12 hours. It is available as 80-mg tablets. The recommended starting dose is 40 to 80 mg/d with a maximum dose of 320 mg. Doses of 160 mg and above are given as divided doses before breakfast and dinner. The drug is metabolized by the liver, and the metabolites and conjugates have no hypoglycemic effect. An extended-release preparation is also available.

d. Glimepiride—This sulfonylurea is supplied in tablets containing 1, 2, and 4 mg. It has a long duration of effect with a half-life of 5 hours, allowing once-daily administration. Glimepiride achieves blood glucose lowering with the lowest dose of any sulfonylurea compound. A single daily dose of 1 mg/d has been shown to be effective, and the maximal recommended dose is 8 mg. It is completely metabolized by the liver to relatively inactive metabolic products.

Meglitinide Analogs

Repaglinide is supplied as 0.5, 1, and 2-mg tablets. Its structure is similar to that of glyburide but lacks the sulfonic acid-urea moiety. It also acts by binding to the sulfonylurea receptor and closing the ATP-sensitive potassium channel. It is rapidly absorbed from the intestine and then undergoes complete metabolism in the liver to inactive biliary products, giving it a plasma half-life of less than 1 hour. The drug therefore causes a brief but rapid pulse of insulin. The starting

dose is 0.5 mg three times a day 15 minutes before each meal. The dose can be titrated to a maximum daily dose of 16 mg. Like the sulfonylureas, repaglinide can be used in combination with metformin. Hypoglycemia is the main side effect. In clinical trials, when the drug was compared with glyburide, a long-acting sulfonylurea, there was a trend toward less hypoglycemia. Like the sulfonylureas, it causes weight gain. Metabolism is by the cytochrome P4503A4 isoenzyme. Other drugs that induce or inhibit this isoenzyme may increase or inhibit the metabolism of repaglinide. The drug may be useful in patients with renal impairment or in the elderly.

Mitiglinide is a benzylsuccinic acid derivative that is very similar to repaglinide in its clinical effects. It binds to the sulfonylurea receptor causing a brief pulse of insulin. It is given as a 5 or 10-mg dose just before a meal and reduces the postprandial rise in blood glucose. It has been approved for use in Japan.

δ-Phenylalanine Derivative

Nateglinide is supplied in tablets of 60 and 120 mg. This drug binds the sulfonylurea receptor and closes the ATP-sensitive potassium channel. The drug is rapidly absorbed from the intestine, reaching peak plasma levels within 1 hour. It is metabolized in the liver and has a plasma half-life of about 1.5 hours. Like repaglinide, it causes a brief rapid pulse of insulin, and when given before a meal, it reduces the postprandial rise in blood glucose. The 60-mg dose is used in patients with mild elevations in HbA$_{1c}$. For most patients, the recommended starting and maintenance dosage is 120 mg three times a day before meals. Like the other insulin secretagogues, its main side effects are hypoglycemia and weight gain.

2. DRUGS THAT ACT ON INSULIN TARGET TISSUES

Metformin

Metformin (1,1-dimethylbiguanide hydrochloride) is used, either alone or in conjunction with other oral agents or insulin, in the treatment of patients with type 2 diabetes.

Metformin acts primarily through AMPK (Figure 17–8), which it activates by uncoupling mitochondrial oxidative phosphorylation and increasing cellular AMP levels. Metformin's therapeutic effects primarily derive from its effects on the liver, where increased AMPK activity reduces hepatic gluconeogenesis and lipogenesis. Metformin is a substrate for organic cation transporter 1, which is abundantly expressed in hepatocytes and in the gut.

Metformin has a half-life of 1.5 to 3 hours, does not bind to plasma proteins, and is not metabolized in humans, being excreted unchanged by the kidneys.

Metformin is the first-line therapy for patients with type 2 diabetes. The current recommendation is to start this drug at diagnosis. A side benefit of metformin therapy is its tendency to improve both fasting and postprandial hyperglycemia and hypertriglyceridemia in obese patients with diabetes without the weight gain associated with insulin or sulfonylurea therapy. Metformin is ineffective in patients with type 1 diabetes. Patients with renal failure (calculated GFR less than 50 mL/min) should not get this drug because failure to excrete this drug may produce high blood and tissue levels of metformin that would stimulate lactic acid overproduction. Likewise, patients with liver failure or abusers of ethanol should not receive this drug; lactic acid production from the gut and other tissues, which rises during metformin therapy, can result in lactic acidosis when defective hepatocytes cannot remove the lactate or when alcohol-induced reduction of nucleotides interferes with lactate clearance. Finally, metformin is relatively contraindicated in patients with cardiorespiratory insufficiency, because they have a propensity to develop hypoxia that would aggravate the lactic acid production already occurring from metformin therapy. The age cutoff for prescribing metformin has not been defined and remains a function of the overall health of the patient. In general, there is concern that after the age of 65 to 70 years the potential for progressive impairment of renal function or development of a cardiac event while taking metformin raises the risk enough to outweigh the benefits of prescribing the drug for patients with type 2 diabetes.

Metformin is dispensed as 500, 850, and 1000-mg tablets. A 500 and 750-mg extended-release preparation is also available. Eighty-five percent of the maximal glucose-lowering effect is achieved by a daily dose of 1500 mg, and there is little benefit from giving more than 2000 mg daily. It is important to begin with a low dose and increase the dosage very gradually in divided doses—taken with meals—to reduce minor gastrointestinal upsets. A common schedule would be one 500-mg tablet three times a day with meals or one 850-mg or 1000-mg tablet twice daily at breakfast and dinner. The maximum recommended dose is 850 mg three times a day. Up to 2000 mg of the extended-release preparation can be given once a day.

The epithelial cells of the gut efficiently absorb metformin, where it accumulates at high concentrations and causes toxicity due to uncoupling of mitochondrial oxidative phosphorylation and increased lactate production. The most frequent side effects of metformin are gastrointestinal symptoms (anorexia, nausea, vomiting, abdominal discomfort, diarrhea), which occur in up to 20% of patients. These effects are dose-related, tend to occur at onset of therapy, and often are transient. However, in 3% to 5% of patients, therapy may have to be discontinued because of persistent diarrheal discomfort. In a retrospective analysis, it has been reported that patients who switched from immediate-release metformin to a comparable dose of extended-release metformin experienced fewer gastrointestinal side effects.

Absorption of vitamin B_{12} appears to be reduced during chronic metformin therapy but usually the vitamin B_{12} levels remain in the normal range. Screening of serum vitamin B_{12} levels should be considered if the patient develops a macrocytic anemia or if the patient develops peripheral neuropathy symptoms. Hypoglycemia does not occur with therapeutic doses of metformin, which permits its description as a euglycemic or antihyperglycemic drug rather than an oral hypoglycemic agent. Dermatologic or hematologic toxicity is rare.

Lactic acidosis has been reported as a side effect but is uncommon with metformin in contrast to phenformin. Metformin both increases lactate production by uncoupling mitochondrial oxidative phosphorylation, especially in the gut, and reduces lactate removal by the liver by blocking gluconeogenesis. At therapeutic doses of metformin, serum lactate levels rise only minimally if at all, since other organs such as the kidney can remove the slight excess. However, if tissue hypoxia occurs, the metformin-treated patient is at higher risk for lactic acidosis due to compromised lactate removal. Similarly, when kidney function deteriorates, affecting not only lactate removal by the kidney but also metformin excretion, plasma levels of metformin rise far above the therapeutic range and can increase lactate production and block hepatic uptake sufficiently to provoke lactic acidosis even in the absence of other causes of increased lactic acid production. Acute renal failure can occur rarely following radiocontrast administration. Metformin therapy should therefore be temporarily halted on the day of radiocontrast administration and restarted a day or two later after confirmation that renal function is normal. Almost all reported cases of lactic acidosis have involved subjects with associated risk factors that should have contraindicated its use (kidney, liver, or cardiorespiratory insufficiency, alcoholism, advanced age).

Peroxisome Proliferator–Activated Receptor Agonists

Thiazolidinediones are insulin sensitizers exerting their antidiabetic effects through the activation of PPARγ (see discussion on PPAR nuclear receptors in insulin action and insulin resistance earlier). Observed effects of thiazolidinediones include increased glucose transporter expression (GLUT 1 and GLUT 4); decreased free fatty acid levels; decreased hepatic glucose output; increased adiponectin and decreased resistin release from adipocytes; and increased differentiation of preadipocytes into adipocytes. They have also been demonstrated to decrease levels of plasminogen activator inhibitor type 1, matrix metalloproteinase 9, C-reactive protein, and interleukin-6. Like the biguanides, this class of drugs does not cause hypoglycemia. Troglitazone, the first drug in this class to go into widespread clinical use, was withdrawn from clinical use because of drug-associated fatal liver failure.

Two other drugs in the same class are available for clinical use: **rosiglitazone** and **pioglitazone**. Both are effective as monotherapy and in combination with sulfonylureas, metformin, or insulin. When used as monotherapy, these drugs lower HbA_{1c} by about 1 or 2 percentage points. When used in combination with insulin, they can result in a 30% to 50% reduction in insulin dosage, and some patients can come off insulin completely. The combination of a thiazolidinedione and metformin has the advantage of not causing hypoglycemia. Patients inadequately managed on sulfonylureas can do well on a combination of sulfonylurea and rosiglitazone or pioglitazone. About 25% of patients in clinical trials fail to respond to these drugs, presumably because they are significantly insulinopenic.

In addition to glucose-lowering, the thiazolidinediones have effects on lipids and other cardiovascular risk factors. Rosiglitazone therapy is associated with increases in total cholesterol, LDL cholesterol (15%), and HDL cholesterol (10%). There is a reduction in free fatty acids of about 8% to 15%. The changes in triglycerides were generally not different from placebo. Pioglitazone in clinical trials lowered triglycerides (9%) and increased HDL cholesterol (15%) but did not cause a consistent change in total cholesterol and LDL cholesterol levels. A prospective randomized comparison of the metabolic effects of pioglitazone and rosiglitazone in patients who had previously taken troglitazone (now withdrawn from clinical use) showed similar effects on HbA$_{1c}$ and weight gain. Pioglitazone-treated subjects, however, had lower total cholesterol, LDL cholesterol, and triglyceride levels when compared with rosiglitazone. A study in patients with type 2 diabetes who were not on lipid-lowering therapy has recently confirmed this difference in lipid-lowering effects of the two thiazolidinediones. Small prospective studies have also shown that treatment with these drugs leads to improvement of biochemical and histological features of nonalcoholic fatty liver disease. The thiazolidinediones also may limit vascular smooth muscle proliferation after injury and there are reports that troglitazone and pioglitazone reduce neointimal proliferation after coronary stent placement. Also, in one double-blind, placebo-controlled study, rosiglitazone was shown to be associated with a decrease in the ratio of urinary albumin to creatinine.

The dosage of rosiglitazone is 4 to 8 mg daily and of pioglitazone 15 to 45 mg daily, and the drugs do not have to be taken with food. Rosiglitazone is primarily metabolized by the CYP 2C8 isoenzyme and pioglitazone is metabolized by CYP 2C8 and CYP 3A4.

Safety concerns and some troublesome side effects have emerged about this class of drugs that limit their use.

A meta-analysis of 42 randomized clinical trials with rosiglitazone suggested that this drug increases the risk of angina pectoris or myocardial infarction. A meta-analysis of clinical trials with pioglitazone did not show a similar finding. Although conclusive data are lacking, the European Medicines Agency has suspended the use of rosiglitazone in Europe. In the United States, the FDA has mandated that it can be prescribed to new patients only if they are unable to achieve glucose control on other medications or are unable to take pioglitazone.

Edema occurs in about 3% to 4% of patients receiving monotherapy with rosiglitazone or pioglitazone. The edema occurs more frequently (10%-15%) in patients receiving concomitant insulin therapy and may result in congestive heart failure. The drugs are contraindicated in diabetic individuals with New York Heart Association class III and IV cardiac status. Thiazolidinediones have also rarely been reported as being associated with new onset or worsening macular edema which resolved or improved once the drug was discontinued.

In experimental animals, rosiglitazone stimulates bone marrow adipogenesis at the expense of osteoblastogenesis resulting in a decrease in bone mineral density. An increase in fracture risk in women (but not men) has been reported with both rosiglitazone and pioglitazone. The fracture risk is in the range of 1.9 per 100 patient-years with the thiazolidinedione. In at least one study of rosiglitazone, the fracture risk was increased in premenopausal as well as postmenopausal women. This increased risk for fractures is perhaps the most important reason for limiting the use of this class of drugs.

Other side effects include anemia, which occurs in 4% of patients treated with these drugs; it may be due to a dilutional effect of increased plasma volume rather than a reduction in red cell mass. Weight gain occurs, especially when the drug is combined with a sulfonylurea or insulin. Some of the weight gain is fluid retention, but there is also an increase in total fat mass. In preclinical studies with pioglitazone, bladder tumors were observed in male rats receiving clinically relevant doses of the medication. In a planned five-interim analysis of data from a long term observational cohort there was no overall increased risk of bladder cancer with pioglitazone therapy. However, increased bladder cancer risk was observed with increasing dose and duration of pioglitazone use, reaching statistical significance after 24 months of exposure.

Troglitazone, the first drug in this class, was withdrawn from clinical use because of drug-associated fatal liver failure. The two currently available agents, rosiglitazone and pioglitazone, have thus far not caused hepatotoxicity. The FDA has, however, recommended that patients should not initiate drug therapy if there is clinical evidence of active liver disease or pretreatment elevation of the alanine aminotransferase (ALT) level that is 2.5 times greater than the upper limit of normal. Obviously, caution should be used in initiation of therapy in patients with even mild ALT elevations. Liver biochemical tests should be performed prior to initiation of treatment and periodically thereafter.

3. DRUGS THAT AFFECT GLUCOSE ABSORPTION

Alpha-Glucosidase Inhibitors

Drugs of this family are competitive inhibitors of intestinal brush border α glucosidases. Two of these drugs, acarbose and miglitol, are available for clinical use in the United States. Voglibose, another α glucosidase inhibitor, is available in Japan, Korea, and India. Acarbose and miglitol are potent inhibitors of glucoamylase, α-amylase, and sucrase. They are less effective on isomaltase and are ineffective on trehalase or lactase. Acarbose binds 1000 times more avidly to the intestinal disaccharidases than do products of carbohydrate digestion or sucrose. A fundamental difference exists between acarbose and miglitol in their absorption. Acarbose has the molecular mass and structural features of a tetrasaccharide, and very little (~2%) crosses the microvillar membrane. Miglitol, however, is structurally similar to glucose and is absorbable. Both drugs delay the absorption of carbohydrates and reduce postprandial glycemic excursion.

   a. Acarbose is available as 50 and 100-mg tablets. The recommended starting dose is 50 mg twice daily, gradually increasing to 100 mg three times daily. For maximal benefit on postprandial hyperglycemia, acarbose should be given with the first mouthful of food ingested. In diabetic patients it reduces postprandial hyperglycemia by 30% to 50%, and its overall effect is to lower the HbA$_{1c}$ by 0.5% to 1%. The principal adverse effect, seen in 20% to 30% of patients, is flatulence. This is caused by undigested carbohydrate reaching the lower bowel, where gases are produced by bacterial flora. In 3% of cases, troublesome diarrhea occurs. This gastrointestinal discomfort tends to discourage excessive carbohydrate consumption and promotes improved compliance of patients with type 2 diabetes with their diet prescriptions.

   When acarbose is given alone, there is no risk of hypoglycemia. However, if combined with insulin or sulfonylureas, it may increase risk of hypoglycemia from these agents. A slight rise in hepatic aminotransferases has been noted in clinical trials (5% vs 2% in placebo controls, and particularly with doses >300 mg/d). This generally returns to normal on stopping this drug. In the UKPDS, approximately 2000 patients on diet, sulfonylurea, metformin, or insulin therapy were randomized to acarbose or placebo therapy. By 3 years, 60% of the patients had discontinued the drug, mostly because of gastrointestinal symptoms. In the 40% of patients who remained on the drug, acarbose was associated with a 0.5% lowering of HbA$_{1c}$ compared with placebo.

   b. **Miglitol** is similar to acarbose in terms of its clinical effects. It is indicated for use in diet- or sulfonylurea-treated patients with type 2 diabetes. Therapy is initiated at the lowest effective dosage of 25 mg three times a day. The usual maintenance dose is 50 mg three times a day, although some patients may benefit from increasing the dose to 100 mg three times a day. Gastrointestinal side effects occur as with acarbose. The drug is not metabolized and is excreted unchanged by the kidney. Theoretically, absorbable α-glucosidase inhibitors could induce a deficiency of one or more of α-glucosidases involved in cellular glycogen metabolism and biosynthesis of glycoproteins. This does not occur in practice because—unlike the intestinal mucosa, which is exposed to a high concentration of the drug—circulating plasma levels are 200-fold to 1000-fold lower than those needed to inhibit intracellular α glucosidases. Miglitol should not be used in renal failure because its clearance is impaired in this setting.

4. INCRETINS

The gut makes several incretins, gut hormones that amplify postprandial insulin secretion, including glucagon-like peptide-1 (GLP-1, Figure 17–9) and glucose-dependent insulinotropic polypeptide (GIP). Therapeutic drugs in this class include GLP-1 receptor agonists and **dipeptidyl peptidase 4** (DPP-4) inhibitors, which increase levels of both GLP-1 and GIP.

When GLP-1 is infused in patients with type 2 diabetes, it stimulates insulin secretion and lowers glucose levels. GLP-1, unlike the sulfonylureas, has only a modest insulin stimulatory effect under normoglycemic conditions. This means that GLP-1 administration has a lower risk of causing hypoglycemia than the sulfonylureas. GLP-1, in addition to its insulin stimulatory effect, also has a number of other pancreatic and extrapancreatic effects (see Table 17–4).

GLP-1 Receptor Agonists

GLP-1 is rapidly proteolyzed by DPP-4 and by other enzymes such as endopeptidase 24.11. It is also cleared rapidly by the kidney. As a result, the half-life of GLP-1 is only 1 to 2 minutes. The native peptide, therefore, cannot be used therapeutically. Instead, the approach taken has been to develop metabolically stable analogs or derivatives of GLP-1 that are not subject to the same enzymatic degradation or renal clearance. Two GLP-1 receptor agonists, exenatide and liraglutide, are currently available for clinical use.

   a. **Exenatide or exendin 4** is a GLP-1 receptor agonist isolated from the saliva of the Gila monster (a venomous lizard) that is resistant to DPP-4 action and is cleared from the plasma by glomerular filtration. When given to patients with type 2 diabetes by subcutaneous injection twice a day, this compound lowers blood glucose and HbA$_{1c}$ levels. Exenatide appears to have the same effects as GLP-1 on glucagon suppression and gastric emptying. In clinical trials, adding exenatide to the therapeutic regimen of patients with

type 2 diabetes who are already taking metformin or a sulfonylurea (or both) further lowered the HbA$_{1c}$ value by 0.4% to 0.6% over a 30-week period. These patients also lost 3 to 6 lb in weight. In an open-label extension study up to 80 weeks, the HbA$_{1c}$ reduction was sustained, and there was further weight loss (to a total loss of ~10 lb).

The main side effect was nausea, affecting over 40% of patients. The nausea was dose-dependent and declined with time. The risk of hypoglycemia was higher in subjects on sulfonylureas. The delay in gastric emptying may affect the absorption of some other drugs; therefore, antibiotics and oral contraceptives should be taken 1 hour before exenatide doses. Low-titer antibodies against exenatide develop in over one-third (38%) of patients, but the clinical effects are not attenuated. High-titer antibodies develop in a subset of patients (~6%), and in about half of these cases, an attenuation of glycemic response has been seen.

The FDA has received 30 postmarketing reports of acute pancreatitis in patients taking exenatide. The pancreatitis was severe (hemorrhagic or necrotizing) in six instances and two of these patients died. Many of the patients had other risk factors for pancreatitis, but the possibility remains that the drug was causally responsible for some cases. Patients taking exenatide should be advised to seek immediate medical care if they experience unexplained, persistent, severe abdominal pain. The drug should be discontinued if pancreatitis is suspected. The FDA also reported 16 cases of renal impairment and 62 cases of acute renal failure in patients taking exenatide. Some of these patients had preexisting kidney disease and others had one or more risk factors for kidney disease. A number reported nausea, vomiting, and diarrhea and it is possible that these side effects cause volume depletion and contributed to the development of renal failure.

Exenatide is dispensed as two fixed-dose pens (5 and 10 μg). It is injected 60 minutes before breakfast and before dinner. Patients should be prescribed the 5-μg pen for the first month and then, if tolerated, the dose should be increased to 10 μg twice daily. The drug is not recommended in patients with glomerular filtration rate less than 30 mL/min.

   b. **Liraglutide** is a soluble fatty acid acylated GLP-1 analog—with replacement of lysine with arginine at position 34 and the attachment of a C16 acyl chain to a lysine at position 26. The fatty-acyl GLP-1 retains affinity for GLP-1 receptors, but the addition of the C16 acyl chain allows for noncovalent binding to albumin, both hindering DPP-4 access to the molecule and contributing to a prolonged half-life and duration of action. The half-life is approximately 12 hours allowing the drug to be injected once a day.

In clinical trials lasting 26 and 52 weeks, adding liraglutide to the therapeutic regimen (metformin, sulfonylurea, thiazolidinedione) of patients with type 2 diabetes further lowered the HbA$_{1c}$ value. Depending on the dose and design of the study, the HbA$_{1c}$ decline was in the range of 0.6% to 1.5%. The patients had sustained weight loss of 1 to 6 lb.

Like exenatide, the most frequent side effect is nausea and vomiting affecting approximately 10% of subjects. There was also an increase in incidence of diarrhea. About 2% to 5% of subjects withdrew from the studies because of the GI symptoms. Pancreatitis may also occur—in the clinical trials there were seven cases of pancreatitis in the liraglutide-treated group with one case in the comparator group (2.2 vs 0.6 cases per 1000 patient-years). Liraglutide stimulates C-cell neoplasia and causes medullary thyroid carcinoma in rats. Human C cells express very few GLP-1 receptors and the relevance to human therapy is unclear but because of the animal data, the drug should not be used in patients with personal or family history of medullary thyroid carcinoma or multiple endocrine neoplasia syndrome type 2.

The dosing is initiated at 0.6 mg daily increased after 1 week to 1.2 mg daily. An additional increase in dose to 1.8 mg is recommended if needed for optimal glycemic control. Titration should of course be based on tolerability. There is limited experience using the drug in renal failure but no dose adjustment is recommended.

DPP-4 Inhibitors

An alternative to the use of GLP-1 receptor agonists involves inhibition of the enzyme DPP-4 with prolongation of the action of endogenously released GLP-1 and GIP. Two oral DPP-4 inhibitors, sitagliptin and saxagliptin, are available for the treatment of type 2 diabetes in the United States. An additional DPP-4 inhibitor, Vildagliptin, is available in Europe.

a. Sitagliptin in clinical trials was shown to be effective in lowering glucose when used alone and in combination with metformin and pioglitazone. In various clinical trials, improvements in HbA_{1c} ranged from 0.5% to 1.4%. The usual dose of sitagliptin is 100 mg once daily, but the dose is reduced to 50 mg daily if the calculated creatinine clearance is 30 to 50 mL/min and to 25 mg for clearances less than 30 mL/min. Unlike exenatide, sitagliptin does not cause nausea or vomiting. It also does not result in weight loss. The main adverse effect appears to be a predisposition to nasopharyngitis or upper respiratory tract infection. A small increase in neutrophil count of approximately 200 cells/mL has also occurred. Since its FDA approval and clinical use, there have been reports of serious allergic reactions to sitagliptin, including anaphylaxis, angioedema, and exfoliative skin conditions, including Stevens-Johnson syndrome. There have also been reports of pancreatitis (88 cases including two cases of hemorrhagic or necrotizing pancreatitis). The frequency of these events is unclear. DPP-4 is a pleiotropic enzyme that inactivates a variety of peptide hormones, neuropeptides, and chemokines and DPP-4 inhibitors have been shown to prolong the action of neuropeptide Y and substance P. Whether its inhibition over a long-term period will have negative consequences is not known.

b. Saxagliptin when added to the therapeutic regimen (metformin, sulfonylurea, thiazolidinedione) of patients with type 2 diabetes further lowered the HbA_{1c} value by about 0.7% to 0.9%. The dose is 2.5 or 5 mg once a day. The 2.5-mg dose should be used in patients with calculated creatinine clearance less than 50 mL/min. It lowers HbA_{1c} by about 0.6% when added to metformin, glyburide, or thiazolidine in various 24-week clinical trials. The drug is weight neutral. The main adverse reactions were upper respiratory tract infection, naspharyngitis, headache, and urinary tract infection. There is also small reversible dose-dependent reduction in absolute lymphocyte count which remains within normal limits. Hypersensitivity reactions such as urticaria and facial edema occurred in 1.5% of patients on the drug compared to 0.4% with placebo. The metabolism of saxagliptin is through CYP 3A4/5; so strong inhibitors or inducers of CYP 3A4/5 will affect the pharmacokinetics of saxagliptin and its active metabolite.

c. Vildagliptin, like the other DPP-4 inhibitors, lowers HbA_{1c} by about 0.5% to 1% when added to the therapeutic regimen of patients with type 2 diabetes. The dose is 50 mg once a day or twice a day. The adverse reactions include upper respiratory tract infections, nasopharyngitis, dizziness, and headache. Rare cases of hepatic dysfunction including hepatitis have been reported. Liver function testing is recommended, quarterly the first year, and periodically thereafter.

5. OTHERS

Pramlintide is a synthetic analog of islet amyloid polypeptide (IAPP) that when given subcutaneously (1) delays gastric emptying, (2) suppresses glucagon secretion, and (3) decreases appetite. It is approved for use both in type 1 and insulin-treated type 2 patients. In 6-month clinical studies with type 1 and insulin-treated type 2 patients, those on the drug had approximately a 0.4% reduction in HbA_{1c} and lost about 1.7 kg compared to placebo. The HbA_{1c} reduction was sustained for 2 years, but some of the weight was regained. The drug is given immediately before the meal by injection. Hypoglycemia is the most concerning adverse event, and it is recommended that the short-acting or premixed insulin doses be reduced by 50% when the drug is started. Since the drug slows gastric emptying, recovery from hypoglycemia can be a problem because of delay in absorption of the fast-acting carbohydrate. Nausea was the other main side effect, affecting 30% to 50% of subjects. It tended to improve with time. In patients with type 1 diabetes, pramlintide is initiated at the dose of 15 μg before each meal and titrated by 15 μg increments to a maintenance dose of 30 or 60 μg before each meal. In patients with type 2 diabetes, the initiation dose is 60 μg premeals increased to 120 μg in 3 to 7 days if no significant nausea occurs.

A combination of pramlintide and recombinant human leptin (metreleptin) is currently being evaluated in clinical trials for weight loss.

Drug Combinations

A number of drug combinations, glyburide-metformin (Glucovance), glipizide-metformin (Metaglip), repaglinide-metformin (Prandi-Met), rosiglitazone-metformin (Avandamet), pioglitazone-metformin (ACTOplus Met), sitagliptin-metformin (Janumet), saxagliptin-metformin extended release (kombiglyze XR), rosiglitazone-glimepiride (Avandaryl), and pioglitazone-glimepiride (Duetact) are available. These combinations, however, limit the clinician's ability to optimally adjust dosage of the individual drugs and for that reason are of questionable merit.

6. INSULIN

Insulin is indicated for individuals with type 1 diabetes as well as for those with type 2 diabetes whose hyperglycemia does not respond to diet therapy and other diabetes drugs.

Human insulin is now produced by recombinant DNA techniques (biosynthetic human insulin). Animal insulins are no longer available in the United States. With the availability of highly puri-fied human insulin preparations, immunogenicity has been mark-edly reduced, thereby decreasing the incidence of therapeutic complications such as insulin allergy, immune insulin resistance, and localized lipoatrophy at the injection site. The insulins are also quite stable and refrigeration while in use is not necessary. During travel, reserve supplies of insulin can be readily transported with-out significant loss of potency, provided they are protected from extremes of heat or cold.

Insulins in Europe and United States are available only in a concentration of 100 U/mL (U100). Low-dose (0.3 mL) dispos-able insulin syringes allow for accurate dosing of as low as 1 or 2 U. If extremely low doses of insulin are needed, diluted insulin can be prepared using diluent available from the insulin manufac-turer. For use in rare cases of severe insulin resistance in which large quantities of insulin are required, a U500 (500 U/mL) regu-lar human insulin is available from Eli Lilly.

Insulin preparations differ with regard to their time of onset and duration of biologic action (Figure 17–11; Table 17–14).

TABLE 17–14 Summary of bioavailability characteristics of the injectable insulins.

Insulin Preparations	Onset of Action	Peak Action	Effective Duration
Insulins lispro, aspart, glulisine	5-15 min	1-1.5 h	3-4 h
Human regular	30-60 min	2 h	6-8 h
Human NPH	2-4 h	6-7 h	10-20 h
Insulin glargine	1.5 h	Flat	~24 h
Insulin detemir	1 h	Flat	17 h

The short-acting preparations are regular insulin and the rapidly acting insulin analogs (Table 17–15). They are dispensed as clear solutions at neutral pH and contain small amounts of zinc to improve their stability and shelf life. The long-acting preparations are neutral protamine hagedorn (NPH) insulin and the long-acting insulin analogs. NPH insulin is dispensed as a turbid sus-pension at neutral pH with protamine in phosphate buffer. The long-acting insulin analogs are dispensed as clear solutions; insulin glargine is at acidic pH and insulin detemir is at neutral pH. The rapidly acting insulin analogs and the long-acting insulins are designed for subcutaneous administration, while regular insulin can also be given intravenously. While insulin aspart has been approved for intravenous use (eg, in hyperglycemic emergencies), there is no advantage in using insulin aspart over regular insulin by this route.

It is important to recognize that values given for time of onset of action, peak effect, and duration of action are only approximate and that there is great variability in these parameters from patient to patient and even in a given patient depending on the size of the

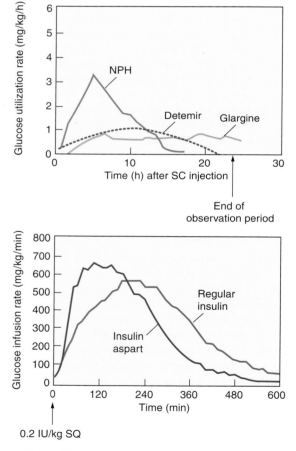

FIGURE 17–11 Extent and duration of action of various types of insulin (in a fasting diabetic). Duration of action may be extended considerably when the dose of a given insulin formulation increases above the average therapeutic doses depicted here.

TABLE 17–15 Insulin preparations available in the United States.[a]

Short Acting Insulin Preparations
Insulin lispro (Humalog, Lilly)
Insulin aspart (Novolog, Novo Nordisk)
Insulin glusisine (Apidra, Sanofi Aventis)
Regular insulin (Lilly, Novo Nordisk)
Long acting Insulin Preparations
NPH insulin (Lilly, Novo Nordisk)
Insulin glargine (Lantus, Sanofi Aventis)
Insulin detemir (Levemir, Novo Nordisk)
Premixed Insulins
    % NPH/% regular
        70/30 (Lilly, Novo Nordisk)
    75% insulin lispro/protamine (NPL) 25% insulin lispro
        Humalog mix 75/25 (Lilly)
    50% NPL/50% insulin lispro
        Humalog mix 50/50 (Lilly)
    70% insulin aspart/protamine/30% insulin aspart
        Novolog Mix 70/30 (Novo Nordisk)

[a]All types of insulin available in the United States are recombinant human or human insulin analog origin. All the insulins are dispensed at U100 concentration. There is an additional U500 preparation of regular insulin.

dose, the site of injection, the degree of exercise, the avidity of circulating anti-insulin antibodies, and other less well-defined variables.

Short-Acting Insulin Preparations

A. Regular insulin Regular insulin is a short-acting, soluble crystalline zinc insulin whose hypoglycemic effect appears within 30 minutes after subcutaneous injection, peaks at about 2 hours, and lasts for about 5 to 7 hours when usual quantities (ie, 5-15 U) are administered. Intravenous infusions of regular insulin are particularly useful in the treatment of diabetic ketoacidosis and during the perioperative management of insulin-requiring diabetics. Regular insulin is indicated when the subcutaneous insulin requirement is changing rapidly, such as after surgery or during acute infections—although the rapidly acting insulin analogs may be preferable in these situations.

For very insulin-resistant subjects who would otherwise require large volumes of insulin solution, a U500 preparation of human regular insulin is available. Because a U500 syringe is not available, a U100-insulin syringe or tuberculin syringe is used to measure doses. The physician should carefully note dosages in both units and volume to avoid overdosage.

B. Rapidly acting insulin analogs *Insulin lispro* (Humalog) is an insulin analog produced by recombinant technology, wherein two amino acids near the carboxyl terminal of the B chain have been reversed in position; proline at position B28 has been moved to B29 and lysine has been moved from B29 to B28. **Insulin aspart** (Novolog) is a single substitution of proline by aspartic acid at position B28. **Insulin glulisine** (Apidra) differs from human insulin in that the amino acid asparagine at position B3 is replaced by lysine and the lysine in position B29 by glutamic acid. These changes reduce the tendency to form hexamers in these three analogs, in contrast to human insulin. When injected subcutaneously, the analogs quickly dissociate into monomers and are absorbed very rapidly, reaching peak serum values in as soon as 1 hour—in contrast to regular human insulin, whose hexamers require considerably more time to dissociate and become absorbed. The amino acid changes in these analogs do not interfere with their binding to the insulin receptor, with the circulating half-life, or with their immunogenicity, which are all identical to those of human regular insulin.

Clinical trials have demonstrated that the optimal times of preprandial subcutaneous injection of comparable doses of the rapid-acting insulin analogs and of regular human insulin are 20 minutes and 60 minutes before the meal, respectively. Although this more rapid onset of action has been welcomed as a great convenience by patients with diabetes who object to waiting as long as 60 minutes after injecting regular human insulin before they can begin their meal, patients must be taught to ingest adequate absorbable carbohydrate early in the meal to avoid hypoglycemia during the meal. Another desirable feature of rapidly acting insulin analogs is that their duration of action remains at about 4 hours irrespective of dosage. This contrasts with regular insulin, whose duration of action is prolonged when larger doses are used.

The rapidly acting analogs are also commonly used in pumps. In a double-blind crossover study comparing insulin lispro with regular insulin in insulin pumps, persons using insulin lispro had lower HbA$_{1c}$ values and improved postprandial glucose control with the same frequency of hypoglycemia. The concern remains that in the event of pump failure, users of the rapidly acting insulin analogs will have more rapid onset of hyperglycemia and ketosis.

The structural differences between insulin lispro and human insulin may be sufficient to prevent insulin lispro from binding to human insulin antibodies in some patients, and there have been case reports of successful use of insulin lispro in those rare patients who have a generalized allergy to human insulin or who have severe antibody-mediated insulin resistance.

Long-Acting Insulin Preparations

a. **Neutral Protamine Hagedorn (NPH)**, or isophane, insulin is an intermediate-acting insulin in which the onset of action is delayed by combining two parts of soluble crystalline zinc insulin with one part protamine zinc insulin. The mixture has equivalent concentrations of protamine and insulin, so that neither is in excess (isophane). Its onset of action is delayed by 2 to 4 hours, and its peak response is generally reached in about 8 to 10 hours. Because its duration of action is often less than 24 hours (with a range of 10-20 hours), most patients require at least two injections daily to maintain a sustained insulin effect.

Flocculation of suspended particles may occasionally frost the sides of a bottle of NPH insulin or clump within bottles from which multiple small doses are withdrawn over a prolonged period. This instability is a rare phenomenon and might occur less frequently if NPH human insulin were refrigerated when not in use and if bottles were discarded after 1 month of use. Patients should be vigilant for early signs of frosting or clumping of the NPH insulin, because it indicates a pronounced loss of potency. Several cases of diabetic ketoacidosis have been reported in patients with type 1 diabetes who had been inadvertently injecting this denatured insulin.

b. **Insulin glargine** is an insulin analog in which the asparagine at position 21 of the A chain of the human insulin molecule is replaced by glycine and two arginines are added to the carboxyl terminal of the B chain. The arginines raise the isoelectric point of the molecule close to neutral, making it more soluble in an acidic environment. In contrast, human insulin has an isoelectric point of pH 5.4. Insulin glargine is a clear insulin that, when injected into the neutral pH environment of the subcutaneous tissue, forms microprecipitates that slowly release the insulin into the circulation. It lasts for about 24 hours without any pronounced peaks and is given once a day to provide basal coverage. This insulin cannot be mixed with the other insulins because of its acidic pH. When this insulin was given as a single injection at bedtime to type 1 diabetes patients, fasting hyperglycemia was better controlled when compared with bedtime NPH insulin. The clinical trials also suggest that there may be less nocturnal hypoglycemia with this insulin when compared with NPH insulin.

In one clinical trial involving patients with type 2 diabetes, insulin glargine was associated with a slightly more rapid progression of retinopathy when compared with NPH insulin. The frequency was 7.5% with the analog and 2.7% with the NPH. This observation however, was not confirmed in a 5-year open label prospective study of 1024 subjects randomized to NPH or insulin glargine. There was no increase in the risk of progression of retinopathy with the analog insulin.

In in vitro studies, insulin glargine has a sixfold greater affinity for the IGF-1 receptor compared with the human insulin. There has also been a report that insulin glargine has increased mitogenicity compared with human insulin in a human osteosarcoma cell line. Circulating levels of insulin glargine, however, are low, and the clinical significance of these observations is not yet clear. An observational study from Germany of 127,031 patients who had exposure to regular insulin, short-acting insulin analogs, and insulin glargine reported a strong correlation between increased insulin dose and cancer risk. Moreover insulin glargine, dose for dose, appeared to carry a higher risk than regular insulin. Additional studies are needed to confirm or refute this observation. Because of lack of safety data, use of insulin glargine during pregnancy is not recommended.

c. **Insulin detemir** is an insulin analog in which the tyrosine at position 30 of the B chain has been removed and a 14-C fatty acid chain (tetradecanoic acid) is attached to the lysine at position 29 by acylation. The fatty acid chain makes the molecule more lipophilic than native insulin, and the addition of zinc stabilizes the molecule and leads to formation of hexamers. After injection, self-association at the injection site and albumin binding in the circulation via the fatty acid side chain lead to slower distribution to peripheral target tissues and prolonged duration of action. The affinity of insulin detemir is four- to fivefold lower than that of human soluble insulin and, therefore, the U100 formulation of insulin detemir has a concentration of 2400 nmol/mL compared to 600 nmol/mL for NPH. The duration of action for insulin detemir is about 17 hours at therapeutically relevant doses. It is recommended that the insulin is injected once or twice a day to achieve a stable basal coverage. Apparently this insulin has been reported to have lower within-subject pharmacodynamic variability compared to NPH insulin and insulin glargine. In vitro studies do not suggest any clinically relevant albumin binding interactions between insulin detemir and fatty acids or protein-bound drugs. Because there is a vast excess (~400,000) of albumin-binding sites available in plasma per insulin detemir molecule, it is unlikely that hypoalbuminemic disease states will affect the ratio of bound to free insulin detemir.

Insulin Mixtures

Because intermediate-acting insulins require several hours to reach adequate therapeutic levels, their use in patients with type 1 diabetes requires supplements of regular insulin or insulin lispro or insulin aspart preprandially. For convenience, regular or NPH insulin may be mixed together in the same syringe and injected subcutaneously in split dosage before breakfast and supper. It is recommended that the regular insulin be withdrawn first, then the NPH insulin. No attempt should be made to mix the insulins in the syringe, and the injection is preferably given immediately after the syringe is loaded. Stable premixed insulins (70% NPH and 30% regular) are available as a convenience to patients who have difficulty mixing insulin because of visual problems or insufficient manual dexterity.

With increasing use of rapid-acting insulin analogs as a preprandial insulin, it has become evident that combination with an intermediate-acting or long-acting insulin is essential to maintain postabsorptive glycemic control. It has been demonstrated that insulin lispro can be acutely mixed with NPH insulin without affecting its rapid absorption. Premixed preparations of insulin lispro and NPH insulin however are unstable because of exchange of insulin lispro with the human insulin in the protamine complex. Consequently, over time, the soluble component becomes a mixture of regular and insulin lispro at varying ratios. In an attempt to remedy this, an intermediate insulin composed of isophane complexes of protamine with insulin lispro was developed and given the name NPL (neutral protamine lispro). Premixed combinations of NPL and insulin lispro are now available for clinical use (Humalog Mix 75/25 and Humalog Mix 50/50). These mixtures have a more rapid onset of glucose-lowering activity compared with 70% NPH/30% regular human insulin mixture and can be given within 15 minutes before or after starting a meal. Similarly, a 70% insulin aspart protamine/30% insulin aspart (NovoLogMix 70/30) is now available. The main advantages of these new mixtures are that (1) they can be given within 15 minutes of starting a meal and (2) they are superior in controlling the postprandial glucose rise after a carbohydrate-rich meal. These benefits have not translated into improvements in HbA$_{1c}$ levels when compared with the usual 70% NPH/30% regular mixture.

The longer-acting insulin analogs (insulin glargine or insulin detemir) cannot be acutely mixed with either regular insulin or the rapid-acting insulin analogs.

Methods of Insulin Administration

a. **Insulin syringes and needles**—Disposable plastic syringes with needles attached are available in 1-mL, 0.5-mL, and 0.3-mL sizes. Their finely honed 30- to 31-gauge attached needles have greatly reduced the pain of injections. They are light, not susceptible to damage, and convenient when traveling. Moreover, their clear markings and tight plungers allow accurate measurement of insulin dosage. The *low-dose* syringes have become increasingly popular, because most patients take less than 30 U at one injection and also it is available with half unit markings. Two lengths of needles are available: short (8 mm) and long (12.7 mm). Long needles are preferable in obese patients to reduce the variability of insulin absorption.

b. **Sites for injection**—Any part of the body covered by loose skin can be used as an injection site, including the abdomen, thighs, upper arms, flanks, and upper-outer quadrants of the buttocks. In general, regular insulin is absorbed more rapidly from upper regions of the body such as the deltoid area or the abdomen rather than from the thighs or buttocks. Exercise appears to facilitate insulin absorption when the injection site is adjacent to the exercising muscle. Rotation of sites continues to be recommended to avoid delayed absorption when fibrosis or lipohypertrophy occurs due to repeated use of a single site. However, considerable variability of absorption rates from different regions, particularly with exercise, may contribute to the instability of glycemic control in certain patients with type 1 diabetes if injection sites are rotated indiscriminately over different areas of the body. Consequently, diabetologists recommend limiting injection sites to a single region of the body and rotating sites within that region. It is possible that some of the stability of glycemic control achieved by infusion pumps may be related to the constancy of the region of infusion from day to day. For most patients, the abdomen is the recommended region for injection because it provides a considerable area in which to rotate sites, and there may be less variability of absorption with exercise than when the thigh or deltoid areas are used. The effect of anatomic regions appears to be much less pronounced with the analogs.

c. **Insulin pen injector devices**—Insulin pens eliminate the need for carrying insulin vials and syringes. Cartridges of insulin lispro, insulin aspart, and insulin glargine are available for reusable pens (Lilly, Novo Nordisk, and Owen Mumford). Disposable prefilled pens are also available for insulin lispro, insulin aspart, insulin glulisine, insulin detemir, insulin glargine, NPH, 70% NPH/30% regular, 75% NPL/25% insulin lispro, and 70% insulin aspart protamine/30% insulin aspart. Thirty-one-gauge needles (5, 6, and 8-mm long) for these pens make injections almost painless.

d. **Insulin pumps**—Several small portable open loop pumps for the delivery of insulin are in the market. These devices contain an insulin reservoir and a pump programmed to deliver regular insulin subcutaneously; they do not contain a glucose sensor. With improved methods for self-monitoring of *blood* glucose at home (see later), these pump systems are becoming increasingly popular. In the United States, Medtronic MiniMed, Insulet, Animas, and Roche insulin infusion pumps are available for subcutaneous delivery of insulin. These pumps are small (about the size of a pager) and easy to program. They have many features, including the ability to record a number of different basal rates throughout a 24-hour period and adjust the time over which bolus doses are given. They are able also to detect pressure build-up if the catheter is kinked. The catheter connecting the insulin reservoir to the subcutaneous cannula can be disconnected so the patient can remove the pump temporarily (eg, for bathing). Ominpod (Insulet Corporation) is an insulin infusion system in which the insulin reservoir and infusion set are integrated into one unit (pod), so it does not use a catheter. The pod, placed on the skin, delivers subcutaneous basal and bolus insulin based on wirelessly transmitted instructions from a personal digital assistant.

The great advantage of **continuous subcutaneous insulin infusion (CSII)** is that it allows for establishment of a basal profile tailored to the patient. The patient, therefore, is able to eat with less regard to timing because the basal insulin infusion should maintain a constant blood glucose level between meals. Also, the ability to adjust the basals makes it easier for the patient to manage glycemic excursions that occur with exercise. The pumps also have software that can assist the patient to calculate boluses based on glucose reading and carbohydrates to be consumed. They also keep track of the time elapsed since last insulin bolus and the patient is reminded of this when he or she attempts to give additional correction bolus before the effect of the previous bolus has worn off (*insulin on board* feature). This feature reduces the risk of overcorrecting and subsequent hypoglycemia.

CSII therapy is appropriate for patients who are motivated, mechanically adept, educated about diabetes (diet, insulin action, treatment of hypo- and hyperglycemia), and willing to monitor their blood glucose four to six times a day. Known complications of CSII include ketoacidosis, which can occur when insulin delivery is interrupted, and skin infections. Another major disadvantage is the cost and the time demanded of physicians and staff in initiating therapy. Almost all patients use the rapid-acting insulin analogs in their pumps. Clinical trials have shown that when compared with regular insulin, subjects using rapid-acting insulin analogs in pumps had lower HbA$_{1c}$ values and improved postprandial glucose control with the same frequency of hypoglycemia. There does remain a concern that in the event of pump failure, the insulin analogs could result in more rapid onset of hyperglycemia and ketosis.

e. **Inhaled insulin**—Exubera, the first inhaled insulin preparation approved by the FDA is no longer available; the manufacturer stopped marketing it because of lack of demand. In clinical trials, Exubera was as effective as subcutaneous regular insulin in controlling postprandial glucose excursions. Physicians, however, were reluctant to prescribe Exubera for a number of reasons, including a lack of long-term safety data on pulmonary function, availability of other insulin delivery systems, cost, lack of insurance coverage, and awkward dosing. The manufacturer also subsequently reported that there were six cases of lung cancer in patients who were on inhaled insulin and one case in the comparator-treated patients. All the patients who developed lung cancer had a history of prior cigarette smoking. There is currently only one pharmaceutical company that is still conducting clinical trials with inhaled insulin (Technosphere insulin, MannKind Corporation).

f. **Pancreas transplantation**—This transplantation done at the time of renal transplantation is becoming more widely accepted. Patients undergoing simultaneous pancreas and kidney transplantation have an 85% chance of pancreatic graft survival and a 92% chance of renal graft survival after 1 year. About 1200 pancreas transplants are performed yearly in the United States. About 75% of the transplants are perfomed at the same time as the kidney transplant with both organs from the same donor. About 15% of the pancreas transplants are performed after a previously successful kidney transplant and 10% are performed without a kidney transplant. Solitary pancreatic transplantation in the absence of a need for renal transplantation should be considered only in those rare patients who fail all other insulin therapeutic approaches and who have frequent severe hypoglycemia or who have life-threatening complications related to their lack of metabolic control.

g. **Islet cell transplantation**—This is a minimally invasive procedure, and investigators in Edmonton, Canada, reported initial insulin independence in a small number of patients with type 1 diabetes, who underwent this procedure. Using islets from multiple donors and steroid-free immunosuppression, percutaneous transhepatic portal vein transplantation of islets was achieved in more than 20 subjects. Several centers around the world have successfully replicated this experience. Unfortunately, although all of the initial cohorts achieved insulin independence posttransplantation, some for more than 2 years of follow-up, a decline in insulin secretion occurred with time, and the subjects have again required supplemental insulin. However, patients with successful transplants had complete correction of severe hypoglycemic reactions, leading to a marked improvement in overall quality of life. Islet transplant trials with different immunosuppressive regimens are currently underway. Even if long-term insulin independence is demonstrated, wide application of this procedure for the treatment of type 1 diabetes is limited by the dependence on multiple donors and the requirement for potent long-term immunotherapy.

STEPS IN THE MANAGEMENT OF THE DIABETIC PATIENT

History and Examination

A complete history is taken and physical examination is performed for diagnostic purposes and to rule out the presence of coexisting or complicating disease. Nutritional status should be noted, particularly if catabolic features such as progressive weight loss are present despite a normal or increased food intake. The family history should include not only the incidence but also the age at onset of diabetes in other members of the family, and it should be noted whether affected family members were obese, whether they required insulin, and whether they developed complications from their diabetes. Other factors that increase cardiovascular risk, such as a smoking history, presence of hypertension or hyperlipidemia, or oral contraceptive pill use should be documented.

A careful physical examination should include baseline height and weight, pulse rate, and blood pressure. If obesity is present, it should be characterized as to its distribution, and a waist-to-hip ratio should be recorded. All peripheral arterial pulses should be examined, noting whether bruits or other signs of atherosclerotic disease are present. Neurologic and ophthalmologic examinations should be performed, with emphasis on investigation of abnormalities that may be related to diabetes, such as neovascularization of the retina or stocking/glove sensory loss in the extremities.

Laboratory Diagnosis

See also Laboratory Testing in diabetes mellitus earlier. Laboratory diagnosis should include documentation of the presence of fasting hyperglycemia (plasma glucose ≥126 mg/dL [7 mmol/L]), postprandial (post-glucose tolerance test) values consistently ≥200 mg/dL (11.1 mmol/L) or HbA_{1c} ≥6.5%. An attempt should be made to characterize the diabetes as type 1 or type 2, based on the clinical features present and on whether ketonuria accompanies the glycosuria. For the occasional patient, measurement of ICA, ICA 512, GAD, and insulin antibodies can help in distinguishing between type 1 and type 2 diabetes. Many newly diagnosed patients with type 1 diabetes still have significant endogenous insulin production, and C-peptide levels may not reliably distinguish between type 1 and type 2 diabetes. Other baseline laboratory measurements that should be made part of the record include hemoglobin A_{1c}, lipid profile, serum creatinine and electrolytes, complete blood count, electrocardiogram, and urine albumin measurement (type 2 patient).

Patient Education and Self-Management Training

Since diabetes is a lifelong disorder, education of the patient and the family is probably the most important obligation of the clinician who provides initial care. The best persons to manage a disease that is affected so markedly by daily fluctuations in environmental stress, exercise, diet, and infections are the patients themselves and their families. It must be remembered that education is necessary not only for patients with newly diagnosed diabetes and their families, but also for patients with diabetes of any duration who may never have been properly educated about their disorder or who may not be aware of advances in diabetes management. The *teaching curriculum* should include explanations by the physician or nurse of the nature of diabetes and its potential acute and chronic hazards and how they can be recognized early and prevented or treated. Self-monitoring of blood glucose should be emphasized, especially in insulin-requiring diabetic patients, and instructions must be given on proper testing and recording of data. Patients must also be helped to accept the fact that they have diabetes; until this difficult adjustment is made, efforts to cope with the disorder are likely to be futile. Counseling should be directed at avoidance of extremes such as compulsive rigidity or self-destructive neglect.

Patients on insulin should have an understanding of the actions of basal and bolus insulins. They should be taught how to determine whether the basal dose is appropriate and how to adjust the rapidly acting insulin dose for the carbohydrate content of a meal. Patients and their families or friends should also be taught to recognize signs and symptoms of hypoglycemia and how to institute appropriate therapy for hypoglycemic reactions. Strenuous exercise can precipitate hypoglycemia, and patients should know how much to reduce their insulin dosage in anticipation of strenuous activity or to take supplemental carbohydrate. Injection of insulin into a site farthest away from the muscles most involved in exercise may help ameliorate exercise-induced hypoglycemia, since insulin injected in the proximity of exercising muscle may be more rapidly mobilized. Exercise training also increases the effectiveness of insulin and insulin doses should be adjusted accordingly. Because infections, particularly pyogenic ones with fever and toxemia, provoke a marked increase in insulin requirements, patients must be taught how to appropriately administer supplemental rapid-acting insulin as needed to correct hyperglycemia during infections.

Type 2 diabetes on noninsulin medications should be informed about the time of onset, peak action, duration of action, and any adverse effects of pharmacologic agents being used. They should also learn to inquire about possible drug interactions whenever any new medications are added to their regimens.

The targets for blood glucose control should be elevated appropriately in elderly patients since they have the greatest risk if subjected to hypoglycemia and the least long-term benefit from more rigid glycemic control. Patients should be provided advice on personal hygiene, including detailed instructions on foot and dental care. All infections (especially pyogenic ones) provoke the release of high levels of insulin antagonists such as catecholamines or glucagon and thus bring about a marked increase in insulin requirements. Patients who are oral agents may decompensate and temporarily require insulin. All patients receiving therapy that can cause hypoglycemia should wear a MedicAlert bracelet or necklace that clearly states that insulin or an oral sulfonylurea drug is being taken. Patients should be told about community agencies, such as

American Diabetes Association chapters, that can serve as a continuing source of instruction.

Finally, vigorous efforts should be made to persuade new diabetics who smoke to give up the habit, since large vessel peripheral vascular disease and debilitating retinopathy are less common in nonsmoking diabetic patients.

Specific Therapy

With the publication of data from the DCCT and the UKPDS, there has been a shift in the guidelines regarding acceptable levels of control. The ADA recommends that for patients with either type 1 and type 2 diabetes, the goal is to achieve preprandial blood glucose values of 80 to 120 mg/dL and an average bedtime glucose of 100 to 140 mg/dL and HbA$_{1c}$ of <7% (nondiabetic range: 4%-6%). Obviously, these goals should be modified by taking into account the patient's ability to carry out the treatment regimen, the risk of severe hypoglycemia, and other patient factors that may reduce the benefit of such tight control.

A. Type 1 diabetes   Patients with type 1 diabetes require replacement therapy with exogenous insulin. This should be instituted under conditions of an individualized diabetic diet with multiple feedings and normal daily activities so that an appropriate dosage regimen can be developed.

At the onset of type 1 diabetes, many patients recover some pancreatic β cell function and may temporarily need only low doses of exogenous insulin to supplement their own endogenous insulin secretion. This is known as the *honeymoon period*. Within 8 weeks to 2 years, however, most of these patients show either absent or negligible pancreatic β cell function. At this point, these patients should be switched to a more flexible insulin regimen with a combination of rapid-acting insulin analogs or regular insulin together with intermediate-acting or long-acting insulin. At a minimum, the patient should be on a three-injection regimen and frequently may need four or more injections. Twice-daily split-dose insulin mixtures cannot maintain near-normalization of blood glucose without hypoglycemia (particularly at night) and are not recommended. Self-monitoring of blood glucose levels is required for determining the optimal adjustment of insulin dosage and the modulation of food intake and exercise in type 1 diabetes.

Certain caveats should be kept in mind regarding insulin treatment. Considerable variations in absorption and bioavailability exist, even when the same dose is injected in the same region on different days in the same individual. Such variation often can be minimized by injecting smaller quantities of insulin at each injection and consequently using multiple injections. Furthermore, a given insulin dosage may demonstrate considerable variability in pharmacokinetics in different individuals, either because of insulin antibodies that bind insulin with different avidity or for other as yet unknown reasons. A properly educated patient should be taught to adjust insulin dosage by observing the pattern of recorded self-monitored blood glucose levels and correlating it with the approximate duration of action and the time to peak effect after injection of the various insulin preparations (see Table 17–14).

A combination of rapid-acting insulin analogs and long-acting insulins (insulin glargine or insulin detemir) allows for more physiologic insulin replacement. In clinical studies, combinations of rapid-acting insulin analogs (insulin lispro or insulin aspart) with meals together with intermediate-acting (NPH) or longer-acting insulin (insulin glargine) for basal coverage have now been shown to have improved HbA$_{1c}$ values with less hypoglycemia when compared with a regimen of regular insulin with meals and NPH at night. Table 17–16 illustrates some regimens that might be appropriate for a 70-kg person with type 1 diabetes eating meals of standard carbohydrate intake and moderate to low fat content.

Multiple injections of NPH insulin can be mixed in the same syringe as the insulin lispro, insulin aspart, and insulin glulisine. Insulin glargine is usually given once in the evening to provide 24-hour coverage. This insulin *should not be mixed* with any of the other insulins and must be given as a separate injection. There are occasional patients in whom insulin glargine does not seem to last for 24 hours, and in such cases it needs to be given twice a day.

Continuous subcutaneous insulin infusion by portable battery-operated *open loop* devices currently provides the most flexible approach, allowing the setting of different basal rates throughout the 24 hours and permitting patients to delay or skip meals and vary meal size and composition (see Methods of Insulin Administration, earlier). The dosage is usually based on providing 50% of the estimated insulin dose as basal and the remainder as intermittent boluses prior to meals. For example, a 70-kg man requiring 35 U of insulin per day may require a basal rate of

TABLE 17–16 Examples of intensive insulin regimens using rapid-acting insulin analogs (insulin lispro, aspart, or glulisine) and NPH, or insulin glargine in a 70-kg man with type 1 diabetes.[a-c]

	Prebreakfast	Prelunch	Predinner	Bedtime
Rapid-acting insulin analog	5 U	4 U	6 U	—
NPH insulin	3 U	3 U	2 U	8-9 U
OR				
Rapid-acting insulin analog	5 U	4 U	6 U	—
Insulin glargine	—	—	—	15-16 U

[a]Assumes that patient is consuming approximately 75 g carbohydrate at breakfast, 60 g at lunch, and 90 g at dinner.

[b]The dose of rapid-acting insulin analogs can be raised by 1 or 2 U if extra carbohydrate (15-30 g) is ingested or if premeal blood glucose is >170 mg/dL. The rapid-acting insulin analogs can be mixed in the same syringe with NPH insulin.

[c]Insulin glargine cannot be mixed with any of the available insulins and must be given as a separate injection.

0.7 U/h throughout the 24 hours with the exception of 3 AM to 8 AM, when 0.8 U/h might be appropriate (for the *dawn phenomenon*). The meal bolus would depend on the carbohydrate content of the meal and the premeal blood glucose value. One unit per 15 g of carbohydrate plus 1 U for 50 mg/dL of blood glucose above a target value (eg, 120 mg/dL) is a common starting point. Further adjustments to basal and bolus dosages would depend on the results of blood glucose monitoring. Most patients use the rapid-acting insulin analogs in the pumps.

One of the more difficult therapeutic problems in managing patients with type 1 diabetes is determining the proper adjustment of insulin dose when the early morning blood glucose level is high before breakfast (Table 17–17). Prebreakfast hyperglycemia is sometimes due to the *Somogyi effect*, in which nocturnal hypoglycemia evokes a surge of counterregulatory hormones to produce high blood glucose levels by 7 AM. However, a more common cause of prebreakfast hyperglycemia is the waning of the evening or bedtime insulin and/or the dawn phenomenon. That is, reduced tissue sensitivity to insulin between 5 AM and 8 AM (dawn), due to spikes of growth hormone released hours before, at onset of sleep. Table 17–17 shows that diagnosis of the cause of prebreakfast hyperglycemia can be facilitated by self-monitoring of blood glucose at 3 AM in addition to the usual bedtime and 7 AM measurements. This is required for only a few nights, and when a particular pattern emerges from monitoring blood glucose levels overnight, appropriate therapeutic measures can be taken. Prebreakfast hyperglycemia due to the Somogyi effect can be treated by reducing the dose of either intermediate- or long-acting insulin analog at bedtime. For hyperglycemia due to waning of overnight basal insulin and/or dawn phenomenon, an increase in the evening dose of the basal insulin or shifting it from dinnertime to bedtime (or both) can be effective. A bedtime dose either of insulin glargine or insulin detemir provides more sustained overnight insulin levels than human NPH and may be effective in managing refractory prebreakfast hyperglycemia. If this fails, insulin pump therapy may be required with a higher basal insulin infusion rate (eg, from 0.8 U/h to 0.9 U/h from 6 AM until breakfast).

B. Type 2 diabetes

Therapeutic recommendations are based on the relative contributions of β cell insufficiency and insulin insensitivity in individual patients. The possibility that the individual patient has a specific etiological cause for their diabetes should always be considered, especially when the patient does not have a family history of type 2 diabetes or does not have any evidence of central obesity or insulin resistance. Such patients should be evaluated for other types of diabetes such as LADA or MODY. Patients with LADA should be prescribed insulin when their disease is diagnosed and treated like patients with type 1 diabetes. It is also important to note that many type 2 patients have a progressive loss of β cell function and will require additional therapeutic interventions with time.

Weight reduction—One of the primary modes of therapy in the obese patient with type 2 diabetes is weight reduction. Normalization of glycemia can be achieved by reducing adipose stores, with consequent restoration of tissue sensitivity to insulin. A combination of caloric restriction, increased exercise, modification of behavior, and consistent reinforcement of good eating habits is required if a weight reduction program is to be successful. Knowledge of the symptoms of diabetes and an understanding of the risks and complications of diabetes often increase the patient's motivation for weight reduction. Even so, significant weight loss is seldom achieved and is even more difficult to maintain in the morbidly obese patient. Weight control is variable in moderately obese patients, depending on the enthusiasm of the therapist and the motivation of the patient.

For selected patients, medical or surgical options for weight loss should be considered (also see Chapter 20). Sibutramine, a combined serotonin-norepinephrine reuptake inhibitor, is moderately effective in promoting weight loss. It has however been associated with increased risk of heart attack and stroke and has been withdrawn from clinical use.

Orlistat is a reversible inhibitor of gastric and pancreatic lipases and prevents the hydrolysis of dietary triglycerides. These triglycerides are then excreted in the feces. In a 1-year study in obese patients with type 2 diabetes, those taking orlistat had lost more weight, had lower HbA$_{1c}$ values, and had improved lipid profiles. The main adverse reactions were gastrointestinal, with oily spotting, oily stool, flatus, and fecal

TABLE 17–17 Typical patterns of overnight blood glucose levels and serum-free immunoreactive insulin levels in prebreakfast hyperglycemia due to various causes in patients with type 1 diabetes.

	Blood Glucose Levels (mg/dL)			Serum-Free Immunoreactive Insulin Levels (μU/mL)		
	10 PM	3 AM	7 AM	10 PM	3 AM	7 AM
Somogyi effect	90	40	200	High	Slightly high	Normal
Dawn phenomenon	110	110	150	Normal	Normal	Normal
Waning of circulating insulin levels plus dawn phenomenon	110	190	220	Normal	Low	Low
Waning of circulating insulin levels plus dawn phenomenon plus Somogyi effect	110	40	380	High	Normal	Low

urgency and frequency. Malabsorption of fat-soluble vitamins also occurs. Patients should take a multivitamin tablet containing fat-soluble vitamins at least 2 hours before or 2 hours after the administration of orlistat. Cases of severe liver injury have been reported with this drug although a cause and effect relationship has not been established.

Bariatric surgery (Roux-en-Y, gastric sleeve, biliopancreatic diversion/duodenal switch, or gastric banding) typically result in substantial weight loss, and long-term follow-up has shown that many patients with diabetes who undergo these procedures maintain the weight reduction.

Nonobese patients with type 2 diabetes frequently have increased visceral adiposity—the so-called metabolically obese normal-weight patient. There is less emphasis on weight loss but exercise remains an important aspect of treatment.

Antihyperglycemic agents—The current recommendation is to start metformin therapy at diagnosis and not wait to see if the patient can achieve target glycemic control with weight management and exercise. **Metformin** is advantageous because, apart from lowering glucose without the risk of hypoglycemia, it also lowers triglycerides and promotes some modest weight loss. The drug, however, cannot be used in patients with renal failure, and some patients have gastrointestinal side effects at even the lowest doses. Under these circumstances the choice of the initial agent depends on a number of factors, including comorbid conditions, adverse reactions to the medications, ability of the patient to monitor for hypoglycemia, drug cost, and patient and physician preferences. **Sulfonylureas** have been available for many years, and their use in combination with metformin is well established. They do, however, have the propensity to cause hypoglycemia and weight gain. **Thiazolidinediones** improve peripheral insulin resistance and lower glucose without causing hypoglycemia. They also have been reported to improve nonalcoholic fatty liver disease. In addition, they have beneficial effects on the lipid profile and some other cardiovascular risk factors. They decrease microalbuminuria, and reduce neointimal tissue hyperplasia after coronary artery stent placement. Thiazolidinediones, however, can cause fluid retention and are contraindicated in patients with heart failure. They also very commonly increase weight, which patients find distressing, affecting adherence. The drugs are associated with increased fracture risk in women and this adverse effect significantly limits their use. Pioglitazone is the preferred choice because of concerns regarding rosiglitazone and the risk of ischemic heart disease. Both drugs are contraindicated in patients with active liver disease and in patients with liver enzyme levels ≥2.5 times the upper limit of normal. The **α-glucosidase inhibitors** have modest glucose-lowering effects and have gastrointestinal side effects. They have a lower risk of hypoglycemia than the sulfonylureas and promote weight loss. The GLP-1 receptor agonists (exenatide and liraglutide) have a lower risk of hypoglycemia than the sulfonylureas, and they promote weight loss. However, they need to be given by injection, cause nausea, may cause pancreatitis, and are contraindicated in patients with gastroparesis. The DPP-4 inhibitors (sitagliptin and saxagliptin) also have a low risk of hypoglycemia, and they do not cause nausea or vomiting. They can also be used in patients with kidney impairment. There are, however, reports of serious allergic reactions, including anaphylaxis, angioedema, and

Stevens-Johnson syndrome. There is concern that sitagliptin, like the GLP-1 receptor agonists, may cause pancreatitis.

When patients are not well controlled on their initial therapy (usually metformin) then a second agent should be added. In those patients where the problem is hyperglycemia after a carbohydrate-rich meal (such as dinner), a short-acting secretagogue before meals may suffice to put the glucose levels into the target range. Patients with severe insulin resistance or nonalcoholic fatty liver disease or microalbuminuria may be candidates for pioglitazone. Subjects who are very concerned about weight gain may benefit from a trial of a GLP-1-receptor agonist or DPP-4 inhibitor. If two agents are inadequate, then a third agent is added, although data on efficacy with such combined therapy are limited. When the combination of oral agents (and injectable GLP-1 receptor agonists) fail to achieve target glycemic control in patients with type 2 diabetes or if there are contraindications to their use, then insulin treatment should be instituted. Various insulin regimens may be effective. One proposed regimen is to continue the oral combination therapy and then simply add a bedtime dose of NPH or long-acting insulin analog (insulin glargine or insulin detemir) to reduce excessive nocturnal hepatic glucose output and improve fasting glucose levels. If the patient does not achieve target glucose levels during the day, then daytime insulin treatment can be initiated. A convenient insulin regimen under these circumstances is a split dose of 70/30 NPH/regular mixture (or Humalog Mix 75/25 or NovoLogMix 70/30) before breakfast and before dinner. If this regimen fails to achieve satisfactory glycemic goals or is associated with unacceptable frequency of hypoglycemic episodes, then a more intensive regimen of multiple insulin injections can be instituted as in patients with type 1 diabetes. Metformin principally reduces hepatic glucose output, and it is reasonable to continue with this drug when insulin therapy is instituted. The thiazolidinediones, which improve peripheral insulin sensitivity, can be used together with insulin, but this combination is associated with more weight gain and peripheral edema. The sulfonylureas also have been shown to be of continued benefit. There is limited information on the benefits of continuing the GLP1-receptor agonists or the DPP-4 inhibitors once insulin therapy is initiated. Weight-reducing interventions should continue even after initiation of insulin therapy and may allow for simplification of the therapeutic regimen in the future.

IMMUNOPATHOLOGY OF INSULIN THERAPY

At least five molecular classes of insulin antibodies are produced during the course of insulin therapy: IgA, IgD, IgE, IgG, and IgM. Human insulin is much less antigenic than the older formulations of animal (especially beef) insulins, but because of its hexameric presentation at therapeutic injection doses, it is also treated as a foreign substance by the immune system and results in detectable—albeit low—titers of insulin antibodies in most patients.

A. Insulin allergy   Insulin allergy, a hypersensitivity reaction of the immediate type, is a rare condition in which local or systemic urticaria occurs immediately after insulin injection. This reaction is due to histamine release from tissue mast cells sensitized by adherence of IgE antibodies to their surface. In severe cases, anaphylaxis can occur. The appearance of a subcutaneous nodule at the site of insulin injection, occurring several hours after the injection and lasting for up to 24 hours, has been attributed to an IgG-mediated complement-binding Arthus reaction. Because sensitivity was often due to noninsulin protein contaminants, the highly purified insulins have markedly reduced the incidence of insulin allergy, especially of the local variety. Antihistamines, corticosteroids, and even desensitization may be required, especially for systemic hypersensitivity in an insulin-dependent patient. A protocol for allergy testing and insulin desensitization is available from the Lilly Company. A trial of insulin analogs should also be considered. There is a case report of successful use of insulin lispro in the face of generalized allergy to human insulin.

B. Immune insulin resistance All patients who receive insulin (including insulin analogs) develop a low titer of circulating IgG antibodies, and this neutralizes the rapid action of insulin to a small extent. With the animal insulins, a high titer of circulating antibodies is sometimes developed, resulting in extremely high insulin requirements, often to more than 200 U/d. This is now very rarely seen with the switch to the highly purified human insulins and has not been reported with use of the analogs.

C. Lipodystrophy at injection sites Rarely, a disfiguring atrophy of subcutaneous fatty tissue occurs at the site of insulin injection. Although the cause of this complication is obscure, it seems to represent a form of immune reaction, particularly because it occurs predominantly in females and is associated with lymphocyte infiltration in the lipoatrophic area. This complication has become even less common because of the development of highly purified insulin preparations of neutral pH. Injection of highly purified preparations of insulin directly into the atrophic area often results in restoration of normal contours.

Lipohypertrophy, on the other hand, is not a consequence of immune responses; rather, it seems to be due to the pharmacologic effects of depositing insulin in the same location repeatedly. It is prevented by rotation of injection sites. There is a case report of a male patient who had intractable lipohypertrophy (fatty infiltration of injection site) with human insulin but no longer had the problem when he switched to insulin lispro.

ACUTE COMPLICATIONS OF DIABETES MELLITUS

Hypoglycemia

Hypoglycemic reactions (see later and Chapter 18) are the most common complications that occur in patients with diabetes who are treated with insulin. Hypoglycemia may result from delay in taking a meal, from unusual physical exertion without supplemental calories, or from an increase in insulin dose. In addition, it can occur in any patient taking oral agents that stimulate pancreatic β cells (eg, sulfonylureas, meglitinide, D-phenylalanine analogs), particularly if the patient is elderly, has renal or liver disease, or is taking certain other medications that alter metabolism of the sulfonylureas (eg, phenylbutazone, sulfonamides, or warfarin). It occurs more frequently with the use of long-acting sulfonylureas.

The signs and symptoms of hypoglycemia may be divided into those resulting from stimulation of the autonomic nervous system and those arising from neuroglycopenia (insufficient glucose for normal central nervous system function). When the blood glucose falls to around 54 mg/dL, the patient starts to experience both sympathetic (tachycardia, palpitations, sweating, tremulousness) and parasympathetic (nausea, hunger) nervous system symptoms. If these autonomic symptoms are ignored and the glucose levels fall further (to around 50 mg/dL), then neuroglycopenic symptoms appear, including irritability, confusion, blurred vision, tiredness, headache, and difficulty speaking. A further decline in glucose (below 30 mg/dL) can then lead to loss of consciousness or even a seizure.

With repeated episodes of hypoglycemia, there is adaptation and autonomic symptoms do not occur until the blood glucose levels are much lower and so the first symptoms are often due to neuroglycopenia. This condition, which is referred to as **hypoglycemic unawareness**, results from failure of the sympathetic nervous system to respond to hypoglycemia (Table 17–18). This adaptation of the central nervous system to recurrent hypoglycemic episodes is due to upregulation of the GLUT 1 transporters at the blood-brain barrier and increased glucose transport into the brain despite subnormal levels of plasma glucose. It has been shown that hypoglycemic unawareness can be reversed by keeping glucose levels high for a period of several weeks. Except for sweating, most of the sympathetic symptoms of hypoglycemia are blunted in patients receiving β-blocking agents for angina pectoris or hypertension. Though not absolutely contraindicated, these drugs must be used with caution in insulin-requiring diabetics, and β_1-selective blocking agents are preferred.

Hypoglycemia in insulin-treated patients with diabetes occurs as a consequence of three factors: behavioral issues, impaired counterregulatory systems, and complications of diabetes.

TABLE 17–18 Hypoglycemic "unawareness" in type 1 diabetes mellitus.

I. Sleeping patient (nocturnal hypoglycemia)
II. Hypoglycemia with unawareness while awake
A. Manifestations
a. Neuroglycopenic symptoms first (weakness, lethargy, confusion, incoordination, blurred vision)
b. Autonomic symptoms are delayed and blunted (tremor, anxiety, palpitations, sweating, hunger)
B. Mechanisms
1. Defective autonomic response:
a. Adaptation to chronic hypoglycemia (increased brain glucose transporter I)
b. Due to diabetic autonomic neuropathy
C. Management
1. Identify patients at risk and reevaluate glycemic goals
2. Advise frequent self-monitoring of blood glucose; use of continuous glucose monitoring systems
3. Learn to detect subtle symptoms of neuroglycopenia
4. Avoid recurrent hypoglycemia
5. Injectable glucagon made available to family

TABLE 17–19 Counterregulatory responses to hypoglycemia.

Normal Counterregulation	Defective Counterregulation in Type 1 Diabetes[a]
Glucagon rises rapidly to three to five times baseline after insulin-induced hypoglycemia, provoking hepatic glycogenolysis.	Glucagon response to insulin-induced hypoglycemia is lost after onset of type 1 diabetes.
Adrenergic discharge (1) raises hepatic glucose output by glycogenolysis and (2) provides warning to subject of impending hypoglycemic crisis.	Blunted or absent adrenergic response may occur as a result of: (1) Neural damage associated with advanced age or autonomic neuropathy (2) Neural dysfunction (iatrogenic) from frequent hypoglycemia

[a]Type 2 diabetics are less well characterized as to their defective counterregulation of glucagon loss, but appear to have the same frequency and causes of adrenergic loss as do type 1 diabetics.

Behavioral issues include injecting too much insulin for the amount of carbohydrates ingested. Drinking alcohol in excess, especially on an empty stomach, can also cause hypoglycemia. In patients with type 1 diabetes, hypoglycemia can occur during or even several hours after exercise, and so glucose levels need to be monitored and food and insulin adjusted. Some patients do not like their glucose levels to be high, and they treat every high glucose level aggressively. These individuals who *stack* their insulin, that is, give another dose of insulin before the first injection has had its full action, can develop hypoglycemia.

Counterregulatory issues resulting in hypoglycemia include impaired glucagon response and impaired sympatho-adrenal responses (Table 17–19). Patients with diabetes of greater than 5 years duration lose their glucagon response to hypoglycemia. As a result, they are at a significant disadvantage in protecting themselves against falling glucose levels. Once the glucagon response is lost, their sympatho-adrenal responses take on added importance. Unfortunately, aging, autonomic neuropathy, or hypoglycemic unawareness due to repeated low glucose levels further blunts the sympatho-adrenal responses. Occasionally, Addison disease develops in persons with type 1 diabetes mellitus; when this happens, insulin requirements fall significantly, and unless insulin dose is reduced, recurrent hypoglycemia will develop.

Complications of diabetes that increase the risk for hypoglycemia include autonomic neuropathy, gastroparesis, and renal failure. The sympathetic nervous system is an important system alerting the individual that the glucose level is falling by causing symptoms of tachycardia, palpitations, sweating, and tremulousness. Failure of the sympatho-adrenal responses increases the risk of hypoglycemia. In patients with gastroparesis, insulin given before a meal promotes maximal glucose uptake into cells before the food is absorbed, causing the glucose levels to fall. Finally, in renal failure, hypoglycemia

can occur presumably because of decreased insulin clearance as well as loss of the renal contribution to gluconeogenesis in the postabsorptive state.

Treatment

To treat insulin-induced hypoglycemia, the diabetic patient should carry glucose tablets or juice at all times. For most episodes, ingestion of 15 g of carbohydrate is sufficient to reverse the hypoglycemia. The patient should be instructed to check the blood glucose in 15 minutes and treat again if the glucose level is still low.

A parenteral glucagon emergency kit (1 mg) should be provided to every patient with diabetes who is on insulin therapy. Family or friends should be instructed how to inject it subcutaneously or intramuscularly into the buttock, arm, or thigh in the event that the patient is unconscious or refuses food. The drug can occasionally cause vomiting and the unconscious patient should be turned on his or her side to protect the airway. Glucagon mobilizes glycogen from the liver raising the blood glucose by about 36 mg/dL in about 15 minutes. After the patient recovers consciousness additional oral carbohydrate should be given. Glucagon is contraindicated in sulfonylurea-induced hypoglycemia where it paradoxically causes insulin release. People with diabetes on hypoglycemic drug therapy should also wear a MedicAlert bracelet or necklace or carry a card in his or her wallet.

Medical personnel treating severe hypoglycemia can give 50 mL of 50% glucose solution by rapid intravenous infusion. If intravenous therapy is not available, 1 mg of glucagon can be injected intramuscularly. If the patient is stuporous and glucagon is not available, small amounts of honey or maple syrup or glucose gel (15 g) can be inserted within the buccal pouch, although, in general, oral feeding is contraindicated in unconscious patients. Rectal administration of maple syrup or honey (30 mL per 500 mL of warm water) has been effective.

Most patients who arrive at emergency departments in hypoglycemic coma appear to recover fully; however, profound hypoglycemia or delays in therapy can result in permanent neurologic deficit or even death. Furthermore, repeated episodes of hypoglycemia may have a cumulative adverse effect on intellectual functioning. The physician should carefully review with the patient the events leading up to the hypoglycemic episode. Associated use of other medications, as well as alcohol or narcotics, should be noted. Careful attention should be paid to diet, exercise pattern, insulin or sulfonylurea dosage, and general compliance with the prescribed diabetes treatment regimen. Any factors thought to have contributed to the development of the episode should be identified and recommendations made in order to prevent recurrences of this potentially disastrous complication of diabetes therapy.

If the patient is hypoglycemic from use of a long-acting oral hypoglycemic agent (eg, chlorpropamide or glyburide) or from high doses of a long-acting insulin, admission to hospital for treatment with continuous intravenous glucose and careful monitoring of blood glucose is indicated.

Coma

Coma is a *medical emergency* calling for immediate evaluation to determine its cause so that proper therapy can be started. Patients with diabetes may be comatose because of hypoglycemia, diabetic ketoacidosis, hyperglycemic hyperosmolar coma, or lactic acidosis. When evaluating a comatose diabetic patient, these must be considered *in addition* to the myriad causes included in the differential diagnosis of coma (eg, cerebrovascular accidents, head trauma, intoxication with alcohol, or other drugs).

After emergency measures have been instituted (airway protection; laboratory tests; intravenous dextrose unless fingerstix blood glucose shows hyperglycemia), a careful history (from family, friends, or paramedics), physical examination, and laboratory evaluation are required to resolve the differential diagnosis. Patients in deep coma from a hyperosmolar nonketotic state or from hypoglycemia are generally flaccid and have quiet breathing—in contrast to patients with acidosis, whose respirations are rapid and deep if the pH of arterial blood has dropped to 7.1 or below. When hypoglycemia is a cause of the coma, the state of hydration is usually normal. Although the clinical laboratory remains the final arbiter in confirming the diagnosis, a rapid *estimate* of blood glucose and ketones can be obtained by the use of bedside glucose and ketone meters (see Laboratory Findings in diabetes mellitus, earlier). Table 17–20 is a summary of some laboratory abnormalities found in diabetic patients with coma attributable to diabetes or its treatment.

1. DIABETIC KETOACIDOSIS

This acute complication of diabetes mellitus may be the first manifestation of previously undiagnosed type 1 diabetes or may result from increased insulin requirements in type 1 diabetes patients during the course of infection, trauma, myocardial infarction, or surgery. The National Data Group reports an annual incidence of five to eight episodes of diabetic ketoacidosis per 1000 diabetic patients. In all cases, precipitating factors such as infection should be searched for and treated appropriately. Poor compliance, either for psychological reasons or because of inadequate patient education, is probably the most common cause of diabetic ketoacidosis, particularly when episodes are recurrent. In adolescents with type 1 diabetes, recurrent episodes of severe ketoacidosis often indicate the need for counseling to alter this behavior.

Diabetic ketoacidosis has been found to be one of the more common serious complications of insulin pump therapy, occurring in approximately 1 per 80 patient-months of treatment.

Patients with type 2 diabetes may also develop ketoacidosis under severe stress such as sepsis, trauma, or major surgery.

Pathogenesis

Acute insulin deficiency results in rapid mobilization of energy from stores in muscle and fat depots, leading to an increased flux of amino acids to the liver for conversion to glucose and of fatty acids for conversion to ketones (acetoacetate, β-hydroxybutyrate, and acetone). In addition to this increased availability of precursor, there is a direct effect of the low insulin-glucagon ratio on the liver that promotes increased production of ketones as well as of glucose. In response to both the acute insulin deficiency and the metabolic stress of ketosis, the levels of insulin-antagonistic hormones (corticosteroids, catecholamines, glucagon, and GH) are consistently elevated. Furthermore, in the absence of insulin, peripheral utilization of glucose and ketones is reduced. The combination of increased production and decreased utilization leads to an accumulation of these substances in blood, with plasma glucose levels reaching 500 mg/dL (27.8 mmol/L) or more and plasma ketones reaching levels of 8 to 15 mmol/L or more. β-Hydroxybutyrate is the predominant ketone and its ratio to acetoacetate increases from 1:1 to as much as 5:1.

The hyperglycemia causes osmotic diuresis leading to depletion of intravascular volume. As this progresses, impaired renal blood flow reduces the kidney's ability to excrete glucose, and hyperosmolality worsens. Severe hyperosmolality (>330 mOsm/kg) correlates closely with central nervous system depression and coma.

In a similar manner, impaired renal excretion of hydrogen ions aggravates the metabolic acidosis that occurs as a result of the accumulation of the ketoacids, β-hydroxybutyrate, and acetoacetate.

TABLE 17–20 Summary of some laboratory abnormalities in patients with coma directly attributable to diabetes or its treatment.

	Urine			Plasma		
	Glucose	**Acetone**	**Glucose**	**Bicarbonate**	**Acetone**	**Osmolality**
Diabetic ketoacidosis	++ to ++++	++++	High	Low	++++	+++
Hyperglycemic nonketotic coma	++ to ++++	0 or +[a]	High	Normal or slightly low[b]	0	++++
Hypoglycemia	0[c]	0 or +	Low	Normal	0	Normal
Lactic acidosis	0 to +	0 or +	Normal, low, or high	Low	0 or +	Normal

[a]A small degree of ketonuria may be present if the patient is severely stressed or has not been eating because of illness.

[b]A patient may be acidotic if there is severe volume depletion with cardiovascular collapse or if sepsis is present.

[c]Leftover urine in bladder might still contain sugar from earlier hyperglycemia.

The accumulation of ketones may cause vomiting, which exacerbates the intravascular volume depletion. In addition, prolonged acidosis can compromise cardiac output and reduce vascular tone. The result may be severe cardiovascular collapse with generation of lactic acid, which then adds to the already existent metabolic acidosis.

Clinical Features

A. Symptoms and signs The appearance of diabetic ketoacidosis is usually preceded by a day or more of polyuria and polydipsia associated with marked fatigue, nausea, and vomiting. Eventually, mental stupor ensues and can progress to frank coma. On physical examination, evidence of dehydration in a stuporous patient with rapid and deep respirations and the *fruity* breath odor of acetone strongly suggest the diagnosis. Postural hypotension with tachycardia indicates profound dehydration and salt depletion. Abdominal pain and even tenderness may be present in the absence of abdominal disease, and mild hypothermia is usually present.

B. Laboratory findings Typically, the patient with moderately severe diabetic ketoacidosis has a plasma glucose of 350 to 900 mg/dL (19.4-50 mmol/L), serum ketones are positive at a dilution of 1:8 or greater, hyperkalemia of 5 to 8 mEq/L, slight hyponatremia of approximately 130 mEq/L, hyperphosphatemia of 6 to 7 mg/dL, and an elevated blood urea nitrogen and creatinine. Acidosis may be severe (pH ranging from 6.9-7.2 with a bicarbonate concentration ranging from 5-15 mEq/L); pCO_2 is low (15-20 mm Hg) secondary to hyperventilation.

The fluid depletion is typically about 100 mL/kg. The hyperkalemia occurs despite total body potassium depletion, because of the shift of potassium from the intracellular to extracellular spaces in systemic acidosis. The average total body potassium deficit resulting from osmotic diuresis, acidosis, and gastrointestinal losses is about 3 to 5 mEq/kg body weight. Similarly despite the elevated serum phosphate, total body phosphate is generally depleted. Serum sodium is generally reduced, due to loss of sodium ions by polyuria and vomiting (7-10 mEq/kg), and because severe hyperglycemia shifts intracellular water into the interstitial compartment (for every 100 mg/dL of plasma glucose above normal, serum sodium decreases by 1.6 mEq/L). Serum osmolality can be directly measured by standard tests of freezing point depression or can be estimated by calculating the molarity of sodium, chloride, and glucose in the serum. A convenient formula for estimating *effective* serum osmolality is:

$$\text{mOsm/kg} = 2[\text{measured Na}^+] + \frac{\text{Glucose (mg/dL)}}{18}$$

The effective serum osmolality in humans is generally between 280 and 300 mOsm/kg. These calculated estimates are usually 10 to 20 mOsm/kg lower than values recorded by standard cryoscopic techniques. Central nervous depression or coma occurs when the effective serum osmolality exceeds 320 to 330 mOsm/L.

Blood urea nitrogen and serum creatinine are invariably elevated because of dehydration. Urea exerts an effect on freezing point depression as measured in the laboratory, but it is freely permeable across cell membranes and therefore not included in calculations of effective serum osmolality. Serum creatinine may also be falsely elevated due to interference from acetoacetate with some automated creatinine assays. However, most laboratories can correct for these interfering chromogens by using a more specific method, if asked to do so.

The nitroprusside reagents (Acetest and Ketostix) used for the bedside assessment of ketoacidemia and ketoaciduria measure only acetoacetate and its by-product, acetone. The sensitivity of these reagents for acetone, however, is quite poor, requiring over 10 mmol/L, which is seldom reached in the plasma of ketoacidotic subjects—although this detectable concentration is readily achieved in urine. Thus, in the plasma of ketotic patients, only acetoacetate is measured by these reagents. The more prevalent β-hydroxybutyrate has no ketone group and is therefore not detected by the conventional nitroprusside tests. This takes on special importance in the presence of circulatory collapse during diabetic ketoacidosis, wherein an increase in lactic acid can shift the redox state to increase β-hydroxybutyrate at the expense of the readily detectable acetoacetate. Bedside diagnostic reagents would then be unreliable, suggesting no ketonemia in cases where β-hydroxybutyrate is a major factor in producing the acidosis. Under these circumstances, β-hydroxybutyrate can be directly measured at the bedside using the Precision Xtra meter (Abbott Diagnostics). Many clinical laboratories now offer β-hydroxybutyrate measurement.

In about 90% of cases, serum amylase is elevated. However, this often represents salivary as well as pancreatic amylase and correlates poorly with symptoms of pancreatitis, such as pain and vomiting. Therefore, in patients with diabetic ketoacidosis, an elevated serum amylase does not justify a diagnosis of acute pancreatitis; serum lipase may be useful if the diagnosis of pancreatitis is being seriously considered.

Treatment

Patients with mild DKA are alert and have pH between 7.25 and 7.30; those with moderate DKA have pH between 7.0 and 7.24 and are alert or slightly drowsy; and those with severe DKA are stuporous and have pH <7.0. Those with mild DKA can be treated in the emergency room, but those with moderate or severe DKA require admission to the intensive care unit or step-down unit.

The therapeutic goals are to restore plasma volume and tissue perfusion; reduce blood glucose and osmolality toward normal; correct acidosis; replenish electrolyte losses; and identify and treat precipitating factors. Gastric intubation is recommended in the comatose patient to prevent vomiting and aspiration that may occur as a result of gastric atony, a common complication of diabetic ketoacidosis. In patients with preexisting cardiac or renal failure or those in severe cardiovascular collapse, a central venous pressure catheter or a Swan-Ganz catheter should be inserted to evaluate the degree of hypovolemia and to monitor subsequent fluid administration.

Plasma glucose should be recorded hourly and electrolytes and pH at least every 2 to 3 hours during the initial treatment period. A bedside glucose meter should be used to titrate the insulin therapy.

1. **Fluid replacement.** In most adult patients, the fluid deficit is 4 to 5 L. Once the diagnosis of diabetic ketoacidosis is established in the emergency department, administration of at least 2 L of isotonic saline (0.9% saline solution) in an adult patient in the first 2 to 3 hours is necessary to help restore plasma volume and stabilize blood pressure while acutely reducing the hyperosmolar state. In addition, by improving renal plasma flow, fluid replacement also restores the renal capacity to excrete hydrogen ions, thereby ameliorating the acidosis as well. After the first 2 L of fluid have been given, the fluid should be changed to 0.45% saline solution given at a rate of 300 to 400 mL/h, because water loss exceeds sodium loss in uncontrolled diabetes with osmotic diuresis. Failure to give sufficient volume replacement (at least 3-4 L in 8 hours) to restore normal perfusion is one of the most serious therapeutic shortcomings affecting satisfactory recovery. In the same way, excessive fluid replacement (>5 L in 8 hours) may contribute to acute respiratory distress syndrome or cerebral edema. When blood glucose falls to approximately 250 mg/dL, the fluids should be changed to a 5% glucose solution to maintain plasma glucose in the range of 250 to 300 mg/dL. This prevents the development of hypoglycemia and also reduces the likelihood of cerebral edema, which may result from a too rapid decline of blood glucose.

2. **Insulin.** Immediately after the initiation of fluid replacement, a rapid bolus of 0.15 U of regular insulin per kilogram of body weight should be given intravenously to prime the tissue insulin receptors. This inhibits both gluconeogenesis and ketogenesis while promoting utilization of glucose and keto acids. Following the initial bolus, an insulin infusion is initiated at a rate of 0.1 U/kg/h. When a continuous infusion of insulin is used, 25 U of regular human insulin should be placed in 250 mL of isotonic saline and the first 50 mL of solution flushed through to saturate the tubing before connecting it to the intravenous line. The insulin infusion should be piggybacked into the fluid line so that the rate of fluid replacement can be changed without altering the insulin delivery rate. If the plasma glucose level fails to fall at least 10% in the first hour, a repeat loading dose is recommended. Rarely, a patient with insulin resistance is encountered; this requires doubling the insulin dose every 2 to 4 hours if severe hyperglycemia does not improve after the first two doses of insulin and fluid replacement. The insulin dose should be adjusted with the goal of lowering the glucose concentration by about 50 to 70 mg/dL/h. If clinical circumstances prevent use of insulin infusion, then the insulin can be given intramuscularly. An initial 0.15 U/kg of regular insulin is given intravenously, and at the same time, the same size dose is given intramuscularly. Subsequently, regular insulin is given intramuscularly hourly at a dose of 0.1 U/kg until the blood glucose falls to around 250 mg/dL, when the insulin can be given subcutaneously. Insulin therapy, either as a continuous infusion or as injections given every 1 to 2 hours, should be continued until arterial pH has normalized.

3. **Potassium.** Total body potassium loss from polyuria and vomiting may be as high as 200 mEq. However, because of shifts of potassium from cells into the extracellular space as a consequence of acidosis, serum potassium is usually normal to slightly elevated prior to institution of treatment. As the

acidosis is corrected, potassium flows back into the cells, and hypokalemia can develop if potassium replacement is not instituted. If the patient is not uremic and has an adequate urine output, potassium chloride in doses of 10 to 30 mEq/h should be infused during the second and third hours after beginning therapy. Replacement should be started sooner, if the initial serum potassium is inappropriately normal or low, and should be delayed, if serum potassium fails to respond to initial therapy and remains above 5 mEq/L, as in cases of renal insufficiency. Cooperative patients with only mild ketoacidosis may receive part or all of their potassium replacement orally.

An electrocardiogram can be of help in monitoring the patient's potassium status: high peaked T waves are a sign of hyperkalemia, and flattened T waves with U waves are a sign of hypokalemia.

Foods high in potassium content should be prescribed when the patient has recovered sufficiently to take food orally. Tomato juice has 14 mEq of potassium per 240 mL, and a medium-sized banana has about 10 mEq.

4. **Sodium bicarbonate.** The use of sodium bicarbonate in management of diabetic ketoacidosis has been questioned because clinical benefit was not demonstrated in one prospective randomized trial and because of the following potentially harmful consequences: (1) development of hypokalemia from rapid shift of potassium into cells if the acidosis is overcorrected, (2) tissue anoxia from reduced dissociation of oxygen from hemoglobin when acidosis is rapidly reversed (leftward shift of the oxygen dissociation curve), and (3) cerebral acidosis resulting from lowering of cerebrospinal fluid pH. It must be emphasized, however, that these considerations are less important when severe acidosis exists. It is therefore recommended that bicarbonate be administered to diabetic patients in ketoacidosis if the arterial blood pH is 7.0 or less with careful monitoring to prevent overcorrection.

One to two ampules of sodium bicarbonate (one ampule contains 44 mEq/50 mL) should be added to 1 L of 0.45% saline. (**Note:** Addition of sodium bicarbonate to 0.9% saline would produce a markedly hypertonic solution that could aggravate the hyperosmolar state already present.) This should be administered rapidly (over the first hour). It can be repeated until the arterial pH reaches 7.1, but *it should not be given if the pH is 7.1 or greater*, because additional bicarbonate increases the risk of rebound metabolic alkalosis as ketones are metabolized. Alkalosis shifts potassium from serum into cells, which can precipitate a fatal cardiac arrhythmia. As noted earlier, serious consideration should be given to placement of a central venous catheter when administering fluids to severely ill patients with cardiovascular compromise.

5. **Phosphate.** Phosphate replacement is seldom required in treating diabetic ketoacidosis. However, if severe hypophosphatemia of less than 1 mg/dL (<0.35 mmol/L) develops during insulin therapy, a small amount of phosphate can be replaced per hour as the potassium salt. Correction of hypophosphatemia helps restore the buffering capacity of the plasma, thereby facilitating renal excretion of hydrogen. It also corrects the impaired oxygen dissociation from hemoglobin by regenerating 2,3-diphosphoglycerate. However, three randomized studies in which phosphate was replaced in only half of a group of patients with diabetic ketoacidosis did not show any apparent clinical benefit from phosphate administration. Moreover, attempts to use potassium phosphate as the sole means of replacing potassium have led to a number of reported cases of severe hypocalcemia with tetany. To minimize the risk

of inducing tetany from too rapid replacement of phosphate, the average deficit of 40 to 50 mmol of phosphate should be replaced intravenously at a rate *no greater than 3 to 4 mmol/h* in a 60- to 70-kg person. A stock solution (Abbott) provides a mixture of 1.12 g KH_2PO_4 and 1.18 g K_2HPO_4 in a 5-mL single-dose vial (this equals 22 mmol of potassium and 15 mmol of phosphate). One-half of this vial (2.5 mL) should be added to 1 L of either 0.45% saline or 5% dextrose in water. Two liters of this solution, infused at a rate of 400 mL/h, corrects the phosphate deficit at the optimal rate of 3 mmol/h and provides 4.4 mEq of potassium per hour. Additional potassium should be administered as potassium chloride to provide a total of 10 to 30 mEq of potassium per hour, as noted earlier. If the serum phosphate remains below 2.5 mg/dL after this infusion, a repeat 5-hour infusion can be given.

6. **Hyperchloremic acidosis during therapy.** Because of the considerable loss of keto acids in the urine during the initial phase of therapy, substrate for subsequent regeneration of bicarbonate is lost, and correction of the total bicarbonate deficit is hampered. A portion of the bicarbonate deficit is replaced with chloride ions infused in large amounts as saline to correct the dehydration. In most patients, as the ketoacidosis clears during insulin replacement, a hyperchloremic, low-bicarbonate pattern emerges with a normal anion gap. This is a relatively benign condition that reverses itself over the subsequent 12 to 24 hours once intravenous saline is no longer being administered.

TRANSITION TO SUBCUTANEOUS INSULIN REGIMEN

Once the diabetic ketoacidosis is controlled and the patient is awake and able to eat, subcutaneous insulin therapy can be initiated. Initially, the patient may still have significant tissue insulin resistance and may require a total daily insulin dose of ~0.6 U/kg. Half of the total daily dose can be given as a long-acting basal insulin and the other half as short-acting insulin premeals. The patient should get injection of the basal insulin and a dose of the rapid-acting insulin analog with the first meal and the insulin infusion discontinued an hour later. The overlap of the subcutaneous insulin action and insulin infusion is necessary to prevent relapse of diabetic ketoacidiosis. The increased tissue insulin resistance is only present for a few days at most and as the patient improves the doses of both basal and bolus insulins should be reduced to avoid hypoglycemia. In fact, a patient with new diagnosis of type 1 diabetes who still has significant β cell function may not require any basal insulin and only very low doses of rapid-acting insulin analogs before meals.

Complications and Prognosis

Low-dose insulin infusion and fluid and electrolyte replacement combined with careful monitoring of patients' clinical and laboratory responses to therapy have dramatically reduced the mortality rates of diabetic ketoacidosis to less than 5%. However, this complication remains a significant risk in the aged who have mortality rates over 20% and in patients in profound coma in whom treatment has been delayed. Acute myocardial infarction and infarction of the bowel following prolonged hypotension worsen the

outlook. Prior kidney dysfunction worsens prognosis because the kidney plays a key role in compensating for pH and electrolyte abnormalities. Symptomatic cerebral edema occurs primarily in the pediatric population. Risk factors for development include severe baseline acidosis, rapid correction of hyperglycemia, and excess volume administration in the first 4 hours. Onset of headache or deterioration in mental status during treatment should lead to consideration of this complication. Intravenous mannitol at a dosage of 1 to 2 g/kg given over 15 minutes is the mainstay of therapy. Excess crystalloid infusion can precipitate pulmonary edema. Acute respiratory distress syndrome is a rare complication of treatment for DKA.

Disposition

After recovery and stabilization, patients should receive intensive detailed instructions about how to avoid this potentially disastrous complication of diabetes mellitus. They should be taught to recognize the early symptoms and signs of ketoacidosis.

Urine ketones or capillary blood β-hydroxybutyrate should be measured in patients with signs of infection or in those using an insulin pump when capillary blood glucose is unexpectedly and persistently high. When heavy ketonuria and glycosuria persist on several successive examinations, supplemental regular insulin should be administered, and liquid foods such as lightly salted tomato juice and broth should be ingested to replenish fluids and electrolytes. Patients should be instructed to contact the physician if ketonuria persists and, especially, if vomiting develops, or if appropriate adjustment of the infusion rate on an insulin pump does not correct the hyperglycemia and ketonuria. Table 17–21 summarizes the guidelines for patients regarding ketone testing and what to do with the results. In adolescents, recurrent episodes of severe diabetic ketoacidosis often indicate poor compliance with the insulin regimen, and these patients should receive intensive family counseling.

2. HYPERGLYCEMIC, HYPEROSMOLAR STATE

This form of hyperglycemic coma is characterized by severe hyperglycemia, hyperosmolality, and dehydration in the absence

TABLE 17–21 Guidelines for treatment of ketones in patients with type 1 diabetes.

Check ketones if blood glucose persistently over 250 mg/dL or if nauseated or vomiting	
Blood ketones <1.5 mmol/L or urine ketones absent or small	Blood ketones >1.5 or urine ketones moderate or large
Drink plenty of fluids	Call medical team for advise or go to urgent care or emergency room
Give fast-acting insulin by syringe	Drink plenty of fluids
Monitor glucose levels	Give fast-acting insulin by syringe
	Monitor ketone levels

Note: Blood ketones <0.6 mmol/L are normal.

of significant ketosis. It occurs in patients with mild or occult diabetes and patients are typically middle-aged or elderly. Lethargy and confusion develop as serum osmolality exceeds 300 mOsm/kg, and coma can occur if osmolality exceeds 330 mOsm/kg. Underlying renal insufficiency or congestive heart failure is common, and the presence of either worsens the prognosis. A precipitating event such as pneumonia, cerebrovascular accident, myocardial infarction, burns, or recent operation can often be identified. Certain drugs, such as phenytoin, diazoxide, glucocorticoids, and thiazide diuretics, have been implicated in its development, as have procedures associated with glucose loading such as peritoneal dialysis.

Pathogenesis

A partial or relative insulin deficiency may initiate the syndrome by reducing glucose utilization by muscle, fat, and liver, while promoting hyperglucagonemia and increasing hepatic glucose output. The result is hyperglycemia that leads to glycosuria and osmotic diuresis with obligatory water loss. The presence of even small amounts of insulin is believed to prevent the development of ketosis by inhibiting lipolysis in the adipose stores. Therefore, even though a low insulin-glucagon ratio promotes ketogenesis in the liver, the limited availability of precursor free fatty acids from the periphery restricts the rate at which ketones are formed. If a patient is unable to maintain adequate fluid intake because of an associated acute or chronic illness or has suffered excessive fluid loss (eg, from burns or therapy with diuretics), marked dehydration results. As plasma volume contracts, renal insufficiency develops; this, then, limits renal glucose excretion and contributes markedly to the rise in serum glucose and osmolality. As serum osmolality exceeds 320 to 330 mOsm/kg, water is drawn out of cerebral neurons, resulting in mental obtundation and coma.

Clinical Features

A. Symptoms and signs   The onset of the hyperglycemic, hyperosmolar, nonketotic state may be insidious, preceded for days or weeks by symptoms of weakness, polyuria, and polydipsia. A history of reduced fluid intake is common, whether due to inappropriate absence of thirst, gastrointestinal upset, or, in the case of elderly or bedridden patients, lack of access to water. A history of ingestion of large quantities of glucose-containing fluids, such as soft drinks or orange juice, can occasionally be obtained; these patients are usually less hyperosmolar than those in whom fluid intake was restricted. The absence of toxic features of ketoacidosis may retard recognition of the syndrome and thus delay institution of therapy until dehydration is profound. Because of this delay in diagnosis, the hyperglycemia, hyperosmolality, and dehydration in hyperglycemic, hyperosmolar, nonketotic coma is often more severe than in diabetic ketoacidosis.

Physical examination reveals the presence of profound dehydration (orthostatic fall in blood pressure and rise in pulse, supine tachycardia, or even frank shock, dry mucous membranes, decreased skin turgor). The patient may be lethargic, confused, or comatose. Kussmaul respirations are absent unless the precipitating event for

the hyperosmolar state has also led to the development of metabolic acidosis (eg, sepsis or myocardial infarction with shock).

B. Laboratory findings   Severe hyperglycemia is present, with blood glucose values ranging from 800 to as high as 2400 mg/dL (44.4-133.2 mmol/L). In mild cases, where dehydration is less severe, dilutional hyponatremia as well as urinary sodium losses may reduce serum sodium to about 120 to 125 mEq/L—this protects, to some extent, against extreme hyperosmolality. Once dehydration progresses further, however, serum sodium can exceed 140 mEq/L, producing serum osmolalities of 330 to 440 mOsm/kg (normal, 280 to 295 mOsm/kg; see the section Diabetic Ketoacidosis for a convenient method for estimating serum osmolality). Ketosis is usually absent or mild; however, a small degree of ketonuria may be present if the patient has not been eating because of illness. Acidosis is not a part of the hyperglycemic, hyperosmolar state, but it may be present (often lactic acidosis) because of other acute underlying conditions (eg, sepsis, acute renal failure, myocardial infarction). Prerenal azotemia is the rule with blood urea nitrogen frequently over 100 mg/dL.

The physician must initiate a careful search for the event that precipitated the episode of hyperglycemic, hyperosmolar state if it is not obvious after the initial history and physical examination. Chest x-rays and cultures of blood, urine, and other body fluids should be obtained to look for occult sources of sepsis. Cardiac enzymes and serial electrocardiograms can be ordered to look for evidence of silent myocardial infarction.

Treatment

There are some differences in fluid, insulin, and electrolyte replacement in this disorder, as compared with diabetic ketoacidosis. However, in common with the treatment of ketoacidotic patients, careful monitoring of the patient's clinical and laboratory response to therapy is essential.

1. Fluid replacement. The fluid deficit may be as much as 100 to 200 mL/kg or about 9 L. If circulatory collapse is present, fluid therapy should be initiated with isotonic saline. In all other cases, initial replacement with hypotonic (usually 0.45%) saline is preferable, because these patients are hyperosmolar with considerable loss of body water and excess solute in the vascular compartment. As much as 4 to 6 L of fluid may be required in the first 8 to 10 hours. Careful monitoring of fluid quantity and type, urine output, blood pressure, and pulse is essential. Placement of a central venous pressure catheter should be strongly considered to guide replacement of fluid, especially if the patient is elderly or has underlying renal or cardiac disease. Because insulin therapy decreases plasma glucose and therefore serum osmolality, a change to isotonic saline may be necessary at some time during treatment. Once blood glucose reaches 250 mg/dL, 5% dextrose in 0.45% or 0.9% saline solution should be substituted for the sugar-free fluids. When consciousness returns, oral fluids should be encouraged.

2. Electrolyte replacement. Hyperkalemia is less marked, and much less potassium is lost in the urine during the osmotic diuresis of hyperglycemic, hyperosmolar, nonketotic coma than in diabetic ketoacidosis. There is, therefore, less severe total potassium depletion, and less potassium replacement is needed to restore potassium stores to normal. However, because the initial serum potassium usually is not elevated and because it declines rapidly as insulin therapy allows glucose and potassium to enter cells, it is recommended that potassium replacement be initiated earlier than in ketotic patients: 10 mEq of potassium chloride can be added to the *initial* liter of fluid administered if the initial serum potassium is not elevated and if the patient is making urine. When serum phosphate falls below 1 mg/dL during insulin therapy, phosphate replacement can be given intravenously with the same precautions as those outlined for ketoacidotic patients (see earlier). If the patient is awake and cooperative, part or all of the potassium and phosphate replacement can be given orally.

3. Insulin therapy. In general, less insulin is required to reduce the hyperglycemia of nonketotic patients than is the case for patients in diabetic ketoacidosis. In fact, fluid replacement alone can decrease glucose levels considerably. An initial insulin bolus of 0.15 U/kg is followed by an insulin infusion rate of 0.1 U/kg/h titrated to lower blood glucose by 50 to 70 mg/dL/h. Once the patient has stabilized and the blood glucose falls to around 250 mg/dL, insulin can be given subcutaneously.

Complications and Prognosis

The severe dehydration and low output state may predispose the patient to complications such as myocardial infarction, stroke, pulmonary embolism, mesenteric vein thrombosis, and disseminated intravascular coagulation. Fluid resuscitation remains the primary approach to the prevention of these complications. Low-dose heparin prophylaxis is reasonable but benefits of routine anticoagulation remain doubtful. Rhabdomyolysis is a recognized complication of the hyperosmolar state, and it should be looked for and treated.

The overall mortality rate of hyperglycemic, hyperosmolar, nonketotic coma is over 10 times that of diabetic ketoacidosis, chiefly because of its higher incidence in older patients, who may have compromised cardiovascular systems or associated major illnesses. When patients are matched for age, the prognoses of these two forms of hyperosmolar coma are reasonably comparable.

Disposition

After the patient is stabilized, the appropriate form of long-term management of the diabetes must be determined. Insulin treatment should be continued for a few weeks, but the patients usually recover sufficient endogenous insulin secretion to make a trial of diet or diet plus oral agents worthwhile. When the episode occurs in a patient who has known diabetes, then education of the patient and caregivers should be instituted. They should be taught how to recognize situations (gastrointestinal upset, infection) that predispose to recurrence of hyperglycemic, hyperosmolar state as well as detailed information on how to prevent the escalating dehydration (small sips of sugar-free liquids, increase in usual hypoglycemic therapy, or early contact with the physician) that culminates in hyperosmolar coma.

3. LACTIC ACIDOSIS

When severely ill diabetic patients present with profound acidosis and an anion gap over 15 mEq/L but relatively low or undetectable levels of keto acids in plasma, the presence of excessive plasma lactate (>5 mmol/L) should be considered, especially if other causes of acidosis such as uremia are not present.

Pathogenesis

Lactic acid is the end product of the anaerobic metabolism of glucose. Normally, the principal sources of this acid are the erythrocytes (which lack the enzymes for aerobic oxidation), skeletal muscle, skin, and brain. The chief pathway for removal of lactic acid is by hepatic (and to some degree renal) uptake for conversion first to pyruvate and eventually back to glucose, a process that requires oxygen. Lactic acidosis occurs when excess lactic acid accumulates in the blood. This can be the result of overproduction (tissue hypoxia), deficient removal (hepatic failure), or both (circulatory collapse). Lactic acidosis is not uncommon in any severely ill patient suffering from cardiac decompensation, respiratory or hepatic failure, septicemia, or infarction of the bowel or extremities. Type A lactic acidosis is associated with tissue hypoxia from hypovolemia or endotoxic shock and need not be associated with hyperglycemia. Type B lactic acidosis is defined as that which occurs in the absence of clinical evidence for tissue hypoxia and is associated with diabetes per se or with biguanide therapy.

With the discontinuance of phenformin therapy in the United States, lactic acidosis in patients with diabetes mellitus has become uncommon, but it still must be considered in the acidotic diabetic patient if the patient is seriously ill, and especially if the patient is receiving metformin therapy as well. Most cases of metformin-associated lactic acidosis occur in patients in whom there were contraindications to the use of metformin, in particular renal failure.

Clinical Features

A. Symptoms and signs   The main clinical features of lactic acidosis are marked hyperventilation and mental confusion, which may progress to stupor or coma. When lactic acidosis is secondary to tissue hypoxia or vascular collapse, the clinical presentation is variable, reflecting that of the prevailing catastrophic illness. In the rare instance of idiopathic or spontaneous lactic acidosis, the onset is rapid (usually over a few hours), the cardiopulmonary status is stable, and mentation may be relatively normal.

B. Laboratory findings   Plasma glucose can be low, normal, or high in diabetic patients with lactic acidosis, but usually it is moderately elevated. Plasma bicarbonate and arterial pH are quite low. An anion gap is present (calculated by subtracting the sum of the plasma bicarbonate and chloride from the plasma sodium; normal is 12-15 mEq/L). Ketones are usually absent from plasma, but small amounts may be present in urine if the patient has not been eating recently. Other causes of anion gap metabolic acidosis should be excluded—for example, uremia, diabetic or alcoholic ketoacidosis, and salicylate, methanol, ethylene glycol, or paraldehyde intoxication. In the absence of azotemia, hyperphosphatemia may be a clue to the presence of lactic acidosis.

The diagnosis is confirmed by demonstrating, in a sample of blood that is promptly chilled and separated, a plasma lactate concentration of 6 mmol/L or higher (normal is ~1 mmol/L). Failure to rapidly chill the sample and separate the plasma can lead to falsely high plasma lactate values as a result of continued glycolysis by the red blood cells. Frozen plasma remains stable for subsequent assay.

Treatment

The cornerstone of therapy is aggressive treatment of the precipitating cause. An adequate airway and good oxygenation should be ensured. If hypotension is present, fluids and, if appropriate, pressor agents must be given to restore tissue perfusion. Appropriate cultures and empiric antibiotic coverage should be instituted in any seriously ill patient with lactic acidosis in whom the cause is not immediately apparent. Alkalinization with intravenous sodium bicarbonate to keep the pH above 7.2 has been recommended in the emergency treatment of severe lactic acidosis. However, there is no evidence that the mortality rate is favorably affected by administering bicarbonate, and the matter is at present controversial, particularly because of the hazards associated with bicarbonate therapy. Hemodialysis may be useful in those cases associated with metformin toxicity. Dichloroacetate, an anion that facilitates pyruvate removal by activating pyruvate dehydrogenase, reverses certain types of lactic acidosis in animals, but in a prospective controlled clinical trial involving 252 patients with lactic acidosis, dichloroacetate failed to alter either hemodynamics or survival.

CHRONIC COMPLICATIONS OF DIABETES MELLITUS (TABLE 17-22)

In most patients with diabetes, a number of pathologic changes occur at variable intervals during the course of the disease. These changes involve the vascular system for the most part; however, they also occur in the nerves, the skin, and the lens. In addition to these complications, patients with diabetes have an increased incidence of certain types of infections and may handle their infections less well than the general population.

Classifications of Diabetic Vascular Disease

Diabetic vascular disease is conveniently divided into two main categories: microvascular disease and macrovascular disease.

A. Microvascular disease   Disease of the smallest blood vessels, the capillary and the precapillary arterioles, is manifested mainly by thickening of the capillary basement membrane. Microvascular disease involving the retina leads to diabetic retinopathy, and disease involving the kidney causes diabetic nephropathy. Small vessel disease may also involve the heart, and cardiomegaly with heart failure has been described in diabetic patients with patent coronary arteries.

TABLE 17-22   Chronic complications of diabetes mellitus.

Eyes
　Diabetic retinopathy
　　Nonproliferative (background)
　　Proliferative
　Cataracts
　　Subcapsular (snowflake)
　　Nuclear (senile)
Kidneys
　Intercapillary glomerulosclerosis
　　Diffuse
　　Nodular
　Infection
　　Pyelonephritis
　　Perinephric abscess
　　Renal papillary necrosis
　Renal tubular necrosis
　　Following dye studies (urograms, arteriograms)
Nervous System
　Peripheral neuropathy
　　Distal, symmetric sensory loss
　Motor neuropathy
　　Foot drop, wrist drop
　　Cranial nerves III, IV, VI, VII
　　Diabetic amyotrophy
　Autonomic neuropathy
　　Postural hypotension
　　Resting tachycardia
　　Loss of sweating
　　Gastroparesis
　　Diabetic diarrhea
　　Urinary bladder atony
　　Impotence (may also be secondary to pelvic vascular disease)
Skin
　Diabetic dermopathy (shin spots)
　Necrobiosis lipoidica diabeticorum
　Candidiasis
　Foot and leg ulcers
　　Neurotropic
　　Ischemic
Cardiovascular System
　Heart disease
　　Myocardial infarction
　　Cardiomyopathy
　Peripheral vascular disease
　　Ischemic ulcers: gangrene
　Cerebrovascular disease
Bones and Joints
　Diabetic cheiroarthropathy
　Dupuytren contracture
　Charcot joint
　Osteomyelitis
Unusual Infections
　Necrotizing fasciitis
　Necrotizing myositis
　Mucor meningitis
　Emphysematous cholecystitis
　Malignant otitis externa

B. Macrovascular disease Large vessel disease in diabetes is essentially an accelerated form of atherosclerosis. It accounts for the increased incidence of myocardial infarction, stroke, and peripheral gangrene in diabetic patients. Just as in the case of atherosclerosis in the general population, the exact cause of accelerated atherosclerosis in the diabetic population remains unclear. Abnormalities in vessel walls, platelets and other components of the clotting system, red blood cells, and lipid metabolism have all been postulated to play a role. In addition, there is evidence that coexistent risk factors such as cigarette smoking and hypertension may be important in determining the course of the disease.

Prevalence of Chronic Complications by Type of Diabetes

Although all of the known complications of diabetes can be found in both types of the disease, some are more common in one type than in the other. In type 1 diabetes, end-stage renal disease develops in up to 40% of patients, compared with less than 20% of patients with type 2 diabetes. Although blindness occurs in both types, it occurs more commonly as a result of severe proliferative retinopathy, vitreous hemorrhages, and retinal detachment in type 1 disease, whereas macular edema and ischemia are the usual cause in type 2. Similarly, although diabetic neuropathy is common in both type 1 and type 2 diabetes, severe autonomic neuropathy with gastroparesis, diabetic diarrhea, resting tachycardia, and postural hypotension is much more common in type 1.

In patients with type 1 diabetes, complications from end-stage renal disease are a major cause of death, whereas patients with type 2 diabetes are more likely to have macrovascular diseases leading to myocardial infarction and stroke as the main causes of death. Cigarette use adds significantly to the risk of both microvascular and macrovascular complications in diabetic patients.

Molecular Mechanisms by Which Hyperglycemia Causes Microvascular and Macrovascular Damage

Epidemiological data and prospective intervention studies such as the DCCT have confirmed the central role of glucose in the development of chronic diabetic complications.

Four molecular mechanisms of glucose-induced damage have been proposed: (1) increased polyol pathway flux; (2) increased intracellular advanced glycation end product (AGE) formation; (3) activation of protein kinase C; and (4) increased hexosamine pathway flux.

Increase flux through the polyol pathway consumes NADPH. Because this cofactor is needed to regenerate reduced glutathione, NADPH depletion is predicted to exacerbate intracellular oxidative stress and cause cellular injury. Inhibitors of aldose reductase, the first enzyme in the polyol pathway have been shown to improve diabetic neuropathy.

Intracellular autoxidation of glucose results in production of intracellular dicarbonyls (glyoxal, 3-deoxyglucosone, methylglyoxal), also referred to as AGE precursors. These precursors damage

target tissues by modifying intracellular and extracellular proteins and matrix components. Intracellular protein modifications may alter cellular functions. Modifications of extracellular matrix proteins result in abnormal interactions with other matrix proteins and integrins. The modified plasma proteins bind to receptors on endothelial cells, mesangial cells, and macrophages causing expression of cytokines and growth factors including interleukin 1, IGF-1, TNF-α, transforming growth factor-β (TGF-β), macrophage colony stimulating factor, granulocyte-macrophage stimulating factor, platelet-derived growth factor, thrombomodulin, tissue factor, vascular cell adhesion molecule 1 (VCAM 1), and vascular endothelial growth factor (VEGF). Induction of VEGF has been implicated in the vascular hyperpermeability associated with diabetes.

Protein kinase C isoforms β and δ are activated by diacylglycerol whose levels are increased by elevated intracellular glucose. Activation of these isoforms leads to alterations in expression of endothelial nitric oxide synthase, endothelin 1, VEGF, TGF-β, PAI-1, and activation of nuclear factor κB and NADPH oxidases. Inhibitors of the protein kinase β isoform improve retinopathy and nephropathy in experimental models.

Hyperglycemia increases hexosamine pathway flux by providing more fructose-6-phosphate for the rate-limiting enzyme of the pathway glutamine: fructose-6-phosphate amidotransferase. Activity of this pathway leads to increased donation of N-acetylglucosamine moieties to serine and threonine moieties of complication-promoting factors such as PAI-1 or TGF-β.

It has been proposed that all four of these pathways are associated with overproduction of superoxide by mitochondria. High ambient glucose leads to increased substrate flux through glycolysis and the tricarboxylic acid cycle. This leads to increased potential difference across the inner mitochondrial membrane and generation of superoxide by the electron transport chain. The increased production of superoxide reduces glyceraldehyde-3-phosphate dehydrogenase (GAPDH) activity, which in turn leads to upstream increase in intracellular glucose and accumulation of glycolytic intermediates such as glyceraldehyde 3-phosphate and fructose 6-phosphate. The increased intracellular glucose leads to increased flux through the polyol pathway and also is the primary initiating event in the formation of both intracellular and extracellular AGEs. The glycolytic intermediates are important initiators of the hexosamine pathway (fructose 6-phosphate) or the protein kinase C pathway (glyceraldehyde-3-phosphate).

Genetic Factors in Susceptibility to Development of Chronic Complications of Diabetes

Although no genetic susceptibility genes have been identified as yet, two unrelated observations indicate that approximately 40% of people with diabetes may be unusually susceptible to the ravages of hyperglycemia or other metabolic sequelae of an inadequate insulin effect.

(1) In one retrospective study of 164 juvenile-onset diabetic patients with a median age at onset of 9 years, 40% were incapacitated or dead from end-stage renal disease with

proliferative retinopathy after a 25-year follow-up, whereas the remaining subjects were either mildly affected (40%) or had no clinically detected microvascular disease (20%). This study was completed long before the availability of glycemic self-monitoring methodology, so it is unlikely that any of these patients were near optimal glycemic control.

(2) Data from renal transplantation indicate that only about 40% of normal kidneys developed evidence of moderate to severe diabetic nephropathy within 6 to 14 years of being transplanted into diabetic subjects with end-stage renal failure, whereas as many as 60% were only minimally affected. These observations support the hypothesis that although approximately 60% of people suffer only minimal consequences from hyperglycemia and other metabolic hazards of insulin insufficiency, 40% or so suffer severe, potentially catastrophic microvascular complications if the disease is poorly controlled. The genetic mechanisms for this increased susceptibility are as yet unknown but could be related to one or more of the molecular mechanisms outlined above. Identification of the genetic mechanism(s) would be very helpful in justifying more intensive insulin therapy in the group susceptible to complications in an effort to achieve near-normalization of blood glucose. The remaining 60% of less susceptible individuals might then be spared the inconveniences of strict glycemic control as well as the risks of hypoglycemia inherent in present methods of intensive insulin therapy.

SPECIFIC CHRONIC COMPLICATIONS OF DIABETES MELLITUS (TABLE 17–22)

1. OPHTHALMOLOGIC COMPLICATIONS

Diabetic Retinopathy

For early detection of diabetic retinopathy, adolescent or adult patients who have had type 1 diabetes for more than 5 years and *all* patients with type 2 diabetes should be referred to an ophthalmologist for examination and follow-up. In patients with type 1 diabetes, after 10 to 15 years, 25% to 50% of patients show some signs of retinopathy. This prevalence increases to 75% to 95% after 15 years and approaches 100% after 30 years of diabetes. In patients with type 2 diabetes, 60% have nonproliferative retinopathy after 16 years. When hypertension is present in a patient with diabetes, it should be treated vigorously because hypertension is associated with an increased incidence and accelerated progression of diabetic retinopathy.

A. Pathogenesis and clinical features   Two main categories of diabetic retinopathy exist: nonproliferative and proliferative. Diabetic macular edema can occur at any stage.

Nonproliferative (background) retinopathy represents the earliest stage of retinal involvement by diabetes and is characterized by such changes as microaneurysms, dot hemorrhages, exudates, and retinal edema. During this stage, the retinal capillaries leak proteins, lipids, or red cells into the retina. When this process occurs in the macula (clinically significant macular edema), the area of greatest concentration of visual cells, there is interference with visual acuity; this is the most common cause of visual impairment in type 2 diabetes.

Proliferative retinopathy involves the growth of new capillaries and fibrous tissue within the retina and into the vitreous chamber. It is a consequence of small vessel occlusion, which causes retinal hypoxia; this in turn stimulates new vessel growth. New vessel formation may occur at the optic disc or elsewhere on the retina. Proliferative retinopathy can occur in both types of diabetes but is more common in type 1, developing about 7 to 10 years after onset of symptoms, with a prevalence of 25% after 15 years' duration. Prior to proliferation of new capillaries, a preproliferative phase often occurs in which arteriolar ischemia is manifested as cotton-wool spots (small infarcted areas of retina). Vision is usually normal until vitreous hemorrhage or retinal detachment occurs. Proliferative retinopathy is a leading cause of blindness in the United States, particularly because it increases the risk of retinal detachment.

B. Treatment   Extensive scatter xenon or argon photocoagulation and focal treatment of new vessels reduce severe visual loss in those cases in which proliferative retinopathy is associated with recent vitreous hemorrhages or in which extensive new vessels are located on or near the optic disk. Macular edema, which is more common than proliferative retinopathy in patients with type 2 diabetes (up to 20% prevalence), has a guarded prognosis, but it has also responded to scatter therapy with improvement in visual acuity if detected early. Injection of bevacizumab (Avastin), an antivascular endothelial growth factor (anti-VEGF), into the eye has been shown to stop the growth of the new blood vessels in diabetic eye disease. Avoiding tobacco use and correction of associated hypertension are important therapeutic measures in the management of diabetic retinopathy. There is no contraindication to using aspirin in patients with proliferative retinopathy.

Cataracts

Two types of cataracts occur in diabetic patients: subcapsular and senile. **Subcapsular cataract** occurs predominantly in patients with type 1 diabetes, may come on fairly rapidly, and has a significant correlation with the hyperglycemia of uncontrolled diabetes. This type of cataract has a flocculent or *snowflake* appearance and develops just below the lens capsule.

Senile cataract represents a sclerotic change of the lens nucleus. It is by far the most common type of cataract found in either diabetic or nondiabetic adults and tends to occur at a younger age in diabetic patients, particularly when glycemic control is poor.

Two separate abnormalities found in diabetic patients, both of which are related to elevated blood glucose levels, may contribute to the formation of cataracts: (1) glycosylation of the lens protein, and (2) an excess of sorbitol, which is formed from the increased quantities of glucose found in the insulin-independent lens. Accumulation of sorbitol leads to osmotic changes in the lens that ultimately result in fibrosis and cataract formation.

Glaucoma

Glaucoma occurs in approximately 6% of persons with diabetes. It is generally responsive to the usual therapy for open-angle disease.

Closed-angle glaucoma can result from neovascularization of the iris in diabetic persons, but this is relatively uncommon except after cataract extraction when accelerated new vessel growth involving the angle of the iris obstructs outflow.

2. RENAL COMPLICATIONS

Diabetic Nephropathy

A. Pathogenesis and clinical findings About 4000 cases of end-stage renal disease due to diabetic nephropathy occur annually among diabetic patients in the United States. This represents about one-third of all patients being treated for renal failure. The cumulative incidence of nephropathy differs between the two major types of diabetes. Patients with type 1 diabetes, who have not received intensive insulin therapy and have had only fair to poor glycemic control, have a 30% to 40% chance of having nephropathy after 20 years—in contrast to the much lower frequency in patients with type 2 diabetes, who are not receiving intensive therapy, in whom only about 15% to 20% develop clinical renal disease. However, because so many more individuals are affected with type 2 diabetes, end-stage renal disease is much more prevalent in people with type 2 diabetes in the United States and especially throughout the rest of the world. There is no question that improved glycemic control and more effective therapeutic measures to correct hypertension can reduce the incidence of end-stage renal disease in both types of diabetes in the future.

Diabetic nephropathy is initially manifested by proteinuria; subsequently, as kidney function declines, urea and creatinine accumulate in the blood. Thickening of capillary basement membranes and of the mesangium of renal glomeruli produces varying degrees of glomerulosclerosis and renal insufficiency. Diffuse glomerulosclerosis is more common than nodular intercapillary glomerulosclerosis (Kimmelstiel-Wilson lesions); both produce heavy proteinuria.

Sensitive radioimmunoassay methods have permitted detection of microgram concentrations of urinary albumin. Conventional 24-hour urine collections, in addition to being inconvenient for patients, also show wide variability of albumin excretion, since several factors such as sustained erect posture, dietary protein, and exercise tend to increase albumin excretion rates. For these reasons, an albumin-creatinine ratio in an early morning spot urine collected upon awakening is preferable. In the early morning spot urine, a ratio of albumin (μg/L) to creatinine (mg/L) of <30 μg/mg creatinine is normal, and a ratio of 30 to 300 μg/mg creatinine suggests abnormal microalbuminuria. At least two of early morning spot urine collections over a 3- to 6-month period should be abnormal before a diagnosis of microalbuminuria is justified.

Subsequent renal failure can be predicted by persistent urinary albumin excretion rates exceeding 30 μg/min. Glycemic control as well as a low-protein diet (0.8 g/kg/d) may reduce both the hyperfiltration and the elevated microalbuminuria in patients in the early stages of diabetes and those with incipient diabetic nephropathy. Increased microalbuminuria correlates with increased levels of blood pressure and antihypertensive therapy decreases microalbuminuria. Evidence from some studies—but not the

UKPDS—supports a specific role for ACE inhibitors in reducing intraglomerular pressure in addition to lowering systemic blood pressure. An ACE inhibitor (captopril, 50 mg twice daily) in normotensive diabetics impedes progression to proteinuria and prevents the increase in albumin excretion rate. Since microalbuminuria has been shown to correlate with elevated nocturnal systolic blood pressure, it is possible that normotensive diabetic patients with microalbuminuria have slightly elevated systolic blood pressure during sleep, which is lowered during antihypertensive therapy. This action may contribute to the reported efficacy of ACE inhibitors in reducing microalbuminuria in normotensive patients.

If treatment is inadequate, then the disease progresses with proteinuria of varying severity, occasionally leading to nephrotic syndrome with hypoalbuminemia, edema, and an increase in circulating LDL cholesterol as well as progressive azotemia. In contrast to all other renal disorders, the proteinuria associated with diabetic nephropathy does not diminish with progressive renal failure (patients continue to excrete 10 to 11 g daily as creatinine clearance diminishes). As renal failure progresses, there is an elevation in the renal threshold at which glycosuria appears.

Patients with diabetic nephropathy should be evaluated and followed by a nephrologist.

B. Treatment Hemodialysis has been of limited success in the treatment of renal failure due to diabetic nephropathy, primarily because of progression of large vessel disease with resultant death and disability from stroke and myocardial infarction. Growing experience with chronic ambulatory peritoneal dialysis suggests that it may be a more convenient method of providing adequate dialysis with a lower incidence of complications.

Renal transplantation, especially from related donors, is often successful. For patients with compatible donors and no contraindications (such as severe cardiovascular disease), it is the treatment of choice.

Necrotizing Papillitis

This unusual complication of pyelonephritis occurs primarily in diabetic patients. It is characterized by fever, flank pain, pyuria, and sloughing of renal papillae in the urine. It is treated by intravenous administration of appropriate antibiotics.

Renal Decompensation After Radiographic Dyes

The use of radiographic contrast agents in diabetic patients with reduced creatinine clearance has been associated with the development of acute renal failure. Contrast-induced nephropathy is defined as an increase in serum creatinine of at least 0.5 mg/dL or 25% compared with baseline after exposure to intravenous contrast. The increase in serum creatinine occurs shortly after the procedure and peaks 3 to 5 days later before improving over the next 1 to 3 weeks. Although frequently transient, it can cause permanent impairment of renal function. Diabetic patients with normal renal function do not appear to be at increased risk for contrast nephropathy. If a contrast study is considered essential, patients with a serum creatinine of 1.5 to 2.5 mg/dL should be adequately hydrated before the procedure. Hydration with saline has been the cornerstone of contrast nephropathy prevention: intravenous saline 1 mL/kg/h is started 12 hours before the procedure and continued for 12 hours afterward. Some studies suggest that sodium bicarbonate infusions are more effective, and an alternate option is to infuse sodium bicarbonate: 150 mL of sodium bicarbonate (1 mEq/mL) is added to 1 L of 5% dextrose and infused at 3.5 mL/kg/h for 1 hour before the procedure; 1.2 mg/kg/h during the procedure and for 6 hours afterward. N-acetylcysteine has also been shown in some trials to decrease the incidence of contrast nephropathy. One regimen consists of using oral N-acetylcysteine 600 mg twice a day starting the day before the procedure for a total of four doses. A combination of N-acetylcysteine and intravenous saline or intravenous sodium bicarbonate may be more beneficial. Radiographic contrast material should not be given to a patient with a serum creatinine greater than 3 mg/dL unless the potential benefit outweighs the high risk of acute renal failure.

3. NEUROLOGIC COMPLICATIONS (DIABETIC NEUROPATHY)

Peripheral and autonomic neuropathy are the two most common complications of both types of diabetes. Up to 50% of patients with type 2 diabetes are affected. The pathogenesis of both types of neuropathy is poorly understood. Some lesions, such as the acute cranial nerve palsies and diabetic amyotrophy, have been attributed to ischemic infarction of the involved peripheral nerve. The much more common symmetric sensory and motor peripheral neuropathies and autonomic neuropathy are felt to be due to metabolic complications.

Unfortunately, there is no consistently effective treatment for any of the neuropathies. However, several long-term clinical trials have definitively shown that normalization of blood glucose levels can prevent development and progression of this devastating complication.

Peripheral Neuropathy

A. Distal symmetric polyneuropathy   This is the most common form of diabetic peripheral neuropathy in which loss of function appears in a stocking-glove pattern and is due to an axonal neuropathic process. Longer nerves are especially vulnerable—hence the impact on the foot. Both motor and sensory nerve conduction is delayed in the peripheral nerves, and ankle jerks may be absent.

Sensory involvement usually occurs first and is generally bilateral, symmetric, and associated with dulled perception of vibration, and temperature. Pain, when present, can range from mild discomfort to severe incapacitating symptoms (see later). The sensory deficit may eventually be of sufficient degree to prevent patients from feeling pain. Patients with symptoms of sensory neuropathy should be examined with a 5.07 Semmes-Weinstein filament. Those who cannot feel the filament must be considered at risk for unperceived neuropathic injury.

The denervation of the small muscles of the foot results in clawing of the toes and displacement of the submetatarsal fat pads anteriorly. These changes, together with the joint and connective tissue changes, alter the biomechanics of the foot, increasing plantar pressures. This combination of decreased pain threshold, abnormally high foot pressures, and repetitive stress (eg, walking) can lead to calluses and ulcerations in the high-pressure areas such as over the metatarsal heads. Peripheral neuropathy also predisposes to the development of Charcot arthropathy. Other predisposing factors for this condition include autonomic neuropathy and trauma. The acute Charcot foot presents with pain and swelling, and if the condition is untreated, it leads to a rocker bottom deformity and ulceration. The early radiologic changes are of joint subluxation and periarticular fractures. As the process progresses, there is frank osteoclastic destruction leading to deranged and unstable joints particularly in the midfoot.

Not surprisingly, the key issue for healing of neuropathic ulcers in a foot with good vascular status is mechanical unloading. Additionally, any infection should be treated with debridement and appropriate antibiotics. Healing times of 8 to 10 weeks are typical. In the occasional patient, where healing appears refractory, platelet-derived growth factor (becaplermin) should be considered for local application. A postmarket epidemiologic study showed increased cancer deaths in patients who had used three or more tubes of becaplermin on their leg or feet ulcers, and there is now a boxed warning in the drug label. Once ulcers are healed, therapeutic footwear is key to preventing recurrences. Custom-molded shoes are reserved for patients with significant foot deformities. Other patients with neuropathy may require accommodative insoles that distribute the load over as wide an area as possible. Patients with foot deformities and loss of protective threshold should seek regular care from a podiatrist. They should be educated about appropriate footwear, and those patients with loss of protective threshold should be instructed to inspect their feet daily for reddened areas, blisters, abrasions, or lacerations.

B. Isolated peripheral neuropathy   Involvement of the distribution of only one nerve (mononeuropathy) or of several nerves (mononeuropathy multiplex) is characterized by sudden onset with subsequent recovery of all or most of the function. This neuropathology has been attributed to vascular ischemia or traumatic damage. Cranial and femoral nerves are commonly involved, and motor abnormalities predominate. The patient with cranial nerve involvement usually presents with diplopia. Clinical examination reveals signs of single third, fourth, or sixth nerve weakness, and the pupil is spared. A full recovery of function occurs in 6 to 12 weeks. Diabetic amyotrophy presents with onset of severe pain in the front of the thigh. Within a few days or weeks of the onset of pain, the patient develops weakness and wasting of the quadriceps. Usually as the weakness appears, the pain tends to improve. Management includes analgesia and improved diabetic control. The symptoms improve over 6 to 18 months.

C. Painful diabetic neuropathy   Hypersensitivity to light touch and occasionally severe *burning* pain, particularly at night, can become physically and emotionally disabling. Amitriptyline, 25 to 75 mg at bedtime, has been recommended for pain associated with diabetic neuropathy. Dramatic relief has often resulted within 48 to 72 hours. This rapid response is in contrast to the 2 or 3 weeks required for an antidepressant effect. Patients often attribute benefit to having a full night's sleep after amitriptyline, compared to many previously sleepless nights occasioned by neuropathic pain. Mild to moderate morning drowsiness is a side effect that generally improves with time or can be lessened by giving the medication several hours before bedtime. This drug should not be continued if improvement has not occurred after 5 days of therapy. If amitriptyline's anticholinergic effects are too troublesome, then nortriptyline can be used. Desipramine in doses of 25 to 150 mg/d seems to have the same efficacy as amitriptyline. Tricyclic antidepressants in combination with phenothiazine or fluphenazine have been shown in two studies to be efficacious in painful neuropathy, with benefits unrelated to relief of depression. Gabapentin (900-1800 mg/d in three divided doses) has also been shown to be effective in the treatment of painful neuropathy and should be tried if the tricyclic drugs prove ineffective. Pregabalin, a congener of gabapentin, has been shown in an 8-week study to be more effective than placebo in treating painful diabetic peripheral neuropathy. However, this drug was not compared with an active control. Also, because of its abuse potential, it has been categorized as a Schedule V controlled substance. Duloxetine, a serotonin and norepinephrine reuptake inhibitor, has been approved for the treatment of painful diabetic neuropathy. In clinical trials, this drug reduced the pain sensitivity score by 40% to 50%. Capsaicin, a topical irritant, has been found to be effective in reducing local nerve pain; it is dispensed as a cream (Zostrix 0.025%, Zostrix-HP 0.075%) to be rubbed into the skin over the painful region two to four times daily. Gloves should be used for application, because hand contamination could result in discomfort if the cream comes in contact with eyes or sensitive areas such as the genitalia. Five percent lidocaine patch applied over an area of maximal pain has been reported to be of benefit and this therapy is currently in clinical trials.

Diabetic neuropathic cachexia is a syndrome characterized by a symmetric peripheral neuropathy associated with profound weight loss (up to 60% of total body weight) and painful dysesthesias affecting the proximal lower limbs, the hands, or the lower trunk. Treatment is usually with insulin and analgesics. The prognosis is usually good, and patients typically recover their baseline weight with resolution of the painful sensory symptoms within 1 year.

Autonomic Neuropathy

Neuropathy of the autonomic nervous system is common in patients with diabetes of long duration and can be a very disconcerting clinical problem. It can affect many diverse visceral functions including blood pressure and pulse, gastrointestinal activity, bladder function, and erectile function. Treatment is directed specifically at each abnormality.

Involvement of the gastrointestinal system may be manifested by nausea, vomiting, and postprandial fullness (from gastric atony); symptoms of reflux or dysphagia (from esophageal involvement); constipation and recurrent diarrhea, especially at night (from involvement of the small bowel and colon); and fecal incontinence (from anal sphincter dysfunction). Gallbladder function is altered, and this enhances stone formation.

Gastroparesis should be considered in type 1 diabetic patients in whom unexpected fluctuations and variability in their blood glucose levels develops after meals. Radiographic studies of the stomach and radioisotopic examination of gastric emptying after liquid and solid meals are of diagnostic value in these patients. Metoclopramide has been of some help in treating diabetic gastroparesis. It is a dopamine antagonist that has central antiemetic effects as well as a cholinergic action to facilitate gastric emptying. It is given in a dose of 10 mg orally three or four times a day, 30 minutes before meals and at bedtime. Drowsiness, restlessness, fatigue, and lassitude are common adverse effects. Tardive dyskinesia and extrapyramidal effects can occur especially when the drug is used for longer than 3 months and the FDA has cautioned against its chronic use. Erythromycin appears to bind to motilin receptors in the stomach and has been found to improve gastric emptying in doses of 250 mg three times daily over the short term, but its effectiveness seems to diminish over time. Tegaserod (Zelnorm), the partial 5-HT4 agonist, has been withdrawn from the US market by the FDA, so it is no longer used for this indication. In selected patients, injections of botulinum toxin into the pylorus can reduce sphincter resistance and enhance gastric emptying. Gastric electrical stimulation has been reported to improve symptoms and quality of life indices in patients with gastroparesis refractory to pharmacologic therapy.

Diarrhea associated with autonomic neuropathy has occasionally responded to broad-spectrum antibiotic therapy, although it often undergoes spontaneous remission. Refractory diabetic diarrhea is often associated with impaired sphincter control and fecal incontinence. Therapy with loperamide, 4 to 8 mg daily, or diphenoxylate with atropine, two tablets up to four times a day, may provide relief. In more severe cases, tincture of paregoric or codeine (60-mg tablets) may be required to reduce the frequency of diarrhea and improve the consistency of the stools. Clonidine has been reported to lessen diabetic diarrhea; however, its usefulness is limited by its tendency to cause orthostatic hypotension in these patients who already have autonomic neuropathy. Constipation usually responds to stimulant laxatives such as senna. Metamucil and other bulk-providing agents may relieve either the diarrhea or the constipation phases, which often alternate.

Inability to completely empty the bladder can sometimes occur. Bethanechol in doses of 10 to 50 mg three times a day has occasionally improved emptying of the atonic urinary bladder. Catheter decompression of the distended bladder has been reported to improve its function, and considerable benefit has been reported after surgical severing of the internal vesicle sphincter.

Use of Jobst fitted stockings, tilting the head of the bed, and arising slowly from the supine position are useful in minimizing symptoms of orthostatic hypotension. Some patients may require the addition of a mineralocorticoid such as fludrocortisone acetate (0.1-0.2 mg twice daily). Fludrocortisone therapy, however, can result in supine hypertension and hypokalemia. Midodrine (10 mg three times a day), an alpha adrenergic agonist, can be tried if Jobst stockings and sleeping upright prove ineffective in providing symptomatic relief.

Erectile dysfunction due to neuropathy differs from the psychogenic variety in that the latter may be intermittent (erections occur under special circumstances), whereas diabetic erectile dysfunction is usually persistent. To distinguish neuropathic or psychogenic erectile dysfunction from the erectile dysfunction caused by aortoiliac occlusive disease or vasculopathy, papaverine is injected into the corpus cavernosum of the penis. If the blood supply is competent, a penile erection occurs (Chapter 12). Urinary incontinence, with large volumes of residual urine, and retrograde ejaculation can also result from pelvic neuropathy.

There are medical, mechanical, and surgical approaches available for treatment of erectile dysfunction. Penile erection depends on relaxation of the smooth muscle in the arteries of the corpus cavernosum, and this is mediated by nitric oxide-induced cyclic 3′,5′-guanosine monophosphate (cGMP) formation. cGMP-specific phosphodiesterase type 5 (PDE5) inhibitors impair the breakdown of cGMP and improve the ability to attain and maintain an erection. Sildenafil (Viagra), vardenafil (Levitra), and tadalafil (Cialis) have been shown in placebo-controlled clinical trials to improve erections in response to sexual stimulation. The recommended dose of sildenafil for most patients is one 50-mg tablet taken approximately 1 hour before sexual activity. The peak effect is at 1.5 to 2 hours, with some effect persisting for 4 hours. Patients with diabetes mellitus using sildenafil reported 50% to 60% improvement in erectile function. The maximum recommended dose is 100 mg. The recommended dose of both vardenafil and tadalafil is 10 mg. The doses may be increased to 20 mg or decreased to 5 mg based on efficacy and side effects. Tadalafil has been shown to improve erectile function for up to 36 hours after dosing. In clinical trials, only a few adverse effects have been reported—transient mild headache, flushing, dyspepsia, and in some altered color vision. Priapism can occur with these drugs and patients should be advised to seek immediate medical attention if an erection persists for longer than 4 hours. The PDE5 inhibitors potentiate the hypotensive effects of nitrates, and their use is contraindicated in patients who are concurrently using organic nitrates in any form. Caution is advised for men who have suffered a heart attack, stroke, or life-threatening arrhythmia within the previous 6 months; men who have resting hypotension or hypertension, and men who have a history of cardiac failure or have unstable angina. Rarely, a decrease in vision or permanent visual loss has been reported after PDE5 inhibitor use.

Intracorporeal injection of vasoactive drugs causes penile engorgement and erection. Drugs most commonly used include papaverine alone, papaverine with phentolamine, and alprostadil (prostaglandin E₁). Alprostadil injections are relatively painless, but careful instruction is essential to prevent local trauma, priapism, and fibrosis. Intraurethral pellets of alprostadil avoid the problem of injection of the drug.

External vacuum therapy (Erec-Aid System) is a nonsurgical treatment consisting of a suction chamber operated by a hand pump that creates a vacuum around the penis. This draws blood into the penis to produce an erection that is maintained by a specially designed tension ring inserted around the base of the penis and which can be kept in place for up to 20 to 30 minutes. Although this method is generally effective, its cumbersome nature limits its appeal.

In view of the recent development of nonsurgical approaches to therapy of erectile dysfunction, resort to surgical implants of penile prostheses is becoming less common.

4. CARDIOVASCULAR COMPLICATIONS
Heart Disease

Microangiopathy occurs in the heart and may explain the existence of congestive cardiomyopathies found in diabetic patients without demonstrable coronary artery disease. Much more commonly, however, heart failure in patients with diabetes is a consequence of coronary atherosclerosis. Myocardial infarction is three to five times more common in diabetic patients than in age-matched controls and is the leading cause of death in patients with type 2 diabetes. Cardiovascular disease risk is increased in patients with type 1 diabetes as well, although the absolute risk is lower than in patients with type 2 diabetes. Women with diabetes lose the protection against myocardial infarction that is usually present during the childbearing years. The increased risk of atherosclerosis in people with diabetes may reflect the combination of hyperlipidemia, abnormalities of platelet adhesiveness, coagulation factors, hypertension, and oxidative stress and inflammation.

Large intervention studies of risk factor reduction in diabetes are lacking, but it is reasonable to assume that reducing these risk factors would have beneficial effects. Lowering LDL cholesterol reduces first events in patients without known coronary disease and secondary events in patients with known coronary disease. These intervention studies included some patients with diabetes, and the benefits of lowering LDL cholesterol were apparent in this group. The National Cholesterol Education Program clinical practice guidelines have designated diabetes as a coronary risk equivalent and have recommended that patients with diabetes should have an LDL cholesterol goal of <100 mg/dL. Lowering LDL cholesterol to 70 mg/dL may have additional benefit and is a reasonable target for most patients with type 2 diabetes who have multiple risk factors for cardiovascular disease.

The ADA also recommends lowering blood pressure to 130/80 mm Hg or less. The Antihypertensive and Lipid-Lowering Treatment to Prevent Heart Attack Trial (ALLHAT) randomized 33,357 subjects (age 55 years or older) with hypertension and at least one other coronary artery disease risk factor to receive treatment with chlorthalidone, amlodipine, or lisinopril. Chlorthalidone appeared to be superior to amlodipine and lisinopril in lowering blood pressure, in reducing the incidence of cardiovascular events, in tolerability, and in cost. The study included 12,063 individuals with type 2 diabetes. The Heart Outcomes Prevention Evaluation (HOPE) study randomized 9297 high-risk patients who had evidence of vascular disease or diabetes plus one other cardiovascular risk factor to receive ramipril or placebo for a mean period of 5 years. Treatment with ramipril resulted in a 25% reduction of the risk of myocardial infarction, stroke, or death from cardiovascular disease. The mean difference in blood pressure between the placebo and ramipril groups was 2.2 mm Hg systolic and 1.4 mm Hg diastolic, and the reduction in cardiovascular event rate remained significant after adjustment for this small difference in blood pressure. The mechanism underlying this protective effect of ramipril is unknown. Patients with type 2 diabetes who already have cardiovascular disease or microalbuminuria should therefore be considered for treatment with an ACE inhibitor. More clinical studies are needed to address the question of whether patients with type 2 diabetes, who do not have cardiovascular disease or microalbuminuria, would specifically benefit from ACE inhibitor treatment.

Aspirin (81-325 mg daily) inhibits thromboxane synthesis by platelets and is effective in reducing cardiovascular morbidity and mortality in patients who have a history of myocardial infarction or stroke (secondary prevention). It is unclear if aspirin prevents primary cardiovascular events in people with diabetes. The current recommendation is to give aspirin to those people with diabetes who are at increased risk for cardiovascular events (greater than 10% 10 year risk of cardiovascular events). Typically this includes most 50-year-old men and 60-year-old women with one or more additional risk factors (smoking, hypertension, dyslipidemia, family history of premature cardiovascular disease, and albuminuria). Contraindications for aspirin therapy include age less than 21 years (because of risk of Reye syndrome), aspirin allergy, bleeding tendency (eg, anticoagulant therapy), recent gastrointestinal bleeding, or active hepatic disease. The Early Treatment Diabetic Retinopathy Study (ETDRS) showed that aspirin does not influence the course of proliferative retinopathy. There was no statistically significant difference in the severity of vitreous/preretinal hemorrhages or their rate of resolution between the aspirin and placebo groups. Thus, it appears that there is no contraindication to aspirin use to achieve cardiovascular benefit in diabetic patients who have proliferative retinopathy.

Peripheral Vascular Disease

Atherosclerosis is markedly accelerated in the larger arteries. It is often diffuse, with localized enhancement in certain areas of turbulent blood flow, such as at the bifurcation of the aorta or other large vessels. Clinical manifestations of peripheral vascular disease include ischemia of the lower extremities, impotence, and intestinal angina.

The incidence of **gangrene of the feet** in people with diabetes is 30 times that in age-matched controls. The factors responsible for the development of this condition, in addition to peripheral vascular disease, are small vessel disease, peripheral neuropathy with loss of both pain sensation and neurogenic inflammatory responses, and secondary infection. In two-thirds of patients with ischemic gangrene, pedal pulses are not palpable. In the remaining one-third who has palpable pulses, reduced blood flow through these vessels can be demonstrated by plethysmographic or Doppler ultrasound examination. Prevention of foot injury is imperative. Agents that reduce peripheral blood flow such as tobacco and propranolol should be avoided. Control of other risk factors such as hypertension is essential. Cholesterol-lowering agents are useful as adjunctive therapy when early ischemic signs are detected and when dyslipidemia is present. Patients should be advised to seek immediate medical care if a diabetic foot ulcer develops. Improvement in peripheral blood flow with endarterectomy and bypass operations is possible in certain patients.

5. SKIN AND MUCOUS MEMBRANE COMPLICATIONS

Chronic pyogenic infections of the skin may occur, especially in poorly controlled diabetic patients. Eruptive xanthomas can result from hypertriglyceridemia, associated with poor glycemic control. Candidal infection can produce erythema and edema of intertriginous areas below the breasts, in the axillas, and between the fingers. It causes vulvovaginitis in most chronically uncontrolled diabetic women with persistent glucosuria and is a frequent cause of pruritus. While antifungal creams containing miconazole or clotrimazole offer immediate relief of vulvovaginitis, recurrence is frequent unless glucosuria is reduced.

Necrobiosis lipoidica diabeticorum are oval or irregularly shaped plaques with reddish demarcated borders and a glistening yellowish surface usually located over the anterior surfaces of the legs or the dorsal surfaces of the ankles. Rarely, lesions can occur on the hands, fingers, forearms, face, and scalp. The necrobiosis lesion usually starts out as an oval violaceous patch that slowly expands. The advancing border is red and the central area turns yellow-brown. The thinning of the dermis in the center of the lesion leads to the shiny surface and prominent telangiectasia. It also allows the subcutaneous fat to become more visible hence the yellowish appearance. Pathologically, the lesions show degeneration of collagen, granulomatous inflammation of subcutaneous tissues and blood vessels, capillary basement membrane thickening, and obliteration of vessel lumina. The condition is associated with type 1 diabetes, although it can occur in patients with type 2 diabetes and also in people without diabetes. It occurs in about 0.3% of patients with diabetes, usually in patients in their 30s and 40s, and is about three times more common in women than in men. In some studies an association with microalbuminuria and retinopathy has been reported. Improving glycemic control may help the condition. The first-line treatment includes topical and subcutaneous corticosteroids. Second-line treatments include systemic steroids, cyclosporine, ticlodipine, nicotinamide, clofazimine, fumarate esters, intralesional etanercept, and topical psoralen with ultraviolet A. Pulsed dye lasers can improve the appearance of telangiectasias. Flare-ups are frequent. No treatment is completely effective.

Shin spots are uncommon in adult diabetics. They are brownish, rounded, painless atrophic lesions of the skin in the pretibial area.

6. BONE AND JOINT COMPLICATIONS

Bone and joint complications are generally attributed to metabolic or vascular sequelae of long-standing diabetes.

Diabetic cheiroarthropathy is a syndrome of chronic progressive stiffness of the hand secondary to contracture and tightening of the skin over the joints. It is characterized by inability to flatten the palms against a flat surface (prayer sign). It is believed to be due to glycosylation of collagen and perhaps other proteins in connective tissue. It is associated with poor glycemic control and with longer duration of diabetes.

Dupuytren contractures consist of nodular thickening and contracture of the palmar fascia of the hand, producing flexure contractures of the fingers. It can occur in the absence of diabetes, but is more common in people with diabetes. The etiology is unclear but there may be an inflammatory component. Glucocorticoid injection into discrete nodules can sometimes help but the standard treatment is surgical fasciectomy.

Carpal tunnel syndrome occurs when the median nerve is compressed within the carpal tunnel. It is more common in people with diabetes, especially those who also have diabetic cheiroarthropathy. It is presumably due to glycosylation of collagen and other proteins in the connective tissue.

Patients with adhesive capsulitis of the shoulder (frozen shoulder) complain primarily of stiffness and loss of range of motion. They may also have shoulder pain. It occurs more frequently in people with long-standing diabetes—the incidence being two to four times higher than in the general population. The patients may also have diabetic cheiroarthropathy or Dupuytren contractures. In most cases it is a limited condition that responds to physical therapy. Patients should be warned that recovery may take 6 to 18 months. For a few patients surgery may be necessary. Adhesive capsulitis of the hip has also been described.

Data on bone mineral density and fracture risk in people with diabetes are contradictory. Bone mineral density has been reported to be low, normal, or high in type 2 diabetes patients. Type 2 diabetes patients do appear to be at increased risk for nonvertebral factures. Women with type 1 diabetes have an increased risk of fracture when compared to women without diabetes. It is likely that other factors such as duration of diabetes and diabetes complications such as neuropathy and renal disease affect both the bone mineral density and fracture risk.

Diffuse idiopathic skeletal hyperostosis (DISH) is a skeletal disease characterized by ossification of the anterior longitudinal ligament of the spine and various extraspinal ligaments. It causes stiffness and decreased range of spinal motion. The peripheral joints most commonly affected are the metacarpophalangeal joints, elbows, and shoulders. Diabetes, obesity, hypertension, and dyslipidemia are risk factors for this condition.

Hyperuricemia and gout are disorders associated with the metabolic syndrome. Thus, it is not surprising that type 2 diabetes patients are at increased risk for acute gout as well as chronic tophaceous gout.

Bursitis, particularly of the shoulders and hips, occurs more frequently than expected in patients with diabetes.

7. INFECTION

There are also several unusual infections that occur almost exclusively in diabetic patients (eg, emphysematous cholecystitis, mucormycosis, malignant otitis externa, and necrotizing papillitis). As noted earlier, atherosclerosis with peripheral vascular disease is very common in the diabetic population, and the resultant ischemia undoubtedly plays a role in the frequent and severe lower extremity infections seen in these patients.

MANAGEMENT OF DIABETES IN THE HOSPITALIZED PATIENT

A number of studies have observed that hospitalized patients with diabetes and those with new-onset hyperglycemia (ie, those without a preadmission diagnosis of diabetes) have higher inpatient morbidity and mortality. The morbidity and mortality in diabetics is twice that of nondiabetics. Those with new-onset hyperglycemia have even a higher mortality—almost eightfold greater in one study. These observations have led to increased interest in improving glucose control in the hospitalized diabetic patient.

Most patients with diabetes are hospitalized for reasons other than their diabetes. Up to 10% to 15% of all hospitalized patients have diabetes. Audits suggest that as many as a 30% of hospitalized diabetic patients have inappropriate management of their diabetes such as being given metformin where contraindicated; failure to act on high blood glucose levels; omission of diabetes medication; no record of diabetes complications; inappropriate insulin management; or blood glucose monitoring. Use of outpatient oral therapies or insulin regimens in the hospital is challenging. Patients are not eating according to their normal schedule and are often fasting for procedures. It is, therefore, usual to use insulin, subcutaneous or intravenous, in the hospitalized patient. Insulin is safe to use in patients with cardiac, renal, and liver disease and its dosing can be adjusted to match changing inpatient needs.

Surgery represents a stressful situation during which most of the insulin antagonists (catecholamines, GH, corticosteroids) are mobilized. In the patient with diabetes, this can lead to a worsening of hyperglycemia and perhaps even ketoacidosis. The aim of medical management of people with diabetes during the perioperative period is to minimize these stress-induced changes. Recommendations for management depend both on the patient's usual diabetic regimen and on the type of surgery (major or minor) to be done.

For people with diabetes controlled with diet alone, no special precautions are necessary unless diabetic control is markedly disturbed by the procedure. If this occurs, small amounts of short-acting insulin, as needed, will correct the hyperglycemia. Patients on oral agents should not take them on the day of surgery. If there is significant hyperglycemia, short-acting insulin can be given as needed. If this approach does not provide adequate control, an insulin infusion should be started in the manner indicated below. The oral agents can be restarted once the patient is eating normally after the operation. It is important to order a postoperative serum creatinine level to ensure normal renal function prior to restarting metformin therapy.

Patients taking insulin represent the only serious challenge to management of diabetes when surgery is necessary. The insulin regimen used to control the glucose depends on the kind of diabetes (type 1 or type 2); whether it is minor surgery (<2 hour and patient eating afterward) or major surgery (longer than 2 hours, invasion of body

TABLE 17–23 Recommendations for management of insulin-treated diabetes during surgery.

	Minor surgical procedures (<2 h; eating afterward)	Major surgical procedures (>2 h; invasion of body cavity; not eating immediately after recovery)
Type 2 patients on basal bolus insulin regimen; twice daily premixed insulin	No insulin on the day of operation. Start 5% dextrose infusion; monitor fingerstix blood glucose and give subcutaneous short-acting insulin every 4 or 6 h	Same regimen as minor procedure. If control is not satisfactory, then intravenous insulin infusion
Type 1 patient on basal bolus insulin regimen or on insulin pump	Patients on pump should discontinue the pump the evening before procedure and should be given a 24 h basal insulin. On day of procedure, start 5% dextrose; monitor blood glucose and give subcutaneous short-acting insulin every 4 or 6 h	Initiate insulin infusion on morning of procedure and transition back to usual regimen when eating

cavity, not eating afterward); and the preoperative insulin regimen (basal bolus or premixed insulin twice a day or premeal bolus only or regular before meals and NPH at bedtime). Type 1 patients have to be on some insulin to prevent the development of diabetic ketoacidosis. Many type 2 patients on insulin are fine without insulin for a few hours. Ideally patients with diabetes should undergo surgery early in the morning. Table 17–23 summarizes the approach for these various kinds of patients. One insulin infusion method adds 10 U of regular insulin to 1 L of 5% dextrose in half-normal saline, and this is infused intravenously at a rate of 100 to 180 mL/h. This gives the patient 1 to 1.8 U of insulin per hour, which, except in the most severe cases, generally keeps the blood glucose within the range of 100 to 250 mg/dL (5.5-13.9 mmol/L). The infusion may be continued for several days if necessary. Plasma glucose or blood glucose should be determined every 2 to 4 hours to be sure metabolic control is adequate. If it is not, adjustments in the ratio of insulin to dextrose in the intravenous solution can be made.

An alternative method, which is gaining increasing popularity, consists of separate infusions of insulin and glucose delivered by pumps to permit independent adjustments of each infusion rate, depending on hourly variation of blood glucose values. There are a number of different algorithms available for insulin infusions. Table 17–24 provides guidelines for management with an insulin infusion and an algorithm designed to achieve glycemic control in the range of 120 to 180 mg/dL blood glucose.

After surgery, when the patient has resumed an adequate oral intake, intravenous administration of insulin and dextrose can be stopped half an hour after the first subcutaneous insulin injection. Insulin needs may vary in the first several days after surgery because of continuing postoperative stresses and because of variable caloric intake. In this situation, multiple doses of regular insulin, guided by blood glucose determinations, can keep the patient in acceptable metabolic control.

In the intensive care units, glucose levels are controlled most frequently using insulin infusions. Patients on total parental nutrition (TPN) can have insulin added to the bag. Standard TPN contains 25% dextrose, so 50-mL/h infusion delivers 12.5 g of dextrose per hour.

On the general surgical and medical wards, most patients are managed on subcutaneous insulin regimens. Limited cross-sectional and prospective studies suggest that the best glucose control is achieved on a combination of basal and bolus regimen with 50% of daily insulin needs provided by intermediate or long-acting insulins. Standardized order sets prompt medical personnel to write more physiological insulin orders, reduce errors, and include algorithms for recognition and treatment of hypoglycemia. Table 17–25 is an example of one such order set for a subcutaneous insulin regimen.

Targets for Glucose Control in the Hospitalized Patient

A number of studies have observed that hospitalized patients with diabetes and those with new-onset hyperglycemia (ie, those without a preadmission diagnosis of diabetes) have higher inpatient morbidity and mortality. Also, poor glucose control in diabetics at admission is associated with increased size of myocardial infarction and in some studies increased nosocomial infections after surgery. These observations have led to the question of whether lowering glucose levels close to normal in the hospital improves outcomes.

A prospective trial in surgical ICU patients (Leuven 1 study) reported that aggressive treatment of hyperglycemia (blood glucose <110 mg/dL) reduced mortality (35 deaths vs 63, $p < 0.04$) and morbidity. Only a small number of persons in this study (204 of 1548) had a diagnosis of diabetes preoperatively, and so this study suggests that controlling hyperglycemia per se (independent of a diagnosis of diabetes) was beneficial. The benefits, however, were principally seen in patients who were in the ICU for longer than 5 days, and it was unclear whether the benefits would also apply to most surgical patients who stay in the ICU for only 1 to 2 days.

The same investigators performed a similar prospective trial among 1200 medical ICU patients (Leuven 2 study) and reported that aggressive treatment of hyperglycemia reduced morbidity (reduction in acquired renal injury and increased early weaning from mechanical ventilation) but not mortality. Again, as in the surgical ICU study, only a small number of persons (16.9%) had a diagnosis of diabetes at admission.

The findings of the Leuven studies however have not been confirmed in other prospective studies. Two other ICU-based studies (Glucontrol and VISEP) that attempted to confirm the

TABLE 17–24 Guideline for perioperative diabetes management with an intravenous insulin infusion.

1. Maintenance of IV fluids (IV dextrose infusion must be maintained while the patient is on insulin infusion. Minimum rate of 10 mL/h.)
   - ☐ D5 NS at 100 mL/h
   - ☐ D5 1/2 NS at 100 mL/h
   - ☐ D10 NS at _____ mL/h (for patients with fluid restrictions or renal failure)
   - ☐ Additive: KCl 20 mEq/L (generally 20 mEq/L)
   - ☐ Other_____ at _____mL/h
2. Regular insulin infusion 100 U regular insulin in 100 mL NS (1 U = 1 mL)
   A. Flush first 20 mL of infusion through tubing before connecting to patient.
   B. Before beginning infusion, check blood glucose (BG) with glucose meter.
3. **Start insulin infusion rate as follows (when BG ≥100 mg/dL)**
   - ☐ 0.3 U/h taking <30 U insulin daily (recommended for type 1; Pancreatectomy)
   - ☐ 1 U/h for patients previously diet controlled, taking oral hypoglycemic agent, or <30 U insulin daily
   - ☐ 1.5 U/h for patients taking >30 U insulin daily
   - ☐ Other _____ U/h
4. **Adjust insulin infusion rate as follows:**

☐ Standard adjustment	☐ Sensitive Adjustment (for Type 1; Pancreatectomy)
BG <80 mg/dL; stop infusion and **call MD; see instruction # 5 below**	BG <80 mg/dL; stop infusion and **call MD; see instruction # 5 below**
Do not restart insulin infusion until BG > 100 mg/dL[a]	Do not restart insulin infusion until BG > 100 mg/dL[a]
BG 80-120; decrease drip by 0.5 U/h	BG 80-120; decrease drip by 0.2 U/h
BG 121-180; no change in drip rate	BG 121-180; no change in drip rate
BG 181-250; increase drip by 0.5 U/h	BG 181-250; increase drip by 0.2 U/h
BG >250 bolus 5 U regular insulin IV and increase drip by 0.5 U/h	BG >250 bolus 2 U regular insulin IV and increase drip by 0.2 U/h

5. For a BG <80 mg/dL or >400 mg/dL on insulin infusion, call MD.
   - ☒ BG <80 mg/dL but >60 mg/dL, stop insulin infusion; check BG every 15 min.
   - ☒ BG ≤60 mg/dL, stop insulin infusion; give **50-mL D50W IV push**; check BG every 15 min and repeat treatment until BG ≥100 mg/dL. When BG ≥100 mg/dL, call MD for new insulin infusion rate.
   - ☒ BG >400 mg/dL, call MD to reassess insulin infusion rate.
   - ☒ If TPN or tube feeds are interrupted for longer than 30 min, start D10W at 50 mL/h. Notify MD about change and future action.
6. When converting to subcutaneous (SQ) insulin, give prescribed SQ dose 30 min prior to discontinuing insulin infusion. Use Adult SQ Insulin Order Sheet.
7. If patient eating meals give _____ U aspart SQ after patient eats carbohydrates and continue insulin infusion.
8. Discontinue insulin infusion maintenance IV fluids when insulin infusion discontinued.

[a]Check BG every hour with glucose meter until stable (range 100-180 mg/dL) for two consecutive readings and then every 2 hours.

findings were unable to do so. These two studies, however, were stopped prematurely for the following reasons: an interim analysis (falsely) suggested increased mortality in the test group in the Glucontrol study, and hypoglycemic events increased sevenfold in the intensive treatment group in the VISEP study. A large multi-center, multinational study (NICE-SUGAR) recruited 6104 surgical and medical ICU patients with hyperglycemia (20% had diabetes) and randomized them to tight control (81-108 mg/dL) or less tight control (<180 mg/dL). The tight group achieved blood glucose levels of 115 ± 18 and the conventional group 144 ± 23. There were more deaths (829 vs 751) in the tight glucose control group compared to the less tight glucose control group (p = 0.02). The intensively treated group also had more cases of severe hypoglycemia (206 vs 15 cases), and the excess deaths in the intensive group were due to cardiovascular events.

A study on tight intraoperative glycemic control during cardiac surgery also failed to show any benefit; if anything, the intensively treated group had more events. The United Kingdom Glucose Insulin in Stroke Trial (GIST-UK) failed to show beneficial effect of tight glycemic control in stroke patients; however, the investigators acknowledged that, because of slow recruitment, the study was underpowered.

Based on the evidence available so far, ICU patients with blood glucose levels above 180 mg/dL (diabetes and new-onset hyperglycemia) should be treated aiming for target glucose levels between 140 and 180 mg/dL. Targeting blood glucose control in the intensive care unit close to 100 mg/dL is not beneficial and may even be harmful. When patients leave the ICU, target glucose values between 100 mg/dL and 180 mg/dL may be appropriate, although this view is based on clinical observations rather than conclusive evidence.

DIABETES MELLITUS AND PREGNANCY

Hormone and Fuel Balance During Pregnancy

During pregnancy, the rapidly growing fetus impacts metabolism in the mother and causes profound hormonal and metabolic changes. These changes significantly affect the management of

TABLE 17–25 Example of a standardized subcutaneous insulin order set for inpatient use.

1. Check blood glucose and give insulin before meals, bedtime, and 2 AM.

2. Discontinue previous SQ insulin order.

3. If patient becomes NPO for procedure/stops eating:

- **HOLD** nutritional dose of rapid-acting analog.

- Give correctional dose of rapid-acting analog if BG >130 mg/dL.

- Give glargine dose. If BG has been <70 mg/dL in last 24 h, call MD to consider adjusting glargine dose.

- Call MD for NPO orders if patient on 70/30, NPH insulin or has been NPO >12 h.

A. Basal and nutritional insulin dose (in units):

Time	Breakfast	Lunch	Dinner	Bedtime
Rapid-acting analog				
NPH				
Insulin glargine				
Insulin mixture				

B. Meal time correctional insulin with rapid-acting analog. Check box to choose scale. Add or subtract from nutritional dose of rapid-acting analog.

Blood Glucose Range	☐ Sensitive BMI <25 and/or <50 U/d	☐ Average BMI 25-30 and/or 50-90 U/d	☐ Resistant BMI >30 and/or >90 U/d	☐ Custom
<70 mg/dL Once BG • 100, give	Treat for hypoglycemia per protocol (see order #6). Once BG •100 mg/dL give rapid-acting analog with following change when patient eats:			
	2 U less	3 U less	4 U less	--- U less
70-100	1 U less	2 U less	3 U less	--- U less
101-130	Give nutritional rapid-acting insulin as in # 4A			
131-150	+ 0	+ 1	+ 2	+ ---
151-200	+ 1	+ 2	+ 3	+ ---
201-250	+ 2	+ 4	+ 6	+ ---
251-300	+ 3	+ 6	+ 9	+ ---
301-350	+ 4	+ 8	+ 12	+ ---
351-400	+ 5	+ 10	+ 15	+ ---
>400	+ 6	+ 12	+ 18	+ ---

C. ☒ Bedtime and 2 AM correctional insulin with rapid-acting analog if BG ≥ 200 mg/dL.

BG Range (mg/dL)	Default Value (U)	Custom	
200-250	1	---	U
251-300	2	---	
>300	3	---	

4. Call MD for BG <70 mg/dL or > 400 mg/dL.

5. For BG <70 mg/dL, use Hypoglycemia Protocol below. These hypoglycemia orders remain active for duration of SQ insulin administration. For patient taking PO, give 20 g of oral fast-acting carbohydrate per patient preference:

☒ Give 4 glucose tablets (5 g glucose/tablet). Repeat Q 15 min until BG ≥100 mg/dL.

or

☒ Give 6 oz fruit juice. Repeat Q 15 min until BG ≥100 mg/dL.

☒ Give 25-mL D50W IV push if patient cannot take PO. Repeat Q 15 min until BG ≥100 mg/dL.

☒ Check fingerstick glucose every 15 min and repeat treatment until BG is ≥100 mg/dL.

6. Discontinue above monitoring and intervention orders when SQ insulin is discontinued.

Note: Glargine (Lantus) *cannot* be mixed with any other insulin. Give glargine as a separate injection.

preexisting diabetes, and can precipitate hyperglycemia and diabetes in previously nondiabetic mothers.

Early in pregnancy, the hormones of pregnancy initiate changes that prepare the mother for the increasing nutrient requirements of the fetus late in pregnancy. Fat deposition is accentuated in early pregnancy due to enhanced conversion of glucose to triglyceride after meals in pregnant compared with nonpregnant subjects. Elevated prolactin and placental lactogen drive the production of serotonin by the β cell, which leads to β cell expansion, a process that peaks in mid gestation. β cell mass approximately doubles during pregnancy, and both β cell glucose sensitivity and insulin secretory capacity increase. At the same time, α cell mass and glucagon secretion remain unchanged.

As the pregnancy progresses and nutrient utilization by the fetus increases, plasma concentrations of glucose in the fasting state tend to decline slightly. Since the flow of glucose and other nutrients to the fetus depends on the gradient across the placenta, maintenance of maternal glucose levels becomes increasingly important and is achieved through increasing insulin resistance in the liver, muscle, and adipose tissue. Several pregnancy hormones contribute to insulin resistance, but progesterone, which increases steadily through pregnancy and peaks shortly prior to parturition, provides the major drive. Glucose availability for the fetus increases as increased lipolysis in adipose tissue leads to a shift toward fatty acid utilization by maternal tissues. Ketogenesis is also accentuated in the postabsorptive state during pregnancy, secondary to hormonal effects on the maternal liver cells and increased provision of substrate FFA. The increased FFAs contribute to the marked reduction in insulin-mediated glucose uptake by skeletal muscle characteristic of late pregnancy. At the same time, increased insulin production from the previously expanded β cells balances this insulin resistance and ensures a consistent flow of glucose to the fetus, especially after meals. As a net result, during the third trimester, pregnant women without diabetes run slightly higher blood glucose and ketone levels than nondiabetic subjects, and women with preexisting diabetes that do not adjust therapy appropriately can develop severe hyperglycemia.

Pregnancy in Women with Preexisting Diabetes

A. Prevalence The prevalence of pregestational diabetes in pregnant women is increasing. A study from Southern California showed that between 1999 and 2005, the prevalence of preexisting diabetes, age and race/ethnicity adjusted, increased from 0.81/100 in 1999 to 1.82/100 in 2005 (*p* for trend <0.001). Significant increases were observed in all age groups and all racial/ethnic groups. The incidence of type 2 diabetes increasing and in some countries, pregnant women with type 2 diabetes now outnumber those with type 1 diabetes.

In 1988 0.5% of all pregnancies in the United States were complicated by pregestational diabetes and this type accounted for 65% of the complicated pregnancies compared with 26% in 1980.

B. Maternal, fetal, and neonatal consequences of presence of diabetes during pregnancy If diabetes is poorly controlled in the first weeks of pregnancy, the risks of spontaneous abortion and congenital malformation of the infant are increased. Poor glycemic control later in pregnancy is associated with still births, fetal macrosomia, polyhydramnios, and neonatal hypoglycemia. Preexisting diabetes-related complications, particularly gastroenteropathy, retinopathy, and nephropathy can impact both the pregnant woman and the fetus.

Congenital anomalies. Poorly controlled diabetes in the first weeks of pregnancy raises the risks of spontaneous abortion and congenital anomalies of the infant. The commonest anomalies are cardiac, neural tube defects, and genitourinary abnormalities. Their incidence compared to the normal population and their presumed time of occurrence during embryonic development are listed in Table 17–26. The rate of anomalies is higher in diabetic women with poor preconception control. Observational studies demonstrate a linear relationship between glycated hemoglobin levels and malformation rates. From a systematic review of several observational studies, it was estimated that the relative risk reduction of congenital anomalies for each 1% decrease in HbA$_{1c}$ ranged from 0.39 to 0.59. Attending preconception clinics with intensive diabetic management instituted prior to conception and continued through early pregnancy, results in significant reduction in the frequency of anomalies—to rates near the population norms.

Polyhydramnios. Later in pregnancy, polyhydramnios, a common complication in women with poorly controlled diabetes, may lead to preterm delivery. Polyhydramnios also increases the risk for placenta abruptio and postpartum uterine atony.

TABLE 17–26 Congenital malformations in infants of diabetic mothers.[a]

	Ratio of Incidences Diabetic vs Control Group	Latest Gestational Age for Occurrence (Weeks After Menstruation)
Caudal regression	252	5
Anencephaly	3	6
Spina bifida, hydrocephalus, or other central nervous system defects	2	6
Cardiac anomalies	4	
Transposition of great vessels		7
Ventricular septal defect		8
Atrial septal defect		8
Anal/rectal atresia	3	8
Renal anomalies	5	
Agenesis	6	7
Cystic kidney	4	7
Ureter duplex	23	7
Situs inversus	84	6

[a]Modified and reproduced, with permission, from Kucera J. Rate and type of congenital anomalies among offspring of diabetic women. *J Reprod Med.* 1971;7:61; and Mills JL, Baker L, Goldman AS. Malformations in infants of diabetic mothers occur before the seventh gestational week: implications for treatment. *Diabetes.* 1979;28:292.

Polyhydramnios is an excess volume of amniotic fluid (>1000 mL, often >3000 mL). It is most often associated with fetal macrosomia. The excess volume of amniotic fluid is not related simply to the concentration of glucose or other solutes in amniotic fluid or to excess fetal urine output as measured by change in bladder size on ultrasonography. Other possible factors include decreased fetal swallowing, decidual and amniotic fluid prolactin, and as yet unknown determinants of the complicated multicompartmental intrauterine transfer of water. Polyhydramnios is rare in women with well-controlled diabetes.

Fetal macrosomia. Many fetuses of poorly controlled diabetic mothers are **macrosomic** (birth weight >90th percentile for gestational age), with increased fat stores, increased length, and increased abdomen-to-head or thorax-to-head ratios. The hypothesis that fetal macrosomia results from the causal chain of maternal hyperglycemia → fetal hyperglycemia → fetal hyperinsulinemia → fetal macrosomia has been confirmed by clinical and experimental studies. Macrosomic infants of diabetic mothers have significantly higher concentrations of C peptide (representing endogenous insulin secretion) in their cord sera or amniotic fluid than in those with birth weights appropriate for gestational age. Monkey fetuses with insulin-releasing pellets implanted in utero become macrosomic. Other metabolic substrates that cross the placenta, such as branched-chain amino acids may also play a role in fetal macrosomia, and transplacental lipids could contribute to fat deposition.

Prevention of maternal hyperglycemia throughout pregnancy can reduce the incidence of macrosomia. The glycemic threshold for fetal macrosomia seems to be *postprandial* peak values above 130 mg/dL (7.2 mmol/L). On the other hand, excessively tight glycemic control (average peak postprandial blood glucose levels <110 mg/dL [6.1 mmol/L]) can be associated with insufficient fetal growth and small-for-date infants.

Complications of macrosomia include fetopelvic disproportion leading to shoulder dystocia and its attendant risk for brachial plexus injury and humeral and clavicle fractures. The neonate with macrosomia is also at increased risk for hypoglycemia, hyperbilirubinemia, hypocalcemia, respiratory distress syndrome, and polycythemia.

Adverse maternal outcomes of difficult vaginal delivery include severe perineal lacerations and subsequent urinary and/ or fecal incontinence.

Intrauterine growth retardation. The fetus of a woman with diabetes of long duration and vascular disease may suffer intrauterine fetal growth restriction related to inadequate uteroplacental perfusion. All body diameters may be below normal on ultrasonographic measurements, but the abdominal circumference is especially affected, and oligohydramnios and abnormal Doppler flow measurements of the umbilical cord are common. In these patients provision of adequate rest, meticulous control of hypertension (target <135/85 mm Hg), maintenance of normal blood glucose levels, and intensive fetal surveillance are all essential for success.

Intrauterine death. Prior to the 1970s, the incidence of apparently sudden intrauterine fetal demise in the third trimester of diabetic pregnancies was at least 5%. Except for congenital malformations, the cause of stillbirth is often not obvious. The risk is greater with poor diabetic control, and the incidence of fetal death exceeds 50%, if ketoacidosis develops in the mother. Some instances of fetal demise are associated with preeclampsia-eclampsia, which is more common in pregnancies complicated by diabetes. Fetal death has also been associated with pyelonephritis—this is now largely prevented by screening for and treating asymptomatic bacteriuria. Other than these known risk factors, one can presume (based on experimental studies) that the combination of fetal hyperglycemia and hypoxia leads to acidosis and myocardial dysfunction. Good glycemic control in diabetic women greatly reduces the risk of stillbirth.

Neonatal hypoglycemia. Hypoglycemia is common in the first 48 hours after delivery from previously hyperglycemic mothers and is defined as blood glucose below 36 mg/dL (2.0 mmol/L) regardless of gestational age. The risk is as high for infants of mothers with type 2 diabetes as type 1 diabetes. Neonatal hypoglycemia is most closely linked to poor maternal glucose control and elevated fetal insulin levels during labor and delivery, although data from amniotic fluid insulin studies suggest that the more hyperinsulinemic the fetus in the late third trimester, the higher the risk of neonatal hypoglycemia. Infants of diabetic mothers may also have deficient catecholamine and glucagon secretion, and the hypoglycemia may be related to diminished hepatic glucose production and oxidation of free fatty acids. The symptomatic infant may be lethargic with associated apnea, tachypnea, cyanosis, or seizures. Early feeding with 10% dextrose in water by bottle or gavage by 1 hour of age should be instituted in the at-risk neonate. If this is not successful, treatment with intravenous dextrose solutions is indicated. There are usually no long-term sequelae of episodes of neonatal hypoglycemia. Keeping maternal blood glucose levels below 144 mg/dL and tight glycemic control during labor can reduce the frequency of neonatal hypoglycemia.

Diabetic gastroenteropathy. In early gestation, diabetic gastroparesis can severely exacerbate the nausea and vomiting of pregnancy (hyperemesis gravidarum), which sometimes continues into the third trimester. Drugs stimulating gastric motility such as erythromycin may be useful, but many patients with this complication require hyperalimentation to achieve nutritional intake adequate for fetal development.

Diabetic retinopathy. Background diabetic retinopathy may develop or progress during pregnancy, but it usually regresses postpartum. If background retinopathy is already present in early pregnancy, the rate of progression to neovascularization over the course of the pregnancy (proliferative diabetic retinopathy) is 6% if the background retinopathy is mild; 18% if it is moderate; and 38% if severe preproliferative changes are present. The risk factors for progression to proliferative retinopathy include poor glycemic control before and during early pregnancy, rapid improvement in glycemic control during pregnancy, hypertension, and perhaps the many growth factors derived from placental tissue. These risks are an important reason to institute intensified preconception management of diabetes. During pregnancy, sequential ophthalmologic examinations are essential in women with type 1 or type 2 diabetes, and laser photocoagulation treatment of the retina may be necessary.

Diabetic nephropathy. The risk of worsening of diabetic nephropathy during pregnancy depends on baseline renal function and the degree of hypertension. Total urinary albumin excretion does not increase substantially in normal pregnancy, but total urinary protein collections, which obstetricians have used to define preeclampsia, may show a twofold increase in uncomplicated gestation. Diabetic women with microalbuminuria (30-299 mg/24 h) may have worsening of the albuminuria during pregnancy and 15% to 45% develop the preeclamptic syndrome. Albuminuria usually regresses postpartum. Women with macroalbuminuria (24-hour urinary albumin >300 mg) and well-preserved renal function (serum creatinine <1.2 mg/dL [<106 μmol/L]; creatinine clearance >80 mL/min) at the beginning of pregnancy are likely to have moderate decline in renal function during gestation, and approximately 6% may have renal failure at follow-up several years after pregnancy. The latter figure may not be different from the course of diabetic nephropathy in nonpregnant women with this level of renal dysfunction. If initial renal function in pregnancy is impaired (serum creatinine >1.2 mg/dL [>106 μmol/L]; creatinine clearance <80 mL/min), then 35% to 40% are expected to show further decline during pregnancy, and 45% to 50% have renal failure at follow-up several years later. Thus, careful preconception counseling is important for these patients and their family members.

Management

Pregnant women with preexisiting diabetes should ideally receive care in a multidisciplinary clinic staffed by obstetricians, endocrinologists, diabetes nurse specialists, dietitians, and specialist midwives. There is substantial evidence that this improves the outcomes in women with pregestational diabetes.

Preconception counseling. All diabetic women of reproductive age should be counseled to use adequate birth control and plan their pregnancies. Before any planned pregnancy, the couple should be referred for preconception assessment and counseling. There should be assessment and discussion regarding management of diabetic complications. Baseline measurements should include thyroid function tests including autoantibodies; early morning spot urine albumin/creatinine ratio; urinalysis to rule out asymptomatic bacteriuria; retinal examination; and cardiological assessment in high-risk patients such as those with evidence of microvascular disease. ACE inhibitors and ARBs cannot be used during pregnancy. If necessary, alternative antihypertensive agents that are safe for use in pregnancy (methyldopa, nifedipine, amlodipine, labetolol) should be prescribed. Lipidlowering therapies are also contraindicated, and lipid abnormalities must be managed by dietary measures. There should be discussion of risks and expected management strategies in the pregnancy. The patient should be given glycemic goals with the aim of achieving control as close to normal as possible before conception.

Glucose and insulin management. Women are seen every 2 to 4 weeks in the first and second trimester and then every 1 to 2 weeks until 36 weeks and then weekly to term. The goal of glucose management during pregnancy is to prevent both preprandial and postprandial hyperglycemia. Patients with type 2 diabetes on oral agents are usually switched to insulin treatment during pregnancy. There are small nonrandomized studies suggesting that metformin use is safe in the first trimester. The drug does cross the placenta, but it has not been associated with teratogenesis. Glyburide does not significantly cross the placenta, and studies in gestational diabetes suggest that it may be relatively safe late in pregnancy. Exposure to glyburide early in pregnancy does not appear to be associated with any harm but data are limited. Until randomized control studies of metformin and glyburide use at conception and early pregnancy are available, caution should be exercised regarding their use early in pregnancy.

Perinatal outcome is optimal if patients aim for fasting plasma glucose levels below 100 mg/dL (5.6 mmol/L) and postprandial levels below 130 mg/dL (7.2 mmol/L). For patients with a history of recurrent severe hypoglycemic reactions, somewhat higher blood glucose targets should be selected. Self-monitoring of capillary blood glucose should be performed eight or more times a day. Occasional monitoring in the middle of the night is recommended to monitor for nocturnal hypoglycemia. There is evidence that continuous glucose monitoring systems may be helpful in reducing both hyperglycemia and hypoglycemic excursions. These systems do not replace self-monitoring of blood glucose but allow for fine-tuning of glycemic control and alert the patient to rapid changes in glucose levels. One randomized study showed that pregnancies using continuous glucose monitoring had better glycemic control in the third trimester and lower risk of macrosomia. Clinical trials using continuous glucose monitors during pregnancy are currently underway. Confirmation of long-term control is provided by sequential measurement of glycosylated hemoglobin and fructosamine every 4 to 6 weeks.

Patients should see the nutritionist to assess caloric needs and get instructed on carbohydrate counting. The caloric intake is based on ideal body weight and it is approximated 30 to 35 kcal/kg for normal-weight women; about 24 kcal/kg current weight for overweight women; and 10 to 15 kcal/kg current weight for obese women. All patients should learn how to self-adjust their doses of short-acting insulin based on planned carbohydrate load or premeal blood glucose levels.

Type 1 patients are typically on a basal bolus insulin regimen (see Table 17–16). Currently, NPH is the only intermediate insulin available for basal coverage during pregnancy. Typically a type 1 patient might require up to three small injections of NPH to provide adequate basal coverage using short-acting insulin analogs to control the glucose rise with meals. Studies on insulin glargine use during pregnancy are limited. Retrospective case control studies have not shown any adverse effects of glargine use at the time of conception and during pregnancy. Many type 1 patients elect to use insulin pumps during pregnancy. Since the risk of diabetic ketoacidosis is increased with pump use, it is especially critical that patients have adequate instruction on the use of insulin pumps and can troubleshoot any problems that may arise.

Women with type 2 diabetes can be managed with regular insulin or short-acting insulin analogs before meals and NPH insulin at bedtime. Sometimes NPH insulin is also required in the morning.

Total insulin requirements vary during gestation. There is usually an increase in insulin dose between weeks 3 and 7, then a slight decrease between weeks 7 and 15 followed by a gradual increase until about week 35. The insulin requirements in type 1 diabetes at around 35 weeks (1.0 U/kg/24 h) are almost double the prepregnancy requirements. Women with type 2 diabetes usually start out with higher doses and may eventually require as much as 1.5 to 2 U/kg/24 h. Exercise can improve insulin sensitivity and should be encouraged in type 2 patients. The benefits of exercise are less obvious in women with type 1 diabetes, and there is always a concern about exercise-induced hypoglycemia.

TABLE 17–27   Schedule of obstetric tests and procedures.

Procedure	Risk Based on Glycemic Control, Presence of Vascular Disease	
	Low Risk	**High Risk**
Ultrasound to date gestation	8-12 wk	8-12 wk
Prenatal genetic diagnosis	As needed	As needed
Targeted perinatal ultrasound; fetal echocardiography	18-22 wk	18-22 wk
Fetal kick counts	28 wk	28 wk
Ultrasound for fetal growth	28 and 37 wk[a]	Every 3-8 wk
Antepartum FHR monitoring, backup with biophysical profile	36 wk, weekly	27 wk, 1-3 per wk
Amniocentesis for lung	…	35-38 wk
Induction of labor	41 wk[b]	35-38 wk

[a]Not needed in normoglycemic, diet-treated women with gestational diabetes mellitus.
[b]Earlier for obstetric reasons or for impending fetal macrosomia.

Hypoglycemic reactions are more frequent and sometimes more severe in early gestation but are a risk at any time during pregnancy. Therefore, insulin-treated patients should take snacks between meals and at bedtime to prevent hypoglycemia. Family members should be instructed in the use of glucagon. Hypoglycemic reactions have not been associated with fetal death or congenital anomalies, but they pose a risk to maternal health.

Fetal monitoring (Table 17–27). First-trimester ultrasound is often obtained to document viability, as the rate of miscarriage is higher in women with diabetes, and to estimate gestational age. A second-trimester, detailed ultrasound examination of fetal anatomy is performed at approximately 18 weeks for detection of congenital anomalies. Ultrasound examination in the third trimester (at 28-32 weeks and 38 weeks) is performed to assess fetal growth.

Antepartum fetal testing is recommended using fetal movement counting, biophysical profile, nonstress test (NST), and/or contraction stress test (CST) initiated at 32 to 34 weeks of gestation. Most simply, the infrequency of fetal movement as noted in regular fetal kick counts (fewer than four per hour) may indicate fetal jeopardy. The fetal biophysical profile is a rigorous analysis of fetal activity patterns using ultrasound to assess gross body movements, the tone of the limbs, and chest wall motions as well as reactivity of the fetal heart rate (FHR) and the volume of amniotic fluid. The presence of FHR accelerations and long-range variability on the NST and the absence of late decelerations (lower FHR persisting after the contraction subsides) on the CST indicate that the fetus is well oxygenated. Generally, the NST and CST are sensitive screening tests, and abnormal results of FHR monitoring in these tests overestimate the diagnosis of fetal distress. Therefore, it is wise to obtain additional evidence of fetal jeopardy (by biophysical ultrasonographic assessment) before cesarean delivery is recommended in preterm pregnancies. In term gestation with abnormal fetal testing, there is little to be gained by continuing the pregnancy. In complicated patients with intrauterine growth retardation, oligohydramnios, preeclampsia, or poor blood glucose control, testing may start as early as 26 weeks and is performed more frequently.

Timing of delivery. Unless maternal or fetal complications arise, the goal for delivery in diabetic women should be 38 to 41 weeks in order to reduce neonatal morbidity from preterm deliveries. On the other hand, the obstetrician may wish to induce labor before 39 weeks, if there is concern about increasing fetal weight. Before a preterm delivery decision (<37 weeks) is made or delivery is considered in women with poor glycemic control at 37 to 38 weeks of gestation, fetal pulmonary maturity should be determined. Tests for maturity using amniocentesis assess risk of neonatal respiratory distress syndrome and include the lecithin-sphingomyelin (L/S) ratio, phosphatidylglycerol, and other biochemical or physical assays of surfactant activity. In pregnancies complicated by hyperglycemia, fetal hyperinsulinemia can lead to low pulmonary surfactant apoprotein production. The lowest risk of respiratory distress syndrome is attained by delaying delivery (if possible) until 38 to 41 weeks and minimizing the need for cesarean sections.

Route of delivery. Once fetal lung maturity is likely, the route of delivery must be selected based on the usual obstetric indications. If the fetus seems large (>4200 g) on clinical and ultrasonographic examination of diabetic women, cesarean section probably should be performed because of the possibility of shoulder dystocia and birth trauma. Otherwise, induction of labor is reasonable, because maternal and peripartum risks are fewer following vaginal delivery. Once labor is underway, continuous FHR monitoring is essential. Maternal blood glucose levels greater than 150 mg/dL (8.3 mmol/L) can be associated with intrapartum fetal hypoxia.

Insulin and glucose management during labor and delivery. It is important to avoid maternal hyperglycemia during labor because it increases the risk for fetal acidemia and neonatal hypoglycemia. The goal is to maintain glucose levels between 70 and 110 mg/dL (3.9-6.1 mmol/L). Maternal glucose levels above 180 mg/dL (10 mmol/L) are consistently associated with neonatal hypoglycemia. During the latent phase of labor, maternal metabolic demands are fairly stable but there is significant energy expenditure during active labor and delivery and insulin needs are minimal. Glucose control is typically managed using intravenous dextrose (at 100-125 mL/h) and insulin infusions (Table 17–28).

After delivery of the placenta, the insulin-resistant state rapidly disappears, and insulin requirements are close to prepregnancy levels. Type 1 or type 2 patients who were previously on insulin can go back to their usual prepregnancy insulin regimens and doses once they start eating. Type 2 patients who were on oral agents prepregnancy frequently do not require any medication during the first 24 to 48 hours postpartum. They can stay on insulin while breastfeeding or go on metformin or glyburide which are safe while breastfeeding.

Neonatal management. Planning for the care of the infant should be started prior to delivery, with participation by the pediatrician or neonatologist in decisions about timing and management of delivery. In complicated cases, the pediatrician must

TABLE 17–28   Protocol for intrapartum insulin infusion.[a]

Intravenous Fluids

If blood glucose is >130 mg/dL (>7.2 mmol/L), infuse mainline Ringer lactate at a rate of 125 mL/h.

If blood glucose is <130 mg/dL (<7.2 mmol/L), infuse mainline Ringer lactate to keep vein open and begin Ringer lactate and 5% dextrose at a rate of 125 mL/h controlled by infusion pump.

Insulin Infusion

Mix 100 U of regular human insulin (U100) in 100 mL NaCl 0.9% and piggyback to mainline. The concentration is 1 U/mL. Adjust intravenous insulin hourly according to the following table when the blood glucose is >70 mg/dL (>3.9 mmol/L). Target blood glucose 70 to 110 mg/dL.

Blood Glucose in mg/dL(mmol/L)	Type 1	Type 2	Gestational Diabetes	Custom
<70 (<3.9)	No insulin	No insulin	No insulin	
71-90 (3.9-5)	0.5 U/h	No insulin	No insulin	
91-110 (5.1-6.1)	1	1 U/h	No insulin	
111-130 (6.2-7.2)	1.5	2	1 U/h	
131-150 (7.3-8.3)	2	3	2	
151-170 (8.4-9.4)	2.5	4	3	
171-190 (9.5-10.6)	3	5	4	
>190 (>10.6)	Call MD and check urine ketones			

[a]Protocol useful also for diabetic pregnant women who are "NPO" or being treated with beta-adrenergic tocolysis or corticosteroids. The scale dosages may need to be doubled for the latter. Boluses of short-acting insulin must be used to cover meals.

be in attendance to learn about antenatal problems, to assess the need for resuscitation, to identify major congenital anomalies, and to plan initial therapy for the sick infant if required. Infants of mothers with poorly controlled diabetes have an increased risk of respiratory distress syndrome. Possible reasons include abnormal production of pulmonary surfactant or connective tissue changes leading to decreased pulmonary compliance. However, in recent years, the incidence of respiratory distress syndrome in these pregnancies has declined from 24% to 5%, probably related to better maternal glycemic control, selected use of amniotic fluid tests, and delivery of most infants at term. Other possible problems in infants of diabetic mothers include hypocalcemia less than 7 mg/dL (1.75 mmol/L), hyperbilirubinemia greater than 15 mg/dL (256 μmol/L), polycythemia (central hematocrit >70%), and poor feeding. These complications are presumably related to fetal hyperglycemia and hyperinsulinemia and probably to intermittent low-level fetal hypoxia. Improved control of the maternal diabetic state has reduced their incidence.

Gestational Diabetes

Gestational diabetes (GDM) is defined as glucose intolerance that develops or is first recognized during pregnancy. As insulin resistance increases during pregnancy, euglycemia depends on a compensatory increase in insulin secretion. Failure to compensate with increased insulin secretion leads to gestational diabetes. As the increase in insulin resistance is greatest in the third trimester, GDM usually develops going into this period. The prevalence of GDM in a population is reflective of the prevalence of type 2 diabetes in that population. In low-risk populations, such as those found in Sweden, the prevalence in population-based studies is lower than 2% even when universal testing is offered, while studies in high-risk populations, such as the Native American Cree, Northern Californian Hispanics, and Northern Californian Asians, reported prevalence rates ranging from 4.9% to 12.8%. Other risk factors include a history of macrosomia (birth weight >4000 g), polycystic ovarian syndrome, essential hypertension or pregnancy-related hypertension, history of spontaneous abortions and unexplained still births, family history of diabetes, obesity, age older than 25 years, and history of gestational diabetes (Table 17–29).

Women with GDM are at increased risk for urinary tract infections, pyelonephritis, asymptomatic bacteriuria, and preeclampsia. There is a 10% risk of polyhydramnios. Fetal risks of poor glucose control include stillbirths and macrosomia. There is no increase in risk for congenital anomalies since the glucose intolerance develops later in pregnancy.

Strategies for diagnosis are outlined in Table 17–30. Currently, international consensus is lacking regarding the diagnostic criteria for GDM. The 100 g 3-hour OGTT test is commonly used in the United States and the 75 g 2-hour WHO test is used in many other countries. The risk assessment for GDM (see Table 17–29) should be performed at the first prenatal visit. Those women at high risk should undergo OGTT testing as soon as feasible. If the test is negative, then they should be retested at 24 to 28 weeks of gestation. A fasting plasma glucose of ≥126 mg/dL or random glucose of ≥200 mg/dL confirmed on repeat testing is diagnostic of diabetes and negates the need to perform a glucose challenge test. Lower risk women are screened for GDM using a two-step protocol performed at 24 to 28 weeks. First, a glucose challenge test is performed using a 50 g glucose load. The patient does not have to be fasting. A 1-hour plasma glucose value of 140 mg/dL (7.8 mmol/L) or greater identifies approximately 80% of women with GDM; decreasing the cutoff value to 130 mg/dL (7.2 mmol/L)

TABLE 17–29   Risk factors for gestational diabetes mellitus.

Maternal age >37 y
Ethnicity
Indian subcontinent—11-fold
Southeast Asian—eightfold
Arab/Mediterranean—sixfold
Afro-Caribbean—threefold
Prepregnancy weight >80 kg or BMI>28 kg/m^2
Family history of diabetes in first-degree relative
Previous macrosomia/polyhydramnios
Previous unexplained stillbirth
Polycystic ovarian syndrome

TABLE 17–30   Screening and diagnosis of gestational diabetes.

Perform blood glucose testing at 24-28 wk
Two-step protocol:
  A. Glucose challenge test: 1-h plasma glucose after 50 g
     glucose load.
     ≥140 mg/dL (≥7.8 mmol/L) identifies ~80 of women with GDM;
     ≥130 mg/dL (≥7.2 mmol/L) increases sensitivity to ~90%.
  B. 100 g OGTT: If a woman meets or exceeds threshold on glucose
     challenge test then perform fasting diagnostic 100 g OGTT within
     a week. The test is performed after an at least 8-h overnight
     fast and after at least 3 d of unrestricted diet (≥150 g
     carbohydrate per day). Subject should be seated and should not
     smoke during test.
The test is positive if two of the following glucose levels are found.
  Fasting: ≥95 mg/dL (≥5.3 mmol/L)
  1 h: ≥180 mg/dL (≥10 mmol/L)
  2 h: ≥155 mg/dL (≥ 8.6 mmol/L)
  3 h: ≥140 mg/dL (≥7.8 mmol/L)
If one value is abnormal, repeat test in 4 wk
  One step protocol:
     Perform diagnostic 100 g OGTT testing as soon as feasible. If
     negative, repeat at 24-28 wk.

Adapted from Summary and Recommendations, Fourth International Workshop-Conference on Gestational Diabetes Mellitus. *Diabetes Care.* 1998;21(suppl 2):B162.

increases the sensitivity to approximately 90%. Women with the positive glucose challenge test should undergo a 3-hour 100 g oral glucose tolerance test within the week.

Although there is continuing debate regarding universal screening, recent studies are supportive of this position. An observational study of Caucasian women, where all were tested with the oral glucose tolerance test, found that the prevalence of GDM among women with no risk factors was 2.8%. Excluding this low-risk group would still require 80% of women to be tested and would miss 10% of all cases of GDM. The Hyperglycemia and Pregnancy Outcome (HAPO) study reported a continuous relationship between glucose concentration with the 28-week oral glucose tolerance test and neonatal adiposity, cesarean sections, neonatal hypoglycemia, premature delivery, shoulder dystocia, need for intensive neonatal care, hyperbilirubinemia, and preeclampsia. A study by Landon and colleagues of women with mild GDM on a 100 g 3-hour glucose tolerance test found that treatment reduced the risk of fetal overgrowth, shoulder dystocia, cesarean delivery, and hypertensive disorders. The ADA policy states that screening may be omitted in low-risk women. The United States Preventive Services Task Force on Preventive Health Care has concluded that there is not enough evidence to support or deny universal screening for GDM. Women who have a history of GDM with previous pregnancy should undergo preconception counseling similar to those patients with pregestational diabetes. They should begin to monitor their glucose levels when they begin to try to conceive or as soon as their new pregnancy is confirmed. These women do not need retesting for GDM.

HbA$_{1c}$ values are helpful for assessment of pregestational diabetes but are not helpful for management of GDM where they are normal.

The goal of therapy is prevention of fasting and postprandial hyperglycemia. The Australian Carbohydrate Intolerance Study in Pregnant Women (ACHOIS) trial found that intervention to lower glucose levels to less than 100 mg/dL before meals and less than 126 mg/dL 2 hours after meals reduced the rate of serious perinatal outcomes (defined as death, shoulder dystocia, bone fracture, and nerve palsy) from 4% to 1%. After diagnosis, the patient should be placed on a diabetic meal plan modified for pregnancy. The caloric intake is based on ideal body weight—25 to –35 kcal/kg ideal weight, 40% to 55% carbohydrate, 20% protein, and 25% to 40% fat. Calories are distributed over three meals and three snacks (see Table 17–25). Most patients can be taught to count their carbohydrates and to read food labels. This caloric distribution will help 75% to 80% of patients to become normoglycemic. Patients should also be encouraged to participate in moderate aerobic exercise such as walking or antenatal exercise classes, of at least 15 to 30-minutes duration, three or more times a week. In normal pregnancy, expected weight gain varies according to the prepregnancy weight. The Fifth International Workshop-Conference on GDM recommends a relatively small gain during pregnancy of 7 kg (15 lb) for obese women (BMI ≥30 kg/m^2) and a proportionally greater weight gain (up to 18 kg or 40 lb) for underweight women (BMI <18.5 kg/m^2) at the onset of pregnancy. However, there are no data on optimal weight gain for women with GDM.

If fasting capillary blood glucose levels exceed 90 to 100 mg/dL (5-5.6 mmol/L) or if 1-hour or 2-hour postprandial glucose values are consistently greater, respectively, than 130 or 105 mg/dL (7.2 or 5.8 mmol/L), therapy is begun with insulin. The total insulin dose varies from 0.7 to 2 U/kg. NPH is the preferred long-acting insulin. Insulin glargine and insulin detemir have not been well studied. Insulin aspart or lispro and regular insulin can be used. Hypoglycemia is a risk factor with aggressive management of glucose levels with insulin. Patients and family members should be instructed on monitoring for and treating hypoglycemia.

Metformin and glyburide can be considered as alternative options to insulin therapy. Metformin does cross the placenta but has not been associated with teratogenesis. The advantage of this drug is that it does not result in hypoglycemia. An open label study (the MiG trial) of 751 women with GDM at 20 to 33 weeks' gestation randomized to either metformin or insulin did not show a difference in primary composite outcome of neonatal complications. Forty-six percent of the subjects on metformin did, however, require supplemental insulin. Glyburide does not significantly cross the placenta. Langer and colleagues randomized 404 women with GDM at 11 to 33 weeks' gestation to glyburide therapy or insulin treatment. There was no significant difference in fetal outcomes in the two groups—large for gestational infants, macrosomia, neonatal ICU admission, or fetal abnormalities. Target glycemic control was achieved in 88% of patients on insulin and 82% on glyburide. There was significant reduction in maternal hypoglycemic episodes in the glyburide group compared to the insulin group (2% vs 20%). There were some differences in neonatal outcomes such as more neonatal hypoglycemia in the glyburide arm. The study was not adequately powered, however, to determine the statistical significance of these differences.

Patients are usually scheduled for follow-up visits every 1 to 2 weeks. A 24-hour urine collection may be performed to establish baseline level of proteinuria and creatinine clearance due to the higher likelihood of preeclampsia. It is not necessary to routinely perform ophthalmic examinations in these patients unless there is a strong suspicion of preexisting type 2 diabetes mellitus. Fetal monitoring is warranted in those patients who are not well controlled, requiring insulin therapy, or who have other complications of pregnancy. The most commonly used test is a twice-weekly nonstress test.

If blood glucose levels are close to normal and there are no other complications, the delivery can go to term. It is generally recommended that the pregnancy does not go beyond term. Most patients do not require insulin during delivery. Blood glucose levels should be monitored the following day to ensure that the patient has reverted to normoglycemia. About 95% of patients return to normal glucose status.

Progression to type 2 diabetes later in life occurs in 5% to 50% of women with gestational diabetes. The wide range in incidence is influenced by body weight, family history, glucose levels, and the need for insulin treatment during pregnancy—and the choice of contraception and lifestyle after pregnancy. All patients with gestational diabetes should undergo a 75 g 2-hour glucose tolerance test at 6 to 10 weeks after delivery to guide future medical management. Follow-up protocols after pregnancy and criteria for the diagnosis of diabetes mellitus in the nonpregnant state are presented in Table 17–11.

REFERENCES

The Endocrine Pancreas

Andralojc KM, Mercalli A, Nowak KW, et al. Ghrelin-producing epsilon cells in the developing and adult human pancreas. *Diabetologia.* 2009;52:486. [PMID: 19096824]

Baggio LL, Drucker DJ. Biology of incretins: GLP-1 and GIP. *Gastroenterology.* 2007;132:2131. [PMID: 17498508]

Cabrera O, Berman DM, Kenyon NS, et al. The unique cytoarchitecture of human pancreatic islets has implications for islet cell function. *Proc Natl Acad Sci USA.* 2006;103:2334. [PMID: 16461897]

Gross DN, van den Heuvel AP, Birnbaum MJ. The role of FOXO in the regulation of metabolism. *Oncogene.* 2008;27:2320. [PMID: 18391974]

Hiriart M, Aguilar-Bryan L. Channel regulation of glucose sensing in the pancreatic beta-cell. *Am J Physiol Endocrinol Metab.* 2008;295:E1298. [PMID: 18940941]

Kieffer TJ, McIntosh CH, Pederson RA. Degradation of glucose-dependent insulinotropic polypeptide and truncated glucagon-like peptide 1 *in vitro* and *in vivo* by dipeptidyl peptidase IV. *Endocrinology.* 1995;136:3585. [PMID: 7628397]

McCarthy MI, Hattersley AT. Learning from molecular genetics: novel insights arising from the definition of genes for monogenic and type 2 diabetes. *Diabetes.* 2008;57:2889. [PMID: 18971436]

Meier JJ, Butler AE, Saisho Y, et al. Beta-cell replication is the primary mechanism subserving the postnatal expansion of beta-cell mass in humans. *Diabetes.* 2008;57:1584. [PMID: 18334605]

Ohneda K, Ee H, German M. Regulation of insulin gene transcription. *Semin Cell Dev Biol.* 2000;11:227. [PMID: 10966856]

Oliver-Krasinski JM, Stoffers DA. On the origin of the beta cell. *Genes Dev.* 2008;22:1998. [PMID: 18676806]

Rorsman P, Renstrom E. Insulin granule dynamics in pancreatic beta cells. *Diabetologia.* 2003;46:1029. [PMID: 12879249]

Sinclair EM, Drucker DJ. Proglucagon-derived peptides: mechanisms of action and therapeutic potential. *Physiology (Bethesda).* 2005;20:357. [PMID: 16174875]

Smith, SB, Qu, HQ, Taleb, N, et al. Rfx6 directs islet formation and insulin production in mice and humans. *Nature.* 2010;463:775. [PMID: 20148032]

Steinberg GR, Kemp BE. AMPK in health and disease. *Physiol Rev.* 2009;89:1025. [PMID: 19584320]

Tontonoz P, Spiegelman BM. Fat and beyond: the diverse biology of PPAR gamma. *Annu Rev Biochem.* 2008;77:289. [PMID: 18518822]

Vaxillaire M, Froguel P. Monogenic diabetes in the young, pharmacogenetics and relevance to multifactorial forms of type 2 diabetes. *Endocr Rev.* 2008;29:254. [PMID: 18436708]

Wilson, ME, Scheel, D, German, MS. Gene expression cascades in pancreatic development. *Mech Dev.* 2003;120:65. [PMID: 12490297]

Diagnosis, Classification, and Pathophysiology of Diabetes Mellitus

Action to Control Cardiovascular Risk in Diabetes Study Group. Effects of intensive glucose lowering in type 2 diabetes. *N Engl J Med.* 2008;358:2545. [PMID: 18539917]

ADVANCE Collaborative Group. Intensive blood glucose control and vascular outcomes in patients with type 2 diabetes. *N Engl J Med.* 2008;358:2560. [PMID: 18539916]

American Diabetes Association. Diagnosis and classification of diabetes mellitus. *Diabetes Care.* 2010;33(suppl 1):S62. [PMID: 20042775]

Bell GI, Polonsky KS. Diabetes mellitus and genetically programmed defects in beta-cell function. *Nature.* 2001;414:788. [PMID: 11742410]

Biddinger SB, Kahn CR. From mice to men: insights into the insulin resistance syndromes. *Annu Rev Physiol.* 2006;68:123. [PMID: 16460269]

Bluestone, JA, Herold, K, Eisenbarth, G. Genetics, pathogenesis and clinical interventions in type 1 diabetes. *Nature.* 2010;464:1293. [PMID: 20432533]

Butler, AE, Janson, J, Bonner-Weir, S, et al. Beta-cell deficit and increased beta-cell apoptosis in humans with type 2 diabetes. *Diabetes.* 2003;52:102. [PMID: 12502499]

Cohen RM, Holmes YR, Chenier TC, Joiner CH. Discordance between HbA1c and fructosamine: evidence for a glycosylation gap and its relation to diabetic nephropathy. *Diab Care.* 2003;26:16. [PMID: 12502674]

Diabetes Prevention Trial, Type 1 Diabetes Study Group. Effects of insulin in relatives of patients with type 1 diabetes mellitus. *N Engl J Med.* 2002;346:1685. [PMID: 12037147]

Duckworth W, Abraira C, Moritz T, et al. VADT Investigators. Glucose control and vascular complications in veterans with type 2 diabetes. *N Engl J Med.* 2009;360:129. [PMID: 19092145]

Eisenbarth GS, Gottlieb PA. Autoimmune polyendocrine syndromes. *N Engl J Med.* 2004;350:2068. [PMID: 15141045]

Fonseca, SG, Fukuma, M, Lipson, KL, et al. Wfs1 is a novel component of the unfolded protein response and maintains homeostasis of the endoplasmic reticulum in pancreatic beta-cells. *J Biol Chem.* 2005;280:39609. [PMID: 16195229]

Gaede P, Lund-Andersen H, Parving HH, Pedersen O. Effect of a multifactorial intervention on mortality in type 2 diabetes. *N Engl J Med.* 2008;358:580. [PMID: 18256393]

Gaede P, Vedel P, Larsen N, Jensen GV, Parving HH, Pedersen O. Multifactorial intervention and cardiovascular disease in patients with type 2 diabetes. *N Engl J Med.* 2003;348:383. [PMID: 12556541]

Gallagher, EJ, LeRoith, D, Karnieli, E. The metabolic syndrome—from insulin resistance to obesity and diabetes. *Endocrinol Metab Clin North Am.* 2008;37:559. [PMID: 18775352]

Gandhi, GY, Basu, R, Dispenzieri, A, et al. Endocrinopathy in POEMS syndrome: the Mayo Clinic experience. *Mayo Clin Proc.* 2007;82:836. [PMID: 17605964]

Gottlieb PA, Eisenbarth GS. Diagnosis and treatment of pre-insulin dependent diabetes. *Annu Rev Med.* 1998;49:391. [PMID: 9509271]

Greeley, SA, Tucker, SE, Worrell, HI, et al. Update in neonatal diabetes. *Curr Opin Endocrinol Diabetes Obes.* 2010;17:13. [PMID: 19952737]

Harris R, Donahue K, Rathore SS, Frame P, Woolf SH, Lohr KN. Screening adults for type 2 diabetes: a review of the evidence for the U.S. Preventive Services Task Force. *Ann Intern Med.* 2003;138:215. [PMID: 12558362]

Herold KC, Hagopian W, Auger JA, et al. Anti-CD3 monoclonal antibody in new-onset type 1 diabetes mellitus. *N Engl J Med*. 2002;346:1692. [PMID: 12037148]

Holman RR, Paul SK, Bethel MA, Matthews DR, Neil HA. 10-year follow-up of intensive glucose control in type 2 diabetes. *N Engl J Med*. 2008;359:1577. [PMID: 18784090]

Holman RR, Paul SK, Bethel MA, Neil HA, Matthews DR. Long-term follow-up after tight control of blood pressure in type 2 diabetes. *N Engl J Med*. 2008;359:1565. [PMID: 18784091]

Hull, RL, Westermark, GT, Westermark, P, et al. Islet amyloid: a critical entity in the pathogenesis of type 2 diabetes. *J Clin Endocrinol Metab*. 2004;89:3629. [PMID: 15292279]

International Expert Committee. International Expert Committee report on the role of the A1C assay in the diagnosis of diabetes. *Diab Care*. 2009;32:1327 [PMID: 19502545]

Knowler WC, Barrett-Connor E, Fowler SE, et al. Reduction in the incidence of type 2 diabetes with lifestyle intervention or metformin. *N Engl J Med*. 2002;346:393. [PMID: 11832527]

Kahn, R, Buse, J, Ferrannini, E, et al. The metabolic syndrome: time for a critical appraisal: joint statement from the American Diabetes Association and the European Association for the Study of Diabetes. *Diab Care*. 2005;28:2289. [PMID: 16123508]

Kahn SE. The relative contributions of insulin resistance and beta-cell dysfunction to the pathophysiology of type 2 diabetes. *Diabetologia*. 2003;46:3. [PMID: 12637977]

Monajemi, H, Stroes, E, Hegele, RA, et al. Inherited lipodystrophies and the metabolic syndrome. *Clin Endocrinol (Oxf)*. 2007;67:479. [PMID: 17561981]

Nathan DM, Kuenen J, Borg R, Zheng H, Schoenfeld D, Heine RJ. A1c-Derived Average Glucose Study Group. Translating the A1C assay into estimated average glucose values. *Diab Care*. 2008;31(8):1473. [PMID: 18540046]

Ohkubo Y, Kishikawa H, Araki E, et al. Intensive insulin therapy prevents the progression of diabetic microvascular complications in Japanese patients with non-insulin-dependent diabetes mellitus: a randomized prospective 6-year study. *Diab Res Clin Pract*. 1995;28:103. [PMID: 7587918]

Olefsky JM, Glass CK. Macrophages, inflammation, and insulin resistance. *Annu Rev Physiol*. 2010;72:219. [PMID: 20148674]

O'Rahilly S. Human genetics illuminates the paths to metabolic disease. *Nature*. 2009;462:307. [PMID: 19924209]

Savage, DB, Petersen, KF, Shulman, GI. Disordered lipid metabolism and the pathogenesis of insulin resistance. *Physiol Rev*. 2007;87:507. [PMID: 17429039]

Shichiri M, Kishikawa H, Ohkubo Y, Wake N. Long term results of the Kumamoto Study on optimal diabetes control in type 2 diabetic patients. *Diab Care*. 2000;23(suppl 2):B21. [PMID: 10860187]

Simha V, Garg A. Inherited lipodystrophies and hypertriglyceridemia. *Curr Opin Lipidol*. 2009;20:300. [PMID: 19494770]

Stumvoll M, Gerich J. Clinical features of insulin resistance and beta cell dysfunction and the relationship to type 2 diabetes. *Clin Lab Med*. 2001;21:31. [PMID: 11321936]

The Diabetes Control and Complications Trial Research Group. The effect of intensive treatment of diabetes on the development and progression of long-term complications in insulin-dependent diabetes mellitus. *N Engl J Med*. 1993;329:977. [PMID: 8366922]

The Diabetes Control and Complications Trial/Epidemiology of Diabetes Interventions and Complications Research Group. Retinopathy and nephropathy in patients with type 1 diabetes four years after a trial of intensive therapy. *N Engl J Med*. 2000;342:381. [PMID: 10666428]

The Diabetes Control and Complications Trial/Epidemiology of Diabetes Interventions and Complications (DCCT/EDIC) Study Research Group. Intensive diabetes treatment and cardiovascular disease in patients with type 1 diabetes. *N Engl J Med*. 2005;353:2643. [PMID: 16371630]

The Juvenile Diabetes Research Foundation Continuous Glucose Monitoring Study Group. Continuous glucose monitoring and intensive treatment of type 1 diabetes. *N Engl J Med*. 2008;359:1464. [PMID: 18779236]

Turnbull FM, Abraira C, Anderson RJ, et al. Intensive glucose control and macrovascular outcomes in type 2 diabetes. *Diabetologia*. 2009;52:2288. [PMID: 19655124]

Turner RC, Cull CA, Frighi V, Holman RR. Glycemic control with diet, sulfonylurea, metformin, or insulin in patients with type 2 diabetes mellitus: progressive requirement for multiple therapies (UKPDS 49). *JAMA*. 1999;281:2005. [PMID: 10359389]

UK Prospective Diabetes Study (UKPDS) Group. Effect of intensive blood-glucose control with metformin on complications in overweight patients with type 2 diabetes (UKPDS 34). *Lancet*. 1998;352:854.

UK Prospective Diabetes Study Group. Efficacy of atenolol and captopril in reducing risk of acrovascular and microvascular complications in type 2 diabetes: UKPDS 39. *BMJ*. 1998;317:713. [PMID: 9732338]

UK Prospective Diabetes Study Group. Intensive blood-glucose control with sulphonylureas or insulin compared with conventional treatment and risk of complications in patients with type 2 diabetes (UKPDS 33). *Lancet* .1998;352:837. [PMID: 9742976]

UK Prospective Diabetes Study Group. Tight blood pressure control and risk of macrovascular and microvascular complications in type 2 diabetes (UKPDS38). *BMJ*. 1998;317:703. [PMID: 732337]

U.S. Preventive Services Task Force Recommendation Statement. Screening for type 2 diabetes mellitus in adults. *Ann Intern Med*. 2008;148:846. [PMID: 18519930]

Vaxillaire M, Froguel P. Monogenic diabetes in the young, pharmacogenetics and relevance to multifactorial forms of type 2 diabetes. *Endocr Rev*. 2008;29:254. [PMID: 18436708]

Wajchenberg BL. Subcutaneous and visceral adipose tissue: their relation to the metabolic syndrome. *Endocr Rev*. 2000;21:697. [PMID: 11133069]

Wenzlau, JM, Frisch, LM, Gardner, TJ, et al. Novel antigens in type 1 diabetes: the importance of znt8. *Curr Diab Rep*. 2009;9:105. [PMID: 19323954]

Treatment of Diabetes Mellitus

Ahrén B. Clinical results of treating type 2 diabetic patients with sitagliptin, vildagliptin or saxagliptin—diabetes control and potential adverse events. *Best Pract Res Clin Endocrinol Metab*. 2009;23:487. [PMID: 19748066]

American Diabetes Association. Standards of medical care in diabetes—2010. *Diab Care*. 2010;33(suppl 1):S11. [PMID: 20042772]

American Diabetes Association. Physical activity/exercise and diabetes mellitus (position statement). *Diab Care*. 2004;27(suppl 1):S58. [PMID: 14693927]

Bode BW, Tamborlane WV, Davidson PC. Insulin pump therapy in the 21st century. Strategies for successful use in adults, adolescents and children with diabetes. *Postgrad Med*. 2002;111:69. [PMID: 12040864]

Bolli GB. Physiological insulin replacement in type 1 diabetes mellitus. *Exp Clin Endocrinol Diabetes*. 2001;109(suppl 2):5317. [PMID: 11723567]

Boner G, Cao Z, Cooper ME. Combination antihypertensive therapy in the treatment of diabetic nephropathy. *Diabetes Technol Ther*. 2002;4:313. [PMID: 12165170]

Brunkhorst FM, Engel C, Bloos F, et al. German Competence Network Sepsis (SepNet). Intensive insulin therapy and pentastarch resuscitation in severe sepsis. *N Engl J Med*. 2008;358:125. [PMID: 18184958]

Coursin DB, Connery LE, Ketzler JT. Perioperative diabetic and hyperglycemic management issues. *Crit Care Med*. 2004;32(4 suppl):S116. [PMID: 15064670]

Cryer PE. The barrier of hypoglycemia in diabetes. *Diabetes*. 2008;57:3169. [PMID: 19033403]

Daneman D. Type 1 diabetes. *Lancet*. 2006;367(9513):847. [PMID: 16530579]

Del Pilar Solano M, Goldberg RB. Management of diabetic dyslipidemia. *Endocrinol Metab Clin North Am*. 2005;34:1. [PMID: 15752919]

DeWitt DE, Hirsch IB. Outpatient insulin therapy in type 1 and type 2 diabetes mellitus: scientific review. *JAMA*. 2003;289:2254. [PMID: 12734137]

Drucker DJ, Sherman SI, Gorelick FS, Bergenstal RM, Sherwin RS, Buse JB. Incretin-based therapies for the treatment of type 2 diabetes: evaluation of the risks and benefits. *Diab Care*. 2010;33:428. [PMID: 20103558]

Franz MJ, Bantle JP, Beebe CA, et al. Evidence-based nutrition principles and recommendations for the treatment and prevention of diabetes and related complications. *Diab Care*. 2002;25:148. [PMID: 11772915]

Gaglia JL, Shapiro AM, Weir GC. Islet transplantation: progress and challenge. *Arch Med Res*. 2005;36:273. [PMID: 15925017]

Gandhi GY, Nuttall GA, Abel MD, et al. Intensive intraoperative insulin therapy versus conventional glucose management during cardiac surgery: a randomized trial. *Ann Intern Med.* 2007;146:233. [PMID: 17310047]

Gilliam LK, Hirsch IB. Practical aspects of real-time continuous glucose monitoring. *Diabetes Technol Ther.* 2009;11(suppl 1):S75. [PMID: 19469681]

Gray CS, Hildreth AJ, Sandercock PA, et al. Glucose-potassium-insulin infusions in the management of post-stroke hyperglycaemia: the UK Glucose Insulin in Stroke Trial (GIST-UK). *Lancet Neurol.* 2007;6:397. [PMID: 17434094]

Grundy SM, Cleeman JI, Merz CN, et al. National Heart, Lung, and Blood Institute, American College of Cardiology Foundation, American Heart Association: implications of recent clinical trials for the National Cholesterol Education Program Adult Treatment Panel III guidelines. *Circulation.* 2004;110:227. [PMID: 15249516]

Hirsch IB. Insulin analogues. *N Engl J Med.* 2005;352:174. [PMID: 15647580]

Holst JJ, Gromada J. Role of incretin hormones in the regulation of insulin secretion in diabetic and nondiabetic humans. *Am J Physiol Endocrinol Metab.* 2004;287:E199. [PMID: 15271645]

Jeitler K, Horvath K, Berghold A, et al. Continuous subcutaneous insulin infusion versus multiple daily insulin injections in patients with diabetes mellitus: systematic review and meta-analysis. *Diabetologia.* 2008;51:941. [PMID: 18351320]

Khan MA, St Peter JV, Xue JL. The metabolic syndrome: time for a critical appraisal: joint statement from the American Diabetes Association and the European Association for the Study of Diabetes. *Diab Care.* 2005;28:2289. [PMID: 16123508]

Khan M, et al. A prospective, randomized comparison of the metabolic effects of pioglitazone or rosiglitazone in patients with type 2 diabetes who were previously treated with troglitazone. *Diab Care.* 2002;25:708. [PMID: 11919129]

Krauss RM. Lipids and lipoproteins in patients with type 2 diabetes. *Diab Care.* 2004;27:1496. [PMID: 15161808]

Lee C-H, Olson P, Evans RM. Lipid metabolism, metabolic diseases, and peroxisome proliferator-activated receptors. *Endocrinology.* 2003;144:2201. [PMID: 12746275]

Massicotte A. Contrast medium-induced nephropathy: strategies for prevention. *Pharmacother.* 2008;28:1140. [PMID: 18752385]

Nathan, DM, Buse JB, Davidson MB, et al. American Diabetes Association; European Association for Study of Diabetes. Medical management of hyperglycemia in type 2 diabetes: a consensus algorithm for the initiation and adjustment of therapy: a consensus statement of the American Diabetes Association and the European Association for the Study of Diabetes. *Diab Care.* 2009;32:193. [PMID: 18945920]

Neumiller JJ. Differential chemistry (structure), mechanism of action, and pharmacology of GLP-1 receptor agonists and DPP-4 inhibitors. *J Am Pharm Assoc.* 2009;49(suppl 1):S16. [PMID: 19801361]

NICE-SUGAR Study Investigators. Intensive versus conventional glucose control in critically ill patients. *N Engl J Med.* 2009;360:1283. [PMID: 19318384]

Rucker D, Padwal R, Li SK, Curioni C, Lau DC. Long term pharmacotherapy for obesity and overweight: updated meta-analysis. *BMJ.* 2007;335:1194. [PMID: 18006966]

Snow V, Weiss KB, Mottur-Pilson C. The evidence base for tight blood pressure control in the management of type 2 diabetes mellitus. *Ann Intern Med.* 2003;138:587. [PMID: 12667031]

Stacher G. Diabetes mellitus and the stomach. *Diabetologia.* 2001;44:1080. [PMID: 11596661]

Tahrani AA, Piya MK, Kennedy A, Barnett AH. Glycaemic control in type 2 diabetes: targets and new therapies. *Pharmacol Ther.* 2010;125:328. [PMID: 19931305]

Tamborlane WV, Fredrickson LP, Ahern JH. Insulin pump therapy in childhood diabetes mellitus: guidelines for use. *Treat Endocrinol.* 2003;2:11. [PMID: 15871551]

Van den Berghe G, Wouters P, Weekers F, et al. Intensive insulin therapy in the critically ill patient. *N Engl J Med.* 2001;345:1359. [PMID: 11794168]

Van den Berghe G, Wilmer A, Hermans G, et al. Intensive insulin therapy in the medical ICU. N *Engl J Med.* 2006;354:449. [PMID: 16452557]

Vijan S, Hayward RA. Treatment of hypertension in type 2 diabetes mellitus: blood pressure goals, choice of agents, and setting priorities in diabetes care. *Ann Intern Med.* 2003;138:593. [PMID: 12667032]

Weissberg-Benchell J, Antisdel-Lomaglio J, Seshadri R. Insulin pump therapy: a meta-analysis. *Diab Care.* 2003;26:1079.[PMID: 12663577]

White SA, Shaw JA, Sutherland DE. Pancreas transplantation. *Lancet.* 2009;373:1808. [PMID: 19465236]

Yki-Jarvinen H. Thiazolidinediones. *N Engl J Med.* 2004;351:1106. [PMID:15356308]

Yusuf S, Sleight P, Pogue J, Bosch, J. Davies R, Dagenais G. Effects of an angiotensin-converting enzyme inhibitor, ramipril, on death from cardiovascular causes, myocardial infarction and stroke in high-risk patients. The Heart Outcomes Prevention Evaluation Study Investigators. *N Engl J Med.* 2000;342:145. [PMID: 10639539]

Zinman B, Ruderman N, Campaigne BN, Devlin JT, Schneider SH. American Diabetes Association. Physical activity/exercise and diabetes. *Diabetes Care.* 2004;27(suppl 1):S58. [PMID: 14693927]

Zoungas S, Ninomiya T, Huxley R, et al. Systematic review: sodium bicarbonate treatment regimens for the prevention of contrast-induced nephropathy. *Ann Intern Med.* 2009;151:631. [PMID: 19884624]

Acute Complications of Diabetes Mellitus

Herbel G, Boyle PJ. Hypoglycemia: pathophysiology and treatment. *Endocrinol Metab Clin North Am.* 2000;29:725. [PMID: 11149159]

Henderson G. The psychosocial treatment of recurrent diabetic ketoacidosis: an interdisciplinary team approach. *Diabetes Educator.* 1991;17:119. [PMID: 1899827]

Kitabchi AE, Nyenwe EA. Hyperglycemic crises in diabetes mellitus: diabetic ketoacidosis and hyperglycemic hyperosmolar state. *Endocrinol Metab Clin North Am.* 2006;35:725. [PMID: 17127143]

Luft FC. Lactic acidosis update for critical care clinicians. *J Am Soc Nephrol.* 2001;12(suppl 17):S15. [PMID: 11251027]

Nugent BW. Hyperosmolar hyperglycemic state. *Emerg Med Clin North Am.* 2005;23:629. [PMID: 15982538]

Okuda Y, Adrogue HJ, Field JB, Nohara H, Yamashita K. Counterproductive effects of sodium bicarbonate in diabetic ketoacidosis. *J Clin Endocrinol Metab.* 1996;81:314. [PMID: 8550770]

Salpeter SR, Greyber E, Pasternak GA, Salpeter EE. Risk of fatal and nonfatal lactic acidosis with metformin use in type 2 diabetes mellitus. *Cochrane Database Syst Rev.* 2010;4:CD002967. [PMID: 20091535]

Wagner A, Risse A, Brill HL, et al. Therapy of severe diabetic ketoacidosis. Zero mortality under very-low-dose insulin application. *Diab Care.* 1999;22:674. [PMID: 10332664]

Wrenn KD, Slovis CM, Minion GE, Rutkowski R. The syndrome of alcoholic ketoacidosis. *Am J Med.* 1991;91:119. [PMID: 1867237]

Chronic Complications of Diabetes Mellitus

Antihypertensive and Lipid-Lowering Treatment to Prevent Heart Attack Trial (ALLHAT). Major outcomes in high-risk hypertensive patients randomized to angiotensin-converting enzyme inhibitor or calcium channel blocker vs diuretic: the Antihypertensive and Lipid-Lowering Treatment to Prevent Heart Attack Trial (ALLHAT). *JAMA.* 2002;298:2981. [PMID: 12479763]

American Diabetes Association Position Statement. Preventive foot care in people with diabetes. *Diab Care.* 2004;27(suppl 1):S63.

Boulton AJ. The diabetic foot: from art to science. The 18th Camillo Golgi lecture. *Diabetologia.* 2004;47:1343. [PMID: 15309286]

Boulton AJ, Vinik AI, Arezzo JC, et al. Diabetic neuropathies: a statement by the American Diabetes Association. *Diab Care.* 2005;28:956. [PMID: 15793206]

Brownlee M. The pathobiology of diabetic complications: a unifying mechanism. *Diabetes.* 2005;54:1615. [PMID: 15919781]

Deckert T, Kofoed-Enevoldsen A, Norgaard K, Borch-Johnsen K, Feldt-Rasmussen B, Jensen T. Microalbuminuria: implications for micro- and macrovascular disease. *Diab Care.* 1992;15:1181. [PMID: 1396015]

Horowitz M, O'Donovan D, Jones KL, Feinle C, Rayner CK, Samsom M. Gastric emptying in diabetes: clinical significance and treatment. *Diab Med.* 2002;19:177. [PMID: 11918620]

Marso SP, Hiatt WR. Peripheral arterial disease in patients with diabetes. *J Am Coll Cardiol.* 2006;47:921. [PMID: 16516072]

Mauer SM, Goetz FC, McHugh LE, et al. Long-term study of normal kidneys transplanted into patients with type I diabetes. *Diabetes*. 1989;38:516. [PMID: 2647558]

Mayfield JA, Reiber GE, Sanders LJ, Janisse D, Pogach LM. American Diabetes Association. Preventive foot care in diabetes. *Diab Care*. 2004;27(suppl 1):S63. [PMID: 14693928]

McGill JB. Improving microvascular outcomes in patients with diabetes through management of hypertension. *Postgrad Med*. 2009;121:89. [PMID: 19332966]

Mohamed Q, Gillies MC, Wong TY. Management of diabetic retinopathy: a systematic review. *JAMA*. 2007;298:902. [PMID: 17712074]

Molitch ME, DeFronzo RA, Franz MJ, et al. American Diabetes Association. Nephropathy in diabetes. *Diab Care*. 2004;27(suppl 1):S79. [PMID: 14693934]

Schwartz SG, Flynn HW Jr, Scott IU. Pharmacotherapy for diabetic retinopathy. *Expert Opin Pharmacother*. 2009;10:1123.[PMID: 19405788]

SimÓ R, Hernández C. Advances in the medical treatment of diabetic retinopathy. *Diab Care*. 2009;32:1556. [PMID: 19638526]

Vardi M, Nini A. Phosphodiesterase inhibitors for erectile dysfunction in patients with diabetes mellitus. *Cochrane Database Syst Rev*. 2007;1:CD002187. [PMID: 17253475]

Vinik AI, Mehrabyan A. Diabetic neuropathies. *Med Clin North Am*. 2004;88:947. [PMID: 15308387]

Diabetes Mellitus and Pregnancy

Australian Carbohydrate Intolerance Study in Pregnant Women (ACHOIS) Trial Group. Effect of treatment of gestational diabetes mellitus on pregnancy outcomes. *N Engl J Med*. 2005;352:2477.[PMID: 15951574]

Boinpally T, Jovanovic L. Management of type 2 diabetes and gestational diabetes in pregnancy. *Mt Sinai J Med*. 2009;76:269. [PMID: 19421970]

HAPO Study Cooperative Research Group. Hyperglycemia and adverse pregnancy outcomes. *N Engl J Med*. 2008;358:1991. [PMID: 18463375]

Kim H, Toyofuku Y, Lynn FC, et al. Serotonin regulates pancreatic beta cell mass during pregnancy. *Nat Med*. 2010;16:804. [PMID: 20581837]

Kitzmiller JL, Gavin LA, Gin GD, Jovanovic-Peterson L, Main EK, Zigrang WD. Preconception management of diabetes continued through early pregnancy prevents the excess frequency of major congenital anomalies in infants of diabetic mothers. *JAMA*. 1991;265:731. [PMID: 1990188]

Kitzmiller J.L, Block JM, Brown FM, et al. Managing preexisting diabetes for pregnancy: summary of evidence and consensus recommendations for care. *Diab Care*. 2008;31:1060. [PMID: 18445730]

Landon MB, Spong CY, Thom E, et al. A multicenter, randomized trial of treatment for mild gestational diabetes. *N Engl J Med*. 2009;361:1339.[PMID: 19797280]

Langer O, et al. A comparison of glyburide and insulin in women with gestational diabetes. *N Engl J Med*. 2000;343:1134.

Metzger B, Coustan DR, and the Organizing Committee. Summary and recommendations of the Fourth International Workshop—Conference on Gestational Diabetes. *Diab Care*. 1998;21(suppl 2):B162.

MiG Trial Investigators. Metformin versus insulin for the treatment of gestational diabetes. *N Engl J Med*. 2008;358:2003. [PMID: 18463376]

Murphy HR, Rayman G, Lewis K, et al. Effectiveness of continuous glucose monitoring in pregnant women with diabetes: randomised clinical trial. *BMJ*. 2008;337:1680. [PMID: 18818254]

Reece EA, Leguizamon G, Wiznitzer A. Gestational diabetes: the need for a common ground. *Lancet*. 2009;373:1789. [PMID: 19465234]

Walkinshaw SA. Pregnancy in women with pre-existing diabetes: management issues. *Semin Fetal Neonatal Med*. 2005;10:307. [PMID: 15927547]

Hypoglycemic Disorders

Umesh Masharani, MB, BS, MRCP (UK), and
Stephen E. Gitelman, MD

ACTH	Adrenocorticotrophic hormone	**IGF-II**	Insulin-like growth factor II
ACE	Angiotensin-converting enzyme	**IGFBP3**	IGF-binding protein-3
ADP	Adenosine diphosphate	**Kir**	Inward rectifier potassium channel
ALS	Acid-labile subunit	**NADH**	Nicotinamide adenine dinucleotide (reduced form)
ATP	Adenosine triphosphate		
GDH	Glutamate dehydrogenase	**NICTH**	Nonislet cell tumor hypoglycemia
GIP	Glucose-dependent insulinotropic polypeptide	**NIPHS**	Noninsulinoma pancreatogenous hypoglycemic syndrome
GLP-1	Glucagon-like peptide 1	**PEPCK**	Phosphoenolpyruvate carboxykinase
G-6-Pase	Glucose-6-phosphatase	**RIA**	Radioimmunoassay
HbA$_{1c}$	Hemoglobin A$_{1c}$	**SSTR**	Somatostatin receptor
ICMA	Immunochemiluminometric	**SUR**	Sulfonylurea receptor

Circulating plasma glucose concentrations are kept within a relatively narrow range by a complex system of interrelated neural, humoral, and cellular controls. Under the usual metabolic conditions, the central nervous system is wholly dependent on plasma glucose and counteracts declining blood glucose concentrations with a carefully programmed response. This is often associated with a sensation of hunger and, as the brain receives insufficient glucose to meet its metabolic needs (neuroglycopenia), an autonomic response is triggered to mobilize storage depots of glycogen and fat. In the postabsorptive state, hepatic glycogen reserves and gluconeogenesis from the liver and kidney directly supply the central nervous system with glucose, which is carried across the blood-brain barrier by a specific glucose transport system, while the mobilization of fatty acids from triglyceride depots provides energy for the large mass of skeletal and cardiac muscle, renal cortex, liver, and other tissues that utilize fatty acids as their basic fuel, thus sparing glucose for use by the tissues of the central nervous system.

The normal lower limit of fasting plasma glucose is typically 70 mg/dL (3.9 mmol/L). Lower values may occur during prolonged fasting, strenuous exercise, or pregnancy or may occur as a laboratory artifact. In normal men, plasma glucose does not fall below 55 mg/dL (3 mmol/L) during a 72-hour fast. However, for reasons that are not clear, normal women may experience a fall to levels as low as 30 mg/dL (1.7 mmol/L) despite a marked suppression of circulating insulin to less than 5 μU/mL. They remain asymptomatic in spite of this degree of hypoglycemia, presumably because ketogenesis is able to satisfy the energy needs of the central nervous system. Basal plasma glucose declines progressively during normal pregnancy, and hypoglycemic levels may be reached during prolonged fasting. This may be a consequence of a continuous fetal consumption of glucose and diminished availability of the gluconeogenic substrate alanine. The cause of these diminished alanine levels in pregnancy is unclear. The greatly increased glucose consumption by skeletal muscle that occurs during prolonged strenuous exercise may lead to hypoglycemia (blood glucose <45 mg/dL) despite increases in hepatic glucose production. Whether the hypoglycemia in this circumstance contributes to fatigue or other symptoms in distance runners is unknown.

In vitro consumption of glucose by blood cell elements may give rise to laboratory values in the hypoglycemic range. This can be avoided by adding a small amount of the metabolic inhibitor sodium fluoride to collection tubes used for specimens containing increased numbers of blood cells (as in leukemia, leukemoid reactions, or polycythemia) and keep samples on ice until separated.

PATHOPHYSIOLOGY OF THE COUNTERREGULATORY RESPONSE TO NEUROGLYCOPENIA

The plasma concentration of glucose that signals the need by the central nervous system to mobilize energy reserves depends on a number of factors, such as the status of blood flow to the brain, the integrity of cerebral tissue, the prevailing arterial level of plasma glucose, the rapidity with which plasma glucose concentration falls, and the availability of alternative metabolic fuels.

A hierarchy of responses has been shown to occur as plasma glucose falls in healthy young volunteers, with hormonal counterregulatory responses being triggered at glucose levels slightly higher (~67 mg/dL [3.7 mmol/L]) than those that induce symptoms of hypoglycemia (Figure 18–1). The first symptoms to appear in healthy people are mediated by autonomic neurotransmitters and occur at plasma glucose levels below 60 mg/dL (3.3 mmol/L). The symptoms consist of tremor, anxiety, palpitations, and sweating, which result from sympathetic discharge; and hunger, which is a consequence of parasympathetic vagal response. Ganglionic blockade and cervical cord section or sympathectomy—but not adrenalectomy—ameliorates these symptoms, indicating that they are due to the release of autonomic neurotransmitters and not dependent on adrenal hormones. As plasma glucose falls below 50 mg/dL (2.8 mmol/L), cerebral neuroglycopenia ensues, consisting of impaired cognition, along with weakness, lethargy, confusion, incoordination, and blurred vision. If counterregulatory responses are inadequate to reverse this degree of profound hypoglycemia, convulsions or coma may occur. This can result in brain damage or death, particularly in those who have not adapted to repeated episodes of hypoglycemia.

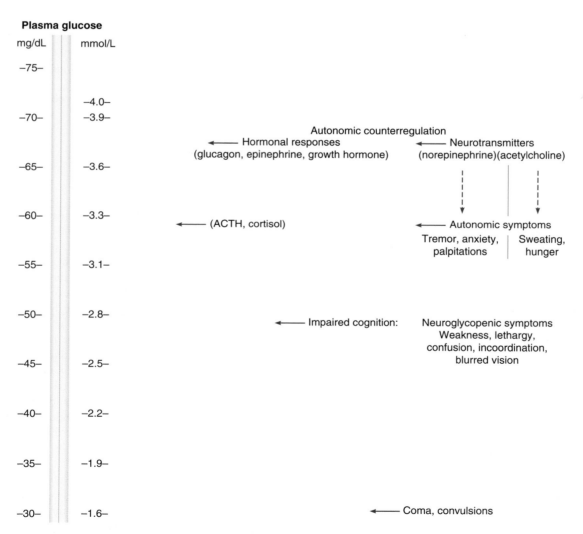

FIGURE 18–1 Hierarchy of autonomic responses to progressive stepwise reduction in plasma glucose concentration in healthy volunteers. (Adapted with permission from Gerich JE, et al. Hypoglycemia unawareness. *Endocr Rev.* 1991;12:356; and from Service FJ. Hypoglycemia disorders. *N Engl J Med.* 1995;332:1144.)

TABLE 18–1 Autonomic nervous system response to hypoglycemia.

Alpha-Adrenergic Effects
Inhibition of endogenous insulin release
Increase in cerebral blood flow (peripheral vasoconstriction)
Beta-Adrenergic Effects
Hepatic and muscle glycogenolysis
Stimulation of plasma glucagon release
Lipolysis to raise plasma-free fatty acids
Impairment of glucose uptake by muscle tissue
Increase in cerebral blood flow (increase in cardiac output)
Adrenomedullary Discharge of Catecholamines
Augmentation of all of the above alpha- and beta-adrenergic effects
Cholinergic Effects
Raises level of pancreatic polypeptide
Increases motility of stomach
Produces hunger
Increases sweating

In elderly people, however, with compromised cerebral blood supply, neuroglycopenic manifestations may be provoked at slightly higher plasma glucose levels. Patients with chronic hyperglycemia (eg, those with poorly controlled, insulin-treated diabetes mellitus) may experience symptoms of neuroglycopenia at considerably higher plasma glucose concentrations than persons without diabetes. This has been attributed to a downregulated glucose transport system across the blood–brain barrier. Conversely, in patients exposed to chronic hypoglycemia (eg, those with an insulin-secreting tumor or those with diabetes who are receiving excessively tight glycemic control with an insulin pump), adaptation to recurrent hypoglycemia occurs by upregulation of the glucose transporters, which results in hypoglycemic unawareness, whereby they show greater tolerance to hypoglycemia without manifesting symptoms. Restoring and maintaining an adequate supply of glucose for cerebral function proceeds by a series of neurogenic events that act directly to raise the plasma glucose concentration and to stimulate hormonal responses that augment the adrenergic mobilization of energy stores (Table 18–1).

Counterregulatory Response to Hypoglycemia

Insulin: Endogenous insulin secretion is lowered both by reduced glucose stimulation to the pancreatic β cell and by sympathetic nervous system inhibition from a combination of alpha-adrenergic neural effects and increased circulating catecholamine levels. This reactive insulinopenia appears to be essential for glucose recovery, because it facilitates the mobilization of energy from existing energy stores (glycogenolysis and lipolysis); increases hepatic enzymes involved in gluconeogenesis and ketogenesis; increases enzymes of the renal cortex, promoting gluconeogenesis; and at the same time prevents muscle tissue from consuming the blood glucose being released from the liver (Chapter 17).

Catecholamines: Circulating catecholamines—and norepinephrine produced at sympathetic nerve endings—provide muscle tissue with alternative sources of fuel by activating beta-adrenergic receptors, resulting in mobilization of muscle glycogen, and by providing increased plasma-free fatty acids from lipolysis of adipocyte triglyceride. Metabolism of these free fatty acids provides energy to promote gluconeogenesis in the liver and kidney, thereby adding to plasma glucose levels already raised by the glycogenolytic effect of catecholamines on the liver. Their cardiovascular and other side effects provide a signal that diabetic patients learn to recognize as a warning of their need to rapidly ingest absorbable carbohydrate.

Glucagon: Plasma glucagon is released by the beta-adrenergic effects of both sympathetic innervation and circulating catecholamines on pancreatic α cells as well as by the direct stimulation of α cells by the low plasma glucose concentration itself. Data are available suggesting that a falling-off of intra-islet insulin concentration in subjects with functioning pancreatic β cells can release pancreatic α cells from insulin inhibition and thus augment glucagon release during hypoglycemia. This glucagon release increases hepatic output of glucose by direct glycogenolysis as well as by facilitating the activity of gluconeogenic enzymes in the liver but not in the kidney. As shown in Figure 18–2, plasma glucagon

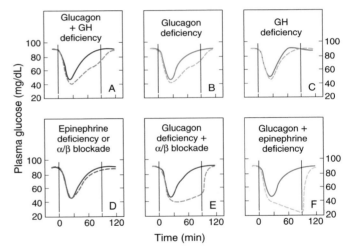

FIGURE 18–2 Solid lines show changes in plasma glucose that occur in normal subjects in response to acute intravenous insulin administration. Note the rapid recovery of glucose levels mediated by intact counterregulatory mechanisms. The dashed lines show the response to insulin-induced hypoglycemia in patients with deficiencies of the counterregulatory mechanisms induced as follows: **A:** Somatostatin infusion (inhibits both glucagon and growth hormone [GH] release). **B:** Somatostatin infusion plus GH infusion (now with functional isolated glucagon deficiency). **C:** Somatostatin infusion plus glucagon infusion (isolated GH deficiency). Note return of glucose response to normal, implying that glucagon is the main counterregulatory hormone. **D:** Bilateral adrenalectomy, leading to epinephrine deficiency, or infusion of phentolamine plus propranolol (alpha and beta blockers, respectively). Note that such deficiencies cause no major abnormality in response to induced hypoglycemia when glucagon is present. **E and F:** Sympathetic modulation (by phentolamine plus propranolol in **E** and by bilateral adrenalectomy in **F**), which seriously impairs the ability to respond to hypoglycemia in the patient made glucagon-deficient by somatostatin infusion. (Reproduced, with permission, from Cryer PE. Glucose counterregulation in man. *Diabetes*. 1981;30:261.)

appears to be the key counterregulatory hormone affecting recovery from *acute* hypoglycemia in nondiabetic humans, with the adrenergic-catecholamine response representing a major backup system. However, in most clinical situations, where hypoglycemia develops *more gradually*, as with inappropriate dosage of insulin or sulfonylureas, or in cases of insulinoma, the role of glucagon may be less influential. When normal volunteers received a prolonged low-dose insulin infusion to produce a gradual decline in plasma glucose levels without waning of insulin levels, the rise of endogenous glucagon contributed much less to counterregulation than after acute hypoglycemia induced by intravenous insulin, which is followed by rapid waning of insulin levels. This finding suggests that glucagon's role in glucose recovery occurs primarily when the level of insulin wanes.

Cortisol: Pituitary corticotrophin (ACTH) is released in association with the sympathetic nervous system stimulation by neuroglycopenia. This results in elevation of plasma cortisol levels, which in turn permissively facilitates lipolysis and actively promotes protein catabolism and conversion of amino acids to glucose by the liver and kidney.

Growth hormone: Pituitary growth hormone is also released in response to falling plasma glucose levels. Its role in counteracting hypoglycemia is less well defined, but it is known to antagonize the action of insulin on glucose utilization in muscle cells and to directly activate lipolysis by adipocytes. This increased lipolysis provides fatty acid substrate to the liver and renal cortex which facilitates gluconeogenesis.

Cholinergic neurotransmitters: Acetylcholine is released at parasympathetic nerve endings, and its vagal effects induce the sensation of hunger that signals the need for food to counteract the hypoglycemia. In addition, postsynaptic fibers of the sympathetic nervous system that innervate the sweat glands to signal hypoglycemia also release acetylcholine—in contrast to all other sympathetic postsynaptic fibers, which without exception release norepinephrine.

Maintenance of Euglycemia in the Postabsorptive State

Glucose absorption from the gastrointestinal tract ceases by 4 to 6 hours after a meal. During the postabsorptive state which immediately follows, glucose must be produced endogenously from previously stored nutrients to meet the requirements of the central nervous system and other glucose-dependent tissues. These include 125 mg/min of glucose required by the brain and spinal cord as well as an additional 25 mg/min by red blood cells and the renal medulla. It was previously thought that the liver is the only organ involved in glucose production during an overnight fast, but recent data indicate that the renal cortex also has the requisite enzymes for production and release of glucose.

Liver: The liver initially provides glucose by the breakdown of stored hepatic glycogen. However, because these reserves are limited to 80 to 100 g, they begin to be depleted several hours into the postabsorptive state. Thereafter, hepatic glucose production is augmented by gluconeogenesis—the formation of glucose from amino acids, lactate, and glycerol. These substrates are delivered to the liver and kidney from peripheral stores. Muscle and other structural tissues supply amino acids, mainly alanine; blood cell elements supply lactate, the end product of glycolytic metabolism; and adipose tissue supplies glycerol from lipolysis of triglyceride. In addition, oxidation of the free fatty acids released from adipose cells during lipolysis supplies the energy required for gluconeogenesis and provides ketone bodies, acetoacetate, and β-hydroxybutyrate, which can serve as alternative metabolic fuels for the central nervous system during periods of prolonged fasting. Studies have shown that an insulin infusion does not reduce hepatic glucose production if elevated levels of fatty acids are maintained by intravenous administration of a fat emulsion and heparin, suggesting that fatty acids may be the major mediator of gluconeogenesis.

The principal mechanisms regulating hepatic glucose output are the availability of gluconeogenic substrates and the regulation of transcription of key regulatory enzymes such as phosphoenolpyruvate carboxykinase (PEPCK) and glucose-6-phosphatase (G-6-Pase). Glucagon and glucocorticoids through signaling intermediates induce the expression of PEPCK and G-6-Pase. Insulin on the other hand suppresses the expression of these enzymes.

Kidney: Although it is generally acknowledged that after fasting for 60 hours the kidney contributes up to 20% to 25% of endogenous glucose production, its role after an overnight fast remains controversial. One group has found that it produces as much as 25% of the postabsorptive glucose requirement, yet a second group using different methodology found a contribution of no more than 5% in the postabsorptive state. Despite these conflicting findings, it is clear that because the renal medulla removes almost as much glucose as the renal cortex produces, the net renal contribution is minimal in the short-term postabsorptive state as compared to the liver.

The kidney does not have glycogen stores and is dependent on gluconeogenesis as its only source of glucose production. Glutamine—rather than alanine—is the predominant amino acid substrate for renal gluconeogenesis. In addition to its contribution to glucose homeostasis after an overnight fast, the kidney also has been shown to be an important contributor to glucose counterregulation in the event of hypoglycemia. Although glucagon does not affect the kidney, the counterregulatory rise in catecholamines has been shown to stimulate gluconeogenesis in the renal cortex. As with the liver, insulin inhibits renal gluconeogenesis and glucose release. Hormonal changes that begin early in the postabsorptive state regulate the enzymatic steps necessary for hepatic glycogenolysis and hepatic and renal gluconeogenesis and ensure the delivery of the necessary substrate (Table 18–2). An appropriate fall in circulating insulin levels with a corresponding rise in glucagon is most important; elevations in the counterregulatory hormones, namely cortisol and growth hormone, contribute to it but are less critical. Thus, numerous endocrine and metabolic events interact to provide a continuous source of fuel for proper functioning of the central nervous system. Malfunction of any of these mechanisms can lead to symptomatic hypoglycemia.

TABLE 18–2 Hormonal changes to maintain euglycemia in the postabsorptive state.

Decreased Insulin Secretion
Increases hepatic glycogenolysis
Increases lipolysis
Increases hepatic gluconeogenesis
Decreases muscle uptake of glucose
Increased Glucagon Secretion
Increases hepatic glycogenolysis
Facilitates hepatic gluconeogenesis
Increased Cortisol Secretion
Facilitates lipolysis
Increases protein catabolism
Augments hepatic gluconeogenesis

CLASSIFICATION OF HYPOGLYCEMIC DISORDERS

A clinical classification of the more common causes of symptomatic hypoglycemia in adults is presented in Table 18–3. This classification is useful in directing diagnostic considerations. Symptomatic fasting hypoglycemia is a serious and potentially life-threatening problem warranting thorough evaluation. Conditions that produce inappropriate fasting hyperinsulinism are the most common cause of fasting hypoglycemia in otherwise healthy adults. These include insulin-secreting pancreatic β cell tumors and iatrogenic or surreptitious administration of insulin or sulfonylureas. In patients with illnesses that produce symptomatic fasting hypoglycemia despite appropriately suppressed insulin levels, the clinical picture is generally dominated by the signs and symptoms of the primary disease, with hypoglycemia often only a

TABLE 18–3 Common causes of symptomatic hypoglycemia in adults.

Fasting
  With hyperinsulinism
Insulin reaction
Sulfonylurea overdose
Surreptitious insulin or sulfonylurea self-administration
Autoimmune hypoglycemia (idiopathic insulin antibodies, insulin receptor autoantibodies)
Pentamidine-induced hypoglycemia
Pancreatic β cell tumors
  Without hyperinsulinism
Severe hepatic dysfunction
Chronic renal insufficiency
Inanition
Hypocortisolism
Alcohol use
Nonpancreatic tumors

Nonfasting
Alimentary
Functional
Noninsulinoma pancreatogenous hypoglycemic syndrome (NIPHS)
Occult diabetes
Ethanol ingestion with sugar mixers

late or associated manifestation. Hypoglycemia, sometimes severe, can also occur postprandially. In patients with gastric surgery, overrapid gastric emptying and accelerated glucose absorption may result in excess insulin secretion, rapid disposal of glucose, and hypoglycemia. An uncommon condition of islet hyperplasia or adult nesidioblastosis called noninsulinoma pancreatogenous hypoglycemia syndrome can result in hypoglycemia 4 to 6 hours after meals.

SPECIFIC HYPOGLYCEMIC DISORDERS

1. DIABETES (SEE ALSO CHAPTER 17)

Iatrogenic hypoglycemia is common in type 1 patients and also in insulin treated type 2 patients. Most type 1 patients aiming for HbA$_{1c}$ levels below 7% have on average one to two symptomatic hypoglycemic episodes per year. Severe hypoglycemia is defined as an episode requiring assistance, and in one study, incidence rates were about 12 per 100 patient years for both type 1 and insulin-treated type 2 patients. Sulfonylureas, repaglinide, and nateglinide can also cause hypoglycemia. Increased risk factors include age (70 years and older), renal failure, hepatic failure, and use of the long-acting sulfonylureas. A number of other drug-drug interactions (clarithromycin, salicylates, sulfonamides) can also potentiate the hypoglycemic effects of sulfonylureas. The annual incidence of sulfonylurea-induced hypoglycemia is approximately 0.2 per 1000 patient years.

As β cell failure progresses (early in type 1 and late in type 2 diabetes), patients lose their glucagon response to hypoglycemia. This combination of insulin deficiency and impaired glucagon response makes it harder for patients to achieve HbA$_{1c}$ levels below 7% without occasional hypoglycemia. These hypoglycemic episodes attenuate the sympathoadrenal response to hypoglycemia, with decreased epinephrine release from the adrenal and decreased sympathetic neural responses (hypoglycemic unawareness). The hypoglycemia unawareness in turn increases the risk for recurrent hypoglycemia. About 20% to 25% of type 1 patients have hypoglycemic unawareness. Other factors that increase the risk for hypoglycemia include poor self-management skills. Patients may take too much insulin for the carbohydrates or take the wrong insulin or do not appropriately time insulin administration with food ingestion. They also may not adjust the insulin for acute exercise or take extra carbohydrates for unexpected exercise or reduce insulin doses for improved insulin sensitivity with exercise training. Alcohol can decrease endogenous glucose production and can cause hypoglycemia, especially if it is consumed on an empty stomach. Diabetes complications—gastroparesis, autonomic neuropathy, and renal failure also increase the risk for hypoglycemia.

There are other consequences of hypoglycemia apart from the autonomic and neurogenic symptoms of acute hypoglycemia. In severe cases, hypoglycemia can cause convulsions and coma. Permanent neurological damage is rare. Although cross-sectional studies and case reports have reported intellectual decline with recurrent hypoglycemia, longitudinal studies have not shown significant cognitive dysfunction in adults. In the Diabetes Control and Complications Trial, there was no evidence for cognitive decline related to hypoglycemia in 18 years of follow-up. Young children however may be more vulnerable to the effects of hypoglycemia on the brain. Hypoglycemia via its autonomic stimulation and catecholamine release increases cardiac output. In patients with cardiac disease it can also precipitate cardiac arrhythmias, angina, myocardial infarction, and congestive heart failure.

Hypoglycemia can also exert a psychological toll. Acute hypoglycemia induces mood changes including fatigue, pessimism, anger, and behavior changes. Nocturnal hypoglycemia can lead to fatigue and decreased sense of well being the following day. Patients who have had severe hypoglycemia may develop a phobia about hypoglycemia and keep their sugars unreasonably high. Some patients develop an anxiety syndrome. Hypoglycemia can also impact personal relationships, occupation, driving, and leisure activities. Surveys show that type 1 patients have increased risk of driving mishaps (crashes, moving violations) when compared to nondiabetic spouses; and that these are related to hypoglycemia.

The goal of therapy is to restore levels of plasma glucose to normal as rapidly as possible. If the patient is conscious and able to swallow, glucose-containing foods such as candy, orange juice with added sugar, and cookies should be quickly ingested. Fructose, found in many nutrient low-calorie sweeteners for diabetics, should not be used. While it can be metabolized by neurons, fructose is not transported across the blood–brain barrier.

If the patient is unconscious, rapid restoration of plasma glucose must be accomplished by giving 20 to 50 mL of 50% dextrose intravenously over 1 to 3 minutes (the treatment of choice) or, when intravenous glucose is not available, 1 mg of glucagon intramuscularly or intravenously. Families or friends of insulin-treated diabetics should be instructed in the administration of glucagon intramuscularly for emergency treatment at home. Glucagon should not be given if the hypoglycemia is due to sulfonylurea use. Under these circumstances, glucagon can stimulate insulin secretion and worsen the hypoglycemia. Attempts to feed the patient or to apply glucose-containing jelly to the oral mucosa should be avoided because of the danger of aspiration. When consciousness is restored, oral feedings should be started immediately. In patients who have taken massive overdoses of sulfonylureas, the response to intravenous dextrose may be poor. For these patients, intravenous boluses of diazoxide (150-300 mg) may be tried but can result in hypotension. Intravenous octreotide (100 μg) has also been reported to be of benefit.

Patients on insulin or sulfonylureas should be instructed on how to recognize and treat hypoglycemia and what measures they can take to prevent such episodes. Type 1 patients and insulin-treated type 2 patients should monitor their blood glucose frequently. Hypoglycemia not infrequently occurs at night and patients should avoid taking large doses of short-acting insulin just before going to bed. Patients should from time to time also monitor blood glucose levels in the middle of the night. Hypoglycemia can also occur many hours after strenuous exercise, and patients should be advised to monitor at these times and cut back their insulin doses and/or eat more carbohydrate. Continuous glucose monitoring systems are increasingly used by type 1 patients to alert them to falling glucose levels and prevent hypoglycemia. Finally, it is important to individualize glycemic goals. Early in the course of both type 1 and type 2 diabetes when there is still some endogenous β cell function, it is easier to achieve HbA$_{1c}$ levels close to normal with low risk of hypoglycemia. As β cell failure progresses, however, aiming for normality may lead to unacceptably high rates of hypoglycemia. Patients who have had frequent hypoglycemia and have hypoglycemia unawareness should be encouraged to temporarily raise their glycemic targets—as little as 2 to 3 weeks of scrupulous avoidance of hypoglycemia reverses hypoglycemia unawareness and improves the attenuated epinephrine response. Diabetes complications, previous incidence of hypoglycemia, and life expectancy should all be considered in the establishment of glycemic goals.

2. FACTITIOUS HYPOGLYCEMIA

Factitious hypoglycemia should be suspected in any patient with access to insulin or sulfonylurea drugs. It is most commonly seen in health professionals and diabetic patients or their relatives. The reasons for self-induced hypoglycemia vary, with many patients having severe psychiatric disturbances or a pathological need for attention. Inadvertent ingestion of sulfonylureas resulting in clinical hypoglycemia has also been reported, due either to patient error or to a prescription mishap on the part of a pharmacist. Patients with diabetes and factitious hypoglycemia have a presentation similar to brittle diabetes.

When insulin is used to induce hypoglycemia, an elevated serum insulin level often raises suspicion of an insulin-producing pancreatic β cell tumor. It may be difficult to prove that the insulin is of exogenous origin. The combination of hypoglycemia, high immunoreactive insulin levels, suppressed plasma C peptide, and suppressed proinsulin level is pathognomonic of exogenous insulin administration in nondiabetic patients. Patients with renal failure may have normal or even high plasma C-peptide levels, but plasma proinsulin levels are suppressed.

When sulfonylurea abuse is suspected, plasma or urine should be screened for its presence. Hypoglycemia with inappropriately elevated levels of serum insulin and C peptide along with detectable sulfonylureas in blood or urine is diagnostic of inadvertent or factitious sulfonylurea overdose. It is important to use assays which measure not only all the sulfonylureas but also repaglinide and nateglinide.

Treatment of factitious hypoglycemia involves psychiatric therapy and social counseling.

3. DRUGS

Numerous pharmacologic agents may potentiate the effects of insulin and predispose to hypoglycemia. Common offenders include fluoroquinolones such as gatifloxacin and levofloxacin, pentamidine, quinine, angiotensin-converting enzyme (ACE) inhibitors, ethanol, salicylates, and beta-adrenergic–blocking drugs. The fluoroquinolones, especially gatifloxacillin, have been associated with both hypoglycemia and hyperglycemia. Hypoglycemia is an early event; hyperglycemia occurs after several days into therapy. It is thought that the drugs act on ATP-sensitive potassium channels in the β cell. Intravenous pentamidine is cytotoxic to pancreatic β cells, resulting in acute insulin release and hypoglycemia. This occurs in about 10% to 20% of patients receiving the drug and may be followed later by persistent insulinopenia and hyperglycemia. Fasting patients taking noncardioselective beta blockade can have an exaggerated hypoglycemic response to starvation. Beta blockade inhibits fatty acid and gluconeogenic substrate release and reduces plasma glucagon levels resulting in hypoglycemia. Also the symptomatic response to hypoglycemia is altered—tachycardia is blocked while hazardous elevations of blood pressure may result during hypoglycemia in response to the unopposed alpha-adrenergic stimulation from circulating catecholamines and neurogenic sympathetic discharge. However, symptoms of sweating, hunger, and uneasiness are not masked by beta-blocking drugs and remain indicators of hypoglycemia in the aware patient.

Therapy with ACE inhibitors increases the risk of hypoglycemia in diabetic patients who are taking insulin or sulfonylureas, presumably because these drugs increase sensitivity to circulating insulin by increasing blood flow to muscle.

Ethanol-associated hypoglycemia has been proposed to occur as a consequence of hepatic alcohol dehydrogenase activity depleting NADH. The resultant change in the redox state (NADH-to-NAD⁺ ratio) limits the conversion of lactate to pyruvate, the main substrate for hepatic gluconeogenesis. In the patient who is imbibing ethanol but not eating, fasting hypoglycemia may occur after hepatic glycogen stores have been depleted (within 8-12 hours of a fast). No correlation exists between the blood ethanol levels and the degree of hypoglycemia, which may occur while blood ethanol levels are declining. It should be noted that ethanol-induced fasting hypoglycemia may occur at ethanol levels as low as 45 mg/dL (10 mmol/L)—considerably below most states' legal standards (80 mg/dL [17.4 mmol/L]) for being *under the influence*. Most patients present with neuroglycopenic symptoms, which may be difficult to differentiate from the neurotoxic effects of the alcohol. These symptoms in a patient whose breath smells of alcohol may be mistaken for alcoholic stupor. Intravenous dextrose should be administered promptly to all such stuporous or comatose patients. Because hepatic glycogen stores have been depleted by the time hypoglycemia occurs, parenteral glucagon is not effective. Adequate food intake during alcohol ingestion prevents this type of hypoglycemia.

4. AUTOIMMUNE HYPOGLYCEMIA

In recent years, a rare autoimmune disorder has been reported in which patients have circulating insulin antibodies and the paradoxic feature of hypoglycemia. More than 200 cases of insulin-antibody-associated hypoglycemia have been reported since 1970, with 90% of cases reported in Japanese patients. HLA class II alleles (DRB1*0406, DQA1*0301, and DQB1*0302) are associated with this syndrome, and these alleles are 10 to 30 times more

prevalent in Japanese and Koreans, which may explain the higher prevalence of this syndrome in these populations. Hypoglycemia generally occurs 3 to 4 hours after a meal and follows an early postprandial hyperglycemia. It is attributed to a dissociation of insulin-antibody immune complexes, releasing free insulin. This autoimmune hypoglycemia, which is due to accumulation of high titers of antibodies capable of reacting with endogenous insulin, has been most commonly reported in methimazole-treated patients with Graves disease from Japan as well as in patients with various other sulfhydryl-containing medications (captopril, penicillamine) and other drugs such as hydralazine, isoniazid, and procainamide. In addition, it has been reported in patients with autoimmune disorders such as rheumatoid arthritis, systemic lupus erythematosus, and polymyositis, as well as in multiple myeloma and other plasma cell dyscrasias where paraproteins or antibodies cross-react with insulin.

High titers of insulin autoantibodies, usually IgG class, can be detected. Insulin, proinsulin, and C-peptide levels may be elevated but the results may be erroneous because of the interference of the insulin antibodies with the immunoassays for these peptides.

In most cases the hypoglycemia is transient and usually resolves spontaneously within 3 to 6 months of diagnosis, particularly when the offending medications are stopped. The most consistent therapeutic benefit in management of this syndrome has been achieved by dietary treatment with frequent, low-carbohydrate, small meals. Prednisone therapy (30-60 mg/d) has been used to lower the titer of insulin antibodies.

Hypoglycemia due to insulin receptor autoantibodies is also an extremely rare syndrome; most cases have occurred in women often with a history of autoimmune disease. Almost all of these patients have also had episodes of insulin-resistant diabetes and acanthosis nigricans. Their hypoglycemia may be either fasting or postprandial and is often severe and is attributed to an agonist action of the antibody on the insulin receptor. Balance between the antagonistic and agonistic effects of the antibodies determines whether insulin-resistant diabetes or hypoglycemia occurs. Hypoglycemia was found to respond to glucocorticoid therapy but not to plasmapheresis or immunosuppression.

5. PANCREATIC β CELL TUMORS

Spontaneous fasting hypoglycemia in an otherwise healthy adult is most commonly due to insulinoma, an insulin-secreting tumor of the islets of Langerhans. Eighty percent of these tumors are single and benign; 10% are malignant (if metastases are identified); and the remainder are multiple, with scattered micro- or macroadenomas interspersed within normal islet tissue. (As with some other endocrine tumors, histologic differentiation between benign and malignant cells is difficult, and close follow-up is necessary to ensure the absence of metastases.)

These adenomas may be familial and have been found in conjunction with tumors of the parathyroid glands and the pituitary (multiple endocrine neoplasia type 1; see Chapter 22). Over 99% of them are located within the pancreas and less than 1% in ectopic pancreatic tissue.

These tumors may appear at any age, although they are most common in the fourth to sixth decades. A slight predominance in women has been reported in some studies. However, others suggest that there is no gender predilection.

Clinical Findings

The signs and symptoms are chiefly those of subacute or chronic neuroglycopenia rather than adrenergic discharge. The typical picture is that of recurrent central nervous system dysfunction at times of exercise or fasting. Symptoms include episodic disorientation, somnolence, personality changes, amnesia, and loss of consciousness. The preponderance of neuroglycopenic symptoms, rather than those more commonly associated with hypoglycemia (adrenergic symptoms), often leads to delayed diagnosis following prolonged psychiatric care, or treatment for seizure disorders or transient ischemic attacks. Some patients learn to relieve or prevent their symptoms by taking frequent feedings. Obesity may be the result; however, obesity is seen in less than 30% of patients with insulin-secreting tumors.

Diagnosis of Insulinoma

Experts in this field emphasize that the most important prerequisite to diagnosing an insulinoma is simply to consider it, particularly when facing a clinical presentation of fasting hypoglycemia with symptoms of central nervous system dysfunction such as confusion or abnormal behavior. Whipple triad consists of history of symptoms consistent with hypoglycemia, associated low plasma glucose and relief of symptoms upon raising the plasma glucose. β cell tumors do not demonstrate suppression of insulin secretion in the presence of hypoglycemia, and a serum insulin level of 6 μU/mL or more with concomitant plasma glucose values below 45 mg/dL (2.5 mmol/L) suggests an insulinoma. Other causes of hyperinsulinemic hypoglycemia must be considered, however, such as surreptitious administration of insulin or sulfonylureas.

One of the most important steps is to carefully review the patient's history. Attention should be paid to the nature of the symptoms and factors that precipitate and resolve the symptoms. Patients typically complain of feeling tired, experiencing blurred vision, and not thinking clearly. Eating or drinking readily absorbable carbohydrates improves the symptoms within approximately 15 minutes. Timing of the symptoms in relation to meals and exercise should be noted. In insulinoma patients, the symptoms are most likely to occur early in the morning before breakfast or if a meal is missed during the day. Patients occasionally present when they attempt to go on a diet to lose weight. Exercise may precipitate the symptoms especially if the activity occurs while fasting or some hours after a meal. Some patients develop symptoms in the middle of the night and may have to eat. Partners of patients often provide useful information, especially if the patient requires assistance in treating the hypoglycemic symptoms. Occasionally the emergency services are called when the patient gets severely confused, presents with focal weakness, loses consciousness, or has a seizure. There may be documentation of low fingerstick glucose at the time when symptoms are present with recovery following administration of

intravenous glucose. With the ready availability of home blood glucose–monitoring systems, patients sometimes present with documented fingerstick blood glucose levels in 40s and 50s at time of symptoms. Access to diabetic medications (sulfonylureas or insulin) should be explored—does a family member have diabetes or does the patient or family member work in the medical field? Medication-dispensing errors should be excluded—has the patient's prescription medication changed in shape or color? Other illnesses that cause hypoglycemia such as renal failure, hepatic failure, Addison disease, or nonislet tumor should be considered. Patients with insulinoma or factitious hypoglycemia usually have a normal physical examination.

If the history is consistent with episodic spontaneous hypoglycemia, patients should be given a home blood glucose monitor and advised to monitor blood glucose levels at the time of symptoms if it is safe and before consumption of carbohydrates. Patients with insulinomas frequently will report fingerstick blood glucose levels in the 40s at the time of symptoms. The diagnosis, however, cannot be made based on a fingerstick blood glucose. It is necessary to have a low laboratory glucose concomitantly with elevated plasma insulin, proinsulin and C-peptide levels, and a negative sulfonylurea screen. When patients give a history of symptoms after only a short period of food withdrawal or with exercise, then an outpatient assessment can be attempted. The patient should be brought by a family member to the office after an overnight fast and observed in the office. Activity such as walking should be encouraged and fingerstick blood glucose measured repeatedly during observation. If symptoms occur or fingerstick blood glucose is below 50 then samples for plasma glucose, insulin, C peptide, proinsulin, sulfonylurea screen, serum ketones, and antibodies to insulin should be sent. If outpatient observation does not result in symptoms or hypoglycemia and if the clinical suspicion remains high, then the patient should undergo an inpatient, supervised, 72-hour fast.

A suggested protocol for the supervised fast is set forth in Table 18–4. In normal men, the blood glucose value does not fall below 55 mg/dL (3.1 mmol/L) during a 72-hour fast, whereas insulin levels fall below 10 μU/mL; in some normal women, however, plasma glucose may fall below 30 mg/dL (1.7 mmol/L) (lower limits have not been established), but serum insulin levels also fall appropriately to less than 5 μU/mL. These women remain asymptomatic despite this degree of hypoglycemia, presumably because ketogenesis is able to provide sufficient fuel for maintenance of central nervous system function. The fast is timed from the last intake of calories. The term *72-hour fast* is actually a misnomer in most cases, because the fast should be immediately terminated as soon as symptoms and laboratory confirmation of hypoglycemia are evident. About 43% of patients with insulinomas are symptomatic within the first 12 hours, 67% by 24 hours and 93% to 95% by 48 hours. Since a minority of patients (~5%-7%) may not demonstrate hypoglycemia after 48 hours of fasting, it is preferable to continue the fast for up to 72 hours. Patients can drink water and decaffeinated, noncaloric drinks. It is important that patients are active (walking) during the fast since exercise may help precipitate hypoglycemia. An intravenous cannula

TABLE 18–4 Suggested hospital protocol for supervised rapid diagnosis of insulinoma.

(1) Obtain baseline serum glucose, insulin, proinsulin, and C-peptide measurements at onset of fast and place intravenous cannula.
(2) Permit only calorie-free and caffeine-free fluids and encourage supervised activity (such as walking).
(3) Measure urine for ketones at the beginning and every 12 hours and at end of fast.
(4) Obtain capillary glucose measurements with a reflectance meter every 4 hours until values <60 mg/dL are obtained. Then increase the frequency of fingersticks to each hour, and when capillary glucose value is <49 mg/dL, send a venous blood sample to the laboratory for serum glucose, insulin, proinsulin, and C-peptide measurements. Check frequently for manifestations of neuroglycopenia.
(5) If symptoms of hypoglycemia occur or if a laboratory value of serum glucose is <45 mg/dL or if 72 hours have elapsed, then conclude the fast with a final blood sample for serum glucose, insulin, proinsulin, C-peptide, β-hydroxybutyrate or acetone, and sulfonylurea measurements. Then give oral fast-acting carbohydrate followed by a meal. If the patient is confused or unable to take oral agents, administer 50 mL of 50% dextrose intravenously over 3-5 minutes. Do not conclude a fast based simply on basis of a capillary blood glucose measurement—wait for the laboratory glucose value unless the patient is symptomatic and it would be dangerous to wait.

should be placed to allow for blood draws and as a safety precaution, should intravenous dextrose infusion be required. Fingerstick blood glucose levels should be measured at intervals and blood sent to the laboratory if the patient is symptomatic or when fingerstick blood glucose levels are below 50 mg/dL. The decision to stop the fast is not always easy. Patients should be carefully monitored for symptoms of hypoglycemia. If the patient is symptomatic and the laboratory glucose is less than 45 mg/dL then the test can be stopped. If the symptoms are equivocal and the laboratory glucose is in the mid 50s or higher, then the fast should be continued, if the patient is agreeable. At the time of termination of the fast, blood should be sent to the laboratory for plasma glucose, insulin, proinsulin, C peptide, and serum β-hydroxybutyrate levels and a sulfonylurea screen.

Virtually all patients with insulin-secreting islet cell tumors fail to suppress their insulin secretion appropriately when the plasma glucose is less than 45 mg/dL (Table 18–5). It is important to be aware of limitations of the particular insulin assay that is used. When radioimmunoassays (RIAs) with a sensitivity of 5 μU/mL are used, patients with insulinomas have plasma insulin concentrations of 6 μU/mL or more. Immunochemiluminometric assays (ICMA) have sensitivities of less than 1 μU/mL, and with these assays, the cutoff for insulinomas is 3 μU/mL or higher. Previous treatment with insulin may lead to development of autoantibodies to insulin that interfere with the assays, leading to falsely low or elevated values depending on the method used. Proper collection

of samples is also important. If serum is not separated and frozen within 1 to 2 hours, falsely low values result because the insulin molecule undergoes proteolytic degradation. Plasma insulin levels measured by ICMA may be lower in hemolyzed samples. Calculation of ratios of insulin (μU/mL) to plasma glucose (mg/dL) is not helpful in making the diagnosis.

Factitious use of insulin will result in suppression of endogenous insulin secretion and low C-peptide levels. Elevated circulating proinsulin levels in the presence of fasting hypoglycemia is characteristic of most β cell tumors and does not occur in factitious hyperinsulinism. Thus, C-peptide and proinsulin levels (by ICMA) of $\geq$200 pmol/L and $\geq$5 pmol/L, respectively, are characteristic of insulinomas. C peptide is renally cleared and caution should be used in interpreting elevated levels in the setting of renal failure. Proinsulin normally represents less than 10% of total immunoreactive insulin. Insulinoma cells are poorly differentiated, which affects their ability to process proinsulin to insulin. Thus, most patients with insulinoma have elevated levels of proinsulin, representing as much as 30% to 90% of total immunoreactive insulin. Hyperinsulinemia suppresses ketone production. Plasma β-hydroxybutyrate levels in patients with insulinoma are 2.7 nmol/L or less. A progressive increase in β-hydroxybutyrate levels after 18 hours of fasting is strongly predictive that the fast will be negative.

A variety of stimulation tests with intravenous tolbutamide, glucagon, or calcium have been devised to demonstrate exaggerated and prolonged insulin secretion in the presence of insulinomas. However, because insulin-secreting tumors have a wide range of granule content and degrees of differentiation, they are variably responsive to these secretagogues. Thus, absence of an excessive insulin-secretory response during any of these stimulation tests does not rule out the presence of an insulinoma. In addition, the tolbutamide stimulation test is extremely hazardous to patients with responsive tumors because it induces prolonged and refractory hypoglycemia. For that reason, it is no longer included in the diagnostic workup of insulinoma.

The hyperinsulinism associated with insulinoma impairs glycogenolysis. Thus, when patients with insulinoma are given 1 mg IV glucagon at the end of the 72-hour fast, there is an increase in plasma glucose within the first 30 minutes. The glucose rise is 25 mg/dL or more at 20 to 30 minutes, whereas normal subjects

TABLE 18–5 Diagnostic criteria for insulinoma after a 72-hour fast.

Plasma glucose	<45mg/dL
Plasma insulin (RIA)	$\geq$6 uU/mL
Plasma insulin (ICMA)	$\geq$3 uU/mL
Plasma C peptide	$\geq$200 pmol/L
Plasma proinsulin	$\geq$5 pmol/L
β-Hydroxybutyrate	$\leq$2.7 nmol/L
Sulfonylurea screen (including repaglinide and nateglidine)	Negative

Conversion factors: insulin uU/mL × 7.175 = pmol/L; C-peptide ng/mL × 0.33 = nmol/L.

have a lower increment. Intravenous glucagon can also cause an exaggerated release of insulin from insulinomas. Patients are tested after an overnight fast, and serum insulin levels measured every 5 minutes for 15 minutes after 1 mg IV glucagon. An increase in insulin level exceeding 130 μU/mL (twice upper limit of normal) suggests an insulin-secreting tumor. However, only about half of patients with insulinomas have insulin levels above 130 μU/mL and so the test is not so helpful. Also, in some patients the exaggerated insulin secretion can lead to severe hypoglycemia. Nausea is an unpleasant side effect, often occurring several minutes after administration of intravenous glucagon.

The oral glucose tolerance test is of no value in the diagnosis of insulin-secreting tumors. A common misconception is that patients with insulinomas have flat glucose tolerance curves because the tumors discharge insulin in response to oral glucose. In fact, most insulinomas respond poorly, and curves typical of diabetes are more common. In those rare tumors that do release insulin in response to glucose, a flat curve may result; however, this also can be seen occasionally in normal subjects.

Low HbA$_{1c}$ values have been reported in patients with insulinoma, reflecting the presence of chronic hypoglycemia. There is however considerable overlap with normal patients and no HbA$_{1c}$ value is diagnostic.

Tumor localization studies   After the diagnosis of insulinoma has been unequivocally made by clinical and laboratory findings, studies to localize the tumor should be initiated. The focus of attention should be directed at the pancreas only, because virtually all insulinomas originate from this tissue; ectopic cancers secreting insulin are unknown to all major centers, with only one published report describing an atypical insulin-producing tumor believed to have originated from a small cell carcinoma of the cervix.

Because of the small size of these tumors (average diameter of 1.5 cm in one large series), imaging studies do not necessarily identify all tumors. A pancreatic dual phase, thin section, helical CT scan can identify 82% to 94% of the lesions. MRI scans with gadolinium can be helpful in detecting a tumor in 85% of cases. One case report suggests that diffusion-weighted MRI can be useful for detecting and localizing small insulinomas, especially those with no hypervascular pattern. The imaging study used will depend upon local availability and local radiologic skill. If the imaging study is negative, then an endoscopic ultrasound should be performed. In experienced hands, about 80% to 90% of tumors can be detected. Finally, needle aspiration of the identified lesion can be attempted to confirm the presence of a neuroendocrine tumor. If the tumor is not identified or imaging results are equivocal, then the patient should undergo selective calcium-stimulated angiography which has been reported to localize the tumor to particular regions of the pancreas approximately 90% of the time. In this test, angiography is combined with injections of calcium gluconate into the gastroduodenal, splenic, and superior mesenteric arteries and insulin levels are measured in the hepatic vein effluent. The procedure is performed after an overnight fast. Ten percent of calcium gluconate, diluted to a volume of 5 mL normal saline, is bolused into selected arteries at a dose of 0.0125 mmol Ca^{2+}/kg (0.005 mmol/kg for obese patients). Five milliliter blood samples are taken from the hepatic effluent at times 0, 30, 60, 90, 120, and 180 seconds after calcium injection. Fingerstick blood glucose levels are measured at intervals and a dextrose infusion is maintained throughout the procedure. Calcium stimulates insulin release from insulinomas but not normal islets. A step-up in insulin levels at 30 or 60 seconds (twofold or greater) regionalizes the source of the hyperinsulinism to the head of the pancreas for the gastroduodenal artery, the uncinate process for the superior mesenteric artery, and the body and tail of the pancreas for the splenic artery. A less than twofold elevation of insulin in the 120 second sample may represent effects of recirculating calcium and is not considered a positive localization. In a single insulinoma, the response is in one artery alone (Figure 18–3) unless the

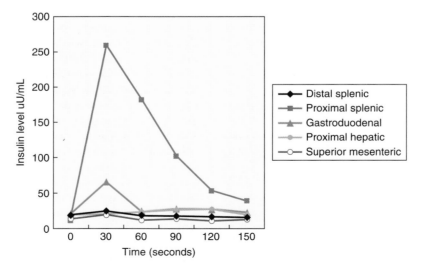

FIGURE 18–3 Responses of serum insulin to selective intra-arterial calcium stimulation in a patient with biochemical confirmation of inappropriate hyperinsulinism. An islet cell tumor was removed from the tail of the pancreas.

tumor resides in an area fed by two arteries or if there are multiple insulinomas as in multiple endocrine neoplasia, type 1. Patients who have diffuse islet hyperplasia (the noninsulinoma pancreatogenous hypoglycemia syndrome [NIPHS]) will have positive responses in multiple arteries. Because diazoxide may interfere with this test, it should be discontinued for at least 48 to 72 hours before sampling. Patients should be closely monitored during the procedure to avoid hypoglycemia (as well as hyperglycemia), which could affect insulin gradients. These studies combined with careful intraoperative ultrasonography and palpation by a surgeon experienced in insulinoma surgery correctly identify up to 98% of tumors.

Treatment of Insulinoma

The treatment of choice for insulin-secreting tumors is surgical resection. While waiting for surgery, patients should be given diazoxide, a potent inhibitor of insulin secretion. It acts by opening the ATP-sensitive potassium channel of the pancreatic β cell and hyperpolarizing the cell membrane. This reduces calcium influx through the voltage-gated calcium channel, thereby reducing insulin release. Divided doses of 300 to 400 mg/d usually suffice, but occasionally a patient may require up to 800 mg/d. A liquid preparation of diazoxide (50 mg/mL) is available in the United States. Side effects include edema due to sodium retention (which generally necessitates concomitant thiazide administration), gastric irritation, and mild hirsutism.

Tumor resection should be performed only by surgeons with extensive experience with removal of islet cell tumors, because these tumors may be small and difficult to recognize. The tumors are enucleated whenever possible unless they have malignant features (eg, hardness or an appearance of infiltration). Preoperative imaging studies, including endoscopic ultrasound, can identify tumors amenable to laparoscopic surgery. Laparoscopic surgery is associated with faster postoperative recovery. Laparoscopic intraoperative ultrasound should be used to confirm the location and depth of the tumor within the gland and also note its relationship to the pancreatic duct and splenic vessels. Open surgery is still necessary for some tumors such as those in the head of the pancreas close to the main pancreatic duct. In the very occasional case where the tumor cannot be found at operation despite the use of intraoperative ultrasound, it is no longer advisable to blindly resect the body and tail of the pancreas since a nonpalpable tumor, missed by ultrasound, is most likely embedded within the fleshy head of the pancreas that is left behind with subtotal resections. Most surgeons prefer to close the incision and treat the patient medically and/or repeat the localization studies.

Diazoxide should be administered on the day of surgery in patients who are responsive to it, because the drug greatly reduces the need for glucose supplements and the risk of hypoglycemia during surgery. Typically, it does not mask the glycemic rise indicative of surgical cure. Blood glucose levels should be monitored frequently during the operation and a 5% or 10% dextrose infusion should be used to maintain euglycemia. Hyperglycemia occurs for a few days postoperatively most likely due to edema and inflammation of the pancreas secondary to its mobilization and manipulation during surgical resection of the insulinoma. However, other possible contributing factors include high levels of counterregulatory hormones induced by the procedure, chronic downregulation of insulin receptors by the previously high circulating insulin levels from the tumor, and, perhaps, suppression of normal pancreatic β cells by long-standing hypoglycemia. Small subcutaneous doses of regular insulin may be prescribed every 4 to 6 hours if plasma glucose exceeds 300 mg/dL (16.7 mmol/L), but in most cases pancreatic insulin secretion recovers after 48 to 72 hours, and very little insulin replacement is required.

Diazoxide therapy is the treatment of choice in patients with inoperable functioning islet cell carcinomas and in those who are poor candidates for operation. A few patients have been maintained on long-term (>10 years) diazoxide therapy with no apparent ill effects. Hydrochlorothiazide, 25 to 50 mg daily, should also be prescribed to counteract the edema and hyperkalemia secondary to diazoxide therapy as well as to potentiate its hyperglycemic effect. Frequent carbohydrate feedings (every 2-3 hours) can also be helpful in maintaining euglycemia, although obesity may become a problem.

When patients are unable to tolerate diazoxide because of side effects such as gastrointestinal upset, hirsutism, or edema, a calcium channel blocker such as verapamil (80 mg given orally every 8 hours) may be tried. This is based, in part, on verapamil's inhibitory effect on insulin release from insulinoma cells in vitro.

A potent long-acting synthetic octapeptide analog of somatostatin (octreotide) has been used to inhibit release of hormones from a number of endocrine tumors, including inoperable insulinomas, but it has had limited success with the latter. Of the five somatostatin receptors (SSTRs) that have been identified in humans, SSTR2, which predominates in the anterior pituitary, has a much greater affinity for octreotide than SSTR5, which predominates in the pancreas. This explains why octreotide is much more effective in treating acromegaly than in treating insulinoma, except in the occasional cases where insulinoma cells happen also to express SSTR2. When hypoglycemia persists after attempted surgical removal of the insulinoma and if diazoxide or verapamil is poorly tolerated or ineffective, a trial of 50 µg of octreotide injected subcutaneously twice daily may control the hypoglycemic episodes in conjunction with multiple small carbohydrate feedings.

Streptozocin has proved to be beneficial in patients with islet cell carcinomas. With selective arterial administration, effective cytotoxic doses have been achieved without the undue renal toxicity that characterized early experience. Benign tumors appear to respond poorly, if at all.

6. NONISLET CELL TUMOR HYPOGLYCEMIA (NICTH)

A variety of nonislet cell tumors have been found to cause fasting hypoglycemia. Most are large and mesenchymal in origin, retroperitoneal fibrosarcoma being the classic prototype. However, hepatocellular carcinomas, adrenocortical carcinomas, renal cell carcinomas, gastrointestinal tumors, lymphomas, leukemias, and a variety of other tumors have also been reported.

Laboratory diagnosis depends on fasting hypoglycemia associated with serum insulin levels below 5 µU/mL. In many cases, the hypoglycemia is due to the expression and release of an incompletely processed insulin-like growth factor II (IGF-II) by the tumor (see also Chapter 21). The primary IGF-II translation product is pre-pro-IGF-II consisting of N-terminal signal peptide of 24 amino acids, 67 amino acid mature IGF-II, and an 89 amino acid extension (E-domain) at the C-terminus. Posttranslational processing of pre-pro-IGF-II involves removal of the N-signal sequence; O-glycosylation of one or more threonine residues of the E-domain and sequential proteolysis of the E-domain. During this process an IGF-II protein with a 21 amino extension of the E-domain (pro-IGF-IIE[68-88]) is relatively stable intermediate that may be secreted from the cell. Most of the mature IGF-II released from the liver is complexed with IGF-binding protein-3 (IGFBP3) and acid-labile subunit (ALS). This ternary protein complex is generally inactive in adults because it is unable to bind properly to tissue receptors. It is only the free IGF-II (<1%) and that bound in binary complexes (predominantly IGFBP2 and IGFBP3) that is accessible to tissue compartment and available to bind the IGF and insulin receptors. However, in patients with nonpancreatic tumors associated with hypoglycemia, incompletely processed mainly nonglycosylated forms of IGF-II are released—in particular pro-IGF-IIE (68-88) form. These incompletely processed molecules are heterogeneous in size and are also referred to as **big IGF-II** and have molecular mass of 10 to 17 kDa in contrast to mature IGF-II at 7.5 kDa. Pro-IGF-II can form binary complexes with IGFBPs but have reduced affinity for forming a tertiary complex with ALS. As a consequence, more of the pro-IGF-II is available for binding to the insulin receptors in the muscle to promote glucose transport and to insulin receptors in liver and kidney to reduce glucose output. The increased production of pro-IGF-II by the tumor may also displace processed IGF-II from IGFBPs, increasing free, unbound IGF-II. The IGF-II may bind to receptors for IGF-I in the pancreatic β cell to inhibit insulin secretion and in the pituitary to suppress growth hormone release. With the reduction of growth hormone, there is a consequent lowering of IGF-I levels as well as IGFBP-3 and ALS.

Size exclusion acid chromatography has been the standard method for detection of Pro-IGF-II in NICTH but the process is time consuming. Immunoblot analysis after separating the proteins on 16.5% tricine-sodium dodecyl sulphate-polyacrylamide gels is a more rapid and equally sensitive method. The IGF-II antibody used recognizes both mature and pro-IGF-II forms. In normal subjects, most of the IGF-II migrates at 7.5 kDA and a small amount in the 10 to 17 kDA region, whereas with NICTH most of the IGF-II migrates in the 10 to 17 kDA region and a small amount at 7 kDA.

The clinical syndrome of nonislet cell tumor hypoglycemia, therefore, is supported by laboratory documentation of serum insulin levels below 5 µU/mL with plasma glucose measurements of 45 mg/dL or lower. Values for growth hormone and IGF-I are also decreased. Levels of IGF-II may be increased but often are normal in quantity despite the presence of the immature, higher molecular weight form of IGF-II, which can only be detected by special laboratory techniques.

Not all the patients with NICTH have elevated pro-IGF-II. Ectopic insulin production has been described (bronchial carcinoid, ovarian carcinoma, and a small cell carcinoma of the cervix). Hypoglycemia due to IGF-I released from a metastatic large cell carcinoma of the lung has also been reported.

Treatment is aimed toward the primary tumor, with supportive therapy using frequent feedings. Diazoxide is ineffective in reversing the hypoglycemia caused by these tumors.

7. ALIMENTARY (REACTIVE) HYPOGLYCEMIA

Some disorders cause hypoglycemia in the postprandial state. This condition occurs in patients following gastric surgery (including Roux-en-Y gastric bypass surgery), in autoimmune hypoglycemia, in islet hyperplasia (noninsulinoma pancreatogenous hypoglycemia syndrome), and occasionally in occult diabetes.

Late dumping syndrome: After major gastric surgery (gastrectomy, vagotomy, pyloroplasty, gastrojejunostomy, and laparoscopic Nissen fundoplication, Billroth II procedure, and Roux-en-Y gastric bypass), some patients develop hypoglycemia post meals especially when they consume foods containing high levels of carbohydrates. This is also referred to as the late dumping syndrome. Late dumping occurs 1 to 3 hours after a meal. Rapid delivery of a meal to the small intestine results in an initial high concentration of carbohydrates in the proximal small bowel and rapid absorption of glucose. This is countered by a hyperinsulinemic response. The high insulin levels are responsible for the subsequent hypoglycemia. The hypoglycemic symptoms include lightheadedness, sweating, confusion, and even loss of consciousness. Gastrointestinal hormones—glucose-dependent insulinotropic polypeptide (GIP) and glucagon-like peptide 1 (GLP-1)—may play a role in the hyperinsulinemic response. An increased GLP-1 response has been noted in patients after total gastrectomy, esophageal resection, partial gastrectomy, and Roux-en-Y surgery. Furthermore, a positive correlation was found between the rise in plasma GLP-1 and insulin release. Decrease in requirement for gastric surgery for peptic ulcer disease and newer gastric operations such as proximal gastric vagotomy have reduced the incidence of postgastrectomy syndromes. However, as Roux-en-Y gastric bypass surgery has become a popular treatment for morbid obesity, there have been a number of reports of severe postprandial neuroglycopenia. The prevalence of the syndrome after Roux-en-Y procedure is not known. The University of Minnesota surgery group identified 14 cases of postprandial hypoglycemia in 3082 procedures (0.4%), but it is unclear how many patients may have eluded detection or failed to maintain follow-up.

Patients typically complain of the symptoms more severe after consumption of large amounts or readily absorbable carbohydrates. The mixed meal test can be used to precipitate the symptoms. The composition of the mixed meal has not been standardized, and it is reasonable to request the patient to consume a meal that leads to symptoms during everyday life. The University of Minnesota

TABLE 18–6 Test meals for evaluation of postprandial hypoglycemia after Roux-en-Y gastric bypass surgery.

High Carbohydrate Meal (79% Carbohydrate, 11% Fat, and 10% Protein; 405 kcal)	Low Carbohydrate Meal (2% Carbohydrate, 74% Fat, and 24% Protein; 415 kcal)
8 oz of orange juice 1 slice of toast with 1 tsp of margarine and 2 tsp of jam	Decaffeinated black coffee or tea (without sugar) 1 egg, a 1-oz sausage patty, and a 0.5-oz slice of cheese

After overnight fast (≥8 hours) give high carbohydrate meal on day 1 and low carbohydrate meal on day 2. Measure plasma glucose and serum insulin levels before (fasting) and 30, 60, 90, 120, 150, and 180 minutes after the meal.

Adapted from Kellogg TA, et al. Postgastric bypass hyperinsulinemic hypoglycemia syndrome: characterization and response to a modified diet. *Surg Obes Relat Dis.* 2008 4:492-499.

investigators formalized a high carbohydrate and a low carbohydrate test meal (Table 18–6) and showed that in patients with postgastric bypass hypoglycemia, the high carbohydrate meal resulted in hyperglycemia and concomitant hyperinsulinemia at about 30 minutes after a meal. Glucose levels then fell to a nadir (range 28-62 mg/dL) at 90 to 120 minutes. Eating the low carbohydrate meal, however, resulted in very little change in plasma glucose levels and only a modest increase in plasma insulin. The prolonged (5 hour) oral glucose tolerance test is not recommended for evaluation because a large number of healthy subjects will have a false-positive result. There have been case reports of insulinoma and noninsulinoma pancreatogenous hypoglycemia syndrome occurring in patients who present with hypoglycemia post-Roux-en-Y surgery. It is unclear how often this occurs. A careful history may identify those patients who have history of hypoglycemia with exercise or when meals are missed, and these individuals may require a formal 72-hour fast to rule out an insulinoma. Those patients with well-documented postprandial hyperinsulinemic hypoglycemia, which does not respond to medical treatment, may need to have selective calcium-stimulated angiography to identify diffuse islet cell hyperplasia (nesidioblastosis).

Several different treatments can be tried for the late dumping syndrome. Dietary modification is the best option but may be difficult to sustain for some patients. More frequent meals with smaller portions of less rapidly assimilated carbohydrate and more slowly absorbed fat or protein can be tried. Alpha glucosidase inhibitors (acarbose and miglitol) can be a useful adjunct to a low carbohydrate diet in some patients. Octreotide 50 μg administered subcutaneously two or three times a day 30 minutes prior to each meal has been reported to improve symptoms in patients with severe dumping refractory to other forms of medical interventions. Information regarding long-term octreotide use is however limited. Various surgical procedures to slow down gastric emptying have been reported to improve symptoms, but long-term efficacy studies are lacking. Recently it has been reported that endoscopic gastrojejunal anastomotic reduction to induce delay in gastric pouch emptying in patients with Roux-en-Y surgery

improves the dumping syndrome symptoms. Partial pancreatectomy is also an option for those postgastric bypass patients with hypoglycemia who have a positive selective calcium stimulation test and in whom medical therapy has failed.

Noninsulinoma pancreatogenous hypoglycemia syndrome (NIPHS): These are patients with hyperinsulinemic hypoglycemia due to generalized islet hyperplasia and nesidioblastosis. These patients predominantly have symptoms 2 to 4 hours after meals and only rarely while fasting. The majority of patients are male (70%), and all have neuroglycopenic symptoms including diplopia, dysarthria, confusion, disorientation, and even convulsions and coma. At the time of hypoglycemia, these patients have elevated insulin; C-peptide and proinsulin levels; and negative sulfonylurea, repaglinide, and nateglinide screens. Typically these patients have a negative 72-hour fast. Imaging studies are also negative. These patients have a positive selective arterial calcium stimulation test—usually positive for multiple arteries. NIPHS patients do not have mutations in the *KIR6.2* and *SUR1* genes, which have been abnormal in some cases of children with a syndrome of familial hyperinsulinemic hypoglycemia (see later) Gradient-guided partial or subtotal pancreatectomy relieves the hypoglycemic symptoms in the majority of patients.

Late hypoglycemia of occult diabetes: This condition is characterized by insulin release from pancreatic β cells, resulting in initial exaggeration of hyperglycemia during a glucose tolerance test. In response to this hyperglycemia, exaggerated delayed insulin release produces late hypoglycemia 4 to 5 hours after ingestion of glucose. These patients are often obese, frequently have a family history of diabetes mellitus and have impaired glucose tolerance. In the obese, treatment is directed at reduction to ideal weight. These patients also often respond to reduced intake of refined sugars with multiple, spaced, small feedings high in dietary fiber. They should be considered to have prediabetes or early diabetes (type 1 or 2) and advised to have periodic medical evaluations.

Postprandial syndrome (functional alimentary hypoglycemia): Patients present with symptoms suggestive of increased sympathetic activity—anxiety, weakness, tremor, sweating, or palpitations after meals. Physical examination and laboratory tests are normal. Previously many of these patients underwent a 5-hour oral glucose tolerance test and the detection of glucose levels in the 50s was determined to be responsible for the symptoms, and the recommendation was to modify the diet. It is now recognized that at least 10% of normal subjects who do not have any symptoms have nadir glucose levels less than 50 mg/dL during a 4- to 6-hour oral glucose tolerance test. In a study comparing responses to an oral glucose tolerance test with the response to a mixed meal test, none of the patients who had plasma glucose levels less than 50 mg/dL on oral glucose testing had low glucose values with the mixed meal. Thus, it is not recommended that these patients undergo either a prolonged oral glucose tolerance test or a mixed meal test. The patients should instead be given home blood glucose monitors (with memories) and instructed to monitor fingerstick glucose levels at the time of symptoms. Only patients who have symptoms when their fingerstick blood glucose is low (<50 mg/dL) and who have resolution of symptoms when the glucose is raised by consumption of readily absorbable carbohydrate need additional evaluation. Patients who do not have evidence for low glucose levels at the time of symptoms are generally reassured by their findings. Counseling and support should be the mainstays of therapy in this group, with dietary manipulation used only as an adjunctive form of therapy.

8. DISORDERS ASSOCIATED WITH LOW HEPATIC GLUCOSE OUTPUT

Reduced hepatic gluconeogenesis can result from a direct loss of hepatic tissue (acute yellow atrophy from fulminant viral hepatitis or toxic damage), from disorders that reduce amino acid substrate for hepatic gluconeogenesis (severe muscle wasting and inanition from anorexia nervosa, chronic starvation, uremia, and glucocorticoid deficit from adrenocortical deficiency), or from inborn errors of carbohydrate metabolism affecting glycogenolytic or gluconeogenic enzymes.

CONGENITAL HYPERINSULINISM

Neonatal hypoglycemia is a very common problem and can be due to a variety of causes (Table 18–7). In the first day of life, normal babies do not tolerate fasting for periods of 8 hours after delivery. Hypoglycemia in this setting is attributed to impaired ketogenesis and gluconeogenesis. This developmental immaturity in the metabolic response to fasting resolves within the first 2 to 3 days of life. Hypoglycemia in the first few days of life may be directly related to maternal factors, such as maternal diabetes, intravenous glucose use during labor and delivery, and various medications. All of these factors induce a transient hyperinsulinism in the newborn. Prolonged neonatal hypoglycemia may result from perinatal stress, the Beckwith-Wiedeman syndrome, and hypopituitarism. The risk for hypoglycemia can persist for weeks to months. Persistent hypoglycemia may result from: (1) a deficiency in one or more counterregulatory hormones; (2) defects in glycogenolysis, gluconeogenesis,

or fatty acid oxidation; or (3) congenital hyperinsulinism, the various forms of which are discussed further below.

As with adults, hyperinsulinism is the most frequent cause of persistent hypoglycemia in infants and children. As compared to adults, where the most common cause of hyperinsulinism is an insulin-secreting adenoma, in infants hyperinsulinism most likely stems from an underlying genetic disorder. This condition has been referenced in various ways, including persistent hyperinsulinemic hypoglycemia of infancy or islet dysregulation syndrome, but hereafter will be referred to as congenital hyperinsulinism. Transient congenital hyperinsulinism is a common disorder in the immediate neonatal period. Persistent disorders are rarer, occurring in approximately 1 in 50,000. This problem was originally attributed to an anomaly in islet development, termed **nesidioblastosis**, a reference to endocrine cell budding from pancreatic ducts. However, this budding has since been noted to represent a normal developmental process during the first year of life. Recent advances in our understanding of the regulation of insulin secretion have begun to elucidate the underlying pathophysiology of this complex disease. Congenital hyperinsulinism has now been attributed to at least seven different gene defects. However, depending on the series cited, no genetic explanation is found in 50% or more of cases. Timely diagnosis and aggressive treatment are essential to prevent long-term neurologic sequelae in the affected individual.

Transient Hyperinsulinism

A. Infants of diabetic mothers   The fetuses of mothers with poorly regulated diabetes are exposed to sustained hyperglycemia, leading to increased fetal insulin secretion, with resultant macrosomia. This increased insulin secretion persists postpartum and usually resolves after several days. As a result, infants of diabetic mothers are at high risk of developing hypoglycemia after birth. They can usually be managed with early, frequent feedings or intravenous glucose until insulin secretion has normalized, often 1 to 2 days after birth.

B. Small for gestational age, asphyxiation, and other conditions in newborns   Various perinatal stresses are known to induce hyperinsulinism. Small-for-gestational age and asphyxiated newborns, usually from toxemic mothers, frequently experience hyperinsulinism and hypoglycemia. Hyperinsulinism is also reported in erythroblastosis fetalis, sepsis, cerebral hemorrhage, and severely stressed newborns. Hypoglycemia usually resolves within a period of several days or weeks but may persist in these settings for 6 to 12 months. Some newborns with Beckwith-Wiedemann syndrome and Soto syndrome (also known as cerebral gigantism) show β cell hyperplasia and experience transient hypoglycemia from hyperinsulinism.

Persistent Hyperinsulinism

Persistent hyperinsulinism, continuing for more than several weeks, results from a group of heterogeneous disorders, rather than a single entity, and the various subtypes are discussed below.

TABLE 18–7   **Types of congenital hyperinsulinism and their causes.**

Transient
  Infants of diabetic mothers
  Miscellaneous
    Small for gestational age, asphyxia, and stress in infants
    Syndromes (eg, Beckwith-Wiedemann, Soto)
Persistent
  Defects in ATP-dependent potassium channel
    Sulfonylurea receptor (SUR)
    Kir6.2
    Focal vs diffuse disease
  Metabolic defects
    Glutamate dehydrogenase
    Glucokinase
    Short-chain L-3-hydroxyacyl-CoA dehydrogenase (SCHAD)
    Exercise-induced
    Glycosylation disorders

These forms may be classified in a variety of different ways, including usual time of presentation (shortly after birth vs after months to years of life); mode of genetic transmission (autosomal recessive vs dominant); or anatomic (focal vs diffuse). In this section, the forms are grouped into defects in the pancreatic β cell ATP-sensitive potassium channel, defects affecting intracellular metabolism, and several other miscellaneous conditions.

A. Channel defects

1. **Sulfonylurea receptor and Kir6.2**—The most common cause of congenital hyperinsulinism appears to be related to defects in the pancreatic β cell ATP-sensitive potassium channel. This channel consists of a multimer of two proteins, the sulfonylurea receptor (SUR), a member of the ATP-binding cassette superfamily, and Kir6.2, a member of a family of inwardly rectifying potassium channels. With increases in intracellular ATP, the channel closes, leading to depolarization and insulin secretion (see Chapter 17). Defects in either component of the channel result in channel closure, inappropriate β cell depolarization, and secretion of insulin, even in the face of low or normal glucose concentrations.

   The two genes encoding the channel components are located in tandem on chromosome 11p15. Numerous mutations have now been described and appear to occur more frequently in the SUR than the *Kir6.2* gene. They are usually autosomal recessive defects, but dominant defects have also been reported. Sequencing of these molecules is now available commercially and may not be merely of academic interest: patients harboring *SUR* or *Kir6.2* mutations often do not respond well to medical therapy. Thus, knowledge of the underlying defect may influence treatment decisions for a particular patient as well as inform the family about risk to future children. Relative to other forms of congenital hyperinsulinism, patients with defects in the ATP-sensitive potassium channel often present early in life, with more marked clinical symptomatology, including macrosomia. They experience early onset and severe hypoglycemia that requires high rates of glucose infusion to normalize serum glucose concentrations and typically require pancreatectomy to restore euglycemia.

2. **Focal versus diffuse disease**—Two histologically distinct forms of congenital hyperinsulinism have been described, a diffuse form, mentioned above, which constitutes 35% to 70% of cases, depending on the series cited, and a focal form (focal adenomatous hyperplasia). Diagnosis of the focal form is made by pancreatic venous sampling and by perioperative extemporaneous histologic examination. [18F]Fluorodopa positron emission tomography may also be of utility in defining focal lesions. Histologic examination of the focal form reveals focal hyperplasia, with hypertrophied β cells harboring giant nuclei, in contrast to the diffuse form, where all the islets of Langerhans are irregular in size and contain hypertrophied β cells. The molecular explanation for the focal defect is based on a two-hit model, in which the child already harbors a mutant allele from a paternally derived potassium-ATP channel defect. Subsequent somatic loss of heterozygosity for the maternal 11p chromosome is associated with focal disease and may result from a decrease in dosage of an independent growth-suppressing gene(s) in this region. The distinction between these two forms of hyperinsulinism has potentially important implications for therapy, because patients with focal disease may be cured with more limited partial pancreatectomy, whereas those with the diffuse form require more aggressive near-total resection. Such patients can only be fully evaluated and treated at centers equipped with a team of endocrinologists, interventional radiologists, pathologists, and surgeons with expertise in this disorder.

B. Metabolic defects

The second most common form of congenital hyperinsulinism is the hyperinsulinism-hyperammonemia syndrome, which results from activating mutations of the *glutamate dehydrogenase (GDH)* gene. This condition is inherited in autosomal dominant fashion. This enzyme mediates oxidative deamination of glutamate to alpha ketoglutarate. Activating mutations impair GDH sensitivity to guanosine triphosphate, an allosteric inhibitor, and increase sensitivity to leucine, an allosteric activator. With increased GDH activity, increased production of alpha ketoglutarate with subsequent oxidation in the Krebs cycle generates increased ATP, which in turn activates the ATP-sensitive potassium channel and leads to depolarization and insulin secretion. GDH is also expressed in hepatocytes, and increased activity generates ammonia via glutamate oxidation. Thus, one hallmark of this defect is increased ammonia concentrations three to five times normal. The patients with GDH mutations usually have a milder course than those with defects in the ATP-sensitive potassium channel, often presenting outside of the neonatal period. They often have postprandial hypoglycemia, particularly in response to higher protein loads, but may also manifest fasting hypoglycemia. They usually respond well to diazoxide, and many are able to eventually discontinue treatment.

A much rarer form of autosomal dominant hyperinsulinism results from mutations in glucokinase, the first and rate-limiting step in glycolysis, and an enzyme that is considered to play an essential role in glucose sensing by the β cell. Individuals heterozygous for inactivating mutations have a form of maturity onset diabetes of the young. On the other hand, activating mutations have been described in two families that result in increased rates of glycolysis at lower glucose concentrations. The resultant increase in the intracellular ATP/ADP ratio increases insulin secretion at any given serum glucose concentration, resulting in hypoglycemia.

An entity referred to as **exercise-induced hyperinsulinism** has been described, in which hyperinsulinism is noted following exercise. An underlying genetic cause has not yet been proven, although it is suspected that this represents another metabolic defect. This problem appears to be milder than the others described earlier, and it neither presents in the neonatal period nor results in fasting hypoglycemia. A recent report suggested an autosomal dominant pattern of inheritance in multiple members of two families. Hyperinsulinism was induced by exercise and by pyruvate infusion, suggesting that this disorder results from abnormal transport or metabolism of pyruvate in β cells.

Another autosomal recessive form of congenital hyperinsulinism results from mutations in the gene encoding the short chain L-3-hydroxyacyl-CoA dehydrogenase. This enzyme mediates the penultimate step in fatty acid beta oxidation and as such represents the first link between defects in fatty acid metabolism and insulin secretion. However, it is not yet clear how this defect results in congenital hyperinsulinism.

Congenital disorders in glycosylation have also been linked with congenital hyperinsulinism. The mechanism is unclear, although hypoglycosylation of the SUR with a resultant defect in trafficking to the cell membrane has been offered as a possible explanation. Nonetheless, these patients appear to be responsive to diazoxide, suggesting that at least some functional ATP-sensitive potassium channels reach the cell surface. Affected individuals have multisystem disorders, including neurologic defects.

Despite the evolving elucidation of defects known to be associated with congenital hyperinsulinism, the underlying diagnosis remains unknown in up to one-half of infants diagnosed with this condition.

Clinical Presentation

The cardinal symptoms of hyperinsulinism are recurrent episodes of hypoglycemia and can occur any time after birth until several years of age, or manifest even later in life, depending on the nature and severity of the defect. As in adults, the symptoms of hypoglycemia are secondary to adrenergic responses or neuroglycopenia. However, in neonates and infants, symptoms are difficult to detect and may be less specific. They may include tremors, cyanosis, hypothermia, apnea or irregular breathing, lethargy, apathy, limpness, refusal to eat, high-pitched cries, and seizures of any type. Even if newborns appear asymptomatic, hypoglycemia can be as severe as in symptomatic neonates.

Diagnosis

The differential diagnosis for hypoglycemia in a neonate is quite long and includes deficiencies in counterregulatory hormones (eg, growth hormone, ACTH, glucocorticoids); defects in gluconeogenesis, glycogen synthesis, and breakdown; and disorders in fatty acid metabolism. Hyperinsulinism is suspected in hypoglycemic newborns or infants who require unusually high glucose infusion rates (12-30 mg/kg/min) to maintain blood glucose levels in the target range. Macrosomia may be another clue to hyperinsulinism, although it is not always present. The crucial diagnostic step is to obtain a *critical* blood sample for glucose, insulin, growth hormone, cortisol, blood gas, lactate, free fatty acids, and ketones (β-hydroxybutyrate) during hypoglycemia. Urinary ketones should be measured in the first urine after hypoglycemia. Insulin levels must often be measured during several episodes of hypoglycemia because insulin levels at times of hypoglycemia are not always diagnostically elevated. In fact, insulin levels that are inappropriately measurable during episodes of hypoglycemia are still consistent with the diagnosis. As in adults, the hallmarks of hyperinsulinism include measurable plasma insulin in the face of hypoglycemia (glucose <40 mg/dL), low or unmeasurable ketones and free fatty acids, and hyperresponsiveness to glucagon challenge, with the glycemic response to 0.5 to 1 mg of parenteral glucagon of more than 30 mg/dL (with glucose monitored every 15 minutes for up to 45 minutes after glucagon injection). Low IGF-binding protein (IGFBP) 1 levels also suggests this diagnosis, as insulin suppresses IGFBP1 secretion from the liver.

Treatment

A. Medical therapy   Management of children with congenital hyperinsulinism remains one of the most challenging problems for pediatric endocrinologists, and affected children should be transferred to a tertiary center that has experience in managing such children. Patients may require high glucose infusion rates to maintain euglycemia, and thus a secure central line is usually necessary. They also require frequent glucose monitoring, extensive ongoing laboratory assessment to establish the underlying diagnosis, and a series of medical and/or surgical interventions to effect a cure.

Hypoglycemia in infancy has to be treated aggressively in order to prevent long-term neurologic sequelae. Relative to adults, younger children (up to age 5 to 6 years) appear to be particularly vulnerable to such damage. Those with hyperinsulinism are particularly at risk, because ketone bodies are not present as an alternative fuel source. The therapeutic goal is to achieve glucose levels above 60 mg/dL while the infant is on an appropriate feeding schedule for age. Infants receiving appropriate therapy must be able to support a fast for at least 4 to 6 hours without hypoglycemia. In selected cases in which food refusal or intercurrent illness is a problem, hypoglycemia can be prevented by placing a gastrostomy tube to administer food on a regular basis.

For acute management of hypoglycemia, stabilization of blood glucoses may require infusion rates of glucose up to 20 to 30 mg/kg/min, well above the 4 to 8 mg/kg/min needed to stabilize most neonates. Some centers employ aggressive enteral feeding, using frequent feeds or continuous feeding via nasogastric or gastrostomy tube, with or without cornstarch, as a means to avoid hypoglycemia. The following drugs are also used in the medical management of hyperinsulinemic hypoglycemia.

1. **Diazoxide**—Diazoxide is the drug of choice in neonates who cannot be weaned from intravenous glucose. Diazoxide increases blood glucose by stabilizing the ATP-sensitive potassium channel in the open state, thereby inhibiting membrane depolarization and insulin secretion. Functionally intact SUR and Kir6.2 proteins are necessary for the full action of the drug, and thus, patients with channel defects often do not respond, whereas those with other forms of hyperinsulinism do exhibit salutary responses. Diazoxide also increases catecholamine release, which suppresses insulin release and inhibits insulin's actions peripherally. The initial recommended dose is 10 to 15 mg/kg/d divided every 8 hours, up to a maximal dose of 20 mg/kg/d. Positive responses are usually seen within 48 hours if they are going to occur. Diazoxide has several important side effects that should be considered. Fluid retention can be managed by simultaneous administration of chlorothiazide. Hypertrichosis and coarse facial changes may become quite striking and can be reduced only by decreasing the dose or discontinuing the diazoxide altogether. Hyperuricemia, leukopenia, and thrombocytopenia are rare, but routine serum studies must be monitored while therapy continues. Diazoxide is also an antihypertensive drug, but these effects are rarely encountered with oral administration.

   Depending on the study cited, diazoxide appears to be efficacious in only one-fourth to one-half of the patients with hyperinsulinism and appears to be less likely to work in those patients presenting in the immediate newborn period, a population that often has more marked defects in ATP-sensitive potassium channel activity. Thus, in those patients with persistent hyperinsulinism, determining whether mutations are present in *SUR* or *Kir6.2* genes may help anticipate the response to medical therapy and predict the need for more definitive surgical intervention.

2. **Somatostatin analogs**—This is usually a second-line approach, for those unresponsive to diazoxide. Somatostatin acts via a G protein–coupled receptor to lower intracellular calcium and to hyperpolarize the β cell membrane, thereby inhibiting insulin release. Somatostatin has a half-life of only 1 to 3 minutes, but the synthetic analog octreotide may be administered at intervals of up to 8 hours or via continuous subcutaneous infusion and is efficacious in some patients with congenital hyperinsulinism. A starting dose of 5 to 10 μg/kg/d, administered either as an intermittent bolus or via continuous subcutaneous infusion in a pump, often produces salutary initial responses, but because of tachyphylaxis, the dose sometimes has to be increased to as much as 40 μg/kg/d. Some physicians advocate octreotide in patients who fail to respond to diazoxide therapy alone. However, optimal control of blood glucose often cannot be achieved by adding octreotide, and partial pancreatectomy is necessary. Nonetheless, the medication may help stabilize blood glucose concentrations in the preoperative period and may prove efficacious postoperatively in those patients who have persistent hyperinsulinism even with reduced β cell mass. There are some reports of long-term success (>5 years) with octreotide alone.

Short-term side effects are mostly self-limited within the first several weeks of therapy. Octreotide has nonspecific effects on the gastrointestinal tract, including decreased perfusion of the splanchnic circulation, gallbladder contractility, and bile secretion. Short-term effects may include vomiting, abdominal distension, and steatorrhea, with later risk of cholelithiasis. Possible inhibitory effects of octreotide on other hormonal axes, including effects on the pituitary somatotrope, adrenal, and thyroid, raise concerns about its long-term use, although some centers report successful and uneventful use for years without significant problems.

3. **Glucagon**—Glucagon has a place in the management of hyperinsulinism during initial stabilization of the hypoglycemic infant in the intensive care unit or prior to surgery. This agent stimulates hepatic glycogenolysis and is very effective in these patients because their glycogen stores are replete. A variety of doses has been shown to be effective, including a bolus of 0.2 mg intravenously in cases of severe hypoglycemia followed by a continuous infusion at a dose of 2 to 10 mg/kg/h. An intramuscular glucagon injection may also be used as an emergency treatment of recurrent hypoglycemic episodes at home. Attempts have been made to administer glucagon continuously via subcutaneous infusion with limited success.

4. **Calcium antagonists**—Because calcium influx is required for insulin secretion, calcium antagonists could play a potential role in the treatment of hyperinsulinism. Calcium channel blockers also decrease the transcriptional response of insulin to glucose. However, only rare and limited success has been achieved with this class of drugs, perhaps because of failure to block calcium channels selectively within the β cells.

B. Surgical therapy Partial pancreatectomy is undertaken when maintenance of euglycemia cannot be achieved with medical treatment alone. The initial surgical procedure of choice has traditionally been a 95% pancreatectomy. However, such procedures are now being reconsidered, with the appreciation that some of these infants may have a focal rather than diffuse process and may require only selective resection of the affected pancreatic tissue in order to effect a cure. Unfortunately, only a limited number of medical centers around the world are now equipped to conduct the pre- and perioperative evaluation to distinguish focal from diffuse disease, which includes selective venous sampling and histological analysis.

Even with more aggressive resections, β cell mass reduction does not always lead to euglycemia, and medical therapy may have to be continued following surgery. If this fails to restore euglycemia, a second surgical intervention may be required in which near-total pancreatectomy (99%) is performed. Potential surgical complications include intraoperative injury to the common bile duct and adhesions with intestinal obstruction. Additional complications include exocrine pancreatic insufficiency, often requiring oral supplements at mealtimes, and diabetes mellitus.

Outcome

Neurologic sequelae are the major concern with severe hypoglycemia during infancy and childhood. Multiple episodes of hypoglycemia are more often associated with sequelae than one severe hypoglycemic episode with convulsions. At least one-third of patients with congenital hyperinsulinism suffer from developmental delay based on follow-up via a telephone survey.

Patients with the familial form of congenital hyperinsulinism who harbor mutations in the SUR receptor may be at additional neurologic risk. The SUR is expressed in the brain, and defects in this molecule could potentially interfere with neural development. The role of this receptor in the brain, however, has yet to be elucidated.

Affected individuals also appear to be at higher risk for later development of diabetes. This problem may be related to reduced β cell mass following pancreatectomy or from β cell apoptosis following chronic depolarization in subjects who harbor channel defects.

REFERENCES

Amiel SA. Hypoglycemia: from the laboratory to the clinic. *Diabetes Care.* 2009;32:1364. [PMID: 19638523]

Banarer S, McGregor VP, Cryer PE. Intraislet hyperinsulinemia prevents the glucagon response to hyperglycemia despite an intact autonomic response. *Diabetes.* 2002;51:958. [PMID: 11916913]

Bolli GB, Fanelli CG. Physiology of glucose counterregulation to hypoglycemia. *Endocrinol Metab Clin North Am.* 1999;28:467. [PMID: 10500926]

Boyle PJ, Kempers SF, O'Connor AM, Nagy RJ. Brain glucose uptake and unawareness of hypoglycemia in patients with insulin-dependent diabetes mellitus. *N Engl J Med.* 1995 Dec 28;333(26):1726-1731. [PMID: 7491135]

Cryer PE. Mechanisms of hypoglycemia-associated autonomic failure and its component syndromes in diabetes. *Diabetes.* 2005;54:3592. [PMID: 16306382]

Cryer P E, Axelrod L, Grossman A, et al. Evaluation and management of adult hypoglycemic disorders: an Endocrine Society Clinical Practice Guideline. *J Clin Endocrinol Metab.* 2009;94:709. [PMID: 19088155]

de Groot JW, Rikhof B, van Doorn J, et al. Non-islet cell tumour-induced hypoglycaemia: a review of the literature including two new cases. *Endocr Relat Cancer.* 2007;14:979. [PMID: 18045950]

De Leon DD, Stanley CA. Mechanisms of disease: advances in diagnosis and treatment of hyperinsulinism in neonates. *Nat Clin Pract Endocrinol Metab.* 2007;3:57. [PMID: 17179930]

de Lonlay P, Fournet JC, Rahier J, et al. Somatic deletion of the imprinted 11p15 region in sporadic persistent hyperinsulinemic hypoglycemia of infancy is specific for focal adenomatous hyperplasia and endorses partial pancreatectomy. *J Clin Invest.* 1997;100:802. [PMID: 9259578]

Diabetes Control and Complications Trial/Epidemiology of Diabetes Interventions and Complications Study Research Group. Long-term effect of diabetes and its treatment on cognitive function. *N Engl J Med.* 2007;356:1842. [PMID: 17476010]

Doppman JL, Chang R, Fraker DL, et al. Localization of insulinomas to regions of the pancreas by intra-arterial stimulation with calcium. *Ann Intern Med.* 1995;123:269. [PMID: 7611592]

Dunne MJ, Cosgrove KE, Shepherd RM, Aynsley-Green A, Lindley KJ. Hyperinsulinism in infancy: from basic science to clinical disease. *Physiol Rev.* 2004;84:239. [PMID: 14715916]

Ekberg K, Landau BR, Wajngot A, et al. Contributions by kidney and liver to glucose production in the post-absorptive state and after 60 h of fasting. *Diabetes.* 1999;48:292. [PMID: 10334304]

Fanelli C, Pampanelli S, Epifano L, et al. Long-term recovery from unawareness, deficient counterregulation and lack of cognitive dysfunction during hypoglycemia following institution of rational, intensive insulin therapy in IDDM. *Diabetologia.* 1994;37:1265. [PMID: 7895957]

Glaser B, Hirsch HJ, Landau H. Persistent hyperinsulinemic hypoglycemia of infancy: long-term octreotide treatment without pancreatectomy. *J Pediatr.* 1993;123:644. [PMID: 8410523]

Grant CS. Insulinoma. *Best Pract Res Clin Gastroenterol.* 2005 Oct;19(5):783-798. [PMID: 16253900]

Hardy OT, Hernandez-Pampaloni M, Saffer JR, et al. Accuracy of [18F]fluorodopa positron emission tomography for diagnosing and localizing focal congenital hyperinsulinism. *J Clin Endocrinol Metab.* 2007;92:4706. [PMID: 17895314]

Hoe FM, Thornton PS, Wanner LA, Steinkrauss L, Simmons RA, Stanley CA. Clinical features and insulin regulation in infants with a syndrome of prolonged neonatal hyperinsulinism. *J Pediatr.* 2006;148:207. [PMID: 16492430]

Hussain K, Cosgrove KE. From congenital hyperinsulinism to diabetes mellitus: the role of pancreatic beta-cell KATP channels. *Pediatr Diabetes.* 2005;6:103. [PMID: 15963039]

Kellogg TA, Bantle JP, Leslie DB, et al. Postgastric bypass hyperinsulinemic hypoglycemia syndrome: characterization and response to a modified diet. *Surg Obes Relat Dis.* 2008;4:492. [PMID: 18656831]

Kumar U, Sasi R, Suresh S, et al. Subtype selective expression of the five somatostatin receptors (hSSTR 1–5) in human pancreatic islet cells. *Diabetes.* 1999;48:77. [PMID: 9892225]

Leibowitz G, Glaser B, Higazi AA, Salameh M, Cerasi E, Landau H. Hyperinsulinemic hypoglycemia of infancy (nesidioblastosis) in clinical remission: high incidence of diabetes mellitus and persistent beta-cell dysfunction at long-term follow-up. *J Clin Endocrinol Metab.* 1995;80:386. [PMID: 7852494]

Lupsa BC, Chong AY, Cochran EK, Soos MA, Semple RK, Gorden P. Autoimmune forms of hypoglycemia. *Medicine (Baltimore).* 2009;88:141. [PMID: 19440117]

Marks V, Teale JD. Drug-induced hypoglycemia. *Endocrinol Metab Clin North Am.* 1999;28:555. [PMID: 10500931]

Marks V, Teale JD. Hypoglycemia: factitious and felonious. *Endocrinol Metab Clin North Am.* 1999;28:579. [PMID: 10500932]

Mathur A, Gorden P, Libutti SK. Insulinoma. *Surg Clin North Am.* 2009 Oct;89(5):1105-21. [PMID: 19836487]

Meier JJ, Butler AE, Galasso R, Butler PC. Hyperinsulinemic hypoglycemia after gastric bypass surgery is not accompanied by islet hyperplasia or increased beta-cell turnover. *Diabetes Care.* 2006;29:1554. [PMID: 16801578]

Rave K, Flesch S, Kuhn-Velten WN, Hompesch BC, Heinemann L, Heise T. Enhancement of blood glucose lowering effect of a sulfonylurea when coadministered with an ACE inhibitor: results of a glucose-clamp study. *Diab Metabol Res Rev.* 2005;21:459. [PMID: 15915547]

Seckl MJ, Mulholland PJ, Bishop AE, et al. Hypoglycemia due to an insulin-secreting small cell carcinoma of the cervix. *N Engl J Med.* 1999;341:733. [PMID: 10471459]

Service FJ. Diagnostic approach to adults with hypoglycemic disorders. *Endocrinol Metab Clin North Am.* 1999;28:519. [PMID: 10500929]

Service FJ, Natt N. The prolonged fast. *J Clin Endocrinol Metab.* 2000;85:3973. [PMID: 11095416]

Service GJ, Thompson GB, Service FJ, Andrews JC, Collazo-Clavell ML, Lloyd RV. Hyperinsulinemic hypoglycemia with nesidioblastosis after gastric-bypass surgery. *N Engl J Med.* 2005;353:249. [PMID: 16034010]

Stumvoll M, Meyer C, Mitrakou A, Nadkarni V, Gerich JE. Renal glucose production and utilization: new aspects in humans. *Diabetologia.* 1997;40:749. [PMID: 9243094]

Thompson GB, Service FJ, Andrews JC. Noninsulinoma pancreatogenous hypoglycemia syndrome: an update in 10 surgically treated patients. *Surgery.* 2000;128:937. [PMID: 11114627]

Thornton PS, Alter CA, Katz LE, Baker L, Stanley CA. Short- and long-term use of octreotide in the treatment of congenital hyperinsulinism. *J Pediatr.* 1993;123:637. [PMID: 8410522]

Tucker ON, Crotty PL, Conlon KC. The management of insulinoma. *Br J Surg.* 2006;93:264. [PMID: 16498592]

Weinzimer SA, Stanley CA, Berry GT, Yudkoff M, Tuchman M, Thornton PS. A syndrome of congenital hyperinsulinism and hyperammonemia. *J Pediatr.* 1997;130:661. [PMID: 9108870]

Disorders of Lipoprotein Metabolism

Mary J. Malloy, MD and John P. Kane, MD, PhD

ABCA1	ATP-binding cassette transporter A1	**Idol**	Inducible degrader of the LDL receptor
ABCG1	ATP-binding cassette transporter G1	**LCAT**	Lecithin-cholesterol acyltransferase
ACAT	Acyl-CoA:cholesterol acyltransferase	**LDL**	Low-density lipoproteins
Apo	Apolipoprotein	**LMF1**	Lipase maturation factor 1
ARH	Autosomal recessive hypercholesterolemia	**Lp(a)**	Lipoprotein(a)
CETP	Cholesteryl ester transfer protein	**LPL**	Lipoprotein lipase
CHD	Coronary heart disease	**LRP-1**	LDL receptor-related protein-1
CK	Creatine kinase	**MCP-1**	Monocyte chemoattractant protein-1
FCH	Familial combined hyperlipidemia	**NAFLD**	Nonalcoholic fatty liver disease
FFA	Free fatty acids	**NASH**	Nonalcoholic steatohepatitis
FH	Familial hypercholesterolemia	**PCPE-2**	Procollagen C-proteinase enhancer-2
GPIHDLBP	Glycosylphosphatidylinositol-anchored HDL-binding protein	**PCSK9**	Proprotein convertase subtilisin/kexin type 9
HDL	High-density lipoproteins	**PDGF**	Platelet-derived growth factor
HMG-CoA	Hydroxymethylglutaryl-CoA	**SR-BI**	Scavenger receptor, class B, type I
IDL	intermediate density lipoproteins	**VLDL**	Very low density lipoproteins

The clinical importance of lipoprotein disorders derives chiefly from the role of lipoproteins in atherogenesis and its associated risk of coronary and peripheral vascular disease. The greatly increased risk of acute pancreatitis associated with severe hypertriglyceridemia is an additional indication for intervention. Disordered lipid metabolism is also a critical element in nonalcoholic fatty liver disease. Characterization of dyslipidemia is important for selection of appropriate treatment and may provide clues to underlying primary clinical disorders.

ATHEROSCLEROSIS

Atherosclerosis is the leading cause of death in the United States. Abundant epidemiologic evidence establishes its multifactorial character and indicates that the effects of the multiple risk factors are at least additive. Risk factors include hyperlipidemia, hypertension, smoking, diabetes, physical inactivity, decreased levels of high-density lipoproteins (HDL), hyperhomocysteinemia, and hypercoagulable states. Atheromas are complex lesions containing cellular elements, collagen, and lipids. The progression of the lesion is chiefly attributable to its content of unesterified cholesterol and cholesteryl esters. Cholesterol in the atheroma originates in circulating lipoproteins. Atherogenic lipoproteins include low-density (LDL), intermediate density (IDL), very low density lipoproteins (VLDL), and Lp(a) species, all of which contain the B-100 apolipoprotein (Apo B-100). Chylomicron remnants containing apoB-48 are also atherogenic. All of these are subject to oxidation by reactive oxygen species in the tissues and also by lipoxygenases secreted by macrophages in atheromas. Oxidized lipoproteins cause impairment of endothelial cell-mediated vasodilation and stimulate endothelium to secrete monocyte chemoattractant protein-1 (MCP-1) and adhesion molecules that recruit monocytes to the lesion. Tocopherols (vitamin E) are natural antioxidants that localize in the surface monolayers of lipoproteins, exerting resistance to oxidation.

Increased oxidative stress such as that induced by smoking depletes the tocopherol content. Oxidation of lipoproteins stimulates their endocytosis via scavenger receptors on macrophages and smooth muscle cells, leading to the formation of foam cells. Recent studies strongly support a role of vitamin D in prevention of atherosclerosis, probably by influencing inflammatory activity of macrophages.

Hypertension increases access of lipoproteins to the subintima. Smoking accelerates atherogenesis by reducing HDL and increasing thrombogenesis by platelets—in addition to its pro-oxidant effect. Activated platelets release platelet-derived growth factor (PDGF), stimulating proliferation and migration of cells of smooth muscle origin into the lesion.

Activated macrophages secrete cytokines that drive an inflammatory and proliferative process. Metalloproteases secreted by macrophages weaken the atheroma so that fissuring and rupture can occur. Exposure of blood to subintimal collagen and tissue factor stimulates thrombogenesis, precipitating acute coronary events. The inverse relationship between HDL levels and atherogenesis probably reflects the role of certain species of HDL in cholesterol retrieval and in protecting lipoproteins against oxidation.

Reversal of Atherosclerosis

Angiographic intervention trials have shown that regression of atherosclerotic lesions can occur with lipid-lowering therapy. Large trials have demonstrated striking reductions in the incidence of new coronary events in individuals with hyperlipidemia who have had no prior clinical coronary disease (primary prevention) as well as in patients with antecedent disease (secondary prevention). Thus, timely hypolipidemic therapy appropriate to the lipid disorder decreases the incidence of coronary disease and reduces the need for angioplasty, stenting, and bypass surgery. Side-effects of treatment have been minimal in comparison with the magnitude of this benefit.

Average levels of LDL in the United States and northern Europe are higher than in many other nations, where the levels appear to approach the biologic norm. This probably accounts in large part for the higher incidence of coronary disease in industrialized Western nations and suggests that dietary changes that reduce lipoprotein levels would be beneficial.

OVERVIEW OF LIPID TRANSPORT

The Plasma Lipoproteins

Because lipids are relatively insoluble in water, they are transported in association with proteins. The simplest complexes are those formed between unesterified, or free, fatty acids (FFA) and albumin, which serve to carry the FFA from peripheral adipocytes to other tissues.

The remainder of the lipids are transported in spherical lipoprotein complexes (Table 19–1), with core regions containing hydrophobic lipids. The principal core lipids are cholesteryl esters and triglycerides. Triglycerides predominate in the cores of chylomicrons, which transport newly absorbed lipids from the intestine, and in VLDL, which originate in liver. The relative content of cholesteryl ester is increased in the cores of remnants derived from these lipoproteins. Cholesteryl esters are the predominant core lipid in LDL and HDL. Surrounding the core in each lipoprotein is a monolayer containing amphiphilic phospholipids and unesterified (free) cholesterol. Apolipoproteins, noncovalently bound to the lipids, are located on this surface monolayer (Figure19–1).

B Apolipoproteins

Several lipoproteins contain very high molecular weight B proteins that behave like intrinsic proteins of cell membranes. Unlike the smaller apolipoproteins, the B proteins do not migrate from one lipoprotein particle to another. VLDL contain the B-100 protein, which is retained in the formation of LDL from VLDL remnants by liver. The intestinal B protein, B-48, is found only in chylomicrons and their remnants. Apo B-100 has a ligand domain for binding to the LDL receptor that is conformed as VLDL are transformed into LDL.

Other Apolipoproteins

In addition to the B proteins, the following proteins are present in lipoproteins (see Table 19–1.)

C apolipoproteins are lower molecular weight proteins that equilibrate rapidly among the lipoproteins. There are four distinct species: C-I, C-II, C-III, and C-IV. Apo C-II is a requisite cofactor for lipoprotein lipase.

TABLE 19–1 Lipoproteins of human serum.

	Density Interval (g/cm^3)	Core Lipids	Diameter (nm)	Apolipoproteins in Order of Quantitative Importance
High density (HDL)	1.21-1.063	Cholesteryl ester	7.5-10.5	A-I, A-II, C, E (many others)
Low density (LDL)	1.063-1.019	Cholesteryl ester	21.5	B-100
Intermediate density (IDL)	1.019-1.006	Cholesteryl ester, triglyceride	25-30	B-100, some C and E
Very low density (VLDL)	<1.006	Triglyceride cholesteryl ester	39-100	B-100, C, E
Chylomicrons	<1.006	Triglyceride	60-500	B-48, C, E, A-I, A-II, A-IV
Lp(a)	1.04-1.08	Cholesteryl ester	21-30	B-100, (a)

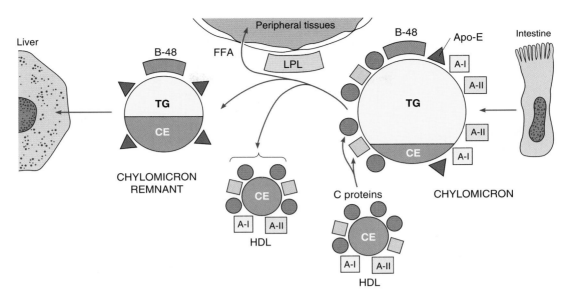

FIGURE 19–1 Metabolism of chylomicrons (A-I, A-II, B-48, and C proteins, apolipoproteins; CE, cholesteryl esters; TG, triglyceride). See text for details.

Three isoforms of Apo E—E-2, E-3, and E-4—are the products of allelic genes. Unlike Apo E-3 and Apo E-4, Apo E-2 does not contain a functional ligand for the LDL receptor. The Apo E-4 alleles are associated with early-onset Alzheimer disease and increased risk of coronary disease.

Apo A-I is the major apolipoprotein of HDL. It is also present in chylomicrons and is the most abundant of the apolipoproteins of human serum (about 125 mg/dL). It is a cofactor for lecithin-cholesterol acyltransferase (LCAT).

Apo A-II is an important constituent of HDL. It contains cysteine, which permits the formation of disulfide-bridged dimers with Apo E.

Apo A-IV is chiefly associated with chylomicrons.

Apo A-V plays a significant role in the removal of triglycerides from plasma.

The (a) protein is a glycoprotein that has a high degree of sequence homology with plasminogen, resulting in binding affinity for tissue plasminogen activator. It is found as a disulfide-bridged dimer with Apo B-100 in LDL-like species of lipoproteins (Lp[a] lipoproteins).

Absorption of Dietary Fat; Secretion of Chylomicrons

Dietary triglycerides are hydrolyzed in the intestine to β-monoglyceride and fatty acids by pancreatic lipase, which is activated by bile acids and a protein cofactor. The partial glycerides and fatty acids form micelles that are absorbed by intestinal epithelium. The fatty acids are reesterified with β-monoglycerides to form triglycerides, and free cholesterol is esterified with fatty acids by acyl-CoA:cholesterol acyltransferase-2 (ACAT-2). Droplets of triglyceride with small amounts of cholesteryl esters, associated with B-48, acquire a monolayer of phospholipid and free cholesterol. Apo A-I and Apo A-II are added, and the nascent chylomicron

emerges into the extracellular lymph space (see Figure 19–1). The new chylomicron begins to exchange surface components with HDL, acquiring Apo C and Apo E and losing phospholipids. This process continues as the chylomicron is carried via the intestinal lymphatics to the thoracic duct and thence into the bloodstream.

Formation of Very Low Density Lipoproteins

The liver exports triglycerides to peripheral tissues in the cores of VLDL (Figure 19–2). These triglycerides are synthesized in liver from free fatty acids abstracted from plasma and from fatty acids synthesized de novo. Release of VLDL by liver is augmented by any condition that results in increased flux of FFA to liver in the absence of compensating ketogenesis. Obesity, increased caloric intake, ingestion of ethanol, and estrogens stimulate release of VLDL and are important factors in hypertriglyceridemia.

Metabolism of Triglyceride-Rich Lipoproteins in Plasma

A. Hydrolysis by lipoprotein lipase Fatty acids derived from the triglycerides of chylomicrons and VLDL are delivered to tissues through a common pathway involving hydrolysis by the lipoprotein lipase (LPL) system. Members of a family of fatty acid transfer proteins facilitate FFA uptake in tissues. LPL is bound to capillary endothelium in heart, skeletal muscle, adipose tissue, mammary gland, and other tissues.

B. Biologic regulation of lipoprotein lipase When glucose levels in plasma are elevated and the release of insulin is stimulated, LPL is transcriptionally upregulated in adipose tissue, and fatty acids derived from triglycerides of circulating lipoproteins are stored. During prolonged fasting, and in diabetic

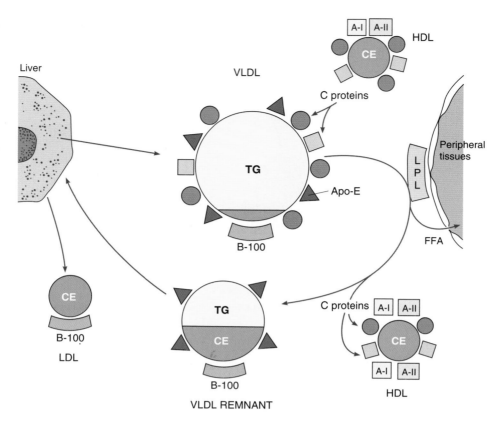

FIGURE 19–2 Metabolism of VLDL (A-I, A-II, B-48, and C proteins, apolipoproteins; CE, cholesteryl esters; TG, triglyceride). See text for details.

ketoacidosis, LPL activity of adipose tissue falls, preventing storage of fatty acids. Heparin is a cofactor for LPL. When it is given intravenously (0.1-0.2 mg/kg), LPL activity is displaced into plasma, permitting its measurement. Apo C-II is an obligatory cofactor.

C. Formation of lipoprotein remnants Hydrolysis by LPL results in depletion of triglycerides in the cores of chylomicrons and VLDL, producing progressive decreases in particle diameter. Lipids from the surface and C proteins are transferred to HDL. The remnant lipoproteins thus formed contain their original complement of Apo B, significant amounts of Apo E, and little Apo C. They have lost about 70% of their triglycerides and are enriched in cholesteryl esters.

D. Fate of lipoprotein remnants Chylomicron remnants are removed from blood quantitatively by high-affinity, receptor-mediated endocytosis in the liver. The receptors include the LDL (B-100:E) receptors and the LDL receptor-related protein-1 (LRP-1). Endocytosis of chylomicron remnants by both requires the presence of Apo E-3 or Apo E-4. The lipids enter hepatic pools, and B-48 protein is degraded. Cholesterol derived from chylomicron remnants exerts feedback control of cholesterol biosynthesis in liver. Some VLDL remnants are removed from blood via the B-100:E receptors (see later) and are degraded. Those that escape uptake are transformed into LDL. Thus, the rate of removal of VLDL remnants is a determinant of LDL production.

Formation of LDL involves the removal of residual triglycerides by hepatic lipase, facilitated by Apo E. LDL contain cholesteryl esters in their cores and retain Apo B-100. In normal individuals, a major fraction of VLDL is converted to LDL, and all of the LDL Apo B comes from VLDL. In certain hypertriglyceridemic states, conversion of VLDL to LDL is decreased. In the absence of impaired conversion, increased secretion of VLDL results in increased production of LDL. This precursor-product relationship explains the clinical phenomenon referred to as the **beta shift**, an increase of LDL (beta-lipoprotein) as hypertriglyceridemia resolves. An example of this occurs temporarily following institution of insulin treatment in uncontrolled diabetes with lipemia. Insulin induces LPL activity, resulting in rapid conversion of VLDL to LDL. Because of its longer half-life, LDL accumulates in plasma. Elevated levels of LDL may persist beyond the time when levels of triglyceride-rich lipoproteins have returned to normal. A similar phenomenon may occur when patients with familial combined hyperlipidemia (FCH) are treated with fibric acid derivatives.

E. Half-lives of lipoproteins Normally, the half-life of chylomicrons is 5 to 20 minutes; that of VLDL is 0.5 to 1 hour; and that of LDL is about 2½ days. At triglyceride levels of 800 to 1000 mg/dL, LPL is at kinetic saturation. Increased input of triglycerides into plasma at those levels rapidly augments the hypertriglyceridemia.

F. Effect of dietary fat restriction Individuals consuming a typical North American diet transport 75 to 100 g or more of triglyceride per day in chylomicrons, whereas the liver exports 10 to 30 g in VLDL. When LPL is saturated and triglycerides are measured in thousands of milligrams per deciliter, acute restriction of dietary fat produces a significant reduction in levels. This intervention is especially important in the lipemic patient with impending pancreatitis. If symptoms suggest that pancreatitis is imminent, oral intake should be eliminated, gastric acid should be suppressed with H_2 blockade, and the patient should not be fed by mouth until the symptoms subside and triglycerides decrease to less than 800 to 1000 mg/dL.

Catabolism of Low-Density Lipoproteins

LDL catabolism is mediated by high-affinity receptors on the cell membranes of virtually all nucleated cells but most importantly hepatocytes. Ligands for these LDL receptors exist in Apo B-100 and Apo E. After endocytosis, Apo B is degraded, and the receptor returns to the cell membrane. The cholesteryl esters of LDL are hydrolyzed to free cholesterol for production of cell membrane bilayers. Free cholesterol down regulates hydroxymethylglutaryl-CoA (HMG-CoA) reductase and other rate-limiting enzymes in the biosynthetic pathway for cholesterol. Cholesterol in excess of need for membrane synthesis is esterified by ACAT-2 for storage. In addition to suppression of cholesterol biosynthesis, the entry of cholesterol via the LDL pathway leads to downregulation of LDL receptors, an effect also observed with dietary saturated fat. Further regulatory mechanisms involve shortening of the residence time of LDL receptors in cell membranes The PCSK9 protein increases the proteolytic degradation of LDL receptors, decreasing the ability of cells to endocytose LDL. Another mechanism that leads to receptor degradation involves ubiquitination of the receptors by Idol (inducible degrader of the LDL receptor).

Metabolism of High-Density Lipoproteins

When isolated by ultracentrifugation, HDL appear to comprise two major classes: HDL_2 and HDL_3. Similar quantities of HDL_3 are isolated from serum of men and women, but about twice as much HDL_2 is found in premenopausal women. Immunochemical studies indicate that there are as many as 20 discrete species of HDL that are obscured by ultracentrifugation. One of these, the 67-kDa prebeta-1 HDL, is the primary acquisitor of cholesterol in the retrieval pathway from peripheral tissues.

A. Sources of HDL   Both liver and intestine produce HDL apolipoproteins, which organize with lipids into the native species of HDL in lymph and plasma. Excess free cholesterol and phospholipids liberated from the surface monolayers of chylomicrons and VLDL as hydrolysis of triglycerides proceeds are transferred to HDL by phospholipid transfer protein. Free cholesterol acquired by HDL is esterified by LCAT. This enzyme transfers 1 mol of fatty acid from a lecithin molecule to the hydroxyl group of unesterified cholesterol, forming cholesteryl esters. LCAT is secreted by liver. In severe hepatic parenchymal disease, levels in plasma are low and esterification of cholesterol is impeded, leading to the accumulation of free cholesterol in lipoproteins and in membranes

of erythrocytes. This transforms them into the target cells classically associated with hepatic disease.

B. Metabolic roles for HDL   HDL serve as carriers for the C apolipoproteins, transferring them to nascent VLDL and chylomicrons. HDL as well as LDL deliver cholesterol to the adrenal cortex and gonads in support of steroidogenesis. HDL play a major role in the centripetal transport of cholesterol. Unesterified cholesterol, exported by the ATP-binding cassette transporter A1 (ABCA1), is acquired from the membranes of peripheral tissues by prebeta-1 HDL and is esterified by LCAT, passing through other HDL species before the cholesteryl esters are incorporated into HDL of alpha-electrophoretic mobility. Cholesterol effluxed from macrophages by the ATP-binding cassette transporter G1 (ABCG1) is acquired by larger HDL. The cholesteryl esters are then transferred to LDL and to triglyceride-rich lipoproteins mediated by cholesteryl ester transfer protein (CETP). Remnants of chylomicrons and a significant fraction of VLDL remnants and LDL are taken up by liver. Cholesteryl esters are also transferred from HDL to hepatocytes by scavenger receptor, class B, type I (SR-BI) receptors.

C. Catabolism of HDL   The pathways of catabolism of HDL are not yet known. Radiochemical studies indicate that Apo A-I and Apo A-II are removed from plasma synchronously and that a portion of the degradation occurs in liver and in kidney.

The Cholesterol Economy

Cholesterol is an essential constituent of the plasma membranes of cells and of myelin. It is required for adrenal and gonadal steroidogenesis and for production of bile acids by liver. Cells synthesize cholesterol, commencing with acetyl-CoA. Formation of HMG-CoA is the initial step. The first committed step, mediated by HMG-CoA reductase, is the formation of mevalonic acid, which is then metabolized via a series of isoprenoid intermediaries to squalene. The latter cyclizes to form a series of sterols leading to cholesterol. A small amount of the mevalonate is converted to the isoprenoid substances ubiquinone, dolichol, and isopentenyl pyrophosphate. This pathway also yields the isoprenoid intermediaries geranyl and farnesyl pyrophosphates that are involved in prenylation of proteins. Prenylation provides an anchor so that proteins such as the low molecular weight G proteins can bind to membranes. Cholesterol synthesis is tightly regulated by cholesterol or its metabolites, which down regulate HMG-CoA reductase. Thus, cells can produce cholesterol not provided by circulating lipoproteins. Hepatocytes and intestinal epithelial cells use cholesterol for secretion of lipoproteins. In addition, cells constantly transfer cholesterol to circulating lipoproteins, chiefly HDL. Cholesterol is converted to bile acids in liver via a pathway initiated by cholesterol 7α-hydroxylase. Most of the bile acids are reabsorbed from the intestine, but the small amount that is lost in stool provides a means of elimination of cholesterol. Activity of cholesterol 7α-hydroxylase is decreased in hypothyroidism, as are the expression of LDL receptors and hepatic lipase.

At usual levels of cholesterol intake, about one-third of the amount ingested is absorbed. Most is transported to liver in chylomicron remnants, suppressing hepatic cholesterogenesis. Individuals may differ substantially in the effect of dietary cholesterol on levels of serum lipoproteins.

DIFFERENTIATION OF DISORDERS OF LIPOPROTEIN METABOLISM

Laboratory Analyses of Lipids and Lipoproteins

Because chylomicrons normally may be present in plasma up to 10 hours after a meal, they contribute as much as 600 mg/dL (6.9 mmol/L) to the triglycerides measured during that period. This alimentary lipemia can be prolonged if alcohol is consumed with the meal. Thus, serum lipids and lipoproteins should be measured after a 10-hour fast. If blood glucose is not to be measured, patients may have fruit and black coffee with sugar (which provide no triglyceride) for breakfast.

A. Inspection   Much useful information is gained from inspection of the serum, especially before and after overnight refrigeration. Opalescence is due to light scattering by large triglyceride-rich lipoproteins. Serum begins to appear hazy when the level of triglycerides reaches 200 mg/dL (2.3 mmol/L). Chylomicrons are readily detected, because they form a white supernatant layer after refrigeration. Uncommon cases in which binding of immunoglobulins to lipoproteins takes place can be detected by the formation of a curd-like lipoprotein aggregate or a snowy precipitate as serum cools. If one of these disorders is suspected, blood should be kept at 37°C during the formation of the clot and separation of the serum, because the critical temperatures for precipitation of the cryoglobulin complex may be higher than room temperature.

B. Laboratory techniques   Several chemical techniques provide reliable measures of cholesterol and triglycerides, an essential minimum for differentiation of disorders of lipoproteins. Unesterified and esterified cholesterol are usually measured together, so that the reported value is the total content of cholesterol in serum. A more complete characterization of lipoproteins is achieved by measurement of the cholesterol and triglyceride contents of individual lipoprotein fractions, separated by preparative ultracentrifugation, a technique usually available only in research laboratories. An efficient quantitative method employs vertical rotor ultracentrifugation, affording assessment of lipoprotein concentrations and particle diameters. LDL particle size can also be assessed by electrophoresis. The content of HDL can be measured using a technique in which they are the only lipoproteins that remain in solution after treatment of the serum with heparin and manganese. Although rapid, the results of this technique tend to be unacceptably variable unless rigid quality control is exercised. Prognostic implications of small changes in HDL cholesterol make such controls necessary. An important determinant of the content of cholesteryl esters in HDL is the

amount of triglyceride-rich lipoproteins to which the HDL are exposed in plasma. Cholesteryl esters from HDL transfer into triglyceride-rich lipoproteins, leading to an inverse dependence of HDL cholesterol on plasma triglycerides. HDL cholesterol cannot be interpreted without knowledge of the level of serum triglycerides. For example, a level of HDL that would normally contain 45 mg/dL (1.17 mmol/L) of cholesterol might contain 37 mg/dL (0.96 mmol/L) when the triglycerides were 200 mg/dL (2.3 mmol/L) and 30 mg/dL (0.78 mmol/L) when they reach 500 mg/dL (5.7 mmol/L).

More sophisticated tests of composition of isolated lipoprotein fractions are of use in certain instances, including the ratio of cholesterol to triglycerides. Enrichment of VLDL by cholesteryl esters is typical of familial dysbetalipoproteinemia that is due to homozygosity for Apo E-2. The Apo E genotype can be determined by PCR analysis. Clinically useful immunoassays are available for Apo B and Lp(a).

Epidemiologic evidence suggests that LDL particles of smaller than normal diameter are associated with an increased risk of atherosclerosis. Small, dense LDL particles are a constant finding when triglyceride levels are elevated even marginally. Laboratory measurement of LDL diameters is therefore unnecessary in patients with hypertriglyceridemia.

Clinical Differentiation of Abnormal Patterns of Plasma Lipoproteins

A. Preliminary screening   Serum cholesterol and triglyceride levels are continuously distributed in the population; therefore, some arbitrary levels must be established to define significance. Epidemiologic studies in Europe and the United States have shown a progressive increase in risk of coronary disease as levels of cholesterol increase. Physicians should at least encourage patients at risk to eat diets low in saturated fats, trans fats, and cholesterol to minimize the burden of LDL in plasma.

The National Cholesterol Education Program has developed guidelines for treatment of hypercholesterolemia in adults. Since this 2001 report, the results of major clinical trials have suggested that more aggressive lipid management is justified. For patients at high risk (coronary heart disease [CHD] or CHD risk equivalents, including diabetes), a suggested LDL-cholesterol goal is less than 70 mg/dL (1.8 mmol/L). Triglyceride levels above 150 mg/dL (1.7 mmol/L) merit investigation. One abnormality commonly associated with increased risk of coronary disease that is not detected if screening is limited to hyperlipidemia is hypoalphalipoproteinemia, or deficiency of HDL. Many affected individuals have normal levels of cholesterol and triglycerides and no clinical features to alert the physician. HDL deficiency underscores the importance of controlling other risk factors and avoiding factors that reduce HDL, such as smoking, the use of some drugs, and obesity.

B. Identification of abnormal patterns   The second step in investigation of hyperlipidemia is determination of the species of lipoproteins involved. In some cases, this may include multiple species; in others, qualitative properties of the lipoproteins are of diagnostic importance. Secondary hyperlipidemias of similar pattern may be the sole cause of the lipoprotein abnormality or may aggravate primary disorders of lipoprotein metabolism. The differentiation of specific primary disorders usually requires additional clinical and genetic information.

The following diagnostic protocol, based on initial measurement of cholesterol, triglycerides, and HDL in serum after a 10-hour fast, supplemented by observation of serum and by additional laboratory measurements where essential, serves as a guide in identifying abnormal patterns. The term **hyperlipidemia** denotes high levels of any class of lipoprotein; **hyperlipemia** denotes high levels of any of the triglyceride-rich lipoproteins.

Case 1: Serum Cholesterol Levels Increased; Triglycerides Normal

If the serum cholesterol level is modestly elevated (up to 260 mg/dL [6.72 mmol/L]), elevated levels of HDL may account for the observed increase in serum cholesterol. This is usually not associated with disease processes. The LDL cholesterol (in mg/dL) may be estimated by subtracting the HDL cholesterol and the estimated cholesterol contribution of VLDL from the total cholesterol level. The VLDL cholesterol is approximated as one-fifth of the serum triglyceride level.

$$\text{LDL cholesterol} = \text{total cholesterol} - \left(\frac{\text{TG}}{5} + \text{HDL cholesterol} \right)$$

Very high levels of HDL measured by the precipitation technique can signal the presence of the abnormal lipoprotein of cholestasis (Lp-X). This disorder is characterized by elevated alkaline phosphatase activity. Rarely, deficiency of CETP or hepatic lipase can cause high levels of HDL.

Case 2: Predominant Increase of Triglycerides; Moderate Increase in Cholesterol May Be Present

Here it is apparent that the primary abnormality is an increase in triglyceride-rich VLDL (hyperprebetalipoproteinemia) or chylomicrons (chylomicronemia), or both (mixed lipemia). Because both contain free cholesterol in their surface monolayers and a small amount of cholesteryl ester in their cores, the total cholesterol may be increased, although to a much smaller extent than triglycerides. Low levels of LDL often seen in hypertriglyceridemia may offset the increase in cholesterol due to the triglyceride-rich lipoproteins, especially in primary chylomicronemia. Because VLDL and chylomicrons compete as substrates in a common removal pathway, chylomicrons are nearly always present when triglyceride levels exceed 1000 mg/dL (11.5 mmol/L).

Case 3: Cholesterol and Triglyceride Levels Both Elevated

This pattern can be the result of either of two abnormal phenotypes. One is a combined increase of VLDL and LDL. This pattern

is termed combined hyperlipidemia and is one of the three phenotypic patterns encountered in kindreds with the disorder FCH. The second phenotype is an increase of remnant lipoproteins derived from VLDL and chylomicrons. These particles have been partially depleted of triglyceride by LPL and enriched with cholesteryl esters by the LCAT system, such that the total content of cholesterol in serum is similar to that of triglycerides. This pattern is almost always an expression of familial dysbetalipoproteinemia. Diagnosis of this disorder is confirmed by a genotype demonstrating absence of the normal E-3 and E-4 alleles.

CLINICAL DESCRIPTIONS OF PRIMARY AND SECONDARY DISORDERS OF LIPOPROTEIN METABOLISM

THE HYPERTRIGLYCERIDEMIAS

Atherogenicity

Epidemiologic evidence supports the atherogenicity of VLDL and their remnants. They have been demonstrated in atherosclerotic plaques from humans. Impaired capacity of the VLDL of some individuals to accept cholesteryl esters from the LCAT reaction may also contribute to atherogenesis by impeding centripetal transport of cholesterol.

Cause of Pancreatitis

Very high levels of triglycerides in plasma are associated with a risk of acute pancreatitis, probably from the local release of FFA and lysolecithin from lipoprotein substrates in the pancreatic capillary bed. When the concentrations of these lipids exceed the binding capacity of albumin, they could lyse membranes of parenchymal cells, initiating a chemical pancreatitis. Many patients with lipemia have intermittent episodes of epigastric pain during which serum amylase does not reach levels commonly considered diagnostic for pancreatitis. This is especially true in patients who have had previous attacks. The observation that these episodes frequently evolve into classic pancreatitis suggests that they represent incipient pancreatic inflammation. The progression of pancreatitis can be prevented by rapid reduction of triglycerides, usually accomplished by restriction of all dietary fat. In some cases, parenteral feeding, excluding fat emulsions, may be required for a few days. The clinical course of pancreatitis in patients with lipemia is typical of the general experience with this disease.

Clinical Signs (Figure 19–3)

When triglyceride levels in serum exceed 3000 to 4000 mg/dL (34.5-46 mmol/L), light scattering by these particles in the blood lends a whitish cast to the venous vascular bed of the retina, a sign known as **lipemia retinalis.** Markedly elevated levels of VLDL or

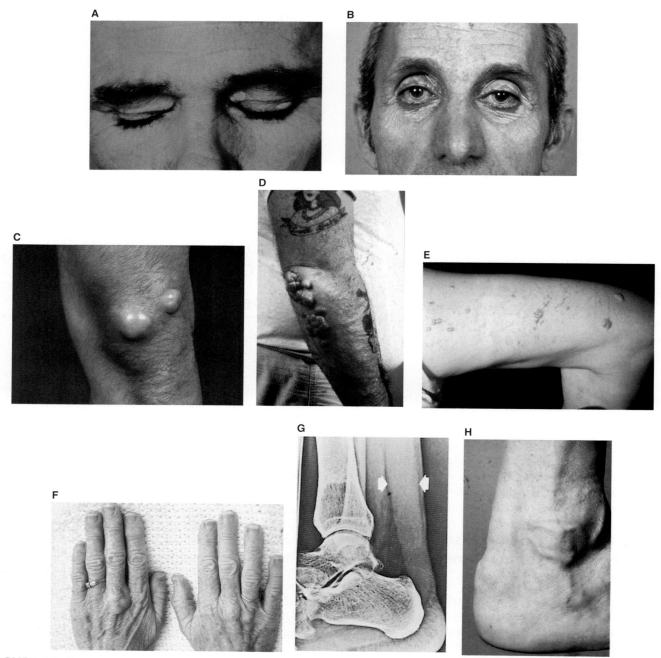

FIGURE 19–3 Clinical manifestations of hyperlipidemias. **A.** Xanthelasma involving medial and lateral canthi. **B.** Severe xanthelasma and arcus corneae. **C.** Tuberous xanthomas. **D.** Large tuberous xanthoma of elbow. **E.** Eruptive xanthomas, singly and in rosettes. **F.** Xanthomas of extensor tendons of the hands. **G.** Xeroradiogram of Achilles tendon xanthoma. **H.** Xanthoma of Achilles tendon. (Normal Achilles tendons do not exceed 7 mm in diameter in the region between the calcaneus and the point at which the tendon fibers begin to radiate toward their origins.)

chylomicrons may be associated with the appearance of eruptive cutaneous xanthomas (see Figure 19–3E). These lesions, filled with foam cells, appear as yellow morbilliform eruptions 2 to 5 mm in diameter, often with erythematous areolae. They usually occur in clusters on extensor surfaces such as the elbows, knees, and buttocks. They are transient and disappear within a few weeks after triglyceride levels are reduced.

Effects of Hypertriglyceridemia on Laboratory Measurements

Light scattering from high levels of triglyceride-rich lipoproteins can cause erroneous results in most chemical determinations involving photometric measurements. Amylase activity in serum may be inhibited; therefore, lipemic specimens should be diluted for measurement of this enzyme. Because the lipoproteins are not permeable to ionic or polar molecules, their core regions constitute a second phase in plasma. When the volume of this phase becomes appreciable, electrolytes and other hydrophilic species are underestimated with respect to their true concentration in the aqueous phase. A practical rule for correcting these values is as follows: For each 1000 mg/dL (11.5 mmol/L) of triglyceride, the measured concentrations of all hydrophilic molecules and ions should be adjusted upward by 1%.

PRIMARY HYPERTRIGLYCERIDEMIA

1. DEFICIENCY OF LIPOPROTEIN LIPASE ACTIVITY

Clinical Findings

A. Symptoms and signs The activity of LPL is dependent upon the integrity of the enzyme and its cofactor, Apo C-II. In addition, defects in Apo A-V, GPIHDLBP, and LMF1 proteins can result in severe impairment of LPL activity. The LMF1 protein is essential for the secretion of both LPL and hepatic lipase in their active conformations. Because the clinical expressions of these defects are similar, they are considered together. On a typical North American diet, lipemia is usually severe (triglycerides of 2000-25,000 mg/dL) (23-287.5 mmol/L). Hepatomegaly and splenomegaly are frequently present. Foam cells laden with lipid are found in liver, spleen, and bone marrow. Splenic infarct has been described and may be a source of abdominal pain. Hypersplenism with anemia, granulocytopenia, and thrombocytopenia can occur. Recurrent epigastric pain and overt pancreatitis are frequently encountered. Eruptive xanthomas may be present. These disorders may be recognized in early infancy or may go unnoticed until an attack of acute pancreatitis occurs or lipemic serum is noted on blood sampling as late as middle age. Patients with these disorders are usually not obese and have normal carbohydrate metabolism unless pancreatitis impairs insulinogenic capacity. Estrogens intensify the lipemia by stimulating hepatic production of VLDL. Therefore, in pregnancy and lactation or during the administration of estrogenic steroids, the risk of pancreatitis increases.

B. Laboratory findings There is a preponderance of chylomicrons in serum such that the infranatant layer of serum refrigerated overnight may be nearly clear with a supernatant chylomicron layer. Many patients have a moderate increase in VLDL, however, and in pregnant women or those receiving estrogens, a pattern of mixed lipemia is usually present. Levels of LDL in serum are decreased, probably representing the predominant catabolism of VLDL by pathways that do not involve the production of LDL. Levels of HDL cholesterol are also decreased.

A presumptive diagnosis of these disorders can be made by restricting oral intake of fat to 10 to 15 g/d. Triglycerides drop precipitously, usually reaching 200 to 600 mg/dL (2.3-6.9 mmol/L) within 3 to 4 days. Confirmation of deficiency of LPL is obtained

by measurement of the lipolytic activity of plasma 10 minutes after injection of heparin (0.2 mg/kg) intravenously. Analysis of lipolysis is done with and without 0.5 mol/L sodium chloride, which inhibits LPL but does not suppress the activity of hepatic lipase. Absence of the Apo C-II cofactor can be demonstrated most readily by electrophoresis or isoelectric focusing of the proteins of VLDL.

Treatment

Treatment of primary chylomicronemia is entirely dietary. Intake of fat should be reduced to 10% or less of total calories. In an adult, this represents 15 to 30 g/d. Because the defect involves lipolysis, both saturated and unsaturated fats must be curtailed. The diet should contain at least 5 g of polyunsaturated fat as a source of essential fatty acids, and fat-soluble vitamins must be provided. Administration of 500 mg daily of marine omega-3 fatty acids is also recommended. Adherence to this diet invariably maintains triglycerides below 1000 mg/dL (11.2 mmol/L) in the absence of pregnancy, lactation, or the administration of exogenous estrogens. Because this is below the level at which pancreatitis usually occurs, compliant patients are at low risk. Pregnant women with these disorders require particularly close monitoring.

2. ENDOGENOUS AND MIXED LIPEMIAS

Etiology and Pathogenesis

Endogenous lipemia (elevated VLDL) and mixed lipemia probably both result from several genetically determined disorders. Because VLDL and chylomicrons are competing substrates in the intravascular lipolytic pathway, saturating levels of VLDL impede the removal of chylomicrons. Therefore, as the severity of endogenous lipemia increases, a pattern of mixed lipemia may supervene. In other cases, the pattern of mixed lipemia appears to be present continuously. Although specific pathophysiologic mechanisms remain obscure, certain familial patterns are known. In all forms, factors that increase the rate of secretion of VLDL aggravate the hypertriglyceridemia (ie, obesity with insulin resistance, appearance of fully developed type 2 diabetes mellitus, alcohol, and exogenous estrogens). Studies of VLDL turnover indicate that either increased production or impaired removal of VLDL may be operative in different individuals. A substantial number of patients with mixed lipemia have partial defects in catabolism of triglyceride-rich lipoproteins, often due to heterozygosity for mutations in LPL. Most patients with significant endogenous or mixed lipemia have centripetal obesity.

Clinical Findings

Clinical features of these forms of hypertriglyceridemia depend on their severity and include eruptive xanthomas, lipemia retinalis, recurrent epigastric pain, and acute pancreatitis.

Endogenous lipemia is frequently an element in a constellation of metabolic abnormalities termed the **metabolic syndrome**. Insulin resistance, usually associated with central obesity, is a core feature of this syndrome. Patients may or may not have hyperglycemia. Low levels of HDL cholesterol largely reflect increased transfer of CE into circulating VLDL. Hypertension and hyperuricemia are frequently present.

Treatment

The first element of treatment is severe restriction of total fat intake. The objective of long-term dietary management is reduction to ideal body weight. Because alcohol causes significant augmentation of VLDL production, abstinence is important. If weight loss is achieved, the triglycerides almost always show a marked response, often approaching normal values. When the fall in triglycerides is not satisfactory, a fibrate or nicotinic acid (in the absence of insulin resistance), singly or in combination, usually produces further reductions. When insulin resistance is present, metformin—with or without a thiazolidinedione—may be a useful adjunct. Pioglitazone is the drug of choice in this class because it is more effective in reducing triglycerides and, unlike rosiglitazone, it does not increase LDL cholesterol.

3. FAMILIAL COMBINED HYPERLIPIDEMIA

Etiology

This inherited disorder, which is the most common form of hyperlipidemia, occurs in 1% to 2% of the population. The underlying process involves overproduction of VLDL. Some affected individuals have increased levels of both VLDL and LDL (combined hyperlipidemia); some have predominantly increased levels of either VLDL or LDL. The level of Apo B-100 is increased. Patterns in the serum of an individual may change with time. It is known that the offspring of an individual having any one of the three phenotypic patterns and a normal individual can have one of the other patterns. Affected children often have hyperlipidemia. If the child is obese, hypertriglyceridemia is likely present, whereas a child of normal weight may have only an elevated LDL.

Clinical Findings

Neither tendinous nor cutaneous xanthomas other than xanthelasma occur. This disorder appears to be inherited as a Mendelian dominant trait involving alternative loci. Modifying genes have been published but major loci have not been identified. Factors that increase the severity of hypertriglyceridemia in other disorders aggravate the lipemia in this syndrome as well.

Treatment

The risk of coronary disease is significantly increased, and patients should be treated aggressively with diet and drugs. Because LDL levels often increase with fibrate therapy in these patients and because resins increase triglycerides, the recommended treatment is an HMG-CoA reductase inhibitor. The addition of niacin or fenofibrate may be required if triglycerides remain elevated or if HDL deficiency is also present. Fenofibrate may be used cautiously with rosuvastatin.

4. FAMILIAL DYSBETALIPOPROTEINEMIA (TYPE III HYPERLIPOPROTEINEMIA)

Etiology and Pathogenesis

A permissive genetic constitution for this disease (homozygosity for Apo E-2) occurs in about 2% of the US population but the expression of hyperlipidemia apparently requires environmental and possibly additional genetic determinants. The molecular basis is the presence of isoforms of Apo E that are poor ligands for high-affinity receptors. In its fully expressed form, the lipoprotein pattern is dominated by the accumulation of remnants of VLDL and chylomicrons. Two populations of VLDL are usually present: normal prebetalipoproteins and remnants with beta-electrophoretic mobility. Remnant particles of intermediate density are also present. Levels of LDL are decreased, reflecting interruption of the transformation of VLDL remnants to LDL. The primary defect is impaired hepatic uptake of remnants of triglyceride-rich lipoproteins. The remnant particles are enriched in cholesteryl esters such that the level of cholesterol in serum is often as high as that of triglycerides. Absence of the E-3 and E-4 alleles in genomic DNA confirms the diagnosis. Additional mutations of Apo E are now known to result in dysbetalipoproteinemia. Some of these cause hyperlipidemia in the heterozygous state, a disorder termed **dominant dysbetalipoproteinemia**.

Clinical Findings

Hyperlipidemia and clinical signs are not usually evident before age 20. In younger patients with hyperlipidemia, hypothyroidism or obesity is likely to be present. Adults frequently have tuberous or tuberoeruptive xanthomas (Figure 19–3C). Both tend to occur on extensor surfaces, especially elbows and knees. Tuberoeruptive xanthomas are pink or yellowish skin nodules 3 to 8 mm in diameter that often become confluent. Tuberous xanthomas—shiny reddish or orange nodules up to 3 cm or more in diameter—are usually moveable and nontender. Another type, planar xanthomas of the palmar creases, strongly suggests dysbetalipoproteinemia. The skin creases assume an orange color from deposition of carotenoids. They occasionally are raised above the level of adjacent skin and are not tender. (Planar xanthomas are also seen in cholestasis.)

Some patients have impaired glucose tolerance, which is usually associated with higher levels of blood lipids. Obesity is commonly present and tends to aggravate the lipemia. Patients with the genetic constitution for dysbetalipoproteinemia often develop severe hyperlipidemia if they are hypothyroid. Atherosclerosis of the coronary and peripheral vessels occurs with increased frequency, and the prevalence of disease of the iliac and femoral vessels is especially high.

Treatment

Management includes a weight reduction diet providing a reduced intake of cholesterol, fat, and alcohol. When the hyperlipidemia does not respond satisfactorily to diet, a fibrate or niacin in low doses (if the patient does not have insulin resistance) is usually effective. These agents can be used together in resistant cases. Some patients respond to the more potent reductase inhibitors alone, and the addition of niacin normalizes the lipid levels in most.

SECONDARY HYPERTRIGLYCERIDEMIA

1. DIABETES MELLITUS

In patients with diabetes, levels of VLDL in plasma are frequently elevated. The severe lipemia associated with absence or marked insufficiency of insulin is attributable to decreased transcription of the *LPL* gene. The administration of insulin usually restores triglyceride levels to normal within a few days. However, if massive fatty liver is present, weeks may be required for the VLDL to return to normal while the liver secretes its triglycerides. Conversion of massive amounts of VLDL to LDL as the impedance of VLDL catabolism is relieved leads to marked accumulation of LDL that may persist for weeks, leading to a spurious diagnosis of primary hypercholesterolemia.

The moderately elevated VLDL seen in type 2 diabetes under average control probably reflects chiefly an increased flux of FFA to liver that stimulates production of triglycerides and their secretion in VLDL. In addition to VLDL, LDL levels are also somewhat increased in diabetic individuals under poor control, probably accounting in part for their increased risk of CHD. Some have much higher levels of VLDL, suggesting that an additional genetic factor predisposing to lipemia is present. Still another cause of lipemic diabetes is the compromised insulinogenic capacity that can result from acute pancreatitis. The deficiency may be severe enough to require exogenous insulin, often only in small doses. In diabetic individuals who develop nephrosis, the secondary lipemia of nephrosis compounds their hypertriglyceridemia. In hyperglycemia, lipoproteins become glycosylated, leading to their uptake by macrophages.

Lipemia may be very severe, with elevated levels of both VLDL and chylomicrons when control is poor. Lipemic patients usually have ketoacidosis when they are insulin-deficient, but lipemia can occur in its absence. Patients with type 1 diabetes who have been chronically undertreated with insulin may have mobilized most of the triglyceride from peripheral adipose tissue, so that they no longer have sufficient substrate for significant ketogenesis. These emaciated individuals may have severe lipemia and striking hepatomegaly.

In type 1 diabetes, the rigid control of blood glucose levels, which can be attained with continuous subcutaneous insulin infusion, is associated with sustained normalization of levels of both LDL and VLDL. The lipemia of type 2 diabetes usually responds well to control of the underlying disorder. In obese insulin-resistant individuals, weight loss is essential. Diets containing slowly absorbed carbohydrates are well tolerated, allowing a decrease in the burden of chylomicron triglycerides in plasma (see Chapter 17).

2. UREMIA

Uremia is associated with modest isolated increases in VLDL. The most important underlying mechanisms are probably insulin resistance and impairment of catabolism of VLDL. Many uremic patients are also nephrotic. The additional effects of nephrosis on lipoprotein metabolism may produce a combined hyperlipidemia. Patients who have had renal transplants may be receiving glucocorticoids, which induce elevation of LDL.

3. HUMAN IMMUNODEFICIENCY VIRUS INFECTION

HIV infection per se is associated with hypertriglyceridemia (see Chapter 25). A syndrome of partial lipodystrophy and insulin resistance, often with marked lipemia, occurs with multidrug treatment that includes certain inhibitors of viral proteases. Acute pancreatitis can ensue. Limited clinical experience suggests that fibric acid derivatives are of some value. Alcohol must be avoided.

4. CORTICOSTEROID EXCESS

In endogenous Cushing syndrome, and with corticosteroid treatment, insulin resistance is present and levels of LDL are increased. It appears that the hyperlipidemia is primarily due to increased secretion of VLDL, which is then catabolized to LDL. More severe lipemia ensues when steroidogenic diabetes appears, reducing catabolism of triglyceride-rich lipoproteins via the LPL pathway.

5. EXOGENOUS ESTROGENS

When estrogens are administered to normal women, triglyceride levels may increase by as much as 15%, reflecting increased production of VLDL. Paradoxically, estrogens increase the efficiency of catabolism of triglyceride-rich lipoproteins. Whereas estrogens tend to induce insulin resistance, it is not clear that this is an important mechanism, because certain nortestosterone derivatives decrease plasma triglycerides despite the induction of appreciable insulin resistance.

Certain individuals, usually those with preexisting mild lipemia, develop marked hypertriglyceridemia when receiving estrogens even in relatively small doses. Thus, triglycerides should be monitored during estrogen therapy. Contraceptive combinations with predominantly progestational effects produce less hypertriglyceridemia than purely estrogenic compounds. Transdermal delivery of estrogen probably results in lesser increases in VLDL secretion because it avoids the hepatic first-pass effect.

6. ALCOHOL INGESTION

Ingestion of appreciable amounts of alcohol does not necessarily result in significantly elevated levels of triglycerides, but many alcoholics are lipemic. Alcohol profoundly increases triglycerides in patients with primary or secondary hyperlipemias. In Zieve syndrome, the alcohol-induced lipemia is associated with hemolytic anemia and hyperbilirubinemia. Because LCAT originates in liver, severe hepatic parenchymal dysfunction may lead to deficiency in the activity of this enzyme. A resultant accumulation of unesterified cholesterol in erythrocyte membranes may account for the hemolysis seen in Zieve syndrome.

Alcohol is converted to acetate, exerting a sparing effect on the oxidation of fatty acids that are then incorporated into triglycerides. This results in hepatomegaly due to fatty infiltration and in marked enhancement of secretion of VLDL. In many individuals, there is sufficient adaptive increase in the removal capacity for triglycerides so that plasma levels are normal.

7. NONALCOHOLIC FATTY LIVER DISEASE AND NONALCOHOLIC STEATOHEPATITIS

These conditions are characterized by hepatic steatosis and abnormalities of liver enzymes in the absence of alcohol ingestion. The cause is not yet understood, but it is likely that misdirection of fatty acids from oxidative pathways to hepatic triglyceride synthesis is involved. Five to ten percent of patients with nonalcoholic fatty liver disease (NAFLD) progress to more severe liver disease, including cirrhosis, end-stage liver disease, and hepatocellular carcinoma. In NAFLD, spontaneous improvement can occur, but liver disease is the third most common cause of death. About 80% of patients with NAFLD or nonalcoholic steatohepatitis (NASH) have features of the metabolic syndrome, including abdominal obesity, hypertension, insulin resistance/glucose intolerance, and hypertriglyceridemia. They are at increased risk for atherosclerosis. Weight reduction with exercise and diet in overweight or obese patients is a central element in treatment. Bariatric surgery has proven effective in a large percentage of morbidly obese patients with NASH. Studies to date reveal only marginal benefit attributable to metformin and thiazolidinediones, although pioglitazone shows some promise. Treatment of coexisting dyslipidemia, diabetes, and hypertension is important. Statins, fenofibrate, and marine omega-3 fatty acids do not appear to increase the risk of further hepatic injury in most patients. Mixed tocopherols are beneficial.

8. NEPHROSIS

The hyperlipidemia of nephrosis is biphasic. Before serum albumin levels fall below 2 g/dL, LDL increases selectively. The synthesis and secretion of VLDL appear to be coupled to that of albumin. The increased flux of VLDL from liver increases production of LDL. As albumin falls below 1 to 2 g/dL, lipemia ensues. Impaired hydrolysis of triglycerides by LPL is due to lack of albumin as an FFA receptor. FFA bind to lipoproteins when albumin levels are low, impairing their ability to undergo lipolysis.

Because coronary disease is prevalent in patients with long-standing nephrotic syndrome, treatment of the hyperlipidemia is indicated, although few studies of the effect of treatment have been reported. The hyperlipidemia is resistant to diet. Fibrates may precipitate myopathy even in small doses. Bile acid–binding resins, niacin, and reductase inhibitors are useful.

9. GLYCOGEN STORAGE DISEASE

In type I glycogenosis, insulin secretion is decreased, leading to increased flux of FFA to liver and increased secretion of VLDL. The low levels of insulin in plasma are the probable cause of reduced activity of LPL. The fatty liver in these patients tends to progress to cirrhosis.

Frequent small feedings help maintain blood glucose levels and ameliorate the lipemia. Nocturnal nasogastric drip feeding is of considerable benefit. Other forms of hepatic glycogen storage disease may be associated with elevated levels of VLDL and LDL in serum.

10. HYPOPITUITARISM AND ACROMEGALY

Part of the hyperlipidemia of hypopituitarism is attributable to secondary hypothyroidism, but hypertriglyceridemia persists after thyroxine replacement. Deficiency of growth hormone is associated with elevated levels of both LDL and VLDL. Decreased insulin levels may be the major underlying defect; however, deficiency of growth hormone may impair the disposal of FFA by oxidation and ketogenesis in the liver, favoring synthesis of triglycerides. Mild hypertriglyceridemia is often associated with acromegaly, probably resulting from insulin resistance. Although growth hormone acutely stimulates lipolysis in adipose tissue, FFA levels are normal in acromegaly.

11. HYPOTHYROIDISM

Whereas significant hypothyroidism produces elevated levels of LDL in nearly all individuals, only a few develop hypertriglyceridemia. The increase in LDL results in part from decreased conversion of cholesterol to bile acids and downregulation of LDL receptors. Lipemia, when present, is usually mild, although serum triglycerides in excess of 3000 mg/dL (34.5 mmol/L) can occur in myxedema reflecting decreased activity of hepatic lipase. Increased content of cholesteryl esters and Apo E in the triglyceride-rich lipoproteins suggests accumulation of remnant particles. Hypothyroidism often causes expression of hyperlipidemia in individuals with dysbetalipoproteinemia.

12. IMMUNOGLOBULIN-LIPOPROTEIN COMPLEX DISORDERS

Both polyclonal and monoclonal hypergammaglobulinemias may cause hypertriglyceridemia. IgG, IgM, and IgA have each been involved. Monoclonal antibodies associated with myeloma, macroglobulinemia, lymphomas, and lymphocytic leukemias have been implicated. Lupus erythematosus and other autoimmune disorders have been associated with the polyclonal type. Binding of heparin by immunoglobulin, with resulting inhibition of LPL, can cause severe mixed lipemia. More commonly, the triglyceride-rich lipoproteins have an abnormally high density, probably as a result of bound immunoglobulin, although some may be remnant-like particles. These complexes usually have gamma mobility on electrophoresis.

Xanthomatosis associated with immunoglobulin complex disease includes tuberous and eruptive xanthomas, xanthelasma, and planar xanthomas of large areas of skin. The latter are otherwise seen only in patients with cholestasis. Deposits of lipid-rich hyaline material can occur in the lamina propria of the intestine, causing malabsorption and protein-losing enteropathy. Circulating immunoglobulin-lipoprotein complexes can fix complement, leading to hypocomplementemia. In such patients, administration of whole blood or plasma can cause anaphylaxis. Hence, washed red cells or albumin are recommended when blood volume replacement is required.

Treatment is directed at the underlying disorder. The critical temperature of cryoprecipitation of some of these complexes is close to body temperature. Therefore, if plasmapheresis is indicated to remove offending immunoglobulins, it should be done at a temperature above the critical temperature measured in serum.

THE PRIMARY HYPERCHOLESTEROLEMIAS

FAMILIAL HYPERCHOLESTEROLEMIA

Etiology and Pathogenesis

Familial hypercholesterolemia (FH), which in its heterozygous form occurs in approximately 1 in 500 individuals, is a codominant trait with high penetrance. Because half of first-degree relatives are affected, all members of a family should be screened. A selective increase in LDL exists from birth and tends to increase during childhood and adolescence such that cholesterol in adult heterozygotes usually varies from about 260 to 400 mg/dL (6.7-10.4 mmol/L). Some individuals—especially those in kindreds in which hypertriglyceridemia is present—may have higher than normal levels of VLDL and IDL. In a few patients with FH, the expression is blunted by independent genetic determinants.

The underlying defect is a deficiency of normal LDL receptors on cell membranes. A number of genetic defects affecting the structure, translation, modification, or transport of the receptor protein have been identified.

Some individuals have combined heterozygosity. In cases in which a kinetic mutant is combined with an ablative mutant, the hypercholesterolemia is greater than that seen in simple heterozygosity, usually in the range of 500 to 800 mg/dL (13-20.8 mmol/L). Those patients who are homozygous for null alleles have extremely severe hypercholesterolemia (approaching 1000 mg/dL [26 mmol/L] or greater) and fulminant atherosclerosis.

Production rates for LDL are moderately increased in heterozygotes and are higher in homozygotes because of increased conversion of VLDL to LDL. In the heterozygote, a greater fraction of LDL is removed by nonreceptor-dependent mechanisms than in normal subjects. In homozygotes, all removal of LDL proceeds through such pathways.

Clinical Findings

Tendon xanthomas are frequently present, causing a broadening or fusiform mass in the tendon. They can occur in almost any tendon but are most readily detected in the Achilles and patellar tendons and in the extensor tendons of the hands (Figure 19–3F, 19–3G,

and 19–3H). Patients who are physically active may complain of achillodynia. Arcus corneae (Figure 19–3B) may occur as early as the third decade. Xanthelasma (Figure 19–3A) may also be present. Both arcus and xanthelasma are seen in some individuals who do not have hyperlipidemia, however. Coronary atherosclerosis tends to occur prematurely in heterozygotes. It is particularly prominent in individuals who are relatively deficient in HDL. It is probable that this represents a coincident inheritance of both traits. Homozygous FH is catastrophic. Xanthomatosis progresses rapidly. Patients may have tuberous xanthomas (Figure19–3C and 19–3D) and elevated plaque-like xanthomas of the extremities, buttocks, interdigital webs, and aortic valves. Coronary disease may be evident in the first decade of life.

Serum cholesterol in excess of 300 mg/dL (7.8 mmol/L) in the absence of significant hypertriglyceridemia and conditions known to cause secondary hypercholesterolemia makes the diagnosis of heterozygous FH likely. The presence of affected first-degree relatives is supportive of this diagnosis, especially if no other phenotypes of hyperlipidemia are present in the family that would suggest FCH. The finding of tendon xanthomas is nearly pathognomonic—beta-sitosterolemia, cerebrotendinous xanthomatosis (cholestanolosis), ligand-defective Apo B, and autosomal recessive hypercholesterolemia (ARH) are exceptions. Although the cholesterol content of umbilical cord blood is usually elevated, the diagnosis is most easily established by measuring serum cholesterol after the first year of life.

Treatment

Treatment of heterozygotes with HMG-CoA reductase inhibitors may normalize LDL levels. However, achieving optimal levels may require one of the binary or ternary combinations involving reductase inhibitors, niacin, bile acid sequestrants, or ezetimibe. Levels of LDL cholesterol less than 100 mg/dL (2.6 mmol/L) can be obtained with combinations of these drugs in most patients. Treatment of homozygotes is extremely difficult. Partial control may be achieved with LDL apheresis in conjunction with niacin, ezetimibe, and a potent statin. Striking reduction of LDL levels is observed after liver transplantation, illustrating the important role of hepatic receptors in LDL clearance.

FAMILIAL COMBINED HYPERLIPIDEMIA

In some individuals in kindreds with FCH (see "Primary Hypertriglyceridemia," earlier), LDL and IDL are the only lipoproteins that are elevated. This pattern may vary in an individual over time. Predominant elevation of VLDL or combined elevations of LDL and VLDL may be observed in the patient or the patient's relatives. Some affected children express hyperlipidemia. In contrast to most cases of FH, the cholesterol level may be as low as 250 mg/dL (6.5 mmol/L) and xanthomas are absent in FCH. Studies of kindreds with the FCH phenotype suggest codominant transmission. Coronary atherosclerosis is accelerated, accounting for about 15% of all coronary events in the United States. The underlying mechanism involves increased secretion of VLDL.

Treatment of the hypercholesterolemia should begin with diet and either niacin or a reductase inhibitor. It may be necessary to use a combination of these agents, or fenofibrate with a statin, to normalize levels of LDL and triglyceride.

Lp(a) HYPERLIPOPROTEINEMIA

Lp(a) normally comprises a very minor fraction of circulating lipoproteins, but it may be present in high concentrations in some individuals. It contains Apo B-100 and the (a) protein, a homolog of plasminogen that can inhibit fibrinolysis. It has been demonstrated in atherosclerotic plaques, and several large studies implicate it as an independent risk factor for coronary disease. The Ile4399Met polymorphism is particularly associated with increased risk. Plasma levels of Lp(a) can be measured by immunoassay. Levels above the stated normal range of a given method present an independent risk of coronary disease and stroke. Levels of Lp(a) primarily reflect genetic determinants but can also be elevated in disorders such as nephrosis because the (a) gene contains an inflammatory response element in its promoter. Niacin is currently the only effective treatment, although not all patients respond. Decreasing plasma levels of LDL appears to reduce the risk attributed to the elevated Lp(a), at least to some extent.

FAMILIAL LIGAND-DEFECTIVE Apo B-100

Mutations involving the ligand domain in Apo B-100 impair the ability of LDL to bind to its receptor. Two prevalent mutations at codon 3500 or 3531 occur in about one in 500 individuals and may be found in compound states with familial hypercholesterolemia. The hypercholesterolemia with ligand defects alone is generally less severe than in FH because the removal of VLDL remnants is normal, resulting in a lower production of LDL. Patients may have tendon xanthomas and are at increased risk of coronary disease. Response to reductase inhibitors varies, but many show some resistance because upregulation of receptors cannot correct the defect completely although it can decrease LDL production because IDL particles are endocytosed by liver via interaction of the LDL receptor with Apo E.

CHOLESTEROL 7α-HYDROXYLASE DEFICIENCY

Loss of function mutations in cholesterol 7α-hydroxylase result in diminished catabolism of cholesterol to bile acids and accumulation of cholesterol in hepatocytes. Downregulation of LDL receptors causes elevated LDL in plasma. VLDL may also be increased. Homozygous patients have early coronary disease and marked resistance to reductase inhibitors as single agents and may have premature cholesterol gallstone disease. Heterozygous patients have moderately elevated LDL. The hyperlipidemia responds well to niacin with a reductase inhibitor.

SECONDARY HYPERCHOLESTEROLEMIA
HYPOTHYROIDISM

In hypothyroidism, LDL and IDL are elevated. Some patients may have lipemia, as described in the section on secondary hyperlipemia. Hyperlipidemia may occur with no overt signs or symptoms of decreased thyroid function. Biliary excretion of cholesterol and bile acids is depressed. Cholesterol stores in tissues appear to be increased, although the number of LDL receptors on cells is decreased. Activity of hepatic lipase is markedly decreased, and atherogenesis is accelerated by myxedema. The hyperlipidemia responds dramatically to treatment with thyroxine.

NEPHROSIS

As described in the section on secondary hypertriglyceridemias, nephrosis produces a biphasic hyperlipoproteinemia. The earliest alteration of lipoproteins in nephrosis is elevation of LDL. Increased secretion of VLDL by liver is probably involved. Because the lipids of the lipoprotein surfaces are altered by enrichment with sphingomyelin, lysolecithin, and FFA, the catabolism of LDL could be impaired. Perhaps the low metabolic rate in affected patients introduces metabolic changes similar to those associated with hypothyroidism. The hyperlipidemia may be an important element in the markedly increased risk of atherosclerosis in these patients. The treatment of choice is a reductase inhibitor or bile acid–binding resin with niacin.

IMMUNOGLOBULIN DISORDERS

One of the lipoprotein abnormalities that can be associated with monoclonal gammopathy is elevation of LDL. A gamma lipoprotein that is a stable complex of immunoglobulin and lipoprotein may be observed on electrophoresis. Cryoprecipitation, often in the temperature range encountered in peripheral tissues when the environmental temperature is low, may occur. Patients may have symptoms from the vascular effect of complement fixation resulting from complex formation and may have hyperviscosity syndrome from the elevated immunoglobulins per se. Planar xanthomas may be present.

Treatment is directed at the underlying process. Plasmapheresis is often effective. If cryoprecipitation occurs at critical temperatures near or above room temperature, the procedure must be carried out in a special warm environment. Transfusion of whole blood or serum may be dangerous in these patients because of rapid production of anaphylatoxins from fresh complement in the serum, resulting from interaction with circulating antibody-antigen complexes. This risk can be minimized by the use of packed red blood cells and albumin in place of whole blood.

ANOREXIA NERVOSA

About 40% of patients with anorexia nervosa have elevated LDL, and levels of cholesterol may reach 400 to 600 mg/dL (10.4-15.6 mmol/L). The hyperlipidemia, which persists despite correction of hypothyroidism, is probably a result of decreased fecal excretion of bile acids and cholesterol. Serum lipoproteins return to normal when proper nutrition is restored.

CHOLESTASIS

The hyperlipidemia associated with obstruction of biliary flow is complex. Levels of cholesterol in these patients exceeding 400 mg/dL (10.4 mmol/L) usually are associated with extrahepatic obstruction or with intrahepatic tumor. Several types of abnormal lipoproteins are present. The most abundant, termed Lp-X, is a bilayer vesicle composed of unesterified cholesterol and lecithin, with associated apolipoproteins but no Apo B. Lp-X is apparent on electrophoresis as a band of zero to gamma mobility that shows metachromatic staining with Sudan black. It is these vesicular particles that cause the serum phospholipid and unesterified cholesterol content to be extremely high. Another abnormal species, called Lp-Y, contains appreciable amounts of triglycerides and Apo B. The LDL in cholestasis also contains an unusually large amount of triglycerides.

Patients may have planar xanthomas, especially at sites of minor trauma, and xanthomas of the palmar creases. Occasionally, eruptive xanthomas are present. Xanthomatous involvement of nerves may lead to symptoms of peripheral neuropathy, and the abnormal lipoproteins may be atherogenic. Whereas bilirubin levels are nearly normal in some patients with chronic cholestasis, all have elevated serum alkaline phosphatase activity.

Neuropathy or evidence of atherosclerosis is the chief indication for treatment of the hyperlipidemia. Bile acid–binding resins are of some value, whereas fibric acid derivatives may cause an increase in cholesterol. Plasmapheresis is the most effective treatment. Large doses of vitamin E are indicated to overcome severe impairment of absorption. Deficiency of other fat-soluble vitamins also occurs.

THE PRIMARY HYPOLIPIDEMIAS

Although the clinician is confronted less frequently by the problem of a striking deficiency in plasma lipids, it is important to recognize the primary and secondary hypolipidemias. A serum cholesterol less than 110 mg/dL (2.9 mmol/L) is noteworthy. Because levels of triglycerides in normal fasting serum may be as low as 25 mg/dL (0.29 mmol/L), significance is limited to cases in which they are virtually absent.

PRIMARY HYPOLIPIDEMIA DUE TO DEFICIENCY OF HIGH-DENSITY LIPOPROTEINS

1. TANGIER DISEASE
Etiology and Pathogenesis

Severe deficiency of HDL occurs in Tangier disease. Heterozygotes lack clinical signs but have about one-half or less of the normal complement of HDL and Apo A-I in plasma. Homozygotes lack normal HDL, and Apo A-I and Apo A-II are present at extremely low levels. Serum cholesterol is usually below 120 mg/dL (3.12 mmol/L) and may be half this value. Mild hypertriglyceridemia is usually present, and LDL is greatly enriched in triglycerides. Mutations in the ATP-dependent transporter ABCA1 underlie this disorder, causing defective efflux of cholesterol from peripheral cells.

Clinical Findings

The clinical features of this rare autosomal recessive disease include large, orange-colored, lipid-filled tonsils, accumulation of cholesteryl esters in the reticuloendothelial system, and an episodic and recurrent peripheral neuropathy with predominant motor weakness in the later stages. The course of the disease is benign in early childhood, but the neuropathy may appear as early as age 8 years. Cholesteryl ester accumulates most prominently in peripheral nerve sheaths. Carotenoid pigment may be apparent in pharyngeal and rectal mucous membranes. Splenomegaly and corneal infiltration may also be present. There is some increase in risk of coronary atherosclerosis.

Treatment

Because some of the lamellar lipoprotein material in plasma is believed to originate in chylomicrons, restriction of dietary fats and cholesterol is suggested.

2. FAMILIAL HYPOALPHALIPOPROTEINEMIA
Etiology and Pathogenesis

This phenotypic pattern is a partial deficiency of HDL that may involve heterogeneous mechanisms. These presumed constitutional disorders must be differentiated from the condition in which moderately low levels of HDL are seen in individuals consuming a diet very low in fat. White and Asian men on such diets usually have HDL cholesterol levels of 38 to 42 mg/dL (1-1.1 mmol/L) by ultracentrifugal analysis, in contrast to a median value of 49 mg/dL (1.3 mmol/L) when consuming a typical North American diet. Such levels are common in Asiatic populations and among vegetarians, where the risk of coronary disease is usually small. HDL cholesterol must also be interpreted in the light of the amount of triglyceride-rich lipoproteins in plasma. Because cholesteryl esters are progressively transferred to the cores of triglyceride-rich lipoproteins as triglyceride levels rise, HDL cholesterol decreases as an inverse function of the triglyceride level.

Etiologic Factor in Coronary Disease

Familial hypoalphalipoproteinemia is fairly common and is an important risk factor in atherosclerosis. This abnormality may be the only apparent risk factor in many cases of premature coronary or peripheral vascular disease and accelerates the appearance of coronary disease in patients with FH or other hyperlipidemias.

Hypoalphalipoproteinemia shows a strong familial incidence. Mutations in several genes have been associated, including *Apo A-I* (the principal protein of HDL), *PCPE-2* (a protease involved in the maturation of Apo A-1), and the WW domain oxidoreductase (a transcriptional regulator involved in HDL metabolism). Although several mechanisms and modes of transmission may be involved, many kindreds show distributions consistent with autosomal dominance. HDL cholesterol levels are usually below 35 mg/dL (0.9 mmol/L).

Treatment

Increases in HDL cholesterol in several coronary intervention trials have been independently associated with plaque regression. Only limited means of raising HDL levels are at hand. Findings that HDL is composed of as many as 20 discrete species further complicate this problem. It is not yet known which of these species may be involved in protecting against atherosclerosis or whether their levels can be increased. Although alcohol ingestion may increase total HDL, it appears that the effect is primarily on the HDL$_3$ ultracentrifugal fraction, which correlates poorly with decreased risk. No recommendation for increased alcohol consumption should be made.

Heavy exercise is associated with increases in HDL in some individuals but must be approached with caution in patients who may have coronary disease. Niacin increases total HDL in many subjects, chiefly the HDL$_2$ ultracentrifugal fraction. Smaller increments in HDL occur with reductase inhibitors and fibric acid derivatives.

The most important reason for measuring HDL cholesterol is to identify patients who are at increased risk. Thus, just as with patients who have premature vascular disease or a family history of early arteriosclerosis, patients with low HDL should be treated more aggressively for elevated levels of the atherogenic lipoproteins. Furthermore, vigorous efforts should be directed at the control of other risk factors such as hypertension. Smoking and obesity are known to decrease HDL significantly.

3. DEFICIENCY OF LECITHIN-CHOLESTEROL ACYLTRANSFERASE

This rare autosomal recessive disorder is not expressed in clinical or biochemical form in the heterozygote. In the homozygote, clinical characteristics are variable. The diagnosis is usually made in adults, although corneal opacities may begin in childhood. Proteinuria may be an early sign. Deposits of unesterified cholesterol and phospholipid in the renal microvasculature lead to progressive loss of nephrons and ultimate renal failure. Many patients have mild to moderate normochromic anemia with target cells. Hyperbilirubinemia or peripheral neuropathy may be present. Red blood cell lipid composition is abnormal, with increased content of unesterified cholesterol and lecithin. Most have elevated plasma triglycerides (200-1000 mg/dL [2.3-11.2 mmol/L]), and levels of serum cholesterol vary from low normal to about 500 mg/dL (13 mmol/L), only a small fraction of which is esterified. The large triglyceride-containing lipoproteins are unusually rich in unesterified cholesterol and appear to have abnormal surface monolayers. LDL are rich in triglycerides, and abnormal vesicular lipoproteins are present in the LDL density interval. Two abnormal HDL species are present: bilayer disks and small spherical particles. Marked restriction of dietary fat and cholesterol delays the onset of renal disease.

PRIMARY HYPOLIPIDEMIA DUE TO DEFICIENCY OF Apo B–CONTAINING LIPOPROTEINS

1. RECESSIVE ABETALIPOPROTEINEMIA

Etiology and Pathogenesis

This disorder could represent a number of mutations involving the processing of Apo B or the secretion of Apo B–containing lipoproteins. The predominant cause is mutations involving the microsomal triglyceride transfer protein. Patients heterozygous for mutations have no abnormalities of lipoproteins or clinical signs. In homozygotes, all forms of Apo B are essentially absent. No chylomicrons, VLDL, or LDL are found in plasma, leaving only HDL. Plasma triglycerides are usually less than 10 mg/dL (0.12 mmol/L) and fail to rise after a fat load. Total cholesterol is usually less than 90 mg/dL (2.3 mmol/L). There is a defect in the incorporation of newly synthesized triglycerides into chylomicrons. However, at low levels of fat intake, about 80% of the ingested triglycerides are absorbed, probably by direct absorption of fatty acids via the portal vein.

Clinical Findings

Clinical features include a paucity of adipose tissue associated with malabsorption of long-chain fatty acids due to failure of the intestine to secrete chylomicrons. Red blood cells may be acanthocytic, with a high cholesterol-phospholipid ratio. There may be progressive degeneration of the central nervous system, including cerebellar degeneration and posterior and lateral spinal tract disease. Retinal degeneration may be severe. Levels of fat-soluble vitamins in plasma may be very low. The neurologic and opthalmologic defects are due to deficiency of vitamin E (normally transported largely in LDL). Patients are apparently normal at birth and develop steatorrhea with impaired growth in infancy. The neuromuscular disorder often appears in late childhood with ataxia, night blindness, decreased visual acuity, and nystagmus. Cardiomyopathy with arrhythmias has been reported and may be a cause of death.

Treatment

Treatment includes administration of fat-soluble vitamins and essential fatty acids. Very large doses of mixed tocopherols (vitamin E; 1000-10,000 IU/d) limit the progressive central nervous system degeneration. Although vitamin A seems to correct the night blindness, it does not alter the course of retinitis pigmentosa. Vitamins D and K may also be indicated. Restriction of dietary fat minimizes steatorrhea.

2. FAMILIAL HYPOBETALIPOPROTEINEMIA

This disorder is usually attributable to defects at the Apo B locus, resulting in decreased production of protein or in the production of truncated gene products. LDL and Apo B in heterozygotes are often present at about half of normal levels. If a mutant allele resulting in the complete interdiction of Apo B synthesis is present in the homozygous state, the clinical and biochemical features may be indistinguishable from those of recessive abetalipoproteinemia, and treatment is the same as for that disorder. Very short truncations of Apo B-100 only allow the formation of abnormally dense, small LDL. Longer truncations permit the formation of larger lipoproteins, even including VLDL-like particles. Mutations in the ANGPTL3 gene can cause deficiency of LDL, HDL, and triglycerides.

Clinical features may be absent in patients who produce at least low levels of LDL-like particles. However, signs and symptoms of tocopherol deficiency may be present. Treatment with mixed tocopherols (800 IU/d) is recommended for all patients.

3. CHYLOMICRON RETENTION DISEASE

This disorder presents in the neonate and appears to be based on the selective inability of intestinal epithelial cells to secrete chylomicrons. Affected individuals have severe malabsorption of triglycerides with steatorrhea. Levels of LDL and VLDL are about half of normal, presumably secondary to malnutrition. Tocopherol levels may be very low and may be associated with neurologic abnormalities. Clinical symptoms diminish somewhat with time if the patient is managed with a low-fat diet and tocopherol supplementation.

SECONDARY HYPOLIPIDEMIA

Hypolipidemia may be secondary to a number of diseases characterized by chronic cachexia (eg, advanced cancer). Myeloproliferative disorders can lead to extremely low levels of LDL, probably owing to increased uptake related to rapid proliferation and membrane synthesis. A wide variety of conditions leading to intestinal malabsorption produce hypolipidemia. In these situations, levels of chylomicrons, VLDL, and LDL in serum are low but never absent. Because most of the lipoprotein mass of fasting serum is of hepatic origin, massive parenchymal liver failure (eg, in Reye syndrome) can cause severe hypolipidemia. A precipitous fall in lipoprotein levels during drug treatment of hyperlipidemia can signal hepatic toxicity. Secondary hypobetalipoproteinemia occurs in oroticaciduria.

The hypolipidemias associated with immunoglobulin disorders result from diverse mechanisms. Affected patients usually have myeloma or macroglobulinemia but may have lymphomas or lymphocytic leukemia. Any of the major classes of immunoglobulins may be involved. In many cases, the immunoglobulins are cryoprecipitins; thus, the diagnosis may be missed if blood is not drawn and serum prepared at 37°C and observed for cryoprecipitation. Immunoglobulin-lipoprotein complexes may precipitate in various tissues. When this occurs in the lamina propria of the intestine, a syndrome of malabsorption and protein-losing enteropathy may result. Monoclonal IgA in myeloma may precipitate with lipoproteins, causing xanthomas of the gingiva and cervix. Xanthomas in the skin are usually planar and may involve intracutaneous hemorrhage, producing a classic purple xanthoma. Planar xanthomas occurring in cholestasis may be confused with this condition because the abnormal lipoprotein of cholestasis (Lp-X), like the circulating lipoprotein complex of immunoglobulin and lipoprotein, has gamma mobility on electrophoresis.

OTHER DISORDERS OF LIPOPROTEIN METABOLISM

THE LIPODYSTROPHIES

Classification

Classification of the lipodystrophies is based on their familial or acquired origin and the regional or generalized nature of the fat loss. To date, mutations in eight gene loci have been associated with phenotypes of lipodystrophy. Insulin resistance is a common feature.

Familial generalized lipodystrophy (Seip-Berardinelli syndrome) is a rare recessive trait associated with mutations in the gene for seipin. It may be diagnosed at birth and is associated with macrosomia. Genital hypertrophy, hypertrichosis, acanthosis nigricans, hepatomegaly, insulin resistance, hypertriglyceridemia, and glucose intolerance are regularly observed.

Familial lipodystrophy of limbs and trunk (Köbberling-Dunnigan syndrome) appears to be transmitted as a dominant trait associated with mutations in the *lamin A* gene. Because sequence anomalies in other regions of the gene are associated with muscular dystrophy, cardiac conduction defects, cardiomyopathy, or axonal neuropathies, overlapping phenotypes may occur. It affects women predominantly and is not evident until puberty. The face, neck, and upper trunk are usually spared. Growth is normal, but otherwise this syndrome shares features of the generalized form noted earlier. It is frequently associated with Stein-Leventhal syndrome and often progresses to fatal cirrhosis.

Acquired forms of lipodystrophy, generalized (Lawrence syndrome) and partial (Barraquer-Simmons syndrome), usually begin in childhood, affect females predominantly, and often follow an acute febrile illness. The generalized type commonly shares the features described earlier, invariably involving the trunk and extremities but sometimes sparing the face. A sclerosing panniculitis, as seen in Weber-Christian syndrome, may appear at the outset. The partial type usually begins in the face and then involves the neck, upper limbs, and trunk. In this disorder, reduced levels of C3 complement are frequently encountered. Most patients have proteinuria, and some develop overt vascular nephritis.

Associated Disorders

Because a number of patients with disorders resembling both familial and acquired types of lipodystrophy have tumors or other lesions of the hypothalamus, appropriate neurologic evaluation should be obtained. Similarly, the physician should be alert to the association of HIV disease and collagen-vascular disorders, including scleroderma and dermatomyositis, with some cases of acquired lipodystrophy.

RARE DISORDERS

Autosomal Recessive Hypercholesterolemia

In autosomal recessive hypercholesterolemia (ARH), LDL levels are markedly elevated, resulting in total cholesterol levels between 400 and 700 mg/dL (10.4 and 18.1 mmol/L). It is attributed to mutations in the gene for the ARH protein that is involved in endocytosis of the LDL receptor. Very large xanthomas (tuberous, tendinous, and planar) are frequently present. Arcus and xanthelasma are also common. Statins and bile acid sequestrants appear to be effective.

PCSK9 Variants

The protease, PCSK9, plays a role in processing the LDL receptor. Gain of function mutations in this gene are associated with hypercholesterolemia, presumably due to reduction in the number of effective receptors. More commonly, loss of function mutations that result in longer residence time of the LDL receptor are associated with low levels of LDL cholesterol.

Werner Syndrome, Progeria, Infantile Hypercalcemia, Sphingolipidoses, and Niemann-Pick Disease

These disorders may be associated with hypercholesterolemia, but levels of triglycerides may be normal. Among the sphingolipidoses, HDL deficiency is typical of Gaucher disease, in which hypertriglyceridemia may also occur. Niemann-Pick disease is attributable in most cases to mutations in the *NCP1* gene and may be associated with hypercholesterolemia or hypertriglyceridemia. However, a similar disorder results from mutations in the *NCP2* locus. The *NCP1* gene product is involved in the postlysosomal transport of lipids. The neurological manifestations of Niemann-Pick disease type C are mitigated by an inhibitor of glycosphingolipid synthesis, miglustat.

Wolman Disease and Cholesteryl Ester Storage Disease

These recessive lipid storage disorders involve the absence and partial deficiency, respectively, of lysosomal acid lipase, resulting in abnormal cholesteryl ester and triglyceride stores in liver, spleen, adrenals, small intestine, and bone marrow. Most patients have elevated levels of both LDL and VLDL. Wolman disease may be fatal in infancy but appears to respond to hematopoietic cell transplant. Cholesteryl ester storage disease responds at least partially to combined statin-ezetimibe therapy.

Cerebrotendinous Xanthomatosis

In this recessive disorder, impaired synthesis of bile acids due to mutations in the *sterol 27-hydroxylase* gene results in increased production of cholesterol and cholestanol that accumulate in tissues. Plasma levels of cholesterol and cholestanol are normal or elevated. Cataracts, tendinous xanthomas, progressive neurologic dysfunction, and premature coronary atherosclerosis are hallmarks of this disease. Its central nervous system effects include dementia, spasticity, and ataxia. Death usually ensues before age 50 from neurologic degeneration or coronary disease. Treatment with chenodeoxycholic acid appears useful. Resins must be avoided because they aggravate the underlying defect.

Phytosterolemia

Mutations in the cassette half transporters ABCG5 or ABCG8 underlie this disorder, which is characterized by normal or elevated plasma cholesterol levels; high concentrations of plant sterol in serum, adipose tissue, and skin; and prominent tendinous and tuberous xanthomas. Substantially larger fractions of phytosterols and cholesterol are absorbed from the intestine than in normal individuals. Serum cholesterol levels may be as high as 700 mg/dL (18.2 mmol/L), reflecting an increase in LDL that contain phytosterol esters in addition to cholesteryl esters. Diagnosis is established by quantitation of phytosterols in plasma by gas-liquid chromatography. Premature coronary disease is common, as is polyarthritis and leukocytoclastic vasculopathy. Treatment consists of a diet restricted in plant sterols and cholesterol and the use of bile acid–binding resins, reductase inhibitors, and ezetimibe.

Cholesteryl Ester Transfer Protein Deficiency

Mutations have been identified that impair the function of CETP, resulting in the retention of cholesteryl esters in HDL. Total HDL cholesterol is increased by 30% to 50% in heterozygotes and by as much as 200 mg/dL in homozygotes. The risk of atherosclerosis may be moderately increased in homozygotes.

TREATMENT OF HYPERLIPIDEMIA

Initial therapy in all forms of hyperlipidemia is an appropriate diet. In most cases, a universal diet (see later) is indicated. In many subjects with lipemia or with mild hypercholesterolemia, compliance with diet is sufficient to control lipoprotein levels. Most patients with severe hypercholesterolemia or lipemia require drug therapy. Diet must be continued to achieve the full potential of the medications. LDL cholesterol and triglycerides should be below 70 mg/dL (1.8 mmol/L) and 130 mg/dL (1.5 mmol/L), respectively, in patients with known atherosclerosis. C-reactive protein, lipoprotein-associated phospholipase A2, and other emerging biomarkers are useful in predicting risk.

Caution Regarding Drug Therapy

Women of childbearing age should be advised of the potential risk of teratogenicity of statins and possibly other hypolipidemic agents. Treatment should be given only if pregnancy is being actively avoided. Nursing mothers should not be treated. Estrogen-containing contraceptives should be avoided or used with caution in patients with hypertriglyceridemia.

In children, hyperlipidemias other than FH and severe cases of the metabolic syndrome usually do not require medication before age 16 years. Factors in the decision to start drug treatment include: the child's age and levels of lipoproteins; the severity and age at onset of symptomatic coronary disease in the child's family; and the presence in the child of other risk factors, especially diabetes or compound dyslipidemias [including hypoalphalipoproteinemia, hyper-Lp(a)lipoproteinemia, FH, and FCH]. Dietary treatment is indicated for all children with hyperlipidemia and should be started after the second year. The exception is primary chylomicronemia, in which an appropriate diet should be instituted as soon as the disease is detected.

DIETARY FACTORS IN THE MANAGEMENT OF LIPOPROTEIN DISORDERS

Restriction of Caloric Intake

The secretion of VLDL by liver is greatly stimulated by caloric intake in excess of requirements for physical activity and basal metabolism. Therefore, the total caloric content of the diet is of greater importance than its specific composition in treating endogenous hyperlipemia. There is a positive correlation between serum levels of VLDL triglyceride and various measures of obesity, but many obese patients have normal serum lipids. On the other hand, most patients with hypertriglyceridemia—except those with lipoprotein lipase deficiency—are obese. As obese patients lose weight, VLDL stabilize at lower levels. There is a modest correlation of LDL levels with body weight in the general population.

Restriction of Fat Intake

In primary chylomicronemia, all types of fats must be restricted rigidly. In the acute management of mixed lipemia with impending pancreatitis, elimination of dietary fat leads to a rapid decrease in triglycerides.

The cholesterol-lowering effect of a significant reduction in total fat is well known. It has also been shown that a 10% to 15% fall in cholesterol is achieved when individuals who have been consuming a typical North American diet restrict their intake of saturated fats to 8% of total calories. Most saturated and trans fatty acids cause increased levels of LDL cholesterol by downregulating hepatic LDL receptors. Whereas polyunsaturated fatty acids do not have this effect, they may reduce levels of HDL and are potentially carcinogenic. Monounsaturated fatty acids increase HDL but do not increase LDL. Moderate use of monounsaturated fats such as olive oil, oleic acid–rich safflower oil, or canola oil is indicated.

Marine Omega-3 Fatty Acids

The omega-3 fatty acids are ligands for peroxisome proliferator–activated receptor alpha. Those found in fish oils have special properties relevant to the treatment of hypertriglyceridemia and may protect against fatal arrhythmias in ischemic myocardium. Substantial decreases in triglyceride levels can be induced in some patients with severe endogenous or mixed lipemia at doses of 3 to 4 g/d of eicosapentaenoic (EPA) and docosahexaenoic (DHA) acids, combined. This should be given in divided doses with meals. EPA and DHA are potent inhibitors of platelet reactivity.

Reduction of Cholesterol Intake

The amount of cholesterol in the diet affects serum cholesterol levels, but individual responses vary. Restriction of dietary cholesterol to less than 200 mg/d (5.2 mmol/d) in normal individuals can result in a decrease of up to 10% to 15% in serum cholesterol, primarily reflecting a decrease in LDL. Dietary cholesterol and saturated or trans fat content have independent effects.

Role of Carbohydrate in Diet

When a high-carbohydrate diet is consumed, hypertriglyceridemia often develops within 48 to 72 hours, and levels of triglycerides rise to a maximum in 1 to 5 weeks. Persons with higher basal triglycerides and those consuming hypercaloric diets show the greatest effect. In persons with type 2 diabetes, a high-carbohydrate diet tends to increase insulin resistance. Substitution of monounsaturated fats for the carbohydrate improves insulin resistance and lipoprotein levels.

Alcohol Ingestion

Ingestion of alcohol is a common cause of secondary hypertriglyceridemia owing to overproduction of VLDL. Some individuals with familial hypertriglyceridemia are particularly sensitive to the effects of alcohol, and abstinence may normalize their triglycerides. Occasionally, chronic alcohol intake may also be associated with hypercholesterolemia. Increased cholesterol synthesis and decreased conversion to bile acids have been observed. Alcohol may account for alimentary lipemia persisting beyond 12 to 14 hours. This possibility should be excluded by the history or a repeat lipid analysis. A positive correlation has been found between alcohol intake and HDL cholesterol levels in some individuals. Because alcohol-induced changes in HDL appear primarily to involve the HDL$_3$ subfraction, there is no justification for the use of alcohol to increase the protective effect of HDL against atherosclerosis. If the low HDL cholesterol is secondary to hypertriglyceridemia, alcohol must be avoided.

Antioxidants

Both alpha and gamma tocopherols (vitamin E) have recognized roles in the elimination of free radicals. Vitamin C assists this activity by restoring the tocopheroxyl radical to active tocopherol. These vitamins have been shown to restore normal vascular reactivity in hyperlipidemic patients, and some epidemiologic evidence suggests that they have an antiatherogenic effect. It is therefore reasonable to include at least 50 IU of mixed tocopherols and 250 mg of vitamin C in the diet each day. Larger doses may partially vitiate the effects of certain hypolipidemic drug regimens and have not been shown to have antiatherogenic potential. Selenium may also be important because it is a cofactor for one species of superoxide dismutase. Diets rich in fruits and vegetables appear to be important, providing isoflavones, quinols, and a number of carotenoid species.

B Vitamins

A significant percentage of Americans carry at least one allele for mutations in the methylene tetrahydrofolate reductase gene that diminishes its efficiency by reducing its affinity for folic acid. This, and certain other mutations, may lead to significantly elevated levels of a metabolite of methionine—homocysteine—that has toxic effects on endothelium. Supplementation with 0.4 to 2 mg of folic acid mitigates this problem. Vitamins B_6 and B_{12} participate in the metabolism of homocysteine. Thus, a B complex supplement should be used. Dietary protein should be restricted to the amount required for replacement of essential amino acids (about 0.5-1 g/kg) in patients with hyperhomocysteinemia. Oral administration of betaine, a methyl donor, can mitigate homocysteine levels in severely affected patients (2 g 3 times daily).

Other Dietary Substances

Several other nutrients have been studied in relation to atherosclerosis. Caffeine and sucrose have negligible effects on serum lipids, and their statistical relationship to CHD is generally unimpressive when data are corrected for cigarette smoking. However, when coffee is prepared by protracted boiling of the grounds, a lipid substance (cafestol) is extracted that contributes to hypercholesterolemia. Lecithin has no effect on plasma lipoproteins. A minor reduction in LDL cholesterol is associated with the addition of oat bran and certain other brans to the diet.

The Universal Diet

Dietary treatment is an important aspect of the management of all forms of lipoprotein disorders and may in some cases be all that is required. Knowledge of the dietary factors mentioned earlier allows selection of appropriate modifications for an individual. However, a basic diet is useful in the treatment of most patients, the elements of which are as follows:

(1) A normal BMI should be achieved and maintained.
(2) Fat should provide less than 35% and saturated fat less than 7% of total calories. Monounsaturated oils should predominate and be used for all high-temperature cooking.
(3) Cholesterol should be reduced to less than 200 mg/d.
(4) Complex carbohydrates should predominate among total carbohydrates.
(5) Alcohol should be avoided in patients with hypertriglyceridemia or those requiring weight loss.
(6) Intake of trans fatty acids should be avoided.
(7) Peroxidized fats resulting from protracted heating should be avoided.

Caloric restriction and reduction of adipose tissue mass are particularly important for patients with increased levels of VLDL and IDL. During periods of substantial weight loss, levels of VLDL and LDL tend to be lower than they would be under isocaloric conditions, even at ideal body weight.

DRUGS USED IN TREATMENT OF HYPERLIPOPROTEINEMIA

BILE ACID SEQUESTRANTS

Mechanism of Action and Efficacy

Cholestyramine, colestipol, and colesevelam are cationic resins that bind bile acids in the intestinal lumen. They are not absorbed and, therefore, increase the excretion of bile acids in the stool up to 10-fold. LDL levels decrease as a consequence of increased expression of high-affinity receptors on hepatic cell membranes. These agents are useful only in disorders involving elevated LDL. Patients who have increased levels of VLDL may have further increases in triglycerides during treatment with resins. In combined hyperlipidemia, where the resins may be given to reduce LDL, a second agent such as niacin may be required to control the hypertriglyceridemia. Levels of LDL fall 15% to 30% in compliant patients with heterozygous familial hypercholesterolemia who are receiving maximal doses of the resins. These agents can contribute an incremental effect in the management of insulin resistance by an incretin-mediated mechanism. When given as a single agent, a modest reduction in new coronary events can result. When given in combined regimens with a statin and/or niacin, regression of coronary artery plaques has been demonstrated by quantitative angiography.

Drug Dosage

In disorders involving moderately high levels of LDL, 20 g of cholestyramine or colestipol daily may reduce cholesterol levels effectively. Treatment should commence at one-half this dosage to minimize gastrointestinal side effects. Maximum doses (30 g colestipol, 32 g cholestyramine, 3.75 g colesevelam daily) are required in more severe cases. These agents are only effective if taken with meals.

Side-Effects

Because the resins are not absorbed, systemic side-effects are absent. Patients frequently complain of a bloated sensation and constipation, both of which may be relieved by the addition of psyllium to the resin mixture. Malabsorption of fat or fat-soluble vitamins with a daily dose of resin up to 30 g occurs only in individuals with preexisting bowel disease or cholestasis. Hypoprothrombinemia has been observed in patients with malabsorption due to these causes. Cholestyramine and colestipol bind thyroxine, digitalis glycosides, and warfarin and impair the absorption of iron, thiazides, beta-blockers, ezetimibe, and other drugs. Absorption of all these (except ezetimibe) is ensured if they are administered 1 hour before the resin. Colesevelam does not bind digoxin, warfarin, or reductase inhibitors. Because they change the composition of bile micelles, bile acid sequestrants theoretically may increase the risk of cholelithiasis, particularly in obese subjects. In practice, this risk appears to be very small. The resins should not be used as single agents in patients with hypertriglyceridemia and should be avoided in those with diverticulitis.

NIACIN (NICOTINIC ACID)

Mechanism of Action and Efficacy

Niacin (but not its amide) is able to effect major reductions in triglyceride-rich lipoproteins and, to a lesser extent, in LDL. It inhibits secretion of VLDL. It increases sterol excretion acutely, mobilizes cholesterol from tissue pools until a new steady-state is established, and decreases cholesterol biosynthesis. That it can cause a continued decrease in hepatic cholesterol production even when given with bile acid–binding resins is probably an important feature of the complementary action of these agents. Levels of HDL, particularly HDL_2, are usually significantly increased, reflecting a decrease in their fractional catabolic rate. Niacin stimulates production of tissue plasminogen activator, an effect that may be of value in preventing thrombotic events. Small, dense LDL are converted to particles of larger diameter during treatment. Niacin is the only available agent that can reduce levels of Lp(a) significantly. Niacin, as a single agent, was given in only one large intervention study which found a significant decrease in nonfatal, recurrent coronary events. In four angiographic studies in which niacin was given with a resin, a statin, or both, significant regression or decreased progression of coronary lesions was reported.

Drug Dosage

The dose of crystalline niacin required varies with the diagnosis. Optimal effect on LDL in heterozygous FH is usually achieved only when 4.5 to 6 g of niacin daily is combined with a resin or reductase inhibitor. For other forms of hypercholesterolemia, dysbetalipoproteinemia, hypertriglyceridemia, and hypoalphalipoproteinemia, 1.5 to 3.5 g/d often has a dramatic effect. Because niacin causes cutaneous flushing, it is usually started at a dosage of 100 mg 3 times daily with meals, increasing to the desired dose within 7 to 10 days. Many patients have no or only occasional flushing when stabilized on a given dose, but most must reach about 3 g/d before flushing ceases. Because the flush is prostaglandin mediated, 0.3 g of aspirin given 20 to 30 minutes before each dose when treatment is initiated or the dose increased (or equivalent doses of other cyclooxygenase inhibitors) may mitigate this symptom. It is important to counsel the patient that the flushing is a harmless cutaneous vasodilation and that the drug should be taken with meals 2 or 3 times daily. A daily dose of 6.5 g is the maximum under any circumstances. Niaspan, a prescription extended-release niacin, appears to be safe in doses up to 2 g daily.

Side-Effects

Some patients have reversible elevations of serum glutamic aminotransferase or alkaline phosphatase activities up to 3 times the upper limit of normal that do not appear to be clinically significant. In a group of patients treated continuously for up to 15 years, no significant liver disease developed despite such enzyme abnormalities. Rarely, patients develop a chemical hepatitis signaled by malaise, anorexia, and nausea. Aminotransferase levels are significantly elevated, and levels of lipoproteins may fall precipitously. Treatment should be stopped immediately. About one-fifth of patients have mild hyperuricemia that tends to be asymptomatic unless the patient has had gout. In such cases, allopurinol can be added to the regimen. A few patients have moderate elevations of blood glucose during treatment. Again, this is reversible except in some patients who have latent type 2 diabetes. The use of niacin should be considered carefully in patients with insulin resistance. Diabetic patients receiving insulin can often be treated successfully. A more common side-effect is gastric irritation, which responds well to H_2 blockers and antacids. Antacids that contain aluminum should be avoided. Rarely, patients develop acanthosis nigricans, which usually clears if the drug is discontinued. Some patients can have cardiac arrhythmias, mostly atrial, while taking niacin. Reversible macular edema has been described rarely.

Niacin should be avoided in patients with peptic ulcer or hepatic parenchymal disease. Liver function, uric acid, and blood glucose should be evaluated before commencing treatment and periodically thereafter.

Most over-the-counter sustained-release preparations should be avoided because of the risk of fulminant hepatic failure. However, if the daily dose is limited to 2 g or less, this rare consequence is probably unlikely.

FIBRIC ACID DERIVATIVES

Mechanism of Action and Efficacy

Gemfibrozil and fenofibrate, which are ligands for peroxisome proliferator–activated receptor alpha, decrease lipolysis in adipose tissue, reduce levels of circulating triglycerides, and cause modest reductions in LDL. However, in some patients, reductions in VLDL levels are attended by increased LDL levels. They cause moderate increases in levels of HDL, including the protein moiety. One primary prevention, and one secondary prevention trial using gemfibrozil as monotherapy showed reduction in new coronary events.

Drug Dosage

The fibrates may be useful in the treatment of patients with severe endogenous lipemia, familial dysbetalipoproteinemia, and some patients with combined hyperlipidemia who are intolerant of niacin. The usual dose of gemfibrozil is 600 mg twice daily. That of fenofibrate varies with the preparation.

Side-Effects

Skin eruptions, gastrointestinal symptoms, and muscle symptoms have been described as well as blood dyscrasias and elevated levels of aminotransferases and alkaline phosphatase. These drugs enhance the effects of the coumarin and indanedione anticoagulants and increase lithogenicity of bile. Concomitant use of fibrates with certain reductase inhibitors increases the risk of myopathy. Fenofibrate is most compatible with pravastatin or rosuvastatin with respect to cytochrome metabolism. Fibrates should be avoided during pregnancy and lactation and are contraindicated if hepatic or renal disease is present.

HMG-CoA REDUCTASE INHIBITORS (TABLE 19–2)

Mechanism of Action and Efficacy

Several closely related structural analogs of HMG-CoA act as competitive inhibitors of HMG-CoA reductase, a key enzyme in the cholesterol biosynthetic pathway. Of these, lovastatin, pravastatin, simvastatin, fluvastatin, atorvastatin, pitavastatin, and rosuvastatin are approved for use in the United States. Inhibition of cholesterol biosynthesis induces an increase in high-affinity LDL receptors in the liver, increasing removal of LDL from plasma and decreasing production of LDL. The latter results from increased uptake of lipoprotein precursors of LDL by hepatic receptors. Modest increases in HDL cholesterol and limited decreases in VLDL levels can be achieved. These drugs have no appreciable effect in patients with severe hypertriglyceridemia. Some of the cholesterol-independent effects of reductase inhibitors appear to involve enhanced stability of atherosclerotic lesions and decreased oxidative stress and vascular inflammation, with improved endothelial function. Institution of treatment with a reductase inhibitor should begin immediately in all patients with acute coronary syndromes regardless of cholesterol level. One angiographic trial with statin monotherapy and three with combined regimens including statins yielded significant reduction in the size of coronary atheromas. A number of primary and secondary trials with statins as monotherapy have demonstrated significant reduction in endpoints including primary or recurrent myocardial infarction, coronary revascularization, atherosclerotic stroke, or cardiac death. In these trials, reduction of LDL cholesterol levels to or below currently accepted goals produced an approximate 35% reduction in new coronary events over the 3 to 5 year duration of the trials. Longer term follow-up suggests that the impact on new coronary events will deepen over time, consistent with observations on individuals with familial hypobetalipoproteinemia or loss of function variants in the *PCSK9* gene.

Drug Dosage

These drugs are the most effective individual agents for treatment of hypercholesterolemia. Their effects are amplified significantly when combined with niacin, ezetimibe, or resin. Daily dosage ranges are presented in Table 19–2. Patients with heterozygous FH usually require higher doses. Because information on long-term safety is lacking, use of these agents in children should be restricted to those with homozygous FH and selected heterozygotes that are at particularly high risk. Women who are lactating, pregnant, or likely to become pregnant should not be given these drugs.

Side-Effects

These agents are generally well tolerated. Side-effects, often transient, include rashes and changes in bowel function. Myopathy with markedly elevated creatine kinase (CK) levels occurs infrequently. Rarely, myopathy can progress to rhabdomyolysis with myoglobinuria and renal shutdown. There is an increased incidence of myopathy in patients receiving certain reductase inhibitors with cyclosporine, fibric acid derivatives, macrolides, HIV protease inhibitors, nefazodone, verapamil, and ketoconazole. Other drugs that compete for metabolism by cytochrome P450 3A4 can be expected to have the same effect. Because pravastatin and rosuvastatin do not compete with these agents for metabolism by cytochrome P450 enzymes, they appear to be compatible with them. Fluvastatin is chiefly metabolized by cytochrome P450 2C9. Thus, competitors for that pathway may cause accumulation of this reductase inhibitor. The myopathy is rapidly reversible on cessation of therapy. Minor elevations of CK activity in plasma are noted more frequently, especially with unusual physical activity. CK levels should be measured before starting therapy and monitored at regular intervals in selected patients. Older patients, those taking higher doses and multiple other drugs, those who have diabetes, those with renal insufficiency, and those with baseline elevated CK levels should be observed more frequently. A form of statin-associated myopathy can occur in the absence of CK elevations.

Moderate, often intermittent elevations of serum aminotransferases (up to 3 times normal) occur in some patients. If the patient is asymptomatic, therapy may be continued if activity is measured frequently (at 1- to 2-month intervals) and the levels are stable. In about 2% of patients, some of whom have underlying liver disease or a history of alcohol use, aminotransferase activity may exceed 3 times the normal limit. This usually occurs after 3 to 16 months of continuous therapy and may portend more severe hepatic toxicity such as that described in the section on niacin. The reductase inhibitor should be discontinued promptly in these

TABLE19–2 Reductase inhibitors.

Drugs (in Increasing Order of Potency)	Dose Range
Fluvastatin	20-80 mg
Pravastatin	10-80 mg
Lovastatin	10-80 mg
Simvastatin	5-80 mg
Atorvastatin	5-80 mg
Resuvastatin	5-40 mg
Pitavastatin	1-4 mg

TABLE 19–3 The primary hyperlipoproteinemias and their drug treatment.

	Single Drug[a]	Drug Combination
Primary Chylomicronemia Chylomicrons (VLDL may be increased)	Niacin, fibrate[b] if VLDL increased	Niacin plus fibrate[b] if VLDL increased
Familial Hypertriglyceridemia VLDL and perhaps chylomicrons increased	Niacin, fibrate	Niacin plus fibrate
Familial Combined Hyperlipoproteinemia VLDL increased LDL increased VLDL, LDL increased	Niacin, fibrate, reductase inhibitor Reductase inhibitor, niacin, ezetimibe Reductase inhibitor, niacin, fibrate	Two or three of the single drugs
Familial Dysbetalipoproteinemia VLDL remnants, chylomicron remnants increased	Niacin, fibrate, reductase inhibitor	Fibrate plus niacin or niacin plus reductase inhibitor
Familial Hypercholesterolemia LDL increased	Reductase inhibitor, ezetimibe, niacin, resin	Two or three of the single drugs
Familial Ligand-Defective Apo B LDL increased	Reductase inhibitor, niacin, ezetimibe	Niacin plus reductase inhibitor or ezetimibe
Lp(a) Hyperlipoproteinemia Lp(a) increased	Niacin	

[a]Single-drug therapy should be tried before drug combinations are used.

[b]Fibric acid derivative.

patients. These agents are contraindicated in the presence of active liver disease and should be used with caution in patients with a history of liver disease. They should be discontinued temporarily during hospitalization for major surgery.

CHOLESTEROL ABSORPTION INHIBITORS

Mechanism of Action and Efficacy

Ezetimibe, the first of this class, inhibits the absorption of cholesterol and phytosterols by enterocytes. By interrupting the enterohepatic circulation of sterols secreted in bile, it increases sterol elimination. No outcome studies with this agent as monotherapy have been reported.

Drug Dosage

Ezetimibe is useful in treating primary hypercholesterolemias and phytosterolemia. Concomitant use of fibric acid derivatives can increase the blood concentration of this drug. Resins can decrease its absorption. It should be avoided in pregnant or lactating women and in patients with liver disease, and used with caution in patients receiving cyclosporine. A single dose of 10 mg daily reduces cholesterol by 15% to 20%.

Side-Effects

Very few side-effects have been reported. The prevalence of elevated liver enzymes may be modestly increased when ezetimibe is given with a reductase inhibitor. Biopsy-proven myopathy has been described rarely.

COMBINED DRUG THERAPY (TABLE 19–3)

Combinations of drugs may be useful (1) when LDL and VLDL levels are both elevated; (2) in cases of hypercholesterolemia in which significant increases of VLDL occur during treatment with a bile acid–binding resin; (3) where a complementary effect is required to normalize LDL levels, as in familial hypercholesterolemia or familial combined hyperlipidemia; and (4) when a hyperlipidemia is accompanied by primary HDL deficiency or an elevated level of Lp(a).

Niacin with Other Agents

The combination of a fibrate with niacin may be more effective than either drug alone in managing marked hypertriglyceridemia. Niacin usually normalizes triglycerides in individuals who have increased levels of VLDL while taking resins. The combination of niacin and resins is more effective than either agent alone in decreasing LDL levels in FH. The combination is also very useful in the treatment of FCH. The absorption of niacin from the intestine is unimpeded by the resin. Niacin is complementary with ezetimibe in treating combined hyperlipidemia.

HMG-CoA Reductase Inhibitors with Other Agents

The addition of resin or niacin to a reductase inhibitor further decreases plasma levels of LDL in patients with primary hypercholesterolemias. Liver function and plasma CK activity should be monitored frequently when the combination includes niacin.

These three drugs used together are more effective, frequently at lower doses, than any of their binary combinations in reducing LDL. Ezetimibe is synergistic with reductase inhibitors. The compatibility of rosuvastatin or pravastatin with fenofibrate makes these combinations useful in combined hyperlipidemia.

REFERENCES

Atherosclerosis

Libby P, Ridker PM, Hansson GK; Leducq Transatlantic Network on Atherothrombosis. Inflammation in atherosclerosis: from pathophysiology to practice. *J Am Coll Cardiol* 2009; 54:2129-38. [PMID: 19942084]

Packard CJ. Lipoprotein-associated phospholipase A2 as a biomarker of coronary heart disease and a therapeutic target. *Curr Opin Cardiol* 2009;24:358-62. [PMID: 19417639]

Shao B, Heinecke JW. HDL, lipid peroxidation, and atherosclerosis. *J Lipid Res* 2009; 50:599-601. [PMID: 19141435]

Lipoproteins

Adiels M, Olofsson S-O, Taskinen M-R, Boren J. Overproduction of very low-density lipoproteins is the hallmark of the dyslipidemia in the metabolic syndrome. *Arterioscler Thromb Vasc Biol* 2008; 28:1225-36. [PMID: 18565848]

Benn M, Nordestgaard BG, Grande P, Schnohr P, Tybjaerg-Hansen A. PCSK9 R46L, low-density lipoprotein cholesterol levels, and risk of ischemic heart disease: 3 independent studies and meta-analyses. *J Am Coll Cardiol* 2010; 55:2843-5. [PMID: 20579540]

de la Llera-Moya M, Drazul-Schrader D, Asztalos BF, Cuchel M, Raeder DJ, Rothblat GH. The ability to promote efflux via ABCA1 determines the capacity of serum specimens with similar high-density lipoprotein cholesterol to remove cholesterol from macrophages. *Arterioscler Thromb Vasc Biol* 2010; 30:796-801. [PMID: 20075420]

Erqou S, Thompson A, Di Angelantonio E, et al. Apolipoprotein(a) isoforms and the risk of vascular disease: systematic review of 40 studies involving 58,000 participants. *J Am Coll Cardiol* 2010; 55:2168-70. [PMID: 20447543]

Kruit JK, Brunham LR, Verchere CB, Hayden MR. HDL and LDL cholesterol significantly influence beta-cell function in type 2 diabetes mellitus. *Curr Opin Lipidol* 2010; 21:178-85. [PMID: 20463468]

Rothblat GH, Phillips MC. High-density lipoprotein heterogeneity and function in reverse cholesterol transport. *Curr Opin Lipidol* 2010; 21:229-38. [PMID: 20480549]

Vaisar T, Pennathur S, Green PS, et al. Shotgun proteomics implicates protease inhibition and complement activation in the antiinflammatory properties of HDL. *J Clin Invest* 2007; 117:746-56. [PMID: 17332893]

Treatment

Ballantyne CM, Raichlen JS, Nicholls SJ, et al. Asteroid Investigators. Effect of rosuvastatin therapy on coronary artery stenoses assessed by quantitative coronary angiography: a study to evaluate the effect of rosuvastatin on intravascular ultrasound-derived coronary atheroma burden. *Circulation* 2008; 117:2458-66. [PMID: 18378607]

Brunzell JD, Davidson M, Furberg CD, et al. Lipoprotein management in patients with cardiometabolic risk: consensus conference report from the ADA and the American College of Cardiology Foundation. *J Am Coll Cardiol* 2008;51:1512-1524. [PMID: 18402913]

Forrester JS. Redefining normal low-density lipoprotein cholesterol: a strategy to unseat coronary disease as the nation's leading killer. *J Am Coll Cardiol* 2010; 56:630-6. [PMID: 20705220]

Grundy SM, Cleeman JI, Merz CM, et al for the Coordinating Committee of the National Cholesterol Education Program. Implications of recent clinical trials for the National Cholesterol Education Program Adult Treatment Panel III guidelines. *Circulation* 2004;110:227-39. [PMID: 15358046]

Sanyal AJ, Chalasani N, Kowdley KV, et al. NASH CRN. Pioglitazone, vitamin E, or placebo for nonalcoholic steatohepatitis. *N Engl J Med* 2010;362:1675-85. [PMID: 20427778]

Steinberg D, Glass CK, Witztum JL. Evidence mandating earlier and more aggressive treatment of hypercholesterolemia. *Circulation* 2008;118:672-9. [PMID: 18678783]

Obesity

Alka M. Kanaya, MD and Christian Vaisse, MD, PhD

α-MSH	α-Melanocyte–stimulating hormone		NHANES	National Health and Nutrition Examination Survey
ACTH	Adrenocorticotropic hormone		NHLBI	National Heart, Lung, and Blood Institute
AGRP	Agouti-related peptide		NTRK2	Neurotrophic tyrosine kinase, receptor, type 2
ARC	Arcuate nucleus of the hypothalamus		NPY	Neuropeptide Y
BDNF	Brain-derived neurotrophic factor		OSA	Obstructive sleep apnea
BMI	Body mass index		PAI-1	Plasminogen-activated inhibitor
CCK	Cholecystokinin		PC-1	Proconvertase 1
CCK-1R	CCK 1 receptor		PCOS	Polycystic ovarian syndrome
CSF	Colony-stimulating factor		POMC	Pro-opiomelanocortin
FFA	Free fatty acid		PVN	Paraventricular nucleus
FTO	Fat mass- and obesity-associated gene		PYY	Peptide YY
GI	Gastrointestinal		RYGB	Roux-en-Y gastric bypass
GLP1	Glucagon-like peptide 1		SH2B1	Adapter protein 1
IL-6	Interleukin 6		SOS	Swedish Obese Subjects
LepR	Leptin receptor		SIM1	Single minded 1
LHA	Lateral hypothalamic area		STAT	Signal transducer and activator of transcription
MC4R	Melanocortin-4 receptor		T2DM	Type 2 diabetes mellitus
MCP-1	Monocyte-chemoattractant protein-1		TMEM18	Transmembrane protein 18
NAFLD	Nonalcoholic fatty liver disease		TNFα	Tumor necrosis factor-α
NCEP	National Cholesterol Education Program		WHO	World Health Organization
NEGR1	Neuronal growth regulator 1			

DEFINITION AND EPIDEMIOLOGY

Definition

Obesity and overweight categories have been defined by examining longitudinal study data that associate a given weight with future adverse health effects. The currently accepted surrogate measure of body fatness is body mass index (BMI) which is measured as weight in kilograms divided by height in meters squared. For adults, a BMI <18.5 kg/m^2 is underweight, 18.5 to 24.9 kg/m^2 is healthy weight, 25.0 to 29.9 kg/m^2 is overweight, and ≥30 kg/m^2 is obese. For children and adolescents, a BMI between the 85th and 95th percentile for age and sex is considered at risk of overweight, and BMI at or above the 95th percentile is considered overweight or obese.

However, BMI does not account for ethnic differences in skeletal structure or musculature. Body frame size varies dramatically by race/ethnicity from small-framed East Asian adults to larger framed Pacific Islanders. Moreover, conventional cut-points for adult overweight (BMI ≥25 kg/m^2) and obesity (BMI ≥30 kg/m^2) do not correspond to similar absolute or relative metabolic risk in all ethnic group. As a result, the World Health Organization (WHO) and International Obesity Task Force proposed a lower BMI cut-point to define obesity in South and East Asian adults: 23 kg/m^2 for overweight and 25 kg/m^2 for obesity.

Prevalence and Projections

National surveys performed by the Centers for Disease Control and Prevention in the United States have found a significant increase in the prevalence of overweight and obesity over the past 30 years. In 2003 to 2004, according to data from the National Health and Nutrition Examination Survey (NHANES), 32.2% of adults were obese. Trends among adults have been tracked by repeat NHANES surveys, showing that the percent of overweight or obese have climbed from 47.0% in 1976 to 1980 to 66.2% in 2003 to 2004, and the prevalence of obesity alone has more than doubled from 15.0% to 32.9% overall. The prevalence of obesity was 45.0% among non-Hispanic blacks, 36.8% among Mexican Americans, and 30.6% among non-Hispanic whites.

The trends in obesity have been most striking among children and adolescents with two- to threefold increases in rates over the past three decades in all age groups. In the NHANES 2003 to 2004 survey, a total of 17.1% of US children and adolescents were overweight (BMI ≥95th percentile). Among children aged 2 to 5 years, the obesity prevalence increased from 5% in the 1976 to 1980 NHANES to 12.4% in 2003 to 2006 NHANES. Similarly, the prevalence in age 6 to 11 years increased from 6.5% to 17.0%, and for ages 12 to 19 years increased from 5% to 17.6% in the most recent national survey.

While the United States leads most of the world with high prevalence of overweight and obesity, these conditions are becoming more prevalent worldwide even in developing countries. In China, overweight prevalence in adults increased from 14.6% to 21.8% between 1992 and 2002, with greatest increases seen among men, urban residents, and high-income groups. In India, the prevalence of overweight ranged from 9.4% in rural men to 38.8% in urban women in 2003 to 2005.

Globally, according to a pooled analysis, in 2005 there were an estimated 937 million (95% CI, 922-951 million) overweight adults and 396 million (388-405 million) obese adults. Using conservative projections, by 2030 the number of overweight adults was estimated to be 1.35 billion and 573 million obese individuals without adjusting for secular trends. The authors warned that if recent secular trends continue unabated, the absolute numbers may total 2.16 billion overweight and 1.12 billion obese adult individuals. Among US residents, projections forecast that by 2030, 86.3% adults will be overweight or obese (51.1%) with black women (96.9%) and Mexican American men (91.1%) being most affected. Wang et al estimate that by 2048, all American adults would become overweight or obese, and in children, the prevalence of overweight (BMI ≥95th percentile) would almost double to 30%.

Possible Explanations for the Increased Obesity Rates

Several hypotheses have been proposed to explain the rapid rise in overweight/obesity in developed and developing countries. The simple explanations start with changes in lifestyle behaviors, primarily the lack of regular physical activity and increased caloric intake that tip the energy balance equilibrium. The reality of the factors promoting the obesity epidemic is clearly more complex and involves multiple layers of determinants including social norms and values, several sectors of influence from governmental to media to the food/entertainment industries, behavioral settings

including the work/home/neighborhood environment, to individual factors that include genetic, socioeconomic, cultural, and psychosocial factors. In a novel social network analysis of the Framingham cohort, investigators found that weight status (gain, loss, or stability of weight) for an individual was highly influenced by his/her friends and family extending out to three degrees of separation. A multifaceted approach will be required to meaningfully curb the obesity epidemic globally.

PATHOPHYSIOLOGY AND GENETICS OF OBESITY

Regulation of Food Intake and Energy Expenditure

Obesity is an increase of energy stored as fat that occurs when caloric intake exceeds caloric expenditure. What causes this imbalance is less clear, but recent advances in our understanding of the physiological systems responsible for the maintenance of energy stores in response to variable access to nutrition and demands for energy expenditure have provided some insights into the pathophysiology of obesity. The physiological system controlling food intake and energy expenditure is composed of (1) long-term and short-term afferent signals that allow for sensing the energy status of the individual; (2) integrating brain centers, most importantly within the hypothalamus, where the level of the efferent response is determined; and (3) efferent signals including those regulating the intensity of hunger and the level of energy expenditure.

One common misconception is that this physiological system is dedicated to the prevention of obesity. Instead this system's essential role is in the prevention of starvation (ie, ensuring adequate energy intake to compensate for the energy requirements of basal metabolism, physical activity, growth, and reproduction). As a result, this physiological system is more strongly biased toward prevention of energy deficiency rather than excess storage.

Informing the Brain of the Energy Status: Leptin and Short-Term Gastrointestinal Signals

Leptin.   The major afferent signal allowing the brain to sense the level of energy stores is the hormone leptin. Discovered in 1994, this cytokine-like 167 amino acid protein is released by adipocytes. Under basal conditions the circulating levels of serum leptin are correlated with fat mass (r = 0.8) and decrease after weight loss. Decreasing leptin levels inform the brain of diminishing fat storage resulting from negative energy balance. This results in compensatory effects on appetite and energy expenditure, aimed at replenishing the stores and reestablishing energy balance. The role of leptin is best understood from the phenotype of rare cases of humans with complete leptin deficiency. Despite early-onset, extremely severe obesity, these patients show behaviors and physiological signs of starvation. This includes hyperphagia, decreased immune function, and hypogonadotropic hypogonadism. The latter reflects deficiency of the leptin signal informing the brain that sufficient energy stores are available for reproduction. Hormonal replacement of leptin-deficient patients corrects all these abnormalities, abolishing the hyperphagia leading to normalization of weight and maturation of the reproductive axis.

Leptin's action is mediated by the leptin receptor (LepR). This receptor is a member of the class I cytokine receptor family which also includes the growth hormone, prolactin and erythropoietin receptors (see Chapter 1). These receptors have a single transmembrane domain and homodimerize upon binding of the ligand. Leptin binding to LepR leads to phosphorylation of the JAK2 receptor-associated kinase followed by recruitment and phosphorylation of the signal transducer and activator of transcription STAT3. Upon activation STAT3 dimerizes and translocates to the nucleus, where it activates transcription of target genes. The LepR is expressed in almost every tissue but only one of five isoforms, LepRb, contains the STAT3 recruitment domain. This isoform is expressed specifically in leptin-responsive brain regions.

In summary, leptin functions as a long-term signal of energy balance by informing the brain of changes in the level of energy stored as fat. A perceived decrease in leptin levels increases the amount of food consumed and minimizes energy expenditure. Leptin levels do not change with meals, and leptin does not acutely change meal size.

Signals from the gastrointestinal tract.

In addition to leptin, which represents a long-term adiposity signal, a number of other hormones, most of which are secreted by the gastrointestinal (GI) system, regulate appetite on a short-term basis (ie, in response to a meal) (Table 20–1). These hormones act on **satiation** (the feeling of fullness that contributes to the decision to stop eating) rather than on **satiety** (the prolongation of the interval until hunger or a drive to eat reappears). Some of these hormones have been shown to act on the same brain centers as leptin does. Altered secretion of or response to these GI hormones may directly contribute to the pathogenesis or the maintenance of obesity. Cholecystokinin (CCK) is secreted by duodenal I cells into the bloodstream. Its secretion is stimulated by the presence of fat and protein in the duodenum. CCK stimulates gut motility, contraction of the gallbladder, pancreatic enzyme secretion, gastric emptying, and acid secretion. CCK acts locally, stimulating vagal sensory nerves through the CCK 1 receptor (CCK-1R) and informs the brain that fat and proteins are being processed and will soon be absorbed. This message is conveyed to the hypothalamus via the hindbrain. Circulating CCK levels increase after meals and infusion of a CCK-1R agonist (CCK33), to postprandial levels, suppresses food intake. Conversely, infusion of a CCK-1R antagonist increases calorie intake. CCK is also a proximal mediator of the broader satiation process, attenuating meal-induced changes of more distal GI hormones, such as ghrelin and peptide YY (PYY).

Glucagon-like peptide 1 (GLP1) is a 30 amino acid peptide derived from the proglucagon gene. GLP1 is secreted into the bloodstream by the intestinal L-cells of the ileum and colon in response to the presence of nutrients in the lumen. GLP1 has a very short half-life (2 minutes), and is degraded by dipeptidyl peptidase-4. It increases insulin secretion in a glucose-dependent manner, decreases glucagon secretion, increases beta cell mass, inhibits gastric emptying, and decreases food intake. GLP1 is thought to signal through the hindbrain via stimulation of the GLP1 receptor (GLP1R) on the vagus nerve.

PYY, a 36 amino acid peptide is released into the bloodstream by intestinal endocrine L-cells of the distal gut (ileum and colon) after food ingestion and in response to the presence of fat in the lumen. PYY3-36, the major form of circulating PYY, binds to the hypothalamic NPY-Y2 receptor and reduces food intake. Obese individuals have lower PYY levels after a test meal than nonobese controls.

Ghrelin, a 28 amino acid octanoylated peptide, is secreted into the bloodstream by endocrine cells lining the fundus of the stomach. Ghrelin secretion is stimulated by fasting, increases preprandially, and is suppressed by food intake. Ghrelin is orexigenic, increasing food intake when administered peripherally, and acts in part by directly modulating the activity of the NPY (neuropeptide Y)/AGRP (agouti-related peptide) neurons in the arcuate nucleus of the hypothalamus.

Central Integration of Energy Homeostasis Signals

The major challenge of adapting food intake to energy expenditure lies in the discontinuous availability of the first and the continuous

---

TABLE 20–1   Selected GI and pancreatic peptides that regulate food intake.

	Main Site of Synthesis	Secretion Pattern	Effect on Food Intake
Ghrelin	Gastric X/A-like cells	Increases prior to meal; decreased by food intake	Stimulates food intake
Cholecystokinin (CCK)	Proximal intestinal I cells	Stimulated by duodenal presence of fat and protein	Promotes meal termination and reduces meal size
Peptide YY3-36 (PYY)	Distal-intestinal L cells	Stimulated by presence of fat in the lumen	Reduces appetite and food intake
Glucagon-like peptide 1 (GLP-1)	Distal-intestinal L cells	Stimulated by presence of nutrients in the lumen	Short-term inhibition of food intake
Pancreatic polypeptide (PP)	Pancreatic F cells	Released in proportion to calories ingested	Reduces appetite and food intake

and variable levels of the second required for survival, growth, and reproduction. The current prevailing model is that the concentration of circulating adiposity signals, primarily leptin, influences the response to short-term satiation signals thereby allowing for sufficient energy intake to maintain a constant level of stored energy. Genetic studies in mice and humans have outlined several critical neuronal populations and circuits that translate information provided by afferent circulating hormonal signals into neural responses that regulate appetite and energy expenditure. The primary locus for the integration of peripheral signals that influence energy balance is the hypothalamus (Figure 20–1). Specifically, two adjacent groups of neurons in the arcuate nucleus (ARC) of the hypothalamus, characterized by their production of specific neuromediators, act as the primary site in the brain for receiving the humoral signals that reflect body energy status. The AGRP/NPY neurons are orexigenic. They are inhibited by leptin and their activity is also modulated by GI hormones, such as ghrelin and PYY. The proopiomelanocortin (POMC) neurons are anorexigenic and are activated by leptin. In these neurons, POMC is processed by the specific proteases proconvertase-1 and proconvertase-2 to the anorexigenic neuropeptide α-melanocyte–stimulating hormone (α-MSH). Interactions between these neurons within the ARC allows for cross talk and modulation of the neuronal output.

These first-order neurons send projections to second-order neurons in other regions of the hypothalamus, specifically the paraventricular nucleus (PVN) and the lateral hypothalamic area (LHA), as well as to the hindbrain. Both α-MSH and AGRP act on a common receptor, the melanocortin-4 receptor (MC4R) expressed on PVN neurons. α-MSH binds to and activates the melanocortin 4 receptor (MC4R) and by competing with α-MSH for the MC4R, AGRP inhibits MC4R-bearing neurons. The MC4R neurons then innervate neurons in other areas of the hypothalamus and brain stem to produce an integrated inhibition of appetite and increase in energy expenditure.

Leptin Resistance in Obesity

While recombinant leptin can correct the exceptionally rare cases of obesity due to genetic leptin deficiency, all other obese patients have leptin levels that are proportional to their fat mass. In addition, recombinant leptin injections in obese patients do not lead to weight loss. Therefore, despite the presence of elevated leptin concentrations, which should reduce food intake and body fat, obese patients appear to be insensitive or resistant to leptin. Both genetic and environmental factors have been shown to contribute to this leptin resistance, and a number of specific alterations in the downstream leptin effector pathways have been suggested to participate in this obesity-associated leptin resistance. Understanding the nature of this leptin resistance may allow for the development of novel obesity treatments but its molecular basis is probably heterogenous and different in each patient.

Genetics of Obesity

Excess caloric intake and the tendency toward a more sedentary lifestyle are certainly to blame for the increased prevalence of obesity,

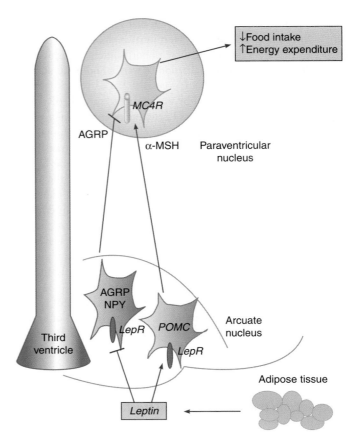

FIGURE 20–1   Leptin-melanocortin system of energy balance. Information about the body's energy stores is conveyed to the brain by hormones such as leptin. Leptin is secreted by adipocytes in proportion to the body's fat mass. Leptin binds to its receptors on two populations of neurons in the arcuate nucleus of the hypothalamus: the orexigenic AGRP/NPY–expressing neurons, and the anorexigenic POMC-expressing neurons. These two groups of neurons have projections to the paraventricular nucleus of the hypothalamus, as well as to other regions of the brain. The PVN has a dense neuronal population that expresses MC4R. When leptin binds its receptors on POMC neurons, α-MSH, a cleavage product of POMC, is released. Activation of MC4R in the PVN by α-MSH relays a satiety signal and causes a decrease in food intake. AGRP is an antagonist of MC4R, and competes with α-MSH for binding to MC4R. Binding of AGRP to MC4R leads to increased food intake. Leptin activates POMC neurons and inhibits AGRP neurons. Therefore, by activating its receptors on these two neuronal populations, leptin acts in a concerted way to increase MC4R activation by α-MSH and decrease its antagonism by AGRP resulting in a net decrease in food intake. (α-MSH, α-melanocyte–stimulating hormone; AGRP, agouti-related peptide; ARC, arcuate nucleus; MC4R, melanocortin 4 receptor; NPY, neuropeptide Y; POMC, pro-opiomelanocortin; PVN, paraventricular nucleus; LepR, leptin receptor).

but individuals exposed to the same environmental pressures have different levels of vulnerability. Indeed, genetic epidemiologic studies, such as twin studies and adoption studies have implicated genetic factors in the susceptibility to obesity. These studies have shown that genetic factors account for 40% to 70% of the population variation in BMI and that the heritability of obesity increases

TABLE 20–2 Common variants increasing the risk of obesity.[a]

Chromosomal Localization	Nearby Genes	Odds Ratio of Obesity in Adults
16q12	FTO	1.25
18q21	MC4R	1.14
2	TMEM18	1.20
16p11	SH2B1	1.10
1p31	NEGR1	1.06
11p14	BDNF	1.05

[a]Only variants replicated in multiple studies and with odds ratios of obesity above 1.05 are indicated.

with its severity. Emphasis has, therefore, now shifted from the question of whether human obesity has a genetic component to how many and which genetic variants underlie this susceptibility. While the majority of genes that contribute to the predisposition to obesity are still unknown, both common genetic variants, with small effects on the BMI at the level of the population, and single gene defects, causing Mendelian forms of obesity, have been described.

Large and comprehensive genome-wide association studies find that a number of common genetic variants are associated with obesity (Table 20–2). These variants are near genes that are expressed in the central nervous system further suggesting a role for an alteration of central regulatory pathways in the pathogenesis of obesity. However, since these variants are not located within the protein-coding regions of these genes, the exact mechanism by which they predispose to obesity remains to be elucidated. More importantly, the individual as well as the combined effects of these common variants only explain a small fraction of the inherited variability in obesity (10%-20%), suggesting that rare variants may contribute more significantly to the genetic predisposition to this condition.

Indeed a number of single gene defects that cause human obesity have been uncovered. These defects have provided more insight into the genetic predisposition and pathophysiology of obesity. Certain mutations can cause obesity as part of a complex syndrome, in which developmental phenotypes are prominent (Table 20–3). However, most single gene defects causing Mendelian forms of obesity are in genes of the leptin-melanocortin system (Table 20–4). The description of patients with these mutations has both provided insight into the genetic predisposition to obesity and has confirmed that the hypothalamic leptin-melanocortin system is critical for energy balance in humans. Mutations in leptin and the LepR cause severe obesity associated with hypogonadotropic hypogonadism. Mutations in POMC cause severe obesity, due to absent synthesis of α-MSH in the hypothalamus, and neonatal adrenal insufficiency, due to lack of ACTH production in the anterior pituitary gland. These recessive syndromes are extremely rare. In contrast, mutations in MC4R represent the most common genetic cause of severe obesity accounting for 2.5% of all cases. Patients who carry such mutations do not have specific clinical or biological characteristics that differentiate them from other patients with severe obesity; genetic testing is the only reliable method to identify these patients. At present, such testing is not recommended since the presence or absence of one of these mutations carries no specific implications for the clinical management of these patients.

HEALTH CONSEQUENCES OF OBESITY

Mechanism Underlying Obesity Complications: Adipose Tissue as an Endocrine Organ

The massive public health burden of obesity is due to the psychological, behavioral, and medical consequences of this chronic increase in adipose tissue mass. Pathophysiological mechanisms

TABLE 20–3 Syndromes that cause human obesity.

Name/OMIM	Clinical Features	Prevalence	Genetics
Prader-Willi OMIM#176270	Diminished fetal activity, obesity, muscular hypotonia, mental retardation, short stature, hypogonadotropic hypogonadism, small hands and feet	1/25000	Imprinting + Deletion 15q12
Bardet-Biedl OMIM#209900	Hypogonadism, pigmentary retinopathy, polydactyly, mental retardation, obesity	1/100,000	Recessive >12 genes involved in function of the primary cilium
Alström OMIM#203800	Myocardiopathy, sensory deficit (retinopathy, deafness), obesity dyslipidemia, diabetes	Rare	Recessive ALMS1, 2p13
Börjeson-Forssman-Lehman OMIM#301900	Severe mental defect, epilepsy, morbid obesity, hypogonadism, facial dysmorphy	Very rare	X-linked recessive PHF6, Xq26.3
Cohen OMIM#216550	Mental retardation, characteristic facies, obesity	Very rare	Recessive COH1, 8q22
Carpenter OMIM#201000	Acrocephalosyndactyly, polydactyly, obesity, mental retardation	Very rare	Recessive RAB23, 6p11

TABLE 20–4 Monogenic obesity due to mutations in genes related to the leptin-melanocortin system.

Gene	N = Families	Transmission	Obesity	Other Phenotypes
Leptin	5(2)	Recessive	Very severe, early onset	Hyponadotropic hypogonadism
Leptin receptor	3(1)	Recessive	Very severe, early onset	Hyponadotropic hypogonadism
POMC	5(5)	Recessive	Very severe, early onset	ACTH deficiency
PC-1	2(2)	Recessive	Severe, early onset	Hyperproinsulinemia, hypercortisolism, hypogonadotropic hypogonadism
NTRK2	1	Dominant	Very severe, early onset	Mental retardation
SIM1	3 (3)	Dominant	Very severe, early onset	+/– Mental retardation
MC4R	2.5% of severely obese patients	Dominant	Severe, variable onset	None

underlying the complications of obesity include the psychological and behavioral responses to the image projected in a society in which obesity is considered cosmetically unattractive, the mechanical effects of increased adipose mass on weight-bearing joints as well as other organs, and the metabolic consequences of increased circulating free fatty acids (FFAs).

It is also now clear that the adipose cell is not simply dedicated to inertly storing energy as triglycerides and releasing free fatty acids and glycerol during periods of increased energy needs. In addition to leptin, described earlier, which informs the brain of the level of energy stores, adipose cells secrete a number of factors, known as adipokines, which can play a role in the pathophysiology of obesity and its complications (Figure 20–2). For example, adiponectin is an abundant plasma protein, structurally related to the complement 1q family, that is secreted exclusively from adipose tissue. Adiponectin circulates in serum as a range of multimers from low-molecular-weight trimers to high-molecular-weight

(HMW) dodecamers. Circulating levels of adiponectin are negatively correlated with fat mass and are reduced in obesity. Adiponectin improves whole-body insulin sensitivity through its receptor-mediated actions on the muscle and the liver. Specifically, adiponectin stimulates fatty acid oxidation and glucose uptake in skeletal muscle and suppresses glucose output in the liver.

In addition, a number of factors secreted by adipose tissue, particularly in the context of obesity, are proinflammatory cytokines. It is now generally accepted that obesity is a state of chronic, low-grade inflammation. These inflammatory molecules exert their effects through both paracrine and endocrine pathways. Initially thought to be secreted by adipocytes, most of these factors are actually produced by other cells such as macrophages, which infiltrate the adipose tissue in obesity. Tumor necrosis factor-α (TNF-α) was the first adipose-derived factor suggested to represent a link between adiposity and the insulin resistance associated with type 2 diabetes. Released by activated macrophages, which infiltrate expanding adipose tissue in obesity, this cytokine has been strongly implicated in the pathogenesis of insulin resistance, directly impairing insulin signaling in hepatocytes and adipocytes. Other adipokines involved in obesity-associated inflammation include interleukin 6 (IL-6), monocyte-chemoattractant protein-1 (MCP-1), plasminogen-activated inhibitor (PAI-1), and colony-stimulating factor (CSF).

Metabolic Complications of Obesity: Insulin Resistance and Type 2 Diabetes

Hyperinsulinemia is characteristically associated with obesity. This hyperinsulinemia is linked to insulin resistance (ie, the decrease in insulin-stimulated glucose utilization, which increases proportionally with fat mass). One of the major consequences of this obesity-associated insulin resistance is the requirement for increased insulin secretion. While the majority of obese individuals can secrete sufficient insulin to accommodate the insulin-resistant

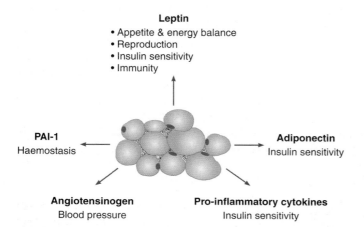

Leptin
• Appetite & energy balance
• Reproduction
• Insulin sensitivity
• Immunity

PAI-1
Haemostasis

Adiponectin
Insulin sensitivity

Angiotensinogen
Blood pressure

Pro-inflammatory cytokines
Insulin sensitivity

FIGURE 20–2 Adipose tissue secretions influencing metabolism.

state, this increased burden on the insulin-producing pancreatic beta cells increases the susceptibility to failure, resulting in type 2 diabetes (T2DM) in genetically predisposed individuals. Indeed, over 80% of T2DM patients are obese. In comparison with a normal-weight individual, BMI greater than 40 (obesity class 3) in a person under 55 years of age increases the risk of T2DM by 18.1-fold in men and 12.9-fold in women. Classification as overweight (BMI 25-30) increases the prevalence of T2DM three- to fourfold in both men and women under 55 years of age. The relative risks associated with excess body weight are weaker in older individuals but are still present (eg, about twofold for overweight and three- to sixfold for obesity class 3).

The increased rate of T2DM is the most worrisome public health issue linked to the increased rates of obesity. The anticipated health outcomes such as premature heart disease, peripheral vascular disease, renal failure, blindness, are deeply concerning and place this among our highest contemporary public health priorities. Some recent studies have estimated that the current generation of American youth will be the first to exhibit shorter life spans than their parents, because of the impact of obesity on T2DM.

Dyslipidemia

Obesity is associated with dyslipidemia characterized by increased levels of very low density lipoprotein (VLDL) cholesterol, triglycerides, and total cholesterol as well as a decrease in HDL cholesterol and an increase in small dense LDL particles. The difference in serum triglyceride concentrations between individuals with BMI less than 21 and those with BMI greater than 30 is about 65 mg/dL (in women) and 62 to 118 mg/dL (in men, depending on age). For HDL cholesterol, each 1-unit BMI change is associated with an HDL-cholesterol decrease of 1.1 mg/dL for young men and 0.7 mg/dL for young women. All of the components of this obesity-associated dyslipidemia have been shown to be atherogenic and play a major role in the development of atherosclerosis and cardiovascular disease in obese individuals.

Weight loss and exercise, even if they do not result in normalization of body weight, can improve this dyslipidemia and thus reduce CVD risk. In addition, obese individuals should be targeted for intense lipid-lowering therapy, when necessary.

The Metabolic Syndrome

The concept of the **metabolic syndrome** was first introduced in 1923 by Kylin who described the clustering of hypertension, hyperglycemia, and gout as a syndrome. Reaven and others redefined this concept as the insulin resistance syndrome, a clustering of glucose intolerance, high triglycerides, low HDL cholesterol, and hypertension. The two most consistent characteristics of persons with the syndrome are insulin resistance and central abdominal obesity. There is strong epidemiologic and pathophysiologic evidence linking visceral adiposity with insulin resistance and diabetes, with dyslipidemia, hyperinsulinemia, and decreased fibrinolysis as possible mediators of the relationship between visceral fat and type 2 diabetes and cardiovascular disease risk.

The earliest attempt to create a definition for this constellation of metabolic disorders was by the WHO wherein an individual with glucose intolerance or insulin resistance was required to have two or more criteria (elevated triglycerides, low HDL cholesterol, high BMI or waist-hip ratio, hypertension, or microalbuminuria) in order to be categorized as having metabolic syndrome. The next attempt at a clinical definition was by the National Cholesterol Education Program (NCEP)-Adult Treatment Panel III in 2001 that required three or more of the following criteria for the metabolic syndrome definition: high fasting glucose, high triglycerides, low HDL, high blood pressure or waist circumference. More recently, the International Diabetes Federation (IDF) proposed further refined criteria that require central abdominal obesity, and two more criteria as proposed by the NCEP. The IDF criteria were the first ones to account for the heterogeneity of body size among different ethnic groups, and the committee recommended different waist circumference cut-points based on ethnicity with a revised definition for South Asians, Chinese, and Japanese recommending similar waist circumference cut-points in men (≥90 cm) and in women (≥80 cm) compared to the European cut-points of ≥94 cm in men and ≥80 cm in women. More recently, the utility of the metabolic syndrome has been questioned, given that there are no treatment options available, and rather each cardiometabolic risk factor (eg, blood pressure control) is treated individually.

Cardiovascular Complications

Higher cardiovascular disease risk has been linked to visceral adiposity with several distinct mechanisms including inflammation, thrombosis, hyperglycemia, atherogenic dyslipidemia, and adipocytokines (hormones and proteins exclusively secreted by adipose tissue). Obesity has been implicated as one of the major risk factors for hypertension, heart failure, and coronary heart disease. Other cardiovascular conditions associated with obesity include peripheral arterial disease and atrial fibrillation.

Altered hemodynamics of obesity due to increases in total blood volume, systemic arterial pressure, and cardiac output increase the workload of the heart and can lead to adverse effects on cardiovascular structure and function. Overweight individuals develop left ventricular dilation and hypertrophy and left atrial enlargement. These structural abnormalities increase the risk of heart failure and of atrial fibrillation. In the Framingham Heart Study, every 1-unit increase in BMI increased the risk of heart failure by 5% in men and 7% in women. However, several recent studies have also found an obesity-cardiovascular disease paradox where overweight and obese individuals with existing heart failure or heart disease have a lower risk of mortality than those who are underweight or normal weight. These findings suggest that obese individuals may have the metabolic reserve to withstand high catabolic needs as exist in heart failure.

Pulmonary Complications

Obesity can cause alveolar hypoventilation, increased pulmonary blood volume, and mechanical effects on the respiratory system. Obstructive sleep apnea (OSA) is associated with obesity and other features of the metabolic syndrome, with the most closely correlated factor being hypertension. Intermittent upper airway obstruction results in hypoxia, sympathetic nervous system surges, and airway inflammation. Patients with sleep apnea have higher risk of systemic and pulmonary hypertension, heart failure, dysrhythmias, myocardial infarction, and overall mortality. Mechanisms that have been implicated in the development of cardiovascular disease in obstructive sleep apnea include increased oxidative stress and inflammation that cause endothelial dysfunction. While significant weight loss can improve OSA and associated metabolic features, mechanical therapies used to treat sleep apnea with constant positive airway pressure have not been found to improve hypertension or other metabolic features.

Gastrointestinal Complications

Nonalcoholic fatty liver disease (NAFLD) is commonly seen with insulin resistance or obesity and includes a spectrum of liver disease from steatosis to nonalcoholic steatohepatitis, advanced fibrosis, and rarely, cirrhosis. Fat accumulates within the liver with recruitment of inflammatory cells and fibrosis. The prevalence of NAFLD in obesity is 50% to 85%. Risk factors associated with NAFLD besides obesity include advancing age, visceral adiposity, atherogenic dyslipidemia, and hypertension. NAFLD is the leading cause of chronic liver disease in the United States, and given the high rates of obesity, approximately one-third of US adults are estimated to have NAFLD.

NAFLD has been observed in overweight children and adolescents with prevalence estimated at 6% to 23% in population-based US samples. In children, there seems to be a clear male predominance for NAFLD which suggests distinct pathophysiologic mechanisms for NAFLD between adults and children. Histologic criteria have been proposed to distinguish adult (type 1) and pediatric (type 2) NAFLD. In a large study of German children, the three main factors that contributed to NAFLD by principal components analysis included an insulin resistance/visceral adiposity factor, a body fat distribution/CRP factor, and lastly a sex steroid hormone factor.

Other GI complications of abdominal obesity include gastroesophageal reflux disease and hiatal hernia. Both of these conditions can cause erosive mucosal changes in the lower esophagus leading to higher risk of Barrett esophagus.

Reproduction and Gynecologic Complications

Obesity has been associated with both female and male infertility. In women, polycystic ovarian syndrome (PCOS) is the main cause of female infertility associated with obesity. Women with PCOS have ovulatory dysfunction and hyperandrogenemia. PCOS is reviewed in more detail in Chapter 13. In men, obesity can cause reduced sperm counts and motility. Hormonal changes with obesity and associated metabolic disorders may lead to poor sperm production. Obesity is also associated with erectile dysfunction through proinflammatory mechanisms and decreased testosterone levels.

Cancer

Several cancers have been linked to obesity, including breast, endometrial, colorectal, prostate, and renal cell carcinomas. Putative mechanisms for breast and endometrial cancer include higher circulating levels of unopposed estrogen and ovarian hyperandrogenism, causing higher levels of testosterone and lower levels of luteinizing hormone. The relationship between obesity and colon cancer is stronger in men than women.

MANAGEMENT OF THE OBESE PATIENT

Screening and Prevention of Complications

Periodic health screening with a measurement of both height and weight to calculate BMI is recommended by many organizations including the National Heart, Lung, and Blood Institute (NHLBI), the US Preventive Services Task Force, and the WHO. Furthermore, the NHLBI also recommends waist circumference measurement routinely to find persons at risk of metabolic complications of overweight. Patients who are found to be in the overweight or obese categories of BMI are recommended to have other risk factors checked as well, including blood pressure, fasting glucose, and lipoprotein levels.

Therapeutic Approaches for Weight Loss

Several behavioral, pharmacologic, and surgical therapies for weight loss have been studied in randomized controlled trials. In general, behavioral interventions with lifestyle change including diet and exercise and pharmacologic therapies work to achieve modest amounts of weight loss while patients adhere to the intervention. Recommended for more severe levels of obesity, bariatric surgery does lead to larger amounts of weight loss, but requires lifelong medical supervision and management of the side effects associated with the surgery.

A. Behavior, diet, and exercise therapies   While many believe that long-term weight loss with lifestyle change is not achievable by most patients, longitudinal studies have found that 20% of overweight individuals are successful at weight loss defined as losing at least 10% of initial body weight and maintaining the loss for at least 1 year. Individuals enrolled in the National Weight Control Registry have lost an average of 33 kg and maintained the loss for more than 5 years. Behaviors that have been most effective for long-term weight loss include high levels of physical activity (~1 hour/day), self-monitoring weight, eating a low-calorie, low-fat diet, eating breakfast regularly, and maintaining a consistent eating pattern throughout the week.

Dietary interventions.   Several commercial, fad, and therapeutic dietary interventions exist for weight loss. Recent dietary trends have focused on relative changes in macronutrient composition of the diet to achieve weight loss, such as low-fat or low-carbohydrate diets. Few have been rigorously tested, and no trials have long-term outcome data (defined as the occurrence of comorbidities or mortality). A recent randomized trial comparing four popular diets (Atkins, Zone, Weight Watchers, and Ornish diet) found that weight change did not significantly differ between participants assigned to any of the four diets, and better dietary adherence predicted higher amount of weight loss. The most difficult diets for participants to adhere to were the very low-fat diet (Ornish) and the low-carbohydrate diet (Atkins). In a recent meta-analysis of five dietary trials for weight loss, low-carbohydrate non–energy-restricted diets were found to be as effective as low-fat, energy-restricted diets for weight loss up to 1 year. The weighted mean difference in weight loss was greater in the low-carbohydrate diets (–3.3 kg, 95% CI –5.3 to –1.4 kg, $p = 0.02$) in the first 6 months, but there was no difference in weight loss after 12 months between the two types of diet (–1.0 kg, 95% CI –3.5 to 1.5 kg, $p = 0.15$). Additionally, there was no clear benefit on cardiovascular risk factors with either type of diet.

Physical activity interventions.

The Institute of Medicine recommends physical activity of 60 min/d for most days of the week for weight loss and/or control of weight. The recommendations for heart disease prevention are 30 min/d of moderate-intensity physical activity on most days per week, or at least 150 min/wk.

In a systematic review of trials of an aerobic physical activity intervention in overweight populations, body weight decreased significantly in seven of nine trials, but weight increased in two trials. The two studies that combined diet with aerobic training had the largest amounts of weight loss (>10 kg each). However, these trials were uncontrolled and of relatively short duration. It remains unclear whether long-term lifestyle change with physical activity can decrease risk of cardiovascular disease or mortality in obese individuals.

Pharmacologic intervention/CAM.

Weight loss medications have had mixed results with most delivering modest amounts of short-term weight loss, often associated with many undesirable side effects. Currently there are four main categories of weight loss medications approved by the FDA: adrenergic agents, serotonergic agents, combination of both adrenergic/serotonergic agents, and lipase inhibitors. Other medications available for off-label use include some antidepressants and anticonvulsant agents. A majority of available obesity treatments work by suppressing appetite centrally. One approved medication, orlistat, prevents digestion and absorption of dietary fat by inhibiting the gut enzyme lipase. There are several different sites of action under investigation for potential medications including specific neurotransmitter targets to decrease appetite and/or promote satiety, endocannabinoid system antagonists and opioid receptor targets to reduce food intake, and peripheral targets that work at the level of the intestines or pancreas to modulate food intake.

Table 20–5 shows specific medications in each category, the amount of weight loss reported in trials compared to placebo from a recent review and meta-analysis, and the common side effects of each agent. The two most frequently studied weight loss medications, sibutramine and orlistat, have had the best efficacy in longer-term trials (52 weeks). However, both of these drugs are associated with significant side effects which limit their use. Other antiobesity medications in the drug development pipeline include lorcaserin, an agonist that targets serotonin 2C receptors to cause satiety, and a multiple monoamine reuptake inhibitor, tesofensine, that reduces reuptake of norepinephrine, serotonin, and dopamine to cause appetite suppression. An endocannabinoid receptor

TABLE 20–5 Medications for treatment of obesity.

Drug	Category	Recommended Dose	Mean Weight Loss vs Placebo (Range in kg)	Side Effects
Phentermine	Adrenergic agent	15-37.5 mg daily	3.6 kg (0.6-6.0 kg)	Dry mouth, headache, insomnia, irritability, tachycardia, ↑BP
Diethylpropion	Adrenergic agent		3.0 kg (−1.6 to 11.5 kg)	Central nervous system stimulation, dizziness, headaches, insomnia, palpitations, tachycardia, mild ↑BP
Orlistat	Lipase inhibitor	60-120 mg 3 times daily	2.89 kg (2.27-3.51 kg)	Diarrhea, flatulence, fecal urgency and incontinence, abdominal pain, dyspepsia
Sibutramine	Norepinephrine/serotonin reuptake inhibitor	10-15 mg daily	4.45 kg (3.62-5.29 kg)	Dry mouth, insomnia, constipation, tachycardia, ↑BP
Off-Label Drugs Associated with Weight Loss				
Buproprion	Antidepressant	300-400 mg daily	2.77 kg (1.1-4.5 kg)	Dry mouth, insomnia, diarrhea, constipation
Fluoxetine	Selective serotonin reuptake inhibitor	60 mg daily	0.90-9.1 kg	Nervousness, sweating, tremors, nausea, vomiting, fatigue, somnolence or insomnia, diarrhea
Topiramate	Anticonvulsant	96 mg/d or 192 mg/d	6.5% more than placebo (4.8%-8.3%)	Paresthesias, difficulty with concentration, change in taste, dizziness, fatigue
Zonisamide	Anticonvulsant	100-600 mg daily	5% decrease compared to placebo	Dizziness, confusion, difficulty with concentration

antagonist, rimonabant, was successful in producing modest weight loss and improving metabolic complications. However, adverse central nervous system side effects of rimonabant including depression and anxiety precluded introduction of this drug into clinical practice.

Complementary and alternative medications such as herbs, vitamins, nutritional supplements, and meal replacement therapies are commonly used by the general public for weight loss. However the efficacy and safety of these herbal remedies has not been well studied. A recent meta-analysis of trials found that compounds containing ephedra, *Cissus quadrangularis*, ginseng, bitter melon, and zingiber had some short-term efficacy with weight loss with mostly mild adverse effects. However, longer-term randomized controlled trials are needed to prove efficacy and safety.

B. Bariatric surgery   Surgical treatment for weight loss has been performed for the past 50 years, and these procedures are increasing in popularity. Approximately 20,000 weight-loss surgeries were performed in 1995 and over 140,000 were done in 2004, a sevenfold increase. There are three main types of bariatric surgeries: restrictive, malabsorptive, and those that have both a restrictive and a malabsorptive component. Purely restrictive surgeries include horizontal gastroplasty, vertical banded gastroplasty, silastic ring vertical gastroplasty, and adjustable gastric banding. Purely malabsorptive surgeries include the oldest of all bariatric procedures, the jejunoileal bypass, biliopancreatic diversion, duodenal switch, and long limb gastric bypass. The combination of restrictive and malabsorptive surgical procedure is the most commonly used bariatric surgery worldwide, the Roux-en-Y gastric bypass procedure (RYGB), which involved stapling the upper stomach into a small 30-mL pouch and attaching it to the jejunum bypassing the lower stomach and duodenum. This procedure can be done with an open surgical approach, or now more commonly with a laparoscopic approach.

Several studies have examined the effects of different types of bariatric surgeries on various outcomes including weight loss, comorbid disease, complication rates, and mortality. There are very few randomized controlled trials comparing different surgical procedures, so most of the outcomes data come from case series, prospective cohort analyses, or nonrandomized trials. The largest and longest double cohort study to date is the Swedish Obese Subjects (SOS) study in which obese adults who voluntarily underwent bariatric surgery were matched to a control group of medically treated patients. After 10 years of follow-up of 1703 participants, those treated with surgery had a 16% weight loss compared to 2% in the controls (p <0.001). They compared the different types of bariatric surgery approaches in this study and found that those who had gastric bypass lost more weight than those who received banding procedures or the vertical banded gastroplasty.

An earlier meta-analysis determined the effect of bariatric surgery on weight loss, mortality, and four comorbid diseases including diabetes, hyperlipidemia, hypertension, and sleep apnea. The mean excess weight loss was 61.2% (58.1%-64.4%), highest in those who had the biliopancreatic diversion or duodenal switch (70.1%) and lowest in those who underwent gastric banding (47.5%). Operative mortality within 30 days of the surgery was 0.1% for purely restrictive procedures and 0.5% for gastric bypass, and 1.1% for biliopancreatic diversion or duodenal switch procedures. Type 2 diabetes resolved in approximately 77% of patients after surgery, hyperlipidemia improved in 70%, hypertension resolved in 62%, and obstructive sleep apnea resolved in 86%.

Much attention has focused on determining the mechanisms involved in the dramatic weight loss associated with bariatric surgery. Previous hypotheses that restrictive procedures reduce the quantity of food ingested at any one time, malabsorptive procedures cause wasting of fat calories, with RYGB employing a combination of both mechanisms, have not been supported by studies. More recent thinking attributes weight loss after bariatric procedures to a substantial decline in hunger and increase in satiety that is regulated through neuroendocrine mechanisms and gut hormones such as ghrelin and PYY. The effect of RYGB surgery on ghrelin levels is controversial since some studies have found increased levels, no change, or decreased levels after surgery. These inconsistent results may be explained by the timing of ghrelin sampling after surgery. After purely restrictive surgeries, ghrelin levels increase, which may help explain the more dramatic weight loss observed following RYGB vs purely restrictive surgeries. PYY levels rise to those of a nonobese person following vertical banded gastroplasty. However, with RYGB, there is an early exaggerated response in PYY secretion, approximately two- to fourfold greater than that observed in lean, obese, or gastric banded patients, which may contribute to the sustained weight loss seen with this type of procedure.

Defining appropriate patient criteria to minimize risks and maximize the benefits from bariatric surgery have been debated. Some studies have concluded that surgical intervention is more effective for weight loss and control of comorbid diseases than nonsurgical treatments in patients with a BMI ≥40 kg/m². In 2004, with extensive scientific input, the National Coverage Advisory Committee panel concluded that bariatric surgery could be offered to Medicare beneficiaries with BMI ≥35 kg/m² who have at least one comorbid disease associated with obesity and have been unsuccessful previously with medical treatment of obesity. Other criteria for patient selection proposed by leading associations include adequate patient commitment with medical follow-up and use of dietary supplements, no other reversible endocrine disorders causing obesity, no current substance abuse, and no severe psychiatric illness.

C. Interventions with efficacy in children   Several studies have investigated behavioral and lifestyle intervention programs for pediatric weight loss. Most randomized controlled trials of overweight children and adolescents have found positive, but small- to -moderate effects, of combined lifestyle interventions on BMI. Family-based behavioral weight loss programs have produced larger effects that persist for several months of follow-up. Less is known about the long-term safety and efficacy of pharmacologic agents for treatment of pediatric obesity.

REFERENCES

Barlow SE, Dietz WH. Obesity evaluation and treatment: expert committee recommendations. The Maternal and Child Health Bureau, Health Resources and Services Administration and the Department of Health and Human Services. *Pediatrics.* 1998;3:E29. [PMID: 1224658]

Berthoud H-R, Morrison C. The brain, appetite, and obesity. *Ann Rev Psychol.* 2008;59:55. [PMID:18154499]

Buchwald H, Avidor Y, Braunwald E, et al. Bariatric surgery: a systematic review and meta-analysis. *JAMA.* 2004;14:1724. [PMID:15479938]

The CDC National Diabetes Fact Sheet. http://www.cdc.gov/diabetes/pubs/estimates.htm#prev3. Accessed December 10, 2003. Data from the National Health Interview Survey and the Third National Health and Nutrition Examination Survey.

Christakis NA, Fowler JH. The spread of obesity in a large social network over 32 years. *N Engl J Med.* 2007;4:370. [PMID:17652652]

Cummings DE, Overduin J. Gastrointestinal regulation of food intake. *J Clin Invest.* 2007;1:13. [PMID:17200702]

Dansinger ML, Gleason JA, Griffith JL, et al. Comparison of the Atkins, Ornish, Weight Watchers, and Zone diets for weight loss and heart disease risk reduction: a randomized trial. *JAMA.* 2005;1:43. [PMID:15632335]

Dickerson LM, Carek PJ. Pharmacotherapy for the obese patient. *Prim Care.* 2009;2:407. [PMID:19501251]

Galic S, Oakhill JS, Steinberg GR. Adipose tissue as an endocrine organ. *Mol Cell Endocrinol.* 2010;2:129. [PMID:19723556]

Grundy SM, Cleeman JI, Daniels SR, et al. Definition of metabolic syndrome: report of the National Heart, Lung, and Blood Institute/American Heart Association conference on scientific issues related to definition. *Circulation.* 2004;3:433. [PMID:14744958]

Hedley AA, Ogden CL, Johnson CL, et al. Prevalence of overweight and obesity among US children, adolescents, and adults, 1999-2002. *JAMA.* 2004;23:2847. [PMID:15199035]

Kahn SE, Hull RL, Utzschneider KM. Mechanisms linking obesity to insulin resistance and type 2 diabetes. *Nature.* 2006;7121:840. [PMID:17167471]

Kenchaiah S, Evans JC, Levy D, et al. Obesity and the risk of heart failure. *N Engl J Med.* 2002;5:305. [PMID:12151467]

Larsson SC, Wolk A. Obesity and colon and rectal cancer risk: a meta-analysis of prospective studies. *Am J Clin Nutr.* 2007;3:556. [PMID:17823417]

Montague CT, O'Rahilly S. The perils of portliness: causes and consequences of visceral adiposity. *Diabetes.* 2000;6:883. [PMID: 10866038]

Morton GJ, Cummings DE, Baskin DG, Barsh GS, Schwartz MW. Central nervous system control of food intake and body weight. *Nature.* 2006;7109:289. [PMID:16988703]

Nordmann AJ, Nordmann A, Briel M, et al. Effects of low-carbohydrate vs low-fat diets on weight loss and cardiovascular risk factors: a meta-analysis of randomized controlled trials. *Arch Intern Med.* 2006;3:285. [PMID:16476868]

Ogden CL, Carroll MD, Curtin LR, et al. Prevalence of overweight and obesity in the United States, 1999-2004. *JAMA.* 2006;13:1549. [PMID:16595758]

Ogden CL, Carroll MD, Flegal KM. High body mass index for age among US children and adolescents, 2003-2006. *JAMA.* 2008;20:2401. [PMID:18505949]

Reaven GM. Banting lecture 1988. Role of insulin resistance in human disease. *Diabetes.* 1988;12:1595. [PMID:3056758]

Romero-Corral A, Montori VM, Somers VK, et al. Association of bodyweight with total mortality and with cardiovascular events in coronary artery disease: a systematic review of cohort studies. *Lancet.* 2006;9536:666. [PMID:16920472]

Sjostrom L, Narbro K, Sjostrem CD, et al. Effects of bariatric surgery on mortality in Swedish obese subjects. *N Engl J Med.* 2007;8:741. [PMID:17715408]

Van Gaal LF, Mertens IL, De Block CE. Mechanisms linking obesity with cardiovascular disease. *Nature.* 2006;7121:875. [PMID:17167476]

WHO. Obesity: preventing and managing the global epidemic. Report of a WHO consultation. World Health Organization Technical Report Series. 2000;1.

Humoral Manifestations of Malignancy

Dolores Shoback, MD, and Janet L. Funk, MD

ACTH	Adrenocorticotropic hormone		**IGF**	Insulin-like growth factor
ANP	Atrial natriuretic peptide		**IGF-BP3**	Insulin-like growth factor binding protein-3
APUD	Amine precursor uptake and decarboxylation (cell)		**IL**	Interleukin
CRH	Corticotropin-releasing hormone		**LH**	Luteinizing hormone
CT	Computed tomography		**MEPE**	Matrix extracellular phosphoglycoprotein
FDG-PET	Fluorodeoxyglucose positron emission tomography		**MRI**	Magnetic resonance imaging
FGF	Fibroblast growth factor		**POMC**	Proopiomelanocortin
FSH	Follicle-stimulating hormone		**PTH**	Parathyroid hormone
GH	Growth hormone		**PTHrP**	Parathyroid hormone-related protein
GHRH	Growth hormone–releasing hormone		**SIADH**	Syndrome of inappropriate antidiuretic hormone (secretion)
hCG	Human chorionic gonadotropin		**TNF**	Tumor necrosis factor
HTLV-1	Human T cell leukemia virus-I		**VIP**	Vasoactive intestinal peptide

ECTOPIC HORMONE AND RECEPTOR SYNDROMES

Some of the most challenging endocrine problems occur in patients with malignancies of diverse cell types, because both endocrine and nonendocrine tumors secrete polypeptide hormones. As it became recognized that a polypeptide hormone could be produced by tumor cells derived from a tissue that normally did not secrete the hormone, the notion of ectopic hormone production developed. Most tumors associated with ectopic hormone syndromes are derived from cells that are normally capable of producing peptide hormones. Initially, it was thought that ectopic hormone production by tumor cells was a rare event. Interestingly, both the frequency and the original conception of this syndrome have been redefined over the last few decades. It has come to be appreciated—through the use of modern biochemical and molecular biologic techniques—that the synthesis of peptide hormones and the transcription of their genes by tumor cells are in fact quite common occurrences. Tumor cells may differ from normal cells in

their ability or inability to process precursor molecules, which may account for the presence or absence of hormone excess states and for the profile of peptide hormone forms and fragments present in the circulation and in tumor cell extracts. However, tumor production of hormone fragments or precursors is much more common than the clinical syndromes of hormone excess.

The classic criteria used to confirm that a tumor is the source of a hormone excess state include the following: (1) evidence of an endocrinopathy in a patient with a tumor; (2) remission of the endocrinopathy after tumor resection; (3) detection of an arteriovenous gradient across the tumor; and (4) documentation of protein and messenger RNA encoding the hormone being produced by tumor tissue.

In addition to classic hormone excess states resulting from the ectopic or inappropriate secretion of a hormone by an endocrine or nonendocrine tumor, endocrinopathies can result from the ectopic expression of a hormone's receptor. This is well illustrated, for example, by the occurrence of Cushing syndrome in pregnancy or in relation to meals, due to the ectopic expression of luteinizing

TABLE 21–1   Polypeptide hormones produced ectopically by benign and malignant tumors and their associated endocrinopathies.

Hormone	Syndrome
Parathyroid hormone-related protein (PTHrP)	Hypercalcemia
Parathyroid hormone (rare)	Hypercalcemia
Adrenocorticotropin (ACTH)	Cushing syndrome
Corticotropin-releasing hormone (CRH)	Cushing syndrome
Antidiuretic hormone (ADH)	Hyponatremia
Insulin and insulin-like growth factors (IGF)	Hypoglycemia
Growth hormone–releasing hormone (GHRH)	Acromegaly
Calcitonin	*No specific syndrome*
Human chorionic gonadotropin (hCG)	Children: precocious puberty Men: erectile dynsfunction, gynecomastia Women: dysfunctional uterine bleeding
Fibroblast growth factor (FGF) 23	Oncogenic osteomalacia
Vasoactive intestinal peptide (VIP)	Diarrhea

hormone (LH) or gastric inhibitory polypeptide receptors in adrenal tissue, respectively. Several other examples of ectopic receptor syndromes have been documented. Some of these will be discussed later, particularly as a cause for unusual forms of adrenocorticotropic hormone (ACTH)-independent Cushing syndrome.

A variety of peptides are produced by both benign and malignant tumors as listed in Table 21–1. The biochemical pathways and machinery leading to the synthesis, processing, and secretion into the circulation of a peptide hormone are present in all cells. In contrast, the multiple enzymatic steps that lead to the production of a highly active steroid hormone (eg, cortisol or 1,25-dihydroxyvitamin D [1,25-$(OH)_2$ D]) are restricted, with rare exceptions, to steroid-producing cells or their precursor cells. Hence, the occurrence of 1,25-$(OH)_2$ D excess caused by a tumor is distinctly unusual, being observed infrequently in hematologic malignancies and only in those with the ability to 1-hydroxylate 25-OH D, the immediate precursor of 1,25-$(OH)_2$ D. Ectopic hormone syndromes—the most common of the paraneoplastic syndromes—thus predominantly reflect peptide hormone excess states. The most common ectopic peptide hormone syndromes are described in greater detail in subsequent sections of this chapter.

APUD Concept of Neuroendocrine Cell Tumors

Over the years since the initial recognition that nonendocrine tumors were the source of the ectopic hormones produced in these

endocrine syndromes, the notion developed that the hormones originated from highly specialized neuroendocrine cells in tumors. These cells were thought to derive from the neural crest and were postulated to be able to synthesize and store biogenic amines and were thus designated as amine precursor uptake and decarboxylation (APUD) cells. Neuroendocrine cells, like calcitonin-secreting C cells and adrenal chromaffin cells, clearly had these properties, and tissues giving rise to ectopic hormone syndromes (eg, lung and gastrointestinal tract) also had APUD cells scattered throughout them. It was originally thought that the tumor cells producing excessive amounts of polypeptide hormones were derived exclusively from APUD cells in the tissue of origin (eg, ACTH-producing cells of the lung).

Newer insights into tumor cell biology have led to a better understanding of the pathogenesis and etiology of the ectopic hormone production states. Studies have shown that not all APUD cells are derived from the neural crest. Some of these cells are of endodermal origin. Furthermore, with careful examination of tumors, it has become clear that peptide hormones are often produced by non-APUD cells. It has, however, been appreciated that the clinically evident hormone hypersecretion states are typically caused by tumors that are in fact derived from APUD cells. These cells are the ones with full capacity to produce and store peptide hormones efficiently in dense secretory granules and then release biologically significant quantities of active hormones in circulating plasma.

HYPERCALCEMIA OF MALIGNANCY

Hypercalcemia is the most common paraneoplastic endocrine syndrome, occurring in 25% of malignancies. In the great majority of patients (98%), the identity of the tumor is apparent at the time of presentation, and the prognosis is poor, as most patients with hypercalcemia of malignancy do not survive beyond 6 months.

Pathogenesis

Elevated serum calcium levels result primarily because of excessive osteoclast-mediated bone resorption. Ectopic hormones produce this effect in bone via two distinct mechanisms: (1) humoral effects of systemically elevated tumor-derived factors and/or (2) local effects of peptide hormones produced by tumor cells within the marrow. When the syndrome of hypercalcemia of malignancy was first described, local effects within bone tumors were thought to be causative. However, in the 1980s, a humoral basis was identified as the most frequent cause (80%), even in settings where focal lytic bone metastases were present. Decreased renal calcium excretion may also contribute to pathogenesis, either because of the hypocalciuric effects of certain humoral mediators of hypercalcemia, such as parathyroid hormone (PTH)-related protein (PTHrP) (discussed later), or because of the decreased glomerular filtration that occurs with hypercalcemia-induced nephrogenic diabetes insipidus.

Humoral Mediators

A humoral cause of hypercalcemia of malignancy was first proposed by Fuller Albright in the 1940s when describing a case occurring in the absence of significant bone metastases. It would take another 50 years for this humoral factor to be identified. It was appreciated early on that the basic biochemical parameters of this syndrome (high serum calcium, low serum phosphorus, elevated nephrogenous cAMP) were suggestive of ectopic PTH production. However, PTH was not the culprit, as serum PTH levels in these cases were actually suppressed. Ultimately, and unlike most other paraneoplastic endocrine syndromes that are caused by well-described hormones of known function, a novel peptide, PTH-related protein (PTHrP), was identified as the humoral mediator of this syndrome in a majority of cases.

As denoted by its name, PTHrP has much in common with PTH. PTHrP was initially so named because of shared biochemical and metabolic effects with PTH. The amino terminal portion of PTHrP bears strong homology to PTH, such that the two peptides bind with similar affinity to PTH receptors (now known as the PTH/PTHrP-1 receptor subtype) in bone and kidney. Therefore, the biochemical markers of PTHrP-mediated hypercalcemia in vivo, when it is produced by tumors in an unregulated fashion, are similar to those of hyperparathyroidism. Some unexplained differences, however, are seen in PTHrP-mediated hypercalcemia of malignancy (vs primary hyperparathyroidism), including normal or suppressed 1,25-$(OH)_2$ D levels and an uncoupling of bone resorption and formation that results in severe bone loss. The reasons for these differences are not understood but are speculated to include: (1) the ability of chronic PTHrP (vs intermittent PTH) stimulation or profound hypercalcemia per se to suppress 1,25-$(OH)_2$ D levels; and (2) the contributions of additional tumor-derived cytokines, such as interleukin (IL)-1α or IL-6, to the process of bone resorption.

Subsequent study of this previously unknown peptide has demonstrated that PTHrP and PTH actually diverge in many critical ways, beginning evolutionarily. Both hormones arose from ancient duplication of a common gene, but evolved separately such that in higher vertebrates, PTH now regulates calcium homeostasis, while PTHrP has critical developmental roles, including endochondral bone growth, tooth eruption, and development of the mammary gland and cardiovascular system. As with other developmentally regulated proteins, PTHrP plays less of a role in adult homeostasis, but can be reexpressed in response to specific changes in gene programming, including pregnancy (calcium regulation by the lactating mammary gland and placenta), injury and inflammation (regulation of vascular tone in ischemia, sepsis, and inflammation-associated bone resorption), and/or tumorigenesis (hypercalcemia of malignancy).

When tumor expression of PTHrP results in inappropriately high levels of PTHrP that reaches bone cells through the circulation or following synthesis in the bone microenvironment, a vicious cycle can ensue. PTHrP stimulates the expression of RANKL (receptor activator of NF-κB ligand) by osteoblasts. RANKL, the primary gatekeeper modulating bone resorption in health and disease, stimulates osteoclast differentiation and function via binding to its receptor, RANK, on osteoclasts and their precursors. Increased numbers of activated osteoclasts are generated both by the local release of PTHrP, in the case of bone metastases, or by high levels of the hormone produced by tumor cells in

extraskeletal sites. Both mechanisms cause enhanced bone resorption. In the case of bone metastases, sequestered growth factors, such as transforming growth factor (TGF)-beta, released locally from the bone matrix during resorption, further enhance tumor cell secretion of PTHrP.

Although PTHrP is by far the most common mediator of hypercalcemia of malignancy, other calciotropic hormones can also cause the syndrome. When hypercalcemia occurs with lymphoma, increased circulating levels of 1,25-$(OH)_2$ D are a common cause, due to increased 1α-hydroxylase activity in lymphoproliferative cells and/or tumor-adjacent macrophages. Other tumor-derived bone-resorbing factors, such as prostaglandins, may also contribute to hypercalcemia of malignancy with certain tumors, like renal cell carcinoma. In contrast, ectopic production of PTH is extremely rare, but has occasionally been reported for neuroendocrine tumors and other solid tumors.

Solid Tumors Associated with Hypercalcemia of Malignancy

The majority of cases of hypercalcemia occurring with solid tumors (80%) are associated with two common tumor types: squamous cell lung carcinoma and breast carcinoma (see Table 21–1). Hypercalcemia is also frequently seen in renal cell carcinoma. Indeed, PTHrP was first isolated and identified by independent research groups each using one of these three tumor types. In contrast, hypercalcemia is rarely seen in other commonly occurring cancers (eg, colon, gastric, thyroid, and small cell lung carcinomas), including some tumors that are frequently metastatic to bone (eg, prostate cancer).

A. Squamous cell carcinomas Squamous cell carcinomas account for more than one-third of all cases of hypercalcemia of malignancy. Humoral effects of tumor-derived PTHrP account for most cases of hypercalcemia in this setting, even when bone metastases are present. Twenty-five percent of patients with squamous cell lung carcinomas develop PTHrP-mediated hypercalcemia, and other sites of squamous cell carcinoma (head, neck, esophagus, cervix, vulva, and skin) are similarly associated with a high incidence of hypercalcemia.

B. Breast carcinoma The majority of patients with breast cancer bone metastases (ie, 70% of those with advanced disease) do not have hypercalcemia. However, hypercalcemia does occur in 30% of advanced-stage breast carcinoma cases and is only rarely seen in the absence of bone metastases. PTHrP is causative, as both a local and/or humoral factor to stimulate bone resorption. Most breast cancer bone metastases (92%-100%) express PTHrP and cause lytic bone destruction. In addition, humoral effects of PTHrP, as evidenced by elevated circulating levels of PTHrP associated with increased nephrogenous cAMP, have been documented in a majority of cases of hypercalcemia occurring in the absence of bone metastases and two-thirds of those cases occurring with bone metastases.

Despite this close association of PTHrP with advanced disease, the prognostic significance of PTHrP expression in primary breast carcinomas, which has been documented in two-thirds of primary tumors in multiple series, is not clear. Reasons for the lack of a simple direct correlation are probably multifactorial and may include: (1) the ability of tumors to modulate PTHrP expression once they metastasize to bone (eg, TGF-beta released from the bone matrix by invading tumor cells is thought to enhance PTHrP expression in the tumor cells, even when the primary tumor is PTHrP-negative); and (2) the tendency for expression of PTHrP to correlate with estrogen receptor and progesterone receptor status, which influences treatment and response to therapy. Additionally, locally produced bone cytokines such as IL-1α, IL-6, and tumor necrosis factor (TNF)-alpha likely act in concert with PTHrP at sites of bone metastases to enhance osteoclast-mediated lytic bone destruction and thus contribute to hypercalcemia. Hypercalcemia seen in late stages of breast cancer is usually unremitting and associated with a survival time of weeks to months.

C. Renal cell carcinoma

Renal cell carcinoma, while less common than squamous cell or breast carcinoma, is also frequently associated with hypercalcemia in advanced cases. While bone metastases are common in advanced disease, hypercalcemia appears to be due primarily to humoral effects of PTHrP. In some series, 100% of renal cell tumors have been reported to stain positively for immunoreactive PTHrP. However, hypercalcemia is reported in less than 20% of cases.

D. Other solid tumors

Hypercalcemia is also associated with other solid tumors, although less frequently. In most of these cases, humoral effects of PTHrP are causative. Bladder carcinoma, large cell and adenocarcinoma of the lung, and endocrine tumors (including islet cell tumors, pheochromocytoma, and carcinoid tumors) have also been reported to secrete PTHrP. PTHrP-mediated hypercalcemia has also been reported for ovarian carcinomas. A case of ectopic PTH production by an ovarian carcinoma has also been reported.

Hematologic Malignancies Associated with Hypercalcemia of Malignancy (Table 21–2)

A. Multiple myeloma

Hypercalcemia and lytic bone lesions are among the diagnostic criteria for multiple myeloma, a hematologic malignancy characterized by infiltration of the bone marrow with malignant plasma cells. Lytic bone lesions and active bone resorption occur adjacent to tumor cells, which secrete multiple factors capable of stimulating osteoclast differentiation and activity. A major effect of these factors, which include macrophage inflammatory peptide-1, TNF-alpha, IL-1, and IL-6, is to induce RANKL expression in osteoblasts. Evidence of RANKL expression by plasma cells also exists. Locally increased RANKL causes bone lysis by binding to its cognate receptor on osteoclasts (RANK) and stimulating their differentiation and activity. More recently, it has been appreciated that defects in bone formation, due to suppression of the Wnt signaling

TABLE 21–2 Hypercalcemia of malignancy.

	Incidence of Hypercalcemia	Etiology of Hypercalcemia	
Solid tumors		**Humoral**	**Local lytic**
Squamous cell (lung, head, neck)	25%	100% (PTHrP)	–
Breast, advanced	30%	65% (PTHrP)	35% (PTHrP)
Renal cell	15%	50%-100% (PTHrP)	50%
Hematologic malignancies			
Multiple myeloma	30%	–	100%
Lymphoma/ leukemia (non-HTLV-1)	<15%	50% (1,25[OH]2D, rarely PTHrP)	50%
HTLV-1 lymphoma/ leukemia	66%	100% (PTHrP)	–

pathway by other tumor factors (eg, Dickkopf-1), also accompany lytic bone disease in multiple myeloma. In 30% of cases, bone lysis leads to hypercalcemia. Because renal disease occurs frequently in myeloma due to the filtration of Bence Jones proteins (light chain fragments of IgG), it is hypothesized that patients with renal impairment may be particularly predisposed to development of hypercalcemia in this setting of increased bone resorption.

B. Lymphoma and leukemia

Hypercalcemia has been reported in up to 15% of patients with lymphoma; is seen primarily in patients with bone involvement; and can occur with a variety of cell types. In most cases, the etiology is evenly divided between: (1) local lytic effects of tumor-derived factors within the marrow, analogous to the mechanisms discussed for myeloma, or (2) humoral effects of tumor-derived 1,25-(OH)$_2$ D. 1, 25(OH)$_2$ D-mediated hypercalcemia of malignancy is unique to lymphoma. Its underlying pathology is analogous to that seen in hypercalcemia in granulomatous disorders where 1α-hydroxylase activity in the abnormal hematopoietic cells or infiltrating macrophages results in unregulated conversion of 25-(OH)$_2$ D to active 1,25-(OH)$_2$ D. Increased intestinal calcium absorption and increased bone resorption are both thought to contribute to hypercalcemia in this setting. In addition, there are also numerous case reports of humoral effects of tumor-derived PTHrP as a cause of hypercalcemia in non-Hodgkin lymphomas (particularly B cell), acute lymphoblastic leukemia, and blast crises in chronic myeloid leukemia. So the clinician confronting such tumors must be cognizant of the different etiologies for the observed hypercalcemia.

Patients diagnosed with adult T cell leukemia or lymphoma induced by HTLV-1 (human T cell lymphotrophic virus-1), the first identified human retrovirus, must be considered separately when evaluating possible causes of hypercalcemia. In these patients, hypercalcemia occurs in two-thirds of cases, responds poorly to treatment, and is due to the humoral effects of tumor-derived PTHrP. Tax1, a transcription factor encoded by the HTLV-1 genome, transforms T cells in these cases by altering the regulation of hundreds of host genes, including transactivation of PTHrP.

Diagnosis

The diagnosis of hypercalcemia is discussed in detail in Chapter 8. Primary hyperparathyroidism and hypercalcemia of malignancy account for more than 90% of all causes of hypercalcemia. Because the incidence of primary hyperparathyroidism is twice that of hypercalcemia of malignancy, primary hyperparathyroidism must always be considered as a potential cause of hypercalcemia in patients with malignancy and can be screened for by simply determining intact PTH levels using a standard two-site immunoradiometric assay. In the setting of hypercalcemia of malignancy with normal renal function, PTH levels are suppressed. Further evaluation can be guided, in part, by the tumor type, which is usually known prior to presentation with hypercalcemia. Elevated PTHrP is detected in a majority of cases of hypercalcemia of malignancy associated with solid tumors, including breast carcinoma with or without bone metastases, and in HTLV-1–induced T cell lymphomas. Measurement of $1,25\text{-}(OH)_2$ D should be considered in all cases of lymphoma-associated hypercalcemia. Lytic bone lesions are usually identified during tumor staging.

Treatment

The treatment of hypercalcemia is discussed in detail in Chapter 8. Because bone resorption is central to all causes of hypercalcemia of malignancy, bisphosphonates are currently a mainstay of therapy. Glucocorticoids may be efficacious in the treatment of hypercalcemia due either to the local lytic effects of neoplastic plasma cells in multiple myeloma or to the increased production of $1,25\text{-}(OH)_2$ D in lymphoma. Recent and ongoing clinical trials are also evaluating the utility of humanized antibodies directed again PTHrP or RANKL in preventing hypercalcemia and other adverse skeletal events in patients with multiple myeloma, breast cancer, and/or other solid tumors. While bisphosphonates are already a mainstay of palliative care for patients with hypercalcemia and have a demonstrated ability to decrease skeletal-related events (metastases and pathologic fractures) and ameliorate bone pain in these patients, their possible use as adjuvants in order to delay or prevent bone metastases in breast and other cancers is currently a very active area of clinical research.

ECTOPIC CUSHING SYNDROME

Many malignant tumors produce the ACTH precursor proopiomelanocortin (POMC) but lack the enzymes necessary to process this precursor to biologically active ACTH. Therefore, only a fraction of such tumors release sufficient ACTH to cause Cushing syndrome. Initially, the tumors recognized to cause this syndrome were of nonpituitary but endocrine origin, such as

islet cell carcinomas and pheochromocytomas. Subsequently, a wide variety of different tumor cell types, both endocrine and nonendocrine, have been associated with the ectopic ACTH syndrome.

The classic description of the ectopic ACTH syndrome was made by Grant Liddle and coworkers in the early 1960s and was based on a series of patients who mostly had highly malignant tumors (eg, small cell carcinoma of the lung). More recently, the ectopic ACTH syndrome has been recognized with increasing frequency with benign tumors, specifically carcinoids. Benign lesions typically present in a more subtle clinical manner, often over months to years, before the tumor is identified. The more gradual development of the clinical syndrome plus the more subtle biochemistry have led to considerable challenges in distinguishing this form of the ectopic ACTH syndrome from pituitary tumors causing Cushing disease. This subtle variant of tumor-induced ACTH excess has been dubbed the *occult* ectopic ACTH syndrome. In addition, it is now recognized that tumors can cause an ectopic ACTH-like syndrome through production of corticotropin-releasing hormone (CRH). Indeed, some of the tumors that make the latter cosecrete ACTH as well. Ectopic CRH production has been seen in bronchial carcinoids, medullary thyroid carcinoma, and metastatic prostatic cancer.

Differential Diagnosis

Cushing syndrome—signs and symptoms resulting from unregulated production of glucocorticoids—is caused by a number of underlying disturbances. These must be differentiated to ensure successful treatment. Causes include pituitary ACTH-dependent Cushing disease, adrenal tumors or ACTH-independent Cushing syndrome, and the ectopic ACTH syndrome. In several large series, 50% to 80% of patients with Cushing syndrome have a pituitary cause. Adrenal adenomas (and very rarely carcinomas) account for 5% to 30% of cases of Cushing syndrome. The ectopic ACTH syndrome comprises approximately 10% to 20% of cases of Cushing syndrome.

A wide variety of tumors cause ectopic ACTH syndrome (Table 21–3). In the classic and initial descriptions of this syndrome, there was a preponderance of malignant tumors, particularly small cell carcinomas of the lung. It is now clear that most cases of ectopic ACTH syndrome are due to benign tumors. Most recently, microscopic carcinoid *tumorlets*, particularly in the lung, have been recognized to cause occult ectopic ACTH syndrome. These tumors may be exceptionally difficult to diagnose by standard techniques.

The diagnosis of Cushing syndrome requires a rigorous approach. Cushing syndrome should be suspected first on solid clinical grounds and then established biochemically. This is accomplished by demonstrating the presence of hypercortisolism—a frankly elevated 24-hour urinary free cortisol level or the lack of suppression of plasma cortisol levels after a 1-mg overnight dexamethasone suppression test (see Chapter 9). In Cushing syndrome due to any cause and often in ectopic ACTH syndrome, random cortisol levels are elevated. Once hypercortisolism is established, plasma ACTH levels are measured. These levels are

TABLE 21–3 Tumors responsible for the ectopic ACTH syndrome in two large contemporary series.

Tumor Type	Number of Patients (% of total) NIH Series (USA) (1983-2004)[a]	Number of Patients (% of total) St. Bartholomew's Hospital (UK) Cushing Disease Database (1969-2001)[b]
Carcinoid		
Thymic	5/90 (5.5%)	2/40 (5%)
Pulmonary	35/90 (39%)	12/40 (30%)
Appendiceal	1/90 (1%)	–
Pancreatic	1/90 (1%)	3/40 (7.5%)
Pulmonary tumorlets	1/90 (1%)	–
Neuroendocrine tumors	13/90 (14%)	2/40 (5%)
Gastrinoma	6/90 (6.7%)	–
Small cell lung cancer	3/90 (3.3%)	7/40 (17.5%)
Pheochromocytoma	5/90 (5.5%)	1/40 (2.5%)
Medullary thyroid cancer	2/90 (2.2%)	3/40 (7.5%)
Small cell colon	–	2/40 (5%)
Miscellaneous	1/90 (1%)	5/40 (12.5%)
Unknown	17/90 (18.9%)	5/40 (12.5%)

[a]Ilias I, Torpy, DJ, Pacak, K, et al. Extensive clinical experience: Cushing's syndrome due to ectopic corticotrin secretion: twenty years' experience at the National Institute of Health. *J Clin Endocrinol Metab.* 2005;90:4955.

[b]Isidori AM, Kaltsas GA, Pozza C. Extensive clinical experience: the ectopic adrenocorticotropin syndrome: clinical features, diagnosis, management, and long-term follow-up. *J Clin Endocrinol Metab.* 2006;91:371.

markedly elevated in classic forms of the ectopic ACTH syndrome, typically secondary to malignant lung neoplasms. There is, however, considerable overlap between the milder cases of the ectopic ACTH syndrome, caused by benign and slowly growing tumors, and Cushing disease due to a pituitary tumor. In the former case, the tumors are often small and clinically silent—hence the descriptor *occult* ectopic ACTH syndrome. For these reasons, rigorous biochemical criteria must be applied in appropriate clinical situations to make certain that the correct diagnosis is made. Plasma ACTH levels in patients with clinically evident tumors are often strikingly elevated (390-2300 pg/mL [87-511 pmol/L] by radioimmunoassay). Individuals with ectopic ACTH syndrome due to occult tumors have ACTH levels that overlap with pituitary-dependent Cushing disease (42-428 pg/mL [9.3-95 pmol/L]). It is said that patients with plasma ACTH levels greater than 200 pg/mL (44.4 pmol/L) typically have the ectopic ACTH syndrome, although further testing is required to prove this and to localize the tumor.

After hypercortisolism and ACTH excess are established, the degree of suppressibility of ACTH with exogenous glucocorticoid is determined. In classic Cushing disease due to a pituitary tumor, supraphysiologic doses of dexamethasone usually suppress the elevated plasma ACTH and cortisol levels. Tumors responsible for the ectopic ACTH syndrome are classically unresponsive to these same doses of dexamethasone. High-dose dexamethasone suppression testing, as this diagnostic maneuver is called, is accomplished by (1) administering 2 mg of dexamethasone every 6 hours for 2 days and measuring urinary free cortisol or plasma cortisol on the second day, or (2) administering 8 mg of dexamethasone the night before obtaining an 8 AM plasma cortisol level. In both tests, the expected suppression of baseline urinary free cortisol and plasma cortisol should be 50% or greater if the Cushing syndrome is due to a pituitary adenoma (ie, Cushing disease). However, between 15% and 33% of patients with ectopic ACTH syndrome also meet these suppression criteria (false positives), mimicking Cushing disease. In addition, 10% to 25% of patients with Cushing disease fail to suppress with high-dose dexamethasone (false negatives). The overnight test probably has greater sensitivity and accuracy than the classic 2-day test, but neither test is considered useful any longer (see Chapter 9).

Additional provocative tests have been developed to improve the diagnostic discrimination between Cushing disease and ectopic ACTH syndrome using ovine CRH. Pituitary corticotrophs are normally responsive to CRH in Cushing disease and unresponsive when ectopic ACTH production or an adrenal lesion is responsible for the cortisol excess. A positive response to CRH is defined as a 50% or greater increase in plasma ACTH and a 20% or greater increase in the plasma cortisol concentrations in the periphery. An increase in ACTH of 100% and in cortisol of more than 50% greatly reduces the likelihood of ectopic ACTH syndrome; however, false-positive and false-negative tests (up to 10%) have been reported. Moreover, in the rare instance of ectopic production of CRH (without concomitant ACTH) by a tumor, a false-positive result may be seen, leading to the erroneous diagnosis of pituitary-dependent Cushing disease.

For these reasons, most centers prefer inferior petrosal sinus sampling for ACTH before and after CRH administration, and this test is now the gold standard. The inferior petrosal sinuses drain the pituitary gland. Concomitant peripheral and petrosal sinus samples are obtained and the central: peripheral ACTH ratio is calculated. In Cushing disease, the ratio should be greater than or equal to 2.0 in the basal state. After CRH administration, this ratio should be greater than or equal to 3.0 in pituitary-dependent Cushing disease. In the ectopic ACTH syndrome, the basal ratio is typically less than 2 and does not rise after the CRH. In rare instances of ectopic CRH syndrome, the basal ratio may be 2.0. The stimulation by CRH gives close to 100% discrimination between ectopic ACTH production and a pituitary tumor secreting ACTH. Generally, a combination of tests is performed to reach a biochemical diagnosis before extensive radiologic studies are undertaken.

The majority of patients (70% or more) with ectopic ACTH syndrome also cosecrete other hormones or tumor marker peptides, among them are carcinoembryonic antigen, somatostatin, calcitonin, gastrin, glucagon, vasoactive intestinal peptide (VIP), bombesin, pancreatic polypeptide, alpha-fetoprotein, and many others. The presence and secretion of these other hormones (in addition to ACTH) suggests that the source of ACTH is nonpituitary in these patients. Given the variety of peptides and the expense inherent in any screening paradigm, measuring these hormones in patients suspected of ectopic ACTH syndrome is not recommended.

The path to localize the tumor responsible for ectopic ACTH production generally starts with a chest radiograph. Most tumors are in the chest or abdomen. Small cell carcinomas of the lung are usually visible on chest radiograph, whereas bronchial carcinoids are often difficult to detect on plain radiographs. In some situations, these tumors may require a long period (as many as 4 or 5 years) of close follow-up before the tumors are detected. Chest computed tomography (CT) scanning should be employed in all subjects with ectopic ACTH to rule out a chest or mediastinal lesion (such as a thymic carcinoid). Abdominal CT scanning is also performed in these patients to confirm the presence of bilateral adrenal enlargement, a sine qua non of the ectopic ACTH syndrome, and to screen for other possible abdominal tumors responsible for the syndrome (eg, pheochromocytoma, islet cell tumor). In the radiologic evaluation of Cushing syndrome, it is always important to bear in mind that the presence of a pituitary microadenoma on magnetic resonance imaging (MRI) does very little to support the diagnosis of pituitary-dependent Cushing disease—as opposed to an ectopic tumor producing ACTH—because of the great numbers (10%-20%) of normal individuals with incidental pituitary microadenomas (see Chapter 4).

Octreotide scanning, another important diagnostic technique, can successfully localize tumors responsible for ectopic ACTH production because up to 80% of such tumors express somatostatin receptors. Iodinated or, more recently, indium-111(^{111}In)-labeled octreotide scanning has demonstrated medullary carcinomas of the thyroid, small cell lung cancers, islet cell tumors, pheochromocytomas, and other tumors.

The ideal imaging algorithm for occult tumors causing ectopic ACTH syndrome is controversial. Functional imaging with higher than standard doses of the somatostatin analog [^{111}In]-diethylene triamine pentaacetate-D-Phe-pentetreotide (OctreoScan) or with [^{18}F] fluorodeoxyglucose positron emission tomography (FDG-PET) was prospectively evaluated in 17 patients with the ectopic ACTH syndrome (based on inferior petrosal sinus sampling) in whom standard imaging studies were inconclusive. Nieman and colleagues found that FDG-PET did not uncover tumors that were not seen on CT or MRI scans. These investigators, however, found OctreoScans to be useful (enhanced sensitivity) in combination with CT/MRI imaging and advocated this diagnostic approach.

Clinical Features

Cushing syndrome causes truncal obesity, violaceous striae, hypertension, fatigue, glucose intolerance, osteopenia, muscle weakness, moon facies, easy bruisability, buffalo hump, depression, hirsutism, and edema. Patients with ectopic ACTH syndrome may show some, all, or none of these features depending on the underlying tumor. It has been appreciated from the initial descriptions of this syndrome that these patients typically present with myopathy, weight loss, and electrolyte and metabolic disturbances more commonly than with the classic features of slowly developing Cushing disease. Hyperpigmentation is also recognized as more common in the ectopic ACTH syndrome than in Cushing disease. Cortisol excess in older men, especially those at risk for lung tumors, is most commonly due to ectopic ACTH production, whereas ACTH-producing pituitary tumors predominate in young and middle-aged women. Glucose intolerance or frank diabetes and hypokalemic alkalosis are typical metabolic disturbances of the ectopic ACTH syndrome. Because of the extreme elevation in plasma cortisol levels in many of these patients, they are at considerable risk for and often succumb to overwhelming opportunistic infections, often with fungal pathogens.

A critical caveat to remember in the clinical evaluation of patients with ACTH-dependent Cushing disease is that slowly growing and occult tumors producing ACTH may present in exactly the same way as classic Cushing disease due to a pituitary tumor. Therefore, both the clinical findings and the laboratory studies summarized earlier show considerable overlap and may engender confusion in distinguishing these occult tumors from a pituitary lesion.

Increasing numbers of patients who have classic features of Cushing syndrome have been shown to have abnormal expression of receptors in their adrenal glands as the cause of their hypercortisolism. The pathophysiology of this form of Cushing syndrome is ACTH-independent, because other hormones are driving the glucocorticoid hypersecretion. This has been likened by Lacroix and colleagues to a *gain of function* mutation causing constitutive activation of a G protein–coupled receptor. Ectopic expression of receptors for gastric inhibitory peptide, vasopressin (V_2 and V_3), serotonin (5-HT$_7$), and β-adrenergic agonists have been reported. Altered activity or greater expression of eutopic receptors for serotonin (5-HT$_4$), LH, and vasopressin (V_1) in adrenal tissue can also cause cortisol excess. In the case of gastric inhibitory peptide, food-stimulated cortisol hypersecretion has been described. In a case report of excessive LH receptor expression in the adrenals associated with macronodular adrenal hyperplasia, the patient had mild Cushingoid features with pregnancy and the gradual development of full-blown Cushing syndrome with menopause. It is noteworthy that many patients with ectopic or eutopic receptor-mediated Cushing syndrome have macronodular adrenal hyperplasia.

SYNDROME OF INAPPROPRIATE ANTIDIURETIC HORMONE SECRETION

The syndrome of inappropriate antidiuretic hormone (SIADH) secretion is characterized by inappropriate retention of water such that hypertonic or inappropriately concentrated urine is excreted in the presence of hyponatremia. There are many well-recognized causes of this syndrome (Table 21–4).

TABLE 21–4   Causes of SIADH.

Tumors
Small cell carcinoma of lung
Squamous cell carcinoma of lung
Cancers of the head and neck
Carcinoma of the duodenum, pancreas, ureter, prostate, uterus, and nasopharynx
Mesothelioma
Thymoma
Hodgkin lymphoma
Leukemia
Central nervous system disorders
Brain tumors (primary and metastatic)
Brain abscess
Subdural hematoma, subarachnoid hemorrhage
Meningitis, encephalitis
Systemic lupus erythematosus
Demyelinating disorders
Head trauma
Acute intermittent porphyria
Guillian-Barré syndrome
Spinal cord lesions
Pituitary stalk lesion
Transsphenoidal adenectomy
Hydrocephalus
Drugs
Nicotine, phenothiazines, tricyclic antidepressants, nonsteroidal anti-inflammatory agents, cyclophosphamide, vincristine, chlorpropamide, colchicine, selective serotonin reuptake inhibitors (sertraline, fluoxetine), azithromycin, thiazide diuretics
Pulmonary disorders
Tuberculosis
Fungal, bacterial, viral, mycoplasmal pneumonia
Empyema, lung abscess
Chronic obstructive pulmonary disease
Nephrogenic syndrome of inappropriate antidiuresis

Modified, with permission, from Verbalis JG. Disorders of body water homeostasis. *Best Pract Res Clin Endo Metab.* 2003;17:471.

Etiology and Pathogenesis

Tumors are a common cause of SIADH (see Table 21–4). Bronchogenic carcinoma, particularly small cell carcinoma, has been associated with this syndrome since its initial description in 1957. Small cell carcinoma accounts for 80% of lung tumors associated with SIADH, but only 3% to 15% of patients with this tumor have SIADH. Most of these tumors, even from patients without the clinical syndrome, contain ADH by immunostaining. Other tumors that cause the syndrome include breast, pancreatic, and thymic carcinomas in addition to those listed in Table 21–4. These tumors typically produce vasopressin, oxytocin, and the carrier protein neurophysin.

Excessive production of vasopressin by tumors leads to an inability to excrete free water. This is due to the fact that tumors release vasopressin independent of serum osmolality. In addition to the production of vasopressin, many tumors also contain the mRNA for the hormone atrial natriuretic peptide (ANP).

Clinical and Laboratory Features

SIADH is the most common cause of hyponatremia in hospitalized patients. It may present with symptoms due to water intoxication and hyponatremia. Although many patients are asymptomatic, depending on the magnitude and chronicity of their hyponatremia, symptomatic individuals usually have fatigue, headache, nausea, and anorexia initially, which can progress to altered mental status, seizures, coma, and even death. Most patients experience weight gain due to water retention but do not have edema. Significant clinical symptoms usually do not develop unless the serum sodium is 125 mEq/L or less, and there is usually a correlation between the level of symptomatology in these patients and their serum sodium values.

Patients with SIADH exhibit hyponatremia, serum hypoosmolality, a less than maximally dilute urine, and the presence of sodium in the urine. Clinically, the diagnosis of SIADH cannot be made unless there is euvolemia with intact renal, adrenal, and thyroid function. Cirrhosis, nephrosis, and congestive heart failure must be excluded. Generally, the diagnosis is made by the presence of hyponatremia, low serum osmolality, and urine osmolality that is less than maximally dilute. Urinary sodium levels are usually high, and urea nitrogen levels are typically low, as are serum uric acid levels. Rarely is it necessary or even helpful to measure vasopressin levels to make this diagnosis. Although these determinations are available, they are even sometimes misleading, and routine testing is not recommended. It is also rarely, if ever, necessary to perform a water-loading test, which can be dangerous in these patients because of their impaired ability to excrete a free water load and their propensity to become water intoxicated. Once the diagnosis of SIADH is made, all possible causes should be considered (see Table 21–4).

Water restriction and demeclocycline are the traditional therapies. Several studies support the efficacy of vasopressin antagonists in the treatment of SIADH, and this approach may be considered. In acutely symptomatic patients or when the serum sodium is reduced to dangerously low levels, infusion of hypertonic saline and administration of loop diuretics (eg, furosemide) are the treatments of choice. Many patients with SIADH due to neoplasms improve and even remit with effective therapy for their underlying cancer.

NON-ISLET CELL TUMOR-INDUCED HYPOGLYCEMIA

Tumor-induced hypoglycemia is rare, with the most common cause being eutopic insulin production by pancreatic islet cell tumors (insulinomas). Ectopic hormone production leading to tumor-induced hypoglycemia is estimated to occur in only 20% of cases, and is primarily due to overproduction of insulin-like growth factor-2 (IGF-2). Ectopic insulin secretion by tumors has only rarely been reported. Solid tumors of mesenchymal (mesothelioma, leiomyosarcoma, and fibrosarcoma) or epithelial origin (hepatoma) in the chest or abdomen are the most common source of ectopic IGF-2 (85%). These tumors are usually slow-growing and well-differentiated, often weighing over 2 kg at diagnosis.

Subtle signs of fasting hypoglycemia may be the presenting symptom in these cases, or hypoglycemia may be detected during the course of tumor treatment. As discussed fully in Chapter 18, signs and symptoms of fasting hypoglycemia include sweating, intense hunger, anxiety, altered consciousness, and visual and behavioral changes.

The first case suggestive of non-islet cell tumor IGF-induced hypoglycemia was described in 1929. However, the pathogenesis of this condition has been elucidated only in the last few decades in parallel with our increased understanding of IGF biology. *IGF-2* gene expression is increased in these tumors; however, posttranslational processing is disrupted such that the majority of circulating IGF-2 is a precursor pro-IGF-2 protein (big IGF-2). Big IGF-2 is less likely to form normal ternary complexes with IGF-binding proteins (IGF-BP), and therefore is more bioavailable. In addition, it is postulated that big IGF-2 may displace normal IGF-1 and IGF-2 from IGF-BP, as free levels of these hormones are also increased in some patients. In addition, big IGF-2 is thought to feedback inhibit growth hormone (GH) secretion, thus resulting in even lower levels of IGF-BP. This vicious cycle thus enhances the bioavailability of free IGF peptides whose affinity for the insulin receptor is only 10-fold lower than that of insulin itself. The typical hormonal profile of patients with this syndrome thus includes suppressed levels of insulin, C-peptide, and total IGF-1; and normal or only slightly elevated levels of total IGF-2, while levels of free IGF-2 are markedly (20-fold) increased.

Stimulated glucose disposal in skeletal muscle by IGF binding to the insulin receptor is thought to be a major contributor to hypoglycemia in this syndrome. Diminished hepatic glucose production may also contribute to hypoglycemia, either due to hepatic insulin receptor–mediated IGF effects and/or direct infiltration of the liver by tumor. While GH levels are suppressed, some acromegalic features, thought to be secondary to IGF-2 binding to the type 1 IGF receptor, can also be present (skin tags, rhinophyma).

Treatment of this paraneoplastic syndrome usually involves curative resection or debulking of the tumor. Preoperatively, patients often require continuous glucose infusions to control their symptoms, and glucagon can be used acutely to raise blood-glucose levels. If the lesion is benign, surgery usually brings relief of the hypoglycemia or even definitive cure. In the absence of a surgical cure, additional palliative measures to control hypoglycemic symptoms have been used with some success, including (1) glucocorticoid treatment to suppress tumor production of IGF-2 and induce hepatic gluconeogenesis, and/or (2) GH treatment to increase serum levels of IGF-BP, as well as to induce hepatic gluconeogenesis.

OTHER HORMONES SECRETED BY TUMORS

1. GROWTH HORMONE–RELEASING HORMONE AND GROWTH HORMONE

Acromegaly, in over 95% of cases, is due to eutopic production of GH by pituitary adenomas. Ectopic GH overproduction is extremely rare, but has been reported for pancreatic islet cell tumors, a bronchial carcinoid tumor, and also by a non-Hodgkin lymphoma. In contrast, ectopic production of GHRH is more common and accounts for 1% of cases of acromegaly. Ectopic secretion of growth hormone–releasing hormone (GHRH) was first described in 1974. Indeed, this hypothalamic hormone was first isolated a decade later from patients with pancreatic GHRH-producing tumors. Extrapituitary tumors produce several biologically active forms of GHRH (37-, 40-, and 44-amino acids) as compared to hypothalamic GHRH (1-40) or (1-44) peptides. Excessive peripheral production of GHRH causes hyperplasia of somatotrophs in the pituitary. Resultant elevated levels of circulating GH and IGF-1, lack of suppression of GH by an oral glucose load, and clinical features of acromegaly in this setting are indistinguishable from those caused by GH-secreting pituitary adenomas (see Chapter 4). Ectopic GHRH as a cause of acromegaly can be simply and specifically diagnosed by documentation of elevated circulating GHRH levels. However, because ectopic GHRH is rarely a cause of acromegaly, this assay is best reserved for atypical presentations associated with additional signs and symptoms specific to those tumors that are the most frequent source of ectopic GHRH (carcinoid and pancreatic tumors). It should also be noted that in rare instances, hypothalamic GHRH-secreting tumors (hamartomas, gliomas, and gangliocytomas) can also produce excessive GHRH and acromegaly. Because the site of GHRH production is within the hypothalamus, these cases do not represent ectopic GHRH secretion. Moreover, from a diagnostic standpoint, circulating GHRH levels in these cases are not elevated.

Carcinoid tumors of the lung, gastrointestinal tract, and thymus are the most frequent peripheral source of GHRH (66%). Interestingly, while 50% of carcinoid tumors are immunoreactive for GHRH, a minority of these tumors are associated with elevated circulating levels of bioactive GHRH. Slow-growing GHRH-producing carcinoid tumors, the majority of which are bronchial in origin, are responsible for an insidious presentation of acromegaly that is often associated with additional symptoms specific to the tumor (eg, wheezing). These tumors can be easily detected by routine imaging. Pancreatic islet cell tumors are the second leading cause of ectopic GHRH secretion. Other tumors associated with this syndrome include small cell lung cancer, adrenal adenoma, pheochromocytoma, medullary thyroid carcinoma, endometrial cancer, and breast cancer. Because somatostatin receptors are often present in GHRH-secreting tumors, octreotide scanning may be helpful in localization of extra-pituitary tumors. In addition to surgical resection, the management of ectopic GHRH-induced acromegaly can also include treatment with somatostatin analogs, particularly those that bind to multiple somatostatin receptor subtypes.

2. CALCITONIN

Calcitonin and its precursor, procalcitonin, are frequently produced by malignancies (10%-30%). Consistent with our lack of knowledge regarding the precise physiologic role of calcitonin, there is often no clinical syndrome associated with its ectopic production. However, after an initial diagnosis, calcitonin levels have been used as a tumor marker to follow responses to treatment. Neuroendocrine tumors are the primary cause of both eutopic (medullary thyroid carcinomas, as discussed in Chapters 7 and 24) or ectopic secretion of calcitonin. While small cell cancer is the lung malignancy most frequently (60%) associated with calcitonin hypersecretion, at least 20% of all lung malignancies may have associated elevated calcitonin levels. This is believed to be due either to tumors arising from the pulmonary neuroendocrine cells (small cell and carcinoid) or to calcitonin expression by neuroendocrine cells within or adjacent to tumor cells, as in large cell lung cancer. Calcitonin is also secreted by neuroendocrine tumors of the pancreas. In patients with these tumors, other hormones such as somatostatin and VIP are often produced as well. Approximately half of the patients with these tumors, in a small series by Fleury and colleagues, had diarrhea, presumably due to the effects of calcitonin alone or in combination with other gut peptides. A significant number of these tumors are malignant with liver metastases. In some cases, symptoms of diarrhea may respond to primary therapy of the tumor.

3. GONADOTROPINS

The gonadotropins (luteinizing hormone [LH], follicle-stimulating hormone [FSH], and human chorionic gonadotropin [hCG]) are composed of two (alpha and beta) subunits. The alpha subunits of these glycoproteins share a common amino acid sequence and differ only in their carbohydrate moieties, while their beta subunits are completely distinct. The first two hormones are pituitary products, and the latter is primarily a product of the trophoblastic cells of the placenta during pregnancy. However, hCG is also expressed in other normal tissues, including the pituitary, which appears to be the primary source of detectable circulating hCG in nonpregnant individuals. While LH and FSH are rarely produced ectopically, elevated circulating hCG levels can be produced by multiple tumor types including those of genitourinary system (ovary, prostate, testes, bladder), lung cancers (particularly small cell cancers), gastrointestinal cancers (colon, pancreas, esophagus), breast cancer, melanomas, teratomas, and hepatoblastomas. Ectopic hCG production must be distinguished from eutopic secretion by trophoblastic tumors (hydatidiform mole, choriocarcinoma). However, in both cases, hCG can serve as an important tumor marker for initial diagnosis and monitoring for tumor size and/or evidence of recurrence.

Trophoblastic tumors often secrete excessive amounts of intact hCG heterodimers. In contrast, nontrophoblastic tumors primarily secrete lesser amounts of the free beta subunit of hCG. Serum hCG levels, which are detectable in 40% of ovarian or bladder cancers, often correlate with a less differentiated tumor cell phenotype and a poorer prognosis. Depending on the age and gender of the patient, the clinical signs and symptoms of hCG excess may vary. Importantly, not all patients manifest signs of their hCG excess. In susceptible individuals, however, elevated hCG may result in clear clinical findings. Children, for example, with malignant hepatoblastoma or pineal teratoma can present with precocious puberty. Women may have dysfunctional uterine bleeding.

Men with high hCG levels may have signs of hypogonadism with impotence and gynecomastia. Because of the thyroid-stimulating effects of high hCG levels, these patients occasionally demonstrate hyperthyroidism.

ONCOGENIC OSTEOMALACIA

Etiology and Clinical Features

Oncogenic osteomalacia is a syndrome seen in association with unusual mesenchymal tumors and rarely with prostate cancer. These patients have hypophosphatemia, renal phosphate wasting, and typically low or inappropriately normal serum levels of 1,25-$(OH)_2$ D. Alkaline phosphatase activity, reflecting bone turnover, is often elevated. Levels of calcium are typically normal, although in some cases PTH levels are elevated. Hypophosphatemia in this syndrome is due to reduced renal phosphate reabsorption. Clinical symptoms include bone pain, proximal muscle weakness, fractures, back pain, waddling gait, and progressive debility. The syndrome often poses a significant diagnostic dilemma to clinicians, because the tumors responsible for it may be very small, obscurely situated, and difficult to identify. Phosphate depletion and low 1,25-$(OH)_2$ D levels lead to poor bone mineralization and osteomalacia. Typically, the diagnosis of osteomalacia is not suspected for years despite the presence of classic symptoms. The humoral basis for the syndrome is supported by the observation that the biochemical abnormalities remit and the osteomalacia heals when the tumor responsible for it is removed.

Pathology and Pathogenesis

Tumors responsible for this form of acquired osteomalacia are usually small and grow slowly. Because the histology of these tumors is unusual and their locations often unanticipated, this syndrome has been dubbed "strange tumours in strange places" by Weiss and colleagues. The range of locations for these tumors includes the lower extremities (45%), head and neck (27%), and upper extremities (17%). In a review of head and neck tumors that cause oncogenic osteomalacia, Gonzalez-Compta and coworkers noted that in 57% and 20% of cases, respectively, tumors were in the sinonasal and mandibular areas. Because these tumors are often small and difficult to find, careful physical examination combined with cranial, chest, and abdominal CT scanning are usually needed for diagnosis. In several instances, MRI skeletal surveys—and in some instances In-111 pentetreotide scanning and PET/CT scans—have been instrumental in localizing the tumors at skeletal sites.

Most tumors causing this syndrome are benign, but malignant lesions have also been reported. The histologic spectrum of tumors has included hemangiomas, hemangiopericytomas, angiosarcomas, chondrosarcomas, prostate cancer, schwannomas, neuroendocrine lesions, mesenchymal tumors, and uncommonly multiple myeloma. Many of these tumors have been classified pathologically as mixed connective tissue tumors and are often located in bone. Osteoclast-like giant cells and stromal cells as well as highly vascular features characterize these tumors. Delays in diagnosis of as long as 19 years have been reported, thereby supporting the hypothesis of slow growth of these tumors.

Many of the tumors responsible for this syndrome overproduce fibroblast growth factor (FGF) 23, a protein important in normal phosphate homeostasis (see Chapter 8). FGF 23 overexpression appears to be responsible for key aspects of oncogenic osteomalacia. FGF 23 levels fall in response to tumor resection, and the above-described biochemical changes and osteomalacia typically resolve after surgery. FGF 23 messenger RNA and protein have been shown to be expressed in many of these tumors. Other genes, however, have also been implicated in the pathogenesis of oncogenic osteomalacia. They include FGF 7, the matrix extracellular phosphoglycoprotein (MEPE), and frizzled related protein 4 (FRP 4).

Investigators in the field have long noted common features between tumor-induced osteomalacia and X-linked hypophosphatemic rickets. The latter condition is a dominant disorder characterized by rickets or osteomalacia, hypophosphatemia, low normal 1,25-$(OH)_2$ D, and typically elevated FGF 23 levels. Despite these similarities, there are several unresolved differences between the two syndromes. One is that levels of 1,25-$(OH)_2$ D are inappropriately normal in patients with X-linked hypophosphatemic rickets and frankly low in oncogenic osteomalacia. In addition, patients with X-linked hypophosphatemic rickets demonstrate osteosclerosis and enthesopathy (calcification of tendons and ligaments) which are not seen in oncogenic osteomalacia.

X-linked hypophosphatemic rickets is due to defective functioning or synthesis of the PEX gene product, or PHEX, a protein that is homologous to neutral, membrane-bound endopeptidases. PHEX is thought to activate or inactivate a circulating factor involved in phosphate metabolism, termed **phosphatonin.** It has long been proposed that the normal function of phosphatonin was to block renal phosphate reabsorption. FGF 23 has been shown to inhibit phosphate uptake in kidney cells. PHEX, the endopeptidase product of the PEX gene, can degrade FGF 23, but FGF 23 is not thought to be a substrate in vivo for PHEX. It has also been shown that PHEX may stabilize MEPE. Thus, there remain several crucial details to establish regarding the pathogenesis of oncogenic osteomalacia and X-linked hypophosphatemic rickets and the varied features of the two disorders.

GUT HORMONES

Gut hormones, including VIP, somatostatin, gastrin-releasing hormone, and pancreatic polypeptide can be produced ectopically, particularly by neuroendocrine tumors (carcinoid, pancreatic islet, and small cell lung cancer). Of these, only ectopic VIP is manifest clinically. Excess VIP can cause an impressive syndrome of voluminous secretory diarrhea, achlorhydria, and hypokalemia. This constellation of symptoms (Verner-Morrison syndrome) has been termed **pancreatic cholera** when caused by a pancreatic VIP-secreting islet cell tumor. A variety of nonendocrine and neuroendocrine tumors can express and release VIP, including small cell carcinomas of the lung, carcinoids, pheochromocytoma, medullary carcinomas of the thyroid, and some colonic adenocarcinomas.

REFERENCES
Hypercalcemia of Malignancy

Bedard PL, Body JJ, Piccart-Gebhart MJ. Sowing the soil for cure? Results of the ABCSG-12 trial open a new chapter in the evolving adjuvant bisphosphonate story in early breast cancer. *J Clin Oncol.* 2009;27:4043. [PMID: 19652062]

Edwards CM, Zhuang J, Mundy GR. The pathogenesis of the bone disease of multiple myeloma. *Bone.* 2008;42:1007. [PMID: 18406675]

Liao J, McCauley LK. Skeletal metastasis: established and emerging roles of parathyroid hormone related protein (PTHrP). *Cancer Metastasis Rev.* 2006;25:559. [PMID: 17165129]

Syndrome of Inappropriate Antidiuretic Hormone Secretion

Decaux G. The syndrome of inappropriate secretion of antidiuretic hormone (SIADH). *Semin Nephrol.* 2009;29:239. [PMID: 19523572]

Ellison DH, Berl T. Clinical practice. The syndrome of inappropriate antidiuresis. *N Engl J Med.* 2007;356:2064. [PMID: 17507705]

Feldman BJ, Rosenthal SM, Vargas GA, et al. Nephrogenic syndrome of inappropriate antidiuresis. *N Engl J Med.* 2005;352:1884. [PMID:15872203]

Kumar S, Berl T. Vasopressin antagonists in the treatment of water-retaining disorders. *Semin Nephrol.* 2008;28:379. [PMID: 18519088]

Cushing Syndrome

Boscaro M, Arnaldi G. Approach to the patient with possible Cushing's syndrome. *J Clin Endocrinol Metab.* 2009;94:3121. [PMID: 19734443]

Ilias I, Torpy DJ, Pacak K, Mullen N, Wesley RA, Nieman LK. Cushing's syndrome due to ectopic corticotropin secretion: twenty years' experience at the National Institutes of Health. *J Clin Endocrinol Metab.* 2005;90:4955. [PMID: 15914534]

Isidori AM, Kaltsas GA, Grossman AB. Ectopic ACTH syndrome. *Front Horm Res.* 2006;35:143. [PMID: 16809930]

Kumar J, Spring M, Carroll PV, Barrington SF, Powrie JK. 18Flurodeoxyglucose positron emission tomography in the localization of ectopic ACTH-secreting neuroendocrine tumours. *Clin Endocrinol (Oxf).* 2006;64:371. [PMID: 16584507]

Lacroix A, Baldacchino V, Bourdeau I, Hamet P, Tremblay J. Cushing's syndrome variants secondary to aberrant hormone receptors. *Trends Endocrinol Metab.* 2004;15:375. [PMID: 15380809]

Salgado LR, Fragoso MC, Knoepfelmacher M, et al. Ectopic ACTH syndrome: our experience with 25 cases. *Eur J Endocrinol.* 2006;155:725. [PMID: 17062889]

Hypoglycemia

de Groot JW, Rikhof B, van Doorn J, et al. Non-islet cell tumour-induced hypoglycaemia: a review of the literature including two new cases. *Endo Rel Canc.* 2007;14:979.[PMID: 18045950]

Fukuda I, Hizuka N, Ishikawa Y, et al. Clinical features of insulin-like growth factor-II producing non-islet-cell tumor hypoglycemia. *Growth Horm IGF Res.* 2006;16:211. [PMID: 16860583]

Gonadotropins

Stenman UH, Alfthan H, Hotakainen K. Human chorionic gonadotropin in cancer. *Clin Biochem.* 2004;37:549. [PMID: 15234236]

Cole LA. New discoveries on the biology and detection of human chorionic gonadotropin. *Reproductive Biol Endocrinol.* 2009;7:8. [PMID: 19171054]

GHRH and Growth Hormone

Biermasz NR, Smit JW, Pereira AM, Frölich M, Romijn JA, Roelfsema F. Acromegaly caused by growth hormone-releasing hormone-producing tumors: long-term observational studies in three patients. *Pituitary.* 2007;10:237. [PMID: 17541749].

Gola M, Doga M, Bonadonna S, Mazziotti G, Vescovi PP, Giustina A. Neuroendocrine tumors secreting growth hormone-releasing hormone:

pathophysiological and clinical aspects. *Pituitary.* 2006;9:221. [PMID: 17036195]

van Hoek M, Hofland LJ, de Rijke YB, et al. Effects of somatostatin analogs on a growth hormone-releasing hormone secreting bronchial carcinoid, in vivo and in vitro studies. *J Clin Endocrinol Metab.* 2009;94:428. [PMID: 19017754]

Calcitonin

Becker KL, Nylén ES, White JC, Müller B, Snider RH Jr. Clinical review 167: procalcitonin and the calcitonin gene family of peptides in inflammation, infection, and sepsis: a journey from calcitonin back to its precursors. *J Clin Endocrinol Metab.* 2004;89:1512. [PMID: 15070906]

Fleury A, Fléjou JF, Sauvanet A, et al. Calcitonin-secreting tumors of the pancreas: about six cases. *Pancreas.* 1998;16:545. [PMID: 9598818]

Oncogenic Osteomalacia

Berndt T, Kumar R. Phosphatonins and the regulation of phosphate homeostasis. *Annu Rev Physiol.* 2007;69:341. [PMID: 17002592]

Carpenter TO, Ellis BK, Insogna KL, Philbrick WM, Sterpka J, Shimkets R. Fibroblast growth factor 7: an inhibitor of phosphate transport derived from oncogenic osteomalacia-causing tumors. *J Clin Endocrinol Metab.* 2005;90:1012. [PMID: 15562028]

Hannan FM, Athanasou NA, Teh J, Gibbons CL, Shine B, Thakker RV. Oncogenic hypophosphataemic osteomalacia: biomarker roles of fibroblast growth factor 23, 1,25-dihydroxyvitamin D3 and lymphatic vessel endothelial hyaluronan receptor 1. *Eur J Endocrinol.* 2008;158:265. [PMID: 18230836]

Hesse E, Moessinger E, Rosenthal H, et al. Oncogenic osteomalacia: exact tumor localization by co-registration of positron emission and computed tomography. *J Bone Miner Res.* 2007;22:158. [PMID: 17014386]

Imel EA, Peacock M, Pitukcheewanont P, et al. Sensitivity of fibroblast growth factor 23 measurements in tumor-induced osteomalacia. *J Clin Endocrinol Metab.* 2006;91:2055. [PMID: 16551733]

Jan de Beur SM, Streeten EA, Civelek AC, et al. Localisation of mesenchymal tumours by somatostatin receptor imaging. *Lancet.* 2002;359:761. [PMID: 11888589]

Kenealy H, Holdaway I, Grey A. Occult nasal sinus tumours causing oncogenic osteomalacia. *Eur J Intern Med.* 2008;19:516. [PMID: 19013380]

Razzaque MS. FGF23-mediated regulation of systemic phosphate homeostasis: is Klotho an essential player? *Am J Physiol Renal Physiol.* 2009;296:F470. [PMID: 19019915]

Weiss D, Bar RS, Weidner N, Wener M, Lee F. Oncogenic osteomalacia: strange tumours in strange places. *Postgrad Med J.* 1985;61:349. [PMID: 4022870]

Woznowski M, Quack I, Stegbauer J, Büchner N, Rump LC, Schieren G. Oncogenic osteomalacia, a rare paraneoplastic syndrome due to phosphate wasting—a case report and review of the literature. *Clin Nephrol.* 2008;70:431. [PMID: 19000546]

Gut Hormones

Song S, Shi R, Li B, Liu Y. Diagnosis and treatment of pancreatic vasoactive intestinal peptide endocrine tumors. *Pancreas.* 2009;38:811. [PMID: 19650770]

Multiple Endocrine Neoplasia

22

David G. Gardner, MD

ACTH	Adrenocorticotropic hormone	MEN	Multiple endocrine neoplasia
CT	Computed tomography	MRI	Magnetic resonance imaging
GDNF	Glial cell line-derived neurotrophic factor	PCR	Polymerase chain reaction
GDNFR	Glial cell line-derived neurotrophic factor receptor	PTH	Parathyroid hormone
GNAS	Gene encoding the alpha subunit of a stimulatory G protein	*RET*	Rearranged during transfection proto-oncogene
MCT	Medullary carcinoma of thyroid	VIP	Vasoactive intestinal peptide
		ZES	Zollinger-Ellison syndrome

A group of heritable syndromes characterized by aberrant growth of benign or malignant tumors in a subset of endocrine tissues have been given the collective term multiple endocrine neoplasia (MEN). The tumors may be functional (ie, capable of elaborating hormonal products that result in specific clinical findings characteristic of the hormone excess state) or nonfunctional. There are three major syndromes: MEN1 is characterized by tumors involving the parathyroid glands, the endocrine pancreas, and the pituitary; MEN 2A includes medullary carcinoma of the thyroid (MCT), pheochromocytoma, and hyperparathyroidism; and MEN 2B, like MEN 2A, includes MCT and pheochromocytoma, but hyperparathyroidism is typically absent.

MULTIPLE ENDOCRINE NEOPLASIA TYPE 1

MEN1, also known as Wermer syndrome, is inherited as an autosomal dominant trait with an estimated prevalence of 2 to 20 per 100,000 in the general population. Approximately 10% of MEN1 mutations arise de novo. The term **sporadic MEN1** has been applied to this group. MEN1 has a number of unusual clinical manifestations (Table 22–1) that occur with variable frequency among individuals within affected kindreds. The earliest age at which manifestations of MEN1 have been reported is 5 years; penetrance is maximal by the fifth decade of life.

Hyperparathyroidism is the most common feature of MEN1, with an estimated penetrance of 95% to 100% over the lifetime of an individual harboring the *MEN1* gene. The diagnosis of hyperparathyroidism is usually made through a combination of clinical and laboratory criteria similar to those used in the identification of sporadic disease (see Chapter 8). It is typically the first clinical manifestation of MEN1, although this varies as a function of the patient population being examined. Hyperparathyroidism in MEN1 is due to hyperplasia of all four parathyroid glands (or more, if supernumerary glands are present). However, involved glands may undergo metachronous enlargement, and selective resection of these glands often results in sustained clinical remissions. MEN1 is a rare cause of hyperparathyroidism, accounting for only 2% to 4% of cases in the general population.

Enteropancreatic tumors in MEN1 (~50% of all MEN1 patients) can be either functional (ie, capable of producing a secreted product with biologic activity) or nonfunctional. Gastrinomas, frequently associated with Zollinger-Ellison syndrome (ZES), represent approximately 40% to 60% of the enteropancreatic tumors associated with this syndrome. Of equal importance, roughly 25% of patients with ZES are found in MEN1 kindreds. Insulinomas constitute approximately 20% of the islet cell tumors, and the remainder represent a collection of functional (eg, glucagon- or vasoactive intestinal peptide [VIP]-producing tumors) and nonfunctional tumors. It is noteworthy that the gastrinomas of MEN1 are often small, multicentric, and

TABLE 22–1 Clinical manifestations of MEN1.

Manifestation	(%)
Hyperparathyroidism	95
Enteropancreatic tumors	30-80
Pituitary adenomas	20-25
Carcinoid tumors	10-20
Adrenal adenomas	25-40
Subcutaneous lipomas	30
Facial angiofibromas	85
Collagenomas	70

ectopically located outside the pancreatic bed, most often in the duodenal submucosa. This latter feature can have a major impact on the therapeutic approach to these patients (discussed later). Gastrinomas in MEN1 are frequently malignant, as are their sporadic counterparts; however, for reasons that are only poorly understood, the biologic behavior of these tumors is less aggressive than those found in sporadic diseases.

The diagnosis of gastrinomas is based on demonstration of hypergastrinemia in the presence of gastric acid hypersecretion. This latter criterion excludes other more common causes of hypergastrinemia (eg, achlorhydria). When the diagnosis is in question, the secretin stimulation test, which stimulates gastrin secretion from gastrinomas but not from normal tissue, may be employed. *Note:* The availability of secretin for parenteral administration is now quite limited. Histamine receptor blockers and proton pump inhibitors reflexively increase serum gastrin levels and should be discontinued 30 hours and 7 days, respectively, prior to testing to exclude gastrinoma. Others have advocated measurements of multiple gastrointestinal hormones following a standardized mixed meal as the most efficient means of detecting the presence of neuroendocrine tumors in MEN1.

Because of their small size, gastrinomas can be difficult to localize in MEN1. Computed tomography (CT) and magnetic resonance imaging (MRI) may be useful in identifying larger lesions but are typically not helpful in identifying smaller ones. These imaging procedures are useful, however, in demonstrating hepatic metastases when present. The most promising localization techniques studied to date include endoscopic and intraoperative ultrasound, selective arterial secretin injection (followed by hepatic vein sampling for gastrin), and radiolabeled octreotide scanning. Each of these has been employed successfully to identify tumors in studies involving small groups of patients. It is important to recognize, however, that almost half of gastrinomas are not found with preoperative localization studies.

Insulinomas in MEN1 are detected using conventional biochemical testing (see Chapter 18). They can also be difficult to localize given their potential for multicentricity. Endoscopic ultrasound and selective arterial infusions of calcium with hepatic vein sampling (for insulin) have been used successfully to identify lesions in small groups of patients.

Glucagonomas, VIPomas, and somatostatinomas are diagnosed based on two fold or greater elevations in plasma glucagons, VIP, or somatostatin levels, respectively, in the presence of one or more pancreatic nodules. Nonfunctional tumors are typically diagnosed following imaging studies after exclusion of elevated levels of the plasma secretory products described above, or, more rarely, following measurement of pancreatic polypeptide levels.

Pituitary adenomas occur in approximately 25% of patients harboring the *MEN-1* gene. The majority secrete prolactin, with or without secretion of excess growth hormone, followed by those secreting growth hormone alone, nonfunctional tumors, and those secreting excessive amounts of adrenocorticotropic hormone (ACTH) (Cushing disease). A prolactinoma variant of MEN1 has been described (Burin variant). This variant is characterized by an increased frequency of prolactinomas, carcinoids, and hyperparathyroidism and infrequent appearance of gastrinomas in affected kindreds. It does not appear to be associated with a specific mutation of the *MEN1* gene. In one instance it has been linked to a germline mutation in the gene encoding the cyclin-dependent kinase inhibitor p27^{Kip1}, but this has not been confirmed in other patients. Pituitary tumors in MEN1 are rarely malignant, but recent studies suggest that they may be larger and more aggressive than their sporadic counterparts. There is a high incidence of macroadenoma, they display a propensity for making more than a single pituitary hormone, and there is a suggestion that these tumors do not respond as well to medical therapy as do their sporadic counterparts. Diagnosis and management are similar to that of their sporadic counterparts (see Chapter 4).

Adrenal adenomas, including cortisol-producing adenomas, are seen in MEN1, theoretically making the differential diagnosis of Cushing syndrome in this setting complex (ie, adrenal adenoma vs basophilic adenoma of the pituitary gland vs ectopic ACTH secretion from a carcinoid tumor, which is also commonly associated with this syndrome). Empirically, most hypercortisolemia in this setting is due to pituitary disease. Adrenal adenomas are often found together with islet cell tumors in affected patients, and at least in some series they appear to lack the MEN1 genetic defect. This has led to the suggestion that they represent a secondary rather than a primary manifestation of the underlying genetic defect. This, however, remains controversial. Pheochromocytomas harboring an MEN1 rather than an MEN2 mutation have been described in seven patients. Thyroid disease has been said to be more common in MEN1; however, with the possible exception of thyroid adenomas, this link remains obscure. Subcutaneous lipomas, skin collagenomas, and multiple facial angiofibromas (particularly on the upper lip and vermillion border of the lip) are seen in 30% to 90% of family members in affected kindreds. Although clinically of little importance, when present, they may prove useful in identifying affected individuals within a kindred and lead to more effective screening (discussed later). Carcinoid tumors are seen with increased frequency in MEN1. They are almost exclusively foregut carcinoids and may be found in the thymus, in the lung (bronchial carcinoids), or in the gastric mucosa. It is likely that chronic hypergastrinemia (eg, that resulting from coexistent ZES and proton pump inhibitor therapy) contributes to the increased incidence of gastric carcinoids in MEN1. For unclear reasons, thymic carcinoids appear more commonly in males, bronchial carcinoids in females. They occasionally secrete hormonal products (eg, ectopic ACTH), are often malignant, and may behave aggressively. Leiomyomas have rarely been described in MEN1. Disease-specific mortality is due to pancreatic islet carcinoma and malignant thymic carcinoid.

Pathogenesis

MEN1 is inherited as an autosomal dominant trait. Traditional linkage studies localized the defective gene to the long arm of chromosome 11q13. Parallel analyses of DNA from endocrine tumors taken from MEN1 patients demonstrated allelic loss in this area, frequently resulting from large DNA deletions. This raised the possibility that the defective gene was a tumor suppressor gene involved in the control of cellular growth. In this paradigm (Figure 22–1), the inherited defective allele is silent in the presence of a normal, functioning allele on the second chromosome. A subsequent somatic mutation (often a deletion that removes the normal allele) results in a null genotype in which the suppressor gene locus is either absent or defective on both alleles. The high frequency with which such deletions occur is thought to account for the dominant nature of this particular genetic defect. Release of the tumor suppressor gene's growth regulatory activity results in a hyperplastic growth response in cells harboring the

somatic mutation. This promitogenic state probably provides the substrate for subsequent somatic mutations that result in acquisition of a more aggressive, and at times malignant, phenotype, as occurs in gastrinomas associated with ZES. Recent studies have succeeded in identifying the gene, termed the *menin* gene, which appears to be responsible for MEN1 (Figure 22–2). Mutations have been identified throughout the entire 610-amino-acid length of the *menin* coding sequence and include nonsense mutations, missense mutations, and deletions. Over 400 independent mutations have been described in MEN1 kindreds to date. Nevertheless, 5% to 10% of presumed MEN1 mutations are not detectable using available methodology. Menin is a ubiquitously expressed tumor suppressor gene product which has been shown to interact with several components of the trithorax family histone methyltransferase complex, including the mixed lineage leukemia (MLL) proteins. Menin, through this complex, controls expression of the cyclin-dependent kinase inhibitors $p27^{Kip1}$ and $p18^{Ink4c}$. This complex also methylates the lysine 4 residue of histone 3 (H3K4), a modification which has been linked to transcriptional activation. Loss of function of menin (eg, through those mutations associated with MEN1) results in downregulation of $p27^{Kip1}$ and $p18^{Ink4c}$ and deregulated cell growth. Menin also suppresses expression of the developmentally programmed transcription factor, HLXB9, which may also lead to increased growth in menin-deficient cells. Mice heterozygous for deletion of the *menin* gene locus (*Men1*+/–)

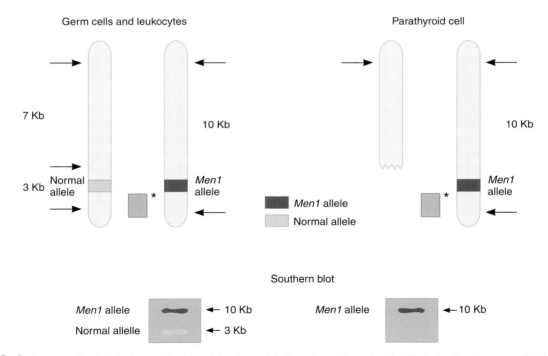

FIGURE 22–1 An example of allelic loss in *Men1* involving large deletion of genetic material. Afflicted patient's germ cells (shown on left) harbor both a normal and defective gene at the *Men1* locus. Each of these is detected using selective restriction enzyme digestion and Southern blot analysis of the genomic DNA. Affected somatic cells (eg, parathyroid chief cells) undergo a second mutation, typically a deletion of the normal allele, resulting in detection of only the mutant allele by Southern analysis. Sporadic disease is thought to follow sequential mutation or deletion of each *Men1* allele in the somatic cell. Solid bar (light purple) with asterisk represents radiolabeled probe used in Southern analysis; arrows indicate points of restriction enzyme digestion.

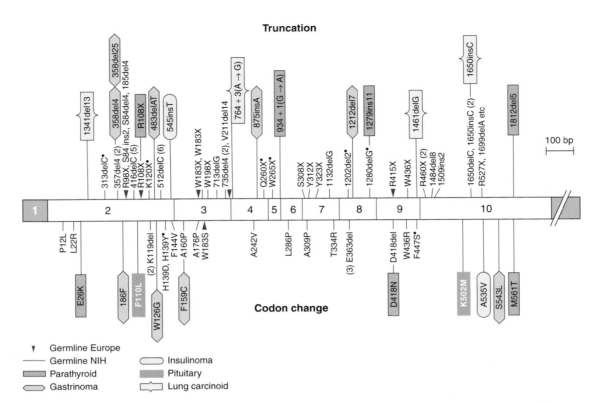

FIGURE 22–2 Some of the more common germline menin mutations from 56 MEN1 kindreds and somatic mutations from 24 endocrine tumors. Mutations above the bar cause protein truncations through stop codons or frameshifts leading to premature stop codons; two cause splice errors. Mutations below the bar cause missense or single-amino-acid codon changes. (Reproduced, with permission, from Marx S, et al. Multiple endocrine neoplasia type 1: clinical and genetic topics. *Ann Intern Med.* 1998;129:484.)

develop parathyroid dysplasia, adenomas, and carcinomas; pancreatic islet tumors, anterior pituitary tumors, and adrenal cortical tumors, all of which display loss of heterozygosity at the *Men* locus.

The *Men1* gene is also the gene most frequently mutated in a variety of sporadic endocrine tumors. Parathyroid adenomas (20%), gastrinomas (40%), insulinomas (15%), VIP-secreting tumors (60%), nonfunctioning pancreatic tumors (15%), glucagonoma (60%), adrenal cortical tumors (<5%), angiofibromas (10%), lipomas (30%), bronchial carcinoids (35%), and pituitary tumors (<5%) often harbor somatic mutations at the *Men1* locus. It is important to note that screening for germline mutations at the *Men1* locus fails to detect mutations 5% to 10% of the time despite evidence for loss of heterozygosity at 11q13. It is thought that the relevant mutations may be in regulatory regions surrounding the *Men1* gene. Haplotype testing or genetic linkage analysis can be useful in these cases to identify relevant *Men1* carriers. Unlike MEN2 (see later), there is no clear association between specific *Men1* gene mutations and the nature or extent of endocrine gland involvement, although nonsense mutations at Tyr^{312} and Arg^{460} have been shown to be more common with the Burin variant.

Treatment

Therapy of hyperparathyroidism in MEN1 is directed toward surgical extirpation of hyperplastic parathyroid tissue, typically with resection of three and one-half glands. This leaves one-half gland in situ in an attempt to preserve residual parathyroid function and avoid hypoparathyroidism. Alternatively, patients may be subjected to total parathyroidectomy with transplantation of the most normal appearing tissue to the nondominant forearm. There have been no head-to-head comparisons made between these approaches. Total parathyroidectomy (with transplant) is associated with a higher frequency of hypoparathyroidism, whereas subtotal parathyroidectomy has a higher rate of recurrence. Prophylactic near-total thymectomy is often performed at the time of neck exploration to remove potential intrathymic parathyroid glands as well as thymic carcinoid tumors.

Both persistence and recurrence of hyperparathyroidism occur more frequently in MEN1 than in sporadic disease. Persistence of hyperparathyroidism, defined as a failure to normalize serum calcium and parathyroid hormone (PTH) levels following the initial surgery, with removal of 3 to 3.5 parathyroid glands, occurs in 12% of cases of MEN1. Recurrent disease, defined as reappearance of hyperparathyroidism following at least 3 months of normocalcemia, is seen in as many as 44% of these cases 8 to 12 years following surgery. The high frequency of persistent hyperparathyroidism in MEN1 probably reflects the high frequency of supernumerary glands (prevalence as high as 30%) and ectopically located parathyroid tissue in patients carrying the *Men1* gene. The increased frequency of recurrent disease is thought to result from the continued presence of the underlying mitogenic stimulus that drives parathyroid gland growth in this syndrome. Reoperation for recurrent disease in the neck is successful about 90% of the time, whereas autograft removal is successful in about 60% of patients.

Therapy of gastrinomas in MEN1 remains controversial. Suppression of gastric acid production with proton pump inhibitors (eg, omeprazole) remains a mainstay of therapy. Conservative medical management of these tumors has been predicated on their assumed low-grade malignant behavior, the dominance of complications related to gastric acid hypersecretion in contributing to morbidity and mortality, and the failure of most attempts at surgical resection to alter the natural course of the disease. More recently, recognition of the potential for more aggressive behavior in some of these tumors—in a recent study, 14% of these tumors demonstrated aggressive growth—and the fact that many of these tumors are ectopically located in duodenal submucosa and peripancreatic lymph nodes rather than the pancreatic bed has renewed interest in the possibility of surgical cure. A number of small studies have reported encouraging results when measures to both localize and remove gastrinoma tissue in the pancreas, duodenum, and regional lymph nodes have been used. Although the nature of the underlying genetic lesion and the multicentricity of these tumors may place limits on the prospects for cure of this disease in most patients, the slow growth characteristics of these tumors permit long periods of symptom-free survival following reduction of the tumor burden. For patients with liver or other metastatic disease, symptoms related to hypergastrinemia may be controlled with the proton pump antagonists, as described earlier. More conventional cancer therapy (eg, systemic chemotherapy, radiation therapy, or selective chemoembolization of hepatic metastases) is palliative and reserved for advanced stages of the disease. Islet tumors more than 3 cm carry an increased risk of malignancy and are usually resected regardless of functional status.

It is important to remember that calcium stimulates gastric acid secretion. This may occur through gastrin-dependent and gastrin-independent pathways. In MEN1 patients with both hyperparathyroidism and ZES, correction of the hyperparathyroidism and attendant hypercalcemia frequently results in a reduction in both basal and maximal acid output and a decline in serum gastrin levels. Secretin stimulation tests often normalize following parathyroidectomy. More importantly, there is a reduction in the dose of medication (eg, proton pump inhibitor) required to control symptoms of ZES following parathyroid surgery in approximately 60% of patients.

Unlike gastrinomas, insulinomas are rarely localized outside the pancreatic bed. Therefore, a more aggressive approach can be directed toward the pancreas in planning surgical resection. Enucleation of the identifiable lesions in the pancreatic head and blind resection of the pancreatic body and tail are often more successful in correcting hyperinsulinemia than in restoring normal gastrin levels in patients with ZES. Nonsurgical candidates (eg, those with serious coexisting disease or those in whom candidate tumors cannot be identified) can be managed with conventional medical therapy (eg, diazoxide or verapamil). (See Chapter 18.)

Nonfunctional tumors, the most common pancreatoduodenal neuroendocrine tumors in MEN1, are managed somewhat differently than the functional tumors. Surgical efforts to minimize spread of metastases are weighed against the need to avoid incurring surgical complications, including mortality, with little clinical benefit. In general, surgery is not recommended for tumors less than 2 cm in diameter. Life expectancy of MEN1 patients with nonfunctional tumors (~43 years) is similar to that of those with gastrinomas and considerably shorter than those with other types of functional tumors (~61 years).

Screening

MEN1 accounts for less than 1% of all pituitary tumors, 2% to 4% of cases of primary hyperparathyroidism, and about 25% of all gastrinomas. Thus, although routine screening for *Men1* gene mutations is not indicated for sporadic cases of hyperparathyroidism or patients with pituitary tumors, screening of all cases of ZES is likely to be cost-effective in identifying carriers. The frequency of germline mutations in the *Men1* gene in patients with tumors thought to be sporadic based on family analysis is about 5% for gastrinomas and 1% to 2% for other manifestations (eg, hyperparathyroidism, prolactinomas). Excluding those patients with ZES, screening for MEN1 outside affected MEN1 kindreds should be limited to those individuals for whom the index of suspicion for the syndrome is high (eg, familial history of endocrine tumors or hypersecretory states; history of multiple endocrine tumors or multigland involvement with hyperparathyroidism in the propositus). Identification of the carrier state should be performed with the intent of acquiring information that allows the clinician to focus screening on the relevant patient population (eg, members of an affected kindred who do not share the *Men1* gene mutation need not be subjected to follow-up screening). Unlike the situation in MEN2 (see later), carrier analysis should not be used to support a major therapeutic intervention. Such interventions (eg, pancreatic exploration) may be associated with significant morbidity, and there is no evidence that they prolong patient survival. Patients with hyperparathyroidism should be screened for MEN1—even in the absence of a positive family history or any history of multiple endocrine tumors—if parathyroid hyperplasia is identified at the time of parathyroidectomy or if there is a history of recurrent hyperparathyroidism following parathyroidectomy. Patients with ZES should be screened for MEN1 given its high frequency (~25%) in such individuals. Patients with isolated pituitary lesions have a low probability of having coexistent MEN1 and probably do not require screening unless there are other clinical features suggesting the syndrome. Genetic screening is available commercially at a number of locations (see www.genetests.org).

Although most clinicians agree that screening for MEN1 in high-risk groups is worthwhile, details of the individual screening protocols vary considerably—from more focused, cost-effective approaches to broad-based screening designed to detect occult disease. One example of a moderately cost-effective protocol is presented in Figure 22–3. A complete examination and full family history should be obtained on all patients. In individuals within

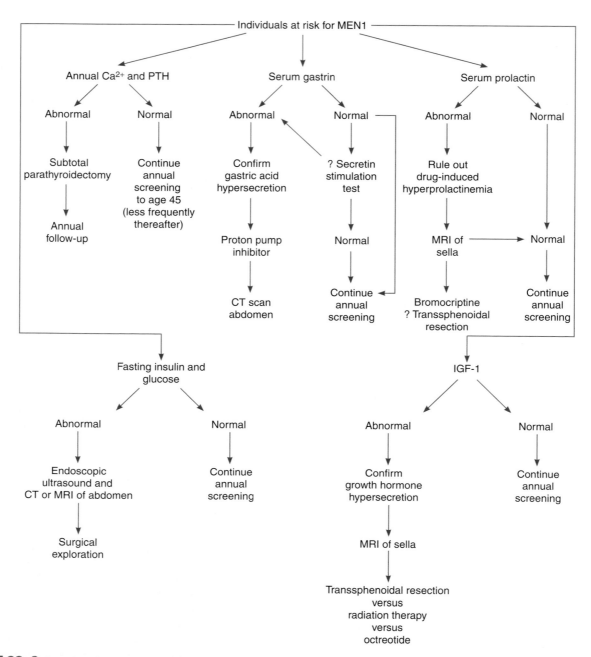

FIGURE 22–3 Screening for MEN1. Testing is targeted to individuals with a high probability of harboring the *MEN1* gene (eg, first-degree relatives of affected kindred members). If genetic testing is available and the specific mutation has been confirmed, screening would be limited to those individuals harboring the defective gene. Screening for other pancreatic (eg, insulinomas) or pituitary tumors (eg, somatotroph adenomas) is based on the prevalence of the specific lesion in the affected kindred or the presence of signs or symptoms suggesting a particular lesion (IGF, insulin-like growth factor).

affected kindreds, ionized (or albumin-corrected) calcium and PTH levels should be checked at yearly intervals. Fasting serum gastrin levels should also be determined annually—or more frequently if ZES is a prominent component of the phenotype in the affected kindred. In kindreds in whom the disease is particularly aggressive, the secretin stimulation test (if available) can lend to

additional diagnostic sensitivity. Determination of fasting glucose, insulin, and proinsulin levels may prove useful, particularly if symptoms of hypoglycemia are present. Pancreatic polypeptide measurements may identify an unsuspected pancreatic neuroendocrine tumor. Levels of chromogranin A, a secretory product of parathyroid glands and other neuroendocrine tissues, can also be helpful in assessing nonspecific endocrine gland hypersecretion. Routine screening for other functional or nonfunctional islet cell tumors is probably not justified without clinical findings (eg, watery diarrhea, hypokalemia). As noted earlier, these lesions are typically multifocal and may be very small, which makes detection difficult even with sophisticated imaging studies. The same holds true for the pituitary lesions. In the absence of obvious clinical findings (eg, evidence of a hyper- or hyposecretory state or symptoms referable to a mass lesion in the sella turcica), routine screening should be confined to periodic measurements of serum prolactin and perhaps insulin-like growth factor-I. The former has been found to be useful in identifying pituitary disease in females harboring the *Men1* gene defect. Imaging studies (eg, MRI of the pituitary and anterior mediastinum, CT of the abdomen) should be performed at presentation and repeated at 3-year intervals. A thorough family history that excludes pituitary disease in the kindred may mitigate the need for pituitary imaging studies over the long term.

Follow-up screening in patients known to have MEN1 should include yearly fasting gastrin, calcium, albumin, PTH, chromogranin A, and pancreatic polypeptide levels from age 10 on. Some clinicians have argued that these patients should have annual CT or MRI studies of the abdomen and prolactin measurements plus MRI of the sella every other year; in addition, consideration should be given to performing an annual CT of the chest (see Glascock and Carty). Others have argued for imaging studies on presentation and every 3 years thereafter (see Schussheim et al).

Penetrance of MEN1 is greater than 95% by age 45. Screening should be continued at periodic intervals at least to age 45. If there is no evidence of typical endocrine organ involvement by that age, screening frequency might be reduced. It is important to note, however, that the risk is not reduced to zero at age 45. A minority of patients presents with their first manifestation of the syndrome well after age 45. Surgical resection of diseased tissue (eg, parathyroidectomy) should be followed with continued screening looking both for recurrent disease and involvement of other organ systems.

MULTIPLE ENDOCRINE NEOPLASIA TYPE 2

MEN2 is an autosomal dominant disorder with an estimated prevalence of 1 to 10 per 100,000 in the general population. It can be subdivided into two independent syndromes: MEN 2A (Sipple syndrome) and MEN 2B. Manifestations of MEN 2A include MCT, pheochromocytoma, and hyperparathyroidism. MEN 2B includes MCT, pheochromocytoma, and a number of somatic manifestations (Table 22–2; Figure 22–4), but hyperparathyroidism is rare. Penetrance of MEN2 is greater than 80% in individuals harboring the defective gene.

Medullary carcinoma of the thyroid is the most common manifestation of MEN2 and often represents the first clinical presentation in individuals with multiorgan involvement. It also dominates the clinical course of patients affected with the disease.

TABLE 22-2 Clinical manifestations of MEN2.

Manifestation	(%)
MEN 2A	
Medullary carcinoma of thyroid	80-100
Pheochromocytoma	40
Hyperparathyroidism	25
MEN 2B	
Medullary carcinoma of thyroid	100
Pheochromocytoma	50
Marfanoid habitus	75
Mucosal neuromas	100
Ganglioneuromatosis of bowel	>40

Eighty percent to 100% of individuals at risk develop MCT at some point during their lifetime. The classic thyroid lesion of MEN2 is hyperplasia of the calcitonin-producing parafollicular cells, which typically serves as the precursor of MCT. These tumors in MEN2 patients tend to be multicentric and concentrated in the upper third of the thyroid gland, reflecting the normal distribution of parafollicular cells.

As much as one-fourth of all MCT is genetic in origin. Roughly 30% of the heritable fraction is attributable to *MEN 2A*; 65% occurs as an isolated entity (isolated familial MCT), and 5% is found in *MEN 2B* kindreds. Isolated familial MCT is defined as MCT presenting as the only clinical manifestation in more than 10 carriers in a kindred and multiple carriers or affected members over the age of 50 with adequate history and laboratory support

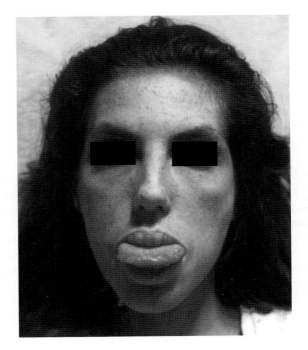

FIGURE 22–4 Patient with MEN 2B syndrome. Note the multiple neuromas on the lips and tongue and the marfanoid facies.

to rule out the presence of pheochromocytoma or hyperparathyroidism. The disease tends to behave more aggressively in MEN 2B than with either MEN 2A or familial MCT, with earlier presentation (often before age 5) and more rapid progression.

Biochemical diagnosis depends heavily on the calcitonin-producing properties of the hyperplastic parafollicular cells or MCT. These lesions respond to pentagastrin or calcium infusions with significant increments in plasma calcitonin levels (see Chapter 8). Occasionally, immunohistochemical staining of poorly differentiated thyroid tumors for calcitonin reveals the identity of the malignancy. The presence of extracellular amyloid is also one of the identifying features of these tumors. This material reacts with anticalcitonin antisera, suggesting that it includes aggregated hormone released from neighboring tumor cells. MCT spreads initially within the thyroid bed and to regional lymph nodes. Distant metastases to liver, lung, and bone occur late in the course of the disease.

Pheochromocytomas develop in approximately 50% of individuals harboring the *MEN2* gene. They are usually located in the adrenal bed, often are bilateral, and are rarely malignant. Diagnosis is based on standard clinical criteria (eg, hypertension, presence of headaches, palpitations, diaphoresis), elevations in plasma or urine catecholamines or catecholamine metabolites (eg, urinary or plasma metanephrine or normetanephrine), and demonstration of an adrenal mass on conventional abdominal imaging. As noted above for MCT, pheochromocytomas in MEN2 are preceded by a hyperplastic phase (adrenal medullary hyperplasia), although, unlike parafollicular cell hyperplasia, the adrenal precursor lesion can be difficult to detect with conventional biochemical testing.

As in MEN1, hyperparathyroidism in MEN2 is due to hyperplasia of the parathyroid glands. It is seen in about 25% of patients harboring the *MEN2A* gene and is reported, but rarely seen, as part of MEN 2B. The disease is usually less aggressive than its counterpart in MEN1 and approximates more closely the behavior of sporadic disease. It responds well to surgical management.

A number of other phenotypic features are associated with the MEN2 syndromes. Cutaneous lichen amyloidosis is a pruritic erythematous skin lesion that is seen coincident with or often preceding the development of MCT in MEN2. Amyloid in these lesions is composed of keratin rather than calcitonin, as seen in MCT. Cutaneous lichen amyloidosis is thought to result from an abnormality in cutaneous innervation that leads to hyperesthesia and pruritis. Repeated scratching of the pruritic area results in epidermal thickening and increased pigmentation. It has been noted more frequently in association with specific mutations of the *MEN2* gene (specifically Cys^{634} to Tyr^{634}). In a second variant, MEN 2A or familial MCT is associated with Hirschsprung disease (congenital megacolon). This is most frequently found with *RET* gene mutations involving Cys^{609}, Cys^{615}, and Cys^{620}(see below). The intestinal ganglioneuromatosis, mucosal neuromas, marfanoid habitus, and medullated corneal nerves seen in MEN 2B appear to be related to the underlying genetic defect The intestinal lesions can disrupt gut motility, resulting in periods of severe constipation or diarrhea.

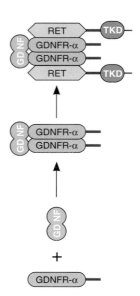

FIGURE 22–5 Structure of GDNFR-α/RET receptor complex. GDNF identifies the ligand, glial cell line–derived neurotrophic factor, and GDNFR-α the GDNF receptor (TKD, tyrosine kinase domain).

Pathogenesis

The pathogenesis of the MEN2 syndromes has been worked out in elegant detail. Traditional genetic linkage studies localized the defective genes in MEN 2A, MEN 2B, and familial MCT to the pericentromeric region of chromosome 10. Subsequent refinement in these analyses indicated that the defective gene was either closely linked to or identical with the *ret* proto-oncogene. RET is a single transmembrane domain, tyrosine kinase-linked protein that forms part of the receptor for the glial cell line–derived neurotrophic factor (GDNF) (see Figure 22–5). This receptor, GDNFR (glial cell line–derived neurotrophic factor receptor), is a glycosyl phosphatidyl inositol-linked cell-surface protein. Additional ligands, neurturin, persephin, and artemin have been shown to associate with and activate RET through their cognate receptors GDNFR$_{α1-4}$. As depicted schematically in Figure 22–6, its most striking structural feature is a series of cysteine residues clustered just outside the membrane-spanning segment. These cysteine residues are thought to exert a tonic inhibitory control on RET activity in the normal cell. RET also has a cadherin-like domain in that portion of the molecule projecting into the extracellular space and a tyrosine kinase-like domain in the intracellular portion of the molecule. RET is expressed endogenously in a variety of cells of neural crest origin, and it appears to play an important role in development. Knockout of the *RET* gene locus in mice results in the absence of myenteric ganglia in the submucosa of the small and large intestine and a variety of genitourinary anomalies, implying an important role in renal development.

Characterization of the *RET* gene in patients with MEN 2A demonstrated a number of mutations in affected kindred members that were not present in their normal counterparts. The mutations were clustered in the cysteines located in RET's extracellular, juxtamembrane domain (see Figure 22–6). Structurally,

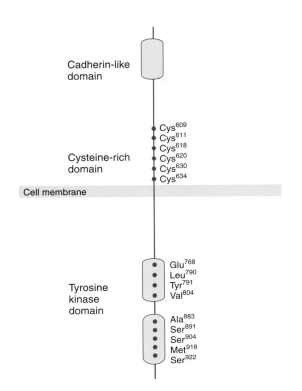

FIGURE 22–6 Structural schematic of wild-type RET, including amino acids that have been shown to be mutated in different disease states. MEN 2A is associated with mutations of Cys^{609}, Cys^{611}, Cys^{618}, Cys^{620}, Cys^{630}, Cys^{634}, and, rarely, Leu^{790} and Tyr^{791}. Familial MCT of the thyroid is frequently associated with mutations at the same Cys residues with the exception of Cys^{634}, as well as mutations at Glu^{768}, Leu^{790}, Tyr^{791}, Val^{804}, and Ser^{891}. MEN 2B mutations typically involve Met^{918} or, more rarely, Ala^{883}, Ser^{922}, or Val^{804}/Ser^{904}. Hirschsprung disease is associated with multiple mutations or deletions extending over the full length of the RET molecule.

these cysteines are encoded by nucleotides in exons 10 and 11 of the *RET* gene. A number of these mutations were simple missense mutations, whereas others involved deletion or insertion of small segments of DNA, but in each case one of the aforementioned cysteines proved to be involved. Selective mutation of one of these six cysteines has now been shown to account for more than 97% of all *RET* mutations associated with MEN 2A. The most frequently mutated residue is Cys^{634}. This amino acid is mutated to arginine (Arg), phenylalanine (Phe), serine (Ser), glycine (Gly), tyrosine (Tyr), or tryptophan (Trp) in approximately 84% of affected MEN 2A kindreds. It has been suggested that mutation of Cys^{634} to Arg^{634} is associated with the phenotypic expression of hyperparathyroidism, whereas mutation of Cys^{634} to any of the amino acids indicated above is linked to pheochromocytoma. It should be noted that the Cys-to-Arg mutation at position 634 is also the most common mutation at this position, accounting for about 64% of all codon changes at this location. Interestingly, a rare but unique mutation involving a four-amino-acid insertion between Cys^{634} and Arg^{635} has been described that results in MCT and a high incidence of hyperparathyroidism but not pheochromocytoma.

Ironically, patients with familial MCT display many of the same cysteine mutations identified in MEN 2A. This implies the existence of independent modulatory genomic factors that restrict the effects of the *RET* mutation to the parafollicular cells of the thyroid in familial MCT. The exception is the mutation of Cys^{634} to Arg^{634}, which is almost uniformly associated with MEN 2A. Several additional mutations have been identified that may be more specific for familial MCT (Figure 22–6). The observation that mutations of Cys^{634} have higher transforming potential than mutations at these other residues has led to the suggestion that MEN 2A represents the more severe phenotype (vs familial MCT) along a spectrum of disease resulting from RET activation. In fact, the noncysteine mutations, which are more common in familial MCT (as high as 60% of familial MCT in one series), are associated with delayed onset of parafollicular C cell disease, but other clinical features (tumor size, bilaterality, the presence of nodal metastases) were not different in patients harboring cysteine versus noncysteine mutations.

Interestingly, patients with MEN 2B do not harbor mutations in the cysteine residues affected in MEN 2A and familial MCT. Instead, the majority possess a single-point mutation involving conversion of Met^{918} to Thr^{918}. This mutation is found in more than 95% of cases of MEN 2B. A minority of patients have been shown to harbor an independent mutation of Ala^{883} to Phe^{883}, Ser^{922} to Tyr^{922}, or a mono-allelic combination of Val^{804} to Met^{804} plus Ser^{904} to Cys^{904}. MEN 2B arises from spontaneous de novo mutations in as many as 50% of affected individuals. For unknown reasons, these mutations are found almost exclusively on the paternal allele.

A number of the germline mutations identified in MEN 2A and familial MCT and the Met^{918} mutation in MEN 2B have been demonstrated as somatic mutations in sporadic MCT (~30%-40%) and pheochromocytoma (<10%). Sporadic parathyroid disease due to these mutations is not known to occur. The presence of the Met^{918} mutation, in particular, is associated with a less favorable clinical outcome in sporadic MCT.

Independent studies have shown a close linkage between the *RET* gene locus and Hirschsprung disease, a disorder characterized by failure of myenteric ganglia to develop normally in the hindgut of affected individuals. This leads to impaired gut motility and, in severe cases, megacolon (a phenotype similar to that reported for the *RET* knockout mice). Examination of *RET* coding sequence in Hirschsprung kindreds revealed a variety of mutations in both the intracellular and extracellular domains, some of which (eg, deletions) would be predicted to eliminate normal expression of the *RET* gene. This, together with findings from the *RET*, *GDNF*, and *GDNFRα-1* knockout mice, suggests that Hirschsprung disease represents the null phenotype for the *RET* locus. Interestingly, several patients have been described who possess features of both MEN2 and Hirschsprung disease. The *RET* mutations in these cases have involved conversion of Cys^{609}, Cys^{618}, or Cys^{620} to Arg. These mutations, while promoting dimerization and increasing tyrosine kinase activity in the RET protein (see below), also appear to have difficulty trafficking to and accumulating in the plasma membrane. It is conceivable that predominance of one or the other of these mechanisms in different cell types could result in a phenotype characterized by both activation (eg, MEN2) and suppression (eg, Hirschsprung disease) of RET activity in the same individual.

By inference, the defect in RET function in MEN2 or familial MCT arises from increased or altered activity of the RET tyrosine kinase. In the case of RET_{MEN2A}, the increase in activity appears to arise from interference with the tonic inhibition of RET tyrosine kinase activity by the clustered cysteine residues in the extracellular domain. This leads to increased dimer formation, autophosphorylation, and tyrosine kinase activity in the mutant RET molecules. In the case of RET_{MEN2B}, there appears to be a change in substrate specificity of the tyrosine kinase that contributes to the phenotype. The activity of RET_{MEN2B}—rather than being restricted to conventional RET substrates (RET substrates are similar to those recognized by the epidermal growth factor receptor)—is capable of phosphorylating substrates normally recognized by members of the Src and Abl families of cytoplasmic tyrosine kinases, signaling pathways which are closely identified with the regulation of cell growth. Thus, it appears that RET_{MEN2B} has acquired the capacity for activation of a potent mitogenic pathway in the expressing endocrine cells merely by altering its selection of substrates for phosphorylation. RET_{MEN2B} also potentiates phosphorylation of Tyr^{1062} more effectively than RET_{MEN2A}. This tyrosine serves as a docking site for multiple effector proteins, including Shc and phosphatidyl inositol 3′-kinase, implying that RET_{MEN2B} may be more effective in triggering downstream signaling pathways.

Treatment

Treatment of heritable MCT should include total thyroidectomy with at least central lymph node dissection. Given the multicentric nature of the disease, subtotal thyroidectomy predictably results in recurrent disease. Basal or stimulated calcitonin levels are used in the postoperative setting to evaluate the presence of residual disease. The precise timing of surgery in patients with subclinical disease (ie, positive by genetic testing but without clinical or laboratory abnormalities) is controversial (see later), but most clinicians would agree that in kindreds with MEN 2B or clinically aggressive MCT, patients should undergo surgery as soon as the genetic defect is demonstrated. Typically, this is before age 6 months in MEN 2B (eg, mutation at Ala^{883} or Met^{918}) and before age 5 years in MEN 2A (eg, mutation at Cys^{611}, Cys^{618}, Cys^{620}, or Cys^{634}). Foci of microscopic MCT are common, and metastatic disease has been described in the first year of life in patients with MEN 2B. The presence of a thyroid nodule or lymph node metastases at the time of diagnosis is strongly associated with persistent or recurrent disease. Mutations associated with familial MCT (eg, Cys^{609}, Glu^{768}, Leu^{790}, Tyr^{791}, Val^{804}, or Ser^{891}) tend to be associated with more indolent disease. Some have suggested that surgery in these patients can be deferred until plasma calcitonin levels (basal or stimulated) are elevated. Patients should always be screened for the presence of pheochromocytoma before undergoing neck exploration. Surgery for metastatic disease is palliative and targeted at reducing tumor burden rather than cure. Localization techniques (eg, MRI or selective venous

sampling for calcitonin) can be helpful in identifying foci of malignant tissue. Recent clinical trials have used a tyrosine kinase inhibitor D6474 (Zactima) to inhibit the RET kinase with an objective remission rate of approximately 30%. Radiation and chemotherapy are of limited utility and are largely confined to later stages of the disease.

Treatment of pheochromocytomas in MEN2 is similar to that for sporadic pheochromocytomas (see Chapter 11). Alpha- and (occasionally) beta-adrenergic blockade is used to control blood pressure and associated hyperadrenergic symptoms and to restore normal intravascular volume in preparation for surgical resection of the tumor. Given the propensity for bilaterality of pheochromocytomas in this disorder, some have favored bilateral adrenalectomy at the time of initial surgery. However, because the incidence of bilaterality is well under 100% and because these tumors are rarely malignant, the most prudent strategy in the face of unilateral adrenal enlargement would appear to be unilateral adrenalectomy at the initial surgery with careful attention at follow-up, looking for the presence of disease in the contralateral adrenal gland. This vigilant approach has the advantage of minimizing morbidity from recurrent pheochromocytoma while sparing the patient the risks associated with lifelong adrenal insufficiency.

Screening

Genetic screening for MEN 2A, MEN 2B, or familial MCT is routinely carried out using polymerase chain reaction (PCR)-based tests designed to identify specific mutations in the RET coding sequence (Figure 22–7; see www.genetests.org for laboratories performing these tests). Known RET mutations account for more than 95% of all instances of MEN2, and selected mutations (eg, Cys^{634} to Arg^{634} in MEN 2A) account for a disproportionate number of affected individuals. Individuals lacking any of the known RET mutations can be tested using conventional haplotype analysis if informative genetic markers and affected family members are available. Biochemical testing using basal or stimulated plasma calcitonin levels has been largely supplanted by genetic screens. The biochemical tests remain useful, however, in identifying residual disease after thyroidectomy.

In view of the fact that a high proportion of cases of MCT are familial to begin with and as much as 6% of patients with apparently sporadic MCT harbor germline RET mutations, genetic testing for RET germline mutations is probably indicated for all patients presenting with MCT. Controversy persists, however, in terms of what should be done for patients once the mutation has been identified. Some investigators citing incomplete clinical penetrance (according to published data, 40% of gene carriers do not present symptomatically prior to age 70) have argued that employing solely genetic criteria in making the decision for operative intervention subjects a small minority of patients to premature thyroidectomy. They argue that genetic testing should be used to identify those patients who require close clinical and biochemical surveillance to assist with the timing of surgery. Ideally, such biochemical testing (eg, pentagastrin stimulation) should be performed on an annual basis. Exceptions to this general approach might include patients with MEN 2B or a particularly aggressive

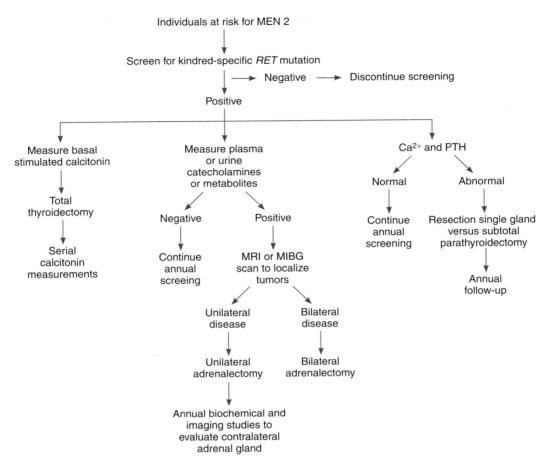

FIGURE 22–7 Screening for MEN 2A. Genetic screening has largely supplanted biochemical testing in identifying individuals at risk. Details of decisions regarding treatment are discussed in the text. Preoperative plasma calcitonin levels are potentially useful for follow-up but should not supplant genetic testing in assessing the need for surgery (MIBG, metaiodobenzylguanidine; *RET*, rearranged during transfection proto-oncogene). (See also Figure 7–48.)

form of familial MCT where the potential for significant morbidity and mortality would justify operation in any patient harboring the genetic defect regardless of the physical or biochemical manifestations of the disease.

The more widely shared view is that the true penetrance of MCT—combined clinical and preclinical disease—in MEN 2A is closer to 100%. This, when coupled with the high degree of sensitivity and specificity of the PCR-based genetic screens, difficulties encountered in obtaining adequate long-term patient follow-up and biochemical screening, and the potential for false-positive pentagastrin stimulation tests—even within MEN2 kindreds—has led to the recommendation that total thyroidectomy should be performed in all individuals harboring an MEN2–associated *RET* mutation. This argument has now been supported by several clinical studies in which parafollicular cell hyperplasia as well as early MCT have been identified in operative specimens taken from genetically affected individuals despite normal pentagastrin stimulation tests. False-positive biochemical tests are also a concern. There are several reports in the literature of patients in

affected kindreds who have undergone total thyroidectomy following positive pentagastrin stimulation tests but did not, in fact, harbor the *MEN2* gene mutation. Histologic examination of excised tissues revealed parafollicular cell hyperplasia, presumably unrelated to MEN2, but no MCT. Collectively, these findings point out the relative deficiencies of biochemical versus genetic testing and offer a compelling argument for early operation as a means of reliably eradicating the disease.

OTHER DISORDERS CHARACTERIZED BY MULTIPLE ENDOCRINE ORGAN INVOLVEMENT

Carney Complex

Carney complex is an autosomal dominant disorder characterized by cardiac, endocrine, cutaneous, and neural tumors. Myxomas of the heart, breast, and skin are seen frequently in this disorder, as is spotty pigmentation of the skin (lentiginosis) and ear canal trichofolliculo-epitheliomas. Additional rare manifestations include psammomatous melanotic schwannoma, breast ductal adenoma, and osteochondromyxoma. Endocrine tumors include primary pigmented micronodular adrenocortical hyperplasia (an ACTH-independent form of Cushing syndrome), follicular thyroid carcinomas, adrenocortical carcinoma, somatotroph (growth hormone–secreting) adenomas of the pituitary gland, large-cell calcifying Sertoli cell tumors of the testes, and ovarian cysts. In approximately half of the known Carney complex kindreds, the genetic lesion maps to 17q22-24, a locus that harbors the type 1 regulatory subunit of protein kinase A. This gene functions as a classic tumor suppressor, and loss of heterozygosity at this locus is associated with the Carney phenotype. A second locus, presumably accounting for the remaining approximately half of Carney complex kindreds, is located at 2p16. The nature of the genetic lesion at this locus remains unknown at present; however, the phenotype is indistinguishable from that found with the 17q22-24 mutations alluded to above.

McCune-Albright Syndrome

The central findings in McCune-Albright syndrome include bony fibrous dysplasia (either monostotic or polyostotic, café au lait spots, and gonadotropin-independent precocious puberty). However, affected individuals also develop tumors or nodular hyperplasia of a number of endocrine glands with associated hypersecretory syndromes. One may see involvement of the pituitary somatotrophs (acromegaly), thyroid gland (hyperthyroidism), or the adrenal cortex (hypercortisolemia). Patients with McCune-Albright syndrome frequently demonstrate hypophosphatemic rickets. This is thought to result from secretion of fibroblast growth factor-23 that is produced in the mesenchymal cells associated with the dysplastic bone lesions. They also have nonendocrine organ involvement that leads to cardiomyopathy with sudden death and liver function abnormalities. The molecular lesion in McCune-Albright syndrome involves a somatic activating mutation of GNAS at the Arg^{201} position, converting the Arg to either Cys or His (see Chapter 1), that leads to ligand-independent activation of adenylyl cyclase and increased intracellular concentrations of cyclic AMP. This somatic mutation is thought to occur early in development, leading to genetic mosaicism for the mutant allele. The phenotype of an individual patient is determined by the tissue distribution of the mutation-bearing cells and the percentage of cells within a given tissue that harbor the mutation. Interestingly, GNAS mutations have been described in a subset of patients harboring intramuscular myxomas (Mazabraud syndrome) with or without associated fibrous dysplasia, a feature that is reminiscent of the Carney complex (see above), another genetic disease which seems to target the cyclic AMP-signaling pathway.

Neurofibromatosis Type 1

Neurofibromatosis type 1 (von Recklinghausen disease) is an autosomal dominant genetic disorder characterized by a variety of skin manifestations, including caféaulait spots, subcutaneous neurofibromas, and axillary and inguinal freckles as well as neural gliomas (eg, optic nerve) and hamartomas of the iris (Lisch nodules). In addition, patients may have a number of endocrine neoplasias, including pheochromocytoma, hyperparathyroidism, MCT, and somatostatin-producing carcinoid tumors of the duodenal wall. The genetic lesion in neurofibromatosis type 1 is located at 17q11.2, a locus that harbors the neurofibromin gene. Neurofibromin is a homolog of the p21 Ras-dependent GTPase-activating proteins and is thought to function in a tumor suppressor mode through regulation of Ras-dependent signaling activity.

Von Hippel-Lindau Disease

Von Hippel-Lindau disease is a heritable autosomal dominant disorder characterized by retinal and cerebellar hemangioblastomas, renal cell carcinoma, islet cell tumors, pheochromocytomas, and renal, pancreatic, and epididymal cysts. The presence of pheochromocytomas and most of the islet cell tumors is confined to the type 2 variant of the disease, which accounts for 25% to 35% of affected kindreds. The genetic lesion has been localized to 3p25. The von Hippel-Lindau protein, which is normally encoded by this locus, participates in the formation of a multiprotein complex involved in the regulation of hypoxia-induced gene transcriptional activity, fibronectin matrix assembly, and ubiquitin ligases.

MEN X

This is a rare syndrome, inherited in autosomal recessive fashion, in which affected patients display a tumor spectrum that overlaps those of MEN1 and MEN2. This syndrome has been linked to a germ line nonsense mutation in the human CDN1B gene encoding the cyclin-dependent kinase inhibitor p27^{Kip1}.

REFERENCES

MEN1

Doherty GM. Multiple endocrine neoplasia type 1: duodenopancreatic tumors. *Surg Oncol.* 2003;12:135. [PMID: 12946484]

Gibril F, Schumann M, Pace A, Jensen RT. Multiple endocrine neoplasia type 1 and Zollinger Ellison syndrome. *Medicine.* 2004;83:43. [PMID: 12946484

Glascock MJ, Carty SE. Multiple endocrine neoplasia type1: fresh perspective on clinical features and penetrance. *Surg Oncol* 2002;11:143. [PMID: 12356510]

Hughes CM, Rozenblatt-Rosen O, Milne TA, et al. Menin associates with a trithorax family histone methyltransferase complex and with the Hoxc8 locus. *Mol Cell.* 2004;13:567. [PMID: 14992727]

Kivlen MH, Bartlett DL, Libutti SK, et al. Reoperation for hyperparathyroidism in multiple endocrine neoplasia type 1. *Surgery.* 2001;130:991. [PMID: 11742328]

Lakhani VT, You YN, Wells SA. The multiple endocrine neoplasia syndromes. *Ann Rev Med.* 2007;58:253. [PMID: 17037976]

Lemos MC, Thakker RV. Multiple endocrine neoplasia type 1 (MEN1): analysis of 1336 mutations reported in the first decade following identification of the gene. *Hum Mut.* 2008;29:22. [PMID: 17879353]

Milne TA, Hughes CM, Lloyd R, et al. Menin and MLL cooperatively regulate expression of cyclin-dependent kinase inhibitors. *Proc Natl Acad Sci (USA).* 2005;102:749. [PMID: 15640349]

Schussheim DH, Skarulis MC, Agarwal SK, et al. Multiple endocrine neoplasia type 1: new clinical and basic findings. *Trends Endocrinol Metab* 2001;12:173. [PMID: 11295574]

Triponez, Dosseh D, Goudet P, et al. Epidemiology data on 108 MEN1 patients from the the GTE with isolated non-functioning tumors of the pancreas. *Ann Surg.* 2006;243:265. [PMID: 16432361]

Trouillas J, Labat-Moleur F, Sturm N, et al. Pituitary tumors and hyperplasia in multiple endocrine neoplasia type 1 syndrome (MEN1): a case control study in a series of 77 patients versus 2509 non-MEN1 patients. *Am J Surg Path.* 2008;32:534. [PMID: 18300794]

MEN2

Brandi ML, Gagel RF, Angeli A, et al. Consensus guidelines for diagnosis and therapy of MEN type 1 and type 2. *J Clin Endocrinol Metab.* 2001;86:5658. [PMID: 11739416]

Elisei R, Romei C, Cosci B, et al. RET genetic screening in patients with medullary thyroid cancer and their relatives: experience with 807 individuals at one center. *J Clin Endocrinol Metab.* 2007;92:4725. [PMID: 17895320]

Machens A, Holzhausen HJ, Thanh PN, et al. Malignant progression from C-cell hyperplasia to medullary thyroid carcinoma in 167 carriers of the Ret germline mutations. *Surgery.* 2003;134:425. [PMID: 14555929]

Punales MKC, daRocha AP, Meotti C, Gross JL, Maia AL. Clinical and oncological features of children and young adults with multiple endocrine neoplasia type 2A. *Thyroid.* 2008;18:1. [PMID: 18991485]

Runeberg-Roos P, Saarma M. Neurotrophic factor receptor RET: structure, cell biology and inherited disease. *Ann Med.* 2007;39:572. [PMID: 17934909]

Verga U, Fugazzola L, Cambiaghi S, et al. Frequent association between MEN 2A and cutaneous lichen amyloidosis. *Clin Endocrinol* 2003;59:156. [PMID: 12864791]

Other Disorders

Riminucci M, Collins MT, Fedarko NS, et al. FGF-23 in fibrous dysplasia of bone and its relationship to renal phosphate wasting. *J Clin Invest.* 2003;112:642. [PMID: 12952917]

Spiegel AM, Weinstein LS. Inherited diseases involving G proteins and G protein-coupled receptors. *Annu Rev Med.* 2004;55:27. [PMID: 14746508]

Stratakis CA, Kirschner LS, Carney JA. Clinical and molecular features of the Carney complex: diagnostic criteria and recommendations for patient evaluation. *J Clin Endocrinol Metab.* 2001;86:4041. [PMID: 11549623]

Geriatric Endocrinology

**Susan L. Greenspan, MD, Mary Korytkowski, MD, and
Neil M. Resnick, MD**

ADA	American Diabetes Association	**LHRH**	Luteinizing hormone–releasing hormone
BG	Blood glucose	**NHANES**	National Health and Nutrition Examination Survey
BMD	Bone mineral density	**NPH**	Neutral protamine Hagedorn
BMI	Body mass index	**NSAIDS**	Nonsteroidal anti-inflammatory drugs
CHF	Congestive heart failure	**OGTT**	Oral glucose tolerance test
CRH	Corticotropin-releasing hormone	**PTH**	Parathyroid hormone
CVD	Cardiovascular disease	**RANK-L**	Receptor activator of nuclear factor kappa B ligand
DHEA	Dehydroepiandrosterone	**SERM**	Selective estrogen receptor modulator
DPP IV	Dipeptidyl peptidase IV	**SIADH**	Syndrome of inappropriate antidiuretic hormone
FFA	Free fatty acids	**T_3**	Triiodothyronine
GFR	Glomerular filtration rate	**T_4**	Thyroxine
GIP	Glucose insulinotropic peptide	**TLI**	Therapeutic lifestyle intervention
GLP1	Glucagon-like peptide 1	**TSH**	Thyroid-stimulating hormone
GLUT	Glucose transporter	**UKPDS**	United Kingdom Prospective Diabetes Study
HHNS	Hyperglycemic hyperosmolar nonketotic syndrome		
IGT	Impaired glucose tolerance		
LH	Luteinizing hormone		

Individuals over age 65 comprise the fastest-growing segment of the United States population; each day this group increases by more than 1000 people. This increase has led to a remarkable situation—of all the people who have ever lived to the age of 65, more than two-thirds are still alive. Thus, it is becoming increasingly important for the endocrinologist to understand how endocrine physiology and disease may differ in the elderly.

Before considering specific endocrinologic conditions in the elderly, however, it is worthwhile to review some general principles that account for many of the age-related changes in disease presentation in the elderly. First, aging itself—in the absence of disease—is associated with only a gradual and linear decline in the physiologic reserve of each organ system (Figure 23–1). Because the reserve capacity of each system is substantial, age-related declines have little effect on baseline function and do not significantly interfere with the individual's response to stress until the eighth or ninth decade. Second, because each organ system's function declines at a different physiologic rate and because 75% of the elderly have at least one disease, endocrine dysfunction in the elderly often presents disparately, with initial symptoms derived from the most compromised organ system. For example, hyperthyroidism in an elderly patient with preexisting coronary and conduction system disease may present with atrial fibrillation and a slow ventricular response, whereas in another equally hyperthyroid patient with a prior stroke, it may present with confusion or depression; neither patient may tolerate hyperthyroidism long enough for the classic thyroid-related manifestations (eg, goiter) to become apparent. Third, elderly patients often have multiple diseases and take many medications that may mimic or mask the usual presentation of endocrine disease.

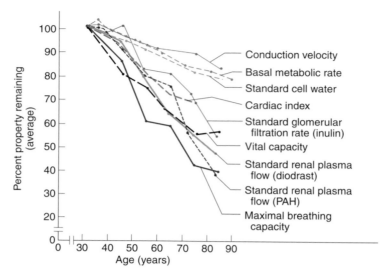

FIGURE 23–1 Influence of age on physiologic function in humans. (Reproduced, with permission, from Shock NW. Discussion on mortality and measurement. In: Strehler BL, et al, eds. *The Biology of Aging: A Symposium*. American Institute of Biological Sciences; 1960.)

THYROID FUNCTION AND DISEASE

The prevalence of thyroid disease in the elderly is approximately twice that in younger individuals, with hypothyroidism ranging from 2% to 7% and hyperthyroidism affecting up to 2% of older individuals. The Whickham Survey of 21,000 adults in Great Britain and its follow-up study, conducted between 1972 and 1993, reported that the incidence of overt hypothyroidism was increased 10-fold in women age 75 and older when compared to women in their twenties. In the NHANES 1999 to 2002 survey (N=4392) the overall prevalence of hypothyroidism was 3.7% (includes overt and mild) including a prevalence of 5.5% for individuals age 50 to 79 years and 12.1% for those age 80 and older. Individuals age 80 and older had five times greater probability for developing hypothyroidism (OR=5.0, p=0.0002) compared to those 12 to 49 years of age. In addition, some studies suggest that up to 9% of hospitalized elderly patients have overt thyroid disease. **Subclinical hypothyroidism**—normal serum levels of thyroid hormones (thyroxine, T_4; triiodothyronine, T_3) with an elevated level of thyroid-stimulating hormone (thyrotropin) (TSH)—is more prevalent, with estimates of 6% to 13% in the elderly (Figure 23–2), and is higher in women than in men. The NHANES III data (N=16,533) suggests that the distribution of TSH shifts to a higher concentration with age and therefore the prevalence of subclinical hypothyroidism may be overshadowed (see Figure 23–3). In the elderly, the progression from subclinical to overt hypothyroidism is roughly 2% to 5% per year. Subclinical hyperthyroidism—normal serum thyroxine with suppressed serum TSH levels—may be found in approximately 2% of elderly subjects (Figure 23–2). The rate of progression to overt hyperthyroidism is less clear. Finally, the overall prevalence of thyroid hormone use in older adults is approximately 7% (10% in women and 2% in men).

There are few major age-related changes in the physiology of the hypothalamic-pituitary-thyroid axis (Chapters 4 and 7). There are slight age-related increases in serum TSH levels (see Figure 23–3)

and decreases in total T_4. TSH release remains pulsatile, although the nocturnal rise in serum TSH appears to be blunted with age. There is a slight age-related decline in serum T_3, but values usually remain within normal limits. The effect of age on the release of TSH by thyrotropin-releasing hormone is less clear, but most recent studies show little clinically relevant change in either sex. The 24-hour radioiodine uptake is also not significantly altered with age. Thyroid antibodies are common in older women (prevalence up to 25%, Figure 23–4), but their presence does not serve as a specific screening test for thyroid disease. The presence of thyroid antibodies (occult thyroid dysfunction) may skew the upper limit of TSH in the African American, Caucasian, and Mexican American ethnic groups (see Figure 23–4).

DISORDERS OF THE THYROID GLAND

The United States Preventive Services Task Force concluded that there was insufficient evidence to recommend routine screening for thyroid disease in adults. Furthermore, there is no consensus regarding screening in the elderly. A scientific review panel suggests case finding for screening older patients at high risk (eg, family history, personal history, radiation, and other risk factors). The American Thyroid Association recommends that adults be screened by serum TSH determination every 5 years. A consensus statement from the American Association of Clinical Endocrinologists, the American Thyroid Association, and the Endocrine Society recommends routine screening for subclinical thyroid dysfunction in adults. However, it is reasonable to measure TSH at any time in older individuals who present with atypical symptoms of thyroid disease such as exacerbation of cardiac symptoms, change in mental status, falling, or onset of depression. Despite the sensitivity of the TSH assay, further evaluation with a free T_4 or total T_4 is often required because up to 98% of elderly subjects with mildly suppressed TSH levels do not have thyrotoxicosis.

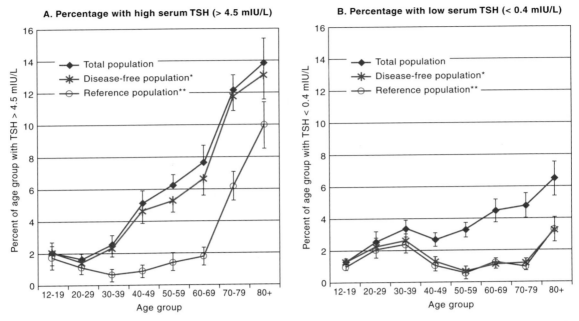

FIGURE 23–2 Percentage with high or low serum thyroid-stimulating hormone (TSH) in the total US population, the disease-free (excludes those people who have reported having thyroid disease, goiter, or taking thyroid medications*) and reference population (excludes those people who reported having thyroid disease, goiter, or taking thyroid medications and those who do not have risk factors such as pregnancy or taking estrogen, androgens, or lithium and who are without the presence of thyroid antibodies or biochemical evidence of hypothyroidism or hyperthyroidism**) by age. **A:** High serum TSH. In the disease-free population, the percentage of people with high serum TSH concentration (>4.5 μIU/mL) is slightly lower than that of the total population but significantly higher than the percentage in the reference population. **B:** Low serum TSH. The percentage of people with low serum TSH in the disease-free population, on the other hand, is significantly lower than the percentage in the total population and similar to the pattern seen in the reference population. Note the elevated prevalence of low TSH in the populations without thyroid disease or risk factors at ages 20 to 39 years and again after age 79 years. The higher prevalence of individuals with low TSH or high TSH in the total population is related directly to the people reporting thyroid disease, goiter, or taking thyroid medication and probably reflects inadequate management of clinical thyroid disease. (Reproduced, with permission, from Hollowell JG, et al. Serum TSH, T₄, and thyroid antibodies in the US population [1988 to 1994]: National Health and Nutrition Examination Survey [NHANES III]. *J Clin Endocrinol Metab.* 2002;87:489. Copyright 2002 by The Endocrine Society.)

1. HYPERTHYROIDISM

Clinical Features

With age, the prevalence of Graves disease decreases (although it remains the most common cause of hyperthyroidism), and the prevalence of multinodular goiter and toxic nodules increases. Elderly hyperthyroid patients tend to present with symptoms or complications related to the most vulnerable organ system—usually the cardiovascular system (atrial fibrillation, congestive heart failure, angina, and acute myocardial infarction) or the central nervous system (apathy, depression, confusion, or lassitude). The hypercatabolic state also causes muscle wasting, particularly of the quadriceps, thereby increasing the risk of falls. Occasionally, hyperthyroid elderly patients present with gastrointestinal symptoms, but these differ from those seen in younger patients because they include constipation, failure to thrive, anorexia, and weight loss. Because of degeneration of the sinus node and fibrotic changes in the cardiac conduction system, older patients are less likely than younger ones to present with palpitations (Table 23–1). However, a very low serum TSH concentration is associated with a threefold higher risk of atrial fibrillation in the subsequent decade. Hyperthyroidism is also associated with bone loss and fractures.

The physical signs of hyperthyroidism also differ in the elderly (see Table 23–1). Sinus tachycardia is less frequent; the thyroid feels normal in size or is not palpable in two-thirds of patients; and lid lag is uncommon. Ophthalmopathy is less common, not only because Graves disease occurs less often, but also because, even with Graves disease, ophthalmopathy occurs less frequently in the elderly. However, although they are less common in the elderly, some findings appear to be highly suggestive of hyperthyroidism. These include increased frequency of bowel movements, weight loss despite increased appetite, fine finger tremor, eyelid retraction, and increased perspiration. Lid lag is uncommon but if found, it is highly suggestive of hyperthyroidism (specific).

Diagnosis

As in younger patients (Chapter 7), the diagnosis is usually confirmed by standard thyroid function tests, beginning with a depressed TSH level as measured by a sensitive immunoradiometric or chemiluminescent assay. There are potential pitfalls, however. Hospitalized elderly patients who are acutely ill (but euthyroid) may have a suppressed serum TSH. Further, other thyroid function tests should help rule out hyperthyroidism. T₃ toxicosis may be

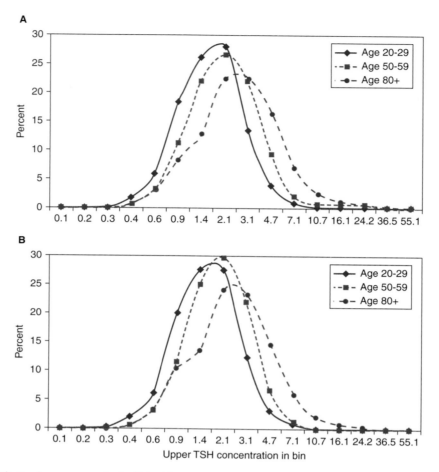

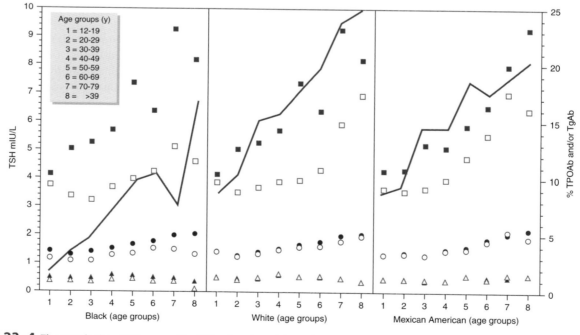

FIGURE 23–3 TSH distribution by age groups in the United States. **A:** Disease-free population. **B:** Reference population, NHANES III (1988-1994).

FIGURE 23–4 The panels show TSH percentiles (5th, triangles; 50th, circles; and 97.5th, squares) for the eight age groups for each ethnicity: left, B; middle, W; right, M. Solid symbols represent the TSH percentiles for antibody-positive subjects, and open symbols represent the TSH percentiles for antibody-negative subjects. In each panel, the solid line links the prevalence of TPOAb and/or TgAb of each age group.

TABLE 23–1 Percentages of patients with symptoms and physical findings attributable to thyrotoxicosis.

	Old₁	Old₂	Young
Number	25	85	247
Mean age	81.5	68.6	40[a]
Range	75-95	60-82	5-73
Symptoms (%)			
Weight loss	44	35	85
Palpitations	36	42	89
Weakness	32	28	70
Dizziness, syncope	20	...	...
Nervousness	20	38	99
No symptoms	8	...	...
Memory loss	8	...	...
Tremor	8	...	...
Local symptoms[b]	8	11	...
Pruritus	4	4	...
Heat intolerance	4	63	89
Physical Findings			
Pulse >100/min	28[c]	58	100
Atrial fibrillation	32	39	10
New-onset atrial fibrillation	20[d]	...	...
Lid lag	12	35	71
Exophthalmos	8	8	...
Fine skin	40	81	97
Tremor	36	89	97
Myopathy	8	39	...
Hyperactive reflexes	24	26	...
Gynecomastia	(1 male)	1	10
None	8	...	...
Thyroid Examination (%)			
Impalpable or normal	68	37	...
Diffusely enlarged	12	22	100
Multinodular goiter	12	20	...
Isolated nodule	8	21	...

Modified and reproduced, with permission, from Tibaldi JM, et al.

Thyrotoxicosis in the very old. *Am J Med.* 1986;81:619.

[a]Approximated from graph of patients' ages.

[b]Dysphagia, enlarging neck mass, etc.

[c]Includes five patients with normal sinus rhythm and two who had atrial fibrillation.

[d]This was transient in four of five patients with conversion to normal sinus rhythm.

Note:

Old₁= Tibaldi JM, et al. Thyrotoxicosis in the very old. *Am J Med.* 1986;81:619.

Old₂= Davis PJ, Davis FB. Hyperthyroidism in patients over the age of 60 years. Clinical features in 85 patients. *Medicine (Balti-more).* 1974;53:161.

Young = Ingbar SH, et al. The thyroid gland. In: Williams RH, ed. *Williams Textbook of Endocrinology.* Saunders; 1981.

more difficult evaluation to diagnose because concomitant nonthyroidal illness is common and can depress serum T_3.

Furthermore, iodide-induced hyperthyroidism, reflecting the Jod-Basedow phenomenon (see Chapter 7), is becoming more common in elderly patients with multinodular goiter because of increased exposure to radiocontrast studies; the resultant hyperthyroidism is generally transient.

Finally, because of screening tests with sensitive TSH assays, subclinical hyperthyroidism (normal T_4, T_3, free T_4 with a suppressed TSH) is being recognized more commonly. This is often found in older subjects with autonomous function of a multinodular goiter or

nodule. Osteoporosis and atrial fibrillation are complications of subclinical hyperthyroidism that may be an indication for treatment. Recent studies suggest a possible increase in all-cause mortality in patients with subclinical hyperthyroidism with an increase beyond the age of 60, especially in aging men (Figure 23–5). If patients are not treated, careful follow-up is recommended.

Treatment

Beta-blocking agents are useful in alleviating symptoms, but radioactive iodine is the therapy of choice in elderly patients because it is efficient, uncomplicated, and inexpensive. Antithyroid drugs can be used prior to radioactive iodine treatment to render the patient euthyroid and to avoid radiation-induced thyroiditis, but they are not definitive treatment and are more toxic in this age group. Surgery has a more limited role because of its increased morbidity.

Following radioactive iodine treatment, patients become euthyroid over a period of 6 to 12 weeks. They should receive careful follow-up, because hypothyroidism develops in 80% or more of patients who have been adequately treated. Once hyperthyroidism has abated, the metabolic clearance rate of other medications may decrease, and doses may require readjustment. Older patients with subclinical hyperthyroidism require follow-up, especially if presented with an iodine load.

2. HYPOTHYROIDISM

Hypothyroidism in the elderly is most often due to Hashimoto thyroiditis, prior thyroid surgery, or radioactive iodine ablative therapy. Medications, including amiodarone, lithium, and interferon-α, can lead to hypothyroidism. The risk of developing hypothyroidism is significantly increased in older women when serum antithyroid antibodies or serum TSH are elevated.

Clinical Features

It is easy to overlook hypothyroidism in an older person, because many euthyroid elderly patients have the same symptoms. Moreover, elderly patients with hypothyroidism are more likely than younger patients to present with cardiovascular symptoms (eg, congestive heart failure or angina) or neurologic findings (eg, cognitive impairment, confusion, depression, paresthesias, deafness, psychosis, or coma). Finally, in the older hypothyroid patient, the physical findings are frequently nonspecific, although puffy face, delayed deep tendon reflexes, and myoedema support the diagnosis.

Diagnosis

Serum TSH is the most sensitive indicator of primary hypothyroidism and should be checked first. The diagnosis should then be confirmed with a low serum T_4 or free T_4. Measurement of serum T_3 is unnecessary and potentially misleading, because T_3 is the thyroid hormone most likely to decrease in nonthyroidal illness. Serum TSH should not be used alone to diagnose hypothyroidism because it does not always differentiate symptomatic from

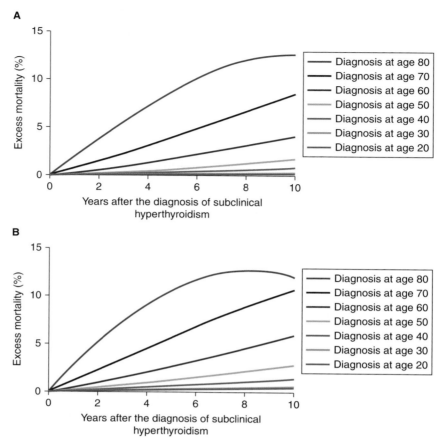

FIGURE 23–5 A: Excess mortality from all causes after the diagnosis of subclinical hyperthyroidism for US women and **B:** US men with subclinical hyperthyroidism. These data are based on a hypothetical approach using mathematical modeling, that is, these data are not based on individual patient data, but derive from aggregated data reported in original cohort studies and life tables.

subclinical hypothyroidism. Furthermore, levels of TSH may be higher at night as a result of the nocturnal rise in serum TSH. Moreover, the pulsatile nature of TSH, resulting in serum TSH slightly above the normal ranges, may lead to a diagnosis of subclinical hypothyroidism in a euthyroid subject. Finally, in hypothyroid patients, serum TSH levels can be reduced to within the normal range by treatment with dopaminergic drugs and corticosteroids. In such patients, determination of free T_4 may help differentiate those with true hypothyroidism from those with nonthyroidal illness (Chapter 7).

Treatment

The doses of thyroid hormone required for adequate replacement decrease with age. Elderly patients should be started on approximately 25 to 50 µg of levothyroxine, and the dose should be increased by approximately 25 µg every 4 to 6 weeks until the serum TSH comes into the normal range. In patients with cardiovascular disease, even lower initial doses can be used (12.5 µg) and increased at a slower rate. Desiccated thyroid hormone and preparations containing T_3 should be avoided, because T_3 is rapidly absorbed and cleared and may be cardiotoxic. The metabolic clearance of other drugs changes as hypothyroidism is corrected, and their dosages may require readjustment. On average, the dose of

levothyroxine in the elderly is roughly 1 µg/kg/d compared with 1.7 µg/kg/d in young adults. Overtreatment documented by a suppressed serum TSH should be avoided because of the potential adverse effects to the skeleton and cardiovascular system.

It is still not known whether treating subclinical hypothyroidism is beneficial. A Cochrane review of 12 small trials that included treatment of subclinical hypothyroidism with thyroid hormone did not find improved survival, decreased cardiac morbidity, or differences in quality of life or symptoms. Two-thirds of patients with subclinical hypothyroidism were chemically euthyroid for at least 4 years, and the absence of antimicrosomal antibodies may identify patients at lowest risk of progression. The presence of antithyroperoxidase antibodies is associated with a higher risk of progression to overt hypothyroidism of 4.3%/year versus 2.6%/year in antibody-negative patients.

If patients are not treated, they need to be followed closely for progression of disease. Elderly patients previously treated with radioactive iodine are more likely to progress to overt hypothyroidism.

3. MULTINODULAR GOITER

The prevalence of multinodular goiter increases with age. However, if swallowing and breathing are not compromised and thyroid function tests are normal, the goiter can be observed without treatment. Levothyroxine therapy rarely shrinks the gland, and although it may prevent further enlargement, the risk of inducing iatrogenic hyperthyroidism is significant. This is compounded by the fact that multinodular goiters may independently develop areas of autonomous function.

4. THYROID NODULES AND CANCER

Thyroid nodules are more common in the elderly. The prevalence of nodules increases with age and is generally higher in women than in men. Furthermore, the prevalence of thyroid nodules detected by ultrasound may be as high as 40% in older women. Ninety percent of these nodules are benign, but the prognosis for elderly patients with malignant nodules may be worse than that for younger patients with malignant nodules. The approach is similar to the workup in a younger patient. The prognosis correlates with the size of the tumor. The outcome in elderly patients may therefore be substantially improved by early evaluation of nodules in patients who are good surgical candidates.

Papillary carcinoma is more common in young and middle-aged patients. However, it has a poorer prognosis in the elderly, possibly because it is detected at a more advanced stage. Follicular carcinoma accounts for 15% of thyroid cancers and usually occurs in middle-aged and older patients. Anaplastic thyroid carcinoma is found almost exclusively in middle-aged and older patients. It presents as a rapidly growing hard mass that is locally invasive, often associated with metastatic lesions, and has a very poor prognosis (Chapter 7).

CARBOHYDRATE INTOLERANCE AND DIABETES MELLITUS

Introduction

Diabetes is an important health condition for the aging population. More than 20% of individuals over the age of 60 years have diabetes, and another 14% have impaired glucose tolerance (IGT). It is anticipated that these numbers will continue to increase in the coming decades. It is therefore almost certain that those involved in the care of patients in this age group will encounter those with some disorder of glucose tolerance.

Both IGT and diabetes are associated with enhanced morbidity and mortality due to macrovascular and cardiovascular disease (CVD); an increase in risk for microvascular complications (retinopathy, neuropathy) that impair the ability to maintain independence; changes in cognitive function; and depression. Older individuals with diabetes have more functional disability and coexisting illnesses such as hypertension, coronary heart disease (CHD), and stroke than those without diabetes. Older adults with diabetes are also at greater risk for urinary incontinence, injurious falls, and issues related to polypharmacy.

Early diagnosis and appropriate intervention can help to avoid some of the adverse consequences of hyperglycemia, while also improving health-related quality of life (HRQL) in this age group. In 2003, the American Geriatric Society published guidelines that are useful in guiding the care of the older person with diabetes. These recommendations are now included as part of the standards of care published annually by the American Diabetes Association.

Aging and the Physiology of Carbohydrate Intolerance

Normal aging is associated with a gradual increase in both fasting (1 mg/dL [0.6 mmol/L] per decade) and glucose-stimulated blood glucose (BG) (5 mg/dL [0.28 mmol/L] per decade) levels, even in lean, physically active individuals with normal body weight. Normoglycemic elderly subjects have higher glucose and insulin levels during an oral glucose tolerance test (OGTT) than body mass index (BMI)-matched young subjects. These changes in BG are more profound in those who have risk factors for abnormal glucose tolerance.

Type 2 diabetes is characterized by defects in both insulin secretion and sensitivity. Although the majority of people with type 2 diabetes are insulin-resistant, insulin resistance by itself is not sufficient to lead to hyperglycemia. Age-related impairments in beta cell function that include reduced conversion of proinsulin to insulin and abnormal insulin secretion are important contributors to the development of hyperglycemia in elderly individuals. Lean elderly patients with type 2 diabetes have a greater impairment in insulin secretion than insulin sensitivity while obese patients have both impaired insulin secretion and sensitivity in muscle and liver (Figure 23–6).

Several abnormalities of beta cell function contribute to the decline in insulin secretory capacity with advancing age. These include an accumulation of intracellular lipid within the beta cell; a decrease in glucose transporter (GLUT) 2 number; and a reduced sensitivity to the incretin hormones, glucagon-like peptide 1 (GLP1), and glucose insulinotropic peptide (GIP) that acts to augment the postprandial insulin response. Genetic susceptibility also plays a role. In individuals without diabetes who carry five or more risk alleles that are associated with development of diabetes, impairments in insulin secretion are observed at an earlier age than those with fewer alleles. Evidence of autoimmunity with antibodies directed against beta cell proteins has been demonstrated as a cause of impaired insulin secretion in up to 12% of elderly individuals.

These impairments in beta cell function can be unmasked by an increase in insulin resistance that occurs with normal aging. The insulin resistance that accompanies aging is associated with the accumulation of intracellular fat and a progressive decline in the number and function of mitochondria resulting in reduced oxidative glucose metabolism and phosphorylation activity. Insulin resistance is augmented by weight gain; reductions in lean body mass and increases in fat mass; physical inactivity; and use of some medications (ie, glucocorticoids and atypical antipsychotics). Insulin resistance occurs in muscle, where there is a reduction in insulin-mediated glucose uptake following a meal; in adipose tissue where impaired regulation of hormone-sensitive lipase results in increases in circulating levels of free fatty acids (FFA); and liver where there is overproduction of glucose in the fasting state and failure to adequately suppress glucose production after a meal.

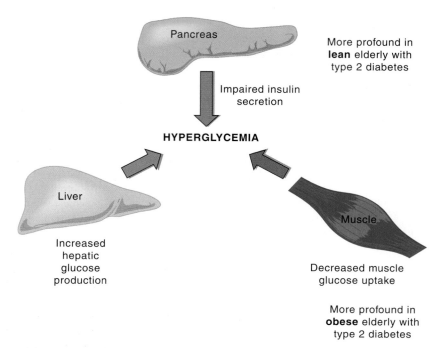

FIGURE 23–6 The pathogenesis of type 2 diabetes mellitus in obese elderly and lean elderly.

Metabolic Syndrome

The metabolic syndrome refers to a clustering of metabolic abnormalities outlined in Table 23–2 that are associated with an increase in risk for type 2 diabetes and CVD. This syndrome is more common in the elderly, increasing from approximately 7% of the population in the third decade to 44% in the seventh decade. Lifestyle interventions targeting modifications in dietary intake, regular exercise, and weight reduction are effective in reducing the progression to overt type 2 diabetes among individuals above age 60 years.

Establishing the Diagnosis of Diabetes Mellitus

A. Diagnostic criteria The majority of elderly individuals with diabetes will have type 2 diabetes. The typical symptoms usually associated with hyperglycemia may either not be present or may have developed so gradually that they may not be perceived as being abnormal. The use of diuretics can mask polyuria and polydipsia as manifestations of hyperglycemia. An age-related decrease in thirst may blunt these usual symptoms. It is therefore important that laboratory measurement of BG be performed on at least an annual basis in individuals above the age of 60.

A diagnosis of diabetes can be established by one of three established criteria outlined in Table 23–3. Oral glucose tolerance testing is performed infrequently in clinical practice and is not required to establish the diagnosis, particularly in elderly individuals. Measurement of an A1c is now accepted as an alternative tool in establishing a diagnosis of diabetes, with values ≥6.5% consistent with a diagnosis of diabetes. A1c values of 6.0% to 6.4% identify those at high risk for development of type 2 diabetes. A reasonable approach would be to measure an A1c in any elderly person with abnormal glucose values.

B. Glycemic goals Both the ADA and the American Geriatrics Society recommend that functional, cognitively intact older adults who have significant anticipated life expectancy be treated to similar glycemic goals as younger adults. This means guiding therapy to achieve HbA1c of <7% for the majority of people with diabetes.

TABLE 23–2 National Cholesterol Education Program criteria for diagnosis of metabolic syndrome.

Diagnosis requires three of the following:
Abdominal obesity
Waist circumference >40 in (>102 cm) men
Waist circumference > 35 in (>88 cm) women
Triglycerides ≥150 mg/dL or drug treatment
HDL-C <40 men or <50 women or drug treatment
Blood pressure ≥130/85 mm Hg or drug treatment
Fasting glucose ≥ 110 mg/dL or drug treatment

Modified with permission from Alberti KG, Zimmet PZ. *Diabet Med.* 1998 Jul;15(7): 539-553.

TABLE 23–3 Criteria for diagnosis of type 2 diabetes.

• Fasting glucose ≥126 mg/dL (7.0 mmol/L)
• Any glucose ≥200 mg/dL (11.1 mmol/L) with symptoms
• 2-h PG ≥200 mg/dL (11.1 mmol/L) during a 75-g OGTT
Newly proposed criterion: A1c ≥6.5%

Note: Any single abnormal measure requires confirmation with a second test.

Achieving this level requires that fasting glucose levels be maintained between 80 and 130 mg/dL, and 2-hour postprandial BG at <180 mg/dL. These recommendations are not absolute. While the goal is to maintain an A1c values as close to normal (<6%) as possible, this goal can be modified in patients who are at high risk for hypoglycemia, who are older, who have comorbid conditions that limit life expectancies. These contingencies have particular relevance to the elderly population who may experience variability in appetite or food intake, or often have other medical problems requiring medications (eg, beta blockers, anxiolytics) that can increase vulnerability to hypoglycemia. On the other hand, uncontrolled diabetes is also associated with undesirable effects in elderly individuals, including fluid and electrolyte abnormalities, problems with urinary incontinence and cognitive function, indicating the need for a reasonable degree of glycemic control even with advanced age. Efforts to achieve A1c levels of <7% are reasonable in some elderly patients, provided that the risk for weight gain and hypoglycemia is minimized. Therapy can be modified to achieve A1c targets of 8% in others as a way of minimizing risk for treatment-associated concerns. However, symptomatic hyperglycemia that can increase risk for an acute hyperglycemic crisis should be avoided in all patients.

C. Glycemic control and complications Because the complications of diabetes mellitus are related to the duration of disease, elderly patients who live long enough suffer the same complications of nephropathy, neuropathy, and retinopathy as their younger counterparts. The United Kingdom Prospective Diabetes Study (UKPDS) examined the relationship between improved glycemic control and the prevention of complications in 3067 patients with type 2 diabetes (mean age 54 years) assigned to intensive (goal of fasting blood glucose <108 mg/dL) or conventional therapy. After a median follow-up of 10 years, the incidence of microvascular complications (retinopathy, neuropathy, and nephropathy) was reduced by 25% with intensive treatment. There was no difference in the incidence of macrovascular complications, but there was a tendency for fewer myocardial infarctions in the intensive therapy group. A 10-year follow-up report from the UKPDS demonstrated a significant favorable legacy effect of early intensive therapy in preventing both microvascular and macrovascular complications.

Elderly diabetic patients have an impaired counterregulatory response to hypoglycemia which can interfere with recovery from a hypoglycemic event. In addition, the ability to sense hypoglycemia declines, as does the ability to take corrective action. Coupled with the diminished cortical reserve due to the higher prevalence of age-associated conditions such as stroke, lacunar infarction, amyloid angiopathy, and Alzheimer disease, the older brain is less able to recover fully from hypoglycemic insult.

Cardiovascular Disease

CVD is a major cause of morbidity and mortality in elderly people with diabetes. For this reason, interventions recommended for the secondary prevention of recurrent coronary events in individuals without diabetes are recommended for all individuals with diabetes independent of known heart disease. This includes control of blood pressure, treatment of hyperlipidemia, and use of low-dose aspirin therapy in those without contraindications. While tight glycemic control has been demonstrated to reduce the risk for microvascular and neuropathic complications, the role of tight glycemic control for prevention of macrovascular disease and CVD has been addressed in several recent clinical trials.

Three recent large, randomized, prospective clinical trials with relevance to an elderly population were conducted in an effort to define the effect of lowering A1c to levels lower than those currently recommended by the ADA on cardiovascular outcomes in patients with type 2 diabetes. The average age of these subjects, all of whom had a history of a CVD event or were at high risk for an event, ranged from 60 to 66 years.

In the Action to Control Cardiovascular Risk in Diabetes (ACCORD) study, the goal of intensive glycemic therapy was to achieve an A1c <6% versus <8% with conventional treatment. The glycemic control study was stopped 18 months early due to the observation of a 22% increase in the relative risk for CVD death with intensive therapy. In the Action in Diabetes and Vascular Disease (ADVANCE) study, the goal of intensive therapy was to achieve an A1c <6.5% using the sulfonylurea, gliclazide (not available in the United States). A reduction in microvascular complications, primarily risk for proteinuria, was observed with intensive therapy, but there were no group differences for CVD events. In the Veterans Affairs Diabetes Trial (VADT), the goal of intensive therapy was to achieve an A1c <6%. There were no significant group differences in the composite outcome of CVD events; however, there were more CVD deaths (36 vs 29) and more sudden deaths in intensively treated subjects (11 vs 4) (p = NS). Severe hypoglycemia within the preceding 90 days was a predictor of CVD events and mortality.

What do these results mean to the practicing physician? It is important to note that all three trials included participants with long-standing type 2 diabetes and varying degrees of established atherosclerosis at time of study entry. In addition, the glycemic targets in these trials were well below what is recommended by the ADA (7%) and may not be appropriate in elderly individuals where the risk for hypoglycemia and related adverse sequelae is greater. Other CVD risk factors (eg, hypertension and hyperlipidemia) were treated to a moderate or high degree, resulting in rates of CVD events that were lower than predicted with standard therapy. This places emphasis on the importance of treating nonglycemic CVD risk factors in patients with diabetes.

Treatment Strategies for Achieving Glycemic Goals in The Elderly

The therapeutic goals for any patient with diabetes, including the elderly, are to avoid symptoms of hyperglycemia and hypoglycemia, to minimize risk for acute and chronic diabetes-related complications, and to achieve an optimal health-related quality of life. While the majority of newly diagnosed elderly individuals will have type 2 diabetes, many individuals with type 1 diabetes are enjoying longer survival, making it likely that these patients will require care during advancing years. Insulin therapy, either alone or in

TABLE 23–4 Oral hypoglycemic agents available for treatment of type 2 diabetes.

Class	Mechanism Action	Side Effects	Agents
Sulfonylureas Short-acting insulin secretagogues	Stimulates insulin production	Hypoglycemia	Glyburide Glipizide Glimeperide Repaglinide Nateglinide
Biguanides (metformin)	↓Gluconeogenesis ↑ Insulin sensitivity	Nausea, diarrhea, rarely lactic acidosis	Metfomin
Thiazolidinediones	Reduce insulin resistance	Edema, CHF Decrease bone density Increase LFTs	Rosiglitazone Pioglitazone
α-Glucosidase inhibitors	Decrease rate of carbohydrate absorption	Bloating, abdominal discomfort, diarrhea	Acarbose miglitol
DPP IV inhibitors	Prolongs action GLP1 Increases insulin release Decreases glucagon	URI Nausea	Sitagliptin Saxagliptin

combination with oral agents, is often required to maintain desired glycemic control in the face of progressive beta cell dysfunction in those with type 2 diabetes. For these reasons, knowledge of insulin and noninsulin injectable medications is as important as that of the five different classes or oral hypoglycemic agents (Table 23–4) indicated for the treatment of type 2 diabetes.

A. Therapeutic lifestyle intervention   The essential components of therapeutic lifestyle intervention (TLI) include dietary modifications and exercise. Weight reduction is recommended for overweight and obese individuals. Recommendations to obtain an adequate amount of sleep as either one uninterrupted sleep cycle or with daily naps may help reduce risk for progression to overt diabetes in those with impairments in glucose intolerance.

Dietary interventions for treatment of diabetes promote appropriate dietary caloric intake with an appropriate distribution of calories among carbohydrates, protein, and fat. There is contradictory information in the literature regarding the optimal diet that should be recommended for patients with diabetes. Studies comparing different diets for achieving weight loss have yielded inconsistent results. In general, obese patients can be encouraged to follow a weight reduction regimen that is most acceptable to their taste, as this is more likely to result in a reasonable degree of compliance.

The Mediterranean diet which emphasizes the intake of fresh fruits and vegetables, whole grains, beans, nuts, and olive oil, may have some advantages over traditional low-fat diets in the elderly population. In one European study of more than 2000 subjects aged 70 to 90 years, the integration of a Mediterranean style diet with other healthy lifestyle interventions reduced all-cause mortality by more than 50%. The Mediterranean diet not only promotes weight loss, but also has demonstrated favorable effects on circulating lipids and BG levels.

In the ongoing Look AHEAD Study, subjects with type 2 diabetes between the ages of 45 and 74 years were able to achieve a 9% weight loss and 21% increase in fitness level with 30 minutes of exercise and 1200 to 1800 calorie intake each day. Exercise

prescriptions and encouragement to maintain a reasonable level of physical activity are as important in the elderly as in the younger population. There is no longer a requirement to perform cardiac stress testing before recommending an exercise program. To optimize compliance with exercise prescriptions, it is important to encourage activities that are enjoyed, that can be performed safely, and that can be incorporated into a daily routine. Some insurance companies now provide health club memberships as a way of encouraging activity. Many elderly individuals have difficulty with aerobic activity as a form of exercise. For those who are housebound or who have difficulty walking for any distance due to presence of spinal stenosis, peripheral neuropathy, claudication or other medical problems, stationary bicycling, arm lifts with weights, or leg lifts can be encouraged. Progressive resistance training has been proposed as a more reasonable and beneficial form of exercise in these patients.

B. Pharmacologic therapy   TLI is rarely adequate at achieving and maintaining glycemic control without pharmacologic therapy in the majority of patients with type 2 diabetes, including the elderly. This means that some form of pharmacologic therapy will almost always be required. While there is no absolute contraindication to use of any of the oral or injectable agents available for treating diabetes, there are special considerations for prescribing and monitoring of these agents in older adults. As a general rule, medications should be started at the lowest dose and gradually titrated upward as tolerated until glycemic targets are reached. In some cases, it becomes necessary to add on a second agent before maximal doses are reached with one agent as a way of minimizing adverse reactions. For example, the incidence of gastrointestinal side-effects increases with increasing doses of the biguanide, metformin. There are many patients who may be unable to tolerate the maximal dose of 2 g of metformin each day, but who are able to tolerate 1 to 1.5 g/d. In these instances, it may be desirable to continue metformin at a lower dose and add an insulin secretogogue to achieve the desired level of glycemic control. A discussion of pharmacologic therapy in this review is presented with consideration of this strategy in an elderly population (see Table 23–4).

Initiation of metformin together with TLI is recommended at the time of diagnosis of type 2 diabetes. Side-effects with use of metformin that have particular relevance to elderly patients include anorexia, nausea, abdominal cramping, and diarrhea that preclude the use of this drug in approximately 5% of all individuals. Reductions in vitamin B_{12} levels have also been observed. Given the high prevalence of vitamin B_{12} deficiency in the elderly population, it is reasonable to monitor its levels and/ or recommend vitamin B_{12} supplementation at a dose of 50 μg/d or more.

The most feared complication of therapy with metformin is lactic acidosis. This can be avoided by following prescribing guidelines that recommend against use of metformin in those with renal insufficiency, defined as a serum creatinine ≥1.5 mg/dL in men, ≥1.4 mg/dL in women; or a creatinine clearance of <60 mL/min. The observed age-related decline in glomerular filtration rate (GFR), as a measure of creatinine clearance, raises concerns for using metformin in the elderly; however, the formulas used to estimate GFR (eGFR) do not always provide accurate results in this population. When there is doubt as to whether metformin can be initiated or continued in a patient with a normal serum creatinine but a reduced eGFR, measurement of a creatinine clearance with 24-hour urine collections can provide a more accurate measure of renal function. In patients assessed as having normal renal function at the time metformin is started; renal function needs to be reassessed with changes in clinical status. Caution is suggested in patients >80 years of age, although there are no data demonstrating a higher incidence of lactic acidosis in this population, provided that renal function is normal.

There may in fact be advantages to metformin therapy. In a study of patients age 72 years with type 2 diabetes and congestive heart failure (CHF), those treated with metformin experienced lower morbidity and mortality when compared to those treated with sulfonylurea monotherapy. There are also epidemiologic data that suggest that treatment with metformin is associated with a lower incidence of cancer and cancer-related deaths.

Alternative or additional pharmacologic therapy is required for patients for whom metformin therapy is contraindicated, who do not tolerate the medication, or who do not achieve the desired level of glycemic control. Insulin secretogogues include long-acting sulfonylureas and shorter-acting meglitinides, which have similar efficacy in lowering A1c levels by 1.5%. The sulfonylureas reduce both fasting and postprandial glucose levels while the shorter-acting meglitinides reduce postprandial glucose excursions. Both renal insufficiency and increasing age are risk factors for hypoglycemia with use of these agents in the elderly when used as either monotherapy or combination therapy. Glipizide and glimepiride are less likely to cause prolonged hypoglycemia in the elderly than glyburide, which has active metabolites. The shorter-acting meglitinides administered immediately prior to a meal can be useful in reducing the risk for hypoglycemia in the elderly who experience variability in appetite or the timing of meals.

TABLE 23–5 Symptoms of hypoglycemia.

Sympathoadrenal Activation
  Sweating
  Sensation of warmth
  Anxiety
  Tremor
  Nausea
  Palpitations
  Tachycardia
  Hunger
Neuroglycopenic
  Fatigue
  Dizziness
  Headache
  Visual disturbance
  Difficulty speaking
  Inability to concentrate
  Loss of memory
  Confusion
  Loss of consciousness
  Seizures

When insulin secretogogues are prescribed, it is important that patients and their family members be educated in how to both recognize and treat a low-BG reaction (Table 23–5). Many individuals are unaware of what these symptoms are and can mistake this for simple fatigue or a cardiac event, resulting in potentially dangerous delays in therapy. It is important that patients be instructed to carry a glucose source with them at all times. This can be in the form of hard candy or glucose tablets.

The two thiazolidinediones available for clinical use are pioglitazone and rosiglitazone. Both agents reduce HA1c levels by 0.8% to 1.5%, with pioglitazone having more favorable effects on circulating triglycerides. Caution is warranted when using this class of medications in elderly individuals due to their potential to cause weight gain, edema, CHF, and reductions in bone mineral density (BMD) with increased fracture risk. In one report investigating outcomes with glitazones in individuals age >65, treatment with rosiglitazone was associated with a 60% increased risk of new-onset CHF, a 40% increased risk for MI, and a 29% increase in mortality. As both the incidence and prevalence CHF increase with age in those with diabetes, caution is required when using these agents in elderly patients. If a decision is made to use these agents, close monitoring for onset of edema, weight gain, and shortness of breath is important. Regular monitoring of 25-hydroxyvitamin D levels and BMD measurements is also indicated to address fracture risk.

The alpha-glucosidase inhibitors, acarbose and miglitol, delay absorption of carbohydrate from the small intestine by inhibiting the enzymes that convert carbohydrates into monosaccharides. This results in a reduction in postprandial glucose excursions, with reductions in A1c of 0.5% to 0.8% when used alone or in combination with other oral agents or insulin. The main limitation to the use of these agents is the high incidence of GI side effects that are directly related to their mechanism of action. Abdominal bloating and distension, diarrhea, and cramping occur in approximately

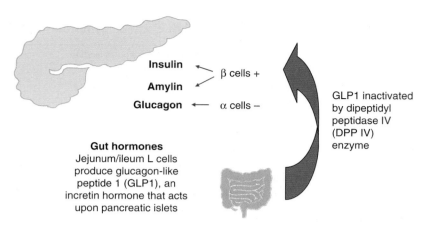

FIGURE 23–7 Hormonal regulation of insulin secretion and glucose homeostasis.

50% of patients. Initiating therapy at a low dose of 25 mg once a day given with the main meal and allowing gradual upward titration can improve compliance with this group of medications. It is important that patients be instructed to use glucose tablets to treat hypoglycemia that may occur when taking this class of medications with sulfonylureas or insulin, as there can be delayed absorption of glucose from food sources.

There are now two relatively new classes of medications that address the role of the incretin hormone, GLP1, in glucose homeostasis: injectable GLP1 analogs and orally administered dipeptidyl peptidase IV inhibitors (DPP IV). GLP1 is a hormone that is normally secreted by L cells in the distal ileum in response to a meal (Figure 23–7). GLP1 acts directly on beta cells to enhance endogenous insulin secretion, and on alpha cells to reduce glucagon levels. Endogenously secreted GLP1 is degraded by the DPP IV, which contributes to its short circulating half-life. Exenatide is the first GLP1 mimetic approved for clinical use. Liraglutide is another agent in this class that has recently been approved for use. Sustained reductions in A1c of approximately 1% have been observed with use of these agents. The major side-effects include anorexia, nausea and vomiting, abdominal pain, diarrhea, and weight loss. However, these side-effects often abate over time and with exenatide are minimized by starting with doses of 5 μg administered twice a day for a month before increasing to 10 μg twice a day. Hypoglycemia is possible when used in combination with a sulfonylurea. There are at least 36 postmarketing reports of acute pancreatitis with use of exenatide, but the incidence of this disorder does not appear to be greater than in the general population with type 2 diabetes. Nevertheless, a high index of suspicion is recommended in patients who report abdominal pain with use of these agents. It is anticipated that a once-weekly preparation of exenatide will become available for clinical use in the next 1 to 2 years.

There are two DPP IV inhibitors available for clinical use, sitagliptin and saxagliptin. By prolonging the duration of action of endogenously secreted GLP1, these agents reduce A1c by 0.6% to 0.9%. The DPP IV inhibitors are weight neutral and do not cause

hypoglycemia when used as monotherapy. The major side-effects of these agents are an increase in upper respiratory and lower urinary tract infections, headache, skin rash, sinusitis, and back pain. The higher incidence of infectious complications may have significance in the elderly population who are more likely to have asymptomatic bacteriuria. However, there is no absolute contraindication to use of these agents in the elderly. Dose adjustments are required in the presence of renal insufficiency with each of the available agents. The relatively benign side-effect profile can make them attractive for use; however, these agents are expensive and may have effects that are currently unknown. DPP IV is a ubiquitous enzyme that is also expressed in lymphocytes, raising concern for alterations in immune function.

When glycemic targets cannot be achieved with the agents discussed earlier, insulin therapy becomes necessary. In patients with isolated morning hyperglycemia, the addition of a bedtime dose of neutral protamine Hagedorn (NPH) can be effective in controlling fasting glucose levels. When both fasting and daytime BG levels are elevated, a long-acting insulin administered once daily can be more effective in lowering glucose levels throughout the day (Table 23–6). When BG levels remain elevated despite the use of basal insulin alone, premeal doses of a short- or rapid-acting insulin can be added.

When adding NPH insulin at bedtime to oral agents, a low starting dose of 5 to 10 U allows an elderly patient to become accustomed to insulin injections with a low risk for hypoglycemia.

TABLE 23–6 Insulin preparations.

Insulin	Onset	Peak	Duration
Lispro/aspart/ glulisine	5-15 min	1-2 h	4-6 h
Regular	30-60 min	2-3 h	6-10 h
NPH	2-4 h	4-10 h	12-18 h
Glargine	2-4 h	Flat	20-24 h
Detemir	2 h	Flat	6-24 h

The dose can then be titrated gradually over a period of several weeks until glucose levels are in the desired range. A commonly used strategy is to advise patients to increase by 1 or 2 U every 4 days until they achieve a fasting glucose of less than 140 mg/dL.

When initiating basal/bolus insulin, the starting dose of insulin can be calculated as 0.2 to 0.3 U/kg/d, with 50% of the dose administered as basal insulin and 50% as premeal insulin in divided doses prior to meals. For patients already receiving basal insulin who require the addition of premeal insulin, the dose of premeal insulin can be calculated as follows:

- If the BG is mildly elevated with the majority of readings below 200 mg/dL, the dose of basal insulin can be reduced by 50% with distribution of the remaining 50% into three premeal insulin doses.
- If the majority of BG levels are >200 mg/dL, premeal insulin doses can be started as approximately 25% to 30% of the current basal dose given before each meal. For example, if a patient is receiving 24 U of glargine or NPH each day, the starting dose of regular or humalog before each meal would be 6 to 8 U.

Many elderly individuals can be given instructions in how to advance their insulin doses or how to adjust the dose of insulin according to results of BG measurements. Correction insulin refers to the administration of supplemental doses of short or rapid-acting insulin when BG exceeds glycemic targets. A reasonable glycemic target may be to maintain all BG between 100 and 150 mg/dL. In these cases, the individual patient can be instructed to reduce their premeal insulin dose by 1 to 2 U if their BG is <100 mg/dL, and to increase by 1 U for every 50 mg/dL above 150 mg/dL.

There will be a minority of elderly patients who are unable to achieve adequate control of postprandial glucose excursions with insulin alone. Pramlintide, a synthetic analog of the beta cell hormone amylin, is effective at reducing postprandial BG levels when used in combination with insulin. This injectable medication is approved for use in combination with insulin for patients with both type 1 and type 2 diabetes. Side-effects of pramlintide include nausea and vomiting, which are more common in people with type 1 diabetes, and hypoglycemia. Nausea and vomiting can be minimized by starting at doses of 15 µg before each meal with gradual upward titration to 60 for people with type 1 diabetes. Those with type 2 diabetes can be started at a dose of 60 µg and titrated to 120 µg before meals. The risk for hypoglycemia can be reduced by reducing prandial insulin doses by 50% when pramlintide is initiated.

In summary, there are five classes of oral agents and two noninsulin injectable therapies, in addition to insulin, that are effective at achieving glycemic control as monotherapy or as part of combination therapy. The side-effect profile, risk for hypoglycemia, and cost need to be considered when choosing a regimen for an individual patient.

Screening for Diabetes-Related Complications in the Elderly

The care of older adults with diabetes is complicated by their clinical and functional heterogeneity. Some older individuals developed diabetes years earlier and may have significant complications.

Others may be newly diagnosed but may already have complications related to the disease. Some older adults with diabetes are frail with limited physical or cognitive abilities due to the presence of other underlying chronic conditions. Life expectancies are highly variable for this population, but often longer than clinicians realize. Providers caring for older adults with diabetes must take this heterogeneity into consideration when setting and prioritizing treatment goals.

Screening for microvascular diabetes-related complications is as important in older adults as it is in younger individuals, with attention directed to complications that can result in functional impairments if these remain untreated. While the natural history of diabetic retinopathy is different in those above age 70, recommendations for periodic eye examinations to detect not only changes related to diabetic retinopathy, but also for cataracts, macular degeneration, or glaucoma are important in allowing for early detection of disorders that can progress to cause visual impairment.

Annual measurement of serum creatinine and urine microalbumin allow for identification of nephropathy and chronic kidney disease due to other causes that can have their progression modified by dietary interventions and use of medications to lower blood pressure. Annual measurement of a lipid profile with interventions to treat those identified as having dyslipidemia can modify risk for cardiovascular events, which are associated with morbidity, decreased quality of life, and mortality.

Regular foot examinations with identification of anatomic abnormalities and sensory deficits that can reduce mobility are recommended. Medicare will cover the cost of special shoe wear for individuals with diabetes complicated by neuropathy or foot deformity. Pedorthic shoe wear is characterized by increased depth with a wider toe box that reduces pressure points that predispose to ulcer formation. Many prescriptions for shoe wear also include orthotics that allow for more even pressure distribution, thus improving the ability to walk without concern for foot injury.

A. Acute hyperglycemic complications Hyperglycemic hyperosmolar nonketotic syndrome (HHNS) is more common in elderly patients than diabetic ketoacidosis (DKA). HHNS can occur in patients with and without a history of type 2 diabetes. It is characterized by severe elevations in BG (>600-800 mg/dL), plasma hyperosmolarity (>320 mOsm/L), severe dehydration, and absent to mild acidosis. The development of HHNS in the elderly population can be attributed, in part, to an impaired thirst mechanism and an age-related increase in the renal threshold for reabsorption of glucose leading to an osmotic diuresis and intravascular volume contraction. Predisposing factors include myocardial infarction, pneumonia, infections, use of certain medications (eg, diuretics, phenytoin, glucocorticoids), or any acute medical illnesses. Patients often present with an altered mental status (lethargy, coma), marked volume depletion, orthostatic hypotension, and prerenal azotemia. Urine and serum ketones can be mildly elevated but usually not to the degree observed with diabetic ketoacidosis.

HHNS is a life-threatening disorder that requires prompt therapy with intravenous fluids and close monitoring of cardiac status. In addition to therapy directed toward treatment of the precipitating event (if known), extracellular fluid volume deficits, which can be profound, are replaced initially with normal saline followed by half-normal (0.45%) saline. Half of the fluid and electrolyte deficits can be replaced in the first 24 hours and the remainder over the next 48 hours.

Once volume replacement is addressed, low-dose intravenous infusions of insulin (5 U bolus followed by 1-5 U/h) can be initiated. The administration of insulin prior to volume correction can exacerbate intravascular fluid depletion and further compromise renal function as glucose shifts to the intracellular compartment. Potassium deficits can be addressed once urine output is established. Following resolution of the hyperglycemia, patients require careful evaluation of the cause of the deterioration as well as attention to the need for ongoing management of hyperglycemia with insulin or oral agents.

Care of the Elderly Patient with Diabetes in the Hospital

Hyperglycemia frequently accompanies acute illnesses that prompt hospitalization in patients with and without a history of diabetes. Newly recognized hyperglycemia adversely affects patient outcomes to a greater extent than established diabetes, with longer hospital length of stay, higher mortality, and increased likelihood of discharge to an extended care or rehabilitation facility. For these reasons, attention to glycemic control is as important during periods of hospitalization as it is in the outpatient setting.

The ability to achieve tight glycemic control in the hospital is hampered by rapid changes in clinical status, as well as by hospital routines that can increase risk for undetected hypoglycemic events that are associated with adverse patient outcomes. Current guidelines suggest glycemic targets of 140 to 180 mg/dL in both critically ill and non-critically ill-hospitalized patients. In critical care settings, this can be achieved with validated IV insulin infusion protocols. In non-critically ill patients, scheduled subcutaneous basal-bolus insulin is preferred. Less stringent glycemic targets may be appropriate for patients who have multiple comorbidities and reduced life expectancy, but in general, glucose levels should be maintained at values below 200 mg/dL to minimize fluid and electrolyte abnormalities, reduce renal complications, and avoid infections.

The practice of using *sliding scale insulin* as the only glycemic management strategy in hospitalized patients is discouraged. These regimens are associated with both hypoglycemia and hyperglycemia as they encourage reaction to a single BG value rather than a rational management strategy. Oral and injectable noninsulin glucose-lowering agents have a limited role for hospital use but may be appropriate for selected non-critically ill patients.

OSTEOPOROSIS AND CALCIUM HOMEOSTASIS

OSTEOPOROSIS

Despite the high prevalence, severe morbidity, and expense of osteoporosis, until recently most of our knowledge was derived from studies of younger postmenopausal women. Yet it is the older woman who typically experiences the ravages of the disease. Twenty-five percent of women have vertebral fractures by age 70; by age 80, the figure is closer to 50%. More than 90% of hip fractures occur in patients over age 70, and by age 90, one woman in three will have sustained such a fracture. Hip fractures are associated with significant morbidity, an increased risk of institutionalization, and an up to 20% increase in mortality rates. Despite the significant differences between perimenopausal and older women, diagnostic and therapeutic approaches for older women are derived largely from studies of newly postmenopausal women. The relevance of such studies for older women has only recently been questioned.

Definition and Risk of Fracture

The definition of osteoporosis has changed over the years. In 1991, a consensus development conference defined osteoporosis as "a disease characterized by low bone mass and microarchitectural deterioration of bone tissue, leading to enhanced bone fragility and a consequent increase in fracture risk." The World Health Organization issued classification criteria for postmenopausal women based on measurements of BMD or bone mineral content. Osteoporosis is defined as a BMD T-score of –2.5 standard deviations below the young adult mean value (Table 23–7). This permits numerical standardization of the definition. In 2008 the World Health Organization developed the FRAX algorithm that estimates the likelihood for a patient to sustain a hip or a major osteoporotic fracture (clinical spine, forearm, hip, or shoulder) over the next 10 years. The model is designed to include men and women, age 40 to 90, who have not previously been treated with medications for osteoporosis. FRAX uses population-based cohorts for Europe, North America, Asia, and Australia, and for the United States risk assessments are available for Caucasian, African American, Hispanic, and Asian groups. In addition to specific risk factors (Table 23–8), the model uses age, gender, height, weight, and femoral neck BMD or T-scores.

TABLE 23–7 World Health Organization diagnostic criteria for osteoporosis.

Diagnosis	Criteria
Normal	Bone mineral density or content –1 SD and above of the young adult mean value (T-score at –1.0 and above)
Osteopenia (low bone mass)	Bone mineral density or content between –1 SD and –2.5 SD of the young adult mean value (T-score between –1 and –2.5; includes individuals in whom prevention of bone loss would be most useful)
Osteoporosis	Bone mineral density or content at or below –2.5 SD of the young adult mean value (T-score at or below –2.5)

Modified and reproduced, with permission, from Kanis JA: The diagnosis of osteoporosis. *J Bone Miner Res*. 1994;9:1137.

TABLE 23–8 Risk factors included in the WHO FRAX model for the 10-y risk of a fracture.

Current age	Parent fractured hip
Gender	Glucocorticoids (≥5 mg/d prednisone for ≥3 mo)
Weight	Rheumatoid arthritis
Height	Secondary osteoporosis
Previous fracture	Alcohol three or more drinks per day
Current smoking	Femoral neck bone mineral density or T-score

Risk Factors for Osteoporosis and Fractures

Multiple factors contributed to the risk of low bone mass, osteoporosis, or fractures. Lifestyle factors include low calcium or vitamin D intake, high caffeine or salt intake, alcohol, smoking, falls, thin/frail habitus, and inactivity. Common endocrine disorders in the elderly include hyperthyroidism, hyperparathyroidism, and diabetes. Multiple myeloma and lymphoma can present with fractures. Emphysema, congestive heart failure, depression, end-stage renal disease, and malabsorption also contribute to it. Medications in the elderly that contribute to bone loss include glucocorticoids (≥5 mg/d of prednisone or equivalent for ≥3 months), anticonvulsants, aromatase inhibitors, androgen deprivation therapy, excess thyroid hormone, lithium, antirejection drugs, and heparin. By age 70, approximately 80% of women have a hip BMD that is osteopenic or osteoporotic, compared with 40% of women in their fifties (Figure 23–8).

Falling is often cited as a major risk factor for hip fracture in older women. Although more than one-third of elderly women fall annually, however, fewer than 5% of falls result in fracture. A fall to the side, a low hip BMD, low BMI (lean body habitus), and high-fall energy have been shown to be significant independent risk factors for hip fracture in community-dwelling elderly. In nursing home subjects, a fall to the side, low hip BMD, and impaired mobility were independent risk factors. Other factors, including a maternal history of hip fracture, previous hyperthyroidism, inability to rise from a chair, poor depth perception, poor contrast vision, and use of anticonvulsants or long-acting benzodiazepines are also associated with hip fractures in elderly women. Furthermore, with multiple risk factors, the risk of hip fracture increases significantly.

Factors Affecting Bone Physiology

There are significant physiologic differences between newly postmenopausal and older women with respect to maintenance of skeletal integrity. Although calcium intake is often inadequate in both age groups, calcium absorption declines with age despite an age-related increase in serum levels of parathyroid hormone (PTH). This increase is not due solely to a decrease in renal reabsorption of calcium but may represent secondary hyperparathyroidism from vitamin D insufficiency. When PTH levels are assessed in elderly community dwelling women, PTH levels increase as vitamin D levels fall below roughly 30 ng/mL (75 nmol/L) (Figure 23–9), similar to what has been observed in younger cohorts.

A. Vitamin D Vitamin D deficiency is common in the elderly, and vitamin D metabolism changes with age. Up to 15% of healthy elderly residents of communities in the sunny southwestern United States have frank vitamin D deficiency; still more have subclinical vitamin D deficiency; and up to 50% of elderly nursing home residents are deficient in vitamin D. This occurs because elderly individuals have decreased sun exposure and an impaired ability to form vitamin D precursors in the skin, a decreased dietary intake of vitamin D, and (possibly) an age-related decline in vitamin D receptors in the duodenum. In addition, the ability to convert vitamin D to its active moiety (1,25[OH]$_2$-D$_3$) is impaired with age. Certain vitamin D receptor polymorphisms have been associated with lower BMD and bone loss in some populations, although further investigations of vitamin D metabolism are needed in the elderly in the United States. Finally optimal vitamin D levels of ≥30 ng/mL (75 nmol/L) have been associated with higher BMD, decreased fracture risk, improved

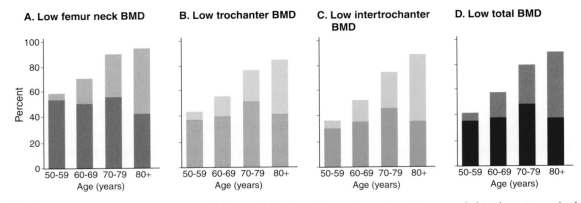

FIGURE 23–8 Prevalence of low femur bone mineral density (BMD) by age for non-Hispanic white women: light color, osteopenia; dark color, osteoporosis. (Source: CDC/NCHS III, phase 1, 1988–1991.) (Reproduced, with permission, from Looker AC, Melton LJ 3rd, Harris TB, Borrud LG, Shepherd JA. Prevalence of low femoral bone density in older US women from NHANES III. *J Bone Min Res.* 2010 Jan;25(1):64–71. [PMID: 19580459])

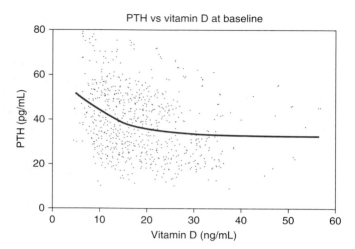

FIGURE 23–9 Baseline parathyroid hormone (PTH) and 25-hydroxyvitamin D levels in 553 community-dwelling elderly women. The line shown is a locally smoothed regression line (LOESS) of PTH given 25-hydroxyvitamin D. Twenty-six observations with PTH above 80 pg/mL are not shown (mean vitamin D level 13.1 ng/mL) to allow details of the LOESS curve to be visible. (Reproduced, with permission, from Greenspan SL, et al. Vitamin D supplementation in older women. *J Gerontol A Biol Sci Med Sci.* 2005;60:754-759. [PMID: 15983179])

lower extremity function, and decreased risk of colon cancer (Figure 23–10).

A. Bone loss and architectural changes The rate of bone loss also differs between newly postmenopausal and older women. Cortical and trabecular bone are lost rapidly at menopause. Older longitudinal studies suggested that bone loss ceased or slowed in older women. However, longitudinal studies suggest that older women lose an average of 0.7% to 1% per year at the hip, and femoral bone loss increases with age. Vertebral BMD changes assessed by anteroposterior measurements can give a misleading assessment of bone mass as a consequence of nonspecific calcifications from osteoarthritis, sclerosis, aortic calcifications, and osteophytes that interfere with and falsely elevate the measurement. Therefore, measurement of femoral BMD is more reliable in the elderly.

In addition, there are changes in bone geometry; cortical bone remodeling in older women is insufficient to compensate for the loss of bone mineral content (Figure 23–11). There are also qualitative changes in trabecular bone, because an age-related reduction in trabecular bone jeopardizes plate integrity or connectivity; trabecular plates not only become perforated and disconnected, but with aging they continue to thin, causing further loss of bone strength and compromising the bone's ability to regain structural integrity with conventional therapy. The loss of trabecular connectivity in the elderly can be visualized by high resolution MicroMRI technology of the wrist (Figure 23–12).

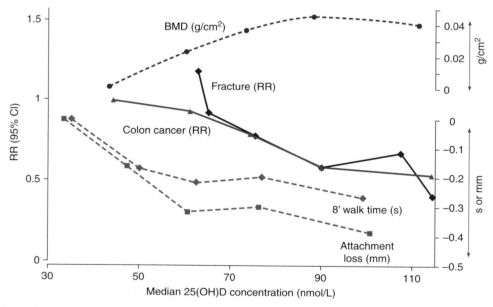

FIGURE 23–10 Relative risks (RRs) of fracture and colon cancer. Solid lines relate to the left axis, and dashed lines relate to the right axis. 25(OH)D, 25-hydroxyvitamin D. For bone mineral density (BMD), the example of older whites was chosen, and the unit is shown in the upper part of the right y axis. For lower extremity, the 8-ft walk test was chosen; the unit is seconds, as shown on the lower half of the right y axis. Alveolar attachment loss (measure of periodontal disease) is given in millimeters for older men, as shown in the lower part of the right y axis. This summary of all outcomes indicates that a desirable serum 25(OH)D concentration for optimal health begins at 75 nmol/L, and the best concentration is 90 to 100 nmol/L. (Reproduced, with permission, from Bischoff-Ferrari HA, et al. Estimation of optimal serum concentrations of 25-hydroxyvitamin D for multiple health outcomes. *Am J Clin Nutr.* 2006;84:18. [PMID: 16825677])

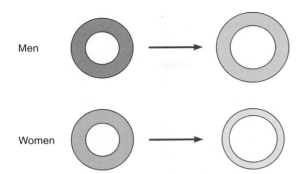

Men

Women

FIGURE 23–11 Schematic representation of cortical bone remodeling with age in males and females. Note that with age-related bone loss, bone is remodeled in men to increase its diameter and partially offset the loss of strength. In women, bone diameter changes little with age, so that bone strength decreases proportionately more than in men. (Reproduced, with permission, from Ruff CB, Hayes WC. Sex differences in age-related remodeling of the femur and tibia. *J Orthop Res*. 1988;6:886.)

Evaluation

Screening older patients by obtaining a BMD measurement is a comfortable, painless, noninvasive, rapid technique for determining an individual's bone mass and relative fracture risk. In general, the relative risk of spine or hip fracture roughly doubles for every standard deviation decrease in BMD below young, gender-matched mean values. Patients may remain dressed and lie on a padded table. Although several methods are available, currently the best technique uses dual-energy x-ray absorptiometry (DXA) of the hip or spine (Figures 23–13 and 23–14). The National Osteoporosis Foundation suggests obtaining a bone mass assessment in all women age 65 or older and all men age 70 or older regardless of risk factors. In addition, younger postmenopausal women and men age 50 to 69 with risk factors (see Risk Factors for Osteoporosis), adults who fracture after age 50, and those with a condition or medication causing bone loss should receive a bone mass measurement. For most elderly women, the hip is the single most useful measurement because nonspecific calcifications can lead to falsely elevated measurements in the posteroanterior view of spine.

Similar to the evaluation in a younger individual who presents with bone loss or fracture, the workup in an older patient can be designed to exclude secondary causes of osteoporosis. Hyperthyroidism and hyperparathyroidism are both more common in older women, can cause bone loss, and can be clinically silent in older individuals. Because 10% of women over age 65 are receiving thyroid hormone replacement therapy and because thyroid hormone overreplacement results in bone loss in postmenopausal women, true physiologic replacement with a normal serum TSH (if possible) should be the goal of treatment. Osteomalacia, vitamin D deficiency, and insufficiency may present as nonspecific muscle or skeletal discomfort and is more common in the elderly. This can best be assessed by checking a 25 hydroxyvitamin D level that should be ≥30 ng/mL or 75 nmol/L. In addition, metastatic carcinoma, multiple myeloma, hepatic and renal disease, and malabsorption (especially secondary to gastrectomy) should be excluded. Hypogonadism in men can be evaluated with a testosterone level. Medications (listed under Risk Factors) can cause bone loss.

Biochemical markers of bone turnover reflect bone formation and resorption. Although these markers are associated with the rate of bone turnover even in elderly women, they cannot be used in lieu of a BMD measurement to assess bone mass or to make a diagnosis. Because factors outside the skeleton contribute to fracture risk in the elderly, however, the search for correctable factors must extend beyond those that affect BMD. Particular attention should be devoted to the patient's home environment and medication use.

Patients who have sustained a fragility fracture as an adult have clinical osteoporosis and require evaluation and treatment. Because two-thirds of vertebral fractures are asymptomatic, patients with 1.5 to 2 in of height loss may need a lateral radiograph to look for vertebral deformities or compression fractures. Older patients presenting with skeletal discomfort should be evaluated by radiography to rule out a fracture. Vertebral osteoporosis usually presents with anterior wedging, involvement of more than one vertebra, prominent vertebral trabeculae, and vertebral deformities usually occurring below T_6 (Figure 23–15). Worrisome signs suggesting that skeletal involvement is not due to osteoporosis alone include nerve root compression, posterior wedging, isolated vertebral involvement (especially above T_4), and pedicle destruction.

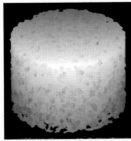
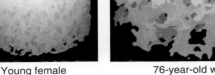
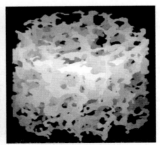

Young female   76-year-old woman   80-year-old woman

FIGURE 23–12 High-resolution MicroMRI images of radial trabecular bone in a young woman at peak bone mass and in 76-year-old and 80-year-old women demonstrating loss of trabecular connectivity (trabecular horizontal struts) with age.

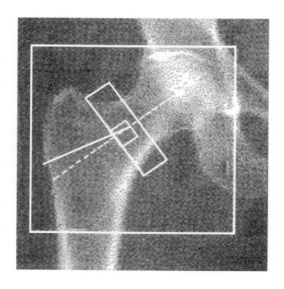

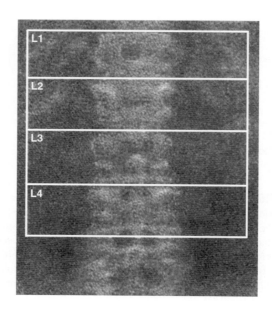

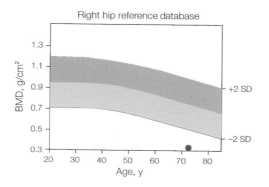

Region	BMD, g/cm²	Peak BMD-matched T-Score	% of mean	Age-matched Z-Score	% of mean
Neck	0.328	–4.69	39	–2.75	52
Trochanter	0.176	–5.22	25	–3.77	32
Intertrochanteric	0.428	–4.34	39	–2.93	49
Total	0.330	–5.02	35	–3.37	45
Ward Triangle	0.180	–4.74	24	–2.04	43

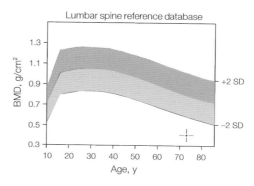

Region	BMD, g/cm²	Peak BMD-matched T-Score	% of mean	Age-matched Z-Score	% of mean
L1	0.305	–5.63	33	–3.62	43
L2	0.406	–5.66	39	–3.42	52
L3	0.382	–6.38	35	–4.03	46
L4	0.495	–5.65	44	–3.23	58
L1-L4	0.410	–5.79	39	–3.53	51

FIGURE 23–13 This patient has a total hip bone mineral density (BMD) of 0.330 g/cm² (black circle on the reference database graph) as measured by dual-energy x-ray absorptiometry, a femoral neck T-score of –4.69 and a total hip T-score of –5.02. The reference database graph displays age- and sex-matched mean BMD levels ±2 SD (shaded areas) derived from the third National Health and Nutrition Examination Survey. T-score indicates the difference in SD between the subject's BMD and the predicted sex-matched mean peak young adult BMD; Z-score, the difference in SD between the subject's BMD and the sex- and age-matched mean BMD; and % of mean, the subject's BMD as a percentage of the mean peak young adult BMD- or age-matched BMD level. (Adapted from bone densitometry report, QDR-4500C bone densitometer, Hologic Inc, Bedford, Massachusetts.)

FIGURE 23–14 This patient has a lumbar spine (L1-L4) bone mineral density (BMD) of 0.410 g/cm² (cross on the reference database graph) measured by dual-energy x-ray absorptiometry and a T-score of –5.79. The reference database graph displays age- and sex-matched mean BMD levels ±2 SDs (shaded areas) derived from a normative database from the manufacturer, Hologic Inc, Bedford, Massachusetts. T-score indicates the difference in SD between the subject's BMD and the predicted sex-matched mean peak young adult BMD; Z-score, the difference in SD between the subject's BMD and the sex- and age-matched BMD level; and percentage of mean, the subject's BMD as a percentage of the mean peak young adult BMD- or age-matched BMD level. (Adapted from bone densitometry report, QDR-4500C bone densitometer; Hologic Inc, Bedford, Massachusetts.)

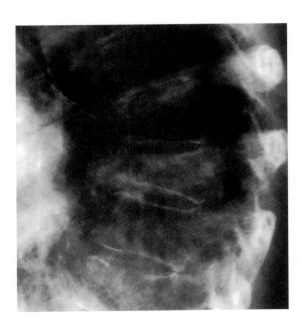

FIGURE 23–15 Lateral thoracic radiograph demonstrating a thoracic anterior wedge fracture. (Reproduced, with permission, from Clinical Crossroads. A 73-year-old woman with osteoporosis. *JAMA.* 1999;281:1531.)

Furthermore, older individuals may complain of persistent groin pain with weight-bearing, while plain radiographs of the hip reveal no fracture. A bone scan may be necessary to confirm the diagnosis of hip fracture. Vertebral fractures can also be assessed with DXA technology by Vertebral Fracture Assessment. Because this can be done at the same point of care when a patient is having a DXA scan, this is convenient for older patients.

Treatment

Because the factors that affect bone physiology—the rate of bone loss, the structure of remaining bone, and the risk of fracture—are substantially different in newly postmenopausal and elderly women, interventions appropriate for younger women may be inappropriate for elderly women. Studies of older individuals that use BMD—or preferably fracture—as an end-point provide the best data.

A. Calcium Controversy surrounds the use of calcium supplementation by itself in postmenopausal women, and few data are available regarding its use in older women. Theoretically, calcium supplementation seems appropriate because calcium intake in the elderly is low, and the ability to adapt to a low calcium diet declines with age. Calcium supplementation reduces the rate of bone loss. A meta-analysis of prospective cohort studies and randomized controlled trials concluded that calcium intake by itself was not associated with hip fracture risk and was neutral for nonvertebral fractures. However, a reduction in hip fractures and improvement in BMD has been demonstrated in very elderly women (mean age 84) treated with vitamin D (800 IU daily) and calcium (1200 mg daily). The National Academy of Sciences

recommends 1200 mg/d of elemental calcium in divided doses. In addition to dairy products, many foods (eg, orange juice, cereals, and nutritional bars) are now fortified with calcium. Calcium carbonate supplements should be given in divided doses with meals to improve absorption in the elderly, who may suffer from achlorhydria. Calcium citrate can be used as an alternative in such patients. A potential problem with prescribing high doses of calcium in the elderly includes inducing or exacerbating constipation. In addition, because compliance with other drug regimens decreases as the number of drugs increases, calcium tablets may be taken at the therapeutic expense of more important medications. Finally, because supplementary calcium does interfere with absorption of zinc, elderly patients receiving calcium supplementation should be encouraged to take a multivitamin containing zinc. Calcium absorption is not impaired by psyllium.

B. Vitamin D Vitamin D deficiency is common in the elderly, and vitamin D is needed for calcium absorption, mineralization of bone, and improvement in muscle strength. The current recommendation from the National Osteoporosis Foundation is 800 to 1000 IU/d. Vitamin D can be administered as a pure supplement of cholecalciferol (available as 400-2000 U tablets), in a daily multivitamin (400-800 IU) or calcium supplement (200-500 IU/tablet). A Cochrane review of 45 trials involving 84,585 participants comparing vitamin D alone or with calcium versus placebo reported vitamin D alone was not effective, but when combined with calcium, did result in hip fracture reduction in institutionalized elderly. Another meta-analysis of randomized controlled trials concluded that 700 to 800 IU/d of vitamin D, but not 400 IU/d of vitamin D, reduced the risk of hip and nonvertebral fractures in elderly patients. Clinical trials utilizing calcitriol (1,25-dihydroxy vitamin D_3) as a therapeutic option for osteoporosis have reported conflicting results. Given that the complications of hypercalcemia are increased, this form of vitamin D should probably be avoided.

C. Exercise Although the rationale for exercise therapy is sound, few data are available on results of exercise in elderly women. One study prescribed exercise for older women and found that forearm bone mineral content increased in those who continued exercising during a 3-year trial. Middle-aged women (mean age 60) participating in high-intensity strength training for 1 year had improvements in femoral bone mass, muscle strength, balance, and activity level compared with controls. A Cochrane review of 111 trials (55,303 participants in the community) reported that multiple component group exercise reduced the rate of falls and risk of falling, as did TaiChi. Walking—generally 30 minutes three times a week—is often suggested for frail individuals.

D. Bisphosphonates Bisphosphonates—nonhormonal agents that inhibit bone resorption—effectively prevent and treat osteoporosis. Bisphosphonates are the mainstay of therapy in the elderly. The aminobisphosphonates, alendronate, risedronate, ibandronate, and zoledronic acid have been shown to increase BMD at the spine (5%-8%) and hip (3%-6%) over 3 years in prospective clinical trials in postmenopausal women. Fractures of the spine were reduced by approximately 40% to 70%. Alendronate, risedronate, and zoledronic acid have reduced nonvertebral fractures (25%-40%), including hip fractures (40%-60%), in women with osteoporosis. Improvements following treatment with alendronate and risedronate have also been demonstrated in older women residing in long-term care facilities. Furthermore zoledronic acid has been shown to reduce clinical fracture 35% and reduce all-cause mortality by 28% in patients following a hip fracture. When taken properly, the oral medications are well-tolerated—an important factor in choosing therapeutic alternatives for the elderly. Moreover the oral medications are available as a daily, weekly (alendronate, risedronate), and once monthly (risedronate, ibandronate) medication and the IV therapies can be given every 3 or 12 months (ibandronate and zoledronic acid respectively). The oral medications have been associated with nausea, heartburn, and epigastric distress. Both the IV and oral bisphosphonates have been associated with arthromyalgias and myalgias which is an important clinical consideration in this age group. Theses agents should not be used in elderly patients with an estimated GFR ≤35 mL/min. Osteonecrosis of the jaw is a rare event in patients using these agents at a dose for osteoporosis. For men, alendronate, risedronate, and zoledronic acid are approved. For glucocorticoid-induced bone loss, alendronate, risedronate, and zoledronic acid are approved for treatment, risedronate is approved for prevention.

E. Estrogen and selective estrogen receptor modulators

There is considerable evidence that estrogen therapy, if initiated at menopause, slows bone loss, temporarily increases bone mass, and may prevent osteoporotic vertebral and hip fractures. If therapy is continued, its efficacy is sustained at least until age 70. In addition, some studies have shown that estrogen increases vertebral and femoral bone mass. However, the Women's Health Initiative found an increased risk of cardiovascular disease, breast cancer, and thromboembolic events along with a significant reduction in hip fractures and other osteoporotic fractures in women receiving conjugated estrogen plus medroxyprogesterone. Because of the increased risks, hormone therapy is currently not recommended as a treatment for osteoporosis because there are other available and effective therapies.

Selective estrogen receptor modulators (SERMs) have estrogen agonist and antagonist actions. Raloxifene has been approved for the prevention and treatment of postmenopausal osteoporosis. Although improvements in BMD are less with raloxifene than estrogen therapy, studies demonstrate a reduction of approximately 50% in vertebral fractures with no mastalgia, vaginal bleeding, or increased endometrial thickness. Studies demonstrated a reduction in cholesterol and raloxifene is also approved for the reduction in the risk of invasive breast cancer in postmenpausal women with osteoporosis. Because there is an increase in venous thromboembolic events, raloxifene should not be used in immobilized elderly or those with clotting abnormalities. Raloxifene has not been shown to reduce nonvertebral or hip fractures.

F. Other therapeutic options

Although calcitonin is an approved therapy for osteoporosis in postmenopausal women, few data are available about its effect on the incidence of fractures. It is expensive and when given by injection is poorly tolerated by the elderly. Nasal calcitonin has been shown to reduce fractures of the spine—but not of the hip—with no improvement in hip bone density. Calcitonin may reduce acute pain associated with vertebral fractures.

Teriparatide, PTH (1-34), the first anabolic agent, has been shown to significantly increase bone density (9.7% for spine bone density in 18 months) and reduce vertebral and nonvertebral fractures in postmenopausal osteoporotic women. Teriparatide is approved for postmenopausal women and men at high risk for fracture and for patients with glucocorticoid-induced osteoporosis. There are little data in the frail elderly. This is given as a subcutaneous daily injection for 2 years only.

Denosumab, an antiresorptive agent, that is a fully monoclonal antibody to receptor activator of nuclear factor kappa B ligand (RANK-L) inhibits binding to RANK and the formation and activation of osteoclasts. Denosumab has been shown to increase BMD at the spine by 9.2% and at the hip by 6.0% over 3 years compared to placebo in a clinical trial in women with an average age of 72 years. Denosumab reduced vertebral fractures by 68%, hip fractures by 40%, and nonvertebral fractures by 20% (all $p<0.05$). This is given as a subcutaneous injection every 6 months and is still under evaluation by the FDA. There are little data in the elderly.

Although results regarding the efficacy of hip protectors for hip fracture reduction in elderly patients have been mixed, hip protectors represent a relatively inexpensive option in frail elders. Poor compliance has been a key component in the lack of efficacy. Furthermore the type and design of the hip pad may also play a role in its efficacy.

Vertebroplasty and kyphoplasty are interventions in which polymethylmethacrylate (vertebroplasty) or polymethylmethacrylate in a balloon (kyphoplasty) are placed in compressed vertebrae for patients with intractable pain from vertebral fractures. There are few trials with these interventions, and it is not known whether the procedures strengthen or weaken adjacent vertebrae. Recent randomized trials with sham-operated controls suggest that vertebroplasty was similar to the control group for pain and pain-related disability associated with an osteoporotic compression fracture.

Summary of Management Recommendations

In summary, there is ample reason to question the validity of extrapolating data from studies of newly postmenopausal women when formulating a treatment plan for older women. However, given the prevalence of the problem, it is reasonable to recommend an adequate daily intake of vitamin D (800-1000 IU), an adequate daily intake of calcium (totaling 1200 mg), and judicious participation in an individually tailored exercise program. The use of bisphosphonates, SERMs, teriparatide (PTH) (1-34), or other treatments needs to be individually considered in elderly women. For elderly men, the use of alendronate, risedronate, zoledronic acid, and teriparatide are available for treatment.

Perhaps more importantly, the risk of falls should be addressed. The risk can be reduced by reviewing medications (including nonprescription agents) and discontinuing (when possible) those with adverse effects on cognition, balance, or blood pressure. Common offenders include long-acting benzodiazepines, tricyclic antidepressants, antipsychotics, antihypertensives, and agents with anticholinergic side-effects. It is also important to correct reversible sensory losses and medical conditions and to educate patients about hazards in their environment, such as throw rugs, extension cords, and poorly illuminated stairways, which could lead to falls and fractures. For patients with gait disorders, physical therapy should be considered.

Patients who have recently sustained a hip fracture should receive the same evaluation and consideration as those without a fracture. Because a hip fracture places the patient at a more than double the risk for a future fracture, and bisphosphonate therapy will reduce that risk, a hip fracture should not serve as a reason to omit evaluation or treatment (see also Chapter 8).

HYPERPARATHYROIDISM

Clinical Features

The prevalence of hyperparathyroidism increases with age. Although its incidence is less than 10 per 100,000 in women under age 40, the incidence increases to 190 per 100,000 in women over age 60. As a result, more than half of all cases of hyperparathyroidism occur in individuals over the age of 65. Most cases are mild. Detection is by routine screening of serum calcium, and few or no symptoms are present. However, with relatively minor elevations of serum calcium (up to 11-12 mg/dL [2.8-3 mmol/L]), some elderly subjects may experience weakness, fatigue, depression, and confusion. Failure to thrive and constipation are commonly seen; renal, gastrointestinal, and skeletal complications occur less often. Other causes of hypercalcemia in the elderly—especially multiple myeloma, malignancy, vitamin D intoxication, and thiazide diuretics—must be considered in the differential diagnosis (see Chapter 8). Familial benign hypocalciuric hypercalcemia, an autosomal dominant disease, can generally be ruled out with a urinary calcium creatinine clearance ratio of less than 0.01. Other causes of secondary hyperparathyroidism due to vitamin D deficiency (common in the elderly) such as malabsorption and chronic kidney disease should also be excluded.

Treatment

For symptomatic patients and those with serum calcium levels 1 mg/dL above the upper limit of normal, parathyroidectomy may be recommended according to current guidelines (see Chapters 8 and 26). Parathyroidectomy is well tolerated in the elderly and is the treatment of choice. Minimally invasive parathyroidectomy uses preoperative localization by neck ultrasound and sestamibi scan and intraoperative measurement of PTH rather than the conventional approach of visualization of all glands. This not only improves the success rate but simplifies the surgical procedure as well. Parathyroidectomy procedures in elderly patients have similar outcomes compared with younger patients with respect to cure rate, morbidity, mortality, and patient satisfaction. For those with more modest elevations, treatment recommendations are less simply stated because it is difficult to differentiate symptoms and signs due to the disease from those seen in older individuals without hyperparathyroidism. Moreover, asymptomatic individuals—especially those with levels of serum calcium under 11 mg/dL (2.8 mmol/L)—have been known to remain asymptomatic for more than a decade. An observational study of 116 patients followed up to 15 years, reported that one-third of subjects had disease progression meeting surgical criteria. Until more data become available, the decision to treat asymptomatic individuals surgically should be made on an individual basis.

In older patients who are not surgical candidates, cinacalcet (a calcimimetic that binds to the calcium-sensing receptor on the cells of the parathyroid gland) can rapidly normalize serum calcium and reduce PTH in patients with primary hyperparathyroidism. Short-term studies demonstrate normalization of serum calcium, a small decrease in serum PTH without a significant impact on BMD. In women, a course of estrogen may be effective. Ethinyl estradiol (30-50 μg/d) or conjugated estrogens (0.625-1.25 mg/d) reduce serum calcium by an average of 0.8 mg/dL (0.2 mmol/L), diminish urinary calcium excretion, and antagonize the skeletal effects of PTH. However, the risks of estrogen (discussed earlier) make this an undesirable choice. In men and women with higher elevations of serum calcium, oral phosphates can be used, but they are less well tolerated in the elderly because of their gastrointestinal side-effects and the potential for ectopic calcification. Furosemide is a less satisfactory alternative in frail elderly patients because it increases the risk of dehydration and resultant hypercalcemia.

CHANGES IN WATER BALANCE

With age, major changes in renal function and homeostatic mechanisms result in significant changes in water balance. Renal blood flow, cortical mass, the number of glomeruli, and tubular function all decline with age, though medullary mass is preserved. On average, the glomerular filtration rate decreases at a rate of 10 mL/min per decade from age 30 onward. Clinically, however, the most relevant change is the age-related decline in creatinine clearance, which is largely due to relative hypertension in the elderly. Because of the decrease in muscle mass associated with aging, however, serum creatinine levels are unchanged and may not accurately reflect the extent of renal functional impairment.

Extrarenal modulators of water balance also change significantly with age. Although there are no changes in the basal level, half-life, volume of distribution, or metabolic clearance of vasopressin, the stimulated responses of vasopressin are significantly altered. Hyperosmolar stimuli increase serum vasopressin levels in older subjects to five times those achieved in younger subjects. This exaggerated antidiuretic hormone response makes elderly patients more susceptible to hyponatremia. On the other hand, the normal vasopressin increase observed in response to overnight dehydration and postural change is impaired in the elderly.

Additionally, basal and stimulated levels of serum renin and aldosterone decline with age. In contrast, basal levels of atrial natriuretic peptide are three times higher in healthy elderly individuals than in young controls. These elevated levels of atrial natriuretic peptide may help identify patients at risk for the development of CHF. Finally, the thirst sensation appears to be somewhat impaired in healthy elderly individuals and is more impaired in those who are frail.

In addition to physiologic changes, many diseases and drugs further increase the vulnerability of the elderly to changes in water balance. These include kidney disease, hypertension, and congestive heart failure as well as medications that alter water balance (eg, narcotics, diuretics, lithium, carbamazepine, amphotericin B, intravenous hypotonic fluids, and hypertonic contrast agents).

HYPERNATREMIA

Clinical Features

The incidence of hypernatremia in elderly patients admitted to the hospital ranges from 1% to 3% and is higher for institutionalized elderly patients. Signs and symptoms are usually nonspecific (eg, lethargy, weakness, confusion, depression, failure to thrive). The cause is usually multifactorial, including impaired thirst mechanism, renal disease, sedative-induced confusion, use of restraints, reduced access to free water intake, excess water loss due to fever, and decreased response to vasopressin. Medications can cause nephrogenic diabetes insipidus; these include lithium, foscarnet, diuretics, amphotericin B, and demeclocycline. Central diabetes insipidus can result from CNS trauma, malignancy, infection, or it may be idiopathic.

Treatment

As in younger patients, initial therapy involves correcting the volume deficit with isotonic saline and then correcting the water deficit with half-normal (0.45%) saline. Roughly 30% of the deficit should be corrected within 24 hours and the remainder within the next 24 to 48 hours (see also Chapter 5).

HYPONATREMIA

Clinical Features

The prevalence of hyponatremia is approximately 2.5% in the general hospital setting—higher in geriatric units—and rises to 25% in nursing home settings. Hyponatremia can be classified by the total body sodium as hypovolemic hyponatremia (decrease in total body sodium, eg, after diarrhea, vomiting, diuretic use), euvolemic hyponatremia (normal total body sodium, as seen with syndrome of inappropriate antidiuretic hormone [SIADH]), hypothyroidism, adrenal insufficiency, and medications) or hypervolemic hyponatremia (excess total body sodium, as seen with CHF or cirrhosis). Presenting symptoms and signs of euvolemic hyponatremia are often nonspecific and include lethargy, weakness, and confusion. The mechanisms predisposing to hyponatremia include

the exuberant response of vasopressin to osmolar stimuli, a decreased ability to excrete a water load, and the sodium-wasting tendency of the older kidney. Furthermore, elderly patients often use medications and have diseases that impair free water excretion. Drugs that can cause hyponatremia include tricyclic antidepressants, phenothiazines, serotonin reuptake inhibitors, angiotensin-converting enzyme inhibitors, morphine, antiseizure medications, nonsteroidal anti-inflammatory drugs (NSAIDs), and acetaminophen. Common hyponatremic syndromes in the elderly include SIADH and thiazide-induced hyponatremia. In the geriatric rehabilitation hospital, approximately half of patients with hyponatremia have SIADH (see Chapters 5 and 21).

Treatment

The treatment of hyponatremia in the elderly depends on the type of hyponatremia. The treatment of euvolemic hyponatremia does not differ from that in younger patients (Chapters 5 and 24). Vasopressin receptor antagonists lead to an increase in electrolyte-free water diuresis, and an increase in serum sodium levels in patients with SIADH and hypervolemic hyponatremia from CHF or cirrhosis. Additional studies are needed, but these agents may become the mainstay of treatment.

HYPORENINEMIC HYPOALDOSTERONISM

Hyporeninemic hypoaldosteronism usually occurs in elderly patients with diabetes and mild renal insufficiency. Patients are usually asymptomatic. Hyperkalemia and metabolic acidosis are found on routine screening. Symptoms of hyperkalemia (eg, heart block) may be provoked by administration of a beta-adrenergic blocking agent, which further compromises extrarenal regulation of potassium homeostasis. After other causes of persistent hyperkalemia are ruled out, patients respond well to administration of small doses of fludrocortisone (0.05 mg/d) or furosemide combined with restriction of dietary potassium.

GLUCOCORTICOIDS AND STRESS

Cortisol levels increase 20% to 50% with age. There is an increase in the nocturnal level of cortisol, an age-related morning increase in cortisol in women (not men), and an advancement in the circadian rhythm (Figure 23–16). Aging is associated with an increase in the cortisol production rate, independent of weight, and this accounts for the increased daily urinary free cortisol levels in older individuals. Dehydroepiandrosterone (DHEA) secretion declines with age and can be partially restored by mineralocorticoid antagonism, but in healthy elders, trials do not support supplementation with DHEA.

In healthy elderly individuals, dynamic testing of the hypothalamic-pituitary-adrenal axis is normal; expected responses to insulin-induced hypoglycemia, metyrapone, dexamethasone, adrenocorticotropic hormone, and corticotropin-releasing hormone (CRH) are preserved (Figure 23–17).

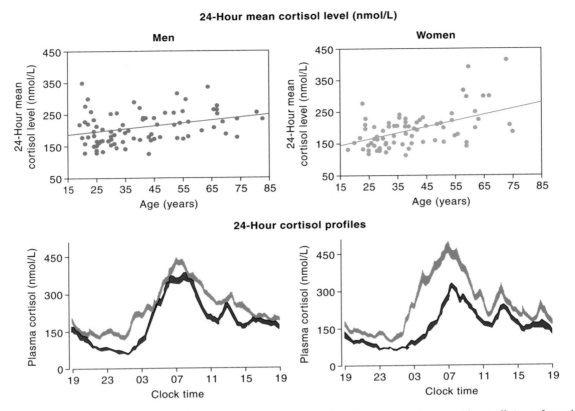

FIGURE 23–16 Upper panels: Age-related changes in 24-hour mean cortisol levels in men and women. The coefficient of correlation for the linear regression was $r = 0.29$ in men ($p < .002$) and $r = 0.50$ in women ($p < .0001$). Sex differences in the slope of the regression failed to reach significance. Lower panels: Mean 24-hour cortisol profiles in men and women 50 years of age and older ($n = 25$ and $n = 22$, respectively; blue lines) compared with those in 20- to 29-year-old subjects ($n = 29$ and $n = 20$, respectively; pink lines). The shading at each time point represents the SEM. (Reproduced, with permission, from van Cauter E, Leproult R, Kupfer DJ. Effects of gender and age on the levels and circadian rhythmicity of plasma cortisol. *J Clin Endocrinol Metab.* 1996;81:2468. Copyright 1996 by The Endocrine Society.)

DISORDERS OF THE HYPOTHALAMIC-PITUITARY-ADRENAL AXIS

1. ABNORMAL RESPONSE TO STRESS

In contrast to the normal responses in the elderly to dynamic testing of the hypothalamic-pituitary-adrenal axis, increased stress elicits abnormal responses. For example, although serum cortisol levels increase to the same extent in young and old patients undergoing elective surgery, the increase may be protracted in the elderly. Compared to younger, physically fit women, older physically fit women have greater cortisol production in the recovery period after a physical exercise challenge. Patients with diabetes mellitus and hypertension have also been found to have an exaggerated and prolonged response to corticotropin-releasing hormone (CRH) stimulation. Older patients with Alzheimer disease may also have a delayed and prolonged response to CRH stimulation. It is not known if these elevated cortisol levels contribute to the increased hypertension, glucose intolerance, muscle atrophy, and impaired immune function observed in the elderly. However, an elevated urinary free cortisol level is an independent predictor of osteoporotic fractures in the elderly.

2. ADRENAL HYPERSECRETION

Although adrenal hypersecretion (Cushing syndrome) is uncommon in the elderly, it is easily overlooked because it mimics normal aging processes. Signs such as hypertension, glucose intolerance, weight gain, and osteoporosis are less specific in elderly than in younger patients, but as in younger patients the diagnosis is established or excluded using the usual criteria (Chapter 9).

3. ADRENAL INSUFFICIENCY

Symptoms of adrenal insufficiency in younger patients (eg, failure to thrive, weakness, weight loss, confusion, and arthralgias) are common complaints in adrenally intact elderly patients; the most specific sign of adrenal insufficiency in the elderly is hyperpigmentation. The laboratory findings of adrenal insufficiency are similar to those in younger patients and include azotemia, hypoglycemia, hyponatremia, hyperkalemia, and eosinophilia. Because the metabolic clearance rate of cortisol decreases with age, older patients generally require lower replacement doses of cortisol (Chapter 9). For critically ill patients, the routine use of glucocorticoids should be reserved for patients diagnosed with adrenal insufficiency or

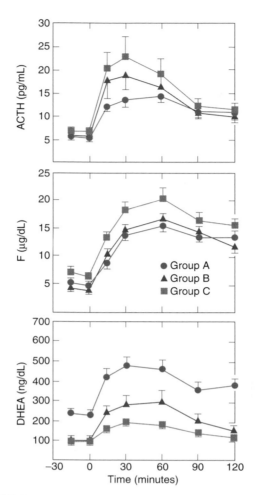

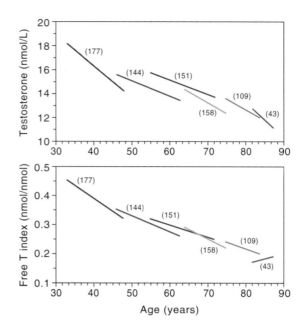

FIGURE 23–18 Longitudinal effects of aging on date-adjusted testosterone (T) and free testosterone index (free T index). Linear segment plots for total T and free T index versus age are shown for men with T and sex hormone–binding globulin (SHBG) values on at least two visits. Each linear segment has a slope equal to the mean of the individual longitudinal slopes in each decade, and is centered on the median age, for each cohort of men from the second to the ninth decade. Numbers in parentheses represent the number of men in each cohort. With the exception of free T index in the ninth decade, segments show significant downward progression at every age, with no significant change in slopes for T or free T index over the entire age range (T, testosterone; SHBG, sex hormone–binding globulin; T/SHBG, free T index). (Reproduced, with permission, from Harman SM, et al. Longitudinal effects of aging on serum total and free testosterone levels in healthy men. *J Clin Endocrinol Metab*. 2001;86:724. Copyright 2001 by The Endocrine Society.)

FIGURE 23–17 Mean values for groups A, B, and C of plasma ACTH (upper panel), F or cortisol (middle panel), and DHEA (lower panel) before and up to 120 minutes after bolus intravenous injection of ovine CRH (1 µg/kg). Group A, 21-49 years, mean age 35.2 years, n = 19. Group B, 50-69 years, mean age 60.7 years, n = 15. Group C, 70-86 years, mean age 77.1 years, n = 15. (Reproduced, with permission, from Pavlov EP, et al. Responses of plasma adrenocorticotropin, cortisol, and dehydroepiandrosterone to ovine corticotropin-releasing hormone in healthy aging men. *J Clin Endocrinol Metab*. 1986;62:767.)

those with hypotension, sepsis, acute respiratory distress syndrome, or lack of responsiveness to standard supportive care. Treatment doses of hydrocortisone (200 mg/d IV in four divided doses) should be weaned as soon as possible.

CHANGES IN REPRODUCTIVE FUNCTION IN MEN

Overall, while sexual activity decreases with age, there are conflicting reports about the physiologic changes in the hypothalamic-pituitary-testicular axis. Longitudinal studies demonstrate an age-related decrease in testosterone and free testosterone and a

higher frequency of hypogonadal values (Figures 23–18 and 23–19). Some studies suggest that circulating testosterone and bioavailable testosterone fall with age by 40% to 65% and are even lower in institutionalized elderly. A decrease in the number or responsiveness of testicular Leydig cells is likely because serum follicle-stimulating hormone and luteinizing hormone (LH) increase with age, and the testosterone response to human chorionic gonadotropin decreases. In addition, there is probably an age-related decrease in the ratio of circulating bioactive to immunoreactive LH. Finally, age-related alterations in pituitary function are suggested by a decreased gonadotropin response to luteinizing hormone–releasing hormone (LHRH) stimulation.

Epidemiologic studies suggest that the declining levels of testosterone are associated with decreased muscle mass and strength, decreased bone mass, increased fat, and insulin resistance. The benefit of testosterone replacement in older hypogonadal men is less clear. Potential adverse events of testosterone replacement include disordered sleep and polycythemia. The clinical impact on the cardiovascular system and prostate disease are also concerns.

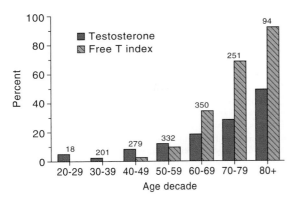

FIGURE 23–19 Hypogonadism in aging men. Bar height indicates the percentage of men in each 10-year interval, from the third to the ninth decades, with at least one testosterone (T) value in the hypogonadal range, by the criteria of total T <11.3 nmol/L (325 ng/dL) [shaded bars], or T/SHBG (free T index) <0.153 nmol/nmol (striped bars). Numbers above each pair of bars indicate the number of men studied in the corresponding decade. The fraction of men who are hypogonadal increases progressively after age 50 by either criterion. More men are hypogonadal by free T index than by total T after age 50, and there seems to be a progressively greater difference, with increasing age, between the two criteria (T, testosterone; SHBG, sex hormone–binding globulin; T/SHBG, free T index). (Reproduced, with permission, from Harman SM, et al. Longitudinal effects of aging on serum total and free testosterone levels in healthy men. *J Clin Endocrinol Metab.* 2001;86:724. Copyright 2001 by The Endocrine Society.)

Androgen supplementation is currently not recommended in healthy older men. Clinical trials are needed to establish a clear benefit and document the safety of testosterone supplementation in elderly men.

The correlation between sexual activity and the age-related hormonal changes described is weak. There are decreased concentrations of spermatozoa in the ejaculate of older men, sperm motility and the volume of ejaculate decrease with age, and the proportion of abnormal spermatozoa also increases. DHEA and DHEA sulfate are steroids of adrenal origin that decrease with age. Levels do not correlate with cognitive function or decline, and DHEA supplementation has not been shown to be beneficial. However, studies in the elderly are ongoing.

Erectile dysfunction (impotence) becomes more prevalent with age, but an endocrinologic cause becomes less likely. The prevalence of erectile dysfunction in men under age 45 is 5%; the prevalence in men over age 75 is 50%. However, more than 90% of men in the latter group have coexistent medical conditions or are taking medications that contribute to the problem. Furthermore, up to 30% of men over age 76 develop erectile dysfunction following prostatectomy, compared with 3% to 11% in younger age groups. Often there are multiple overlapping causes of erectile dysfunction—psychosocial, neurovascular, metabolic (diabetes mellitus), medication-related, and vascular—in the same individual.

The evaluation of erectile dysfunction in the elderly is similar to that in younger individuals (Chapter 12), although more

emphasis must be placed on the effects of drugs (both prescribed and nonprescribed) and vascular causes, and a search for multiple causative factors should be undertaken. Medications associated with erectile dysfunction include diuretics (thiazides, spironolactone); antihypertensives (calcium channel blockers, beta blockers, clonidine), cardiac and cholesterol-lowering drugs, antidepressants (SSRI, tricyclic antidepressants, lithium), phenothiazines, H₂ blockers, hormones (GnRH agonists, 5 alpha-reductase inhibitors, glucocorticoids), anticholinergic agents, and cytotoxic agents. Excess alcohol and smoking also contribute to it. Therapies include phosphodiesterase type 5 inhibitors that relax vascular smooth muscle cells. Because these medications can result in hypotension and increase the risk of myocardial infarction, if used with nitrates, the use must be carefully considered in elderly men with coronary artery disease.

REFERENCES

Thyroid Function and Disease

Aoki Y, Belin RM, Clickner R, Jeffries R, Phillips L, Mahaffey KR. Serum TSH and total T4 in the United States population and their association with participant characteristics: National Health and Nutrition Examination Survey (NHANES 1999-2002). *Thyroid.* 2007;17:1211. [PMID: 18177256]

Biondi B, Cooper DS. The clinical significance of subclinical thyroid dysfunction. *Endocr Rev.* 2008;29:76. [PMID: 17991805]

Gharib H, Tuttle RM, Baskin HJ, Fish LH, Singer PA, McDermott MT. Consensus statement: subclinical thyroid dysfunction: a joint statement on management from the American Association of Clinical Endocrinologists, the American Thyroid Association, and the Endocrine Society. *J Clin Endocrinol Metab.* 2005;90:581. [PMID: 15687817]

Haentjens P, et al. Subclinical thyroid dysfunction and mortality: an estimate of relative and absolute excess all-cause mortality based on time-to-event data from cohort studies. *Eur J Endocrinol.* 2008;159:329. [PMID: 18511471]

Helfand M; U.S. Preventive Services Task Force. Screening for subclinical thyroid dysfunction in nonpregnant adults: a summary of the evidence for the U.S. Preventive Services Task Force. *Ann Intern Med.* 2004;140:128. [PMID: 14734337]

Ochs N, Auer R, Bauer DC, et al. Meta-analysis: subclinical thyroid dysfunction and the risk for coronary heart disease and mortality. *Ann Intern Med.* 2008;148:832. [PMID: 18490668]

Shin SH, Holmes H, Bao R, et al. Outpatient minimally invasive parathyroidectomy is safe for elderly patients. *J Am Coll Surg.* 2009;208:1071. [PMID: 19476894]

U.S. Preventive Services Task Force. Screening for thyroid disease: recommendation statement. *Ann Intern Med.* 2004;140:125. [PMID: 14734336]

Villar HCCE, Saconato H, Valente O, Atallah AN. Thyroid hormone replacement for subclinical hypothyroidism. *Cochrane Database Syst Rev.* 2009;(3):CD000422. [PMID: 17636722]

Walter MA, Briel M, Christ-Crain M, et al. Effects of antithyroid drugs on radioiodine treatment: systematic review and meta-analysis of randomised controlled trials. *BMJ.* 2007;334:514. [PMID: 17309884]

Carbohydrate Intolerance and Diabetes Mellitus

American Diabetes Association. Standards of medical care for patients with diabetes mellitus—2010. *Diab Care.* 2010;33:S11. [PMID: 20042772]

Brown AF, Mangione CM, Saliba D, et al. Guidelines for improving the care of the older person with diabetes mellitus. *J Am Ger Soc.* 2003;51:S265. [PMID: 12694461]

Chalmers J, Cooper ME. UKPDS and the legacy effect. *N Engl J Med.* 2008;359:1618. [PMID: 18843126]

Knoops KTB, de Groot LC, Kromhout D, et al. Mediterranean diet, lifestyle factors, and 10-year mortality in elderly European men and women: the HALE project. *JAMA.* 2004;292:1433. [PMID: 15383513]

Masoudi FA, Inzucchi SE, Wang Y, Havranek EP, Foody JM, Krumholz HM. Thiazolidinediones, metformin, and outcomes in older patients with diabetes and heart failure: an observational study. *Circulation*. 2005;111:583. [PMID: 15699279]

Nathan DM, Buse JB, Davidson MB, et al. Medical management of hyperglycaemia in type 2 diabetes mellitus: a consensus algorithm for the initiation and adjustment of therapy: a consensus statement from the American Diabetes Association and the European Association for the Study of Diabetes. *Diabetologia*. 2009;52:17. [PMID: 18941734]

Osteoporosis and Calcium Homeostasis

Avenell A, Gillespie WJ, Gillespie LD, O'Connell D. Vitamin D and vitamin D analogues for preventing fractures associated with involutional and postmenopausal osteoporosis. *Cochrane Database Syst Rev*. 2009;(2):CD000227. [PMID: 19370554]

Bischoff-Ferrari HA, Dawson-Hughes B, Baron JA, et al. Calcium intake and hip fracture risk in men and women: a meta-analysis of prospective cohort studies and randomized controlled trials. *Am J Clin Nutr*. 2007;86:1780. [PMID: 18065599]

Bischoff-Ferrari HA, Giovannucci E, Willett WC, Dietrich T, Dawson-Hughes B. Estimation of optimal serum concentrations of 25-hydroxyvitamin D for multiple health outcomes. *Am J Clin Nutr*. 2006;84:18. [PMID: 16825677]

Cranney A, Papaioannou A, Zytaruk N, et al: Parathyroid hormone for the treatment of osteoporosis: a systematic review. *CMAJ* 2006;175:52. [PMID: 16818910]

Cummings SR, San Martin J, McClung MR, et al; FREEDOM Trial. Denosumab for prevention of fractures in postmenopausal women with osteoporosis. *N Engl J Med*. 2009;361:756. [PMID: 19671655]

Fraser WD. Hyperparathyroidism. *Lancet*. 2009;374:145. [PMID: 19595349]

Gillespie LD, Robertson MC, Gillespie WJ, et al. Interventions for preventing falls in older people living in the community. *Cochrane Database Syst Rev*. 2009;(2):CD007146. [PMID: 19370674]

Greenspan SL, Schneider DL, McClung MR, et al. Alendronate improves bone mineral density in elderly female long-term care facility residents with osteoporosis. A double-blind, placebo-controlled, randomized trial. *Ann Intern Med*. 2002;136:742. [PMID: 12020142]

Greenspan SL, Myers ER, Kiel DP, Parker RA, Hayes WC, Resnick NM. Fall direction, bone mineral density, and function: risk factors for hip fracture in frail nursing home elderly. *Am J Med*. 1998;104:539. [PMID: 9674716]

Holick MF. Vitamin D deficiency. *N Engl J Med*. 2007;357:266. [PMID: 17634462]

Kallmes DF, Comstock BA, Heagerty PJ, et al. A randomized trial of vertebroplasty for osteoporotic spinal fractures. *N Engl J Med*. 2009;361:569. [PMID: 19657122]

Kanis JA, Oden A, Johnell O, et al. The use of clinical risk factors enhances the performance of BMD in the prediction of hip and osteoporotic fractures in men and women. *Osteoporos Int*. 2007;18:1033. [PMID: 17323110]

Kiel DP, Magaziner J, Zimmerman S, et al. Efficacy of a hip protector to prevent hip fracture in nursing home residents: the HIP PRO randomized controlled trial. *JAMA*. 2007;298:413. [PMID: 17652295]

Lyles KW, Colón-Emeric CS, Magaziner JS et al; HORIZON Recurrent Fracture Trial. Zoledronic acid and clinical fractures and mortality after hip fracture. *N Engl J Med*. 2007;357:1799. [PMID: 17878149]

National Osteoporosis Foundation. *Clinicians' Guide to Prevention and Treatment of Osteoporosis*. Washington, DC: National Osteoporosis Foundation; 2008.

Parikh S, Avorn J, Solomon DH. Pharmacological management of osteoporosis in nursing home populations: a systematic review. *J Am Geriatr Soc*. 2009;57:327. [PMID: 19207148]

Peacock M, Bilezikian JP, Klassen PS, Guo MD, Turner SA, Shoback D. Cinacalcet hydrochloride maintains long-term normocalcemia in patients with primary hyperparathyroidism. *J Clin Endocrinol Metab*. 2005;90:135. [PMID: 15522938]

Rubin MR, Bilezikian JP, McMahon DJ, et al. The natural history of primary hyperparathyroidism with or without parathyroid surgery after 15 years. *J Clin Endocrinol Metab*. 2008;93:3462. [PMID: 18544625]

Wells G, Cranney A, Peterson J, et al. Risedronate for the primary and secondary prevention of osteoporotic fractures in postmenopausal women. *Cochrane Database Syst Rev*. 2008;(1):CD004523. [PMID: 18254053]

Wells GA, Cranney A, Peterson J, et al. Alendronate for the primary and secondary prevention of osteoporotic fractures in postmenopausal women. *Cochrane Database Syst Rev*. 2008;(1):CD001155. [PMID: 18253985]

Changes in Water Balance

Lin M, Liu SJ, Lim IT. Disorders of water imbalance. *Emerg Med Clin North Am*. 2005;23:749. [PMID: 15982544]

Rosner MH. Hyponatremia in heart failure: the role of arginine vasopressin and diuretics. *Cardiovasc Drugs Ther*. 2009;23:307. [PMID: 19554441]

Schrier RW, Bansal S. Diagnosis and management of hyponatremia in acute illness. *Curr Opin Crit Care*. 2008;14:627. [PMID: 19005303]

Glucocorticoids and Stress

Arafah BM. Hypothalamic pituitary adrenal function during critical illness: limitations of current assessment methods. *J Clin Endocrinol Metab*. 2006;91:3725. [PMID: 16882746]

Arlt W. Dehydroepiandrosterone and ageing. *Best Pract Res Clin Endocrinol Metab*. 2004;18:363. [PMID: 15261843]

Giordano R, Bo M, Pellegrino M, et al. Hypothalamus-pituitary-adrenal hyperactivity in human aging is partially refractory to stimulation by mineralocorticoid receptor blockade. *J Clin Endocrinol Metab*. 2005;90:5656. [PMID: 16014406]

Purnell JQ, Brandon DD, Isabelle LM, Loriaux DL, Samuels MH. Association of 24-hour cortisol production rates, cortisol-binding globulin, and plasma-free cortisol levels with body composition, leptin levels, and aging in adult men and women. *J Clin Endocrinol Metab*. 2004;89:281. [PMID: 14715862]

Traustadottir T, Bosch PR, Cantu T, Matt KS. Hypothalamic-pituitary-adrenal axis response and recovery from high-intensity exercise in women: effects of aging and fitness. *J Clin Endocrinol Metab*. 2004;89:3248. [PMID: 15240599]

Reproductive Function in Men

Harman SM, Metter EJ, Tobin JD, et al. Longitudinal effects of aging on serum total and free testosterone levels in healthy men. *J Clin Endocrinol Metab*. 2001;86:724. [PMID: 11158037]

Haren MT, Kim MJ, Tariq SH, Wittert GA, Morley JE. Andropause: a quality-of-life issue in older males. *Med Clin North Am*. 2006;90:1005. [PMID: 16962854]

Liu PY, Swerdloff RS, Veldhuis JD. The rationale, efficacy and safety of androgen therapy in older men: future research and current practice recommendations. *J Clin Endocrinol Metab*. 2004;89:4789. [PMID: 15472164]

McVary KT. Clinical practice. Erectile dysfunction. *N Engl J Med*. 2007;357:2472. [PMID: 18077811]

Mohr BA, Kim MJ, Tariq SH, Wittert GA, Morley JE. Normal, bound and nonbound testosterone levels in normally ageing men: results from the Massachusetts Male Ageing Study. *Clin Endocrinol*. 2005;62:64. [PMID: 15638872]

Endocrine Emergencies

David G. Gardner, MD

ACTH	Adrenocorticotropic hormone	IL	Interleukin
ADH	Antidiuretic hormone (vasopressin)	MRI	Magnetic resonance imaging
APACHE	Acute physiology and chronic health evaluation	PTH	Parathyroid hormone
		PTHrP	Parathyroid hormone–related protein
CT	Computed tomography	SIADH	Syndrome of inappropriate antidiuretic hormone secretion
DDAVP	1-deamino-8-D arginine vasopressin		
DKA	Diabetic ketoacidosis	T_3	Triiodothyronine
FT_4	Free thyroxine	TPP	Thyrotoxic periodic paralysis
GFR	Glomerular filtration rate	TSH	Thyroid-stimulating hormone

Acute or chronic failure of an endocrine gland can occasionally result in catastrophic illness and even death. Thus, it is important to recognize and appropriately manage these endocrine emergencies. This chapter will discuss crises involving the thyroid, anterior pituitary, or adrenal glands; diabetes mellitus; and abnormalities in calcium, sodium, and water balance. Except where indicated, management recommendations are provided for adult patients. Studies in the general area of endocrine emergencies have been limited in size and number. In many instances, recommendations offered in this chapter are based on published expert opinion rather than scientific evidence.

MYXEDEMA COMA

Clinical Setting

Myxedema coma is the end stage of untreated or inadequately treated hypothyroidism. The clinical picture is often that of an elderly obese female who has become increasingly withdrawn, lethargic, sleepy, and confused. The presentation is one of severe hypothyroidism, with or without coma (the term myxedema coma may, therefore, be a misnomer). The history from the patient may be inadequate, but the family may report that the patient has had thyroid surgery or radioiodine treatment in the past or that the patient has previously been receiving thyroid hormone therapy. Myxedema coma is most frequently associated with discontinuation of thyroid hormone therapy and less frequently as the first manifestation of hypothyroidism. Myxedema coma may be

precipitated by an illness such as a cerebrovascular accident, myocardial infarction, or an infection such as a urinary tract infection or pneumonia. Other precipitating factors include gastrointestinal hemorrhage; acute trauma; excessive hydration; or administration of a sedative, narcotic, or potent diuretic drug.

Diagnosis

The physical findings are not specific. The patient may be semicomatose or comatose with dry, coarse skin, hoarse voice, thin scalp and eyebrow hair, possibly a scar on the neck, and slow reflex relaxation time. There is marked hypothermia, with body temperature sometimes falling to as low as 24°C (75°F), particularly in the winter months. It is important to be alert to the presence of complicating factors such as pneumonia, urinary tract infection, ileus, anemia, hypoglycemia, or seizures. Fever may be masked by coexistent hypothermia. Often there are pericardial, pleural, or peritoneal effusions. The key laboratory tests are a low free thyroxine (FT_4) and elevated thyroid-stimulating hormone (TSH). Note that in an emergency situation, serum TSH can be done in 1 hour. The TSH elevation may be less than predicted due to the presence of euthyroid sick syndrome or glucocorticoid or dopamine therapy. If the FT_4 is low and the TSH is low-normal, consider central or pituitary hypothyroidism. Pituitary insufficiency can be confirmed with a low serum cortisol, impaired response to the cosyntropin stimulation test, and/or low follicle-stimulating hormone and luteinizing hormone. It is essential to check blood gases, electrolytes, creatinine, and an electrocardiogram in evaluating

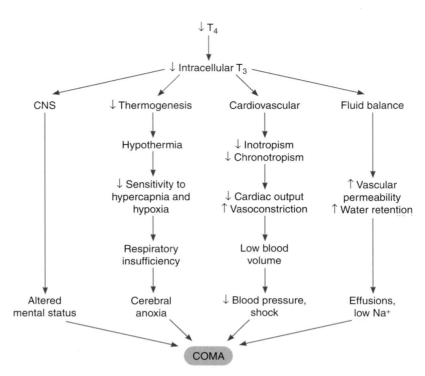

FIGURE 24–1 Pathogenesis of myxedema coma (CNS, central nervous system). (See text for details.)

pulmonary, renal, cardiac, and central nervous system status. The combination of hypothermia, hyponatremia, and hypercapnia should increase suspicion of myxedema coma. It may be necessary to differentiate myxedema coma from the euthyroid sick syndrome associated with coma due to other causes. These patients may present with a low triiodothyronine (T_3), normal or low TSH, but the FT_4 (by dialysis) is normal.

Myxedema coma is a complex problem involving a number of organ systems. The pathogenesis is presented in Figure 24–1. The decrease in serum T_4 results in a lowering of intracellular T_3. This can directly affect central nervous system function with altered mental status. The decrease in intracellular T_3 causes decreased thermogenesis, resulting in hypothermia, which in turn causes decreased central nervous system sensitivity to hypercapnia and hypoxia. The resulting respiratory insufficiency induces cerebral anoxia and coma. At the same time, the decreased intracellular T_3 results in decreased cardiac inotropism and chronotropism, decreased sensitivity to adrenergic stimuli, decreased cardiac output, and generalized vasoconstriction. This leads to a low-output state which, if untreated, culminates in decreased blood pressure and eventually shock and death. Finally, there is a change in fluid balance with increased water retention due to impaired renal perfusion as well as increased vascular permeability. These changes result in effusions and hyponatremia, which in turn contribute to the coma.

Management

Management of myxedema coma involves much more than simply replacing T_4 (Table 24–1). The patient is severely ill and

TABLE 24–1   Management of myxedema coma.

(1) Admit to ICU for ventilatory support and for intravenous medications.
(2) Parenteral thyroxine: Give a loading dose of 300-400 µg IV, then 50-100 µg IV daily. (May also give liothyronine sodium, 10 µg IV every 8 h for the first 48 h if necessary.)
(3) Electrolytes: Water restriction for hyponatremia. Avoid fluid overload.
(4) Limit sedation. Appropriate reduction in drug dosage.
(5) Glucocorticoids: Controversial but necessary in hypopituitarism or polyglandular failure. Dosage: Hydrocortisone sodium phosphate or sodium succinate, 50-100 mg every 6 h initially and tapered downward over 1 wk. (If initial serum cortisol was >30 µg/dL, corticosteroids are unnecessary.)
(6) Hypothermia: Do not externally rewarm.

usually is admitted to the intensive care unit (ICU) for intubation and ventilatory support. Oral medications may be poorly absorbed (due to gastric atony or ileus), and medications should be given intravenously if possible. A loading dose of 300 to 400 µg of T_4 intravenously is given initially to saturate T_4 binding sites in plasma-binding proteins. The patient is then maintained on 50 to 100 µg of T_4 intravenously daily. In addition, small doses of T_3 (eg, 10 µg intravenously every 6-8 hours) may be given over the first 48 hours, but this is usually not necessary, and it may contribute to untoward cardiovascular events. Its use should be restricted to younger patients without history of ischemic heart disease or cardiac arrhythmias. Water restriction is necessary to correct the hyponatremia, and intravenous glucose counteracts the tendency to hypoglycemia. It is essential to treat the precipitating illness (eg, pneumonia or urinary tract infection). The use of hydrocortisone is prudent because patients may have hypopituitarism or autoimmune polyglandular failure. Glucocorticoids are generally given in high doses until baseline cortisol or the results of rapid adrenocorticotropic hormone (ACTH) testing are available. If the initial serum cortisol is more than 30 μg/dL, steroid support is probably unnecessary. However, if serum cortisol is less than 30 μg/dL, hydrocortisone should be given intravenously in a dosage of 50 to 100 mg every 6 hours for the first 48 hours and the dose then tapered over the next 5 to 7 days while the pituitary-adrenal axis undergoes formal testing. Once myxedema coma is suspected in a hypothermic patient, external rewarming should be avoided, because this may cause redistribution of blood flow to subcutaneous tissues and cardiovascular collapse.

Prior to the recognition of the need for intravenous T_4 and for respiratory support, the mortality from myxedema coma was about 80%. Currently, the mortality is about 20% and is mostly due to the underlying or precipitating illness. Predictors of acute mortality include level of consciousness, lower Glasgow scores, and higher (acute physiology and chronic health evaluation) APACHE II scores, all indicative of the severity of the illness at presentation. Higher mortality is also associated with increased age, cardiac complications, and high-dose thyroid hormone replacement (≥500 μg/d of L-T_4 or ≥75 μg/d of L-T_3). The latter presumably reflects the increased metabolic demand attendant to high dose replacement in the setting of limited physiologic reserve. Persistent hypothermia and bradycardia, despite therapy, are associated with a poor prognosis.

THYROID STORM

Clinical Setting

Thyroid storm, or thyrotoxic crisis, is an acute life-threatening exacerbation of thyrotoxicosis. It accounts for 1% to 2% of hospital admissions for thyrotoxicosis. It may occur in a patient with a history of Graves disease who has discontinued antithyroid medication or in a patient with previously undiagnosed hyperthyroidism. The clinical picture is that of an acute onset of hyperpyrexia (with temperature >40°C [104°F]), sweating, marked tachycardia often with atrial fibrillation, nausea, vomiting, diarrhea, agitation, tremulousness, and delirium. The presence of jaundice is considered a poor prognostic sign. Occasionally, the presentation is apathetic without the restlessness and agitation, but with symptoms of weakness, confusion, cardiovascular and gastrointestinal dysfunction, and hyperpyrexia. Some of the factors that may precipitate thyroid storm are listed in Table 24–2.

Diagnosis

The diagnosis is largely based in the clinical findings. Serum T_4, free T_4, T_3, and free T_3 are all elevated, and TSH is suppressed. These findings are not different from what is seen in other patients with hyperthyroidism, but the difference is in the setting. It is

TABLE 24–2 Thyroid storm—precipitating factors.

Withdrawal of antithyroid drugs
Severe infection
Diabetic ketoacidosis
Myocardial infarction
Cerebrovascular accident
Cardiac failure
Surgery
Parturition
Trauma (eg, hip fracture)
Radioiodine (rare)
Drug reaction
Iodinated contrast medium

thought that thyroid storm represents an exacerbation of thyrotoxicosis associated with a shift of T_4 from the bound to the free compartment with an increase in free T_3 and T_4, as well as an exaggerated response to a surge of catecholamines that results from the stress of the precipitating event. The cause of death is usually cardiac arrhythmia and failure. Liver function abnormalities are often seen, as is leukocytosis, even in the absence of infection.

Management

The management of thyroid storm is summarized in Table 24–3. Patients are typically admitted to an ICU for cardiac monitoring. Initially it is important to block further synthesis and secretion of thyroid hormone, first with antithyroid drugs and then with iodide. One may give propylthiouracil, 150 mg every 6 hours orally or rectally, or methimazole, 20 mg every 8 hours orally or rectally. A few hours after initiation of antithyroid drug therapy, iodides may be started. Traditionally, saturated solution of potassium iodide, five drops twice daily, has been used, but currently iopanoic acid in a dose of 0.5 g twice daily orally or intravenously, or iohexol 0.6 g (2 mL of Omnipaque 300) intravenously twice daily is the treatment of choice. These drugs not only inhibit

TABLE 24–3 Management of thyroid storm.

Supportive care
Fluids
Oxygen
Cooling blanket
Acetaminophen
Multivitamins
If indicated, antibiotics, digoxin
Specific measures
Propranolol, 40-80 mg orally every 6 h
Propylthiouracil, 150 mg every 6 h, or methimazole, 20 mg every 8 h; may be administered per rectum if oral route is unavailable
Saturated solution of potassium iodide, 5 drops (250 mg) orally twice daily; or iopanoic acid, 0.5 g IV or orally twice daily; or iohexol, 0.6 g (2 mL of Omnipaque 300) IV twice daily
Dexamethasone, 2 mg every 6 h
Cholestyramine or colestipol, 20-30 g/d

thyroid hormone synthesis but also block the conversion of T_4 to T_3, lowering the thyroid hormone level in the blood. Additional specific therapy includes β-adrenergic blockade with propranolol, 40 to 80 mg orally every 6 hours or 0.5 to 1 mg intravenously over 10 minutes every 3 hours, with continuous cardiac monitoring. In patients with asthma, the $β_1$-selective antagonist esmolol can be given as a bolus dose (0.25-0.5 mg/kg over 10 minutes) followed by continuous intravenous infusion (0.05-0.1 mg/kg/min). The half-life of glucocorticoids is markedly reduced in severe thyrotoxicosis, so that adrenal support may be very useful. Dexamethasone also reduces conversion of T_4 to T_3 (as do the β blockers, especially propranolol). For this purpose, dexamethasone is given in a dosage of 2 mg every 6 hours for 48 hours, followed by tapering of the dose. Finally, cholestyramine or colestipol binds T_4 in the gut interfering with its enterohepatic circulation and may help bring the circulating level of T_4 down more quickly. Supportive therapy includes adequate fluids, oxygen, management of atrial fibrillation or heart failure, parenteral water-soluble vitamins, and a cooling blanket and acetaminophen for hyperpyrexia. Aspirin should be avoided, because it will displace T_4 from thyroid hormone–binding globulin, resulting in an increase in FT_4. Plasmapheresis or dialysis to remove FT_4 has been reported to be useful in nonresponders, but this is rarely necessary.

Therapy for thyroid storm has improved markedly, so the mortality has dropped from 100% in the 1920s to about 20% to 30% in recent series. However, because storm is often associated with other underlying medical problems, it still represents a serious medical complication.

THYROTOXIC PERIODIC PARALYSIS

Clinical Setting

Thyrotoxic periodic paralysis (TPP) is a rare but frightening thyroid emergency. The usual clinical presentation is of an Asian male (male:female ratio approximately 17:1) with symptoms of untreated hyperthyroidism who awakens at night or in the morning with flaccid ascending paralysis. Typically, there is a history of vigorous exercise and/or a large high-carbohydrate meal before retiring. There is usually no family history of periodic paralysis, but there may be a family history of autoimmune thyroid disease. The paralysis initially involves the lower extremities but progresses to the girdle muscles, followed by the upper extremities. Proximal muscle groups are affected to a greater extent than distal. Facial and respiratory muscles are usually spared. Sensory function, bowel and bladder function are not affected. Deep tendon reflexes are depressed or absent. The acute episode may be complicated by cardiac arrhythmias due to the concomitant presence of hypokalemia. The illness has also been reported to occur in Native Americans, African Americans, and in individuals of Mexican or South American descent, but these ethnic groups are affected rarely.

Diagnosis

The differential diagnosis of TPP includes familial periodic paralysis, Guillain-Barré syndrome, and acute intermittent

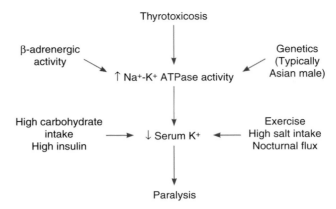

FIGURE 24–2 Pathogenesis of thyrotoxic periodic paralysis. (See text for details.)

porphyria. The diagnosis is based on the absence of a family history, the characteristic presentation, the presence of hyperthyroidism due either to Graves disease or toxic nodular goiter (other types of hyperthyroidism have been implicated as well), and usually a low serum potassium level.

The pathogenesis is summarized in Figure 24–2. Thyrotoxicosis, increased β-adrenergic activity, and an assumed genetic predisposition, perhaps involving the potassium channel Kir2.6, which together with increased Na^+-K^+ ATPase activity leads to increased intracellular potassium concentrations. A high-carbohydrate meal with increased insulin secretion and glycogen deposition, vigorous exercise high salt intake, and the normal nocturnal potassium flux serve to drive serum potassium levels even lower, resulting in flaccid neuromuscular paralysis. Note that there is no loss of total body potassium, merely a shift from the extracellular to the intracellular space. Consequently, aggressive potassium repletion, particularly through the parenteral route, is discouraged because this frequently results in significant hyperkalemia as potassium redistributes across cellular compartments following resolution of the attack. Hypophosphatemia and hypomagnesemia may be present. This is also assumed to reflect intracellular sequestration. The electromyogram, performed while the patient is experiencing weakness, shows myopathic changes with reduced amplitude of compound muscle action potentials. These do not change in amplitude after administration of intra-arterial low-dose epinephrine (distinguishes from familial periodic paralysis). Electrocardiograms show changes associated with hypokalemia, tachycardia, increased QRS voltage, first-degree heart block, and, on occasion, serious ventricular arrhythmias.

Management

The management of this problem is presented in Table 24–4. Propranolol in doses of 60 mg every 6 hours blocks the β-adrenergic stimulation of Na^+-K^+ ATPase. Antithyroid drug therapy should be started immediately, even though it takes time to bring the patient into a euthyroid state. Oral potassium, if indicated, should be administered cautiously. It is particularly

TABLE 24–4 Management of thyrotoxic periodic paralysis.

(1) Oral potassium supplement (if needed); monitor serum K⁺
(2) Oral propranolol (60 mg every 6 h)
(3) Antithyroid drug therapy

Avoid:
IV potassium
IV glucose (ie, crystalloid fluid replacement only)
β-Adrenergic agonists (eg, isoproterenol)

important to be cautious if administering intravenous potassium, which may raise total body potassium to toxic levels as the episode resolves. One should also avoid intravenous glucose, which stimulates insulin secretion and worsens hypokalemia, and β-adrenergic agonists such as isoproterenol, which promote movement of potassium into the intracellular compartment and exacerbate the problem. There is no role for potassium supplementation in preventing attacks. Acetazolamide, which has been shown to reduce frequency of attacks in familial periodic paralysis, may worsen attacks of thyrotoxic periodic paralysis and should be avoided. With appropriate treatment, recovery is rapid, and once the thyrotoxicosis is controlled, the paralysis will not recur.

AMIODARONE-INDUCED THYROTOXICOSIS

Clinical Setting

Amiodarone is a benzofuran derivative that is widely used in the treatment of cardiac arrhythmias. It contains two atoms of iodine per molecule, which represents 37.5% iodine by weight. The compound is stored in adipose tissue and has a half-life in the body of 2 to 3 months, with gradual and continuous release of iodide. The usual daily maintenance dose of amiodarone of 200 to 400 mg/d releases 6,000 to 12,000 μg of iodine daily, which when compared to the normal daily requirement of about 150 μg of iodide represents an enormous iodide load.

The structure of amiodarone resembles that of T_3, and it is thought that part of the cardiac depressant effect of amiodarone may be due to binding to and blocking the T_3 receptor in cardiac muscle. However, the effect of amiodarone on the thyroid gland is different and is due in part to a direct effect of iodine on the thyroid cell—to inhibit or stimulate hormone synthesis—and a cytotoxic effect of amiodarone on the follicular cell—inducing destruction of the cell and release of stored hormone. Thus, the drug may induce hypothyroidism, which is easily managed by thyroxine replacement, or hyperthyroidism, which, because of the underlying heart disease, is much more difficult to manage and may represent a true thyroid emergency. Two mechanisms have been suggested to explain the development of hyperthyroidism: (1) the high iodine level in a multinodular gland, or in the gland of a patient with latent Graves disease, or even in a previously normal gland, can induce hyperthyroidism (see Chapter 7), and

(2) the toxic effect of amiodarone itself may cause acute and chronic thyroiditis with release of T_4 and T_3 into the circulation and severe thyrotoxicosis. Risk factors for amiodarone-induced thyrotoxicosis include the presence of autoimmune thyroiditis and baseline elevation of TSH levels.

The patient with amiodarone-induced thyrotoxicosis may have been on the drug for months. Thyrotoxicosis typically appears 6 to 12 months after the onset of treatment. The underlying heart disease gradually worsens with increasingly frequent episodes of arrhythmia and heart failure. At the same time there may be weight loss, heat intolerance, increased nervousness, and marked muscle weakness. On physical examination, one may find nontender nodular or diffuse thyroid enlargement, tachycardia with or without atrial fibrillation, tremor, hyperreflexia, and, occasionally, lid lag and stare. Laboratory findings are unique because amiodarone inhibits the conversion of T_4 to T_3. Thus, even in the euthyroid patient taking amiodarone, total T_4 may be elevated while FT_4 and TSH are normal. In the hyperthyroid patient, the FT_4 is markedly elevated and TSH is less than 0.01 mU/L (below the detection limit of the assay). Radioiodine uptake in the iodide-loaded patient is low. It has been difficult to distinguish thyrotoxicosis due to follicular cell hyperfunction from that due to follicular cell destruction. Thyroid ultrasound with color Doppler studies may show increased circulation with hyperfunction and decreased blood flow with thyroiditis. Also, the cytokine interleukin (IL)-6 is low in patients with hyperfunction, whereas it is markedly elevated in patients with thyroiditis. However, these tests have not proven sufficiently robust to separate these two disorders.

Management

Management of amiodarone-induced hyperthyroidism is difficult (Table 24–5). Ideally, amiodarone should be discontinued, but often it cannot be stopped because of the underlying heart disease, and even if it is discontinued, the iodine load persists for several months. Further synthesis of T_4 should be blocked with methimazole in a dosage of 40 to 80 mg/d or propylthiouracil in doses of 400 to 800 mg/d. β-Adrenergic blockade, if needed (amiodarone, itself, has some β-blocking activity), should be instituted with propranolol or a comparable drug if cardiac status permits it. Potassium perchlorate in a dosage of 250 mg every 6 hours blocks further iodine uptake and lowers intrathyroidal iodide content. Aplastic anemia has occurred in patients on

TABLE 24–5 Management of amiodarone-induced hyperthyroidism.

(1) Stop amiodarone if possible
(2) Institute β-blocker therapy if possible
(3) Antithyroid drugs: Methimazole, 40-60 mg/d
(4) Potassium perchlorate, 200 mg every 6 h
(5) Cholestyramine or colestipol, 20-30 g/d
(6) Prednisone, 40 mg/d, for acute thyroiditis (consider monitoring IL-6 levels)
(7) Thyroidectomy

high-dose or long-term potassium perchlorate therapy, so that use of this medication has usually been limited to 1 month. Iopanoic acid (0.5 g orally twice daily) can be used to decrease T_4 to T_3 conversion. Cholestyramine or colestipol in a dosage of 20 to 30 g/d binds T_4 and T_3 in the gut and brings blood levels down more quickly. If there is reason to suspect thyroiditis (elevated serum IL-6 or decreased blood flow on ultrasound), corticosteroid therapy often yields dramatic results. Prednisone is given in a dosage of 40 mg/d for 1 month, gradually tapering the dose over the following 2 months. In those cases where a mixed etiology is suspected (ie, hyperfunction plus thyroiditis), a combination of steroids, antithyroid drugs, and β blockers can be used. If medical therapy is unable to control the disease, thyroidectomy results in a permanent cure and may be used as a last resort. Iopanoic acid (see above) can be used to prepare the patient for surgery. Perioperative mortality may be as high as 8% to 9% due to the underlying cardiac disease.

ACUTE ADRENAL INSUFFICIENCY

Clinical Setting

Acute adrenal insufficiency usually occurs as an acute illness in a patient with chronic adrenal insufficiency (see Chapter 9). The chronic adrenal insufficiency may be primary, due to destruction of the adrenal glands associated with autoimmune adrenalitis, adrenal leukodystrophy or, rarely, tuberculosis, fungus, or metastatic malignancy. Chronic adrenal insufficiency may also be secondary to pituitary or hypothalamic disease. Acute adrenal insufficiency may also occur with bilateral adrenal hemorrhage in a previously healthy individual during the course of septicemia with disseminated intravascular coagulopathy or in a patient receiving anticoagulant therapy. In the patient with known adrenal insufficiency, an acute crisis may be precipitated by inadvertent omission of steroid medication or by the concurrent development of a precipitating illness such as severe infection, acute myocardial infarction, cerebrovascular hemorrhage or infarction, surgery without adrenal support, or severe acute trauma. Acute adrenal insufficiency may also be precipitated by the sudden withdrawal of steroids in a patient previously on long-term steroid therapy with associated adrenal atrophy (ie, secondary adrenal insufficiency). Finally, administration of drugs impairing adrenal hormone synthesis such as ketoconazole, aminoglutethimide, etomidate, or mitotane—or drugs increasing steroid metabolism such as phenytoin or rifampin—may precipitate an adrenal crisis.

The patient presents with an acute onset of nausea, vomiting, hyperpyrexia, abdominal pain, dehydration, hypotension, and shock. A clue to the diagnosis of primary adrenal insufficiency is the presence of pigmentation in unexposed areas of the skin, particularly in the creases of the palms and in the buccal mucosa. The differential diagnosis includes consideration of other causes of cardiovascular collapse, sepsis, and intra-abdominal abscess. Failure of the hypotension to respond to pressors is suggestive of adrenal insufficiency and is an indication for a trial of glucocorticoid therapy.

Diagnosis

Primary adrenal insufficiency is characterized by hyponatremia and hyperkalemia. However, in situations of adrenal crisis, the hyponatremia may be obscured by dehydration. Random serum cortisol determinations are not helpful unless the levels are very low (<5 μg/dL [138 nmol/L]) during a period of great stress. The key diagnostic test is failure of serum cortisol to rise above 20 μg/dL (552 nmol/L) 30 minutes after intravenous injection of 250 μg synthetic ACTH (cosyntropin) (see Chapter 9 for details). This test functions best in the diagnosis of primary versus secondary adrenal insufficiency. At a specificity of 95%, sensitivities are 97% and 57%, respectively (see Chapter 3). Interpretation of the test, particularly in the evaluation of secondary adrenal insufficiency, is complicated in the presence of hypoalbuminemia, a marker for reduced protein-bound cortisol in plasma. In this setting, serum-free cortisol levels provide a more accurate assessment of adrenal function. Random serum-free cortisol of >1.8 μg/dL and a Cortrosyn-stimulated value of >3.1 μg/dL in critically ill patients is considered normal. There has been increased interest in using a more physiologic dose of ACTH to perform this stimulation test (1 μg vs 250 μg); however, a recent comparison suggests no particular advantage in the performance characteristics of the low-dose test. Basal serum ACTH is elevated (>52 pg/mL [>11 pmol/L]) in patients with primary adrenal insufficiency but not in patients with secondary adrenal insufficiency due to pituitary or hypothalamic disease. Computed tomography (CT) or sonography of the abdomen reveals adrenal enlargement in patients with adrenal hemorrhage, active tuberculosis, or metastatic malignancy. Atrophy of the adrenals is associated with chronic adrenal insufficiency.

Management

The management of adrenal crisis is outlined in Table 24–6. Hydrocortisone should be administered in a dosage of 100 mg intravenously followed by 50 to 75 mg every 6 hours thereafter. Fluids and Na^+ should be replaced with several liters of 5% glucose in normal saline. After the first 24 hours, the dose of intravenous hydrocortisone can be slowly reduced, but intravenous doses should be given at least every 6 hours because of the short half-life (1 hour) of hydrocortisone in the circulation. When the

TABLE 24–6 Management of adrenal crisis.

(1) Hydrocortisone sodium phosphate or sodium succinate, 100 mg IV stat and then 50-75 mg IV every 6 h for 24 h. Then taper slowly downward over the next 72 h, giving the drug every 4-6 h IV. When patient is tolerating oral feedings, shift to oral replacement therapy, overlapping the first oral and last intravenous doses.

(2) Replace salt and fluid losses with several liters of 5% glucose in normal saline IV.

(3) Patients with primary adrenal insufficiency may require mineralocorticoid (fludrocortisone) when shifted to oral hydrocortisone maintenance therapy.

(4) Diagnose and treat the illness that precipitated the acute crisis.

patient can tolerate oral feedings, hydrocortisone can be given orally, but the first oral dose should overlap the last intravenous dose. Alternatively, hydrocortisone can be administered as a continuous infusion at the rate of 10 mg/h for the first 24 hours, followed by a gradual decrease in the dose. Mineralocorticoid is not necessary during the acute replacement period since enough NaCl and glucocorticoid are being administered to treat the mineralocorticoid deficiency. However, in patients with chronic primary adrenal insufficiency, mineralocorticoid supplementation is necessary when shifting to an oral maintenance program (see Chapter 9). After steroid therapy has been instituted, it is extremely important to evaluate and treat the illness that may have precipitated the acute crisis (eg, infection, myocardial infarction).

Prevention of acute adrenal insufficiency in patients with chronic adrenal insufficiency exposed to mild stress can be addressed merely by doubling the daily steroid dose until the condition resolves followed by rapid titration back to prestress doses. More severe stress (eg, severe infection) requires intravenous hydrocortisone in dosages as outlined above or administration of dexamethasone sodium phosphate, 4 mg intramuscularly every 24 hours for two doses. Dexamethasone would replace glucocorticoids but not mineralocorticoid and would not be adequate in the presence of severe dehydration.

Sepsis

Studies of patients with septic shock have identified a subgroup that may have relative adrenal insufficiency (ie, decreased adrenal reserve). These patients were identified based on a limited increment (ie, the difference between basal and post-ACTH cortisol levels) rather than the absolute level of post-ACTH cortisol. A recent randomized trial (CORTICUS [Corticosteroid Therapy of Septic Shock] study) demonstrated that hydrocortisone therapy did not improve survival or reversal of shock in patients with septic shock, regardless of their response in the Cortrosyn stimulation test. However, hydrocortisone did hasten reversal of shock in those patients in whom shock was reversed. At the present time, the utility of steroid therapy in the management of vasopressor-dependent septic shock remains controversial.

PITUITARY APOPLEXY

Pituitary apoplexy is a rare but frightening syndrome of violent headache, visual and cranial nerve disturbances, and mental confusion, resulting from hemorrhage or infarction of a pituitary tumor or, more rarely, a normal pituitary gland.

Clinical Setting

Pituitary apoplexy usually occurs as a sudden crisis in a patient with a known or, more rarely, previously unrecognized pituitary tumor. However, it may occur in a normal gland during or after parturition. Risk factors include cardiac surgery, dynamic pituitary function testing, head trauma, or anticoagulation therapy. The patient presents with severe headache and visual disturbances, often a bitemporal hemianopia due to compression of the optic chiasm. There may be oculomotor defects, either bilateral or unilateral, due to extension of the hemorrhage into the cavernous sinus(es) where cranial nerves II, III, IV, and VI are located. Often there are meningeal symptoms with stiff neck and mental confusion, so that the differential diagnosis includes subarachnoid hemorrhage and meningitis. Finally, there may be symptoms of acute secondary adrenal insufficiency with nausea, vomiting, hypotension, and collapse. A more subacute/chronic presentation (ie, subclinical hemorrhage followed by partial resolution) may be dominated by symptoms of hypopituitarism.

Diagnosis

The diagnosis of pituitary apoplexy is best approached with magnetic resonance imaging (MRI) of the cranium with pituitary views. Pituitary enlargement and signs of hemorrhage are diagnostic. In the acute setting, hormonal studies are of academic interest only since therapy should include glucocorticoid support regardless of the acute findings. After appropriate acute therapy, evaluation of anterior and posterior pituitary function is indicated to evaluate the possibility of permanent hypopituitarism.

Management

Management involves both hormonal and neurosurgical therapy. High-dose dexamethasone, 4 mg twice daily, provides both glucocorticoid support and relief of cerebral edema. Alternatively, hydrocortisone 50 mg IV every 6 hours can be used. Transsphenoidal pituitary decompression often provides dramatic relief of visual and extraocular motor dysfunction and in the level of consciousness. Pituitary hormone secretion also may resolve particularly in those with normal or elevated prolactin levels. The need for emergent surgery is controversial and should be approached on a case-by-case basis. Conservative medical management in less severely affected patients has been shown to result in recovery of both neurological and endocrine function. After the acute episode has subsided, the patient must be evaluated for the possibility of multiple pituitary hormonal deficiencies (see Chapter 4).

DIABETIC KETOACIDOSIS

Clinical Setting

Diabetic ketoacidosis (DKA) occurs in a setting of absolute or relative insulin deficiency. Estimated annual incidence is 4 to 8 episodes per 1000 patients with diabetes. Specific clinical settings should generate a high index of suspicion for the disorder. Interruptions of normal insulin delivery due to purposeful reduction in insulin dosage or interference with the delivery system (eg, kinking in pump tubing) are frequent precipitating events, as are reduced insulin sensitivity in the setting of systemic infection, myocardial infarction, burns, trauma, or pregnancy. In a significant percentage of patients, DKA is the presenting feature of diabetes. In these instances, clinical suspicion and accurate interpretation of the initial laboratory studies will usually lead to the correct diagnosis. Measurement of HbA$_{1C}$ (hemoglobin A$_{1C}$) levels may help in assessing the chronicity of the diabetes. Mortality in DKA is less than 5% in experienced centers. Prognosis worsens at the extremes of age and in the presence of coma or hypotension.

Diagnosis

DKA is characterized metabolically by two prominent features: hyperglycemia and ketoacidosis (see Chapter 17). Patients with DKA present with evidence of volume contraction (eg, dry mucous membranes, thirst, orthostatic hypotension) and labored breathing (Kussmaul respiration) related to the underlying acidosis. The breath often has a fruity odor, reflecting the presence of acetone. Patients may have abdominal pain mimicking an acute abdomen, nausea, and vomiting. The latter symptoms may be related to elevated gastrointestinal prostaglandins that accrue in the presence of insulin deficiency. Presentation may be dominated by symptoms of the precipitating illness (eg, urinary tract infection, pneumonia, or myocardial infarction).

Plasma glucose levels are elevated, usually to over 250 mg/dL. This reflects impairment in glucose utilization (see discussed earlier), increased gluconeogenesis and glycogenolysis, and reduced renal clearance of glucose in the setting of decreased glomerular filtration rate (GFR). Osmotic diuresis related to glucose excretion results in reduction in intravascular volume and depletion of total

body water, sodium, potassium, phosphate, and magnesium. In general, the relative depletion of water is roughly twice that of the solutes it contains. Hypertonicity in the extracellular fluid compartment, although typically not as severe as that seen in hyperosmotic nonketotic coma (see later), can be significant. Calculated plasma osmolalities greater than 340 mOsm/kg are associated with coma. Plasma osmolality—rather than acidemia—correlates most closely with state of consciousness in DKA (Figure 24–3).

Arterial blood pH is low and, in the absence of coexistent respiratory disease, is partially compensated by a reduction in P_{CO_2}. The acidosis is metabolic in origin and accompanied by an anion gap that is calculated by subtracting the combined concentrations of chloride and bicarbonate from serum sodium concentration. Anion gaps greater than 12 mEq/L are considered abnormal. Keto acids account for most of the unmeasured anions that generate the abnormal gap, although under conditions of extreme volume contraction and hypoperfusion, lactate accumulation may also contribute. Levels of serum and urinary ketones (measured using the nitroprusside reagent) are typically high in DKA. It should be recalled, however, that this reagent reacts strongly only with acetoacetate, less strongly with acetone (which is not a keto acid and does not contribute to the anion gap), and not at all with β-hydroxybutyrate. Thus, paradoxically, the most extreme levels of ketoacidosis may be accompanied by relatively modest levels of ketones measured by this method. As a corollary

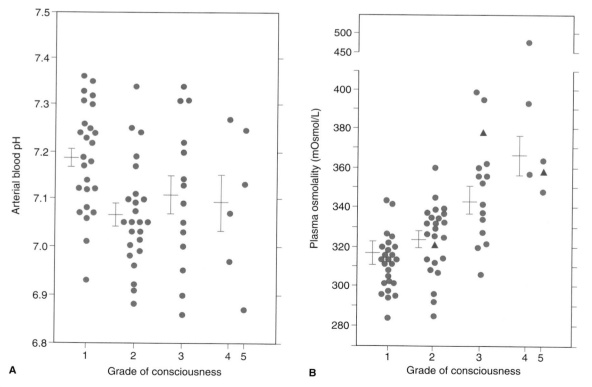

FIGURE 24–3 **A:** Relationship between state of consciousness and blood pH in patients with diabetic ketoacidosis. **B:** Relationship between state of consciousness and plasma osmolality in diabetic ketoacidosis. Note that the state of consciousness correlates with plasma osmolality rather than blood pH. (Reproduced, with permission, from Fulop M, et al. Ketotic hyperosmolar coma. *Lancet.* 1973;2:635.)

of this, resolution of severe DKA may be linked to transient increases in measurable ketone levels as β-hydroxybutyrate is converted to the more readily detectable acetoacetate.

Serum sodium levels may be high, normal, or low, but in all instances total body sodium is depressed. Estimates of depletion range from 7 to 10 mEq/kg body weight. As blood glucose levels rise in DKA, they create an osmotic gradient that draws water, as well as intracellular solutes, into the extracellular space. This results in moderate hyponatremia, which can be corrected to account for the dilutional effect of the transmembrane flux of water by adding 1.6 mEq/L (more recent studies suggest that the correction factor is closer to 2.4 mEq/L) to the sodium concentration for every 100 mg/dL increment in plasma glucose above a basal concentration of 100 mg/dL (see below). The decrease in serum sodium partially offsets the increase in tonicity that accompanies the elevation in plasma glucose. This results in a net increase in plasma osmolality of 2 mOsm/kg H_2O per 100 mg/dL elevation in plasma glucose:

$$\text{Corrected Na}^+ = \text{Measured Na}^+ + 1.6 \left(\frac{\text{Plasma glucose} - 100}{100} \right)$$

Total body potassium levels are also severely depleted in DKA to an average of 5 to 7 mEq/kg body weight. This results from a number of factors, including exchange of intracellular potassium for extracellular hydrogen ion, impaired movement of K^+ into cells in the insulinopenic state, increased urinary potassium excretion secondary to the osmotic diuresis and, in those instances where intravascular volume contraction is present, secondary hyperaldosteronism. Serum potassium levels may be high, normal, or low depending on the severity and duration of DKA, the status of extracellular fluid volume, and the adequacy of renal perfusion and excretory function. A low serum potassium at presentation generally indicates severe potassium deficiency and, in the presence of adequate renal function, is an indication for early and aggressive repletion (see below). Potassium depletion can result in muscle weakness and cardiac arrhythmias, including ventricular fibrillation.

The H^+ excess in DKA titrates endogenous buffer systems including serum bicarbonate, resulting in reduction in concentrations of the latter. Chloride levels may also be low, reflecting the osmotic diuresis alluded to above. Ketone bodies have been estimated to account for one-third to one-half of the osmotic diuresis seen in DKA. Electrolyte depletion is further aggravated by the obligate cation (eg, sodium) excretion required to maintain electrical neutrality. In patients who have maintained adequate hydration during the development of DKA or in those who are aggressively resuscitated with normal saline, chloride levels may be elevated and the anion gap narrowed. This reflects the enhanced clearance of the keto anions in the kidney, converting the system from an anion gap acidosis to a hyperchloremic, nongap acidosis (ie, the hydrogen ion excess persists despite clearance of the anion). Because the excreted keto anions represent a lost source of bicarbonate regeneration, correction of the hyperchloremic acidosis may proceed slowly. The hyperchloremic acidosis is inconsequential from a clinical standpoint.

TABLE 24–7 Management of diabetic ketoacidosis.

Fluid administration
(1) 1-2 L of normal saline over the first hour. Repeat if clinically significant volume contraction persists after the first hour.
(2) Change to half-normal saline, 500-1000 mL/h, depending on volume status. Continue for about 4 h. Decrease rate to 250 mL/h as intravascular volume returns to normal.
(3) Convert fluids to D_5W when plasma glucose falls to 250 mg/dL.

Insulin
(1) Administer 10-20 U of regular insulin IV.
(2) Mix 50 U of regular insulin in 500 mL of normal saline (1 U/10 mL). Discard first 50 mL of infusion to accommodate insulin binding to tubing. Administer through *piggyback* line along with parenteral fluids at a rate of 0.1 U/kg/h.
3. Double the infusion rate after 2 h if there is no improvement in plasma glucose levels.

Potassium
(1) Administer supplemental potassium chloride once renal function is established; provide 20 mEq/L of fluids for patients who are initially normokalemic, 40 mEq/L for those who are hypokalemic at presentation. In the latter case, hold insulin until serum potassium levels begin to increase.
(2) Gauge subsequent replacement based on serum K^+ measurements at 2-h intervals.

Bicarbonate
(1) Sodium bicarbonate only for patients with blood pH less than 7.0.
(2) Add 1 ampule of sodium bicarbonate (44 mEq) to 500 mL of D_5W or half-normal saline. Administer over 1 h.

Total body magnesium and phosphate levels are also depleted by the osmotic diuresis in DKA. Phosphate depletion is amplified by diffusion of the anion from the intracellular to the extracellular compartment in the absence of insulin. Phosphate depletion can result in muscle weakness, rhabdomyolysis, hemolytic anemia, respiratory distress, and altered tissue oxygenation (due to reduction in 2,3-diphosphoglycerate levels in the red blood cell).

Management

Treatment of DKA is focused on two major objectives. The first is restoration of normal tonicity, intravascular volume, and solute homeostasis. The second is correction of the insulinopenic state with suppression of counterregulatory hormone secretion, glucose production, and ketogenesis and improved utilization of glucose in target tissues. The steps outlined in Table 24–7 provide a general approach to the management of this disorder.

Because depletion of intracellular and extracellular fluids may be severe in DKA (typically in the range of 5-10 L), early and aggressive resuscitation with fluids is mandatory. This is usually initiated with administration of 1 to 2 L of isotonic normal saline (0.9% NaCl) over the first hour of therapy. As intravascular volume is restored, renal perfusion increases, with a consequent increase in renal clearance of glucose and a fall in plasma glucose levels. If volume contraction is severe, a second liter of normal saline can be administered. If not, half-normal saline (0.45% NaCl) can be initiated at a rate of 250 to 500 mL/h depending on intravascular volume status. Because water is typically lost in excess of solute in DKA, half-normal saline addresses both the volume depletion and the hypertonicity. It has been suggested that approximately half of the total fluid deficit should be corrected within the first 5 hours of therapy. Half-normal saline can be continued until intravascular volume has been restored or plasma glucose levels fall to 250 mg/dL, at which point D_5W should be started. The latter maneuver reduces the likelihood of insulin-induced hypoglycemia and avoids the theoretical complication of cerebral edema due to osmotically induced fluid shifts from plasma into the central nervous system. This complication is, in fact, seen rarely in adults and uncommonly in children with DKA. It is important to account for ongoing urinary volume and electrolyte losses in assessing fluid requirements.

Once fluid resuscitation has been initiated, insulin should be administered. Only short-acting insulin should be used. A number of different insulin regimens have demonstrated efficacy in the treatment of DKA; however, a commonly used regimen includes a loading dose (10-20 U) of regular insulin intravenously followed by a continuous infusion at a rate of 0.1 U/kg/h. The need for a loading dose is controversial and may not be required in the majority of cases. It is not recommended for children with ketoacidosis. If intravenous access is problematic, maintenance insulin can be given intramuscularly (0.1 U/kg/h). This regimen provides plasma insulin levels in a physiologic range (100-150 mU/mL) with minimal risk of hypoglycemia or hypokalemia. It restores plasma glucose levels at rates equivalent to those obtained with regimens using higher insulin doses. Plasma glucose levels should fall at a rate of 50 to 100 mg/dL/h. Failure to achieve this end point over a 2-hour period should lead to doubling of the infusion rate with reevaluation an hour later. When plasma glucose concentrations reach 250 mg/dL, D_5W is begun to prevent hypoglycemia (see above). Some diabetologists recommend a coincident reduction in insulin dose (to 0.05-0.1 U/kg/h) at this point. The insulin infusion is continued to suppress ketogenesis and allow restoration of normal acid-base balance.

As noted above, total body potassium stores are depleted in DKA (~3-4 mEq/kg), and plasma K^+ levels fall with treatment. Repletion of K^+ is almost always indicated in management of DKA (one notable exception being DKA that occurs in the setting of chronic renal insufficiency); however, the timing of repletion varies as a function of the plasma K^+ level. If the initial K^+ level is less than 4 mEq/L, K^+ depletion is severe, and repletion should begin with the first administration of parenteral fluids if renal function is adequate. Twenty milliequivalents of potassium chloride can be added to the first liter of normal saline if the serum K^+ is in the 3.5 to 4 mEq/L range; 40 mEq should be added for K^+ levels less than 3.5 mEq/L. Particular attention should be devoted to patients in this latter state, because K^+ levels may plummet to very low levels with initiation of insulin therapy. To avoid this, insulin therapy should be postponed in this group until K^+ repletion has begun and serum K^+ levels are on the rise. The general goal of therapy should be to keep the K^+ in a near-normal range. This may require several hundred milliequivalents of potassium chloride administered over several days.

The administration of bicarbonate in the setting of DKA has been controversial. Acidosis, in addition to increasing ventilatory work (Kussmaul respiration), may also suppress cardiac contractile function. Therefore, restoration of normal pH would seem to make sense in the setting of DKA. However, there is considerable risk associated with the use of sodium bicarbonate in this setting, including paradoxical acidification of the central nervous system due to the selective diffusion of CO_2 versus HCO_3^- across the blood–brain barrier and an increase in intracellular acidosis, which may worsen rather than ameliorate cardiac function. Volume overload related to the high tonicity (44.6-50 mEq/50 mL) of the bicarbonate solution, hypokalemia resulting from overly rapid correction of the acidosis, hypernatremia, and rebound alkalosis are also potential complications of bicarbonate therapy. In general, pH of 7.0 or greater is not life-threatening to the average patient with DKA and will resolve with appropriate volume expansion and insulin therapy. For pH less than 7.0, many clinicians would argue for a limited administration of sodium bicarbonate. If bicarbonate is used, careful patient monitoring looking for alterations in mental status or cardiac decompensation is indicated. The goal of therapy should be to maintain pH greater than 7.0, not to return pH to normal.

Similarly, phosphate administration, once considered a key component in the management of DKA (estimated deficit ~5-7 mmol/kg), has come under closer scrutiny. Phosphate depletion definitely occurs in DKA for the reasons outlined above, and in the past repletion of phosphate (much of it as potassium phosphate salts) had been advocated to forestall the development of muscle weakness and hemolysis and to promote tissue oxygenation through generation of 2,3-diphosphoglycerate in erythrocytes. However, the administration of phosphate salts has been associated with the development of hypocalcemia and deposition of calcium phosphate precipitates in soft tissues, including the vasculature. Thus, in general, parenteral phosphate repletion is not routinely provided for patients with DKA unless plasma phosphate falls to very low levels (<1 mmol/L). In this case, 2 mL of a mixture of KH_2PO_4 and K_2HPO_4 solution, containing 3 mmol of elemental phosphorus and 4 mEq of potassium, may be added to 1 L of fluids and introduced over 6 to 8 hours. In no instance should all K^+ repletion be in the form of potassium phosphate salts. In general, renewal of food ingestion and insulin therapy complete restoration of total body phosphate stores and return plasma phosphate levels to normal over a period of several days.

In pediatric patients (age <20 years) the need for volume expansion needs to be weighed against the potential risk of cerebral edema secondary to aggressive fluid administration, although this is controversial (see below). A recent recommendation suggests 10 to 20 mL/kg/h of normal saline during the first 1 to 2 hours with limitation of total fluid administration to 50 mL/kg over the first 4 hours. The remaining fluid deficit is corrected over the next 48 hours. Normal saline or half-normal saline (depending on serum Na^+ levels) usually accomplishes this with a rate of 5 mL/kg/h. The decrease in serum osmolality should not exceed 3 mOsm/kg H_2O/h. An insulin bolus prior to initiating the insulin infusion (0.1 U/kg/h) is usually not required in children.

Finally, it is necessary to actively seek out and treat the precipitants of DKA when they are identified. This includes appropriate cultures of urine and blood (and cerebrospinal fluid, if indicated) and empiric antibiotic therapy directed against the most likely pathogenic organisms (pending the results of the cultures). The presence of fever is typically a good marker for infection or other inflammatory process because it is not a feature of DKA per se. Elevated white blood cell counts, on the other hand, are frequently seen with DKA alone. Hyper-amylasemia is common but rarely reflects pancreatitis—the amylase is usually of salivary origin. Other precipitants should also be sought. Myocardial infarction, which is often clinically silent in diabetic patients, is an uncommon but life-threatening precipitant of DKA in patients with established diabetes.

Complications

Aggressive resuscitation with isotonic or hypotonic fluids is a theoretical but uncommon cause of fluid overload during management of DKA. Careful attention to the cardiovascular examination, chest x-ray, and urine output should aid in preventing this complication.

Hypoglycemia is relatively rare in the current era given the low doses of insulin used in management and appropriate initiation of glucose-containing fluids as plasma glucose levels fall below 250 mg/dL.

Cerebral edema due to rapid correction of plasma hypertonicity has usually been reported with plasma glucose levels below 250 mg/dL. Clinically significant cerebral edema is relatively uncommon in adult patients. Milder forms of cerebral edema have been noted in many patients being treated for DKA but have not been strongly correlated with changes in extracellular tonicity. At present, in a symptomatic adult patient, it would appear prudent to treat hypertonicity exceeding 340 mOsm/kg aggressively with hypotonic fluids to avoid complications related to plasma hyperviscosity. Further correction from that point to normal plasma osmolality (about 285 mOsm/kg) can probably be accomplished in slower fashion over several days. Cerebral edema occurs in 1% to 2% of children with DKA, frequently with devastating results. Approximately one-third of children with clinically significant cerebral edema die during the acute illness, and another third sustain permanent neurologic impairment. The predilection for young children may reflect, in part, immaturity of the autoregulatory mechanism that governs cerebral blood flow. There is increased risk in children less than 5 years of age, and those with low Pco_2 or high blood urea nitrogen at presentation. Cerebral edema in children may be associated with high initial rates of fluid resuscitation (>4 L/m^2/d) and rapid falls in plasma sodium (or corrected sodium) concentration, although it can occur in clinical settings without an apparent cause, and mild degrees of cerebral edema have been noted in DKA even prior to initiation of therapy. In the absence of definitive trial data to guide therapy, lower rates of fluid administration (<2.5 L/m^2/d) with volume resuscitation spread over a longer time interval would seem appropriate if the clinical situation permits. When signs of cerebral edema appear—deterioration in level of consciousness, focal neurologic signs,

hypotension or bradycardia, sudden decline in urine output after an initial period of apparent recovery following treatment for DKA—fluid administration should be reduced and mannitol (0.2-1 g/kg given intravenously over 30 minutes) should be administered with repetition at hourly intervals based on response. CT or MRI scan of the brain can be done once therapy has been initiated to confirm the diagnosis. Hyperventilation has not been shown to alter the course of this complication once it develops.

Patients with DKA are also prone to develop acute respiratory distress syndrome, presumably reflecting the sequelae of a damaged pulmonary endothelium and elevated capillary hydrostatic pressures following fluid resuscitation. Patients who present with rales at the time of initial diagnosis may be at higher risk for the development of this complication. Patients may also be at increased risk for development of pancreatitis as well as systemic infection, including fungal infections (eg, mucormycosis).

Abdominal pain and gastric stasis seen in DKA may put a semi-stuporous patient at risk for aspiration. Up to 25% of patients with DKA have emesis that may be guaiac positive. The latter finding appears to result from hemorrhagic gastritis. Patients who are believed to be at risk with regard to airway protection should have a nasogastric tube in place for evacuation of stomach contents.

Finally, patients with DKA are at risk for recurrence of the disorder if insulin is withdrawn prematurely. The current infusion protocols, because they raise plasma insulin only to physiologic levels, have a very short half-life for control of blood glucose and ketogenesis. Premature cessation of insulin therapy before depot insulin (eg, NPH or glargine insulin) can exert its effect may allow the patient to regress into ketoacidosis. To preclude this possibility, subcutaneous regular and intermediate-acting insulin should be provided on the morning when feeding is to be resumed. The insulin drip should be continued for 1 hour following this injection to provide coverage until the depot insulin becomes effective.

NONKETOTIC HYPEROSMOLAR COMA

Clinical Setting

Hyperosmolar nonketotic coma, like DKA, is a consequence of uncontrolled diabetes mellitus; however, a number of features of this disorder clearly distinguish it from DKA. First, plasma glucose levels in ketoacidosis are usually in the 250 to 400 mg/dL rather than the 700 to 1000 mg/dL range that can be seen with hyperosmolar nonketotic coma. Second, the time course for development of hyperosmolar nonketotic coma typically takes a week or longer, whereas ketoacidosis can develop over 1 to 2 days. Third, ketosis is rare in hyperosmolar nonketotic coma. Circulating insulin levels are probably adequate to control ketogenesis in the latter, although they are incapable of establishing euglycemia. Fourth, hyperosmolar nonketotic coma tends to occur more commonly in the elderly population, often in those receiving chronic care who have difficulty reporting symptoms or maintaining adequate hydration. Like DKA, hyperosmolar nonketotic coma may present as the first manifestation of diabetes mellitus. Mortality remains high in hyperosmolar nonketotic coma (perhaps as high as 20% vs 1%-2% in DKA); in both cases, mortality increases with age.

Precipitants of hyperosmolar nonketotic coma include many of the same complicating illnesses that lead to DKA. Infections (pneumonias are said to be the most common precipitating infection in 40%-60% of cases, with urinary tract infections representing 5%-16% of the total), myocardial infarction, cerebrovascular accident, pancreatitis, burns, heat stroke, and endocrine dysfunction (eg, Cushing syndrome, acromegaly) are frequently associated with hyperosmolar nonketotic coma. Administration of hyperosmolar fluids (eg, tube feedings, total parenteral nutrition, peritoneal dialysis) can precipitate hyperosmolar nonketotic coma, as can medications that impair insulin secretion or action (eg, β-adrenergic blocking agents, phenytoin, corticosteroids, or diazoxide). Diuretics, particularly thiazides, can reduce intravascular volume, reduce the GFR (the dominant mechanism for glucose clearance), and activate counterregulatory hormones (eg, catecholamines), all of which promote development of the hyperosmolar state. Finally, limited access to free water intake, particularly in patients who are dependent on others to provide access to water, is a major determinant in the progression of the hyperosmolar state.

These factors interact in a highly variable fashion to promote the hyperosmolar state associated with hyperosmolar nonketotic coma. In a typical scenario, poorly controlled diabetes—or undiagnosed diabetes presenting for the first time—is aggravated by coincident infection (or other precipitant). This results in significant hyperglycemia as the balance of counterregulatory hormones versus insulin shifts in favor of the former. Hyperglycemia promotes increased insulin resistance and further elevations in blood glucose levels. This leads to an osmotic diuresis in the kidney as plasma glucose levels exceed the threshold for tubular reabsorption. This threshold typically increases with age, leading to even higher plasma glucose levels in the elderly. The osmotic diuresis results in a progressive loss of water and, to a lesser degree, solutes (eg, Na^+, Cl^-, K^+) in the urine. As with DKA, the water loss is buffered initially by an osmotically driven movement of water out of the cells into the extracellular compartment. As the diuresis continues, however, contraction of intravascular volume ensues and glomerular filtration falls, shutting off the body's primary mechanism for controlling plasma glucose levels in this setting. Glucose levels increase dramatically; often to extraordinarily high levels (normal renal excretory function generally limits elevations in plasma glucose to 500-600 mg/dL). Nausea and vomiting, related to the infection, uremia, or hyperosmolality per se, may further aggravate intravascular volume contraction. Factor into this an elderly patient with age-dependent suppression of the thirst mechanism and difficulty communicating a sense of thirst to caregivers, and the stage is set for severe dehydration and the hyperosmolar state of hyperosmolar nonketotic coma.

Diagnosis

The diagnosis is usually based on strong clinical suspicion and laboratory assessments of plasma glucose levels and serum osmolality. The typical patient may be a patient with known type 2 diabetes (often taking an oral hypoglycemic agent), who has shown a subtle but steady deterioration over several days immediately preceding admission. The patient demonstrates significant dehydration, somnolence, stupor, or coma. The course may be marked by a precipitating illness, as described above. Tachycardia and low-grade fever may be present, but blood pressure and respiratory rate are normal. Urine output typically is reduced to low levels as the hyperosmolar state progresses.

The clinical presentation is usually dominated by the central nervous system findings. Patients with hyperosmolar nonketotic coma are lethargic and weak, with an altered sensorium. True coma is less common and usually does not appear until plasma osmolality is significantly elevated (see below). Hallucinations are occasionally present, and seizures, particularly focal seizures, may occur in 25% of patients with hyperosmolar nonketotic coma. Focal findings suggesting cortical ischemia may also be seen. A minority of these reflect true cerebrovascular accidents related to thromboembolic complications (see below). Most represent low-flow states in areas of baseline cerebrovascular ischemia that recover with correction of the metabolic abnormality.

Plasma glucose levels are typically high (occasionally >1000 mg/dL). Measured plasma osmolality is often greater than 350 mOsm/kg. These measurements usually include the contribution of urea, which may accumulate to significant levels in the setting of volume contraction and prerenal azotemia; however, urea does not contribute to the osmotic force that drives fluid movement across cellular membranes because it is freely permeable in these membranes and distributes itself in equivalent concentrations in the intracellular and extracellular compartments. A more accurate measure of the effective osmolality, or tonicity, is obtained from the following formula:

$$\text{Effective osmolality} = 2Na^+ + \frac{\text{Glucose}}{18}$$

where Na^+ and glucose are the concentrations of sodium ion and glucose, respectively. Normal effective osmolalities are in the range of 275 to 295 mOsm/kg. Hyperosmolar nonketotic coma is diagnosed with an effective osmolality greater than 320 mOsm/kg, whereas coma itself is seen with osmolalities greater than 340 mOsm/kg. Coma at effective osmolalities ≤340 mOsm/kg suggests some other cause (eg, meningitis, cerebrovascular accident, or other metabolic abnormality).

Anion gap acidosis is usually not a major component of hyperosmolar nonketotic coma, because ketogenesis is suppressed (see above). If gap acidosis is present, it may suggest lactate accumulation due to tissue hypoperfusion, low-output state, metformin toxicity, or coexistent renal failure or toxic ingestion. Measurement of serum lactate levels, standard renal function tests, or a screen for toxic substances in blood (if a suggestive history is obtained) should help discriminate among these possibilities.

Management

Therapy is in some ways similar to that for DKA except that there is less concern about correction of the acidosis, which is mild or nonexistent with most conventional cases of hyperosmolar nonketotic coma, and greater emphasis is placed on restoration of intravascular volume and serum osmolality. It is also important to address the potentially life-threatening precipitants of nonketotic coma.

Resuscitation of intravascular volume is initiated with parenteral fluids. Over the first hour 1 to 2 L of normal saline are administered. If the patient is profoundly hyperosmolar (>330 mOsm/L), half-normal saline (0.45% NaCl) should be substituted for normal saline. Volume status is reassessed based on blood pressure, urine output, or central venous pressure. If volume contraction persists, normal saline (or half-normal saline if hypertonicity persists) can be continued at a rate of 1 L/h. Once blood pressure and urine output have been restored, hypotonic fluids (eg, half-normal saline) can be substituted for isotonic saline at a rate of 250 to 500 mL/h depending on the need for continued volume resuscitation. The total free water deficit can be approximated using the following formula:

$$\text{Water deficit} = \frac{\text{Plasma osmolality} - 295}{295} \times 0.6(\text{Body weight})$$

where plasma osmolality is in milliosmoles per kilogram, body weight in kilograms, and water deficit in liters. Fluid rates should be adjusted to correct half of the free water deficit in the first 12 hours and the remainder over the ensuing 24 to 36 hours. As with DKA, glucose-containing fluids (eg, D_5W) should be started when plasma glucose levels fall to 250 mg/dL.

Insulin therapy is of secondary importance in the management of hyperosmolar nonketotic coma. It is imperative that insulin therapy not be initiated until volume resuscitation is well under way (eg, following 1-2 L of crystalloid). Insulin promotes movement of glucose, electrolytes, and water into the intravascular compartment. In the absence of adequate volume resuscitation, this can lead to hypotension and cardiovascular collapse. Therapy should be initiated with a loading dose of 10 to 20 U intravenously followed by a drip delivering 0.1 U/kg/h. Conversion back to the outpatient regimen once the acute event has resolved can be accomplished using a strategy similar to that outlined above for DKA.

Electrolytes (ie, Na^+, K^+, Cl^-, PO_4^{3-}, and Mg^{2+}) are significantly depleted in hyperosmolar nonketotic coma due to the osmotic diuresis. These should be repleted as needed (beginning with the first liter of fluids if necessary). Once again, parenteral phosphate should be administered with care, keeping serum phosphate above 1 mg/dL until feeding can reestablish phosphate balance.

Complications

A. Thromboembolic events Coagulopathies related to increased platelet aggregation, hyperviscosity of circulating blood, or disseminated intravascular coagulation can develop in hyperosmolar nonketotic coma. The most appropriate therapy is resuscitation of intracellular volume and treatment of systemic infections. Focal neurologic findings that fail to improve with fluid resuscitation should be further investigated with appropriate consultation and imaging studies, if indicated. Some investigators have recommended low-dose heparin anticoagulation in patients with hyperosmolar nonketotic coma to guard against thromboembolic sequelae. If such therapy is initiated, patients should be closely monitored for development of gastrointestinal bleeding.

B. Cerebral edema This is a serious—although fortunately uncommon—complication of fluid resuscitation in hyperosmolar nonketotic coma (and DKA; see above). It occurs more commonly in children than in adults and frequently follows an overly aggressive management strategy involving administration of large amounts of parenteral fluids. The pathogenesis is not completely defined but probably relates to the increase in cortical capillary hydrostatic pressure and the osmotic gradient engendered by the aggressive use of hypotonic fluids in this setting. Cerebral edema rarely appears with serum glucose levels above 250 mg/dL. Appropriate introduction of glucose-containing fluids into the management strategy when plasma glucose approaches this level is an effective way to guard against this complication.

Clinically, brain edema develops after an initial period of improvement. It is often heralded by the development of headache, altered mental status, and seizure activity. If untreated, this can progress to herniation, with respiratory arrest and death. Recognition of the syndrome and appropriate treatment with mannitol, dexamethasone, and furosemide can be life saving in this setting.

HYPERCALCEMIC CRISIS

Clinical Setting

Severe hypercalcemia, defined arbitrarily as a total Ca^{2+} greater than 14 mg/dL, can occur in the setting of a known hypercalcemic illness but may represent the initial manifestation of such a disorder. Patients present initially with polyuria and polydipsia and, with a more protracted course, develop evidence of intravascular volume contraction with decreased urine output. Alterations in the sensorium dominate the clinical picture and range from behavioral changes and drowsiness to stupor and coma. Bradyarrhythmias and heart block are major cardiac sequelae of hypercalcemia. Hypercalcemia also potentiates digoxin activity, increasing the risk of cardiac glycoside toxicity. Gastrointestinal complaints are prominent. Anorexia, nausea, and vomiting, which further aggravate the volume contraction, are frequently present. Abdominal pain may be of sufficient intensity to mimic an acute abdomen.

Most chronic hypercalcemia is caused by primary hyperparathyroidism and is usually detected as a result of routine laboratory screening. Cancer-related hypercalcemia, most of which is caused by parathyroid hormone–related protein (PTHrP), is a less frequent but important cause of chronic hypercalcemia (see Chapter 21). In acute hypercalcemic crises, malignancy emerges as the major cause of the elevations in serum calcium. Other causes of hypercalcemia (eg, vitamin D intoxication, thiazides, or

TABLE 24–8 Pathogenesis of hypercalcemic crisis.

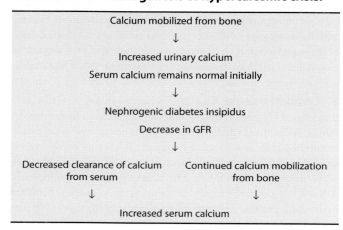

Calcium mobilized from bone

↓

Increased urinary calcium

Serum calcium remains normal initially

↓

Nephrogenic diabetes insipidus

Decrease in GFR

↓

Decreased clearance of calcium   Continued calcium mobilization
from serum   from bone

↓   ↓

Increased serum calcium

TABLE 24–9 Therapy for hypercalcemic crisis.

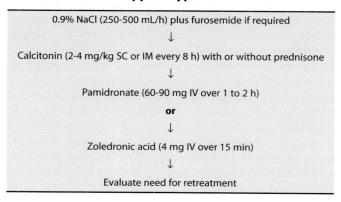

0.9% NaCl (250-500 mL/h) plus furosemide if required

↓

Calcitonin (2-4 mg/kg SC or IM every 8 h) with or without prednisone

↓

Pamidronate (60-90 mg IV over 1 to 2 h)

or

↓

Zoledronic acid (4 mg IV over 15 min)

↓

Evaluate need for retreatment

Addison disease) are either too uncommon or cause such small increments in serum calcium that they rarely need to be considered in the differential diagnosis (see Chapter 8).

Hypercalcemia due to any cause creates a state of nephrogenic diabetes insipidus by uncoupling vasopressin from its receptor-effector system in the kidney (Table 24–8). This results in a water diuresis that eventually promotes intravascular volume contraction and reduced GFR, effectively suppressing the only route of egress for calcium mobilized from bone or transported across the gut lumen. Thus, volume contraction is in large part responsible for the very high levels of serum calcium found in hypercalcemic crisis. By inference, resuscitation of intravascular volume (see below) represents an excellent initial intervention to improve renal perfusion and tubular clearance of Ca^{2+}.

Hypercalcemic crisis should be considered in any patient with disseminated malignancy, particularly squamous carcinomas of the head, neck, and lung. This is especially true when there is a change in the patient's mental status or general clinical condition that cannot be explained by tumor progression, infection, or other metabolic abnormality (eg, uremia). It should also be considered in patients with known primary hyperparathyroidism, particularly in a clinical setting characterized by vomiting, diarrhea, or dehydration (eg, due to thiazide therapy).

Diagnosis

The diagnosis is confirmed by measurement of a total or ionized serum calcium level. The latter may be preferable in the presence of low serum albumin, the predominant Ca^{2+}-binding protein in blood, because hypoalbuminemia may mask an elevation in the free fraction if only total calcium levels are assessed. Albumin-corrected calcium levels can be derived by increasing the total calcium by 0.8 mg/dL for each 1 g/dL decrease in serum albumin, based on a normal albumin level of 4 g/dL. The albumin-adjusted calcium does not always correlate with the measured ionized calcium, however, and should not be relied on for more than a rough estimate of the free calcium fraction, particularly if ionized calcium measurements are available.

On the initial presentation with hypercalcemia, plasma samples should be sent for measurement of intact parathyroid hormone (PTH), PTHrP, and, if the clinical setting is suggestive, 25-hydroxyvitamin D or 1,25-dihydroxyvitamin D levels. Primary hyperparathyroidism is a common disease, and even in a patient with known malignancy it should be excluded as a potentially curable cause of the hypercalcemia.

Management

Intravenous fluids represent the first avenue of approach for management of severe hypercalcemia (Table 24–9). Normalization of intravascular volume improves GFR and increases renal excretion of calcium. Sodium and calcium handling is closely linked in the distal nephron. Fluid resuscitation with normal saline (0.9% NaCl) both restores GFR and promotes natriuresis and calciuresis by regulating transporter mechanisms responsible for sodium and calcium handling in the distal nephron. Over the first hour 500 to 1000 mL of normal saline is given, with rates of 250 to 500 mL/h thereafter depending on the state of volume contraction. The latter can be assessed based on clinical examination, urine output, and assessment of renal function. Several liters of fluid are frequently required before intravascular volume is restored. Continued infusions should be matched with urine outputs to avoid fluid overload. Loop diuretics (eg, furosemide) may be used to accomplish this in patients with an underlying predilection toward fluid retention (eg, congestive heart failure). Saline and loop diuretics can increase urinary calcium excretion by as much as 800 mg/d. This is typically accompanied by a moderate but significant reduction in serum calcium levels (1-3 mg/dL). Careful attention should be devoted to detection of signs of fluid overload. Potassium and magnesium depletion related to the diuresis should be corrected. If loop diuretics are used, it is important that the volume of normal saline administered should at least match urine output. Diuretic-induced volume contraction may lead to reduced GFR and worsening hypercalcemia.

At this point, more definitive and specific therapy should be introduced (see Chapter 8). Severe hypercalcemia is almost always a result of increased mobilization of calcium from bone. Therefore, most effective therapies for hypercalcemia have been directed against the osteoclasts of bone. Bisphosphonates represent the mainstay of therapy. Pamidronate administered at a dose of 60 to 90 mg in 250 mL of saline over 1 to 4 hours (4 hours for outpatients) is effective in reducing serum calcium levels, often into the normal range. A newer generation bisphosphonate, zoledronic acid (4-mg intravenous infusion over 15-30 minutes) has also been used for management of hypercalcemia. In comparison to pamidronate, it is more potent, with a similar safety profile. In addition, it has the advantage of a shorter infusion period and longer duration of antihypercalcemic activity in head-to-head comparisons with pamidronate. The effect of intravenous bisphosphonates can take 2 to 4 days to peak, and the duration of the response is variable, lasting from 1 week to several months. Retreatment for recurrent hypercalcemia is usually successful. Side effects of therapy include inflammation at the infusion site; low-grade fever with flu-like syndrome; osteonecrosis of the mandible and maxilla with long-term or frequent infusions; renal insufficiency; and transient depression of serum calcium, phosphate, and magnesium. Bisphosphonates are also attractive because of their efficacy in controlling pain and fracture in myeloma and osteolytic metastases from breast cancer and other solid tumors. The mechanism here is thought to involve suppression of tumor-induced osteoclastic activity in the neighborhood of the metastases.

Calcitonin has a long history of use in the management of hypercalcemia. It has a direct effect on the osteoclast to suppress bone resorption. It is given either subcutaneously or intramuscularly at a dose of 2 to 4 U/kg body weight every 6 to 12 hours after administration of a test dose to exclude hypersensitivity to the drug. In general, the response to calcitonin, which should be noted after 6 to 12 hours, is modest in magnitude (decrease in serum calcium levels of 1-2 mg/dL) and declines with increasing duration of therapy (tachyphylaxis). Coadministration of glucocorticoids with calcitonin may limit this latter effect and extend the duration of the hypocalcemic effect. Calcitonin is useful largely as adjunctive therapy in controlling hypercalcemia in the acute setting until the effects of more powerful but slower acting agents (eg, bisphosphonates) become available.

Cinacalcet, a calcium receptor agonist, can be useful in the management of PTH-dependent hypercalcemia such as that seen with parathyroid carcinoma. Doses are typically in the range of 30 to 60 mg bid or higher.

Plicamycin is a tumoricidal antibiotic with pronounced hypocalcemic properties at nontumoricidal doses. It presumably targets the osteoclast and its bone-resorptive activity. It is administered as an infusion at a dosage of 15 to 25 μg/kg body weight over 4 to 24 hours. Calcium levels fall, often into the normal range, within 24 to 48 hours in a majority of patients treated. Plicamycin has significant renal and hepatic toxicity, and it induces platelet abnormalities that may result in clinically significant hemorrhage. Toxicity tends to increase with repeated administration, limiting chronic use of the drug. Given the ready availability of less toxic treatment modalities, plicamycin is rarely used in the management of severe hypercalcemia.

Gallium nitrate has shown efficacy in the management of tumoral hypercalcemia in clinical trials. Like the bisphosphonates and plicamycin, gallium is apparently targeted at the osteoclast. Patients are infused with gallium nitrate at a dosage of 200 mg/m^2 over a 5-day period. Gallium's major limitations are the duration of the infusion (often requiring hospitalization) and the potential for significant nephrotoxicity, particularly if it is used in the setting of other nephrotoxic agents.

Other nonselective treatment modalities that are available for management of hypercalcemic crisis include steroids, phosphate, and dialysis. Aside from their potentiation of calcitonin's effects, as described above, steroids are usually effective only in the management of hypercalcemia due to lymphoproliferative disease (eg, multiple myeloma) or vitamin D toxicity (eg, due to ingestion of vitamin D or disseminated granulomatous disease). They are best suited for chronic management of hypercalcemia associated with these disorders. Parenteral phosphate effectively reduces serum calcium levels, although often at the expense of deposition of calcium phosphate salts in parenchymal tissues, and cannot be recommended. Peritoneal or hemodialysis against a low-calcium bath is also very effective in reducing serum calcium levels and is the treatment of choice for severe hypercalcemia in renal failure patients incapable of tolerating or responding to saline diuresis. In clinically tenuous patients not in renal failure undergoing maximal saline diuresis, persistent hypercalcemia may be an indication for hemodialysis as a tool to bridge the interval until more definitive therapy (eg, bisphosphonates) can achieve its maximal effect.

Finally, some effort should be taken to addressing the primary cause of the hypercalcemia. In some instances (eg, disseminated malignancy), therapeutic options may be limited and ineffective in controlling serum calcium levels. In other instances (eg, primary hyperparathyroidism), a definitive surgical approach can be curative and limit further morbidity. Thus, careful investigation of the source of the hypercalcemia is warranted. Such investigation—even in patients with an obvious potential source of hypercalcemia (eg, malignancy)—may identify correctable problems and, at the very least, assist in the development of long-term management strategies once the acute crisis has resolved.

ACUTE HYPOCALCEMIA

Clinical Setting

Hypocalcemia may be seen in a number of disorders affecting the synthesis or action of PTH or vitamin D or following sequestration of calcium into a functionally inaccessible compartment (see Chapter 8). Many of these represent chronic illnesses where hypocalcemic symptoms develop insidiously or where the complication of hypocalcemia is anticipated early and appropriate treatment initiated prior to acute decompensation. However, in selected situations, acute hypocalcemia may dominate the clinical presentation. Appropriate recognition of the high-risk clinical setting should lead to earlier diagnosis and therapeutic intervention with reduced morbidity and mortality.

Probably the most important cause of PTH-deficient hypocalcemia occurs in the postoperative setting following neck surgery for treatment of malignancy or resection of adenomatous or hyperplastic parathyroid glands. This may reflect accidental or purposeful (eg, radical neck dissection) removal of all functioning parathyroid tissue or inadvertent vascular compromise of tissue left in the neck. Residual normal parathyroid tissue can also be functionally atrophied in a patient undergoing surgery for hyperparathyroidism. It can take 1 to 2 days for PTH secretion and calcium levels to return to normal following resection of the adenoma.

Magnesium deficiency can compromise both PTH secretion from the parathyroid gland and PTH action at target tissues in the periphery. Magnesium repletion in patients with low serum magnesium and calcium should be undertaken before launching an exhaustive workup of the hypocalcemia.

Hypocalcemia can be seen in chronic renal insufficiency. Hyperphosphatemia and reduced 1-α hydroxylase activity result in deficient 1,25-dihydroxyvitamin D_3 generation and consequent hypocalcemia. Aggressive management of the hyperphosphatemia (eg, with phosphate binders) and calcitriol are generally useful in promoting normal calcium balance.

Acute sequestration of calcium into bone or nonphysiologic compartments can lead to severe hypocalcemia. Hypocalcemia following removal of a parathyroid adenoma may reflect a hypoparathyroid or aparathyroid state, as discussed above. Alternatively, in patients with severe osteitis fibrosa cystica, the bones, in the absence of PTH-driven bone resorption, serve as a sink for extracellular calcium deposition, as previously unmineralized osteoid becomes calcified. This results in the syndrome termed **hungry bones** or **recalcification tetany**. It is usually distinguished from PTH deficiency by measurements of the hormone (PTH is typically elevated in the hungry bones syndrome). A similar sequestration phenomenon is seen in osteoblastic metastases (eg, in breast or prostatic carcinoma). Typically, osteoclastic activity in these metastases is abrogated through some specific therapeutic intervention, leaving unmineralized matrix to calcify at the expense of extracellular calcium levels.

Sequestration may also occur in nonphysiologic settings such as the peritoneal cavity in acute pancreatitis, where deposition of calcium soaps leads to a subsequent reduction in serum calcium levels. A similar phenomenon occurs in damaged muscle following rhabdomyolysis. Deposition of calcium salts in damaged muscle beds leads to a reduction in serum calcium levels. Interestingly, serum calcium returns to normal or even elevated levels during the recovery phase, reflecting dissolution of the precipitates as the muscle undergoes repair.

Hypocalcemia occurs in the setting of acute systemic illness with a prevalence of nearly 80% in the ICU setting. It has been linked to the cytokine-mediated inflammatory response that frequently dominates this clinical setting. Other potential contributors include increased calcium binding to albumin (eg, as seen with alkalosis), relative PTH deficiency, and decreased renal 1-α-hydroxylase activity. It has also been associated with specific drugs, including antineoplastic agents such as doxorubicin and cytarabine and other agents such as ketoconazole, pentamidine, and foscarnet.

TABLE 24–10   Symptoms and signs of acute hypocalcemia.

Symptoms
Perioral numbness
Tingling paresthesias in distal extremities
Hyperreflexia
Muscle cramps
Carpopedal spasm
Laryngospasm
Seizures
Coma

Signs
Chvostek sign
Trousseau sign
Hypotension
Bradycardia
Prolonged QT interval
Arrhythmias

Diagnosis

Symptomatic hypocalcemia presents with a predictable constellation of signs and symptoms. Most of these findings are related to the increased neuroexcitability that is seen with reductions of extracellular calcium levels (see Table 24–10). Symptoms frequently begin as circumoral paresthesias or paresthesias of the fingers or toes. This is followed by increased muscle cramping and spasm (particularly carpopedal spasm) (see Figure 8–18) and diffuse hyperreflexia. The increased propensity for muscle spasm can provoke generalized tetany which if extended to the laryngeal muscles can lead to laryngospasm and respiratory arrest. Increased excitability in the central nervous system can result in seizures, particularly in patients with a history of seizure disorder.

Physical examination looking for evidence of neuromuscular hyperexcitability is often revealing (see Table 24–10). Chvostek sign is evoked by repetitive tapping of the area overlying the facial nerve approximately 2 cm anterior to the ear lobe below the zygomatic arch. A positive test is contraction of musculature innervated by the facial nerve. The extent of the contraction is roughly proportionate to the severity of the hypocalcemia. Trousseau sign is triggered by inflating a blood pressure cuff on an upper extremity to a level that roughly equates with the systolic blood pressure for 3 to 5 minutes. Spasm of the hand musculature (see carpopedal spasm, above) due to transient ischemia of hyperexcitable nerves innervating the hand is regarded as a positive test. Of the two, a positive Trousseau sign is regarded as more specific for hypocalcemia than is the positive Chvostek sign.

Hypocalcemia can also have significant effects on cardiovascular function, including decreased blood pressure, impaired cardiac contractility, and conduction disturbances. On the electrocardiogram, significant hypocalcemia can manifest as prolongation of the QT interval. In extreme cases this can lead to ventricular arrhythmias, including torsades de pointes. Evidence of sequelae of chronic hypocalcemia may also identify individuals who are at risk for acute hypocalcemia. Subcapsular cataracts and basal ganglia calcification are features associated with long-standing hypocalcemia.

Measurement of total serum calcium, albumin, or ionized calcium, if available, leads quickly to the correct diagnosis. Measurement of plasma PTH, 25-hydroxyvitamin D, and 1,25-dihydroxyvitmin D assists in identifying deficiency of PTH secretion, adequacy of vitamin D stores, or impaired synthesis of bioactive vitamin D, respectively. Mg^{2+} levels should be obtained to exclude hypomagnesemia. Magnesium depletion can present with the same symptoms as hypocalcemia. If present, magnesium repletion should be initiated before additional diagnostic tests are undertaken.

Examination of the medication list looking for drugs with hypocalcemic properties (eg, bisphosphonates, calcitonin, asparaginase, cisplatin, foscarnet) should be performed.

Measurement of serum amylase and lipase should aid in identifying pancreatitis as a source of the hypocalcemia. Creatine kinase and aldolase levels exclude the presence of rhabdomyolysis.

One area of potential confusion is the evaluation of patients in the immediate postparathyroidectomy period. Differentiating a hypoparathyroid or aparathyroid state from hungry bones syndrome can be difficult acutely. As pointed out above, measurement of plasma PTH levels (high in hungry bones syndrome and low in hypoparathyroidism) provides the most definitive separation of the two, but outside of referral centers this typically takes several days and thus is usually not helpful in the acute setting. Measurement of serum phosphate (elevated in hypoparathyroidism and low-normal or low in hungry bones syndrome) or urinary phosphate (often low or absent in hypoparathyroidism) may be useful in identifying the source of hypocalcemia. Fortunately, the treatment of hypocalcemia in these two conditions is largely the same. Thus, establishment of a definitive diagnosis is important mainly for planning the subacute and long-term management of the patient's disease.

Management

In a life-threatening situation (eg, cardiovascular collapse) or in the setting of frank generalized tetany, 10 mL of calcium gluconate (93 mg of elemental calcium) can be administered intravenously over a 5- to 10-minute period and repeated if necessary. Less acute but recurrent hypocalcemic episodes can be managed with continuous calcium infusions. Nine hundred and thirty milligrams (10 ampules) of calcium gluconate can be mixed in 500 mL of D_5W. Infusion rates are established empirically. The initial infusion rate is typically 0.3 mg/kg/h but may be increased to as much as 2 mg/kg/h in patients with high demands for calcium (eg, hungry bones syndrome). Intravenous calcium should be given through a central vein since extravasation of the infusate can lead to tissue sloughing. Caution should also be exercised in infusing calcium in patients with hyperphosphatemia (precipitation of calcium phosphate salts in soft tissues), hypokalemia, or those on digoxin therapy (increased risk of cardiac arrhythmias).

As the acute situation resolves, selected patients become candidates for chronic replacement therapy. Those with minor hypocalcemia may be treated with calcium supplements alone.

Administration of 1 to 3 g of elemental calcium (calcium carbonate contains about 40% elemental calcium by weight) may suffice to restore calcium to the low-normal range and eliminate hypocalcemic symptoms. In those with more refractory hypocalcemia—a category that includes most patients with hypoparathyroidism—the addition of some form of vitamin D or a derivative is required. If ergocalciferol (vitamin D_2) is employed to manage patients with hypoparathyroidism, supraphysiologic doses (50,000 U/d or higher) may be required, reflecting the limited capacity for 1-α hydroxylation of the vitamin D prohormone in the hypoparathyroid state. 1,25-Dihydroxycholecalciferol (calcitriol) works faster than vitamin D_3 and circumvents the 1-α hydroxylase blockade, but it is more expensive and the risk of acute hypercalcemia may be higher. It is given in a dose of 0.25 to 1 μg daily.

In all cases the goal of therapy should be to alleviate hypocalcemic symptoms and restore serum calcium levels to the low-normal range. This can usually be accomplished with some combination of vitamin D and supplemental calcium. The latter allows the practitioner additional flexibility in controlling serum calcium levels without requiring frequent dose modification of the longer-acting vitamin D. Efforts to push calcium levels higher may come at the expense of significant hypercalciuria and increased risk of renal stone formation. Difficulty in maintaining calcium even in the low-normal range without unacceptable hypercalciuria may be managed by addition of a thiazide diuretic (hydrochlorothiazide, 25-100 mg/d) to the regimen. These agents reduce hypercalciuria and, secondarily, raise serum calcium levels. If thiazides are used, careful follow-up is required to guard against the possibility of iatrogenic hypercalcemia. Efforts should be made to restore calcium to the target range and maintain it at this level indefinitely. Chronic hypocalcemia is associated with development of subcapsular cataracts and basal ganglia calcification which, in some cases, leads to the development of a parkinsonism-like syndrome.

HYPONATREMIA

Clinical Setting

Hyponatremia is the most frequent electrolyte problem observed in hospitalized patients (see Chapter 5). It is often asymptomatic when mild to moderate in severity and subacute to chronic in its time course of development. However, significant hyponatremia (<120 mEq/dL) of rapid onset is frequently symptomatic and can be life-threatening.

Hyponatremia typically occurs in one of three clinical settings, each of which is linked to a specific pathophysiologic paradigm (Table 24–11). Hypovolemic hyponatremia is associated with volume contraction. As intravascular volume is reduced by more than about 9%, there is a nonosmotic stimulation of antidiuretic hormone (ADH; vasopressin) release as the body attempts to retain water to support intravascular volume. Hyponatremia of this type is seen with protracted vomiting, diarrhea, or excessive sweating, particularly when fluid losses are replenished with water or hypotonic fluids alone. Volume contraction and hyponatremia

TABLE 24–11 Classification of hyponatremia.

Hypovolemic
  Extrarenal volume loss
  Excessive perspiration
  Losses due to widespread skin involvement (eg, burns)
  Vomiting
  Diarrhea
Renal volume loss
  Diuretic use
  Salt-wasting nephropathy
  Cerebral salt wasting
  Osmotic diuresis with selective repletion of water

Hypervolemic
  Congestive heart failure
  Nephrotic syndrome
  Cirrhosis with ascites
  Chronic renal failure

Normovolemic
  Syndrome of inappropriate antidiuretic hormone secretion
  Intracranial disease
  Pulmonary disease
  Drugs (eg, opioids)
  Severe pain or emotional distress
  Nausea and vomiting
  Postsurgical
  Resetting of the osmostat
Adrenal insufficiency (may be hypovolemic in presence of severe
  mineralocorticoid deficiency)
Hypothyroidism
Water intoxication
  Psychogenic polydipsia
  Nonpsychogenic polydipsia
  Excessive administration of parenteral hypotonic fluids
  Posttransurethral prostatectomy

may also be seen with disorders of renal sodium handling (eg, diuretic use, mineralocorticoid deficiency, or other salt-wasting syndromes). Urinary Na^+ concentration is typically elevated (>20 mEq/L) in these latter disorders, whereas in the former, urinary Na^+ concentration is low, reflecting aggressive resorption of Na^+ in all tubular segments.

Hypervolemic hyponatremia includes those edematous disorders typified by paradoxical retention of Na^+ and water in the face of a total body excess of each. Specific causes of hyponatremia in this group include congestive heart failure, cirrhosis of the liver with ascites, and nephrotic syndrome. Hyponatremia in this setting presumably results from perceived hypoperfusion by baroreceptors in the arterial circulation. Neural impulses transmitting this information to the hypothalamus trigger an increase in ADH release and net water retention.

Normovolemic hyponatremia is probably the most heterogeneous category and the most difficult to define pathophysiologically. It includes the syndrome of inappropriate ADH secretion (SIADH), hypothyroidism, glucocorticoid insufficiency (eg, secondary adrenal insufficiency), psychogenic polydipsia, postoperative hyponatremia, and hyponatremia seen following transurethral resection of the prostate (see Table 24–11).

Diagnosis

Acute hyponatremia, developing over the course of 24 hours or less, presents with headache, nausea, vomiting, lethargy, restlessness, hyporeflexia, seizures, and altered sensorium, which may progress to stupor and coma. Hyponatremic encephalopathy is responsible for 30% of new-onset seizures in the ICU. These findings are thought to result from cerebral edema as the hypotonic extracellular compartment shifts water into the cerebral cortical cells. Such fluid shifts are opposed early through a reduction in intracellular electrolyte concentration and later by depletion of intracellular solutes (eg, amino acids). This acts to reduce the osmotic gradient and limit the net movement of fluid into brain. With chronicity, such solute shifts can reduce brain water content to near-normal. Thus, the acuteness of the reduction in serum Na^+ concentration and the magnitude of the reduction are important markers of potential morbidity in this disorder. Young menstruating women are particularly susceptible to the deleterious effects of cerebral edema in the postoperative setting. They are 25 times more likely than postmenopausal women or men to die or have permanent brain damage. This increased susceptibility may reflect the effects of estrogen and progesterone to promote solute accumulation in the cells of the central nervous system. Such accumulation would be predicted to increase the osmotic drive that leads to cerebral edema in these patients. Other patient groups at particular risk include children and patients with hypoxia or hepatic disease.

The first step in making the diagnosis is to exclude the presence of pseudohyponatremia. The latter results from high circulating concentrations of triglycerides or osmotically active solutes (eg, glucose or proteins) in circulating plasma. Hypertriglyceridemia artifactually lowers serum sodium by physically excluding it from the sizable nonaqueous phase of the sample being measured. This is usually readily detected in the laboratory (eg, by noting the presence of lactescent serum) and is corrected by centrifuging the sample prior to measuring Na^+ concentration in the aqueous phase. Osmotically active solutes, like glucose, draw water from the intracellular to the extracellular compartment, where it may transiently lower existing electrolyte (eg, Na^+) concentrations (see Diabetic Ketoacidosis, above).

Assuming that the presence of hyponatremia is confirmed, an attempt to examine the different diagnostic possibilities listed above should be initiated. Evidence of congestive heart failure, cirrhosis, or nephrotic syndrome is usually apparent on physical examination and confirmable with standard laboratory or imaging studies. Similarly, renal dysfunction should be excluded using conventional renal function tests. Thiazide diuretic use is a frequent cause of hyponatremia and should be investigated early in the evaluation. A careful history of water consumption should be obtained and measurements of water intake in a monitored setting made to exclude psychogenic polydipsia or dipsogenic diabetes insipidus. Hypothyroidism can be excluded with measurement of plasma TSH and free thyroxine levels and glucocorticoid deficiency through an ACTH stimulation test (see Chapters 7 and 9).

Nonosmotic, non-volume-driven ADH secretion is found in SIADH. This is typically a diagnosis of exclusion in non-volume-contracted individuals without evidence of edema, renal insufficiency, hypothyroidism, or adrenal insufficiency. Serum Na$^+$ and osmolality are low in the face of a concentrated urine. Urine Na$^+$ may be modestly elevated (>20 mEq/L), reflecting activation of natriuretic pathways responding to the increase in total body fluid volume. If findings are equivocal, an abnormal water load test (inability to excrete at least 90% of a 20 mL/kg water load in 4 hours or failure to dilute urine osmolality to below 100 mOsm/kg) can be used to confirm the diagnosis. SIADH is seen with a variety of disorders affecting the central nervous system (eg, encephalitis, multiple sclerosis, meningitis, psychosis), the pulmonary system (eg, tuberculosis, pneumonia, aspergillosis), or as a paraneoplastic process associated with a number of solid tumors (eg, small cell carcinoma of the lung, carcinoma of the pancreas, bladder, or prostate). It may also be seen with certain types of drugs (eg, cyclophosphamide, vinca alkaloids, opioids, prostaglandin synthesis inhibitors, tricyclic antidepressants, carbamazepine, clofibrate, and serotonin reuptake inhibitors).

Some difficulty may be encountered in differentiating SIADH from a second hyponatremic syndrome called cerebral salt wasting. The latter is also associated with central nervous system disease, particularly subarachnoid hemorrhage. It is thought to be due to a centrally mediated renal wasting of sodium with consequent volume contraction, volume-dependent activation of ADH secretion, and hyponatremia. It has been suggested that atrial natriuretic peptide or brain natriuretic peptide may play a central role in mediating the natriuresis associated with this disorder. Comparison of the features of these two disorders (Table 24–12) suggests that clinical or biochemical evidence of volume contraction is the major way to differentiate cerebral salt wasting from the euvolemic hyponatremia of SIADH. This is an important distinction, because therapy in cerebral salt wasting involves intravascular volume repletion, whereas in SIADH fluid restriction may represent first-line therapy.

TABLE 24–12 Comparison of laboratory findings in SIADH with CSW.

	SIADH	CSW
Intravascular volume contraction[a]	No	Yes
Serum sodium	↓	↓
Urine sodium	↑	↑↑
Urine volume	N or ↓	↑
Endocrine		
Plasma ADH	↑	N or ↑
Plasma aldosterone	↓	N or ↑
Plasma renin	↓	N or ↓
Plasma ANP	↑	↑
Urea nitrogen, serum	N or ↓	↑
Serum uric acid	↓	N or ↑

[a]Based on clinical assessment or direct measurement of plasma volume.

ADH, antidiuretic hormone; ANP, atrial natriuretic peptide; CSW, cerebral salt wasting; N, normal; SIADH, syndrome of inappropriate antidiuretic hormone secretion.

Management

When the primary stimulus provoking water retention (eg, diuretic use) or consumption (eg, psychogenic polydipsia) can be identified, specific therapy represents the most rational approach for long-term management.

When the cause of hyponatremia is unclear or unaddressable (eg, SIADH), a more generic approach may be adopted. Patients with asymptomatic (eg, mild or chronic) hyponatremia can be managed with water restriction. Calculations of daily water intake should incorporate that included in nonliquid foods consumed by the patient. For patients who are symptomatic, non-acute but unable to adhere to water restriction, treatment with an oral vasopressin antagonist, tolvaptan (15-60 mg/day), or demeclocycline (600-1200 mg/d in divided doses), an antibiotic that uncouples ADH from activation of its receptor, may be sufficient to control serum Na$^+$ levels. Water restriction is not required with demeclocycline therapy and may even be deleterious. Such therapy should be carefully monitored to guard against precipitous dehydration and renal insufficiency. Alternatively, patients can be managed with regular administration of a loop diuretic (eg, furosemide), which leads to excretion of urine approximately half the tonicity of plasma (loop diuretics disrupt the osmotic gradient required for urine concentration). Loop diuretics should be used concomitantly with NaCl supplementation (2-3 g/d) to increase urinary solute excretion and in that way amplify urinary water loss.

Symptomatic acute hyponatremia is an indication for hypertonic saline (3% NaCl) administration. Estimates of excess total body water can be made using the following equation:

$$\text{Excess water} = \frac{295 - \text{Plasma osmolality}}{295} \times 0.6(\text{Body weight})$$

with plasma osmolality in milliosmoles per kilogram, excess water in liters, and body weight in kilograms.

The rise in serum sodium effected by 1 L of 3% saline infusate can be calculated by the following formula from Adrogue and Madias:

$$\Delta Na^+ = \frac{\text{Infusate Na}^+ - \text{Serum Na}^+}{\text{Total body water} + 1}$$

where ΔNa^+ is the change in sodium concentration effected by administration of 1 L of infusate; infusate Na$^+$ is the concentration of Na$^+$ in the infusion (eg, 513 mmol/L for 3% NaCl); and total body water is body weight (kg) × 0.6 (children or nonelderly men), × 0.5 (nonelderly women and elderly men), or × 0.45 (elderly women). The +1 in the denominator accounts for the volume of the infusate. Based on the calculated ΔNa^+, one can adjust the infusion rate to provide the desired increase in serum Na$^+$ over a fixed time interval. An alternative guide to initial therapy estimates that 1 mL/kg of 3% NaCl will increase serum Na$^+$ by approximately 1 mEq/L. Infusion rate algorithms are intended only as a guide and should be adjusted, based on actual Na$^+$ measurements, to raise serum Na$^+$ levels by no more than 0.5 mEq/h (total <8-12 mEq/d) to diminish the risk of central demyelination (see next). If necessary, infusion rates can be adjusted to increase serum sodium by 1 to 2 mEq/h for short periods of time in symptomatic patients; however, the limitation to 8-12 mEq/d should be adhered to, if possible. Furosemide can be administered, if necessary, to avoid intravascular fluid overload; however, given the ability of this drug to promote excretion of a hypotonic urine, the clinician should be aware that the plasma osmolality may increase faster than predicted by the formula set forth above. Once serum Na$^+$ reaches 130 mEq/L, hypertonic saline infusion should be terminated and fluid restriction or normal saline (0.9% NaCl) plus furosemide used for the final correction of serum osmolality.

For moderately symptomatic hyponatremia in a patient requiring parenteral medication, the vasopressin receptor antagonist conivaptan may be used (20 mg IV initially followed by infusion of 20 mg/d for 1-3 days; infusion rate may be increased to 40 mg/d if serum sodium fails to increase appropriately). Moderate fluid restriction is recommended to facilitate reaching serum sodium goal.

It is important to mention that interventions directed at the cause of the hyponatremia (vs treatment of the hyponatremia itself) also require close monitoring. Rapid correction of hyponatremia through administration of glucocorticoids in adrenal insufficiency or volume repletion in thiazide-induced hyponatremia, for example, may be associated with central myelinolysis. Careful monitoring of serum Na$^+$ levels in the posttreatment period is mandatory. If Na$^+$ appears to be rising too rapidly (>1 mEq/h), administration of hypotonic fluids or a small dose of desmopressin acetate (0.25-1 µg parenterally) may be indicated.

Complications

Central pontine myelinolysis was first described in alcoholics and malnourished patients. In the original descriptions it was characterized by demyelination confined to the pons, resulting in quadriplegia and, not infrequently, death. Subsequent observational studies linked it to the treatment of hyponatremia. The classic presentation is of a patient who is aggressively treated for hyponatremia with resolution of the presenting findings (ie, those of cerebral edema), only to develop symptoms of mutism, dysphasia, spastic quadriparesis, pseudobulbar palsy, delirium, and, in many cases, death. Surviving patients often have severe neurologic sequelae. More recent studies using CT and MRI indicate that myelinolysis is not confined to the pons but present in many extrapontine locations as well. Lesions are typically symmetrically distributed and clustered in areas where there is close juxtaposition of gray and white matter.

There has been considerable controversy about the prevalence of this particular syndrome and its relationship to the treatment of hyponatremia. However, both animal and human studies are strongly suggestive of a link between this syndrome and rapid, aggressive correction of hyponatremia. Given the imperfect state of our understanding of this disorder, it would seem prudent to approach the correction of chronic hyponatremia, where solute distribution and water content in the brain are undoubtedly altered because of the chronicity of the disorder, cautiously, with rates of correction no greater that 0.5 mEq/h, as indicated above. The risk of solute redistribution in documented acute hyponatremia (ie, duration <24 hours) is substantially reduced. Clinical

signs of cerebral edema in this setting may be approached more aggressively, although repletion rates greater than 1 mEq/h with a maximal correction of 12 mEq over the first 24 hours should be avoided if possible.

DIABETES INSIPIDUS

Clinical Setting

Diabetes insipidus is a disorder due to absolute or relative deficiency in the circulating levels or bioactivity of ADH (vasopressin) (see Chapter 5).

ADH release is normally suppressed at plasma osmolalities below 285 mOsm/kg, leading to generation of a maximally dilute urine (<100 mOsm/kg). Above 285 mOsm/kg, ADH secretion increases linearly with plasma osmolality. At a plasma ADH level of 5 pg/mL, which corresponds to a plasma osmolality of about 295 mOsm/kg, the urine is maximally concentrated. Despite the fact that plasma ADH levels continue to rise beyond this point, there is no further concentration of the urine. At 295 mOsm/kg, the osmotic threshold for the thirst mechanism is activated. Thirst also rises linearly with increasing plasma osmolality. It provides the body's main defense against hypertonicity, much as suppression of ADH secretion guards against hypotonicity. Provided that the patient remains awake and able to drink and provided that the thirst mechanism remains intact, even complete deficiency of ADH secretion can be adequately compensated by increased water intake.

Defects in ADH secretion (central diabetes insipidus) may occur on a heritable basis, occasionally in association with diabetes mellitus, optic atrophy, and sensorineural deafness (DIDMOAD, or Wolfram syndrome). It may also be seen as a component of a polyendocrine autoimmune syndrome (see Chapter 2). Secondary causes of central diabetes insipidus include head injury (often with stalk section), pituitary surgery, granulomatous disease (sarcoidosis, tuberculosis, histiocytosis X), infections, vascular aneurysms and thrombosis, and tumors (craniopharyngioma; dysgerminoma, meningioma; metastatic disease from breast, lung, or gastrointestinal tumors).

Osmoreceptors for ADH release are believed to reside in the organum vasculosum of the lamina terminalis, whereas those controlling thirst are believed to lie in an independent but neighboring location. Thus, those patients with an isolated defect in ADH secretion (either in the osmoreceptors or the secretory nuclei) are protected from severe dehydration by activation of the thirst mechanism. In those with combined involvement of both ADH secretion and the osmoreceptors controlling thirst (hypodipsic or adipsic diabetes insipidus), the risk of volume contraction and severe dehydration is extreme (see below).

Adequacy of the renal response to ADH requires adequate delivery of glomerular filtrate to distal tubular segments, adequacy of tubular function in the ascending limb of the loop of Henle (to establish and maintain the gradient of medullary tonicity and to generate free water for excretion), and a normal response to vasopressin (ie, intact signal transduction mechanism) in the collecting duct. Unresponsiveness to ADH is due to genetic lesions in the V_2 receptor (X-linked recessive diabetes insipidus) or the functionally linked aquaporin-2 water channel (autosomal recessive diabetes insipidus). It may also be seen in an acquired form with hypokalemia or hypercalcemia, in various forms of intrinsic renal disease (eg, medullary cystic disease) and following therapy with demeclocycline or lithium.

Diagnosis

The presentation of diabetes insipidus in an alert, conscious patient is typically an abrupt onset of polyuria and polydipsia. Hypertonicity is avoided as long as the thirst mechanism remains intact and water intake is able to keep up with urinary losses. In a patient who is unconscious or otherwise incapable of communicating the need for fluids or in patients with coexistent adipsia, polyuria is transient and quickly followed by evidence of severe dehydration and hyperosmolality. Urine volumes in this setting may be normal or even reduced. The clinical findings in hypernatremia associated with diabetes insipidus are dominated by the effects of cellular dehydration and contraction of intravascular volume. In the brain, this can lead to increased traction on dural veins and venous sinuses. This may result in avulsion of vessels from their cranial attachments and intracranial hemorrhage. Other findings include irritability, lethargy, weakness, muscle twitching, hyperreflexia, seizures, and coma.

The diagnosis of polyuria is usually reserved for urine outputs greater than 2.5 L/d. A careful history should be taken to document oral fluid intake (particularly beer or other hypotonic fluids) or parenteral fluid administration (eg, in a postoperative setting). Neurologic or endocrine symptoms that might suggest either a hypothalamic or intrasellar mass, use of medications that could impair water reabsorption (eg, furosemide, demeclocycline, or lithium) or intercurrent conditions that might mimic diabetes insipidus (eg, osmotic diuresis associated with diabetes mellitus or resolving obstructive uropathy) should also be investigated.

Initial evaluation should include measurement of serum sodium, plasma osmolality, and urine osmolality. Diabetes insipidus is typically associated with a high-normal or elevated serum sodium and osmolality in the face of submaximally concentrated urine. Plasma glucose measurement and standard renal function tests should help exclude osmotic diuresis as contributing to the polyuria. Measurement of serum K^+ and Ca^{2+} assists in excluding polyuria resulting from hypokalemia and hypercalcemia, respectively.

In patients with equivocal initial tests, a water deprivation test may be performed. This involves serial measurements of serum Na^+, urine volume, and osmolality in the absence of fluid intake until serum Na^+ is greater than 146 mmol/L or urine osmolality plateaus (<10% change with three successive determinations), and the patient has lost more than 2% of body weight. The test should be stopped if the decrease in body weight reaches 3% or the patient demonstrates orthostatic hypotension. Patients with diabetes insipidus become progressively more hypertonic with water deprivation but fail to increase urine osmolality. Administration of desmopressin promotes water retention and an increase in urine osmolality in patients with central but not nephrogenic diabetes

insipidus. Increases in osmolality of more than 50% indicate central diabetes insipidus, whereas responses of less than 10% suggest nephrogenic diabetes insipidus. Responses between 10% and 50% are equivocal. Plasma ADH levels may be of assistance in defining the nature of the diabetes insipidus in the latter setting. In the presence of high plasma but low urine osmolality, increased plasma ADH levels are associated with nephrogenic diabetes insipidus, whereas subnormal levels are found with central diabetes insipidus. It may be difficult to establish the diagnosis of mild partial central diabetes insipidus. These patients can often achieve maximally concentrated urine during extreme dehydration, reflecting reduced GFR and stimulated vasopressin secretion; however, as plasma osmolality is corrected and intravascular volume is restored, they typically begin to dilute their urine at a plasma osmolality that is well above normal.

Coexistence of glucocorticoid deficiency may mask the presence of central diabetes insipidus. The development of polyuria with the initiation of glucocorticoid replacement should alert the clinician to the possible presence of diabetes insipidus.

In the 48 hours following pituitary surgery or head trauma, transient diabetes insipidus with polyuria is not uncommon. Over the ensuing 2 to 14 days, a period of antidiuresis and hyponatremia may dominate the clinical course. This in turn may be followed by persistent polyuria. The first phase is thought to result from transient dysfunction or stunning of the ADH-producing neurons of the hypothalamus, the second from leakage of ADH from damaged or dying neurons, and the third from permanent loss of ADH-secretory neurons. Not all patients progress through the entire series of events. It is important to recognize the existence of this syndrome and the natural progression of the disorder in evaluating the need for chronic therapeutic intervention.

In pregnancy, there is a resetting of the osmostats controlling both ADH and thirst, resulting in a state of physiologic hypo-osmolality (about 10 mOsm/kg below that seen in the nonpregnant state). In addition, elevations in placental vasopressinase may rarely promote polyuria in patients with otherwise compensated partial central diabetes insipidus. The appropriate treatment for this disorder is desmopressin acetate, an ADH analog that is resistant to degradation by vasopressinase.

Virtually anything that increases the rate of tubular flow (eg, primary polydipsia or central diabetes insipidus) may create a state of functional nephrogenic diabetes insipidus. This is due to washout of the medullary tonicity responsible for generating the osmotic gradient that promotes movement of water from the tubular lumen into the medullary interstitium as well as down regulation of aquaporin-2 water channels as a result of vasopressin deficiency. A therapeutic trial of 1-deamino-8-D arginine vasopressin (DDAVP) for 1 to 2 days often restores medullary tonicity and facilitates the diagnostic workup. Primary polydipsia (eg, psychogenic polydipsia or dipsogenic diabetes insipidus) presents with a dilute urine, but plasma osmolality and serum Na^+ levels are typically low or low-normal and ADH levels are low. Moreover, due to the elevation in tubular flow rates, the response to desmopressin may be limited in magnitude (<10%, which is less than that predicted for central diabetes insipidus). This may make it difficult to differentiate primary polydipsia from partial forms of nephrogenic diabetes insipidus. Plasma ADH levels may be of assistance in making this distinction (elevated in nephrogenic diabetes insipidus and suppressed in psychogenic polydipsia).

Management

Acute diabetes insipidus is characterized by polyuria in the presence or absence of plasma hyperosmolality. As noted above, the presence of hyperosmolality is determined by the adequacy of the patient's thirst mechanism. When a hyperosmolar state with clinical evidence of severe dehydration is present, it is necessary to correct intravascular volume. This is accomplished by administering hypotonic fluids (eg, D_5W), which restore intravascular volume and move plasma osmolality back toward normal. The rate at which the hyperosmolality is corrected is dictated in part by the severity of the clinical symptoms and by the chronicity of the disorder. Chronic hyperosmolality (>24 hours) leads to the accumulation of idiogenic osmoles (eg, taurine and myoinositol) in the central nervous system that serve to offset the osmotically driven movement of water out of that compartment. Aggressive correction of the hyperosmolar state can lead to cerebral edema if the rate of hypotonic fluid administration greatly exceeds the rate at which the neurons in the central nervous system eliminate these idiogenic osmoles. If severe volume contraction is present and blood pressure is reduced, intravascular volume should be repleted initially with normal saline (0.9% NaCl). Following expansion of intravascular volume with normal saline, correction of plasma osmolality with D5W at a rate of 0.5 to 1 mOsm/h—not to exceed 15 mOsm within the first 24-hour period—appears to be reasonably effective in reducing plasma tonicity without incurring an increased risk of cerebral edema. Typically, higher infusion rates are used early in the course when serum osmolalities are highest and reduced as osmolality decreases into the range of 330 mOsm/kg. Correction of the total free water deficit should be spread over about 48 hours. Total water deficit is defined above in the section dealing with DKA. Calculation of hypotonic fluid infusion rates can be made using the formula for change in serum sodium set out in the preceding section, substituting 0 mmol/L for D_5W, 77 mmol/L for 0.45% NaCl, or 154 mmol/L for 0.9% NaCl into the equation, as needed, to calculate the net reduction in serum Na^+. Again, based on the calculated ΔNa^+, one can adjust the rate of delivery of the infusate to provide a specific increment in serum Na^+ concentration over a defined time interval. If signs of cerebral edema (see Hyponatremia, above) appear, hypotonic fluids should be discontinued and appropriate administration of hypertonic fluids (eg, mannitol) initiated.

If the diagnosis of central diabetes insipidus has been established, the patient should receive parenteral desmopressin acetate. The initial dose, in the range of 1 to 2 μg every 24 hours (administered intravenously or intramuscularly), should be given in the evening with the aim of controlling nocturia and maintaining daily urine output under 2 L. If polyuria returns well before the end of the 24-hour dosing interval, the single dose can be increased or split doses can be administered every 12 hours. Ideally, one would like to see some degree of breakthrough polyuria at the end of the dosing interval. This serves to guard against the development of iatrogenic hyponatremia. If this proves difficult to achieve, a dose can be skipped every 48 to 72 hours. Once the patient has been stabilized on a fixed dose of parenteral desmopressin, conversion to a formulation more suitable for the outpatient setting is indicated. Desmopressin acetate is available in liquid form for insufflation through a nasal cannula or as a fixed-dose (10 μg) nasal spray. The former has the advantage of greater flexibility in adjusting the nasal dose, whereas the latter offers greater convenience for some patients. Parenteral desmopressin is generally about 10 times more potent than the nasally administered drug; however, intranasal doses should be titrated for each individual patient. Desmopressin is also available in an oral form. Effective doses can range widely (50-1200 μg/d in divided doses) and should be adjusted for the individual patient.

Treatment of nephrogenic diabetes insipidus is more complex because the problem is one of resistance to—rather than deficiency of—the endogenous hormone. If possible, one should attempt to address the underlying cause of ADH resistance. This can be accomplished by correcting electrolyte abnormalities (eg, hypokalemia or hypercalcemia) or discontinuing medications (eg, demeclocycline, lithium) that are likely to contribute to ADH insensitivity. Failing this, administration of a thiazide diuretic together with salt restriction often reduces the polyuria. This is assumed to result from contraction of intravascular volume with increased proximal reabsorption of fluids and solutes and, consequently, limited availability of fluid in distal nephron segments for free water generation and excretion; however, there may be a second, ADH-independent effect on the aquaporin-2 channels in the collecting duct. Prostaglandins are endogenous antagonists of ADH activity in the collecting duct. Administration of cyclooxygenase inhibitors (eg, indomethacin, 100 mg/d in divided doses) may improve sensitivity to endogenous ADH and reduce polyuria. If the impairment in ADH responsiveness is mild, higher doses of synthetic desmopressin (DDAVP) occasionally prove effective in promoting water retention. Amiloride is the preferred treatment for lithium toxicity. It is thought to prevent the uptake of lithium in collecting duct cells. However, lithium-induced diabetes insipidus may not abate following discontinuation of the drug.

Disorders of thirst in the setting of central diabetes insipidus deserve special mention with regard to therapy. Excessive thirst due to altered osmoreceptor function or behavioral conditioning (eg, before desmopressin treatment) may result in severe hyponatremia once desmopressin treatment is initiated. The patient should be cautioned about excessive consumption of water, and fluid must be restricted if necessary.

Adipsic diabetes insipidus is probably one of the most difficult therapeutic problems faced by endocrinologists. Affected patients have essentially lost all ability to regulate water metabolism on their own. This function must be taken over by the medical team providing their care. Desmopressin is administered in a fixed parenteral dose that is sufficient to reduce urine output to 1.5 to 2 L/d with a fluid intake of 2 to 2.5 L. The difference here is intended to cover the daily insensible losses (about 500-1000 mL) and may need to be adjusted empirically to maintain normal fluid homeostasis. After plasma osmolality and sodium are in the normal range, fluid intake is balanced against urine output. Any net change in urine output over an 8-hour period (this may be extended as the patient's fluid requirements become more predictable) is accommodated by modifying the fluid orders for the ensuing 8 hours. The patient should also be weighed daily. Any alteration in weight is usually reflective of net changes in water retention and can be corrected through modification of fluid intake. Plasma osmolality and serum sodium should be monitored once or twice weekly and appropriate changes in fluid administration made depending on the direction and magnitude of the shift in osmolality. With this system of redundant monitoring, urine volumes and plasma osmolality can be reasonably well controlled for protracted periods of time.

Complications

If left untreated, polyuria secondary to diabetes insipidus can lead to dilation of the collecting system, hydronephrosis, and renal dysfunction. This is the dominant reason for treating polyuria even in patients with an intact thirst mechanism who are capable of controlling plasma osmolality through water ingestion.

Overly rapid correction of the hyperosmolality can result in cerebral edema. The relative risk of this complication should be minimized by careful attention to the rate at which the water deficit is corrected (see earlier).

REFERENCES

Myxedema Coma

Dutta P, Bhansali A, Masoodi SR, et al. Predictors of outcome in myxoedema coma: a study from a tertiary care center. *Crit Care.* 2008;12:R1. [PMID: 18173846]

Kwaku MP, Burman KD. Myxedema coma. *J Intensiv Care Med.* 2007;22:224. [PMID: 17712058]

Ringel MD. Management of hypothyroidism and hyperthyroidism in the intensive care unit. *Crit Care Clin.* 2001;17:59. [PMID: 11219235]

Sarlis NJ, Gourgiotis L. Thyroid emergencies. *Rev Endocr Metab Disord.* 2003;4:129. [PMID: 12766540]

Yamamoto T, Fukuyama J, Fujiyoshi A. Factors associated with mortality of myxedema coma: report of eight cases and literature survey. *Thyroid.* 1999;9:1167. [PMID: 10646654]

Thyroid Storm

Jiang YZ, Hutchinson KA, Bartelloni P, Manthous CA. Thyroid storm presenting as multiple organ dysfunction syndrome. *Chest.* 2000;118:877. [PMID: 10988222]

Yeoung SC, Go R, Balasubramanyam A. Rectal administration of iodide and propylthiouracil in the treatment of thyroid storm. *Thyroid.* 1995;5:403. [PMID: 8563481]

Thyrotoxic Periodic Paralysis

Kung AWC. Thyrotoxic periodic paralysis: a diagnostic challenge. *J Clin Endocrinol Metab.* 2006;91:2490. [PMID: 16608889]

Lin SH. Thyrotoxic periodic paralysis. *Mayo Clin Proc.* 2005;80:95. [PMID: 15667036]

Lin SH, Lin YF. Propanolol rapidly reverses paralysis, hypokalemia and hypophosphatemia in thyrotoxic periodic paralysis. *Am J Kidney Dis.* 2001;37:620. [PMID: 11228188]

Lu K-C, et al. Effects of potassium supplementation on the recovery of thyrotoxic periodic paralysis. *Am J Emerg Med.* 2004;22:544. [PMID: 15666258]

Ryan DP, da Silva MR, Soong TW et al. Mutations in potassium channel Kir2.6 cause susceptibility to thyrotoxic hypokalemic periodic paralysis. Cell 2010;140:88. [PMID: 20074522]

Tassone H, Mouslin A, Henderson SO. The pitfalls of potassium replacement in thyrotoxic periodic paralysis: a case report and review of the literature. *J Emerg Med.* 2004;26:157. [PMID: 1490336]

Amiodarone-Induced Hyperthyroidism

Bartelena L, Wiersinga WM, Tanda ML, et al. Diagnosis and management of amiodarone-induced thyrotoxicosis in Europe: results of an international survey among members of the European Thyroid Association. *Clin Endocrinol.* 2004;61:494. [PMID: 15473883]

Basaria S, Cooper DS. Amiodarone and the thyroid. *Am J Med.* 2005;118,706. [PMID: 15989900]

Conen D, Melly L, Kaufmann C, et al. Amiodarone-induced thyrotoxicosis. *J Am Coll Cardiol.* 2007;49:2350. [PMID: 17572251]

Eaton SE, Euinton HA, Newman CM, Weetman AP, Bennet WM. Clinical experience of amiodarone-induced thyrotoxicosis over a 3-year period: role of colour-flow Doppler sonography. *Clin Endocrinol (Oxf).* 2002;56:33. [PMID: 11849244]

Acute Adrenal Insufficiency

Arafah BM. Hypothalamic-pituitary-adrenal function during critical illness: limitations of current assessment methods. *J Clin Endocrinol Metab.* 2006;91:3725. [PMID: 16882746]

Cooper MS, Stewart PM. Corticosteroid insufficiency in acutely ill patients. *N Engl J Med.* 2003;348:727. [PMID 12594318]

Dorin RI, Qualls CR, Crapo LM. Diagnosis of adrenal insufficiency. *Ann Intern Med.* 2003;139:194. [PMID: 12899587]

Hamarahian AH, Oseni TS, Arafah B. Measurements of serum free cortisol in critically ill patients. *N Engl J Med.* 2004;350:1629. [PMID: 15084695]

Sprung CL Annane D, Keh D et al. Hydrocortisone therapy for patients with septic shock. *N Engl J Med.* 2008;358:111. [PMID: 18184957]

Pituitary Apoplexy

Biousse V, Newman NJ, Oyesiku NM. Precipitating factors in pituitary apoplexy. *J Neurol Neurosurg Psychiatry.* 2001;71:542. [PMID: 11561045]

Nawar RN, AbdelMannan D, Selman WR, Arafah BM. Pituitary tumor apoplexy: a review. *J Intensive Care Med.* 2008;23:75. [PMID: 18372348]

Diabetic Ketoacidosis

Fleckman AM. Diabetic ketoacidosis. *Endocrinol Metab Clin North Am.* 1993;22:181. [PMID: 8325282]

Hom J, Sinert R. Is fluid therapy associated with cerebral edema in children with diabetic ketoacidosis? *Ann Emer Med.* 2008;52:69. [PMID: 18387706]

Kearney T, Dang C. Diabetic and endocrine emergencies. *Postgrad Med J.* 2007;83:79. [PMID: 17308209]

Kitabachi AE, et al. Hyperglycemic crises in adult patients with diabetes. *Diabetes Care.* 2009;32:1335. [PMID: 19564476]

Kitabchi AE, Umpierrez GE, Fisher JN, Murphy MB, Stentz FB. Thirty years of personal experience in hyperglycemic crises: diabetic ketoacidosis and hyperglycemic hyperosmolar coma. *J Clin Endocrinol Metab.* 2008;93:1541. [PMID: 18270259]

Wolfsdorf J, Glaser N, Sperling MA. Diabetic ketoacidosis in infants, children and adolescents. *Diabetes Care.* 2006;29:1150. [PMID: 16644656]

Hyperosmolar Nonketotic Coma

English P, Williams G. Hyperglycemic crises and lactic acidosis in diabetes mellitus. *Postgrad Med.* 2004;80:253. [PMID: 15138313]

Lorber D. Nonketotic hypertonicity in diabetes mellitus. *Med Clin North Am.* 1995;79:39. [PMID: 7808094]

Hypocalcemia

Cooper MS, Gittoes NJL. Diagnosis and management of hypocalcemia. *Br Med J.* 2008;336:1298. [PMID: 18535072]

Dickerson RN. Treatment of hypocalcemia in critical illness. *Nutrition.* 2007;23:358,436. [PMID: 17400132, 17360159]

Hypercalcemic Crisis

Berenson JR. Treatment of hypercalcemia of malignancy with bisphosphonates. *Sem Oncol.* 2002;30(2 suppl 5):12. [PMID: 12584690]

Hyponatremia

Adrogue HJ, Madias NE. Hyponatremia. *N Engl J Med.* 2000;342:1581. [PMID: 10824078]

Ghali J, et al. Efficacy and safety of oral conivaptan: a V1A/V2 vasopressin receptor antagonist, assessed in a randomized, placebo-controlled trial in patients with euvolemic or hypervolemic hyponatremia. *J Clin Endocrinol Metab.* 2006;91:2145. [PMID: 16522696]

Greenberg A, Verbalis JG. Vasopressin receptor antagonists. *Kid Int.* 2006;69:2124. [PMID: 16672911]

Kumar S, Berl T. Sodium. *Lancet.* 998;352:220. [PMID: 98832227]

Sahun M, Villabona C, Rosel P, et al. Water metabolism disturbances at different stages of primary thyroid failure. *J Endocrinol.* 2001;168:435. [PMID: 11241175]

Singh S, Bohn D, Carlotti AP, et al. Cerebral salt wasting: truths, fallacies, theories and challenges. *Crit Care Med.* 2002;30:2575. [PMID: 12441772]

Verbalis JG. Disorders of body water homeostasis. *Best Prac Res Clin Endocr Metab.* 2003;17:471. [PMID: 14687585]

Diabetes Insipidus

Adrogue HJ, Madias NE. Hypernatremia. *N Engl J Med.* 2000;342:1493. [PMID: 10816188]

Mavrakis AN, Tritos NA. Diabetes insipidus with deficient thirst: report of a patient and review of the literature. *Am J Kid Dis.* 2008;51:851. [PMID: 18436097]

Morello J-P, Bichet DG. Nephrogenic diabetes insipidus. *Annu Rev Physiol.* 2001;63:607. [PMID: 11181969]

Singer I, Oster JR, Fishman LM. The management of diabetes insipidus in adults. *Arch Intern Med.* 1997;157:1293. [PMID: 92011003]

AIDS Endocrinopathies

Carl Grunfeld, MD, PhD and Grace Lee, MD

ACTH	Adrenocorticotropic hormone	**LH**	Luteinizing hormone
AIDS	Acquired immunodeficiency syndrome	**M/I**	Glucose disposal adjusted for insulin level
BMD	Bone mineral density	**MRI**	Magnetic resonance imaging
CMV	Cytomegalovirus	**NRTI**	Nucleoside reverse transcriptase inhibitor
CRH	Corticotropin-releasing hormone	**NNRTI**	Nonnucleoside reverse transcriptase inhibitor
CVD	Cardiovascular disease	**PI**	Protease inhibitor
DHEA	Dehydroepiandrosterone	**PPARγ**	Peroxisome proliferator-activated receptor γ
DXA	Dual energy x-ray absorptiometry	**PTH**	Parathyroid hormone
FSH	Follicle-stimulating hormone	**RANK**	Receptor activator of nuclear factor kappa
GH	Growth hormone	**REE**	Resting energy expenditure
GHRH	Growth hormone–releasing hormone	**RXR**	Retinoid X receptor
GnRH	Gonadotropin-releasing hormone	**SREBP**	Sterol regulatory enhancer-binding protein 1
HAART	Highly active antiretroviral therapy	**T₃**	Triiodothyronine
HDL	High-density lipoprotein	**T₄**	Thyroxine
HIV	Human immunodeficiency virus	**TBG**	Thyroxine-binding globulin
IGF	Insulin-like growth factor	**TNF**	Tumor necrosis factor
IL	Interleukin	**TRH**	Thyrotropin-releasing hormone
IMT	Intima media thickness	**VLDL**	Very low density lipoprotein
LDL	Low-density lipoprotein		

Symptoms consistent with endocrine disorders and alterations in endocrine laboratory values are not unusual in individuals infected with the human immunodeficiency virus (HIV). Some of these changes are common to any significant systemic illness; others appear to be more specific to HIV infection or its therapies. Alterations can be found in HIV infection even before clinically significant immunocompromise occurs. As the infected individual becomes immunocompromised, opportunistic infections and neoplasms—as well as the agents used in the treatment of these disorders—can give rise to further changes in endocrine function. Herein we discuss alterations in endocrine function that can accompany HIV infection and acquired immunodeficiency syndrome (AIDS), focusing on evaluation and interpretation of clinical and laboratory findings.

THYROID DISORDERS

In the era of highly active antiretroviral therapy (HAART), clinical thyroid dysfunction is relatively uncommon in stable HIV-infected patients. In several large studies, the prevalence of hypothyroidism was 1% to 2.5% and hyperthyroidism was 0.5% to 1%. The prevalence of subclinical disease was higher, with subclinical hypothyroidism between 3.5% and 20% and subclinical hyperthyroidism <1%, although definitions varied between studies. These data do not support screening for thyroid disease above the standard guidelines. With advanced HIV disease, alterations in thyroid function tests do occur but generally do not result in clinical dysfunction. In patients with AIDS, the effects of opportunistic infections and neoplastic involvement of the thyroid, as well as the effects of some medications used to treat HIV-infected patients, should be considered.

Alterations in Thyroid Function Tests

HIV-infected patients can show alterations in thyroid function tests that are largely asymptomatic. Some of the changes are similar to those seen in the classic euthyroid-sick syndrome, whereas others are unique to the HIV disease state. Advanced HIV is associated with a decrease in thyroid hormone levels, triiodothyronine (T_3) and thyroxine (T_4), similar to that seen in the euthyroid-sick syndrome. When HIV-infected patients were stratified by weight loss and the presence of secondary infection, a decline in T_3 levels corresponded to the severity of disease, consistent with the euthyroid-sick syndrome. Deterioration in nutritional status can also contribute to the decrease in T_3 and T_4, because there is a strong correlation between albumin levels and both free T_4 and total T_3 levels. In the euthyroid-sick syndrome, decreased levels of serum thyroid hormones are due to impaired peripheral T_4 to T_3 conversion by 5′ deiodinase. In HIV-infected patients, decreases in serum free T_4 and free T_3 may be due to decreased extrathyroidal conversion of T_4 to T_3, an increase in serum binding proteins, and/or decreased secretion of TSH.

Despite the similarities in serum thyroid hormone levels between HIV and the euthyroid sick syndrome, significantly ill HIV-infected patients often do not demonstrate the elevated reverse T_3 levels characteristic of the euthyroid sick syndrome. The significance of this difference is unknown.

Another characteristic finding in HIV-infected patients is an elevation in thyroxine-binding globulin (TBG), which rises progressively with advancing immunosuppression. TBG levels correlate inversely with the CD4 lymphocyte count, and in the past were used as a surrogate marker for disease progression. The increase in TBG does not appear to be due to generalized changes in protein synthesis, increases in sialylation and altered clearance of TBG, or changes in estrogen levels. The cause and clinical significance of the increased TBG found in HIV-infected patients are unknown. However, increases in TBG affect total T_4 and T_3 measurements, and this should be considered when interpreting these tests in HIV-infected patients.

Subtle alterations in TSH dynamics have been reported in stable HIV-infected patients. Although their TSH and free T_4 levels remain within the normal range, these individuals demonstrate significantly higher TSH values and lower free T_4 values than uninfected controls. In circadian studies, HIV-infected individuals have higher TSH pulse amplitudes with unchanged pulse frequency as well as a higher peak TSH in response to thyrotropin-releasing hormone (TRH) stimulation. These studies are consistent with a subtle state of compensated hypothyroidism in HIV infection; the mechanisms underlying these alterations have not been elucidated.

The typical pattern of alterations in thyroid function tests in HIV-infected patients is outlined in Table 25–1.

Opportunistic Infections and Neoplasms

Opportunistic pathogens and neoplasms can invade the thyroid in HIV-infected individuals but generally do not cause clinical

TABLE 25–1 Thyroid function tests in HIV-infected patients.

	Basal	After TRH Stimulation
T_3	↓	
T_4	Normal	
Reverse T_3	Normal or ↓	
TBG	↑	
TSH	Normal	↑ Pulse amplitude

↓, decreased; ↑, increased.

thyroid dysfunction. Although the prevalence of thyroid involvement is unknown, autopsy of 100 AIDS patients prior to the era of HAART showed the presence of *Mycobacterium tuberculosis* in 23% of patients' thyroids, followed by cytomegalovirus (CMV) (17%), *Cryptococcus neoformans* (5%), *Mycobacterium avium* (5%), *Pneumocystis carinii* (4%), and other bacteria or fungi (7%).

A few of these pathogens are noteworthy because they have been associated on occasion with both hyper- and hypothyroidism. *Pneumocystis carinii* has been associated with inflammatory thyroiditis accompanied by hypothyroidism in seven cases, hyperthyroidism in three cases, and normal thyroid function in one case. Antithyroid antibodies were negative in all six cases in which they were measured. Radionuclide scanning in seven cases revealed poor visualization of the entire thyroid gland in patients with bilateral disease and nonvisualization of the affected lobe in patients with unilateral disease. Two patients with hyperthyroidism had normalization of thyroid function after treatment of the *P. carinii* infection. Kaposi sarcoma has also been reported to infiltrate the thyroid gland and resulted in significant destruction and hypothyroidism in at least one case. In two cases, lymphoma was associated with thyroid infiltration, causing thyroidal enlargement.

Medication Effects

Several medications used to treat HIV-infected patients can alter the clearance of thyroid hormone by inducing hepatic microsomal enzymes. These medications include rifampin, phenytoin, ketoconazole, and ritonavir. Patients with normal thyroid function should not be clinically affected, although decreases in T_4 may be observed. However, patients receiving L-thyroxine may require increased doses, and patients with decreased pituitary or thyroid reserve may develop clinically apparent hypothyroidism. Isolated, but well-documented reports of need for increased thyroxine doses after starting ritonavir and decreased doses after indinavir have been published; these medications affect glucuronidation, but given the common use of high doses of these drugs in the past, it is surprising how rarely problems present. Interferon-alpha, a therapy used for Kaposi sarcoma and hepatitis C (an increasing coinfection with HIV), has been associated with autoimmune diseases of the thyroid, including hyperthyroidism and hypothyroidism. Medications used in HIV-infected patients that can affect the endocrine system are listed in Table 25–2.

TABLE 25-2 Medications used in HIV-infected patients that can affect the endocrine system.

Thyroid	*Pancreas, Glucose*
Rifampin	Indinavir
Phenytoin	Ritonavir
Ketoconazole	Possibly
Possibly ritonavir	lopinavir/ritonavir
Possibly indinavir	Pentamidine
Interferon-alpha	Trimethoprim-
Adrenals, Electrolytes	sulfamethoxazole
Rifampin	Dedeoxyinosine (ddI)
Ketoconazole	Dedeoxycytosine (ddC)
Ritonavir	Megestrol acetate
Megestrol acetate	Growth hormone
Trimethoprim	*Lipids*
Pentamidine	Ritonavir
Sulfonamides	Efavirenz
Amphotericin B	Nevirapine
Foscarnet	Stavudine
Gonads	Tenofovir
Ketoconazole	
Megestrol acetate	
Bone, Calcium	
Tenofovir	
Adefovir	
Cidofovir	
Foscarnet	
Pentamidine	
Trimethoprim-sulfamethoxazole	
Ketoconazole	
Rifampin, rifabutin	

With the advent of HAART, there have been case report series of newly diagnosed autoimmune diseases such as Graves disease, Hashimoto thyroiditis, and alopecia areata. Immune reconstitution with HAART raises the possibility of subsequent induction of autoimmune diseases. The cases appeared late after immune reconstitution (8-32 months). Possible theories include thymic regeneration or peripheral T lymphocyte expansion causing irregularities in tolerance, leading to autoimmune dysfunction. Other studies, however, could not link autoimmune thyroid disease to HAART, and the low prevalence in the large published studies suggests that increased screening above standard guidelines may not be warranted.

ADRENAL DISORDERS

Opportunistic infections commonly involve the adrenal glands but rarely occupy enough of the gland to cause adrenal insufficiency. Impaired adrenal reserve without overt symptoms of adrenal insufficiency has been described in patients with HIV. Those patients with a subnormal response to dynamic testing represent a group for which there is controversy over when to give baseline replacement glucocorticoids (or mineralocorticoids) or increased doses in stressful situations, especially when baseline levels are normal or elevated. With restoration to health by treatment of opportunistic infections or HIV itself, many of these patients no longer have adrenal insufficiency.

Opportunistic Infections and Neoplasms

Opportunistic organisms are found commonly in the adrenal glands of patients dying of AIDS although they rarely cause clinical adrenal insufficiency. CMV has been associated with significant necrosis of the adrenal gland, although the amount of tissue affected rarely reaches 90%, thought necessary to cause clinical adrenal insufficiency. In one preliminary study, however, the presence of CMV retinitis was associated with an increased rate of adrenal insufficiency compared with AIDS patients without that disorder. Less common opportunistic infections involving the adrenals include *Mycobacterium tuberculosis*, *Mycobacterium avium-intracellulare*, *Cryptococcus neoformans*, *Histoplasma capsulatum*, *P. carinii*, and *Toxoplasma gondii*. In addition, Kaposi sarcoma and lymphoma can involve the adrenals, but rarely to the extent of inducing adrenal insufficiency.

Glucocorticoids

Classic clinical symptoms of adrenal insufficiency are seldom seen, but some clinicians view the weakness and weight loss observed in patients with AIDS as an indicator of adrenal insufficiency. HIV-infected patients usually have normal or, even more commonly, elevated basal cortisol levels. The elevated levels occur most commonly in advanced disease, which may be a stress response, but is confounded by an increase in cortisol-binding globulin. Adrenocorticotropic hormone (ACTH) levels have mostly been found to be normal or elevated in patients with elevated basal cortisol levels, although some reports of low levels exist. Some of these alterations may be mediated by multiple cytokines; both interleukin (IL)-1 and tumor necrosis factor (TNF) can directly stimulate cortisol secretion, while IL-1 and IL-6 can stimulate ACTH and corticotropin-releasing hormone (CRH) release. On the other hand, IL-2 and IL-4 increase sensitivity to cortisol. An increase in cortisol levels may also be a direct response to HIV infection itself. The HIV envelope protein gp120 increases cortisol levels. HIV-1 virus encodes several proteins such as Vpr and Tat that may increase cortisol sensitivity. An increased cortisol to dehydroepiandrosterone (DHEA) ratio correlates with body weight loss and HIV-associated malnutrition.

Subclinical abnormalities in hypothalamic pituitary axis dynamics are often present. Nearly all HIV-infected patients have a normal cortisol response to the standard high-dose (250 µg) ACTH stimulation testing. Other studies have shown that stimulation with low-dose cosyntropin (1 µg) resulted in a diagnosis of glucocorticoid insufficiency in roughly 10% to 20% of outpatients with HIV and up to 50% of critically ill HIV-infected patients. During CRH stimulation testing, a reduced ACTH or cortisol response was seen in up to 50% of stable HIV-infected patients with CD4 counts less than 500/µL. The abnormalities of decreased reserve either at the pituitary or at the adrenal level in HIV infection are similar to those that occur in other infections or serious illnesses.

Although clinically significant abnormalities in glucocorticoid secretion appear to be uncommon, subtle alterations in adrenal biosynthesis may be more common. HIV-infected patients have reduced products of the 17-deoxysteroid pathway (corticosterone, deoxycorticosterone, and 18-hydroxydeoxycorticosterone) with normal or elevated products of the 17-hydroxy pathway (cortisol) before and after ACTH stimulation. It is not known whether this alteration represents an early indication of evolving adrenal insufficiency or is an adaptive response that shifts adrenal synthetic activity to steroids that are crucially needed under conditions such as HIV infection that impose physical stress. Twenty-four-hour urine-free cortisol levels do not predict the subtle adrenal alterations in HIV-infected patients, but may indicate adequate adrenal function.

Glucocorticoid resistance has been described in HIV-infected patients. This syndrome is characterized by symptoms of weakness, fatigue, weight loss, and hyperpigmentation, with elevated cortisol levels and mildly increased ACTH levels. Decreased lymphocyte glucocorticoid receptor affinity for glucocorticoids has been described in these patients. A similar state is seen in glucocorticoid-resistant asthma patients. Increased expression of the beta form of the glucocorticoid receptor, which inhibits the alpha form, has also been reported. Partial glucocorticoid resistance could explain the finding of increased basal cortisol in some HIV-infected patients, but the prevalence and clinical significance of this syndrome are uncertain.

Adrenal Androgens

HIV-infected patients have decreased basal adrenal androgen levels and impaired adrenal androgen responses to ACTH stimulation. Decreased adrenal androgens have been seen at all stages of HIV infection, as well as in HIV-negative intensive care unit patients. Thus, this change may not be specific to HIV infection but may instead be a feature of the physiologic response to illness, which is often accompanied by increased cortisol. In two studies, a fall in DHEA levels predicted progression to AIDS independent of CD4 cell counts. DHEA has been shown in vitro to inhibit HIV replication, which raised the possibility that the decreased DHEA levels observed in HIV-infected patients might influence the effects of the HIV infection. However, the efficacy of DHEA replacement in HIV-infected patients has never been demonstrated. Adrenal androgens may be decreased in women with HIV infection; low-dose testosterone replacement has been shown to induce small improvements in lean mass, depression, and sexual function.

Mineralocorticoids

Although electrolyte disturbances are not uncommon in HIV-infected patients, provocative testing of the mineralocorticoid axis has revealed few abnormalities. In contrast to glucocorticoid levels, basal and ACTH-stimulated aldosterone levels have been found to be normal in almost all HIV-infected patients studied, including both outpatients and inpatients. Nevertheless case reports of hypo- and hyperaldosteronism appear in the literature, although there is no evidence that these disorders are increased in HIV infection. Longitudinal studies suggest that the aldosterone response to ACTH stimulation may diminish with progression to later stages of HIV infection in up to half of HIV-infected patients; however, basal levels of aldosterone and plasma renin

TABLE 25–3 Usual pattern of adrenal hormones in HIV infection.

	Basal	After ACTH Stimulation
Glucocorticoids	Normal or ↑ cortisol; ↓ 17-deoxysteroids	Normal cortisol response
Mineralocorticoids	Normal	Normal
Androgens	↓	↓

↓, decreased; ↑, increased.

activity remain normal, and clinically significant hypoaldosteronism does not develop.

The usual pattern of alterations in adrenal hormones is shown in Table 25–3.

Medication Effects

Several medications used in the treatment of HIV-related disorders can alter glucocorticoid metabolism. Ketoconazole inhibits the cytochrome P450 enzymes P450scc and P450c11, decreasing cortisol synthesis and leading to adrenal insufficiency in patients with decreased adrenal reserve. Rifampin increases hepatic metabolism of steroids and may lead to adrenal insufficiency in patients with marginal adrenal reserve.

Megestrol acetate has intrinsic cortisol-like activity, decreasing serum cortisol and ACTH levels through suppression of the hypothalamic-pituitary-adrenal axis centrally. Patients taking megestrol have decreased cortisol and ACTH levels in response to metyrapone testing. They may become frankly Cushingoid and may show signs of adrenal insufficiency upon its rapid discontinuation. Some HIV protease inhibitors (PIs) block the metabolism of the inhaled steroid fluticasone by CYP3A4 and can lead to Cushing syndrome even in the absence of systemic steroid use. PIs do not seem to have an effect on plasma cortisol levels. However, there is debate in the literature about whether these agents increase or decrease urinary free cortisol or 17-hydroxycorticosteroid excretion.

Medications used to treat HIV-related illnesses can lead to electrolyte disturbances mimicking disorders of mineralocorticoids. Trimethoprim impairs sodium channels in the distal nephron, decreasing potassium secretion, which can result in hyperkalemia. Pentamidine has also been associated with hyperkalemia in rare instances, perhaps through nephrotoxicity. Sulfonamides are associated with interstitial nephritis and hyporeninemic hypoaldosteronism. Finally, amphotericin B causes renal potassium and magnesium wasting.

Medications used in HIV-infected patients that can affect the endocrine system are listed in Table 25–2.

Summary of Adrenal Disorders

In summary, there is little evidence for clinically significant impairment of adrenal steroid excretion in HIV infection. The subtle alterations in the glucocorticoid and androgen synthesis pathways may be an adaptive response to physiologic stress and may occur with other illnesses. Patients with HIV infection who exhibit symptoms consistent with adrenal hormone deficiency should undergo provocative testing in the same manner as uninfected individuals. Patients with both low baseline and abnormal glucocorticoid or mineralocorticoid responses to provocative testing should be treated with physiologic replacement doses of oral glucocorticoids or mineralocorticoids. Patients on replacement should be covered with high doses of glucocorticoids (usually 150-300 mg of hydrocortisone per day or equivalent) during episodes of severe illness. Electrolyte abnormalities should prompt evaluation for medication effects and the presence of renal disease.

The HIV-infected patient with a minimally elevated or frankly high basal cortisol who does not increase significantly after ACTH stimulation poses a difficult problem. Most of these individuals have normal responses to prolonged ACTH stimulation, and seronegative patients with significant illness can have similar patterns that revert to normal after treatment of the illness. Chronic glucocorticoid therapy may have significant adverse consequences in these individuals, who are already immunocompromised. Most HIV-infected patients with this pattern and even many with baseline low levels during acute illness do not appear to require long-term glucocorticoid replacement. Consideration could be given to administering short courses of steroid therapy during significant illness for individuals with indeterminate stimulation results based on clinical judgment and individual patient circumstances.

BONE AND MINERAL DISORDERS

Osteopenia and Osteoporosis

There is evidence of low bone mass and, less commonly, osteoporosis in HIV-infected patients either without therapy or while receiving HAART, but the etiology remains controversial. The incidence of fractures may be increased, but there are too few studies of fracture rate to know with certainty. Therapy with bisphosphonates is effective at increasing bone mineral density (BMD) in HIV-infected patients, but there are no convincing data on fracture prevention.

Prior to the introduction of HIV PIs, low BMD was not commonly observed in HIV-infected patients. The few clinical studies on the effects of HIV on bone mineralization suggested that HIV had relatively little effect on BMD. One study followed 45 HIV-infected men for 15 months and found no change in lumbar spine and hip BMD. However, histomorphometric analysis of bone biopsies from AIDS patients showed some evidence of decreased bone formation and bone turnover; these changes were more marked in more severely affected patients. HIV itself may have an indirect effect on BMD by activating the receptor activator of nuclear factor kappa B ligand (RANK-L), which activates osteoclasts and their precursors. Activated T cells express the receptor for RANK-L—that is, RANK. The cytokines TNF-alpha and IL-1, whose levels may be increased in HIV infection, also have been shown to activate RANK-L.

After the introduction of PI-based HAART, reports of osteoporosis began to emerge. Some cross-sectional studies suggested that patients on PIs had a higher prevalence of osteoporosis and osteopenia compared to HIV-infected patients not taking PIs. However, other studies did not find a specific association of PIs with decreased BMD by dual energy x-ray absorptiometry (DXA). To date, most cross-sectional studies have shown that both HIV-infected men and women, on any form of HAART, have lower BMD or a higher prevalence of osteopenia, compared to gender- and ethnicity-matched control subjects. In one meta-analysis of 20 papers, the prevalence of reduced BMD was 67%, and the prevalence of osteoporosis was 15% in HIV-infected patients, which represents a 6.4-fold greater prevalence of reduced BMD and 3.7-fold greater prevalence of osteoporotic T scores compared to controls. Furthermore, those treated with ARV had a 2.5-fold higher prevalence of reduced BMD than those who were ARV-naive. Lactic acidemia associated with nucleoside reverse transcriptase inhibitor (NRTI) use has been hypothesized to contribute to bone demineralization. However, the role of specific ARV drugs as a cause of bone demineralization remains debated, as many recent studies fail to show an association between osteopenia and individual drugs. Thus, ARV use per se is associated with lower BMD. Divergent effects of PIs on bone cells in vitro have been reported.

Another meta-analysis found that the effect of HIV infection was mostly accounted for by decreased weight. Other studies have found associations of low albumin and past steroid use with low BMD. A randomized longitudinal study showed that continuous ARV therapy, used to suppress HIV, was associated with greater loss of bone mass and perhaps more fractures than intermittent ARV therapy designed to reduce drug exposure. However, the absolute rate of BMD loss by DXA was actually quite small in those on continuous ARV therapy (–0.5%/year at the hip and –0.7%/year at the spine). In a large database analysis, the fracture rate was increased 1.7-fold in HIV-infected Caucasian men and 1.4-fold in HIV-infected Caucasian and African American women compared to their respective controls.

Treatment for HIV-associated osteoporosis with bisphosphonates has been examined. Multiple studies have shown that the bisphosphonates alendronate and zoledronic acid given either with or without calcium and vitamin D supplementation to HIV-infected patients with osteopenia or osteoporosis improved BMD in the lumbar spine and hip after 1 to 2 years of therapy. The effects of treatments for other HIV-related problems on BMD or bone markers have been assessed. Eugonadal men with AIDS wasting syndrome treated with intramuscular testosterone for 3 months had small increases in lumbar spine BMD; however, high doses of testosterone were associated with decreases in HDL cholesterol levels. Recombinant growth hormone (GH) treatment for 24 weeks in HIV wasting syndrome did not affect BMD. Short-term growth hormone–releasing hormone (GHRH), used to treat HIV-infected men with abdominal fat accumulation, was associated with an increase in bone turnover markers; however the effect of GHRH use on BMD remains to be determined.

Osteonecrosis

Osteonecrosis has been reported both in adults and in children infected with HIV, and there is concern about the rising prevalence of osteonecrosis in this population. The most likely reason for the apparent rise in prevalence of the syndrome is increased awareness among clinicians. A study of 339 HIV-infected patients reported a prevalence of asymptomatic osteonecrosis, diagnosed by magnetic resonance imaging (MRI) as 4.4%. The annual incidence has been reported to be between 0.08% and 1.3%, which is much higher than the annual incidence in the general population (0.01%-0.135%).

The clinical presentation and anatomic distribution are similar to HIV-negative patients. The most common location for osteonecrosis is the hip, but other locations include the humeral heads, femoral condyles, and scaphoid and lunate bones. In HIV infection, the majority of large joint involvement is bilateral. Cases of osteonecrosis of the jaw/oral cavity have also been reported.

Plain film x-rays often underdiagnose osteonecrosis as changes on x-ray are confined to advanced stage (III and IV) disease; MRI is more effective at finding early-stage disease. Some data support treatment with bisphosphonates in early disease involving major joints to reduce pain, but there are inadequate randomized, controlled trials to assess whether such therapy prevents progression. Core decompression with and without bone graft has had some success. Total joint replacement may be the only recourse in late disease (eg, following collapse of the femoral head).

An association between osteonecrosis and PIs was initially reported; however, subsequent studies have failed to show a causal relationship with PI use. Other possible etiologies include those that may be more frequent in patients with HIV infection (corticosteroid use, HIV-associated vasculitis, chemotherapy, and irradiation) and other traditional risk factors (ethanol use, sickle cell disease, hemoglobinopathies, and clotting disorders).

Calcium and Phosphate Homeostasis

Calcium, phosphate, and calciotropic hormone disturbances are associated with several HIV-related illnesses and medications. Hypercalcemia with an elevated 1,25-dihyroxyvitamin D level has been associated with both AIDS-related lymphoma and infections with *M. tuberculosis, M. avium-intracellulare, P. jiroveci, C. neoformans,* and *Coccidioides immitis.* This hypercalcemia is likely due to increased extrarenal 1-alpha hydroxylation of 25-hydroxyvitamin D to 1,25-dihydroxyvitamin D by inflammatory macrophages or tumor cells. In CMV infection, activated T cells or proinflammatory cytokines may secrete factors that activate osteoclasts, causing hypercalcemia. The syndrome has also been reported after starting antiretroviral therapy, with improvements in lymphocyte function, as part of the immune reconstitution syndrome. Recombinant human GH treatment has been associated with slight increases in serum calcium levels in some studies.

Mild hypocalcemia has been associated with HIV disease. HIV-infected patients have been shown to have low 1,25-hydroxyvitamin D and 25-hydroxyvitamin D levels, but normal vitamin D–binding protein levels, suggesting an impairment in 1-alpha hydroxylation and a compromised nutritional state. Low 1,25-hydroxyvitamin D levels are associated with advanced disease stage and increased TNF-alpha levels.

Inadequate parathyroid hormone (PTH) responses (ie, functional hypoparathyroidism) may also contribute to the hypocalcemia seen with HIV. PTH levels have been shown to be decreased in HIV-infected patients compared to controls. Parathyroid cells may be targeted by HIV infection: they express CD4 receptors which when activated affect PTH secretion. Invasion of the parathyroid gland by neoplasms and infections can also rarely occur.

Severe hypocalcemia is usually due to medications used to treat opportunistic infections. Variations on Fanconi syndrome are reported increasingly. Hypocalcemia and hypophosphatemia have been reported with tenofovir and adefovir (which are used to treat HIV) and cidofovir (which is used to treat CMV). Hypocalcemia has also been seen during therapy for CMV retinitis with foscarnet. Foscarnet can complex ionized calcium and may have mineral wasting effects at the level of the renal tubule, leading to concurrent hypomagnesemia and hypokalemia. Hypocalcemia and hypomagnesemia have also been reported during pentamidine treatment, and the combination of foscarnet and pentamidine can result in severe, even fatal, hypocalcemia. Trimethoprim-sulfamethoxazole, ketoconazole, and aminoglycosides are also associated with hypocalcemia. Ketoconazole and rifampin can alter vitamin D metabolism but usually do not produce clinically significant effects. Ketoconazole can reduce serum levels of 1,25-dihydroxyvitamin D and lower total—but not ionized—calcium levels. Rifampin and rifabutin can decrease 25-hydroxyvitamin D levels, but usually do not appear to significantly change calcium or PTH levels; one case has been reported of severe osteomalacia attributed to rifabutin.

Medications used in HIV-infected patients that can affect the endocrine system are listed in Table 25–2.

GONADAL DISORDERS

Testicular Function

Testicular atrophy is common in AIDS patients. Histopathologic changes include decreased spermatogenesis, thickened basement membrane, and an interstitial infiltrate. Possible causes of testicular atrophy include opportunistic infection by *M. avium-intracellulare, Toxoplasma,* and CMV, hypogonadism, HIV infection itself, and chemotherapy toxicity. HIV-infected men generally have oligoteratospermia, and as the disease state becomes more severe, the sperm can become grossly abnormal. Hence, male fertility decreases with advancing disease.

Semen washing has been used as a technique for HIV-discordant couples to reduce the risk of viral transmission. The three-step process involves gradient centrifugation, washing, and spontaneous migration to obtain motile sperm. There have been several thousand published cases of semen washing followed by either intrauterine or in vitro fertilization. These observational reports have shown that semen washing is a relatively safe and effective means of establishing pregnancy in HIV-negative women. Still, there is concern that the risk of infection is not completely eliminated after the procedure.

Hypogonadism is a common finding in men, particularly with advanced HIV disease. Prior to the introduction of HAART, hypogonadism was observed in approximately 40% of HIV-infected men. With the widespread use of HAART, the prevalence of hypogonadism has declined to 20%. Early in HIV infection, testosterone levels are normal or even elevated. Elevated basal luteinizing hormone (LH) levels and an increased LH response to gonadotropin-releasing hormone (GnRH) have been observed in these patients, suggesting pituitary dysfunction. In the later stages of HIV infection, low serum testosterone levels are seen, often accompanied by symptoms of decreased libido or erectile dysfunction. Because hypogonadism is associated with loss of lean body tissue and muscle mass, it is thought to contribute to AIDS wasting syndrome. Hypogonadal men infected with HIV tend to have low or normal LH and follicle-stimulating hormone (FSH) levels, similar to that seen in hypogonadotropic hypogonadism. However, GnRH testing in hypogonadal men with HIV has been normal in most cases. Primary hypogonadism with elevated LH and FSH levels has been observed but is far less common.

Several etiologies of the hypogonadism in men infected with HIV have been proposed, and in many cases, the cause of hypogonadism is multifactorial. Chronic illness and weight loss can alter the hypothalamic-pituitary axis. HIV infection increases the levels of the cytokines IL-1 and TNF, which have been shown to suppress hypothalamic pituitary function. Direct pituitary or hypothalamic invasion by toxoplasmosis or CMV is rare. There are divergent data on the extent to which treatment of HIV with ARV drugs increases testosterone levels.

Medications can also alter testicular function. Ketoconazole inhibits gonadal steroidogenesis, resulting in lower testosterone levels, oligospermia, and gynecomastia. Megestrol acetate, a progesterone-like agent, can lead to decreases in testosterone in HIV-infected men, perhaps through central feedback on gonadotropins. Medications used in HIV-infected patients that can affect the endocrine system are listed in Table 25-2.

Most of the studies of testosterone replacement have been performed in the context of AIDS wasting syndrome in which muscle and fat mass are decreased. Testosterone therapy in hypogonadal men with HIV increases lean body mass, but only small improvements in strength are seen. Most studies find that testosterone replacement therapy results in improved sexual functioning, mood, and energy. Testosterone therapy does not appear to exacerbate Kaposi sarcoma, although the studies of this relationship have involved limited numbers of patients.

Ovarian Function

Women represent one of the fastest growing populations with HIV infection. Two key issues include the effects of reproductive function on the natural history of HIV disease, and conversely, the effects of HIV on reproductive function. Recent studies found that women infected with HIV possess 30% to 50% lower HIV-1 RNA levels than men. Limited data suggests that the ovulatory cycle affects HIV infection in women. Early studies suggested no association between the menstrual cycle and HIV-1 RNA levels but may have included women with anovulatory cycles. In ovulating women, HIV-1 RNA levels have been shown to decline from the early follicular phase to the luteal phase. Menopause does not seem to affect the progression of HIV disease or the response to therapy.

In addition to affecting HIV-1 RNA levels, the menstrual cycle may also affect the pharmacokinetics of drugs used to treat HIV infection. Zidovudine levels have been shown to be negatively correlated with estradiol levels, suggesting that the menstrual cycle may affect zidovudine glucuronidation. Further studies are warranted.

Pregnancy does not seem to have a deleterious effect on maternal progression of HIV disease. However, an increase in HIV-1 RNA levels may occur in the early postpartum period. Several, but not all, studies suggest that pregnancy increases the rate of detection of HIV-1 in the genital tract. When HIV-1 is identified in the genital tract, the risk of perinatal transmission has been consistently shown to increase. Simple ARV regimens at the time of delivery have been shown to significantly reduce transmission of HIV to the child.

It is unclear whether HIV infection itself causes menstrual irregularities and/or amenorrhea. Early studies reported menstrual irregularities in HIV-infected women. However, these studies relied on self-report of menstrual symptoms and cycles, and many studies had enrolled an inadequate number of HIV-negative women as controls. Recent studies suggest that HIV may alter menstrual function only slightly. One large study of 802 HIV-infected and 273 HIV-negative women matched for demographic characteristics, body mass index, and substance abuse found that HIV infection increased the odds of having a very short or long cycle. There were no differences in amenorrhea, length of menses, or variability between the two groups. Another study of 197 HIV-infected women and 189 HIV-negative women found that HIV was not associated with menstrual dysfunction.

It is also uncertain whether HIV has an effect on the onset and symptoms of menopause. The average age at menopause in HIV-infected women has been reported to be between 46 and 50 years. While some studies contrast that to reported average age at menopause in controls being slightly greater than 50, the range in multiple population studies is actually 48 to 51. The diagnosis of menopause is complicated by the occurrence of amenorrhea lasting more than 1 year (which meets the clinical definition of menopause) in HIV-infected women who do not have ovarian failure as indicated by normal FSH and LH levels. Factors associated with such amenorrhea include opiate use, low body mass index, and low serum albumin levels suggesting hypothalamic dysfunction and malnutrition as causes rather than menopause. There are conflicting data concerning whether HIV is associated with increased or decreased symptoms of menopause.

With HIV infection, fertility rates decline. Quantifying the rate of decrease in fertility in the United States has been difficult due to confounding factors such as sociodemographics, drug use, weight loss, systemic illness, and sexually transmitted diseases. In Africa, where therapy for HIV was rare, there are numerous studies establishing an association between untreated HIV infection and infertility in virtually all age groups. In sub-Saharan Africa, HIV infection has been shown to account for a population-attributable decline in total fertility of 0.37% for each percentage point of HIV prevalence.

Like men, women infected with HIV have a decline in serum testosterone and adrenal androgen levels with progression of HIV disease and development of complications. Approximately 50% of women with AIDS-related wasting have low androgen levels. Androgen-deficient women may have subtle symptoms of decreased energy, libido, mood, strength, and bone mass. Despite the increased prevalence of androgen deficiency in study subjects with advanced disease, clinical laboratory diagnosis remains difficult in the female population. Total testosterone levels may be increased due to elevations in sex hormone–binding globulin in HIV-infected women, whereas free testosterone levels for women are not well-standardized in clinical laboratories.

Hormonal contraception is affected by ARV therapy. The estrogen component is metabolized by CYP3A4 enzyme. Many of the PIs and some nonnucleoside reverse transcriptase inhibitors (NNRTIs) either inhibit or induce CYP3A4, thus altering ethinyl estradiol and norethindrone levels. Other medications used to treat opportunistic infections such as rifabutin and rifampicin can also induce CYP3A4. There are very few studies on the effects of these medications on ovulation in subjects taking oral contraceptives. The Centers for Disease Control and Prevention recommend using barrier methods or condoms in addition to or in place of oral contraception.

PITUITARY DISORDERS

Opportunistic Infections and Neoplasms

In autopsy series of AIDS patients, nearly 10% of pituitary glands demonstrate some degree of infarction or necrosis; infectious organisms such as CMV, *P. carinii*, *Cryptococcus*, *Toxoplasma*, and *Aspergillus* have been observed. Antemortem pituitary function was not reported in these patients.

Anterior Pituitary Function

Hypopituitarism appears to be rare in AIDS patients; stimulation with TRH, GnRH, or CRH results in normal pituitary responses in almost all patients. Likewise, prolactin levels generally have been found to be normal, with a normal response to TRH stimulation. Some patients have shown a higher maximal pituitary response to stimulation testing compared with uninfected subjects, but the clinical significance of this alteration is not known.

The GH axis has received particular attention in children with HIV who can have poor growth velocity, especially when symptomatically ill. Most of these children demonstrate normal GH levels, although low insulin-like growth factor (IGF)-I levels can be seen. Low IGF-I in the setting of relatively normal GH is often seen in states of malnutrition, which may partially explain this finding. In adults, IGF-I levels may be low in malnourished or symptomatic HIV-infected patients but are usually normal in clinically stable individuals. Circadian GH secretion does not appear to be altered in adults with HIV infection, except in the presence of visceral obesity.

Posterior Pituitary Function

Posterior pituitary function may be altered in HIV infection. Hyponatremia is common in both inpatients and outpatients with HIV. Inappropriately high serum antidiuretic hormone levels have been seen in euvolemic AIDS patients with hyponatremia; however, many of these patients had pulmonary or cerebral infections, which themselves can cause the syndrome of inappropriate antidiuretic hormone secretion. As with any patient, destruction of the posterior pituitary by infection or tumor can lead to central diabetes insipidus; like anterior pituitary destruction, this appears to be rare in HIV infection.

AIDS WASTING SYNDROME

Prior to the introduction of HAART, weight loss and tissue wasting were commonly observed complications of AIDS in up to 30% of patients infected with HIV. A characteristic feature of this syndrome includes wasting of muscle, which is directly associated with increased morbidity and mortality. Muscle is disproportionately lost compared to fat in men. In contrast, women start with higher fat mass, and fat depletion dominates muscle loss until fat reserves are decreased. Weight loss can either be gradual or rapid in nature. Gradual weight loss has been associated with gastrointestinal disease, whereas rapid weight loss is usually seen during opportunistic infections.

The pathogenesis of wasting remains poorly understood. Several etiologies have been proposed including starvation, cachexia, hypermetabolic state, and hypogonadism. Starvation implies solely a limitation of calories, which may occur due to decreased appetite or decreased intake due to gastrointestinal infections with marked diarrhea. Cachexia refers to a state in which muscle is disproportionately lost due to direct effects on muscle. A hypermetabolic state has been proposed as a cause of AIDS wasting syndrome, because resting energy expenditure (REE) has been observed to be increased in HIV infection. However, the increase in REE is also seen in HIV-infected subjects with stable weight. HIV patients with either opportunistic infections or gastrointestinal disease have decreased caloric intake, but do not show the protective decrease in REE that occurs in pure starvation. Hence, the combination of decreased caloric intake and hypermetabolism is the driving force for wasting. The persistent metabolic defects make recovery from wasting incomplete, and recurrent events lead to progressive, step wise wasting.

Hypogonadism is a prominent finding in up to 50% of men and women with AIDS wasting. A direct correlation between testosterone levels and decreased muscle and fat mass exists. Resistance to GH has also been demonstrated in patients with more than a 10% loss in body weight.

Because a 10% loss of weight is associated with increased morbidity and mortality in patients infected with HIV, clinical trials have targeted the restoration of appetite, weight, and lean body mass. The cannabinol derivative dronabinol increased subjective appetite in patients with AIDS wasting syndrome, but had little or no effect to promote weight gain. Megestrol acetate increased appetite and weight, but resulted in mostly gain of fat.

Currently, recombinant GH therapy is the only Food and Drug Administration–approved treatment specifically for AIDS wasting syndrome that increases lean body mass. At high doses (0.1 mg/kg/d), 3 months of GH therapy increased lean body mass by 3 kg and weight by 1 kg. However, patients did experience side-effects including swelling and joint pain. In a lower-dose study (1.4 mg/d), patients had no significant increase in lean body mass after 12 weeks, which suggests that high-dose GH therapy is required. Therapy with recombinant GH is quite costly, especially if given at higher doses.

Androgen therapy has been studied extensively, because almost half of patients with AIDS wasting syndrome exhibit decreased levels of testosterone. In a meta-analysis of six clinical trials, testosterone therapy was shown to increase lean body mass and weight, especially when the therapy was given intramuscularly as opposed to transdermally. However, there have been no studies in which subjects have been randomized to different routes of administration of testosterone. Because testosterone may decrease HDL cholesterol levels, there is some concern about the long-term effects of testosterone therapy on lipid profiles and cardiovascular risk. However, no other side-effects were reported in these small, short-term studies.

Anabolic steroids have similar effects on the AIDS wasting syndrome. Nandrolone decanoate is an injectable testosterone derivative that is approved for treating anemia in patients with chronic renal failure. Two studies of nandrolone decanoate in men found that lean body mass and strength significantly increased. Nandrolone therapy improved lean body mass and weight without evidence of acute toxicity. Therapy using oral anabolic steroids oxandrolone and oxymetholone also increases lean body mass and weight in men and women, but it is associated with significant hepatic transaminitis as well as dyslipidemia.

Another approach has been to use anticytokine therapies to treat patients with AIDS wasting syndrome, but the results have been disappointing. Two studies reported small increases in weight after treatment with thalidomide, a TNF inhibitor. However, TNF levels actually increased and the patients experienced significant side effects including rash, fever, and increased viral load.

ABNORMALITIES OF FAT DISTRIBUTION ASSOCIATED WITH HIV

Shortly after the introduction of HAART with PIs, a constellation of symptoms appeared including abdominal obesity, lipoatrophy in the extremities and face, dorsicocervical fat pads (buffalo hump), gynecomastia, breast enlargement, increased neck circumference, and lipomas along with insulin resistance and dyslipidemia. These changes were clustered into a single syndrome reminiscent of the metabolic syndrome and named HIV lipodystrophy.

In retrospect, some of these changes are not related to HAART with PIs. The appearance of lipoatrophy, fat accumulation in the dorsocervical fat pad, lipomas, and breast hypertrophy was reported in patients on two NRTIs before the introduction of HAART or PIs. The presence of dorsocervical fat pads and lipomas is striking, but their prevalence is low.

Furthermore, the original description of the HIV lipodystrophy syndrome has been refuted, as it has been shown definitively that the major changes in fat (lipoatrophy and abdominal obesity) are not part of the same syndrome, but have different causes. Unfortunately, there is still no widely accepted definition of HIV lipodystrophy that is used in the literature. Depending on the definition of HIV lipodystrophy, the prevalence of these findings varies widely (11%-83%). Part of the confusion is due to differences in methodology used to report fat loss or gain. Many early studies relied on the patient's self-report and/or the clinician's subjective assessment. Later studies quantified fat by anthropometrics or DXA. Neither technique permits the isolation of subcutaneous from visceral fat in the abdomen and trunk; therefore computed tomography and MRI are needed and have been utilized more recently to separately quantify fat in these compartments. Because changes in fat may take years to develop, many studies in the field are cross-sectional rather than prospective in design. In these cross-sectional studies, it is unclear how to match patients to a control group with normal fat distribution, given that most healthy adults are overweight.

Despite these challenges, it has become apparent that peripheral fat loss in the extremities and face does occur with increased frequency in patients taking HAART. In one study, 50% of HIV-infected subjects fell below the lowest decile (10%) of leg fat in controls. However, loss of subcutaneous fat in the abdomen also occurs. In contrast, it is not clear that visceral adipose tissue mass is increased in HIV infection. Furthermore, recent cross-sectional and prospective data showed that increased visceral fat is not linked to loss of subcutaneous fat.

Several etiologies have been proposed for the development of lipoatrophy associated with HIV, but to date no mechanism has been definitively linked to the disorder. The thymidine-based nucleoside analogs, stavudine and zidovudine, have the strongest association with the development of peripheral lipoatrophy. These NRTIs have been proposed to cause lipoatrophy through mitochondrial injury by inhibiting mitochondrial DNA polymerase-γ or depleting mitochondrial DNA. Fortunately, the use of stavudine and zidovudine has decreased. Abacavir is the NRTI with the least effect on fat. Some PIs (eg, indinavir) and NNRTIs (eg, efavirenz) may contribute secondarily to the lipoatrophy observed with NRTI therapy, but there are not enough trials to understand fully the effects of each ARV drug.

The development of central lipohypertrophy is even less well understood. While central lipohypertrophy has been attributed to PI use, the evidence is controversial. In the first reports of appearance of buffalo hump, half of the patients were not on PI therapy or HAART. Recent data suggest that increased visceral fat may be due to restoration to health and normal aging.

Much research has focused on the treatment of the fat changes associated with HIV. Fat loss, especially in the face, can reveal the HIV status of a patient and lead to social stigmatization. The metabolic sequelae can also predispose the patient to the development of hypertriglyceridemia and atherosclerosis. One proposed strategy is to reverse the peripheral lipoatrophy by switching ARV drugs. Substituting another NRTI for a thymidine NRTI, such as stavudine or zidovudine, causes a minimal, albeit statistically significant increase in subcutaneous fat. Lipoatrophy does not fully resolve. In one study, switching from stavudine or zidovudine to abacavir caused a 0.4-kg increase in total limb fat after 24 weeks and a 1.3-kg increase in total limb fat after 104 weeks. However, that gain is insufficient to reach the levels seen in control populations. Complete cessation of therapy without replacement of NRTI results in virologic failure. Switching from PIs to nevirapine, efavirenz, or abacavir did not improve peripheral lipoatrophy. The newer NRTIs, tenofovir and emtricitabine, have been associated with less peripheral lipoatrophy than stavudine.

Thiazolidinediones are potentially attractive agents for treatment of peripheral lipoatrophy and insulin resistance. As ligands for the transcription factor perioxosome proliferator–activated receptor gamma (PPARγ), thiazolidinediones promote adipocyte differentiation. Unfortunately, two randomized studies found no improvement and a third showed minimal improvement in lipoatrophy after thiazolidine treatment for at least 24 weeks. However, the studies did show the expected improvement in insulin resistance.

Reconstructive therapy is available for peripheral lipoatrophy. Injectable skin fillers for the face include bioabsorbable and permanent fillers. Bioabsorbable fillers such as poly-L-acetic acid stimulate collagen production. In one open-label, single-arm study, 43% of patients had an increase in cutaneous thickness greater than 10 mm in the face after 96 weeks of therapy. The effects on collagen production last for approximately 18 months. Hyaluronic acid has also been used to a lesser extent in the treatment of facial lipoatrophy. Side-effects include easy bruisability, redness, and swelling. Permanent fillers are generally not recommended due to the dynamic nature of fat loss in peripheral lipoatrophy. More invasive procedures include autologous fat transplants.

Central lipohypertrophy has been treated with GH and GHRH analogues. At high doses (6 mg/d), GH decreased visceral fat by 21% to 24%. However, a significant number of patients experienced joint swelling, fluid retention, and deterioration in glucose tolerance. A lower dose of GH (3 mg/d) also reduced visceral fat, although to a lesser extent. With further dose reduction, GH (1 mg/d) decreased total fat, but did not significantly alter visceral fat content. A GHRH analogue, tesamorelin, is a recently approved therapy for reduction of visceral obesity in HIV-lipodystrophy that limits the side-effects of excessive GH secretion by increasing the endogenous pulsatility of GH secretion. Tesamorelin (2 mg/d) given for 26 weeks decreased visceral fat by 15%. Unlike GH therapy, tesamorelin did not induce insulin resistance; there were fewer GH-like symptoms of joint and fluid retention. GH therapy is very expensive, and the effects of GH and GHRH reverse when therapy is stopped.

DISORDERS OF GLUCOSE AND LIPID METABOLISM

Shortly after the introduction of HAART, reports of impaired fasting glucose, glucose intolerance, diabetes, and hyperlipidemia appeared in the HIV literature. Given the close temporal relationship to the introduction of PIs, studies focused on the association with PIs. However, other factors such as restoration of health, immune reconstitution, and body composition changes (including lipoatrophy and visceral hypertrophy) may also contribute to the disturbances in metabolism. To clarify these issues, several groups have given HIV antiretroviral drugs to healthy, HIV-seronegative volunteers in order to define direct drug effects. In the sections later, the results in HIV-infected subjects will be compared to those in healthy volunteers to understand the effects of drug versus disease. Metabolic effects are specific to certain drugs and not an effect of the PI class as a whole.

Insulin Resistance, Glucose Intolerance, and Diabetes

With the reports of rapid onset of diabetes after introduction of HAART with a PI, researchers looked for effects of PI on insulin resistance. Subsequent studies looked at hepatic glucose production and insulin secretion.

Several factors contribute to the development of insulin resistance in the setting of HIV. Unlike other infectious states, in which insulin resistance is common, early in the epidemic, AIDS was found to be associated with an increase in insulin sensitivity (Table 25–4). Compared with 10 healthy controls, insulin sensitivity was higher in 10 stable patients with symptomatic HIV. However, with asymptomatic HIV infection, another early study found that there was no change in insulin sensitivity compared with healthy controls. Insulin resistance is common in healthy subjects. Thus, improvement of HIV infection alone may contribute to an observed decrease in insulin sensitivity. More recent studies have found insulin resistance in ARV-naïve, HIV-infected subjects.

Body composition influences insulin sensitivity. Patients studied early in the epidemic, were thin, if not cachectic. In recent studies body weight was higher even in many ARV-naïve patients. Increased visceral fat in the abdomen has been linked to insulin resistance in subjects with or without HIV disease. Upper trunk fat is also independently, strongly associated with insulin resistance.

TABLE 25-4 Effect of HIV and AIDS status on glucose and lipid metabolism prior to the introduction of HAART.

	Insulin Resistance	Total Cholesterol	Triglyceride	VLDL	LDL	HDL
HIV	↔	↓	↑ (8%)	↑ (7%)	↓ (16%)	↓↓↓ (36%)
AIDS	↓	↓	↑↑↑↑ (99%)	↑↑↑↑ (98%)	↓↓↓ (31%)	↓↓↓ (37%)

↔, no effect; ↑ or ↓, 0%-20%; ↓↓, 20%-30%; ↓↓↓, 30%-40%; ↑↑↑↑, >40%. Percentage increases or decreases are denoted when available in the literature.

Likewise, severe lipoatrophy has been linked to insulin resistance regardless of HIV status. The lesser levels of lipoatrophy seen in most HIV-infected patients may also contribute. It should be recognized that each of these factors may contribute in an additive way to insulin resistance.

Much attention has focused on the role of individual therapies in the induction of insulin resistance. Some PIs have been reported to decrease insulin-mediated glucose disposal per unit insulin level (M/I) during the hyperinsulinemic, euglycemic clamp, a technique during which insulin is infused at a steady rate and glucose infused to maintain euglycemia, which directly measures insulin action. In a double-blind, placebo-controlled study in healthy normal volunteers, a single dose of indinavir has been shown to decrease insulin-mediated glucose disposal by 34% (Table 25-5). Indinavir for 4 weeks has also been shown to cause a 17% decrease in insulin-mediated glucose disposal as well as deterioration in glucose tolerance. A single dose of ritonavir decreased insulin sensitivity by 15%. Lopinavir/ritonavir has less of an effect on insulin sensitivity, but the magnitude of this effect is not clear (see Table 25-5). In two studies, lopinavir/ritonavir given for 4 weeks caused no change in insulin sensitivity, whereas in shorter studies, lopinavir/ritonavir given for 1 to 5 days was associated with a 13% to 24% decrease in insulin sensitivity. The study reporting a 13% decrease compared rates in the same subjects on placebo and lopinavir/ritonavir; the study reporting the 24% decrease presented pooled data from some subjects who received both placebo and drug on different occasions, some drug only and some placebo only.

Of note, not all PIs decrease insulin-mediated glucose disposal. In double-blind, placebo-controlled studies, atazanavir and amprenavir had no effect on insulin sensitivity in healthy normal volunteers (see Table 25-5). NNRTIs have not been associated with insulin resistance. In studies where PIs are replaced with NNRTIs, insulin resistance improved.

The mechanism of insulin resistance with PIs includes the acute blockade of the peripheral insulin-regulated glucose transporter (GLUT)4. In vitro studies have shown that PIs (indinavir, ritonavir, and amprenavir) selectively inhibit 2-deoxyglucose transport into 3T3-L1 adipocytes without affecting early insulin-signaling events or the translocation of intracellular GLUT4 to the surface. Indinavir has also been shown to block partially GLUT2, the glucose transporter postulated to be involved in glucose sensing in the pancreas and regulation of insulin secretion. Recently, an analog of the peptidomimetic phenylalanine moiety found in all PIs has been shown to inhibit GLUT4-induced glucose transport in vitro. Because serum levels of PIs vary, some PIs, such as amprenavir, may block GLUT4 in vitro but have no effect in patients.

Increased insulin resistance has also been found in HIV-infected subjects on NRTI therapy. However, it is unclear if the effects of NRTIs are a direct effect of the drug, reactivation of the immune system, restoration of health, or changes in body composition. When stavudine was given to healthy volunteers, there was no decrease in M/I.

In addition to peripheral insulin resistance, impairment in insulin secretion was reported in HIV patients on PI therapy. In HIV-infected subjects treated with either nelfinavir, indinavir, lopinavir/ritonavir, or saquinavir, beta cell function assessed by first-phase insulin secretion showed a 25% decrease. However, insulin secretion in the HIV-infected patients was higher than controls before PI therapy and was reduced only to that of controls after PI therapy. The HIV-infected patients had suppression of HIV RNA levels and increases in CD4 counts. More recently, healthy normal volunteers were given lopinavir/ritonavir for 4 weeks, and no effect was seen on first-phase insulin secretion. Thus, it is not clear whether currently used PIs alter insulin secretion.

Hepatic glucose production is also increased in some patients on PIs. Endogenous glucose production, comprised mostly of hepatic gluconeogenesis and glycogenolysis, is the largest determinant of fasting glucose and can be measured by tracer stable isotope technology. In studies of healthy normal volunteers, indinavir increased endogenous glucose production in the fasting state. During the hyperinsulinemic, euglycemic clamp, indinavir blunted the ability of insulin to suppress endogenous glucose production. Endogenous glucose production was not increased in rats treated with intravenous indinavir during a hyperinsulinemic, euglycemic clamp study. However, the method of stable isotope analysis was different in the rat and human studies, which may explain the discrepancy in results. In humans, full-dose ritonavir has a small detrimental effect on endogenous glucose production, while amprenavir had no effect. The effects of other PIs remain to be determined.

Adipocytokine levels have been explored in HIV infection, and they may explain some of the results in glucose metabolism. Adiponectin, a hormone secreted by adipocytes, has been shown to increase peripheral and hepatic insulin sensitivity. Adiponectin levels inversely correlate with the amount of visceral fat in

TABLE 25–5. Effect of protease inhibitors and nonnucleoside reverse transcriptase inhibitors on glucose and lipid metabolism.[a]

Drug	Fasting Glucose	Insulin[b] Resistance	EGP	Total Cholesterol	TG	LDL	HDL
Indinavir	↑ (HIV negative)	↑↑↑ (−34% M/I) (HIV negative)	↑↑ (HIV negative)	↔	↔ (HIV negative)	↔ (HIV negative) ↑ (HIV infected)[c]	↔↑ (0%-20%)
Ritonavir	↔	↑↑ (−18% M/I) (HIV negative)	↑ (HIV negative)	↑↑	↑↑↑ (150% HIV negative)	↔(HIV negative) ↑(HIV infected)[c]	↓ (0%-5%)
Lopinavir/ ritonavir	↔ (HIV negative)	↔/↑[d] (−13%-24% M/I[d]) (HIV negative)	NA	↔	↑↑ (80% HIV negative)	↔ (HIV negative) ↑ (HIV infected)[c]	↔
Tipranavir/ ritonavir	↔	NA	NA	NA	↑↑ (80% HIV infected)	NA	NA
Atazanavir/ ritonavir	↔ (HIV negative)	↔ (HIV negative)	NA	NA	↑	↔↑	↔↑ (0%-20%)
Darunavir/ ritonavir	NA	NA	NA	NA	↑	↔↑	NA
Amprenavir	↔	↔ (HIV negative)	↔ (HIV negative)	↔↑	↔↑	↑ (HIV infected)	↑ (0%-20%)
Nelfinavir	↔	↔	NA	↔↑	↔↑	↑	↑ (2%-20%)
Saquinavir	NA	NA	NA	NA	NA	NA	NA
Atazanavir	↔	↔ (HIV negative)	NA	↔/↑	↔(HIV negative)	↔(HIV negative) ↔(HIV infected)	↔/↑ (0%-20%)
Efavirenz	NA	NA	NA	↔/↑↑	↔/↑↑	↔/↑	↑↑ (15%-23%)
Nevirapine	↔	↔	NA	↑	↔	↔/↑	↑↑↑ (49%)
Stavudine	NA	NA	NA	NA	↑	NA	NA
Tenofivir	NA	NA	NA	NA	↓	↓	NA

[a]Percentage changes are provided when available from the published literature. Some effects were not precisely quantified in publications. ↑ or ↓, small; ↑↑ or ↓↓, moderate; ↑↑↑ or ↓↓↓, large change. ↔↑ signifies disagreement in the literature.

[b]Insulin resistance is expressed as M/I from euglycemic hyperinsulinemic clamp data as explained in the text. An increase in insulin resistance is reflected in a negative M/I and an upward arrow.

[c]LDL increases in patients with HIV infection who start with low LDL. There is little effect of PI in HIV-negative subjects.

[d]In HIV-negative subjects given one to five doses. No effect after 4 weeks.

EGP, endogenous glucose production; HDL, high-density lipoprotein; LDL, low-density lipoprotein; NA not available; TG, triglyceride.

HIV-negative subjects. In patients with HIV-associated peripheral lipoatrophy, adiponectin levels are reduced. Low adiponectin levels have been proposed to mediate some of the insulin resistance observed in peripheral lipoatrophy and visceral lipohypertrophy. The mechanism which reduces adiponectin levels is unknown. Some have attributed the reduction to PI therapy. In vitro studies of cultured fat cells have suggested that PI treatment suppresses adiponectin mRNA and protein expression. However, two studies in healthy normal volunteers found that in fact adiponectin levels were increased during treatment with the PIs indinavir or lopinavir/ritonavir. The discrepancy in the effect of

PIs on adiponectin levels in vitro and in humans is not well understood.

Levels of leptin, another hormone secreted by adipocytes, correlate with insulin resistance. However, some diseases with very low leptin levels also have insulin resistance. Leptin levels have been shown to be decreased in HIV patients with peripheral lipoatrophy.

Current guidelines set forth by the International AIDS Society-USA (IAS-USA) suggest measuring fasting glucose levels before and during PI therapy. In patients with risk factors for diabetes or with peripheral lipoatrophy or visceral lipohypertrophy, oral glucose tolerance testing may be warranted. Patients with preexisting abnormalities in glucose metabolism or with first-degree relatives with diabetes mellitus should consider avoiding the PIs most associated with insulin resistance; atazanavir and newer PIs may be better choices.

Treatment of PI-induced diabetes should ideally be tailored to the specific alteration in glucose metabolism. Although there are no studies of treatment of PI-induced diabetes per se, there are studies of therapy of patients who have HIV-associated lipoatrophy and lipohypertrophy who also are taking PIs. Thiazolidinediones can ameliorate peripheral insulin resistance induced by PIs. Thiazolidinediones improve insulin resistance in patients with HIV-associated lipoatrophy and lipohypertrophy. Proliferation of lipomas has been reported in one patient with HIV-associated lipoatrophy. Given the recent findings that thiazolidinediones decrease BMD and may increase fracture risk, caution is warranted in HIV-infected patients as they may be at higher risk for bone loss and fracture. Metformin decreases hepatic glucose production and peripheral insulin resistance. Metformin should be used with caution in combination with NNRTI's stavudine and didanosine, which, like metformin, are associated with increased lactic acidosis. Sulfonylureas may prove to be useful in improving insulin secretion. Due to the risk of hypoglycemia, sulfonylureas should be used with caution in treating mild PI-induced diabetes.

Other medications used to treat opportunistic infections are associated with hyperglycemia and hypoglycemia. Pentamidine causes pancreatic beta cell toxicity, acutely leading to hypoglycemia, and over the long-term, it causes diabetes mellitus. Hypoglycemia during pentamidine treatment is associated with increased length of treatment, higher cumulative doses, and renal insufficiency. Patients who develop hypoglycemia in association with pentamidine therapy are at increased long-term risk of developing diabetes mellitus. HIV-infected patients who develop diabetes mellitus following pentamidine therapy have low C peptide levels, suggesting beta cell destruction. Aerosolized pentamidine therapy has also been reported to cause hypoglycemia and diabetes mellitus. Pentamidine, trimethoprim-sulfamethoxazole, and the nucleoside analogs didanosine and zalcitabine have been associated with acute pancreatitis. Megestrol acetate, which has intrinsic glucocorticoid activity, may be associated with diabetes mellitus in HIV-infected patients, perhaps through its glucocorticoid activity, although the rate of hyperglycemia in controlled clinical trials appears to be low. GH can also cause insulin resistance, leading to hyperglycemia and diabetes. Medications used in HIV-infected patients that can affect the endocrine system are listed in Table 25–2.

Lipid Disorders

Alterations in lipid and lipoprotein profiles are common in patients infected with HIV. The observed changes can be due to a number of interrelated issues, including HIV infection itself, antiviral medications, body composition changes, and immune reconstitution. A rational approach to disturbances in lipid metabolism is to assess the status of the HIV infection, medications used to treat HIV, and presence of body composition changes (including peripheral lipoatrophy and central lipohypertrophy). The following section reviews the lipid and lipoprotein profiles individually, with an emphasis on studies prospectively measuring fasting lipid levels.

HIV infection is associated with a mild increase in triglyceride and very low density (VLDL) cholesterol levels (see Table 25–4). Triglyceride and VLDL cholesterol levels rise in association with advancing HIV disease and correlate with HIV RNA levels. The increased triglycerides are thought to be due to interferon-alpha induced decreased clearance of triglycerides and, to a lesser extent, increased VLDL production.

Several antiviral medications can increase triglyceride levels. Full-dose ritonavir can cause a two- to three-fold increase in triglyceride levels, probably by increased VLDL production (see Table 25–5). Ritonavir has been shown in vitro to inhibit the degradation of apolipoprotein B, a protein involved in the formation of VLDL particles. Other studies have suggested that activated sterol regulatory-binding proteins (SREBPs) in the liver are involved in the increase in VLDL production. Because of its ability to inhibit the hepatic enzyme CYP3A4, ritonavir is used to increase the pharmacologic doses of other PIs metabolized through the same cytochrome system. Boosting doses of ritonavir (100 mg twice daily) have also been shown to increase triglycerides, albeit to a lesser extent. The combination lopinavir/ritonavir given to healthy normal volunteers increased triglycerides and VLDL cholesterol levels by 83% and 33%, respectively. Tipranavir/ritonavir produces similar increases to those of lopinavir/ritonavir in HIV-infected individuals. Not all PIs alter triglyceride levels; in healthy normal volunteers, administration of indinavir and atazanavir resulted in no change in triglyceride levels (see Table 25–5). The data are mixed on amprenavir and nelfinavir, with some studies showing an increase in triglycerides and others finding no effect.

The NNRTI efavirenz is associated with increased triglycerides. Again, this is not a class effect as another NNRTI, nevirapine, has not been associated with alterations in triglyceride metabolism.

The effects of NRTIs on lipid metabolism have not been well studied. In some, but not all studies, stavudine use was associated with increased triglyceride levels. The most informative trial compared stavudine with tenofovir and found an increase in triglycerides in the stavudine arm, but not in the tenofovir arm. Given that all subjects got efavirenz, a likely interpretation is that there was a lipid-lowering effect of tenofovir; other data support this interpretation, as adding tenofovir to an effective ARV regimen lowers lipids.

The original clinical syndrome of HIV lipodystrophy has also been reported to be associated with increased triglyceride levels. One study found that 57% of patients with *both* peripheral lipoatrophy and central lipohypertrophy had triglyceride levels above 300 mg/dL. It has long been recognized that visceral obesity in the general population is associated with high triglycerides. However, recent data suggest that lower body fat is protective, as increased levels of lower body fat are associated with lower triglycerides in both HIV-infected patients and controls. Therefore, the loss of lower body fat in HIV-associated lipoatrophy is another reason why triglycerides are high in HIV infection. Hypertriglyceridemia is well known to be multifactorial; genes, diet, alcohol, and physical activity also play a role. In HIV infection, one can add the synergistic effects of the host response to HIV itself, treatment with ritonavir and efavirenz, and HIV-lipoatrophy to the pathogenesis.

After the introduction of HAART, a reported increase in low-density lipoprotein (LDL) cholesterol levels was largely attributed to PI therapy. Recently, it has become increasingly clear that factors other than PIs contribute to this rise in LDL cholesterol levels. In the early stages of HIV infection, LDL cholesterol levels fall (see Table 25–4). With effective therapy, LDL cholesterol levels rise in response to suppression of the infection, independent of the type of therapy. Most, but not all PIs have been associated with increases in LDL cholesterol levels, but average levels are not high. Studies in healthy normal volunteers have provided insight into the direct effects of PIs on cholesterol metabolism apart from those associated with HIV infection. Indinavir, ritonavir, lopinavir/ritonavir, and atazanavir all have no effects on LDL cholesterol levels in healthy normal volunteers (see Table 25–5). In patients with HIV infection, treatment with the NNRTI nevirapine raises LDL cholesterol levels. Studies that involve switching patients from PIs to the NNRTIs nevirapine and efavirenz found that LDL cholesterol levels do not change. Hence, the increase in LDL cholesterol seen in HIV-infected patients is not solely an effect of PI therapy, but likely represents suppression of HIV and restoration to health. Tenofovir may lower LDL levels.

HIV infection and the NNRTIs have significant effects on high-density lipoprotein (HDL) metabolism. Early in the course of HIV infection, prior to the appearance of clinically evident disease, HDL cholesterol levels decline to levels around 25 to 35 mg/dL (see Table 25–4). With advancing HIV disease, HDL cholesterol levels continue to decline to less than 50% of baseline values. The pathogenesis of these changes is not well understood. Shortly after the introduction of PIs, one cross-sectional study reported decreased HDL cholesterol levels in HIV-infected patients. However, subsequent studies have failed to show a decrease in HDL cholesterol levels in either HIV-infected patients or healthy normal volunteers. Indeed, some studies have found modest increases (13%-21%) in HDL cholesterol levels during treatment with indinavir, nelfinavir, amprenavir, and atazanavir therapy in prospective studies of HIV-infected patients. More impressive is the nearly 50% increase in HDL cholesterol seen during treatment with the NNRTI nevirapine. Efavirenz has also been shown to increase HDL cholesterol levels by 15% to 23%. When patients were switched from PIs to the NNRTIs efavirenz and nevirapine, somewhat smaller increases were seen again supporting the concept that HAART with PI induces small increases in HDL. Hence, the increase in HDL cholesterol levels is likely directly due to NNRTI therapy. In some studies, HDL levels have been reported to be lower in patients with HIV-associated lipodystrophy, but the extent to which that decrease is due to HIV is not clear. Visceral obesity and upper trunk fat are associated with lower HDL levels.

A panel of the IAS-USA has suggested guidelines for the diagnosis and treatment of dyslipidemia in HIV-infected subjects. The National Cholesterol Education Program guidelines are recommended for initiating therapy in patients infected with HIV. To monitor for dyslipidemia, a fasting lipid panel should be obtained before initiating or switching therapy. Lipid panels should be repeated 3 to 6 months after starting ARV therapy. In those patients with preexisting cardiovascular disease (CVD) or uncontrollable hyperlipidemia, switching HIV therapy should be considered if the regimen is one linked to the observed dyslipidemia and it is refractory to conventional treatment.

Hypolipidemic therapy should be tailored to the type of dyslipidemia. For patients with triglyceride levels greater than 500 mg/dL, fibrate therapy is recommended. Studies have shown that gemfibrozil and fenofibrate are effective in reducing triglyceride levels in patients infected with HIV, but those who start at high triglyceride levels do not reach normal levels. Fish oil lowers triglycerides, but raises LDL, leading to no net decrease in CVD risk. Niacin is effective and has the advantage of raising HDL levels as well as lowering triglycerides, but niacin-induced insulin resistance may be problematic in HIV-infected patients. HMG-CoA reductase inhibitors may be better second-line agents for lowering triglycerides. As with HIV-negative patients, combination pharmacologic therapy may be required to correct extremely elevated triglyceride levels.

HMG-CoA reductase inhibitors are effective, first-line agents for the treatment of hypercholesterolemia. However, there are multiple drug-drug interactions that are important in HIV-infected patients. Some statins are metabolized by Cyp3A4 which is induced or inhibited by some ARV drugs. In particular, the combination of PI and simvastatin or lovastatin should not be used. PI, especially ritonavir, which is used to boost levels of many HIV ARV drugs to therapeutic levels, inhibit Cyp3A4 which is the major metabolic pathway for simvastatin and lovastatin. Ritonavir-based regimens increase simvastatin levels by 5- to 32-fold and multiple cases of rhabdomyolysis have been reported on such combinations. Atovastatin activity increases twofold, so 80 mg atorvastatin should be avoided. Lopinavir/ritonavir increases rosuvastatin levels two- to fivefold, and tipranvir/ritonavir increases rosuvastatin levels twofold and atorvastatin levels eightfold by unknown mechanisms. If those PI combinations are used, only low doses of rosuvastatin (5 mg) and atorvastatin (10 mg) should be tried. Thus, pravastatin and fluvastatin XL are recommended as first-line statins for patients on PI- or ritonavir-based HAART.

The effects of HIV protease inhibitors on glucose and lipid metabolism are shown in Table 25–5.

HIV, Antiretroviral Therapy, and Risk of Atherosclerosis

The changes in lipid and glucose metabolism seen in HIV raise the question about whether atherosclerosis increases due to HIV or its therapies. Retrospective studies report an increased prevalence of CVD in HIV-infected patients. Some studies also found an association with ARV therapy, particularly PI therapy, in addition to traditional risk factors such as age, gender, smoking, and LDL and HDL cholesterol levels. Smoking is more prevalent in those with HIV infection versus noninfected controls. Cross-sectional studies of the intima media thickness (IMT) of the carotid and femoral arteries by ultrasound have also shown that traditional CVD risk factors provide the dominant contribution to increased plaque. However, after adjusting for traditional CVD risk factors, HIV infection is an independent risk factor for increased IMT, similar in magnitude to male sex, diabetes, and smoking.

CONCLUSION

Some of the changes in HIV infection are similar to those seen in other serious illnesses (euhormone-sick syndrome). However, many of the endocrine and metabolic changes that occur with HIV infection are unique to HIV and require careful consideration in diagnosis and treatment. In addition to the HIV disease state itself, several factors contribute to the development of these changes such as opportunistic infections, immune reconstitution, and ARV medications. As patients are living longer due to the introduction of effective ARV therapy, there is increased interest in the long-term implications of metabolic alterations such as insulin resistance, dyslipidemia, and body composition changes. Given the increased atherosclerotic disease in HIV-infected patients, more aggressive treatment of dyslipidemia is warranted.

REFERENCES

Thyroid Function

Basilio-De-Oliveira CA. Infectious and neoplastic disorders of the thyroid in AIDS patients: an autopsy study. *Braz J Infect Dis*. 2000;4:67. [PMID: 10795071]

Chen F, Day SL, Metcalfe RA, et al. Characteristics of autoimmune thyroid disease occurring as a late complication of immune reconstitution in patients with advanced human immunodeficiency virus (HIV) disease. *Medicine*. 2005;84:98. [PMID: 15758839]

Grunfeld C, Pang M, Doerrler W, et al. Indices of thyroid function and weight loss in human immunodeficiency virus infection and the acquired immunodeficiency syndrome. *Metabolism*. 1993;42:1270. [PMID: 8412739]

Madge S, Kinloch-de-Loes S, Mercey D, Johnson MA, Weller IV. No association between HIV disease and its treatment and thyroid function. *HIV Med*. 2007;8:22. [PMID: 17305928]

Nelson M, Powles T, Zeitlin A, et al. Thyroid dysfunction and relationship to antiretroviral therapy in HIV-positive individuals in the HAART era. *J Acquir Immune Defic Syndr*. 2009;50:113. [PMID: 19092451]

Adrenal Function

Chen F, Kearney T, Robinson S, Daley-Yates PT, Waldron S, Churchill DR. Cushing's syndrome and severe adrenal suppression in patients treated with ritonavir and inhaled nasal fluticasone. *Sex Transm Infect*. 1999;75:274. [PMID: 10615321]

Honour J, Schneider M, Miller R. Low adrenal androgens in men with HIV infection and the acquired immunodeficiency syndrome. *Horm Res*. 1995;44:35. [PMID: 7649525]

Mayo J, Collazos J, Martínez E, Ibarra S. Adrenal function in the human immunodeficiency virus-infected patient. *Arch Intern Med*. 2002;162:1095. [PMID: 12020177]

Norbiato G, Bevilacqua M, Vago T, Clerici M. Glucocorticoid resistance and the immune function in the immunodeficiency syndrome. *Ann NY Acad Sci*. 1998;840:835. [PMID: 9629309]

Stolarczyk R, Rubio SI, Smolyar D, Young IS, Poretsky L. Comparison of 1-micro g and 250-micro g corticotropin stimulation tests for the evaluation of adrenal function in patients with acquired immunodeficiency syndrome. *Metabolism*. 2003;52:647. [PMID: 12759899]

Bone and Mineral Metabolism

Bolland MJ, Grey AB, Gamble GD, Reid IR. Clinical review: low body weight mediates the relationship between HIV infection and low bone mineral density: a meta-analysis. *J Clin Endocrinol Metab*. 2007;92:4522. [PMID: 17925333]

Brown TT, Qaqish RB. Antiretroviral therapy and the prevalence of osteopenia and osteoporosis: a meta-analytic review. *AIDS*. 2006;20:2165. [PMID: 17086056]

Earle KE, Seneviratne T, Shaker J, Shoback D. Fanconi's syndrome in HIV+ adults: report of three cases and literature review. *J Bone Miner Res*. 2004;19:714. [PMID: 15068493]

Fakruddin JM, Laurence J. Interactions among human immunodeficiency virus (HIV)-1, interferon-gamma and receptor of activated NF-kappa B ligand (RANKL): implications for HIV pathogenesis. *Clin Exp Immunol*. 2004;137:538. [PMID: 15320903]

Hasse B, et al. Antiretroviral treatment and osteonecrosis in patients of the Swiss HIV Cohort Study: a nested case-control study. *AIDS Res Hum Retroviruses*. 2004;20:909. [PMID: 15597520]

Huang J, Meixner L, Fernandez S, McCutchan JA. A double-blinded, randomized controlled trial of zoledronate therapy for HIV-associated osteopenia and osteoporosis. *AIDS*. 2009;23:51. [PMID: 19050386]

Mondy K, Powderly WG, Claxton SA, et al. Alendronate, vitamin D, and calcium for the treatment of osteopenia/osteoporosis associated with HIV infection. *J Acquir Immune Defic Syndr*. 2005;38:426. [PMID: 15764959]

Negredo E, Martínez-López E, Paredes R, et al. Reversal of HIV-1-associated osteoporosis with once-weekly alendronate. *AIDS*. 2005;19:343. [PMID: 15718847]

Triant VA, Brown TT, Lee H, Grinspoon SK. Fracture prevalence among human immunodeficiency virus (HIV)-infected versus non-HIV-infected patients in a large U.S. healthcare system. *J Clin Endocrinol Metab*. 2008;93:3499. [PMID: 18593764]

Yombi JC, Vandercam B, Wilmes D, Dubuc JE, Vincent A, Docquier PL. Osteonecrosis of the femoral head in patients with type 1 human immunodeficiency virus infection: clinical analysis and review. *Clin Rheum*. 2009;28:815. [PMID: 19277811]

Gonadal Function

Cejtin HE, Kalinowski A, Bacchetti P, et al. Effects of human immunodeficiency virus on protracted amenorrhea and ovarian dysfunction. *Obstet Gynecol*. 2006;108:1423. [PMID: 17138776]

Conde DM, Silva ET, Amaral WN, et al. HIV, reproductive aging, and health implications in women: a literature review. *Menopause*. 2009;16:199. [PMID: 18800017]

Cu-Uvin S. Effect of the menstrual cycle on virological parameters. *J Acquir Immune Defic Syndr*. 2005;38:S33. [PMID: 15867614]

Dolan SE, Grinspoon S. Androgen deficiency and the role of testosterone administration in HIV-infected women. *J Acquir Immune Defic Syndr*. 2005;38:S48. [PMID: 15867625]

Dolan SE, Wilkie S, Aliabadi N, et al. Effects of testosterone administration in human immunodeficiency virus-infected women with low weight: a randomized placebo-controlled study. *Arch Intern Med*. 2004;164:897. [PMID: 15240605]

Greenblatt RM, Ameli N, Grant RM, Bacchetti P, Taylor RN. Impact of the ovulatory cycle on virologic and immunologic markers in HIV-infected women. *J Acquir Immune Defic Syndr*. 1999;21:293. [PMID: 10608754]

Knapp PE, Storer TW, Herbst KL, et al. Effects of a supraphysiological dose of testosterone on physical function, muscle performance, mood, and fatigue in men with HIV-associated weight loss. *Am J Physiol Endocrinol Metab*. 2008;294:E1135. [PMID: 18430965]

Sauer MV. Sperm washing techniques address the fertility needs of HIV-seropositive men: a clinical review. *Reprod Biomed Online*. 2005;10:135. [PMID: 15705311]

Watts DH. Effect of pregnancy. *J Acquir Immune Defic Syndr*. 2005;38:S36. [PMID: 15867616]

Zheng JH. Data from the United States Food and Drug Administration. *J Acquir Immune Defic Syndr*. 2005;38:S24. [PMID: 15867608]

AIDS Wasting Syndrome

Grunfeld C, Feingold KR. Metabolic disturbances and wasting in the acquired immunodeficiency syndrome. *N Engl J Med*. 1992;327:329-337. [PMID: 1620172]

Grunfeld C, Kotler DP, Dobs A, Glesby M, Bhasin S. Oxandrolone in the treatment of HIV-associated weight loss in men. *JAIDS*. 2006;41:304. [PMID: 16509313]

Kong A, Edmonds P. Testosterone therapy in HIV wasting syndrome: systematic review and meta-analysis. *Lancet Infect Dis*. 2002;2:692. [PMID: 12409050]

Mulligan K, Zackin R, Clark RA, et al. Effect of nandrolone decanoate therapy on weight and lean body mass in HIV-infected women with weight loss: a randomized, double-blind, placebo-controlled, multicenter trial. *Arch Intern Med*. 2005;165:578. [PMID: 15767536]

Schambelan M, Mulligan K, Grunfeld C, et al. Recombinant human growth hormone in patients with HIV-associated wasting. A randomized, placebo-controlled trial. Serostim Study Group. *Ann Intern Med*. 1996;125:873-882. [PMID: 8967667]

Storer TW, Woodhouse LJ, Sattler F, et al. A randomized, placebo-controlled trial of nandrolone decanoate in HIV-infected men with mild to moderate weight loss with recombinant human growth hormone as active reference treatment. *J Clin Endocrinol Metab*. 2005; 90:4474. [PMID: 15914526]

Fat Redistribution Associated with HIV

The Study of Fat Redistribution and Metabolic Change in HIV Infection (FRAM). Fat distribution in men with HIV infection. *JAIDS*. 2005;40:121. [PMID: 16186728]

The Study of Fat Redistribution and Metabolic Change in HIV Infection (FRAM). Fat distribution in women with HIV infection. *JAIDS*. 2006;42:562. [PMID: 16837863]

Falutz J, Allas S, Blot K, et al. Metabolic effects of a growth hormone-releasing factor in patients with HIV. *N Engl J Med*. 2007;357:2359. [PMID: 180757338]

Grunfeld, C., Saag, M., Cofrancesco, J., et al. Regional Adipose Tissue Measured by MRI Over Five Years in HIV-Infected and Control Subjects Indicates Persistence of HIV-Associated Lipoatrophy. *AIDS*. 2010;24:1717-26.

Kotler DP, Muurahainen N, Grunfeld C, et al. Effects of growth hormone on abnormal visceral adipose tissue accumulation and dyslipidemia in HIV-infected patients. *J Acquir Immune Defic Syndr*. 2004;32:239. [PMID: 15076238]

Martin A, Smith DE, Carr A, et al. Reversibility of lipoatrophy in HIV-infected patients 2 years after switching from a thymidine analogue to abacavir: the MITOX Extension Study. *AIDS*. 2004;18:1029. [PMID: 15096806]

Saag MS, Cahn P, Raffi F, et al. Efficacy and safety of emtricitabine vs stavudine in combination therapy in antiretroviral-naive patients: a randomized trial. *JAMA*. 2004;292:180. [PMID: 15249567]

Sutinen J. Interventions for managing antiretroviral therapy-associated lipoatrophy. *Curr Opin Infect Dis*. 2005;18:25. [PMID: 15647696]

Glucose and Lipid Metabolism

Currier J, Scherzer R, Bacchetti P, et al. Regional adipose tissue and lipid and lipoprotein levels in HIV-infected women. *J Acquir Immune Defic Syndr*. 2008;48:35. [PMID: 18197118]

Fichtenbaum CJ, Gerber JG, Rosenkranz SL, et al. Pharmacokinetic interactions between protease inhibitors and statins in HIV seronegative volunteers: ACTG Study A5047. *AIDS*. 2002;16:569. [PMID: 11873000]

Gallant JE, Staszewski S, Pozniak AL, et al. Efficacy and safety of tenofovir DF vs stavudine in combination therapy in antiretroviral-naive patients: a 3-year randomized trial. *JAMA*. 2004;292:191. [PMID: 15249568]

Grunfeld C, Rimland D, Gibert CL, et al. Association of upper trunk and visceral adipose tissue volume with insulin resistance in control and HIV-infected subjects in the FRAM Study. *JAIDS*. 2007;46:283. [PMID: 18167644]

Hertel J, Struthers H, Horj CB, Hruz PW. A structural basis for the acute effects of HIV protease inhibitors on GLUT4 intrinsic activity. *J Biol Chem*. 2004;279:55147. [PMID: 15496402]

Lee GA, Mafong DD, Noor MA, et al. HIV protease inhibitors increase adiponectin levels in HIV-negative men. *J Acquir Immune Defic Syndr*. 2004;36:645. [PMID: 15097312]

Lee GA, Seneviratne T, Noor MA, et al. The metabolic effects of lopinavir/ritonavir in HIV-negative men. *AIDS*. 2004;18:641. [PMID: 15090769]

Lee GA, Rao M, Mulligan K, et al. The effects of ritonavir and amprenavir on insulin-mediated glucose disposal in healthy volunteers: two randomized, placebo-controlled, cross-over trials. *AIDS*. 2007;21:2183. [PMID: 18090045]

Mulligan K, Grunfeld C, Tai VW, et al. Hyperlipidemia and insulin resistance are induced by protease inhibitors independent of changes in body composition in patients with HIV infection. *J Acq Immune Defic Syndr Hum Retrovirol*. 2000;23:35. [PMID: 10708054]

Noor MA, Lo JC, Mulligan K, et al. Metabolic effects of indinavir in healthy HIV-seronegative men. *AIDS*. 2001;15:F11. [PMID: 11399973]

Noor MA, Parker RA, O'Mara E, et al. The effects of HIV protease inhibitors atazanavir and lopinavir/ritonavir on insulin sensitivity in HIV-seronegative healthy adults. *AIDS* 2004;18:2137. [PMID: 15577646]

Pao VY, Lee GA, Taylor S, et al. The protease inhibitor combination lopinavir/ritonavir does not decrease insulin secretion in healthy, HIV-seronegative volunteers. *AIDS*. 2010;24:265. [PMID: 19890203]

Schambelan M, Benson CA, Carr A, et al. Management of metabolic complications associated with antiretroviral therapy for HIV-1 infection: recommendations of an International AIDS Society-USA panel. *J Acquir Immune Defic Syndr*. 2002;31:257. [PMID: 12439201]

Schwarz JM, Lee GA, Park S, et al. Indinavir increases glucose production in healthy HIV-negative men. *AIDS*. 2004;18:1852. [PMID: 15316349]

van der Valk M, Kastelein JJ, Murphy RL, et al. Nevirapine-containing antiretroviral therapy in HIV-1 infected patients results in an antiatherogenic lipid profile. *AIDS*. 2001;15:2407. [PMID: 11740191]

Woerle HJ, Mariuz PR, Meyer C, et al. Mechanisms for the deterioration in glucose tolerance associated with HIV protease inhibitor regimens. *Diabetes*. 2003;52:918. [PMID: 12663461]

Wohl D, Scherzer R, Heymsfield S, et al. The associations of regional adipose tissue with lipid and lipoprotein levels in HIV-infected men. *JAIDS*. 2008;48:44. [PMID: 18360291]

HIV, Antiretroviral Therapy, and the Risk of Atherosclerosis

Currier JS, Kendall MA, Zackin R, et al. Carotid artery intima-media thickness and HIV infection: traditional risk factors overshadow impact of protease inhibitor exposure. *AIDS*. 2005;19:927. [PMID: 15905673]

DAD Study Group, Friis-Møller N, Reiss P, Sabin CA, et al. Class of antiretroviral drugs and the risk of myocardial infarction. *N Engl J Med*. 2007;356:1723. [PMID: 17460226]

Grinspoon SK Grunfeld C, Kotler DP. Initiative to decrease cardiovascular risk and increase quality of care for patients living with HIV/AIDS: executive summary. *Circulation*. 2008;118:198. [PMID: 19455012]

Grunfeld C, Delaney JA, Wanke C, et al. Preclinical atherosclerosis due to HIV infection: carotid intima-medial thickness measurements from the FRAM study. *AIDS*. 2009;23:1841. [PMID: 19455012]

Hsue PY, Lo JC, Franklin A, et al. Progression of atherosclerosis as assessed by carotid intima-media thickness in patients with HIV infection. *Circulation*. 2004;109:1603. [PMID: 15023877]

Endocrine Surgery

Geeta Lal, MD and Orlo H. Clark, MD

ACTH	Adreno-corticotropic hormone	**PHPT**	Primary hyperparathyroidism
CASR	Calcium sensing receptor	**PTH**	Parathyroid hormone
CT	Computed tomography	**RAI**	Radioactive iodine
FBHH	Familial benign hypocalciuric hypercalcemia	**RAIU**	Radioactive iodine uptake
FNAB	Fine needle aspiration biopsy	**RFA**	Radiofrequency ablation
FU	Flouro-uracil	**TACE**	Transarterial chemoembolization
MEN	Multiple endocrine neoplasia	**SPECT**	Single photon emission computed tomography
MRI	Magnetic resonance imaging		
MTC	Medullary thyroid cancer	**TSH**	Thyroid stimulating hormone
		VIP	Vasoactive intestinal peptide
NIH	National institutes of health	**ZES**	Zollinger Ellison syndrome

INTRODUCTION

Many endocrine diseases are appropriately managed surgically. The details of clinical presentation, diagnosis, and medical management are discussed in other sections of this book. This chapter provides an overview of the principles involved in the surgical therapy for these conditions. The indications for surgical intervention, relevant procedures, and the benefits of these procedures are discussed.

THE THYROID GLAND

EMBRYOLOGY AND ANATOMY

The thyroid gland arises in the midline as an endoderm-derived pharyngeal diverticulum around the third week of gestation. The paired median thyroid anlages then descend from their origin at the base of the tongue (foramen cecum) and ultimately form a bilobed thyroid gland anterolateral to the trachea and larynx. The thyroid lobes are connected just below the cricoid cartilage by an isthmus. The connection to the foramen cecum—the thyroglossal duct—separates and is partially resorbed by the sixth week of gestation. Its distal remnant forms the pyramidal lobe. The calcitonin-producing C cells are neuroectodermal in origin, arise from the fourth branchial pouch, and are located in the superoposterior aspect of the gland.

A number of embryologic or developmental abnormalities of the thyroid have been described and are related to the absence or mutations of thyroid differentiation factors, including thyroid transcription factors 1 and 2 (TTF-1 and TTF-2) and transcription factor Pax 8. Thyroglossal duct cysts are usually found in the midline, just inferior to the hyoid bone. A lingual thyroid results from maldescent of the median thyroid anlage and is often accompanied by agenesis of other thyroid tissue. Rests of thyroid tissue may be found anywhere in the central compartment of the neck, including the anterior mediastinum. *Tongues* of thyroid tissue are often seen to extend off the lower thyroid poles, particularly in large goiters. In contrast to the above, thyroid tissue in the lateral neck lymph nodes (lateral aberrant thyroid) almost always represents metastatic thyroid cancer and is not a developmental abnormality.

The adult thyroid gland is reddish-brown in color and weighs approximately 20 g. The thyroid gland is supplied by paired superior and inferior thyroid arteries. The former arise from the external carotid artery and the latter from the thyrocervical trunk. A thyroid ima artery arises directly from the aorta or innominate artery in approximately 2% of individuals and enters the isthmus, replacing an absent inferior artery.

TABLE 26–1 Definitions of various thyroid resections.

Procedure	Description
Nodulectomy or lumpectomy	Removal of lesion with minimal surrounding tissue
Partial thyroidectomy	Removal of lesion and larger rim of normal tissue
Subtotal thyroidectomy	Bilateral removal of >50% of each lobe and an isthmusectomy
Lobectomy or hemithyroidectomy	Complete removal of a lobe and isthmus
Near-total thyroidectomy	Complete removal of one lobe and isthmus and all but 1 g (1 cm) of the contralateral lobe (tissue near ligament of Berry)
Total thyroidectomy	Complete removal of both thyroid lobes, isthmus, and pyramidal lobe

The thyroid is drained by three sets of veins: the superior, middle, and inferior thyroid veins. The first two drain into the internal jugular vein, whereas the last drains into the innominate veins. Both recurrent laryngeal nerves arise from their respective vagus nerves and enter the larynx at the level of the cricothyroid articulation, posterior to the cricothyroid muscle. The left recurrent laryngeal nerve recurs around the ligamentum arteriosum and ascends to the larynx in the tracheoesophageal groove. The right recurrent laryngeal nerve recurs around the subclavian artery and runs 1 to 2 cm lateral to the tracheoesophageal groove at the level of the clavicle and courses obliquely to the larynx. The superior laryngeal nerves also arise from corresponding vagus nerves and divide into internal and external branches. The former provides sensation to the larynx and the latter innervates the cricothyroid muscles. A description of parathyroid embryology and anatomy is presented in the next section.

Prior to discussing indications for thyroidectomy, it is prudent to clarify the definitions of various thyroid resections. A description of these terms is presented in Table 26–1. Of note, nodulectomies are rarely performed, and most surgeons agree that thyroid lobectomy constitutes a minimum resection.

Indications for Surgery

DEVELOPMENTAL THYROID ABNORMALITIES

Thyroglossal duct remnants may become symptomatic, forming cysts, abscesses, and fistulae. There is also a 1% risk of thyroid cancer development in thyroglossal duct cysts. Most are papillary carcinomas, but very rarely a squamous cell carcinoma may develop. Medullary thyroid cancers do not occur at this site.

Treatment of thyroglossal duct remnants consists of the Sistrunk procedure, which involves removal of the cyst and duct

up to the foramen cecum. Because the duct may pass anterior to, posterior to, or through the hyoid bone, it is generally recommended that the midsection of this bone is also resected in order to reduce the risk of recurrence. Surgery may also be needed for enlarged lingual thyroid tissue causing symptoms such as choking, dysphagia, airway obstruction, and hemorrhage. Prior to resection, care must be taken to determine whether the patient has any other functioning thyroid tissue, usually via a thyroid scan or ultrasound.

HYPERTHYROIDISM

Hyperthyroidism may result from increased thyroid hormone production or release of stored thyroid hormone following injury to the thyroid gland such as that seen in subacute thyroiditis. This is an important distinction, because the former group of disorders leads to increased RAIU, whereas the latter are associated with low or normal RAIU. The most common causes of hyperthyroidism are diffuse toxic goiter (Graves disease), toxic multinodular goiter (Plummer disease), or a single toxic nodule, all of which cause increased RAIU. Rarer causes of hyperthyroidism with increased radioactive iodine uptake (RAIU) include a TSH–secreting tumor and a hydatidiform mole. Causes of hyperthyroidism without increased RAIU include subacute thyroiditis, excessive ingestion of medicinal thyroid hormone, struma ovarii, and thyroid hormone–secreting metastatic thyroid cancer. These latter conditions present with the usual symptoms and signs of hyperthyroidism but lack the extrathyroidal manifestations of Graves disease such as ophthalmopathy, pretibial myxedema, and thyroid acropachy.

Diagnostic Tests

Hyperthyroidism is characterized by a suppressed TSH in the presence of elevated free T_4 levels. If free T_4 is normal, free T_3 levels should be measured because they are often elevated early in the course of disease. RAIU can be used to distinguish the various causes of hyperthyroidism. Approximately 90% of patients with Graves disease have elevated levels of thyroid-stimulating antibodies or immunoglobulins (thyroid-stimulating immunoglobulin).

Management of Hyperthyroidism

Hyperthyroidism may be treated medically with antithyroid medications, but relapse is common when the medical treatment is discontinued. Ablation of the thyroid gland with RAI is the mainstay of treatment in North America for patients over 30 years of age. A dose of 8 to 12 mCi of I-131 taken orally is generally required. However, it is associated with a prolonged latency period before effective action, a slightly increased risk of future benign and malignant thyroid tumors, hyperparathyroidism, worsening ophthalmopathy (particularly in smokers), and unavoidable hypothyroidism (3% per year after the first year, independently of dosage). Furthermore, only about 50% of patients treated with RAI are euthyroid at 6 months. It is contraindicated in pregnant women, of concern in children, and should be avoided in women wishing to become pregnant for up to 1 year after treatment.

Surgery overcomes many of the problems associated with RAI and achieves rapid control of hyperthyroidism with minimal side effects in experienced hands.

Absolute indications for thyroidectomy in patients with Graves disease include biopsy-proven suspicious or cancerous nodules, local compressive symptoms, severe reactions to antithyroid medications, reluctance to undergo RAI ablation, or fear of recurrence after RAI. Women who want to become pregnant after treatment or who develop side effects from antithyroid drugs during pregnancy are also candidates for thyroidectomy, as are children. Relative indications for thyroidectomy include patients in whom rapid control of the disease is desired; poorly compliant patients; and patients with severe ophthalmopathy, very large goiters, or low RAIU.

Preoperative Preparation

Patients are usually treated with antithyroid medications to render them euthyroid and to prevent the risk of thyroid storm. Propylthiouracil (100-200 mg 3 times daily) or methimazole (10-20 mg twice daily and then once daily) are the most commonly used medications and are continued up to the day of surgery. In patients who develop agranulocytosis as a complication of these medications, surgery should be deferred until granulocyte counts reach 1000 cells/uL. In addition, patients are also often treated with propranolol (10-40 mg 4 times daily) to control the adrenergic effects of hyperthyroidism. Relatively large doses may be necessary because of increased catabolism of the drug. Lugol solution (iodine and potassium iodide) or saturated solution of potassium iodide is also generally started about 10 days preoperatively to reduce the vascularity of the gland and decrease the risk of precipitating thyroid storm.

Extent of Surgery

The extent of surgery is controversial and depends on multiple factors. For those patients who have experienced severe complications with antithyroid drugs, those who want to eliminate the risk of recurrence, and those with coexistent carcinoma or severe ophthalmopathy, total or near-total thyroidectomy is recommended. However, total thyroidectomy results in inevitable hypothyroidism and is potentially associated with higher complication rates when compared to lesser procedures. Thus, the procedure traditionally preferred by most surgeons for treating patients with Graves disease is a subtotal thyroidectomy. This may be accomplished safely by bilateral subtotal excision or by unilateral lobectomy and isthmusectomy with subtotal contralateral resection (Hartley-Dunhill procedure). Provided an adequate remnant is left behind, the procedure provides rapid relief of thyrotoxicosis while maintaining a euthyroid state without the need for thyroid hormone. However, it is difficult to define what constitutes an adequate remnant, although most surgeons consider a 4- to 7-g remnant sufficient in adults. Rates of postoperative hypothyroidism are variable and are primarily determined by remnant size, thyroid antibody titer, and whether hypothyroidism was reported to be subclinical or overt. Remnants <4 g are associated with a >50% risk of hypothyroidism, and those >8 g are associated with recurrence rates of 15%. Subtotal

resections are associated with recurrence rates of 1.2% to 16.2%, and recurrence may take place many years after thyroidectomy. Therefore, many surgeons now consider avoidance of recurrence, rather than attainment of euthyroidism, as the goal for thyroidectomy in Graves disease. This is gradually leading to total or near-total thyroidectomy becoming the preferred operation for these patients. Patients who experience recurrence after surgery are usually treated with RAI. Patients with hyperthyroidism secondary to toxic multinodular goiter are managed similar to those with Graves disease. Subtotal thyroidectomy is generally advised, however, if no normal remnant can be left, a near-total or total thyroidectomy is recommended. Patients with a solitary toxic nodule >3 cm in size are best treated by ipsilateral lobectomy. Patients with smaller *hot* nodules may be managed by tumor enucleation or RAI ablation.

THYROIDITIS

Thyroiditis, an inflammatory disorder of the thyroid gland, may be classified as acute, subacute, or chronic. Acute suppurative thyroiditis is diagnosed by fine-needle aspiration for cytology, smear, Gram stain, and culture and treated by incision and drainage and antibiotics. Acute thyroiditis is usually self-limited. Thyroidectomy, however, is occasionally needed for clinically coexistent suspicious nodules or cancer, local compressive symptoms, or persistent infection. Recurrent acute thyroiditis is often due to a persistent pyriform sinus fistula. Resection of the entire tract is necessary to prevent recurrence. Subacute and chronic thyroiditis is usually managed medically, but surgical resection is occasionally needed for local symptoms or relapse.

GOITER (NONTOXIC)

Goiters may be diffuse, uninodular, or multinodular. Thyroidectomy is indicated for goiters enlarging despite thyroxine suppression, those causing compressive symptoms (choking, dysphagia, hoarseness, dyspnea, or a positive Pemberton sign—dilation of neck veins and facial erythema on elevation of arms), nodules deemed suspicious by ultrasound, and goiters containing biopsy-proven suspicious or cancerous nodules. Goiters with a significant substernal component (>50%) are considered a relative indication for thyroidectomy. Subtotal thyroidectomy is the preferred treatment for multinodular goiters. A total lobectomy is performed on the side with the dominant nodule, and a subtotal thyroidectomy is performed on the other. A total or near-total thyroidectomy may be performed if there is no normal thyroid tissue present.

THYROID NODULES

Approximately 4% of the North American population develops thyroid nodules. However, the incidence of clinical thyroid cancer is much lower (about 40 patients per million), thus making it imperative to determine which nodules require treatment with thyroidectomy. A thyroid nodule is more likely to be malignant if the patient has a history of therapeutic radiation to the head and neck (6.5-3000 cGy to the thyroid), a family history of thyroid cancer, Cowden syndrome, or MEN 2, and a personal history of thyroid cancer. Other features suggesting cancer include male sex, young (<20) or old (>70) age; a solitary, *cold* solid (or mixed solid-cystic), hard nodule, a nodule with microcalcifications or irregular edges on ultrasonography; the presence of ipsilateral palpable nodes or vocal cord palsy; and a fine-needle aspiration biopsy (FNAB) suspicious for cancer. Approximately 40% of individuals with a history of therapeutic radiation exposure or a family history of thyroid cancer have a thyroid cancer. The cancer is in the index nodule in 60% and in other nodules in 40% of patients.

Diagnostic Tests

Patients with thyroid nodules should be evaluated with TSH measurement and FNAB. If the biopsy suggests a follicular neoplasm, and the TSH level is suppressed or is in the low-normal range, an RAI scan should be performed to rule out a *hot* nodule.

Management

Nodules with any of the worrisome features mentioned above should be removed with—at minimum—an ipsilateral lobectomy and isthmusectomy. If FNAB confirms a malignancy, the patients should undergo thyroidectomy. Patients with benign nodules on FNAB may be treated with exogenous thyroxine. Nodules that continue to enlarge during follow-up may be re-biopsied or removed via a thyroidectomy.

THYROID CANCER

Malignant thyroid tumors include differentiated lesions (which arise from follicular cells); MTC; undifferentiated or anaplastic cancers; and other rare tumors such as lymphomas, squamous cell carcinomas, sarcomas, teratomas, plasmacytomas, paragangliomas, and metastatic thyroid cancers (from melanoma or from breast, kidney, lung, and other head and neck tumors).

1. DIFFERENTIATED THYROID CANCER

This group includes papillary, follicular variant of papillary, follicular, and Hürthle cell tumors. Hürthle cell carcinoma has been considered a subtype of follicular carcinoma by some investigators and a unique differentiated thyroid cancer of follicular cell origin by others.

The characteristics of these tumors are depicted in Table 26–2. The biologic behavior of the follicular variant of papillary thyroid cancer is similar to that of papillary carcinoma. In follicular and Hürthle cell tumors, the diagnosis of malignancy can only be made by the presence of capsular, blood vessel, or lymphatic invasion or when lymph node or distant metastases are present. Familial non-MTCs, especially if there is a family history of more than two affected relatives, have been shown to be more aggressive than their sporadic counterparts.

TABLE 26–2 Characteristics of differentiated thyroid cancers.

Feature	Papillary	Follicular	Hürthle
Frequency	80%	10%-20%	3%-5%
Age group (y)	20-30	40-50	50-60
Multicentric	85%	10%	30%
Lymph node metastases	30%-40%	10%	25%
Distant metastases	2%-14%	33%	15%
RAI uptake	70%	80%	10%
Prognosis (10-y survival)	95%	85%	65%

Surgical Treatment

Occult or minimal papillary carcinomas (<1 cm) have an excellent prognosis and are adequately treated by lobectomy. Lobectomy alone is also considered sufficient treatment for low-risk, unifocal, intrathyroidal cancers in the absence of a history of head and neck irradiation or a family history of thyroid cancer or cervical node metastases. Patients with high-risk cancers (determined by AGES, AMES, or TNM classification; Tables 26–3, 26–4, and 26–5) or bilateral cancers are best treated by total or near-total thyroidectomy. Considerable debate has existed regarding optimal treatment for low-risk differentiated thyroid cancer >1 cm.

Proponents of total thyroidectomy argued that this procedure is advantageous for several reasons: (1) RAI can be used to diagnose and treat recurrent or metastatic disease, (2) serum thyroglobulin becomes a sensitive indicator of recurrent disease, (3) the procedure eliminates the risk of growth of occult cancer in the contralateral lobe and reduces the risk of recurrence, (4) it decreases the 1% risk of progression to undifferentiated cancer, and (5) it decreases the risk of reoperation in case of central neck recurrence. On the other hand, those favoring thyroid lobectomy noted that (1) total thyroidectomy is associated with a higher complication rate and that 50% of local recurrences can be cured with surgery, (2) <5% of recurrences occur in the thyroid bed,

TABLE 26–3 AGES system of classifying high-risk patients.

Variable	Description
Age	Women older than 50 y Men older than 40 y
Grade	Poorly differentiated Fibrous stroma Insular, mucoid, and tall cell variants
Extent	Invasive into adjacent tissues or distant metastases
Size	Tumor with a maximum diameter of >4 cm

Reproduced, with permission, from Clark OH. Papillary thyroid carcinoma: rationale for total thyroidectomy. In: Clark OH, Duh Q-Y, ed. *Textbook of Endocrine Surgery.* Saunders; 1997.

TABLE 26–4 AMES system for classifying high-risk patients.

Variable	Description
Age	Men >40 y, women >50 y
Metastases	Distant metastases
Extent	Invasion of adjacent tissues
Size	>5 cm

(3) multicentricity within the thyroid is not clinically significant, and (4) the prognosis is excellent in patients with low-risk tumors undergoing lobectomy.

Retrospective data indicate that the recurrence rate for patients with low-risk differentiated thyroid cancer is 10% and that the overall mortality rate is approximately 4% at 10 to 20 years. However, among patients who have recurrences, 33% to 50% die from thyroid cancer. Recent studies involving >50,000 patients with papillary cancers demonstrated that total thyroidectomy is associated with improved recurrence and survival rates even in patients with low-risk tumors. Furthermore, the most important information regarding risk for recurrence is available only postoperatively. Revised guidelines from the American Thyroid Association also recommend near-total or total thyroidectomy for thyroid cancers >1 cm unless there are contraindications to this procedure.

TABLE 26–5 TNM[a] staging system for papillary or follicular thyroid cancer.[b]

Papillary or Follicular			
Under 45 y			
Stage I	Any T	Any N	M0
Stage II	Any T	Any N	M1
45 y and older			
Stage I	T1	N0	M0
Stage II	T2	N0	M0
Stage III	T3	N0	M0
	T1	N1a	M0
	T2	N1a	M0
	T3	N1a	M0
Stage IVA	T4a	N0	M0
	T4a	N1a	M0
	T1	N1b	M0
	T2	N1b	M0
	T3	N1b	M0
	T4a	N1b	M0
Stage IVB	T4b	Any N	M0
Stage IVC	Any T	Any N	M1

[a]TNM, tumor, node, metastasis.

[b]Separate stage groupings are recommended for papillary or follicular, medullary, and anaplastic (undifferentiated) carcinoma.

Reproduced, with permission, from American Joint Committee on Cancer. Edge SB et al, eds. *AJCC Cancer Staging Manual*. 7th ed. Springer; 2010, p. 87

It is not usually possible to distinguish follicular and Hürthle cell carcinomas from corresponding adenomas preoperatively. If there are no obvious signs of cancer at surgery (lymphadenopathy or extrathyroidal invasion), a lobectomy is performed, because more than 80% of these tumors are benign. If final pathology confirms cancer, a completion thyroidectomy is usually recommended, except in those patients with minimally invasive tumors. Total or near-total thyroidectomy may be performed at the initial operation in individuals with large (>4 cm) tumors, particularly if nodules are present bilaterally. Total or near-total thyroidectomy is also recommended if marked atypia is seen on FNA, if it is read as *suspicious for papillary carcinoma* or the patient has a family history of thyroid cancer or a personal history of head and neck irradiation.

Postoperative Treatment

Long-term cohort studies by Mazzaferri and Jhiang and others demonstrate that postoperative RAI therapy reduces recurrence rates and leads to improved survival even in patients with low-risk tumors. Several features place patients at increased risk for local recurrences or metastases. These high-risk features include certain histologic subtypes (such as tall cell, columnar, insular, solid variant, and poorly differentiated thyroid cancer), presence of intrathyroidal vascular invasion, or gross or microscopic multifocal disease. According to recently published guidelines from the American Thyroid Association, RAI is currently recommended for patients with known distant metastases, gross extrathyroidal extension of tumor (regardless of size) or tumors >4 cm even in the absence of other high-risk features. Ablation is also recommended for selected patients with 1 to 4 cm tumors with lymph node metastases or other high-risk features. In contrast, RAI is not recommended for patients with unifocal cancers <1 cm in diameter or patients with multifocal tumors (all <1 cm) without additional high-risk features. Thyroxine therapy is not only important as replacement but is given in higher doses to suppress TSH levels (to 0.1 μU/L in low-risk patients and <0.1 μU/L in high-risk patients), thus decreasing the growth stimulus for thyroid cancer cells. The need for TSH suppression must be balanced with the risks of subclinical thyrotoxicosis, such as exacerbation of angina in patients with ischemic heart disease, increased risk for atrial fibrillation, and osteoporosis in postmenopausal women.

2. MEDULLARY THYROID CANCER

This tumor comprises 7% of thyroid malignancies but accounts for approximately 17% of thyroid cancer–related deaths. It arises from the parafollicular (C cells) of the thyroid, which are derived from the neural crest and secrete calcitonin. MTC may be sporadic (75%) or occur in the setting of MEN 2A, MEN 2B, and familial non-MEN MTC. In the hereditary setting, the tumors are often bilateral and multicentric (90%). Approximately 50% of patients with MTC have nodal metastases in the central or lateral neck at presentation. All patients presenting with MTC should be screened for pheochromocytomas, hyperparathyroidism, and mutations of the *RET* proto-oncogene.

In terms of surgical therapy, pheochromocytomas should be treated prior to thyroidectomy to avoid precipitating an intraoperative hypertensive crisis. Total thyroidectomy and bilateral central compartment lymphadenectomy is the treatment of choice due to the high incidence of multicentric disease and ineffectiveness of I-131 therapy for this tumor. An ipsilateral prophylactic lateral neck dissection is recommended for patients with positive central neck nodes and for primary tumors larger that 1 cm.

3. UNDIFFERENTIATED (ANAPLASTIC) THYROID CANCER

This tumor type constitutes approximately 1% of all thyroid cancers and is the most aggressive variant. The peak incidence is in the seventh decade of life. Lymph node involvement is early and common (84%), as is local invasion into the larynx, vocal cords, recurrent laryngeal nerve, esophagus, and major vessels. Distant metastases are present in about 75% of patients. The role of surgery is usually limited to palliation of obstruction by tumor debulking and tracheostomy. In patients without advanced disease, total or near-total thyroidectomy can be performed for cure in a minority of cases. External beam radiation and chemotherapy are usually recommended.

4. THYROID LYMPHOMA AND METASTASES

Most thyroid lymphomas are of the non-Hodgkin B cell type and often develop in patients with long-standing chronic lymphocytic thyroiditis. Chemotherapy and radiotherapy form the mainstay of treatment, with thyroidectomy and node dissection reserved for palliation of airway obstruction or in patients who do not respond to the above therapies. The thyroid gland is a rare site of metastases from tumors of the kidney, lung, breast, and melanoma. In selected patients, thyroidectomy may increase survival.

5. MANAGEMENT OF LYMPH NODES IN THYROID CANCER

Clinically inapparent lymph node metastases may be present in 20% to 90% of papillary thyroid cancers, and a smaller proportion of patients with other tumor subtypes. Several retrospective studies have suggested that lymph node metastases do not have a significant effect on survival in papillary thyroid cancers. Others report that lymph node metastases are associated with poorer survival but only in patients with follicular cancers and papillary cancer >45 years of age. In patients with matted nodes or extranodal invasion, the recurrence rates are higher and the prognosis is worse.

The lymph node regions of the neck are depicted in Figure 26–1. A preoperative neck ultrasound is recommended for patients with malignant findings on FNAB to evaluate the contralateral lobe and lymph node regions. All clinically apparent disease in the central neck should be removed at the time of total thyroidectomy to improve clearance of disease from the central neck. Bilateral central node dissection (level VI) may also improve survival compared to historic controls and decrease the risk of central neck recurrence. Other studies, however, show that central neck dissections are associated with a higher risk of hypoparathyroidism and recurrent nerve injury rates without any reduction in recurrence rates. Given the above, recently published guidelines do not recommend routine prophylactic lymph node dissections but indicate that they may be performed in patients with advanced primary tumors (T_3 or T_4). Prophylactic central neck clearance should also be considered for Hürthle cell cancers which tend to be less RAI-responsive, provided they can be performed by experienced surgeons without increased rates of hypoparathyroidism and recurrent nerve injury.

Papillary and Hürthle cell cancers can also metastasize to lymph nodes in the lateral and posterior compartments (II, III, IV, and V). In patients with biopsy-proven nodal involvement, either clinically or on preoperative ultrasound examination, an ipsilateral modified radical neck dissection is recommended, particularly if these patients may fail RAI therapy based on lymph node number, size, or aggressive primary tumor histology. This procedure removes all the fibrofatty and lymph node tissue while preserving the internal jugular vein, the spinal accessory nerve, the cervical sensory nerves, and the sternocleidomastoid muscle and may reduce the risk of recurrence and subsequent mortality. Because thyroid cancers rarely metastasize to compartment I, these nodes are not routinely removed during a modified radical neck dissection.

In case of MTC, prophylactic central neck lymph node clearance is recommended because these tumors have a worse prognosis and do not take up RAI. The role of prophylactic lateral neck dissection is controversial. Ipsilateral node removal is recommended for MTCs over 1 cm in diameter (or a palpable tumor) and when the central neck nodes are involved with cancer. If ipsilateral nodes are involved, a contralateral neck dissection will also be needed. Therapeutic modified radical neck dissection is indicated for biopsy-proven metastatic disease in clinically involved nodes or those deemed suspicious by imaging.

6. RECURRENT AND METASTATIC THYROID CANCER

Thyroglobulin levels are generally undetectable in patients following total thyroidectomy and RAI ablation. Thyroglobulin levels >2 ng/mL in the absence of thyroglobulin antibodies indicates recurrent or persistent disease. These patients should be imaged with neck ultrasound, CT, or MRI. In general, surgical extirpation is recommended for patients with macronodular disease (>1 cm in diameter), followed by RAI therapy and TSH suppression. Thyroid cancers may metastasize to the lungs, bone, liver, and brain. Microscopic lung metastases in patients with papillary and follicular thyroid cancer are best treated with RAI and macroscopic disease surgically. External beam radiation is useful for unresectable, locally invasive or recurrent disease and to treat bony metastases with minimal to no RAI uptake.

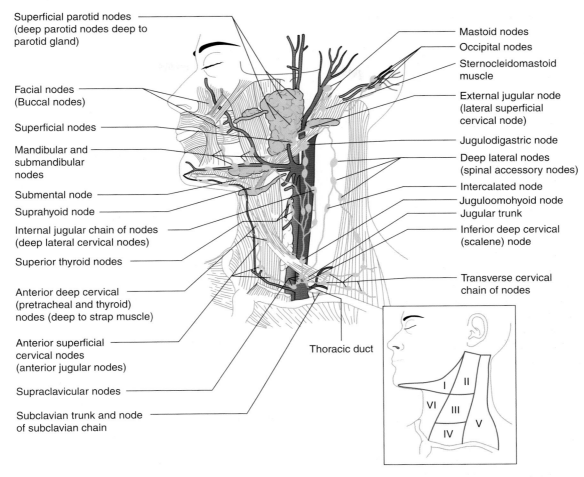

FIGURE 26–1 Lymph node regions of the neck. Level I, submandibular; level II, III, and IV, upper, middle, and lower jugular nodes; level V, posterior triangle nodes; and level VI, central compartment nodes. (Reproduced, with permission, from Roseman BJ, Clark OH. Neck mass. In: Souba W, et al, eds. *ACS Surgery—Principles and Practice*. 6th ed. WebMD Corporation; 2007.)

CONDUCT OF THYROIDECTOMY

A 4- to 5-cm incision is placed in or parallel to a natural skin crease 1 cm below the cricoid cartilage (Figure 26–2A). The subcutaneous tissue and platysma are divided, subplatysmal flaps are raised (Figure 26–2B), and the strap muscles are separated in the midline from the thyroid cartilage to the suprasternal notch. Initial dissection is begun in the midline by identification of delphian nodes and the pyramidal lobe, followed by division of the fascia just cephalad to the isthmus. The trachea is then cleared just caudal to the isthmus. The thyrothymic ligaments and the inferior thyroid veins are ligated and divided. The side with the dominant or suspicious mass is approached first. In case of a proposed lobectomy or the absence of cancer, the isthmus is divided. Tissues are swept lateral to the thyroid by blunt dissection, and the middle thyroid veins are ligated and divided (Figure 26–2C). The superior pole vessels are then individually ligated and divided low on the thyroid gland to decrease the risk of injury to the external branch of the superior laryngeal nerve (Figure 26–2D). The recurrent

laryngeal nerve and the superior parathyroid gland are identified at the level of the cricoid cartilage. Once this is accomplished, the ligament of Berry is divided (Figure 26–2E), and the thyroid is sharply dissected off the trachea. The same procedure is repeated on the other side for a total thyroidectomy.

Several approaches to minimally invasive thyroidectomy such as mini-incision procedures, video-assisted thyroidectomy and total endoscopic thyroidectomy via supraclavicular, axillary incisions, chest and breast approaches have been described (Figure 26–3). These methods are clearly feasible; however, they do require further study to determine their advantages over the more traditional open approach.

Complications of Thyroidectomy

General complications after thyroid surgery include bleeding and wound complications such as infection and keloid formation. Specific complications include injury to the recurrent laryngeal nerve (<1%), or external branch of the superior laryngeal nerve,

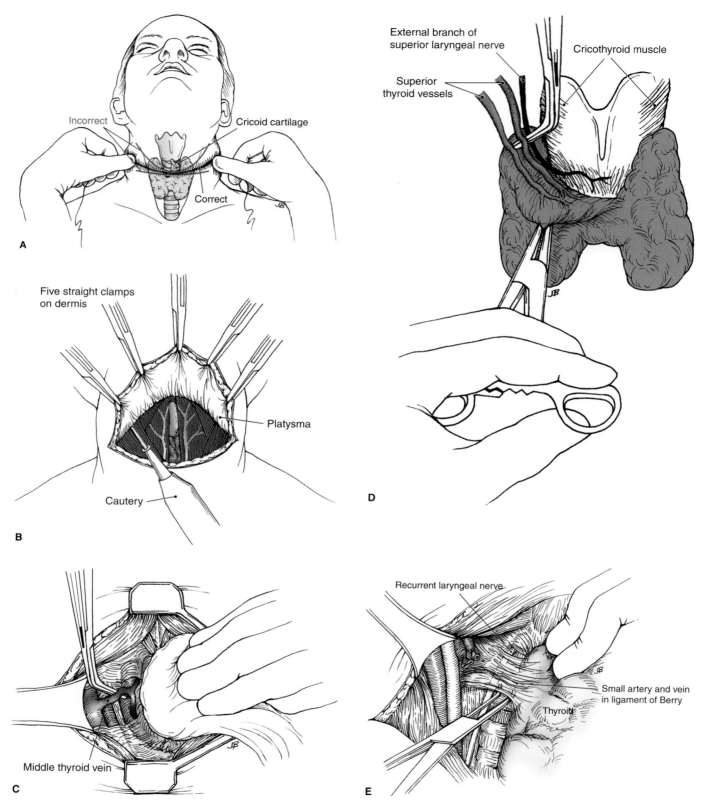

FIGURE 26–2 Conduct of thyroidectomy. **A.** Placement of incision. **B.** Raising subplatysmal flaps. **C.** Dissection of the middle thyroid vein. **D.** Dissection of superior pole vessels. **E.** Dissection at the ligament of Berry. (Reproduced, with permission, from Lal G, Clark OH. Thyroid, parathyroid, and adrenal. In: *Schwartz's Principles of Surgery*. 8th ed. McGraw-Hill; 2004.)

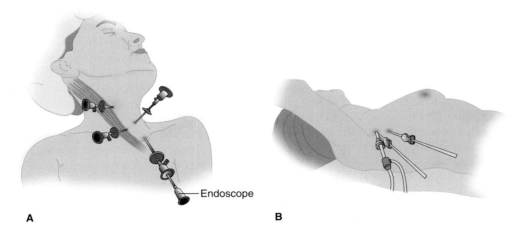

A   **B**

FIGURE 26–3 Endoscopic thyroidectomy can be performed via **(A)** cervical or **(B)** axillary incisions. (Reproduced, with permission, from Inabnet WB, Gagner M. Endoscopic thyroidectomy: supraclavicular approach and Takami HE, Ikeda Y. Endoscopic thyroidectomy via an axillary or anterior chest approach. In: Gagner M, Inabnet WB, eds. *Minimally Invasive Endocrine Surgery*. Lippincott, Williams and Wilkins; 2002).

temporary hypocalcemia (1.6%-15%), permanent hypocalcemia (<2% for total thyroidectomy), and injury to surrounding structures such as the esophagus, major vessels (carotid artery, internal jugular vein), and the cervical sympathetic trunk.

THE PARATHYROID GLAND

EMBRYOLOGY AND ANATOMY

Around the fourth week of gestation, the human embryo forms five pairs of endoderm-lined pharyngeal pouches. The inferior parathyroid glands are derived from the third branchial pouch (with the thymus), whereas the superior glands arise from the fourth branchial pouch. Most individuals have four parathyroid glands that are found as paired structures on the posterior aspect of the thyroid gland. Supernumerary glands occur in up to 22% of people. Fewer than four glands have also been reported in 3% to 5% of individuals. Approximately 85% of parathyroid glands are found within 1 cm of the point of intersection of the recurrent laryngeal nerve and the inferior thyroid artery. The superior parathyroid glands are usually dorsal to the nerve, whereas the inferior glands are usually ventral to it. The glands may also be found in several ectopic locations. Because the inferior glands migrate farther, they are more often situated in ectopic locations such as the thyrothymic ligament, thymus, carotid sheath, and anterior mediastinum. Ectopically located superior glands can be located in the tracheoesophageal groove, carotid sheath, and posterior mediastinum. Intrathyroidal glands have been reported in 0.5% to 3% of individuals and may be superior or inferior. Normal parathyroid glands are generally embedded in fat, appear golden-yellow to light-brown in color, and weigh approximately 40 to 50 mg. The blood supply to the parathyroid glands is primarily via the inferior thyroid arteries, but the superior thyroid arteries may also supply both the upper and the lower glands.

Indications for Surgery

PRIMARY HYPERPARATHYROIDISM

This disorder occurs in 1:500 women and 1:2000 men. It is the most common cause of hypercalcemia in the outpatient population, and along with malignancy-associated hypercalcemia accounts for the majority (>90%) of cases of hypercalcemia. Although most cases of PHPT are sporadic, the disorder may also be inherited as a component of MEN 1, MEN 2A, isolated familial hyperparathyroidism, and familial hyperparathyroidism with jaw tumor syndrome. PHPT is the earliest and most common manifestation of MEN 1, and 80% to 100% of patients develop hypercalcemia by age 40. MEN 1 is characterized by germline mutations in the *MENIN* gene located on chromosome 11. In contrast, hyperparathyroidism develops in only 20% of individuals with MEN 2A and is generally less severe. MEN 2A is characterized by inherited mutations in the *RET* proto-oncogene located on chromosome 10. In sporadic cases, hyperparathyroidism results from a single enlarged gland (adenoma) in 85%, multiple enlarged glands (hyperplasia) in 11%, double adenomas in 3%, and parathyroid carcinoma in 1% of patients. Parathyroid carcinoma should be suspected if patients present with a short history, profound hypercalcemia, and a palpable parathyroid gland. In heritable disorders, hyperparathyroidism is more frequently associated with multiple abnormal parathyroid glands and a higher risk of persistent or recurrent disease. Familial hyperparathyroidism with jaw tumor syndrome is associated with an increased risk of parathyroid cancer and results from germline mutations in the *HRPT2* tumor suppressor gene on chromosome 1.

The classic symptoms of PHPT include painful bones, renal stones, abdominal groans, psychic moans, and fatigue overtones. Other symptoms such as polyuria, nocturia, polydipsia, constipation, and musculoskeletal aches and pains may be present. The disorder may also be associated with hypertension, osteopenia, osteoporosis, nephrolithiasis, gout, pseudogout, peptic ulcer disease, and pancreatitis.

Diagnostic Tests

Other causes of hypercalcemia can generally be excluded by a careful history and physical examination. Laboratory tests that are helpful in making the diagnosis have been discussed in Chapter 8. PHPT is characterized by hypercalcemia (95%), hypophosphatemia (50%), hyperchloremia (30%), serum chloride to phosphate ratio ≥33 (95%), elevated 24-hour urinary calcium, and an increased or inappropriately elevated intact PTH. An elevated alkaline phosphatase level suggests bone disease (osteitis fibrosa cystica). The 24-hour urinary calcium levels may be normal or elevated. Usually, 24-hour urinary studies are obtained unless the patient has previously had documented normocalcemia, to rule out FBHH, a disorder caused by inherited mutations in the *CASR* gene and characterized by low (often <50 mg) 24-hour urinary calcium excretion. Furthermore, the serum calcium to creatinine clearance ratio is <0.01 in patients with FBHH and generally >0.02 in patients with PHPT (see Chapter 8).

Parathyroid tumors may be localized using noninvasive studies such as Tc-99m sestamibi (Figure 26–4A) and ultrasound scanning (Figure 26–4B). MRI and CT scans and invasive localizing studies, including highly selective venous catheterization for PTH, and FNAB of suspected parathyroid masses and arteriograms are generally only used in cases of recurrent or persistent hyperparathyroidism. The utility of noninvasive studies prior to initial neck exploration is controversial; however, most surgeons agree that they are indispensable for recurrent or persistent hyperparathyroidism and for using a minimally invasive approach. 99m-Technetium-labeled sestamibi has more than 80% sensitivity for the detection of hypercellular parathyroid glands, and when it is used in conjunction with SPECT, it has particular utility in identifying ectopic tumors. Neck ultrasound is often complementary and has a sensitivity of 75% in experienced centers. More recently, 4-D CT scans have shown tremendous utility in localizing parathyroid tumors with excellent anatomic detail, in addition to providing functional information. It is important to note that most localizing studies are less sensitive in the setting of multiglandular disease. Since the first use of intraoperative PTH in 1993, it has become widely used to assess the adequacy of parathyroid resection. Although preoperative localization studies and a focused surgical approach are being increasingly used, long-term outcome and cost-effectiveness studies will be necessary before recommending their routine use. However, they should be obtained if a focused parathyroidectomy is planned.

Surgical Management

A. Rationale and guidelines for parathyroidectomy
Patients with classic symptoms and metabolic complications related to PHPT are generally treated by parathyroidectomy. Whether asymptomatic patients should undergo parathyroidectomy is controversial. One aspect of the controversy is the fact that there is no consensus on what constitutes an asymptomatic patient. At the 1990 NIH. Consensus Conference, asymptomatic PHPT was defined as, "the absence of common symptoms and signs of PHPT, including no bone, renal, gastrointestinal or neuromuscular disorders." Nonoperative management was recommended in this group of patients with calcium levels ≤12 mg/dL, based on several observational studies that suggested stability with respect to serum calcium, kidney stones, bone loss, and renal function with time. Parathyroidectomy was recommended for asymptomatic patients <50 years of age and in certain other patients, as outlined in Table 26–6.

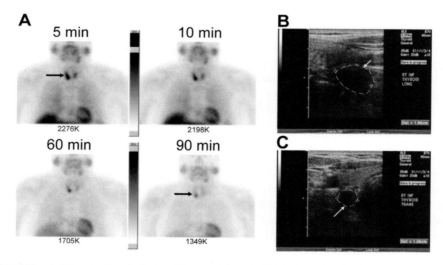

FIGURE 26–4 Parathyroid localization studies. **A.** Sestamibi scan with early (5-10 minute) and delayed (60-90 minute) images showing persistent uptake inferior to the right thyroid lobe (black arrow), suggesting a hypercellular parathyroid gland in this location. **B.** Neck ultrasound (longitudinal view). **C.** Neck ultrasound (transverse view) also showing a probable right inferior parathyroid adenoma (white arrow), which is hypoechoic compared to thyroid tissue.

TABLE 26–6 NIH Consensus Conference and International Workshop indications for surgery in patients with asymptomatic primary hyperparathyroidism.

Criterion	1990	2002	2008
Serum calcium	>12 mg/dL	>1 mg/dL above upper limit of normal	>1 mg/dL above upper limit of normal
Urinary calcium	>400 mg/24 h	>400 mg/24 h	Not indicated
Creatinine clearance	<30% of normal age-matched controls in the absence of another identifiable cause	Reduced by 30% of normal	Reduced to <60 mL/min
Bone mineral density	<2 SD below age- and sex-matched normal value (Z-score)	<2.5 SD below peak bone mass (T-score) at any site	T-score <−2.5 at any site and/or previous fracture
Age	<50 y	<50 y	<50 y

A second NIH Conference was held in 2002 to reevaluate the criteria for parathyroidectomy in asymptomatic patients. The guidelines issued were similar to the previous recommendations except for the following changes. Parathyroidectomy was recommended in the following cases: for milder elevations in serum calcium (ie, if the serum calcium was 1 mg/dL above reported normal range) and if the bone mineral density at any site (forearm, spine, or hip) was more than 2.5 standard deviations below that of gender-matched peak bone mineral density (T score, rather than Z score of <−2.5). The panel recommended caution in using neuropsychological abnormalities, cardiovascular disease, menopause, gastrointestinal symptoms, and serum or urine indices of increased bone turnover as sole indications for parathyroidectomy. These recommendations were revised again in 2008, with elevated urinary calcium excretion (in the absence of nephrolithiasis) no longer being a criterion for surgery. Recommendations from all these conferences are summarized in Table 26–6. It is critical to emphasize that the level of evidence supporting the recommendations is not that of randomized controlled trials.

However, recent investigations suggest that true asymptomatic hyperparathyroidism may be rare. Patients without classic symptoms often present with weakness, fatigue, polydipsia, polyuria, nocturia, bone and joint pain, constipation, and other symptoms. These patients also score lower than healthy controls when assessed by multidimensional health assessment tools such as the SF-36 and other more specific questionnaires. Furthermore, parathyroidectomy not only often improves the classic, but also the nonspecific symptoms described above. In addition, parathyroidectomy has been associated with improved survival (in both asymptomatic and symptomatic patients), is more cost-effective than lifelong follow-up, and is successful in 95% of patients with a minimal (<1%) complication rate. Although bisphosphonates and calcimimetics show promise in the treatment of patients with PHPT, further studies are needed prior to recommending their routine use in this setting. Therefore, most clinicians recommend parathyroidectomy (by surgeons experienced in the procedure) for patients with PHPT, except in those patients where operative risks are prohibitively high.

B. Conduct of parathyroidectomy Issues to consider before deciding on the optimal treatment approach are whether one is dealing with sporadic or familial disease and whether it is the initial operation or reexploration. The presence of concurrent thyroid pathology needing surgical treatment must also be considered. The positioning, incision, and dissection are as described previously for thyroidectomy. A bloodless field is crucial to enable identification of parathyroid glands. The middle thyroid veins are ligated and divided to allow medial retraction of the thyroid lobe. The space between the carotid sheath and thyroid is then opened by sharp and blunt dissection, from the level of the cricoid to the thymus, and the recurrent laryngeal nerve is identified. Most parathyroid glands are found within 1 cm of the junction of the nerve and inferior thyroid artery—the superior glands lie dorsal and the lower glands more ventral or anterior to the nerve. Because parathyroid glands are often embedded in fat, any fat lobule at typical parathyroid locations should be explored.

C. Bilateral versus unilateral approach Traditionally, all four parathyroid glands have been explored without preoperative localizing studies, with a 95% success rate in the hands of an experienced surgeon. Investigators in favor of unilateral exploration have suggested decreased recurrent laryngeal nerve injury, less postoperative hypocalcemia, shorter operative time, and early discharge as advantages of this approach. Potential disadvantages of unilateral exploration include the risk of missing multiple abnormal or ectopic parathyroid glands.

More surgeons today are using a unilateral or focal approach directed by localizing studies with or without intraoperative gamma probe or intraoperative PTH measurements. We have found that when two localizing studies—Tc-99m sestamibi and ultrasound—identify the same solitary parathyroid gland in patients with sporadic PHPT, this was the only abnormal parathyroid gland in 95% of patients. In patients with sporadic PHPT and positive preoperative localization studies, our current approach is to recommend focused parathyroidectomy via a 2.5-cm incision with intraoperative PTH measurement. If the PTH level falls more than 50% within 10 minutes after removal of an abnormal parathyroid gland, the procedure is terminated. If the level does not fall, a PTH measurement is repeated in another 10 minutes, because it may fall slowly in some patients. A bilateral approach is needed in patients with known familial disease, with negative or equivocal localization tests, with secondary or tertiary HPT, or a history of lithium treatment. If parathyroid cancer is suspected intraoperatively, it is resected with the ipsilateral thyroid lobe and regional lymph nodes.

D. Subtotal parathyroidectomy versus total parathyroidectomy with autotransplantation Either subtotal (generally resection of 3½ glands) or total parathyroidectomy with primary parathyroid autotransplantation may be performed in patients with multiglandular disease. In the latter technique, 12 to 20 small fragments (1 × 1 mm) of parathyroid tissue are placed into multiple pockets in the forearm muscle of the nondominant arm. The site is marked with silk sutures and is easily accessible under local anesthesia should the patient develop recurrent hypercalcemia. The recurrence rates for hyperparathyroidism appear to be similar after subtotal or total parathyroidectomy. However, a 5% failure rate has been reported after autotransplantation of parathyroid tissue. Therefore, subtotal parathyroidectomy is preferred. The most normal gland is biopsied first, leaving a 50-mg remnant (the size of a normal parathyroid gland); if it appears viable, the remaining glands are excised. Patients undergoing either of these procedures should have tissue cryopreserved, if possible. Parathyroid glands should not be routinely biopsied at exploration but rather biopsy should be used to confirm parathyroid tissue or help determine if the gland is normal or abnormal. As with thyroid surgery, video-assisted and endoscopic axillary approaches are feasible, but clear benefits compared with the open approach await long-term multicenter studies.

PERSISTENT AND RECURRENT PRIMARY HYPERPARATHYROIDISM

Persistent hypercalcemia occurs after about 5% to 10% of explorations. Recurrent hypercalcemia is rare except in patients with familial disease and occurs after an intervening period (>6 months) of normocalcemia. The most common reasons for persistent or recurrent hyperparathyroidism are a missed gland in normal or ectopic location, unrecognized hyperplasia, supernumerary glands, subtotal tumor resection, parathyroid carcinoma, or parathyromatosis (usually due to implantation of cells due to spillage at the initial procedure). The most common sites of ectopic glands in patients with recurrent or persistent PHPT (Figure 26–5) are paraesophageal (28%), mediastinal (26%), intrathymic (24%), intrathyroidal (11%), carotid sheath (9%), and undescended (high cervical 2%). The management of these patients involves confirmation of the diagnosis—in particular, exclusion of FBHH; review of original operative notes and pathology reports; and localization studies, which are absolutely essential in this group of patients. Preoperative evaluation of the vocal cords is routinely performed. The issue of reexploration in mildly symptomatic patients is controversial. The neck is usually reexplored first, and median sternotomy may be needed in 1% to 2% of patients.

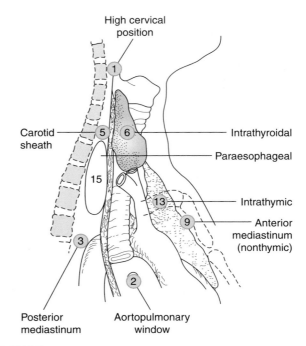

FIGURE 26–5 Ectopic locations of parathyroid tumors found at reoperation after an initial failed neck exploration. The numbers indicate the actual number of glands found at each location (*n* = 54). (Reproduced, with permission, from Shen W, et al. Reoperation for persistent or recurrent primary hyperparathyroidism. *Arch Surg.* 1996;131:861. Copyright 1996 by the American Medical Association.)

Cryopreservation should be performed routinely and autotransplantation selectively. Reexploration by an experienced surgeon is successful in more than 90% of patients, but reoperative parathyroidectomy is generally associated with more complications than an initial operation.

SECONDARY HYPERPARATHYROIDISM

This disorder occurs most often in individuals with end-stage renal failure but may also occur in other conditions resulting in hypocalcemia, such as vitamin D deficiency, idiopathic hypercalciuria, and long-term lithium therapy.

Indications for surgery include serum calcium and phosphate product more than 70, renal osteodystrophy with or without bone pain, severe pruritus, ectopic soft tissue calcifications and tumoral calcinosis, serum calcium >11 mg/dL with markedly elevated PTH, and calciphylaxis.

These patients should undergo dialysis the day prior to surgery to correct electrolyte (specifically potassium) abnormalities. Patients with this disorder require bilateral exploration and either subtotal parathyroidectomy, leaving a 50 to 60 mg histologically confirmed, well-vascularized remnant of hyperplastic parathyroid distant from the recurrent laryngeal nerve; or total parathyroidectomy with autotransplantation of a similar amount of tissue.

Upper thymectomy is usually performed in these patients, because up to 15% of patients have a fifth hyperplastic gland.

SPECIAL CONSIDERATION: FAMILIAL HYPERPARATHYROIDISM

Patients from MEN 1 families should have PHPT treated before coexisting gastrinoma. All glands should be identified, ectopic glands should be sought in the neck and upper mediastinum, and bilateral cervical thymectomy should be routinely performed due to the occurrence of thymic carcinoids. A subtotal parathyroidectomy (preferred by authors) or total parathyroidectomy, as described above, can be performed. MEN 2A patients should undergo screening for the presence of a pheochromocytoma and *RET* mutation prior to thyroid or parathyroid surgery. Because the parathyroids are at risk during thyroidectomy and central neck node dissection, and hyperparathyroidism is less virulent in these patients, only obviously enlarged glands should be removed. Normal-appearing glands should be marked and removed abnormal parathyroid tissue cryopreserved.

COMPLICATIONS OF PARATHYROID SURGERY

General complications are similar to those associated with thyroidectomy. Specific complications include recurrent laryngeal nerve injury, hypomagnesemia, and hypocalcemia. The latter may arise due to suppressed function of the remaining glands after removal of an adenoma; injury to the parathyroid remnant; or bone hunger, which is the influx of calcium and phosphorus into metabolically active bones. Bone hunger can be predicted based on the severity of bone disease and the preoperative alkaline phosphatase level and is generally more severe in individuals with secondary hyperparathyroidism. Hypocalcemia can be treated with oral calcium and vitamin D supplementation (calcitriol, 0.25-0.5 µg twice daily). Intravenous calcium is seldom required but may be necessary in severely symptomatic patients.

THE ADRENAL (SUPRARENAL) GLAND

EMBRYOLOGY AND ANATOMY

The adrenals are paired structures located superior to the kidneys. The adrenal is divided into an outer cortex and an inner medulla. The cortex originates from mesodermal tissue near the gonads on the adrenogenital ridge at approximately the fifth week of gestation. Adrenocortical tissue can thus be found in the ovaries, spermatic cord, and testes. The adrenal medulla originates from the neural crest, which is ectodermal in origin.

Each adrenal is supplied by three sets of arteries: the superior adrenal (from the inferior phrenic artery), the middle adrenal (from the aorta), and the inferior adrenal (from the renal artery).

These vessels branch into as many as 50 arterioles. The left adrenal vein empties into the ipsilateral renal vein, whereas the right adrenal vein drains into the inferior vena cava (see Chapter 9).

Indications for Surgery

PRIMARY HYPERALDOSTERONISM

This disorder accounts for 1% of hypertensive patients and results from an adrenal adenoma (Conn syndrome, 75%), adrenal hyperplasia (24%), or adrenocortical cancer (1%). Glucocorticoid-suppressible hyperaldosteronism is another rare cause of hyperaldosteronism. Patients with primary hyperaldosteronism typically present with hypertension (long-standing and difficult to control despite multiple medications), muscle weakness, polydipsia, polyuria, headaches, and fatigue.

Diagnostic Tests

The diagnosis must be suspected in any hypertensive patient with spontaneous hypokalemia (<3.2 mmol/L) or hypokalemia while on diuretic therapy (despite potassium supplementation). Other abnormalities include hypernatremia, alkalosis, and hypochloremia. Elevated plasma and urine aldosterone levels with suppressed plasma renin activity levels confirm the diagnosis. Plasma aldosterone concentration to plasma renin activity ratios of >1:25 to 30 are highly suggestive of the diagnosis. The diagnosis can be confirmed by documenting failure to suppress plasma aldosterone with oral or intravenous salt loading. Once the biochemical diagnosis is confirmed, it is important to distinguish between patients with a unilateral adenoma from those with hyperplasia because unilateral adrenalectomy is virtually always curative for the former (see Chapter 9 for details). Tumors can be localized with CT scans, MRI, iodocholesterol scans, or selective venous catheterization for aldosterone and cortisol. A unilateral 0.5- to 2-cm adrenal tumor with a normal-appearing contralateral gland essentially confirms an aldosteronoma if the biochemical and clinical profiles are appropriate.

Surgical Management

Patients are prepared for surgery with potassium repletion, sodium restriction, and treatment with spironolactone or eplerenone (aldosterone antagonists). Amiloride or triamterene (potassium-sparing diuretics) as well as other effective antihypertensive medications, including calcium channel blockers and angiotensin-converting enzyme inhibitors, can also be used. Patients with a unilateral hyperfunctioning tumor are best managed with a laparoscopic adrenalectomy. Postoperatively, patients may require saline infusions, fludrocortisone (50-100 µg/d), or, rarely, glucocorticoids if they develop Addison disease. Adrenalectomy improves blood pressure in approximately 80% of patients and leads to resolution of hypokalemia in most. Only 20% to 30% of patients with bilateral hyperplasia benefit from adrenalectomy. Surgical candidates can be selected based on bilateral adrenal vein sampling for aldosterone and cortisol. A unilateral gradient suggests a potential benefit from surgical intervention. The remaining patients are best managed by medical therapy with spironolactone, triamterene, or amiloride.

HYPERCORTISOLISM

Cushing syndrome refers to a complex of symptoms and physical signs resulting from cortisol hypersecretion, independent of etiology. Causes of Cushing syndrome include ACTH–secreting pituitary tumor leading to bilateral adrenal hyperplasia (Cushing disease 70%); primary adrenal adenoma, hyperplasia, or carcinoma (20%); ectopic ACTH-secreting tumors (small cell lung, pancreatic, thyroid, thymic, and other cancers—10%); or the exogenous administration of steroids. Patients present with weight gain, muscular weakness, polyuria, emotional lability, moon facies, acne, hirsutism, central obesity, hypertension, diabetes mellitus, and virilization.

Diagnostic Tests

Diagnostic tests in patients with Cushing syndrome are directed toward confirming the diagnosis and determining the etiology of the disorder. A low-dose (1-mg) overnight dexamethasone suppression test is usually performed. Patients with Cushing syndrome do not generally suppress cortisol levels to <3 ug/dL, although this threshold is controversial. In patients with a negative test but high clinical suspicion, the classic dexamethasone suppression test (2 mg over 48 hours) or a 24-hour urinary free cortisol measurement is performed. Salivary cortisol measurements are increasingly being used at some centers. Once hypercortisolism is confirmed, the plasma ACTH level, if suppressed, indicates a primary adrenal etiology for the disorder. High-dose (8-mg) dexamethasone suppression tests may be performed to delineate the source of increased cortisol secretion (see Chapter 9 for details). Adrenal tumors are localized using CT, MRI, or iodocholesterol scans and pituitary tumors by MRI scanning and selective venous catheterization of petrosal veins after corticotropin-releasing factor stimulation.

Surgical Management

Cushing disease is treated with trans-sphenoidal hypophysectomy and microsurgical excision of the pituitary adenoma. Irradiation may also be used, but the response is delayed, and the treatment often results in panhypopituitarism. Unilateral laparoscopic adrenalectomy is the treatment of choice in patients with adrenal adenomas, whereas open adrenalectomy is recommended for carcinomas. Bilateral laparoscopic adrenalectomy is used to treat patients with Cushing disease who fail to respond to radiation or hypophysectomy and selected patients with Cushing syndrome secondary to ectopic ACTH production. Symptoms of Cushing syndrome can be treated with medications that inhibit steroid production (ketoconazole, metyrapone, aminoglutethimide).

Preoperatively, electrolyte abnormalities are corrected, and all patients are given exogenous steroids (hydrocortisone, 100 mg intravenously every 8 hours). After unilateral adrenalectomy, steroids are tapered off over months. After bilateral surgery, lifelong treatment with hydrocortisone is necessary. Fludrocortisone is sometimes needed, and steroid supplementation must be increased in situations of stress. The prognosis after adrenalectomy for adenoma is excellent. After bilateral adrenalectomy, approximately 20% of patients develop Nelson syndrome (hyperpigmentation, headaches, exophthalmos, and blindness) from continuing growth of the pituitary tumor.

ADRENAL CORTICAL CARCINOMA

This rare neoplasm is slightly more common in women than in men and has a bimodal age distribution, occurring more frequently in children under 5 years of age and in adults in their forties and fifties. Approximately 50% of these tumors are nonfunctioning. The remaining secrete cortisol (30%), androgens (20%), estrogens (10%), aldosterone (2%), or multiple hormones (35%). Most adrenocortical cancers are sporadic, but they can also occur in the setting of the Li-Fraumeni syndrome (*p53*) and MEN 1 (*MENIN*). Adrenocortical cancers are often characterized by the rapid onset of Cushing syndrome with virilizing features. Nonfunctioning tumors usually present with an enlarging abdominal mass and abdominal pain or, less commonly, with weight loss, hematuria, varicocele, and dyspnea.

Diagnosis

The biochemical workup of a unilateral adrenal mass is outlined in the section on adrenal incidentaloma (see Chapter 9). CT or MRI scans are commonly employed to evaluate the size and invasiveness of the mass. The size of the mass remains the single most reliable indicator of malignancy. Carcinomas are more likely to be present in lesions over 6 cm in diameter. Studies based on SEER registry data show that the sensitivity, specificity, and likelihood ratio of tumor size in predicting malignancy as 96%, 51%, and 2, respectively, for tumors ≥4 cm; and 90%, 78%, and 4.1, respectively, for tumors ≥6 cm. Other features suggesting malignancy on CT include irregular shape and margins, heterogeneity, and hemorrhage. On MRI, carcinomas have a moderate signal intensity on T2-weighted image (adrenal tumor to liver ratio 1.2-2.8). FNAB is usually recommended for patients with an isolated adrenal mass and a history of carcinoma of the lung, breast, stomach, kidney, colon, melanoma, or lymphoma and in those with symptoms and signs of underlying malignancy. FNAB is generally not recommended when a primary adrenal carcinoma is suspected as the diagnosis cannot be reliably made via this test and has the potential to seed the biopsy tract. Care must be taken to exclude pheochromocytoma prior to biopsy to avoid precipitating a hypertensive crisis (see Chapters 9 and 11).

Surgical Treatment

Complete surgical excision offers the only chance of prolonged survival or cure. Transabdominal adrenalectomy with en bloc excision of contiguously involved structures (liver, kidney, spleen, or pancreas) is usually recommended. A thoracoabdominal approach may also be used for large (>10 cm) right-sided tumors.

Laparoscopic adrenalectomy is not usually recommended for suspected adrenal cancers. The adrenolytic agent mitotane and other antitumor drugs such as etoposide, cisplatin, and doxorubicin have also been used with partial success for metastatic tumors. Five-year actuarial survival rates of 32% to 48% have been reported in patients who underwent complete resection. Features predicting poor survival include tumor size over 12 cm, six or more mitoses per high-power field, intratumoral hemorrhage, local invasion, and distant metastases.

SEX STEROID EXCESS

Virilization and feminization can be caused by many disorders, including congenital adrenal hyperplasia, adrenal adenomas or carcinomas, ovarian or testicular tumors, hypothalamic or pituitary disease, placental disorders, and exogenous sex steroid administration. Several different variants of congenital adrenal hyperplasia occur, each caused by a specific enzyme defect. Adrenal virilization occurring postnatally usually results from an adenoma or carcinoma. Virilization presents in females with hirsutism, clitoromegaly, alopecia, breast atrophy, and oligomenorrhea. In males, feminizing tumors lead to gynecomastia and testicular atrophy.

Diagnostic Tests

Karyotype analysis to rule out sex chromosome anomalies such as Klinefelter syndrome and determinations of either plasma and or urinary steroid metabolites are needed to establish the diagnosis of a particular enzyme deficiency as discussed in Chapters 9 and 14. The dexamethasone suppression test (2-4 mg/d in divided doses 4 times daily for 7 days) can be used to distinguish congenital adrenal hyperplasia from neoplasia. CT, MRI, and iodocholesterol scans are used to localize the tumors.

Surgical Management

Congenital adrenal hyperplasia is managed medically not surgically. Adrenalectomy is reserved for treatment of adrenal steroid excess caused by an adenoma or carcinoma. The perioperative management is similar to that for patients with Cushing syndrome. Patients with adrenal carcinomas have a poor prognosis.

PHEOCHROMOCYTOMA

This catecholamine-secreting tumor of the adrenal medulla and extra-adrenal chromaffin tissue accounts for 0.1% to 0.2% of all patients with hypertension. It is often called **the 10% tumor** because 10% are bilateral, 10% are malignant, 10% occur in children, 10% are extra-adrenal, and 10% are familial (occurring in association with MEN 2A, MEN 2B, von Hippel-Lindau syndrome, neurofibromatosis, other neurocutaneous syndromes, and the familial paraganglioma and pheochromocytoma syndromes caused by mutations in the succinyl dehydrogenase family of genes [*SDHB, SDHC and SDHD*]) (see Chapter 11).

Headache, palpitations, and diaphoresis constitute the classic triad of pheochromocytoma. Nonspecific symptoms include anxiety, tremulousness, severe headaches, paresthesias, flushing, chest pain, shortness of breath, abdominal pain, nausea, and vomiting as well as others. The most common clinical sign is hypertension, which may be sustained or episodic.

Diagnostic Tests

These are performed in a nonstressed patient. Twenty-four-hour urine collections are tested for catecholamines (epinephrine, norepinephrine, dopamine) and their metabolites (metanephrines and normetanephrines). Plasma metanephrines, catecholamines, and chromogranin A levels are also used to make the diagnosis. Provocative tests such as glucagon infusion and clonidine suppression are rarely necessary. Radiologic investigations such as CT or MRI scans, and metaiodobenzylguanidine scans are used to localize the tumors and assess for possible extra-adrenal tumors (see Chapter 11 for details). Of note, extra-adrenal sites lack phenylethanolamine-*N*-methyltransferase, and hence, secrete primarily norepinephrine rather than epinephrine.

Surgical Treatment

Adrenalectomy is the treatment of choice and can safely be performed laparoscopically. Preoperative preparation typically consists of treatment with an alpha-adrenergic blocker such as phenoxybenzamine (10-40 mg 4 times daily; maximum: 300 mg/d) for at least 7 days preoperatively. Beta blockers such as propranolol (5-40 mg 4 times daily) are added in patients who have persistent tachycardia and arrhythmias but only after adequate alpha blockade has been established in order to avoid the effects of unopposed alpha stimulation (ie, hypertensive crisis and congestive heart failure). Patients should also be volume repleted to avoid postoperative hypotension, which ensues with the loss of vasoconstriction after tumor removal. Nitroprusside is the drug of choice for intraoperative hypertension. After surgery, 95% of patients with paroxysmal hypertension and 65% with sustained hypertension become normotensive. Patients with malignant pheochromocytoma, defined by invasion into surrounding structures or presence of distant metastases, have a poor prognosis. Although risk of malignancy increases with size for all pheochromocytomas, size does not seem to reliably predict malignancy in pheochromocytomas. The risk of malignant tumors is also increased in patients with germline *SDHB* mutations.

ADRENAL INCIDENTALOMA

The term **incidentaloma** is used to denote an adrenal mass discovered during imaging done for other reasons. Adrenal masses have been identified in up to 8% of individuals in autopsy series and in 4.4% of those undergoing abdominal CT scans. The widespread use of ultrasound, CT, and MRI scans over the past two decades has led to an appreciable increase in the number of these lesions identified. Most of these lesions are benign nonfunctioning adenomas. The differential diagnosis of these lesions is summarized in Table 26–7.

TABLE 26–7 Differential diagnosis of an adrenal incidentaloma.

Benign	Malignant
Adrenal cortex Functioning adenoma Nonfunctioning adenoma	Adrenocortical cancer
Adrenal medulla Pheochromocytoma	Malignant pheochromocytoma
Others Cysts Myelolipomas Ganglioneuroma Hematoma	Metastasis

Diagnosis

The workup is used to discern which lesions are functional or malignant and thus, warrant adrenalectomy. Asymptomatic patients with obvious cysts, hemorrhage, myelolipomas, or diffuse metastatic disease do not mandate further testing. All other patients should undergo biochemical testing for hormonally active tumors. At a minimum, this includes serum electrolytes; low-dose (1-mg) dexamethasone suppression testing; and a 24-hour urine collection for catecholamines, metanephrines, and 17-ketosteroids; however, the issue of which tests to order is controversial. Confirmatory tests can be performed based on the results of these screening tests. It is extremely important to identify patients with subclinical Cushing syndrome. Functional tumors and nonfunctional masses over 4 cm (in patients who have an acceptable operative risk) are treated by laparoscopic adrenalectomy, whereas heterogeneous, irregular, or enlarging tumors are treated by open or laparoscopic adrenalectomy. FNAB should be performed only in patients with a history of carcinoma and a suspected isolated adrenal metastasis, or if there is a question as to whether the tumor is of adrenal origin (see Chapter 9 for details). Care must be taken to exclude pheochromocytoma prior to biopsy to avoid precipitating a hypertensive crisis.

Treatment

Laparoscopic adrenalectomy has become the procedure of choice for most of the lesions described above except when malignancy is likely or suspected. Patients with nonfunctioning homogeneous lesions <4 cm in diameter should be followed with serial examinations and CT or MRI scans at 3 to 12 months. Adrenalectomy is indicated for any lesion that grows during the observation period.

TECHNIQUE OF ADRENALECTOMY

There are no randomized controlled trials comparing laparoscopic and open adrenalectomies. However, several retrospective studies have shown that the laparoscopic technique is safe and associated with less postoperative pain, shorter mean hospital stay, lower morbidity, and more rapid complete recovery. Laparoscopic adrenalectomy has become the procedure of choice for most adrenal lesions, and the indications are similar to those for open procedures.

Laparoscopic adrenalectomy is contraindicated in patients with a known adrenocortical cancer or coagulopathy. Two approaches have been described: transperitoneal (lateral and anterior) and posterior retroperitoneal. The former provides a conventional view of the anatomy, and the anterior approach allows for bilateral procedures without repositioning the patient. The posterior approach may be preferable in reoperative cases and obese patients but provides a limited working space. The lateral transperitoneal approach is described in the next paragraph.

The patient is placed in the lateral decubitus position, with the table flexed to open the space between the lower rib cage and the iliac crest. Pneumoperitoneum is created by insufflating carbon dioxide gas and four 10-mm trocars are placed between the midclavicular line medially and the anterior axillary line laterally (Figure 26–6A), approximately two finger-breadths below the costal margin. A 30-degree laparoscope inserted via the midclavicular port is used to aid the dissection, which is carried out via atraumatic instruments inserted via the two most lateral ports. In general, the dissection of the adrenal usually begins superomedially and then proceeds inferiorly in a clockwise fashion (Figure 26–6B and Figure 26–6C). The adrenal gland is dissected from surrounding tissue using an electrocautery or an ultrasonic scalpel (Harmonic Ultrasonic Scalpel). These methods are also useful for control of the small adrenal arteries, but the larger adrenal arteries and adrenal veins need to be clipped or stapled. The adrenal is placed in a specimen (EndoCatch) bag and can be morcellated prior to extraction.

Open adrenalectomy may be performed by the anterior, posterior, retroperitoneal, or thoraco-abdominal approaches. The latter is very useful, particularly for large adrenal cancers.

Complications of Laparoscopic Adrenalectomy

Specific procedure-related complications include trocar site-associated hematoma and subcutaneous emphysema, injury to surrounding organs such as the spleen, pancreas, liver and colon, and bleeding from venous injuries.

THE ENDOCRINE PANCREAS

EMBRYOLOGY AND ANATOMY

The pancreas is a retroperitoneal organ located at the level of L2. It weighs 75 to 100 g, is approximately 15 to 20 cm in length, and is divided into the head and uncinate process, the neck, the body, and the tail. The uncinate process forms part of the head and surrounds the superior mesenteric vessels. The main pancreatic duct (duct of Wirsung) is 2 to 3.5 mm wide, runs in the center of the pancreas, and drains the body, tail, and uncinate process. The lesser duct (duct of Santorini) usually drains the head, communicates

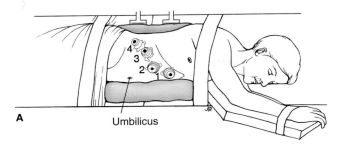

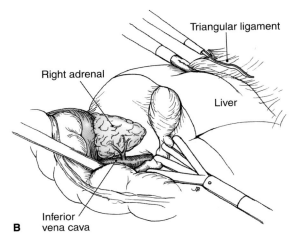

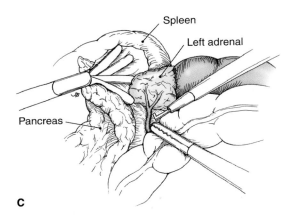

FIGURE 26-6 Technique of laparoscopic adrenalectomy. **A.** Positioning and placement of trocars. **B.** Exposure of the right adrenal is facilitated by division of the triangular ligament. **C.** Dissection and reflection of the spleen and tail of the pancreas aids in identifying the left adrenal. (Reproduced, with permission, from Lal G, Clark OH. Thyroid, parathyroid, and adrenal. In: *Schwartz's Principles of Surgery*. 8th ed. McGraw-Hill; 2004.)

with the duct of Wirsung, and drains separately via a minor papilla located 2 cm proximal to the ampulla of Vater. The common bile duct is found posteriorly in the pancreatic head and joins the main pancreatic duct before draining into the ampulla.

The pancreas originates as dorsal and ventral pancreatic buds from the primitive endoderm at about the fifth week of gestation. The former gives rise to the superior head, neck, body, and tail,

whereas the later forms the inferior head and the uncinate process. The ventral duct fuses with the dorsal bud to form the duct of Wirsung, and the proximal portion of the dorsal duct forms the duct of Santorini. In 10% of individuals, the ducts fail to communicate, resulting in pancreas divisum, where the entire pancreas is drained by the lesser duct.

Indications for Surgery

Endocrine pancreatic tumors arise from the islet cells, which are derived from the neural crest. Common functioning tumors are described next.

INSULINOMA

This β-cell–derived neoplasm is the most common pancreatic endocrine tumor. Insulinomas are evenly distributed throughout the pancreas (one-third each in the head, body, and tail). Most patients (90%) have a benign, solitary lesion. Approximately 10% of patients have malignant insulinomas with metastatic disease to the liver and peripancreatic lymph nodes. The insulinoma syndrome is characterized by the Whipple triad, which includes symptoms of hypoglycemia during fasting, serum glucose <50 mg/dL, and relief of hypoglycemic symptoms by exogenous glucose administration. Hypoglycemic symptoms may result from neuroglycopenia (confusion, seizures, personality change, coma) or due to a catecholamine surge (tachycardia, diaphoresis, trembling). Other causes of hypoglycemia such as reactive hypoglycemia, adrenal insufficiency, end-stage liver disease, nonpancreatic tumors (mesothelioma, sarcoma, adrenal carcinoma, carcinoid), and surreptitious administration of oral hypoglycemics or insulin should be excluded.

Diagnostic Tests

The diagnosis is made during a 72-hour monitored fast if glucose levels fall to <50 mg/dL while insulin levels are more than 20 uU/mL and the insulin to glucose ratio is >0.4 (normal: <0.3). This is considered the gold-standard test. Increased levels of C peptide and proinsulin are also diagnostic, whereas low levels suggest factitious hyperinsulinemia.

Once the diagnosis is confirmed biochemically, noninvasive tests such as double-contrast, fine-cut (5 mm) CT or MRI scans can identify large tumors or liver metastases. Transgastric endoscopic ultrasound is the most successful preoperative localization test (sensitivity 83%-93%). Some pancreatic neuroendocrine tumors also express somatostatin receptors and can be imaged using radiolabeled octreotide. Unfortunately, this is only effective in about 30% of patients with insulinomas (see Chapter 18 for details). Selective arteriography with calcium stimulation of insulin secretion, monitored through a catheter positioned in the right hepatic vein (Imamura-Doppmann test, sensitivity 88%) is an invasive test that is used selectively when other localization studies fail to identify the tumor or in patients following unsuccessful prior surgery.

Treatment

A. Surgical treatment   Operation is the only curative treatment. Prior to surgery, patients are instructed to take several small frequent meals, and diazoxide administration can be helpful in avoiding hypoglycemic attacks. Other medications commonly used include verapamil, diphenylhydantoin, and glucocorticoids. Somatostatin analogues can also be used if the tumors are positive for somatostatin receptors. Glucose levels are monitored perioperatively. The combination of inspection, palpation, and intraoperative ultrasound allows detection of nearly all tumors and their relationship to the pancreatic duct. Small (<2 cm) benign tumors in any part of the pancreas that are not intimately associated with the main pancreatic duct are best treated by enucleation. Larger tumors (up to 5 cm) can be enucleated if located in the pancreatic head but are removed by spleen-preserving distal pancreatectomy if located in the tail. Large tumors in the head that appear malignant are usually resected by a Whipple procedure. When a tumor cannot be identified, blind distal resections should generally not be performed. However, a small distal pancreatic resection may be sufficient to rule out nesidioblastosis (β-cell hyperplasia). Resection of peripancreatic and duodenal nodes is advised in patients with probable malignant tumors. Hepatic resection should be considered for cure or palliation in patients with metastatic tumors. In cases of nonresectable disease, debulking may be reasonable to achieve symptomatic control and may also prolong survival. Other modalities such as RFA, cryotherapy, and TACE may also be considered in this setting. Patients with insulinomas in the setting of MEN 1, in contrast to those with sporadic tumors, require distal pancreatectomy and enucleation of tumors from the head of the pancreas. Surgical resection is curative in about 95% of cases.

B. Medical treatment   Diazoxide and verapamil are often used to decrease insulin secretion from insulinoma. Combination chemotherapy (streptozocin, 5-FU, and doxorubicin) has also been used for unresectable insulinomas.

GASTRINOMA (ZOLLINGER-ELLISON SYNDROME)

This neoplasm leads to abdominal pain, peptic ulceration of the proximal gastrointestinal tract (90%) and diarrhea (50%). The diagnosis should be suspected in patients with recurrent postoperative and postbulbar ulcers, ulcers associated with diarrhea, a family history of ulcer diathesis or MEN 1, and failure to respond to adequate medical therapy. Up to 75% of gastrinomas occur sporadically. In contrast to insulinomas, 60% of gastrinomas are malignant and present with local invasion and metastases. Also, virtually all insulinomas are situated within the pancreas, but up to 70% of gastrinomas are found within the duodenum.

Diagnostic Tests

Fasting serum gastrin levels are generally over 200 pg/mL, and values over 1000 pg/mL are diagnostic of gastrinomas except in

TABLE 26–8 **Causes of hypergastrinemia.**

A. Hypergastrinemia associated with increased gastric acid
1. Gastrinoma, sporadic, or familial (MEN 1)
2. Antral G cell hyperfunction (rare)
3. Retained gastric antrum
4. Short bowel syndrome
5. Gastric outlet obstruction
6. Renal failure (acid can be normal)
7. *Helicobacter pylori* gastritis (acid can be low)
B. Hypergastrinemia associated with little or no gastric acid
1. Pernicious anemia (achlorhydria)
2. Chronic atrophic gastritis
3. Vagotomy
4. Gastric ulcer associated with hypochlorhydria

hypochlorhydric patients. Elevated gastrin levels may also be found in several other disease states (Table 26–8), and other tests are therefore necessary. Basal gastric acid output over 15 mEq/h (>5 mEq/h in patients with previous vagotomy) or a ratio of basal to maximal acid output >0.6 suggests a gastrinoma. An increase of gastrin over 200 pg/mL above the basal level on stimulation with 2 U/kg secretin confirms the diagnosis. In patients with ZES, serum PTH, calcium, and prolactin levels should be measured to rule out MEN 1.

Imaging studies used to localize gastrinomas are similar to those used for investigation of insulinomas. However, endoscopic ultrasound and visceral angiograms are less sensitive for gastrinomas, because many are small and not within the pancreas. Most pancreatic gastrinomas are situated to the right of the superior mesenteric vessels. Octreotide scans or positron emission tomography (PET) with Ga-DOTATOC may be useful. Selective pancreatic angiograms utilizing secretin stimulation and hepatic venous sampling for gastrin levels may also be used.

Treatment

A. Surgical treatment   Patients are treated with proton pump inhibitors preoperatively. Most gastrinomas are located in the gastrinoma triangle, which is surrounded by the cystic duct superiorly, the second and third portions of the duodenum inferiorly, and the junction of the neck and body of the pancreas medially. The Whipple procedure is recommended for large (>6 cm) or clinically malignant tumors in the head of the pancreas. Intraoperative ultrasound, endoscopy with duodenal transillumination, and a longitudinal duodenotomy are necessary to identify many tumors. All peripancreatic and periduodenal lymph nodes should be removed, as primary lymph node gastrinomas have been reported. Single hepatic metastases may be resected. Total gastrectomy is rarely indicated today except in noncompliant patients or those refractory to medical therapy when the gastrinoma cannot be identified or completely removed. Patients with MEN 1 often have multiple gastrinomas. The extent and role of surgery in patients with MEN 1/ZES remains controversial. Some groups advise early and aggressive surgeries to prevent liver disease, whereas others advise resection of MEN 1 gastrinomas >2 cm as small tumors are characterized by a good prognosis. In advanced, surgically incurable tumors, cytoreductive measures including resection or RFA/TACE are reasonable if >90% of the tumor mass can be removed, although this does not appear to prolong survival. Liver transplantation may be a consideration in young patients with diffuse, unresectable pancreatic metastases. In contrast to patients with MEN 1 who have nearly 100% recurrence rates, about 34% of patients with sporadic gastrinomas remain disease-free at 10 years after surgical treatment. Overall survival rates after surgical treatment are reported to be 94% at 10 years.

B. Medical treatment Octreotide may be used to decrease gastrin secretion. The combination of doxorubicin, streptozotocin, and 5-FU can be used as systemic chemotherapy. Somatostatin analogues and interferons have not shown much efficacy.

VIPOMA (VERNER-MORRISON) SYNDROME

This disorder is also known as the WDHA (watery diarrhea, hypokalemia, achlorhydria) or pancreatic cholera syndrome. Patients typically present with high-volume diarrhea (>5 L/d), muscular weakness (due to hypokalemia) and lethargy, hyperglycemia, hypercalcemia, and, rarely, cutaneous flushing.

Diagnostic Tests

Because secretion of VIP can be episodic, multiple fasting levels should be measured. Localizing studies are performed as described earlier for insulinomas and gastrinomas.

Treatment

A. Surgical treatment Fluid and electrolytes should be aggressively repleted prior to surgery. The diarrhea often responds to octreotide. Most of these tumors are located in the body and tail and hence are best managed by a distal pancreatectomy. Small tumors may be enucleated. If the tumor is not localized, the autonomic chain and adrenals should be examined for extrapancreatic tumors. If no tumor is identified, distal pancreatectomy may be considered. Palliative debulking may be performed for metastatic disease to control symptoms if >90% of the tumor mass can be resected. Other ablative therapies such as RFA/TACE or cryotherapy may also be used as cytoreductive measures and liver transplantation may be an option in selected cases.

B. Medical treatment Somatostatin analogues may provide palliation of symptoms particularly if the tumors are octreotide scan positive. They may also have an effect on tumor growth. Interferon-α may be indicated in tumors not responding to somatostatin analogues. Systemic therapy as described for other tumors may also be used.

GLUCAGONOMA

Patients with this tumor have mild diabetes, stomatitis, anemia, malnutrition, hypoproteinemia, and a characteristic severe dermatitis (necrolytic migratory erythema). The latter is thought to be secondary to the hypoaminoacidemia.

Diagnostic Tests

The clinical presentation and biopsy of the rash are sufficient for the diagnosis. Hyperglycemia, hypoproteinemia, and an elevated fasting glucagon level (>150 pg/mL) confirm the diagnosis. Localizing and staging tests are performed, as described above for the more common tumors. Most of these tumors are malignant.

Treatment

A. Surgical treatment Patients need preoperative octreotide, hyperalimentation, and routine deep venous thrombosis prophylaxis. Up to 70% of these tumors present with metastases, and surgery is the only potentially curable treatment. Most tumors are solitary and located in the tail, where they are amenable to distal pancreatectomy. Palliative debulking with distal pancreatectomy and splenectomy (if needed) in the setting of metastatic disease may help refractory symptoms. If splenectomy is planned, appropriate vaccination to reduce the risk of overwhelming postsplenectomy sepsis is recommended preoperatively.

B. Medical treatment As with other neuroendocrine tumors, octreotide and embolization of hepatic metastases may help control symptoms.

SOMATOSTATINOMA

The somatostatinoma syndrome is characterized by steatorrhea, diabetes, hypochlorhydria, and gallstone disease. Most somatostatinomas are malignant (75% have metastases at presentation) and are located in the pancreatic head. The diagnosis is established by fasting somatostatin levels of 100 pg/mL or more. Somatostatinomas are usually treated with the Whipple procedure (ie, pancreaticoduodenectomy). Fluid and electrolyte abnormalities should be corrected preoperatively.

NONFUNCTIONING PANCREATIC TUMORS

Approximately 33% of patients with pancreatic endocrine neoplasms have no evidence of a defined clinical syndrome and are deemed to have nonfunctioning tumors. However, some of these tumors produce pancreatic polypeptide and chromogranin A, particularly in the setting of MEN 1. These patients usually present with abdominal pain, weight loss, and jaundice—similar to ductal adenocarcinoma of the pancreas. The tumors are most commonly present in the head, neck, and uncinate process. The tumors are localized and staged similar to functional tumors.

Octreotide scans are recommended to assess receptor expression status and assess extent of disease. Endoscopic retrograde cholangiopancreatography and percutaneous transhepatic cholangiography are used for the evaluation of jaundice.

Surgical Treatment

Approximately 75% of these tumors are malignant. Surgical resection (pancreaticoduodenectomy or distal pancreatectomy) is the treatment of choice for sporadic tumors, because these tumors are not amenable to enucleation. In the presence of MEN 1, the indications for surgery are controversial. More aggressive groups recommend tumor enucleation in the head and prophylactic subtotal pancreatectomy, whereas more conservative groups recommend close follow up and enucleation of lesions >2 cm. Biliary and gastric bypasses may be necessary for palliation. These tumors often grow slowly. Five-year survival rates after resection are 50%. Resectable liver disease should be treated with surgery and or RFA. In patients with unresectable disease, combination chemotherapy (streptozocin and doxorubicin) with RFA/TACE may provide palliation. Poorly differentiated tumors are characterized by aggressive tumor biology, absence of somatostatin receptors, and poor prognosis. Surgical resection is recommended only for resectable primary tumors. Cytoreductive procedures are generally not recommended in these patients.

Technique of Pancreatic Exploration for Neuroendocrine Tumors

Patients are explored through a midline or bilateral subcostal incision. A detailed description of the Whipple procedure and a distal pancreatectomy is beyond the scope of this chapter, and the reader is referred to surgical atlases. A general description of the necessary maneuvers is presented here. The gastrocolic ligament and the inferior retroperitoneal attachments of the pancreas are divided to permit examination of the body and tail. A Kocher maneuver is performed to facilitate bimanual examination of the head and uncinate process. The duodenum, splenic hilum, small bowel mesentery, gonads (in women), and lymph nodes are assessed for extrapancreatic disease. The liver is examined for metastatic disease. Intraoperative ultrasound may facilitate identification of tumors. Early experience suggests that a laparoscopic approach is also feasible in these tumors, particularly sporadic insulinomas, when the lesion is identified with localization studies.

Complications of Pancreatic Surgery

The most important complications of pancreatic surgery (tumor enucleation, distal pancreatectomy, or Whipple resection) are pancreatic fistula, pseudocyst, or abscess formation, which may lead to necrotizing retroperitoneal infection, and hemorrhage. Other complications include upper gastrointestinal tract bleeding, marginal ulceration, and biliary fistula formation. The mortality of a Whipple procedure is <5% and that of other pancreatic surgical procedures is <1%.

REFERENCES

The Thyroid Gland

Boger MS, Perrier ND. Advantages and disadvantages of surgical therapy and optimal extent of thyroidectomy for the treatment of hyperthyroidism. *Surg Clin North Am.* 2004;84:849. [PMID: 15145239]

Brent GA. Clinical practice. Graves' disease. *N Engl J Med.* 2008;358:2594. [PMID: 18550875]

Chi SY, Hsei KC, Sheen-Chen SM, Chou FF. A prospective randomized comparison of bilateral subtotal thyroidectomy versus unilateral total and contralateral subtotal thyroidectomy for Graves' disease. *World J Surg.* 2005;29:160. [PMID: 15650802]

Cooper DS, Doherty GM, Haugen BR, et al. Revised American Thyroid Association Management Guidelines for patients with thyroid nodules and differentiated thyroid cancer. *Thyroid.* 2009;19:1167. [PMID: 19860577]

Hogan AR, Zhuge Y, Perez EA, Koniaris LG, Lew JI, Sola JE. Pediatric thyroid carcinoma: incidence and outcomes in 1753 patients. *J Surg Res.* 2009;156:167. [PMID: 19631341]

Kupferman ME, Patterson M, Mandel SJ, LiVolsi V, Weber RS. Patterns of lateral neck metastasis in papillary thyroid carcinoma. *Arch Otolaryngol Head Neck Surg.* 2004;130:857. [PMID: 15262763]

Lee J, Grumbach M, Clark OH. The optimal treatment for pediatric Graves' disease is surgery. *J Clin Endocrnol Metab.* 2007;92:801. [PMID: 17341575]

Miccoli P, Pinchera A, Materazzi G, et al. Surgical treatment of low- and intermediate-risk papillary thyroid cancer with minimally invasive video-assisted thyroidectomy. *J Clin Endocrinol Metab.* 2009;94:1618. [PMID: 19223525]

Moo-Young TA, Traugott AL, Moley JF. Sporadic and familial medullary thyroid carcinoma: state of the art. *Surg Clin North Am.* 2009;89:1193. [PMID: 19836492]

Neff RL, Farrar WB, Kloos RT, Burman KD. Anaplastic thyroid cancer. *Endocrin Metab Clin North Am.* 2008;37:525. [PMID: 18502341]

Richards ML. Thyroid cancer genetics: multiple endocrine neoplasia type 2, non-medullary familial thyroid cancer, and familial syndromes associated with thyroid cancer. *Surg Oncol Clin N Am.* 2009;18:39. [PMID: 19056041]

Woodrum DT, Gauger PG. Role of ^{131}I in the treatment of well differentiated thyroid cancer. *J Surg Oncol.* 2005;89:114. [PMID: 15719384]

The Parathyroid Gland

Bilezikian JP, Khan AA, Potts JT Jr, Third International Workshop on the Management of Asymptomatic Primary Hyperparathyroidism. Guidelines for the management of asymptomatic primary hyperparathyroidism: summary statement from the third international workshop. *J Clin Endocrinol Metab.* 2009;94:335.[PMID: 19193908]

Delellis RA. Challenging lesions in the differential diagnosis of endocrine tumors: parathyroid carcinoma. *Endocr Pathol.* 2008;19:221. [PMID: 19058032]

Eastell R, Arnold A, Brandi ML, et al. Diagnosis of asymptomatic primary hyperparathyroidism: proceedings of the third international workshop. *J Clin Endocrinol Metab.* 2009;94:340. [PMID: 19193909]

Henry JF, Sebag F, Cherenko M, Ippolito G, Taieb D, Vaillant J. Endoscopic parathyroidectomy: why and when? *World J Surg.* 2008;32:2509. [PMID: 18758853]

Irvin GL, III. Quick intraoperative parathyroid hormone assay: surgical adjunct to allow limited parathyroidectomy, improve success rate, and predict outcome. *World J Surg.* 2004;28:1287. [PMID: 15517474]

Udelsman R, Pasieka JL, Sturgeon C, Young JE, Clark OH. Surgery for asymptomatic primary hyperparathyroidism: proceedings of the third international workshop. *J Clin Endocrinol Metab.* 2009;94:366. [PMID: 19193911]

Westerdahl J, Bergenfelz A. Unilateral versus bilateral neck exploration for primary hyperparathyroidism: five-year follow-up of a randomized controlled trial. *Ann Surg.* 2007;246:976. [PMID: 18043099]

The Adrenal Gland

Al-Fehaily M, Duh QY. Clinical manifestation of aldosteronoma. *Surg Clin North Am.* 2004;84:887. [PMID: 15145241]

Broome JT, Gauger P. Surgical techniques for adrenal tumors. *Minerva Endocrinol.* 2009;34:185. [PMID: 19471241]

Ilias I, Torpy DJ, Pacak K, Mullen N, Wesley RA, Nieman LK. Cushing's syndrome due to ectopic corticotropin secretion: twenty years' experience at the National Institutes of Health. *J Clin Endocrinol Metab.* 2005;90:4955. [PMID: 15914534]

National Institutes of Health. NIH state-of-the-science statement on management of the clinically inapparent adrenal mass ("incidentaloma"). *NIH Consensus State Sci Statements.* 2002;19:1. [PMID: 14768652]

Sippel RS, Chen H. Subclinical Cushing's syndrome in adrenal incidentalomas. *Surg Clin North Am.* 2004;84:875. [PMID: 15145240]

Sturgeon C, Shen WT, Clark OH, Duh QY, Kebebew E. Risk assessment in 457 adrenal cortical carcinomas: how much does tumor size predict the likelihood of malignancy? *J Am Coll Surg.* 2006;202:423. [PMID: 16500246]

Walz KM. Extent of adrenalectomy for adrenal neoplasm: cortical sparing (subtotal) versus total adrenalectomy. *Surg Clin North Am.* 2004;84:743. [PMID: 15145232]

Zarnegar R, Kebebew E, Duh QY, Clark OH. Malignant pheochromocytoma. *Surg Oncol Clin N Am.* 2006;15:555. [PMID: 16882497]

The Endocrine Pancreas

Abood GJ, Go A, Malhotra D, Shoup M. The surgical and systemic management of neuroendocrine tumors of the pancreas. *Surg Clin North Am.* 2009;89:249. [PMID: 19186239]

Anlauf M, Wieben D, Perren A, et al. Persistent hyperinsulinemic hypoglycemia in 15 adults with diffuse nesidioblastosis: diagnostic criteria, incidence, and characterization of beta-cell changes. *Am J Surg Pathol.* 2005;29:524. [PMID: 15767809]

Doherty GM. Multiple endocrine neoplasia type 1. *J Surg Oncol.* 2005;89:143. [PMID: 15719382]

Ehehalt F, Saeger HD, Schmidt CM, Grützmann R. Neuroendocrine tumors of the pancreas. *Oncologist.* 2009;14:456. [PMID: 19411317]

Fernandez-Cruz L, Martínez I, Cesar-Borges G. Laparoscopic surgery in patients with sporadic and multiple insulinomas associated with multiple endocrine neoplasia type 1. *J Gastrointest Surg.* 2005;9:381. [PMID: 15749601]

Mazzaglia PJ, Berber E, Milas M, Siperstein AE. Laparoscopic radiofrequency ablation of neuroendocrine liver metastases: a 10-year experience evaluating predictors of survival. *Surgery.* 2007;142:10. [PMID: 17629995]

McLean AM, Fairclough PD. Endoscopic ultrasound in the localisation of pancreatic islet cell tumours. *Best Pract Res Clin Endocrinol Metab.* 2005;19:177. [PMID: 15763694]

Starke A, Saddig C, Mansfeld L, et al. Malignant metastatic insulinoma—postoperative treatment and follow-up. *World J Surg.* 2005;29:789. [PMID: 15880279]

Appendix

Normal Hormone Reference Ranges[a,b]

Test	Source	Ages, Conditions, etc	Conventional Units	Conversion Factor	SI Units	Comments
Adrenocorticotropic hormone (ACTH) stimulation test (cosyntropin test): 0.25 mg of synthetic ACTH$_{1-24}$ (cosyntropin) is administered IV or IM, and serum cortisol is measured at 0, 30, and 60 min. Normal response: peak cortisol >20 µg/dL (>540 nmol/L). A dose of 1 µg of ACTH will give a similar response in the normal individual (see Chapter 9).						
ACTH	Plasma	Men	7-50 pg/mL	0.222	1.55-11.1 pmol/L	Collect in silicone-coated EDTA-containing tubes. Keep iced. Avoid contact with glass during collection and separation. Process immediately. Separate and freeze plasma in plastic tube at −20°C.
		Women	5-27 pg/mL		1.11-6 pmol/L	
		Children				
		Prepubertal	7-28 pg/mL		1.55-6.2 pmol/L	
		Postpubertal	2-49 pg/mL		0.44-10.78 pmol/L	
		Post-dexamethasone suppression	2-5 pg/mL		0.4-1.1 pmol/L	
Aldosterone	Serum (fasting)	Sodium intake 300 mmol/d: Adult	–	27.7		Levels in pregnant patients are three to four times higher.
		Upright AM	<28 ng/dL		<776 pmol/L	
		Upright PM	<21 ng/dL		<582 pmol/L	
		Supine AM	3-16 ng/dL		83.1-443 pmol/L	
		Adrenal vein	200-400 ng/dL		5540-11,080 pmol/L	
	Urine	Sodium diet (100-300 mmol/d) Children:	–		–	Collect 24-h specimen in 10 g boric acid to maintain pH <7.5. Refrigerate during collection.
		2-7 y	≤5.7 µg/d			
		8-11 y	≤10.2 µg/d			
		12-16 y	≤15.6 µg/d			
		Adult	≤2.3-21 µg/d			
		Post-fludrocortisone or intravenous saline infusion	≤5.0 µg/d			
Alkaline phosphatase, bone specific	Serum	2-24 mo	25.4-124.0 µg/L	–	–	IRMA; collect following an overnight fast; useful in Paget disease and osteoporosis; assay also known as Ostase; increased levels seen in states of high bone turnover (Paget disease, hyperthyroidism, osteoporosis).
		6-9 y	41-134.6 µg/L			
		10-13 y				
		Males	43.8-177.4 µg/L			
		Females	24.2-154.2 µg/L			
		14-17 y				
		Males	13.7-128 µg/L			
		Females	10.5-75.2 µg/L			
		Adult males				
		18-29 y	8.4-29.3 µg/L			
		30-39 y	7.7-21.3 µg/L			
		40-49 y	7.0-18.3 µg/L			
		60-68 y	7.6-14.9 µg/L			
		Adult females				
		18-29 y	4.7-17.8 µg/L			
		30-39 y	5.3-19.5 µg/L			
		40-49 y	5.0-18.8 µg/L			
		50-76 y	5.6-29 µg/L			

(Continued)

Test	Source	Ages, Conditions, etc	Conventional Units	Conversion Factor	SI Units	Comments
Alpha subunit	Serum	Men	<0.6 ng/mL	–	–	RIA; used to assess gonado-tropin hormone subunit secretion in pituitary adenomas.
		Women				
		Premenopausal	<1.5 ng/mL			
		Postmenopausal	0.9-3.3 ng/mL			
		Hypothyroid	<3.7 ng/mL			
		Pregnant or hCG-producing tumor	1.8-360 ng/mL			
3α-Androstenediol glucuronide	Serum	Prepubertal children	0.1-0.6 ng/mL	2.14	0.2-1.3 nmol/L	Freeze serum and store at −20°C.
		Tanner II-III				
		Male	0.19-1.64 ng/mL		0.41-3.51 nmol/L	
		Female	0.33-2.44 ng/mL		0.71-5.22 nmol/L	
		Adult				
		Male	2.6-15 ng/mL		5.6-32.1 nmol/L	
		Female	0.6-3.0 ng/mL		1.3-6.4 nmol/L	
Androstenedione	Serum	Men		3.49		
		18-30 y	50-220 ng/dL		175-768 nmol/L	
		31-50 y	40-190 ng/dL		140-663 nmol/L	
		51-60 y	50-220 ng/dL		175-768 nmol/L	
		Women				
		Follicular	35-250 ng/dL		122-873 nmol/L	
		Midcycle	60-285 ng/dL		209-995 nmol/L	
		Luteal	30-235 ng/dL		105-820 nmol/L	
		Postmenopausal	20-75 ng/dL		70-262 nmol/L	
		Children				
		1-12 mo	6-78 ng/dL		21-272 nmol/L	
		1-4 y	5-51 ng/dL		17-178 nmol/L	
		5-9 y	6-115 ng/dL		21-401 nmol/L	
		10-13 y	12-221 ng/dL		42-771 nmol/L	
		14-17 y	22-225 ng/dL		77-785 nmol/L	
		Tanner II-III				
		Male	17-82 ng/dL		59-286 nmol/L	
		Female	43-180 ng/dL		150-628 nmol/L	
		Tanner IV-V				
		Male	57-150 ng/dL		199-523 nmol/L	
		Female	7-68 ng/dL		24-237 nmol/L	
Antidiuretic hormone (ADH; vasopressin)	Plasma	If serum osmolality >290 mOsm/kg	1-13 pg/mL	0.925	0.9-12 pmol/L	Collect in EDTA tubes. Keep iced. Centrifuge refrigerated. Store at −70°C within 2 h. 1 μU = 2.5 pg
		If serum osmolality <290 mOsm/kg	<2 pg/mL		<1.85 pmol/L	
Angiotensin II	Plasma	Adults	10-50 ng/L	–	–	Collect in EDTA. Centrifuge refrigerated. Store frozen at −70°C.
C peptide of insulin	Serum	Fasting	0.8-3.1 ng/mL	0.331	0.26-1.03 nmol/L	Freeze serum at −20°C; stable for 1 d at room temperature and 1 wk at −20°C.
Calcitonin	Serum	Male	<10 pg/mL	0.293	<2.93 pmol/L	Fasting, nonlipemic specimen. Refrigerate, spin down immediately. Store at −20°C.
		Female	<5 pg/mL		<1.46 pmol/L	
		Child				
		<6 mo	<41 pg/mL		<12 pmol/L	
		6 mo-3 y	<14 pg/mL		<4.1 pmol/L	
		3-17 y	<6 ng/mL		<1.76 pmol/L	

Calcitonin stimulation test utilizing calcium infusion: 2 mg/kg of calcium in the form of calcium gluconate is administered IV over 1 min. Blood samples for calcitonin are obtained at 1, 2, 5, and 10 min after the infusion. Normal peak values for calcitonin 2 min after calcium infusion: female; <70 ng/L (<20.5 pmol/L); male: <491 ng/L (<144 pmol/L).

(Continued)

Test	Source	Ages, Conditions, etc	Conventional Units	Conversion Factor	SI Units	Comments
Calcium, 24-h urinary	Urine	Calcium Men Women Calcium Men Women	 50-300 mg/24 h 50-250 mg/24 h 30-210 mg/g creatinine 30-275 mg/g creatinine	– –	 –	Collect in 25 mL of 6N HCl. Refrigerate during collection; elevated in primary hyperparathyroidism, Paget disease, multiple myeloma, vitamin D toxicity; reduced in rickets, osteomalacia, familial hypocalciuric hypercalcemia.
Calcium, ionized	Serum	Adults Children 8 mo-10 y 11-17 y	4.8-5.6 mg/dL 4.9-5.4 mg/dL 4.8-5.3 mg/dL	–	–	Refrigerated serum must be collected anaerobically in gel barrier tube; elevated in primary hyperparathyroidism, vitamin D toxicity, cancer; reduced in pseudo-hypoparathyroidism, hypoparathyroidism, and severe vitamin D deficiency.
Calcium, total	Serum	Adults Children <1 mo 1-11 mo 1-3 y 4-19 y	8.6-10.2 mg/dL 8.4-10.6 mg/dL 8.7-10.5 mg/dL 8.5-10.6 mg/dL 8.9-10.4 mg/dL	–	–	Overnight fasting preferred; used to diagnose parathyroid and vitamin D disorders; elevated in primary hyperparathyroidism, vitamin D toxicity; reduced in hypoparathyroidism and vitamin D deficiency.
Catecholamines (fractionated by HPLC)	Plasma	Adults: Norepinephrine Supine Ambulatory Epinephrine Supine Ambulatory Dopamine Supine Ambulatory Total (N+E) Supine Upright Children (age 3-15 y): Epinephrine Supine Norepinephrine Supine Dopamine	 – 112-658 pg/mL 212-1109 pg/mL – <50 pg/mL <95 pg/mL – <10 ng/mL <20 ng/mL 123-671 pg/mL 242-1125 pg/mL – – <464 pg/mL – < 1251pg/mL <60 pg/mL	 0.00591 0.00546 0.00654 0.00591 – – 0.00546 – 0.00591 0.00654	 – 0.66-3.89 nmol/L 1.28-6.55 nmol/L – <0.27 nmol/L <0.52 nmol/L – <0.065 nmol/L <0.13 nmol/L 0.73-3.97 nmol/L 1.43-6.64 nmol/L – – <2.54 nmol/L < 7.4 nmol/L 0.39 nmol/L	Collect by intravenous catheter after patient has rested 30 min. Collect and centrifuge under refrigeration; freeze in plastic tube at –20°C.

(Continued)

Test	Source	Ages, Conditions, etc	Conventional Units	Conversion Factor	SI Units	Comments
	Urine	Norepinephrine	–	5.91	–	24-h urine preservative: 25 mL of 6N HCl. Freeze aliquot promptly at –20°C.
		3-8 y	5-41 µg/24 h	–	29.5-242.3 nmol/24 h	
		9-12 y	5-50 µg/24 h		29.5-295.8 nmol/24 h	
		13-17 y	12-88 µg/24 h		70.9-526 nmol/24 h	
		>17 y	15-100 µg/24 h		89-591 nmol/24 h	
		Epinephrine	–	5.46		
		3-8 y	1-7 µg/24 h	–	5.46-38.2 nmol/24 h	
		9-12 y	<8 µg/24 h		<43.7 nmol/24 h	
		13-17 y	<11 µg/24 h		<60 nmol/24 h	
		>17 y	2-24 µg/24 h		11-131 nmol/24 h	
		Total (N + E)		5.91		
		3-8 y	9-51 µg/24 h		53-301 nmol/24 h	
		9-12 y	9-71 µg/24 h		53-420 nmol/24 h	
		13-17 y	13-90 µg/24 h		77-532 nmol/24 h	
		>17 y	26-121 µg/24 h		154-715 nmol/24 h	
		Dopamine		6.54		
		3-8 y	80-378 µg/24 h	–	523-2472 nmol/24 h	
		9-12 y	51-474 µg/24 h		334-3100 nmol/24 h	
		13-17 y	51-645 µg/24 h		334-4218 nmol/24 h	
		>17 y	52-480 µg/24 h		340-3139 nmol/24 h	
Cholecystokinin	Plasma (fasting)		3.9 ng/mL	0.26	1 pmol/L	–
Chorionic gonadotropin, beta subunit (β-hCG)	Serum	Men	<5 mIU/mL	1.00	<5 mIU/mL	See Chapter 16 for further details and interpretation.
		Women				
		Premenopausal, Nonpregnant	<5 mIU/mL		<5 mIU/mL	
		Postmenopausal	<10 mIU/mL		<10 mIU/mL	
		Females postconception				
		<1 wk	5-50 mIU/mL		5-50 mIU/mL	
		1-2 wk	50-500 mIU/mL	–	50-500 mIU/mL	
		2-3 wk	100-5000 mIU/mL	–	100-5000 mIU/mL	
		3-4 wk	500-10,000 mIU/mL	–	500-10,000 mIU/mL	
		4-5 wk	1000-50,000 mIU/mL		1000-50,000 mIU/mL	
		5-6 wk	10,000-100,000 mIU/mL		10,000-100,000 mIU/L	
		6-8 wk	15,000-200,000 mIU/mL		15,000-200,000 mIU/mL	
		2-3 mo	10,000-100,000 mIU/mL		10,000-100,000 mIU/mL	
Chromogranin A	Serum	Adults	<36.4 ng/mL	1.00	<36.4 µg/L	–
Collagen type 1 C-telopeptide (CTx)	Serum	Adults	–	–	–	–
	–	Men	–	–		Frozen serum, collected between 8 AM and 10 AM. Used to evaluate osteoporosis and Paget disease.
		18-29 y	87-100 pg/mL			
		30-39 y	70-780 pg/mL			
		40-49 y	60-700 pg/mL			
		50-68 y	87-345 pg/mL			
		Women				
		18-29 y	64-640 pg/mL			
		30-39 y	60-650 pg/mL			
		40-49 y	40-465 pg/mL			

(Continued)

Test	Source	Ages, Conditions, etc	Conventional Units	Conversion Factor	SI Units	Comments
Collagen cross-linked N-telopeptide (NTx), serum or urine	1.0 mL refrigerated serum; 2 mL refrigerated urine	Men Serum Second AM voided urine 18-29 y 30-59 y 24-h urine Women Premenopausal Serum Second AM Urine 24-h urine	 10.7-22.9 nmol BCE/L 12-99 nmol BCE/mmol creatinine 9-60 nmol BCE/mmol creatinine 5-87 nmol BCE/mmol creatinine 8.7-19.8 nmol BCE/L 4-64 nmol BCE/mmol creatinine 5-79 nmol BCE/mmol creatinine	–	–	Monitor response to treatment in patients with osteoporosis; diagnose high bone turnover state; possibly elevated in Paget disease of bone, hyperthyroidism, osteoporosis.

Corticotropin-releasing hormone (CRH) test: Ovine CRH in a dose of 1 μg/kg is administered IV. Blood samples for ACTH and cortisol determinations are taken at 15, 30, and 60 min. The peak ACTH response of >10 pg/mL (>2.2 pmol/L) occurs at 15 min. The peak cortisol response of >10 μg/dL (>280 nmol/L) occurs at 30-60 min (see Chapter 4).

Test	Source	Ages, Conditions, etc	Conventional Units	Conversion Factor	SI Units	Comments
Corticotropin-releasing hormone	Plasma	Men and nonpregnant women Pregnant women 1st trimester 2nd trimester 3rd trimester Cord blood	<34 pg/mL <40 pg/mL <153 pg/mL <847 pg/mL <338 pg/mL	2.0	<68 pmol/L <80 pmol/L <306 pmol/L <1694 pmol/L <676 pmol/L	Markedly elevated at term pregnancy.
Cortisol	Serum	Adult Total 8-10 AM 4-6 PM Peak post-ACTH Children Premature (31-35 wk) Term Infants (3 d) 1-17 y Free AM PM	 5-21 μg/dL 2-14 μg/dL >20 μg/dL <15 μg/dL <14 μg/dL 2-17 μg/dL 0.4-1.92 μg/dL 0.2-0.9 μg/dL	27.59	 138-579.4 nmol/L 55.2-386.3 nmol/L 551.8 nmol/L <414 nmol/L <386 nmol/L 55-469 nmol/L 11-53 nmol/L 5-25 nmol/L	Collect and process under refrigeration. Spin down immediately. Salivary cortisol is in equilibrium with free cortisol and may be used as an index to free cortisol. Reference range may vary with method and laboratory.
	Urine (free)	24-h specimen RIA Adults Children 1-4.9 y 5-9.9 y 10-13.9 y 14-17.9 y	 4-50 μg/24 h 0.9-8.2 μg/24 h 1-30 μg/024 h 1-45 μg/24 h 3-55 μg/24 h	2.76	 11-138 nmol/24 h 2.5-22.6 nmol/24 h 2.8-82.8 nmol/24 h 2.8-124.2 nmol/24 h 8.3-151.8 nmol/24 h	Collect 24-h specimen with 8 g of boric acid or 10 mL of 6N HCl as preservative. Liquid chromatography/tandem mass spectrometry.

(Continued)

Test	Source	Ages, Conditions, etc	Conventional Units	Conversion Factor	SI Units	Comments
Dehydroepi-androsterone (DHEA)	Serum (fasting preferred)	Men	180-1250 ng/dL	0.347	62.5-433.8 nmol/L	Separate serum immediately and store at −20°C.
		Women	130-980 ng/dL		45.1-340 nmol/L	
		Pregnancy	135-810 ng/dL		46.8-281 nmol/L	
		Post-ACTH stimulation in men and women	545-1845 ng/dL		189-640.2 nmol/L	
		Children			<1160 nmol/L	
		Premature (31-35 wk)	<3343 ng/dL		<246 nmol/L	
		Term (1 wk)	<761 ng/dL			
		Tanner II-III				
		Male	25-300 ng/dL		8.7-104 nmol/L	
		Female	69-605 ng/dL		23.9-209.9 nmol/L	
		Tanner IV-V				
		Male	100-400 ng/dL		34.7-138.8 nmol/L	
		Female	165-690 ng/dL		57.3-239.4 nmol/L	
Dehydroepi-androsterone sulfate (DHEAS)	Serum (fasting preferred)	Male		0.0272		Stable 72 h at 40°C. Store at −20 °C.
		0-1 mo	<316 μg/dL		<8.6 μmol/L	
		1-6 mo	<58 μg/dL		<1.6 μmol/L	
		7-12 mo	<26 μg/dL		<0.7 μmol/L	
		1-3 y	<15 μg/dL		<0.4 μmol/L	
		4-6 y	<27 μg/dL		<0.7 μmol/L	
		7-9 y	<91 μg/dL		<2.4 μmol/L	
		10-13 y	<138 μg/dL		<0.6 μmol/L	
		14-17 y	38-340 μg/dL		1.0-9.2 μmol/L	
		18-29 y	110-510 μg/dL		3.0-13.9 μmol/L	
		30-39 y	110-370 μg/dL		3.0-10.1 μmol/L	
		40-49 y	45-345 μg/dL		1.2-9.4 μmol/L	
		50-59 y	25-240 μg/dL		0.7-6.5 μmol/L	
		60-69 y	25-95 μg/dL		0.7-2.6 μmol/L	
		70-90 y	<75 μg/dL		<2.0 μmol/L	
		Female		0.0272		
		0-1 mo	15-261 μg/dL		0.4-7.1 μmol/L	
		1-6 mo	<74 μg/dL		<2.0 μmol/L	
		7-12 mo	<26 μg/dL		<0.7 μmol/L	
		1-3 y	<22 μg/dL		<0.6 μmol/L	
		4-6 y	<34 μg/dL		<0.9 μmol/L	
		7-9 y	<92 μg/dL		<2.5 μmol/L	
		10-13 y	<148 μg/dL		<4.0 μmol/L	
		14-17 y	37-307 μg/dL		1.0-10.1 μmol/L	
		18-29 y	45-320 μg/dL		1.2-8.7 μmol/L	
		30-39 y	40-325 μg/dL		1.1-8.8 μmol/L	
		40-49 y	25-220 μg/dL		0.7-6.0 μmol/L	
		50-59 y	15-170 μg/dL		0.4-4.6 μmol/L	
		60-69 y	<185 μg/dL		<5.0 μmol/L	
		70-90 y	<90 μg/dL		<2.5 μmol/L	
Deoxycorticos-terone (DOC)	Serum (fasting preferred)	Male		30.26		Process immediately. Store at −20 °C.
		Adult	3.5-11.5 ng/dL		106-333 pmol/L	
		Female				
		Follicular phase	1.5-8.5 ng/dL		45-257 pmol/L	
		Luteal phase	3.5-13 ng/dL		91-393	
		Pregnancy				
		1st trimester	5-25 ng/dL		151-757 pmol/L	
		2nd trimester	10-75 ng/dL		303-2270 pmol/L	
		3rd trimester	30-110 ng/dL		908-3329 pmol/L	
		Children				
		<1 y	7-57 ng/dL		212-1725 pmol/L	
		1-5 y	4-49 ng/dL		121-1483 pmol/L	
		6-12 y				
		Male	9-34 ng/dL		272-1029 pmol/L	
		Female	2-13 ng/dL		61-393 pmol/L	

(Continued)

Test	Source	Ages, Conditions, etc	Conventional Units	Conversion Factor	SI Units	Comments
11-Deoxycortisol	Serum	Male		0.02887		Process immediately. Store at −20°C. Early morning specimen preferred.
		18-29 y	<119 ng/dL		<3.4 nmol/L	
		30-39 y	<135 ng/dL		<3.9 nmol/L	
		40-49 y	<76 ng/dL		<2.2 nmol/L	
		50-59 y	<42 ng/dL		<1.2 nmol/L	
		Female				
		18-29 y	<107 ng/dL		<3.1 nmol/L	
		30-39 y	<51 ng/dL		<1.5 nmol/L	
		40-49 y	<62 ng/dL		<1.8 nmol/L	
		50-66 y	<37 ng/dL		<1.1 nmol/L	
		Children				
		Cord blood	295-554 ng/dL		8.5-16 nmol/L	
		Premature infants	<235 ng/dL		<6.8 nmol/L	
		Full-term infants	<170 ng/dL		<4.9 nmol/L	
		1-12 mo	10-200 ng/dL		0.3-5.8 nmol/L	
		1-4 y	7-210 ng/dL		0.2-6.1 nmol/L	
		5-9 y	<122 ng/dL		<3.5 nmol/L	
		10-13 y	<245 ng/dL		<7.1 nmol/L	
		14-17 y	<302 ng/dL		<8.7 nmol/L	

Dexamethasone suppression test (low dose) for the diagnosis of Cushing syndrome (see Chapter 9): Obtain a baseline serum cortisol at 0700-0800 h. Administer 1 mg dexamethasone orally at 2300 h that evening and obtain another serum cortisol at 0700-0800 h the following morning. **Interpretation:** A normal response (normal suppressibility) is a reduction of the post-dexamethasone serum cortisol to <1.8 µg/dL (<50 nmol/L).

Dexamethasone suppression test (high dose) for the differential diagnosis of Cushing syndrome (see Chapter 9): Obtain a baseline serum cortisol at 0700-0800 h. Administer 8 mg dexamethasone orally at 2300 h that evening and obtain another serum cortisol at 0700-0800 h the following morning. **Interpretation:** A reduction of the post-dexamethasone serum cortisol to <50% of the baseline cortisol indicates suppressibility.

Dexamethasone-CRH test: Administer dexamethasone, 0.5 mg every 6 h orally for eight doses, followed by CRH, 1 µg/kg IV 2 h after the last dose of dexamethasone. Plasma cortisol is obtained 15 min after CRH. Normal: <1.4 µg/dL (<38.6 nmol/L). (See Chapter 9.)

Test	Source	Ages, Conditions, etc	Conventional Units	Conversion Factor	SI Units	Comments
Dihydrotesterone (male)	Serum	Cord blood	<2-8 ng/dL	0.0344	<0.07-0.28 nmol/L	Separate serum within 1 h after collection and store at −20°C.
		1-6 mo	12-85 ng/dL		<0.41-2.9 nmol/L	
		Prepubertal	<5 ng/dL		<0.2 nmol/L	
		Tanner II-III	3-33 ng/dL		0.1-1.1 nmol/L	
		Tanner IV-V	22-75 ng/dL		0.8-2.6 nmol/L	
		Adult	25-75 ng/dL		0.9-2.6 nmol/L	
Dihydrotesterone (female)	Serum	Cord blood	<2-5 ng/dL	0.0344	<0.07-0.17 nmol/L	
		1-6 mo	<5 ng/dL		<0.2 nmol/L	
		Prepubertal	<5 ng/dL		<0.2 nmol/L	
		Tanner II-III	5-19 ng/dL		0.2-0.7 nmol/L	
		Tanner IV-V	3-30 ng/dL		0.1-1 nmol/L	
		Adult	5-30 ng/dL		0.2-1 nmol/L	
Erythropoietin	Serum	Adult	4.1-19.5 mU/mL	1.00	4.1-19.5 mU/mL	
		Child				
		3 wk-2 mo	5.0-13.0 mU/mL		5.0-13.0 mU/mL	
		3 mo-16 y	9.0-28.0 mU/mL		9.0-28.0 mU/mL	
Estradiol	Serum	Male		3.67		
		1-9 y	<4 pg/mL		<15 pmol/L	
		10-11 y	<12 pg/mL		<44 pmol/L	
		12-14 y	<24 pg/mL		<88 pmol/L	
		15-17 y	<31 pg/mL		<114 pmol/L	
		>17 y	<29 pg/mL		<106 pmol/L	
		Female				
		1-9 y	<16 pg/mL		<59 pmol/L	
		10-11 y	<65 pg/mL		<239 pmol/L	
		12-14 y	<142 pg/mL		<521 pmol/L	
		15-17 y	<283 pg/mL		<1039 pmol/L	
		Follicular	39-375 pg/mL		143-1376 pmol/L	
		Midcycle peak	96-762 pg/mL		352-2797 pmol/L	
		Luteal	48-440 pg/mL		176-1614 pmol/L	
		Postmenopausal	<10 pg/mL		<37 pmol/L	

(Continued)

Test	Source	Ages, Conditions, etc	Conventional Units	Conversion Factor	SI Units	Comments
Estradiol, free		Adult male	<0.45 pg/mL	3.67	<1.7 pmol/mL	
		Adult female				
		Follicular	0.43-5.03 pg/mL		1.6-18.5 pmol/mL	
		Midcycle	0.72-5.89 pg/mL		2.6-21.6 pmol/mL	
		Luteal	0.40-5.55 pg/mL		1.5-20.4 pmol/mL	
		Postmenopausal	<0.38 pg/mL		<1.4 pmol/mL	
Estrone	Serum	Adult male	<68 ng/L	3.70	<251 pmol/L	
		Postpubertal female				
		Follicular phase	10-138 ng/L		37-511 pmol/L	
		Midcycle	49-268 ng/L		181-992 pmol/L	
		Luteal phase	16-173 ng/L		59-640 pmol/L	
		Postmenopausal	<65 ng/L		<240 pmol/L	
Follicle-stimulating hormone	Serum or plasma (heparin)	Adult males (>18 y)	1.6-8 IU/L	1.00	1.6-8 IU/L	
		Adult females (>18 y)				
		Follicular phase	2.5-10.2 IU/L		2.5-10.2 IU/L	
		Midcycle peak	3.1-17.7 IU/L		3.1-17.7 IU/L	
		Luteal phase	1.5-9.1 IU/L		1.5-9.1 IU/L	
		Postmenopausal	23-116 IU/L		23-116 IU/L	
		Boy				
		0-9 y	<3.0 IU/L		<3.0 IU/L	
		10-13 y	0.3-4.0 IU/L		0.3-4.0 IU/L	
		14-17 y	0.4-7.4 IU/L		0.4-7.4 IU/L	
		Girls				
		0-8 y	0.5-4.5 IU/L		0.5-4.5 IU/L	
		9-13 y	0.4-6.5 IU/L		0.4-6.5 IU/L	
		14-17 y	0.8-8.5 IU/L		0.8-8.5 IU/L	
Gastrin	Serum	Adults	<100 pg/mL	0.475	<48 pmol/L	Overnight fast required. Store at −20°C.
		Children 5-7 y	13-64 pg/mL		6.2-30 pmol/L	
Glucagon	Plasma	Adults	<60 pg/mL	0.287	<17.2 pmol/L	Centrifuge immediately under refrigeration. Store in plastic vial with 0.5 mL aprotinin (10,000 KIU/mL) at −20°C. Overnight fast required.
		Children				
		Cord blood	<215 pg/mL		<62 pmol/L	
		Day 1	<240 pg/mL		<69 pmol/L	
		Day 2	<400 pg/mL		<115 pmol/L	
		Day 3	<420 pg/mL		<121 pmol/L	
		Day 4-14	<148 pg/mL		<42 pmol/L	
Growth hormone	Serum	Fasting		46.5		Store at −20°C. **Note:** GH values fluctuate widely, and functional tests must be utilized for diagnosis of GH deficiency or excess. See Chapter 4 for details of suppression and stimulation tests for GH excess or deficiency.
		Children	<13 ng/mL		<604 pmol/L	
		Adults	<10 ng/mL		<465 pmol/L	
		Post-75-g glucose load	<1 ng/mL		<46 pmol/L	
Growth hormone–binding protein	Serum	Adults	400-4260 pmol/L	1.0	400-4260 pmol/L	Store at −20°C.
		Children				
		3-8 y	320-3820 pmol/L		320-3820 pmol/L	
		9-13 y	240-2890 pmol/L		240-2890 pmol/L	
		14-17 y	290-3140 pmol/L		290-3140 pmol/L	
Growth hormone–releasing hormone	Plasma	Adults	<49 pg/mL	1.0	<49 pg/mL	Store at −20°C.
		Children (4-14 y)	6.8-19 pg/mL		6.8-19 pg/mL	
Hemoglobin A₁c	Whole blood	Nondiabetic	<6%			Collection in EDTA. Keep refrigerated.
Homovanillic acid	Urine	3-8 y	0.5-6.7 mg/24 h	5.49	2.7-36.8 µmol/24 h	Preservative: 10 mL of 6N HCl. Avoid alcohol, coffee, tea, tobacco, and strenuous exercise for 2 wk pretest.
		9-12 y	1.1-6.8 mg/24 h		6.0-37.3 µmol/24 h	
		13-17 y	1.4-7.2 mg/24 h		7.7-39.5 µmol/24 h	
		>17 y	1.6-7.5 mg/24 h		8.8-41.2 µmol/24 h	

(Continued)

Test	Source	Ages, Conditions, etc	Conventional Units	Conversion Factor	SI Units	Comments
17-Hydroxy-corticoids	Urine	Males, age 1-20 y	0.5-10 mg/24 h	2.76	1.4-28 µmol/24 h	Preservative: 10 mL of 6N HCl
		Adult males	3-10 mg/24 h		8.3-28 µmol/24 h	
		Females, age 1-20 y	0.5-7 mg/24 h		1.4-19 µmol/24 h	
		Adult females	2-6 mg/24 h		5.5-16.6 µmol/24 h	
5-Hydroxyindole-acetic	Urine	Age 2-10 y	<8 mg/24 h	5.23	<41.8 µmol/24 h	Preservative: 10 mL of 6N HCl. Refrigerate during 24-h collection. For 48 h prior to and during collection, avoid avocados, and alcohol.
		Age >10 y	<6 mg/24 h		<31.4 µmol/24 h	
18-Hydroxy-corticosterone	Serum	Adult		27.51		Refrigerate.
		Supine (8-10 AM)	4-37 ng/dL		110-1018 pmol/L	
		Ambulatory (8-10 AM)	5-80 ng/dL		138-2201 pmol/L	
		Children				
		Premature infants (31-35 wk)	<380 ng/dL		<10,454 pmol/L	
		Term infants (3 d)	<942 ng/dL		<25,914 pmol/L	
17-Hydroxy-pregnenolone	Serum	Adults	20-450 ng/dL	0.0301	0.6-13.5 nmol/L	Process immediately. Store at −20°C.
		Post-ACTH	290-910 ng/dL		8.7-27.4 nmol/L	
		Children				
		Premature infants	<2409 ng/dL		<72.5 nmol/L	
		Term infants	<830 ng/dL		25 nmol/L	
		1-12 mo	14-830 ng/dL		0.4-25 nmol/L	
		1-5 y	10-100 ng/dL		0.3-3 nmol/L	
		6-12 y	11-190 ng/dL		0.3-5.7 nmol/L	
		Tanner II-III				
		Males	20-360 ng/dL		0.6-10.8 nmol/L	
		Females	58-450 ng/dL		1.7-13.5 nmol/L	
		Tanner IV-V				
		Males	32-300 ng/dL		1-9 nmol/L	
		Females	53-540 ng/dL		1.6-16.3 nmol/L	
17-Hydroxy-progesterone	Serum (fasting preferred)	Males		0.0303		
		18-30 y	32-307 ng/dL		1-9.3 nmol/L	
		31-40 y	42-196 ng/dL		1.3-5.9 nmol/L	
		41-50 y	33-195 ng/dL		1-5.9 nmol/L	
		51-60 y	37-129 ng/dL		1.1-3.9 nmol/L	
		Females				
		Follicular phase	<185 ng/dL		<5.6 nmol/L	
		Midcycle phase	<225 ng/dL		<6.8 nmol/L	
		Luteal phase	<285 ng/dL		<8.6 nmol/L	
		Postmenopausal	<45 ng/dL		<1.4 nmol/L	
		Children				
		Premature infants	<360 ng/dL		<10.9 nmol/L	
		Term infants	<420 ng/dL		<12.7 nmol/L	
		1-12 mo	11-170 ng/dL		0.3-5.2 nmol/L	
		1-4 y	4-115 ng/dL		0.1-3.5 nmol/L	
		5-9 y	<90 ng/dL		<2.7 nmol/L	
		10-13 y	<169 ng/dL		<5.1 nmol/L	
		14-17 y	16-283 ng/dL		0.5-8.6 nmol/L	
		Post-ACTH				
		1-12 mo	85-465 ng/dL		2.6-14.1 nmol/L	
		1-5 y	50-350 ng/dL		1.5-10.6 nmol/L	
		6-12 y	75-220 ng/dL		2.3-6.7 nmol/L	
		Tanner II-III				
		Males	12-130 ng/dL		0.4-3.9 nmol/L	
		Post-ACTH	69-310 ng/dL		2.1-9.4 nmol/L	
		Females	18-220 ng/dL		0.5-6.7 nmol/L	
		Post-ACTH	80-420 ng/dL		2.4-12.7 nmol/L	

(Continued)

Test	Source	Ages, Conditions, etc	Conventional Units	Conversion Factor	SI Units	Comments
		Tanner IV-V				
		Males	51-190 ng/dL		1.5-5.8 nmol/L	
		Post-ACTH	105-230 ng/dL		3.2-7 nmol/L	
		Females	36-200 ng/dL		1.1-6.1 nmol/L	
		Post-ACTH	80-225 ng/dL		2.4-6.8 nmol/L	
Insulin, total (free and bound)	Serum	Fasting	≤20 µU/mL (≤0.8 ng/mL)	172.1 (ng/mL → pmol/L)	≤137.6 pmol/L	Cold centrifuge. Freeze at −20°C. Must always be evaluated in light of simultaneous plasma glucose measurement.
Insulin with oral glucose tolerance test	Serum	1 h	50-130 µU/mL (2-5.2 ng/mL)	172.1 (ng/mL → pmol/L)	344-895 pmol/L	Cold centrifuge. Freeze at −20°C.
		2 h	<30 µU/mL (<1.2 ng/mL)		<207 pmol/L	
Insulin-like growth factor-I (IGF-I)	Serum	Male		1.0		Store refrigerated. Elevated in acromegaly and gigantism; reduced in isolated GH deficiency.
		1-7 d	≤31 ng/mL		≤31 µg/L	
		8-14 d	≤43 ng/mL		≤43 µg/L	
		15 d-1 y	25-265 ng/mL		25-265 µg/L	
		1-2 y	45-222 ng/mL		45-222 µg/L	
		3-4 y	36-202 ng/mL		36-202 µg/L	
		5-6 y	32-259 ng/mL		32-259 µg/L	
		7-8 y	65-278 ng/mL		65-278 µg/L	
		9-10 y	52-330 ng/mL		52-330 µg/L	
		11-12 y	80-723 ng/mL		80-723 µg/L	
		13-14 y	142-855 ng/mL		142-855 µg/L	
		15-16 y	176-845 ng/mL		176-845 µg/L	
		17-18 y	152-668 ng/mL		152-668 µg/L	
		19-30 y	126-382 ng/mL		126-382 µg/L	
		31-40 y	106-255 ng/mL		106-255 µg/L	
		41-50 y	86-220 ng/mL		86-220 µg/L	
		51-60 y	87-225 ng/mL		87-225 µg/L	
		61-70 y	75-228 ng/mL		75-228 µg/L	
		71-80 y	31-187 ng/mL		31-187 µg/L	
		81-88 y	68-157 ng/mL		68-157 µg/L	
		>88 y	Not established		Not established	
		Male				
		Tanner stage I	59-296 ng/mL		59-296 µg/L	
		Tanner stage II	56-432 ng/mL		56-432 µg/L	
		Tanner stage III	135-778 ng/mL		135-778 µg/L	
		Tanner stage IV	230-855 ng/mL		230-855 µg/L	
		Tanner stage V	181-789 ng/mL		181-789 µg/L	
		Female				
		1-7 d	≤31 ng/mL		≤31 µg/L	
		8-14 d	≤43 ng/mL		≤43 µg/L	
		15 d-1 y	25-265 ng/mL		25-265 µg/L	
		1-2 y	99-254 ng/mL		99-254 µg/L	
		3-4 y	36-202 ng/mL		36-202 µg/L	
		5-6 y	57-260 ng/mL		57-260 µg/L	
		7-8 y	97-352 ng/mL		97-352 µg/L	
		9-10 y	49-461 ng/mL		49-461 µg/L	
		11-12 y	101-580 ng/mL		101-580 µg/L	
		13-14 y	199-658 ng/mL		199-658 µg/L	
		15-16 y	236-808 ng/mL		236-808 µg/L	
		17-18 y	165-526 ng/mL		165-526 µg/L	
		19-30 y	138-410 ng/mL		138-410 µg/L	
		31-40 y	126-291 ng/mL		126-291 µg/L	
		41-50 y	88-249 ng/mL		88-249 µg/L	

(Continued)

Test	Source	Ages, Conditions, etc	Conventional Units	Conversion Factor	SI Units	Comments
		51-60 y	92-190 ng/mL		92-190 µg/L	
		61-70 y	87-178 ng/mL		87-178 µg/L	
		71-80 y	25-171 ng/mL		25-171 µg/L	
		81-88 y	31-162 ng/mL		31-162 µg/L	
		>88 y	Not established		Not established	
		Female				
		Tanner stage I	45-358 ng/mL		45-358 µg/L	
		Tanner stage II	111-426 ng/mL		111-426 µg/L	
		Tanner stage III	169-644 ng/mL		169-644 µg/L	
		Tanner stage IV	297-627 ng/mL		297-627 µg/L	
		Tanner stage V	142-868 ng/mL		142-868 µg/L	
Insulin-like growth factor-II (IGF-II)	Serum	Children		1.0		Store refrigerated. Elevated in mesenchymal tumors with hypoglycemia; overnight fasting preferred.
		0-4 y	Not established		Not established	
		5-9 y	754-1216 ng/mL		754-1216 µg/L	
		10-13 y	610-1217 ng/mL		610-1217 µg/L	
		14-17 y	649-1225 ng/mL		649-1225 µg/L	
		Adult				
		18-30 y				
		31-40 y	546-1260 ng/mL		546-1260 µg/L	
		41-50 y	460-1240 ng/mL		460-1240 µg/L	
			414-1230 ng/mL		414-1230 µg/L	
		51-60 y	414-1248 ng/mL		414-1248 µg/L	
Insulin-like growth factor–binding protein-III (IGFBP III)	Serum	1-7 d	< 0.7 mg/L	1.0	<0.7 mg/L	Separate serum within 1 h. Free serum in plastic vial at −20°C. Major carrier of IGFs, transporting ~95% of IGF-I and IGF-II. IGF-BP3 is GH-responsive and reflects GH actions: elevated in acromegaly and low in hypopituitarism and GH deficiency. Can be used to discriminate among causes of short stature.
		8-15 d	0.5-1.4 mg/L		0.5-1.4 mg/L	
		16 d-1 y	0.7-3.6 mg/L		0.7-3.6 mg/L	
		2 y	0.8-3.9 mg/L		0.8-3.9 mg/L	
		3 y	0.9-4.3 mg/L		0.9-4.3 mg/L	
		4 y	1.0-4.7 mg/L		1.0-4.7 mg/L	
		5 y	1.1-5.2 mg/L		1.1-5.2 mg/L	
		6 y	1.3-5.6 mg/L		1.3-5.6 mg/L	
		7 y	1.4-6.1 mg/L		1.4-6.1 mg/L	
		8 y	1.6-6.5 mg/L		1.6-6.5 mg/L	
		9 y	1.8-7.1 mg/L		1.8-7.1 mg/L	
		10 y	2.1-7.7 mg/L		2.1-7.7 mg/L	
		11 y	2.4-8.4 mg/L		2.4-8.4 mg/L	
		12 y	2.7-8.9 mg/L		2.7-8.9 mg/L	
		13 y	3.1-9.5 mg/L		3.1-9.5 mg/L	
		14 y	3.3-10 mg/L		3.3-10 mg/L	
		15 y	3.5-10 mg/L		3.5-10 mg/L	
		16 y	3.4-9.5 mg/L		3.4-9.5 mg/L	
		17 y	3.2-8.7 mg/L		3.2-8.7 mg/L	
		18 y	3.1-7.9 mg/L		3.1-7.9 mg/L	
		19-20 y	2.9-7.3 mg/L		2.9-7.3 mg/L	
		21-40 y	3.4-7.8 mg/L		3.4-7.8 mg/L	
		41-60 y	3.3-6.9 mg/L		3.3-6.9 mg/L	
		61-70 y	3.0-6.6 mg/L		3.0-6.6 mg/L	
		71-80 y	2.5-5.7 mg/L		2.5-5.7 mg/L	
		81-85 y	2.2-4.5 mg/L		2.2-4.5 mg/L	
		Males				
		Tanner I	1.4-5.2 mg/L		1.4-5.2 mg/L	
		Tanner II	2.3-6.3 mg/L		2.3-6.3 mg/L	
		Tanner III	3.1-8.9 mg/L		3.1-8.9 mg/L	
		Tanner IV	3.7-8.7 mg/L		3.7-8.7 mg/L	
		Tanner V	2.6-8.6 mg/L		2.6-8.6 mg/L	
		Females				
		Tanner I	1.2-6.4 mg/L		1.2-6.4 mg/L	
		Tanner II	2.8-6.9 mg/L		2.8-6.9 mg/L	
		Tanner III	3.9-9.4 mg/L		3.9-9.4 mg/L	
		Tanner IV	3.3-8.1 mg/L		3.3-8.1 mg/L	
		Tanner V	2.7-9.1 mg/L		2.7-9.1 mg/L	

(Continued)

Test	Source	Ages, Conditions, etc	Conventional Units	Conversion Factor	SI Units	Comments
Islet cell antibody (ICA)	Serum	Adults and children	Negative (<1.25 JDF units)	1.0	Negative (<1.25 JDF units)	Refrigerated serum sample. ICA includes antibodies directed against GAD (glutamic acid decarboxylase), IA-2, insulin, GM2-1, and other cell surface proteins. ICA is present during the prediabetic phase and predicts the development of type 1 diabetes. Titers are compared to a single international reference standard reported in JDF (Juvenile Diabetes Foundation) units.
17-Ketosteroids	Urine	Males		3.47		Collect urine with 10 g of boric acid, 30 mL of 6N HCl or 25 mL 50% acetic acid and refrigerate during collection.
		17-20 y	9-22 mg/d		31.23-76.34 µmol/d	
		>20 y	8-20 mg/d		27.76-69.4 µmol/d	
		Females				
		>16 y	6-15 mg/d		20.82-52.05 µmol/d	
		Children				
		<1 y	<1.0 mg/d		<3.47 µmol/d	
		1-4 y	<2.0 mg/d		<6.94 µmol/d	
		5-8 y	<3.0 mg/d		<10.41 µmol/d	
		9-12 y	3-10 mg/d		10.41-34.7 µmol/d	
		13-16 y	5-12 mg/d		17.35-41.64 µmol/d	
Leptin	Serum	Adult males (BMI 18-25)	1.2-9.5 ng/mL	1.0	1.2-9.5 µg/L	Refrigerated serum sample required for RIA.
		Adult females (BMI 18-25)	4.1-25.0 ng/mL		4.1-25.0 µg/L	
		Children				
		Prepubertal males	1.6-10.8 ng/mL		1.6-10.8 µg/L	
		Tanner II-III males	2.1-11.6 ng/mL		2.1-11.6 µg/L	
		Tanner IV-V males	3.4-10.2 ng/mL		3.4-10.2 µg/L	
		Prepubertal females	1.7-10.6 ng/mL		1.7-10.6 µg/L	
		Tanner II-III females	2.6-11.5 ng/mL		2.6-11.5 µg/L	
		Tanner IV-V females	3.4-13.0 ng/mL		3.4-13.0 µg/L	
Luteinizing hormone	Plasma or serum	Males		1.0		Test measures the sum of LH and hCG; high hCG levels in pregnancy or trophoblastic disease cross-react in the assay, giving falsely high LH levels. Third-generation LH assay is sensitive to 0.03 mIU/mL and is more appropriate for use in children. Freeze specimen at −20°C.
		1-7 y	≤0.10 mIU/mL		≤0.10 IU/L	
		8-9 y	≤0.44 mIU/mL		≤0.44 IU/L	
		10-11 y	≤2.28 mIU/mL		≤2.28 IU/L	
		12-14 y	0.31-5.29 mIU/mL		0.31-5.29 IU/L	
		15-17 y	0.15-5.33 mIU/mL		0.15-5.33 IU/L	
		Adults	1.5-9.3 mIU/mL		1.5-9.3 IU/L	
		Females				
		1-7 y	≤0.45 mIU/mL		≤0.45 IU/L	
		8-9 y	≤3.36 mIU/mL		≤3.36 IU/L	
		10-11 y	≤5.65 mIU/mL		≤5.65 IU/L	
		12-14 y	≤11.00 mIU/mL		≤11.00 IU/L	
		15-17 y	≤15.80 mIU/mL		≤15.80 IU/L	
		Adults				
		Follicular phase	1.9-12.5 mIU/mL		1.9-12.5 IU/L	
		Midcycle peak	8.7-76.3 mIU/mL		8.7-76.3 IU/L	
		Luteal phase	0.5-16.9 mIU/mL		0.5-16.9 IU/L	
		Postmenopausal	5.0-52.3 mIU/mL		5.0-52.3 IU/L	

(Continued)

Test	Source	Ages, Conditions, etc	Conventional Units	Conversion Factor	SI Units	Comments
Metanephrines, fractionated, urine	Urine	Metanephrines		5.07		5 mL aliquot of urine; abstain from medication, tobacco, tea, and coffee for 3 d prior to collection.
		3 mo-4 y	25-117 µg/24 h		126.8-593.2 nmol/24 h	
		5-9 y	11-139 µg/24 h		55.8-704.7 nmol/24 h	
		10-13 y	51-275 µg/24 h		258.6-1394.3 nmol/24 h	
		14-17 y	40-189 µg/24 h		202.8-958.2 nmol/24 h	
		18-29 y	25-222 µg/24 h		126.8-1125.6 nmol/24 h	
		30-39 y	36-190 µg/24 h		182.5-963.3 nmol/24 h	
		40-49 y	58-203 µg/24 h		294.1-1029.2 nmol/24 h	
		≥50 y	90-315 µg/24 h		456.3-1597.1 nmol/24 h	
		Normetanephrines				
		3 mo-4 y	54-249 µg/24 h		273.8-1262.4 nmol/24 h	
		5-9 y	31-398 µg/24 h		157.2-2018 nmol/24 h	
		10-13 y	67-503 µg/24 h		339.7-2550 nmol/24 h	
		14-17 y	69-531 µg/24 h		349.8-2692 nmol/24 h	
		18-29 y	40-412 µg/24 h		202.8-2089 nmol/24 h	
		30-39 y	35-482 µg/24 h		177.4-2444 nmol/24 h	
		40-49 y	88-649 µg/24 h		446.2-3290 nmol/24 h	
		≥50 y	122-676 µg/24 h		618.5-3427 nmol/24 h	
		Metanephrines, total				
		3 mo-4 y	79-345 µg/24 h		400.5-1749 nmol/24 h	
		5-9 y	49-408 µg/24 h		284.4-2069 nmol/24 h	
		10-13 y	110-714 µg/24 h		557.7-3620 nmol/24 h	
		14-17 y	107-741 µg/24 h		542.5-3757 nmol/24 h	
		18-29 y	94-604 µg/24 h		476.6-3062 nmol/24 h	
		30-39 y	115-695 µg/24 h		583.1-3524 nmol/24 h	
		40-49 y	182-739 µg/24 h		922-3747 nmol/24 h	
		≥50 y	224-832 µg/24 h		1136-4218 nmol/24 h	
Metanephrines, fractionated, plasma	Plasma	Metanephrine	≤57 pg/mL		≤0.29 nmol/L	Assay by liquid chromatography, tandem mass spectrometry (LC/MS/MS). Requires minimum of 1.5 mL refrigerated EDTA plasma. Patient should
		Normetanephrine	≤148 pg/mL		≤0.75 nmol/L	
		Total metanephrines	≤205 pg/mL		≤1.04 nmol/L	

(Continued)

Test	Source	Ages, Conditions, etc	Conventional Units	Conversion Factor	SI Units	Comments
						refrain from alcohol, coffee, tea, tobacco, and strenuous exercise. Patient should be seated and relaxed before the sample is collected. Overnight fasting is recommended. Increased in pheochromocytoma, neuroblastoma, and stress.

Metyrapone stimulation test: Metyrapone in a dose of 30 mg/kg is administered orally at midnight. The 8 AM plasma 11-deoxycortisol is >7 µg/dL (>0.2 nmol/L) and plasma ACTH is >100 pg/mL (22 pmol/L). (See Chapter 4.)

Test	Source	Ages, Conditions, etc	Conventional Units	Conversion Factor	SI Units	Comments
Osmolality	Serum	Random specimen	278-305 mOsm/kg	1.00	278-305 mOsm/kg	0.2-mL room temperature serum.
	Urine		50-1200 mOsm/kg		50-1200 mOsm/kg	1-mL refrigerated urine.
Osteocalcin	Serum	Males and females		1.0		Overnight fast preferred. Store refrigerated.
		6-9 y	40.2-108.0 ng/mL		40.2-108.0 ng/mL	
		10-13 y	35.8-165.5 ng/mL		35.8-165.5 ng/mL	
		14-17 y				
		Males	27.8-194.1 ng/mL		27.8-194.4 ng/mL	
		Females	16.3-68.7 ng/mL		16.3-68.7 ng/mL	
		Adults				
		Males	11.3-35.1 ng/mL		11.3-35.4 ng/mL	
		Females	7.2-27.9 ng/mL		7.2-27.9 ng/mL	
Pancreatic polypeptide	Plasma	Adults		0.246		Collect with EDTA present, process immediately, and freeze plasma at −60°C.
		18-29 y	≤480 pg/mL		≤118.1 nmol/L	
		30-39 y	70-400 pg/mL		17.2-98.4 nmol/L	
		40-49 y	70-430 pg/mL		17.2-105.8 nmol/L	
		50-62 y	100-780 pg/mL		24.6-191.9 nmol/L	
		>62 y	Not established		Not established	
		Children				
		Cord blood				
		Term infants	≤163 pg/mL		≤40.1 nmol/L	
		Preterm infants	≤180 pg/mL		≤44.3 nmol/L	
		Term infants (6 d)	≤276 pg/mL		≤67.9 nmol/L	
		1 mo-2 y	≤644 pg/mL		≤158.4 nmol/L	
		3-7 y	≤685 pg/mL		≤168.5 nmol/L	
		>7 y	80-270 pg/mL		19.7-66.4 nmol/L	
Parathyroid hormone	Serum	Adults	10-65 pg/mL	0.100	1.0-6.5 pmol/L	Intact hormone measured by immunochemiluminometric assay. Freeze serum at −20°C.
		Children				
		6-9 y	9-59 pg/mL			
		10-13 y	11-74 pg/mL			
		14-17 y	9-69 pg/mL			
Parathyroid hormone-related protein	Plasma				≤4.7 pmol/L	Immunoradiometric assay. Collect blood in syringe and transfer to cold special collection tube and mix thoroughly. Centrifuge in refrigerated centrifuge and store plasma frozen.
Pregnanetriol	24-h urine	Males	71-1000 mg/d	2.97	211-2970 µmol/d	Refrigerate urine during the collection and collect without preservatives. Gas chromatography/mass spectrometry (GC/MS) method. Accumulates in urine when 17-hydroxyprogesterone levels are high.
		Females	47-790 mg/d		140-1436 µmol/d	
Pregnenolone	Serum	Adult males	10-200 ng/dL	0.0318	0.3-6.4 nmol/L	Useful in the diagnosis of congenital adrenal hyperplasia and in virilizing adrenal tumors.
		Adult females	10-230 ng/dL		0.3-7.3 nmol/L	

(Continued)

Test	Source	Ages, Conditions, etc	Conventional Units	Conversion Factor	SI Units	Comments
Progesterone	Serum	Adults		0.0318		Freeze at −20°C. Early morning specimen is preferred. Liquid chromatography, tandem mass spectrometry (LC/MS/MS) method.
		Males				
		18-29	≤0.3 ng/mL		≤0.954 nmol/L	
		30-39	≤0.2 ng/mL		≤0.636 nmol/L	
		40-49	≤0.2 ng/mL		≤0.636 nmol/L	
		50-59	≤0.2 ng/mL		≤0.636 nmol/L	
		Females				
		Early follicular phase	≤0.6 ng/mL		≤1.908 nmol/L	
		Late follicular phase	≤14.5 ng/mL		≤46.11 nmol/L	
		Midcycle	≤16.1 ng/mL		≤51.2 nmol/L	
		Luteal phase	≤31.4 ng/mL		≤99.9 nmol/L	
		Postmenopausal	≤0.2 ng/mL		≤0.636 nmol/L	
		Children				
		Males				
		5-9 y	≤0.7 ng/mL		≤2.23 nmol/L	
		10-13 y	≤1.2 ng/mL		≤3.82 nmol/L	
		14-17 y	<0.8 ng/mL		≤2.54 nmol/L	
		Females				
		5-9 y	≤0.6 ng/mL		≤1.908 nmol/L	
		10-13 y	≤10.2 ng/mL		≤32.43 nmol/L	
		14-17 y	≤11.9 ng/mL		≤37.84 nmol/L	
Proinsulin	Serum	Adults	≤18.8 pmol/L	1.0	≤18.8 pmol/L	Radioimmunoassay on frozen serum. Useful in the diagnosis of insulinoma.
Prolactin	Serum	Adult		0.045		Freeze serum at −20°C.
		Men	2.0-18.0 ng/mL		0.09-0.81 nmol/L	
		Women				
		Nonpregnant	3.0-30.0 ng/mL		0.14-1.35 nmol/L	
		Pregnant	10.0-209.0 ng/mL		0.45-9.4 nmol/L	
		Postmenopausal	2.0-20.0 ng/mL		0.09-0.9 nmol/L	
		Children				
		Males				
		Tanner I	≤10 ng/mL		≤0.45 nmol/L	
		Tanner II-III	≤6.1 ng/mL		≤0.3 nmol/L	
		Tanner IV-V	2.8-11.0 ng/mL		0.13-0.5 nmol/L	
		Females				
		Tanner I	3.6-12.0 ng/mL		0.03-0.54 nmol/L	
		Tanner II-III	2.6-18.0 ng/mL		0.117-0.81 nmol/L	
		Tanner IV-V	3.2-20.0 ng/mL		0.144-0.9 nmol/L	
Renin	Plasma	Normal sodium diet (75-150 mmol/d)		0.278		Draw in cold tube, separate plasma, and freeze in plastic within 15 min after collection.
		0800 recumbent	0.3-3.0 µg/L/h		0.09-0.9 ng/L/s	
		1200 upright	0.4-8.8 µg/L/h		0.12-2.7 ng/L/s	
		upright/sitting	0.65-5.0 µg/L/h		0.18-1.39 ng/L/s	
Sex hormone–binding globulin	Serum	Adults		1.0		Store refrigerated, collect room temperature serum sample. Immunochemiluminometric assay.
		Males				
		18-29 y	7-49 nmol/L		7-49 nmol/L	
		30-39 y	8-48 nmol/L		8-48 nmol/L	
		40-49 y	9-45 nmol/L		9-45 nmol/L	
		50-59 y	18-47 nmol/L		18-47 nmol/L	
		60-69 y	17-54 nmol/L		17-54 nmol/L	
		70-79 y	23-65 nmol/L		23-65 nmol/L	
		80-91 y	20-63 nmol/L		20-63 nmol/L	

(Continued)

Test	Source	Ages, Conditions, etc	Conventional Units	Conversion Factor	SI Units	Comments
		Females				
		18-29 y	6-112 nmol/L		6-112 nmol/L	
		30-39 y	14-102 nmol/L		14-102 nmol/L	
		40-49 y	11-100 nmol/L		11-100 nmol/L	
		50-59 y	17-78 nmol/L		17-78 nmol/L	
		60-69 y	17-95 nmol/L		17-95 nmol/L	
		70-79 y	21-90 nmol/L		21-90 nmol/L	
		80-91 y	26-77 nmol/L		26-77 nmol/L	
		Children				
		Males and females	18-136 nmol/L		18-136 nmol/L	
		3-9 y	17-123 nmol/L		17-123 nmol/L	
		10-13 y	11-71 nmol/L		11-71 nmol/L	
		14-17 y				
		Tanner stage				
		Males	39-155 nmol/L		39-155 nmol/L	
		I	33-135 nmol/L		33-135 nmol/L	
		II	21-72 nmol/L		21-72 nmol/L	
		III	11-92 nmol/L		11-92 nmol/L	
		IV	11-54 nmol/L		11-54 nmol/L	
		V				
		Females	38-114 nmol/L		38-114 nmol/L	
		I	24-90 nmol/L		24-90 nmol/L	
		II	22-112 nmol/L		22-112 nmol/L	
		III	22-69 nmol/L		22-69 nmol/L	
		IV	18-76 nmol/L		18-76 nmol/L	
		V				
Somatostatin	Plasma	Adults	10-22 pg/mL	0.426	4.26-9.37 pmol/L	Draw in prechilled tube, separate plasma, and freeze immediately.
Testosterone, total	Serum	Male		0.0347		Freeze at −20°C.
		Cord blood	17-61 ng/dL		0.59-2.11 nmol/L	
		1-10 d	≤187 ng/dL		≤6.49 nmol/L	
		1-3 mo	72-344 ng/dL		2.5-11.9 nmol/L	
		3-5 mo	≤201 ng/dL		≤6.97 nmol/L	
		5-7 mo	≤59 ng/dL		≤2.05 nmol/L	
		7-12 mo	≤16 ng/dL		≤0.56 nmol/L	
		1-5.9 y	≤5 ng/dL		≤0.17 nmol/L	
		6-7.9 y	≤25 ng/dL		≤0.87 nmol/L	
		8-10.9 y	≤42 ng/dL		≤1.46 nmol/L	
		11-11.9 y	≤260 ng/dL		≤9.022 nmol/L	
		12-13.9 y	≤420 ng/dL		≤14.57 nmol/L	
		14-17.9 y	≤1000 ng/dL		≤34.7 nmol/L	
		Tanner stage I	≤5 ng/dL		≤0.17 nmol/L	
		Tanner stage II	≤167 ng/dL		≤5.79 nmol/L	
		Tanner stage III	21-719 ng/dL		0.73-24.95 nmol/L	
		Tanner stage IV	5-70 ng/dL		0.17-2.43 nmol/L	
		Tanner stage V	110-975 ng/dL		3.82-33.83 nmol/L	
		Adults				
		18-69 y	250-1100 ng/dL		8.68-38.17 nmol/L	
		70-89 y	90-890 ng/dL		3.12-30.88 nmol/L	
		Female				
		Cord blood	16-44 ng/dL		0.56-1.53 nmol/L	
		1-10 d	≤24 ng/dL		≤0.83 nmol/L	
		1-3 mo	≤17 ng/dL		≤0.59 nmol/L	
		3-5 mo	≤12 ng/dL		≤0.42 nmol/L	
		5-7 mo	≤13 ng/dL		≤0.45 nmol/L	
		7-12 mo	≤11 ng/dL		≤0.38 nmol/L	
		1-5.9 y	≤8 ng/dL		≤0.28 nmol/L	
		6-7.9 y	≤20 ng/dL		≤0.69 nmol/L	
		8-10.9 y	≤35 ng/dL		≤1.21 nmol/L	
		11-17.9 y	≤40 ng/dL		≤1.38 nmol/L	

(Continued)

Test	Source	Ages, Conditions, etc	Conventional Units	Conversion Factor	SI Units	Comments
		Tanner stage I	≤8 ng/dL		≤0.28 nmol/L	
		Tanner stage II	≤24 ng/dL		≤0.83 nmol/L	
		Tanner stage III	≤28 ng/dL		≤0.97 nmol/L	
		Tanner stage IV	≤31 ng/dL		≤1.08 nmol/L	
		Tanner stage V	≤33 ng/dL		≤1.15 nmol/L	
		Adult				
		18-69 y	2-45 ng/dL		0.069-1.56 nmol/L	
		70-94 y	2-40 ng/dL		0.069-1.38 nmol/L	
		Pregnancy				
		1st trimester	20-135 ng/dL		0.69-4.68 nmol/L	
		2nd trimester	11-153 ng/dL		0.38-5.31 nmol/L	
		3rd trimester	11-146 ng/dL		0.38-5.07 nmol/L	
Testosterone, free	Serum	Male		3.47		Freeze at −20°C. Tracer equilibrium dialysis.
		5-9 y	≤5.3 pg/mL		≤18.4 pmol/L	
		10-13 y	0.7-52.0 pg/mL		2.4-180 pmol/L	
		14-17.9 y	18.0-111 pg/mL		62.5-385 pmol/L	
		Adults				
		18-69 y	35-155 pg/mL		121.4-5379 pmol/L	
		70-89 y	30-135 pg/mL		104.1-468.4 pmol/L	
		Female				
		5-9 y	0.2-5.0 pg/mL		0.69-17.3 pmol/L	
		10-13 y	0.1-7.4 pg/mL		0.35-25.7 pmol/L	
		14-17 y	0.5-3.9 pg/mL		1.73-13.5 pmol/L	
		Adults				
		18-69 y	0.1-6.4 pg/mL		0.35-22.2 pmol/L	
		70-89 y	0.2-3.7 pg/mL		0.69-12.8 pmol/L	
		Pregnancy				
		1st trimester	0.5-6.0 pg/mL		1.73-20.8 pmol/L	
		2nd trimester	0.2-3.1 pg/mL		0.69-10.8 pmol/L	
		3rd trimester	0.2-4.1 pg/mL		0.69-14.2 pmol/L	
Thyroglobulin	Serum	Adult	2.0-35 ng/mL	1.00	2.0-35 ng/mL	Freeze at −20°C. Presence of thyroglobulin autoantibodies in the patient's serum may falsely lower the result.
Thyroid antibodies	Serum	Thyroperoxidase antibodies	<35 IU/mL			Serum collected and refrigerated.
		Thyroglobulin antibodies	<20 IU/mL			
Thyroid-stimulating hormone (TSH) ultra sensitive	Serum	Adult		−		Sensitivity: 0.01 mU/mL. TSH levels decline in first several weeks of life, although they remain elevated in some infants. Free T_4 is helpful in the interpretation of TSH.
		Males and nonpregnant females	0.40-4.50 mU/L		0.40-4.50 mU/L	
		Pregnant females				
		1st trimester	0.3-4.5 mU/L		0.3-4.5 mU/L	
		2nd trimester	0.5-4.6 mU/L		0.5-4.6 mU/L	
		3rd trimester	0.8-5.2 mU/L		0.8-5.2 mU/L	
		Children				
		Term infants				
		1-4 d	3.2-35.0 mU/L		3.2-35.0 mU/L	
		5-6 d	Not established		Not established	
		1-4 wk	1.7-9.1 mU/L			
		1-12 mo	0.80-8.20 mU/L			
		1-19 y	0.5-4.30 mU/L			
Thyroid-stimulating hormone receptor antibody (TSH-R Ab [stim])	Serum		≤125% of basal activity	−		Assay based on cyclic AMP generation in CHO cells transfected with human TSH receptor gene.

Test	Source	Ages, Conditions, etc	Conventional Units	Conversion Factor	SI Units	Comments
Thyroid uptake of radioactive iodine (RAIU)	Activity over thyroid gland	Fractional uptake 2 h 6 h 24 h	 4%-12% 6%-15% 8%-30%			Ingestion or administration of iodide will decrease thyroid uptake of RAI.
Thyrotropin-binding inhibitory immunoglobulin (TB-II)	Serum	Adults and children Graves disease	≤16% inhibition 16%-100% inhibition	– 	– 	Sensitivity: 2% inhibition. May be useful in Graves disease, neonatal hypothyroidism, and postpartum thyroid dysfunction.
Thyrotropin-blocking antibody	Serum	Adults	≤10% inhibition	–	–	In vitro bioassay useful in diagnosis of transient hypothyroidism in infants due to maternally transferred antibodies; elevated in some forms of hypothyroidism.
Thyroxine-binding globulin (TBG)	Serum	Men Women Children 3-8 y 9-13 y 14-17 y	12.7-25.1 µg/mL 13.5-30.9 µg/mL 16.1-24.2 µg/mL 12.5-25.8 µg/mL 9.8-23.7 µg/mL	1.00		Quantifies TBG to differentiate TBG abnormalities from thyroid dysfunction.
Thyroxine (T_4)	Serum	Children 1-8 y 9-13 y 14-17 y Adults Pregnancy First trimester Second trimester Third trimester	 5.9-11.5 µg/dL 4.7-10.4 µg/dL 5.0-9.8 µg/dL 4.8-10.4 µg/dL 6.4-15.2 µg/dL 7.4-15.2 µg/dL 7.7-14.7 µg/dL	12.87	 75.9-148 nmol/L 60.5-133.8 nmol/L 64.3-126.1 nmol/L 61.8-133.8 nmol/L 82.4-195.6 nmol/L 95.2-195.6 nmol/L 99.1-189.2 nmol/L	Refrigerate serum. Fasting preferred. Elevated levels in pregnancy due to increased TBG.
Thyroxine, free (FT_4)	Serum	Children (3-20 y) Adults (21-87 y) Pregnancy 1st trimester 2nd trimester 3rd trimester	1.0-2.4 ng/dL 0.8-2.7 ng/dL 0.9-2.0 ng/dL 0.8-1.5 ng/dL 0.8-1.7 ng/dL	12.87	12.87-30.9 pmol/L 10.3-34.7 pmol/L 11.6-25.7 pmol/L 10.3-19.3 pmol/L 10.3-23.6 pmol/L	Direct equilibrium dialysis and radioimmunoassay. Refrigerate serum.
Triiodothyronine (T_3), total	Serum	<1 y 1-9 y 10-13 y 14-18 y Adult Pregnancy 1st trimester 2nd and 3rd trimester	Not established 127-221 ng/dL 123-211 ng/dL 97-186 ng/dL 60-181 ng/dL 81-190 ng/dL 100-260 ng/dL	0.0154	Not established 1.96-3.4 nmol/L 1.89-3.25 nmol/L 1.49-2.86 nmol/L 0.92-2.79 nmol/L 1.25-2.93 nmol/L 1.54-4.00 nmol/L	Refrigerate serum. Immunochemiluminometric assay. Used to diagnose and monitor treatment of hyperthyroidism.
Free T_3 (FT_3)	Serum	Adults Children <1 y 1-9 y 10-13 y 14-18 y	230-420 pg/dL Not established 337-506 pg/dL 335-480 pg/dL 287-455 pg/dL	15.4	3.5-6.47 pmol/L Not established 5.19-7.79 pmol/L 5.16-7.79 pmol/L 4.42-7.01 pmol/L	Nondialysis; ICMA on refrigerated serum.

(Continued)

Test	Source	Ages, Conditions, etc	Conventional Units	Conversion Factor	SI Units	Comments
FT$_3$	Serum	Nonpregnant adults Pregnant women Children <1 y 1-9 y 10-13 y 14-17 y	210-440 pg/dL 200-380 pg/dL Not established 282-518 pg/dL 286-556 pg/dL 242-501 pg/dL	15.4	3.23-6.78 pmol/L 3.08-5.85 pmol/L Not established 4.34-7.98 pmol/L 4.40-8.56 pmol/L 3.73-7.72 pmol/L	Tracer dialysis, RIA on refrigerated serum.
Reverse T$_3$ (RT$_3$)	Serum		0.11-0.32 ng/mL	0.0154	0.169-0.49 nmol/L	Radioimmunoassay to establish the cause of abnormal thyroid function tests as due to nonthyroidal illness.
Vanillylmandelic acid (VMA)	24-h urine Random or spot urine	Adults Children 3-8 y 9-12 y 13-17 y Children Birth-6 mo 7-11 mo 1-2 y 3-8 y 9-12 y 13-17 y Adults	≤6.0 mg/d ≤2.3 mg/d ≤3.4 mg/d ≤3.9 mg/d 5.5-26 mg/g Cr 6.1-20 mg/g Cr 2.5-21 mg/g Cr 1.7-6.5 mg/g Cr 1.4-5.1 mg/g Cr 1.5-3.6 mg/g Cr 1.1-4.1 mg/g Cr	5.88 0.573	≤13.5 nmol/d ≤20 nmol/d ≤22.9 nmol/d ≤35.3 nmol/d 3.2-14.9 mmol VMA/mol Cr 3.5-11.5 mmol VMA/mol Cr 1.4-12.0 mmol VMA/mol Cr 0.97-3.7 mmol VMA/mol Cr 0.80-2.9 mmol VMA/mol Cr 0.86-2.1 mmol VMA/mol Cr 0.63-2.3 mmol VMA/mol Cr	10 mL aliquot of urine, HPLC detection; 24-h urine is collected with 25 mL of 6N HCl added. Patients should avoid alcohol, coffee, tea, tobacco, nicotine, bananas, citrus fruit, and heavy exercise prior to the collection.
Vasoactive intestinal peptide	Serum		<50 pg/mL	0.30	<15 pmol/L	Frozen EDTA plasma.
Vitamin D (25-hydroxy)	Serum		20-100 ng/mL	2.50	50-250 nmol/L	Measures both D$_2$ and D$_3$. Freeze serum in plastic tube at −20°C. Liquid chromatography tandem mass spectrometry (LC/MS/MS)
Vitamin D (1,25 dihydroxy)	Serum	Adults Children 3-7 y	15-60 pg/mL 27-71 pg/mL	2.50	32.5-167 pmol/L 22.5-135 pmol/L	Extraction, chromatography, radioreceptor assay. Freeze serum in plastic tube at −20°C.

[a]Adapted from the *Clinical Laboratories Manual* of the University of California Hospital and Clinics, San Francisco, California, July 4, 2010; and, with permission, from Quest Diagnostics Nichols Institute normal values for endocrine tests. *The Quest Diagnosis Manual. Endocrinology Test Selection and Interpretation.* 4th ed. Fisher D, ed. 2007. The factors used in converting conventional units to SI units were derived in part from the *CRC Handbook of Chemistry and Physics* and conversion tables from other online resources. It is important to emphasize that normal ranges vary among different laboratories, and the clinician must know the normal range for the test of interest in the laboratory performing the test.

[b]Semen analysis is discussed in Chapter 12.

BCE, bone collagen equivalent.

Index

Page numbers followed by "f" and "t" indicate figures and tables, respectively.